THE COMPLETE TEXTBOOK OF
VETERINARY NURSING

Commissioning Editor: *Robert Edwards*
Development Editor: *Veronika Watkins/Clive Hewat*
Project Manager: *Alan Nicholson*
Designer/Design Direction: *Charles Gray*
Illustration Manager: *Merlyn Harvey*

SECOND EDITION

THE COMPLETE TEXTBOOK OF
VETERINARY NURSING

Edited by

Victoria Aspinall
BVSc MRCVS

Director, Abbeydale Vetlink Veterinary Training, Ashcott, Somerset, UK

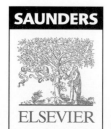
SAUNDERS

ELSEVIER

Edinburgh   London   New York   Oxford   Philadelphia   St Louis   Sydney   Toronto   2011

SAUNDERS
ELSEVIER

First edition 2006

ISBN 978-0-7020-4050-4

British Library Cataloguing in Publication Data
A catalogue record for this book is available from the British Library.

Library of Congress Cataloguing in Publication Data
A catalogue record for this book is available from the Library of Congress.

Notices
Knowledge and best practice in this field are constantly changing. As new research and experience broaden our understanding, changes in research methods, professional practices, or medical treatment may become necessary.

Practitioners and researchers must always rely on their own experience and knowledge in evaluating and using any information, methods, compounds, or experiments described herein. In using such information or methods they should be mindful of their own safety and the safety of others, including parties for whom they have a professional responsibility.

With respect to any drug or pharmaceutical products identified, readers are advised to check the most current information provided (i) on procedures featured or (ii) by the manufacturer of each product to be administered, to verify the recommended dose or formula, the method and duration of administration, and contraindications. It is the responsibility of practitioners, relying on their own experience and knowledge of their patients, to make diagnoses, to determine dosages and the best treatment for each individual patient, and to take all appropriate safety precautions.

To the fullest extent of the law, neither the Publisher nor the authors, contributors, or editors, assume any liability for any injury and/or damage to persons or property as a matter of products liability, negligence or otherwise, or from any use or operation of any methods, products, instructions, or ideas contained in the material herein.

ELSEVIER your source for books, journals and multimedia in the health sciences

www.elsevierhealth.com

Working together to grow libraries in developing countries

www.elsevier.com | www.bookaid.org | www.sabre.org

ELSEVIER   BOOK AID International   Sabre Foundation

The publisher's policy is to use paper manufactured from sustainable forests

Printed in China

Contents

Contributors

Nicola Ackerman BSc (Hons) RVN Cert SAN MBVNA
Senior Medical Nurse, The Veterinary Hospital, Colwill Road, Plymouth, Devon, UK

Lorraine Allan BVSc MRCVS
Lecturer in Veterinary Nursing, Myerscough College, Bilsborrow, Preston, Lancashire, UK

Victoria Aspinall BVSc MRCVS
Director of Abbeydale Vetlink Veterinary Training Ltd, Ashcott, Somerset, UK

Sally Bowden BSc (Hons) Cert Ed RVN Hon MBVNA
Veterinary Nurse Training and Consultancy Services Essex, UK

Emma Brooks VN
Veterinary Nurse, Bristol, UK

Sue Dallas VN
Freelance Lecturer in Veterinary Nursing, Great Ryburgh, Norfolk, UK

Clare Cave VN
Freelance Lecturer in Veterinary Nursing, Woolavington, Bridgwater, Somerset, UK

Sarah Cottingham BSc (Hons) PGDipCABC PGCE VN
Lecturer in Animal Care, Plumpton College, Plumpton, Nr Lewes, Sussex, UK

Suzanne Easton MSc BSc (Hons) PGCE
Senior Lecturer in Diagnostic Imaging, University of the West of England, Bristol, UK

Maggie Fisher BVetMed CBiol MIBiol DipEVPC MRQA MRCVS
Consultant in Veterinary Parasitology, Shernacre Enterprise, Malvern, Worcestershire, UK

Andi Godfrey BSc (Hons)
Freelance Writer, Hereford Road, London, UK

Cecilia Gorrel BSc DDS MA Vet MB MRCVS Hon FAVD Dipl EVDC
Veterinary Dentistry and Oral Surgery Referrals, Pilley, Nr Lyminton, Hampshire, UK

Kirsty Gwynne RVN Cert Ed
Director of Abbeydale Vetlink Veterinary Training Ltd, Ashcott, Somerset, UK

Helen Harris RVN Cert Ed
Programme Manager: Veterinary Nursing, Duchy College, Stoke Climsland, Callington, Cornwall, UK

Paula Hotson Moore VN
Internal Verifier and Lecturer, University of Bristol Veterinary School, Langford, Somerset UK

Alison Jones BVet Med MRCVS
Principal 'Vets on the Park', Lyndale, Moorend Grove, Cheltenham, Gloucestershire, UK

Kirsty Jones RVN Cert Ed
Director of Abbeydale Vetlink Veterinary Training Ltd, Ashcott, Somerset, UK

Jocelyn Lander RVN
Head Nurse, Purton Veterinary Group, Swindon, Wiltshire, UK

Gareth Lawler BSc (Hons) PGCE
Lecturer in Animal Care, Pencoed College, Bridgend, South Wales, UK

Jessica Maughan BSc VN
Locum Nurse, Ruardean Woodside, Gloucestershire, UK

Suzanne May RVN
Head of Centre and Senior Lecturer in Veterinary Nursing, Harper Adams University College, Shropshire, UK

Pip Millard VN
Farm Manager, Badgeworth, Cheltenham, UK

Wendy Miller-Smith RVN Cert Ed CMS
Veterinary Consultant, Closes Court, Kirkcowan, Newton Stewart, Ayrshire, UK

Louise Minshell
Gloucestershire Wildlife Rescue/Oak and Furrows Wildlife Rescue, Gloucester UK

Helen Moreton BSc PhD
Senior Lecturer and Course Manager for MSc Applied Equine Science, Royal Agriculture College, Cirencester, Gloucestershire, UK

Julie Ouston MA Vet MB MRCVS
Director of MYF Training Ltd, Hippodrome House, Aldershot, Hampshire, UK

Catherine Phillips VN
Subject Leader in Veterinary Nursing, Hartpury College, Hartpury, Gloucester, UK

Corinna Pippard Bsc (Hons) PhD
Lecturer, Caernafon, Gwynedd, N Wales

Sharon Reid RVN
Senior Veterinary Nurse, University of Glasgow Small Animal Clinic, Bearsden Road, Bearsden, Glasgow, UK

Amanda Rock BVSc MRCVS
Critical Care Veterinary Surgeon, Liskeard, Cornwall, UK

Anne Rogers BSc (Hons)
Admissions Officer, Cirencester, UK

Trish Scorer VN
Internal Verifier for Abbeydale Vetlink Veterinary Training Ltd, Ashcott, Somerset, UK

Beverley Shingleton VN Cert Ed
Programme Manager for ND in Animal Management, Plumpton College, Plumpton, Nr Lewes, Sussex UK

Dorothy Stables MSc BA (Hons) MTD DN RM RN
Former Lecturer in Applied Biology, St Bartholomew's College of Nursing and Midwifery, City University, London, UK

Michael Stevenson BVM&S
Director of AAS Veterinary Services Ltd, Abbeydale, Gloucester, UK

Anja Walker BSc BVSc MRCVS
Director of Western Counties Equine Clinic, Culmstock, Nr Cullumton, Devon UK

Juliet Whatley VN Cert. Ed
External Verifer, RCVS, London, UK

Jane Williams VNCert Ed.
Lecturer in Veterinary Nursing, Buckfastleigh, Devon, UK

James Yeates BVSc Cert WEL MRCVS
Resident in Animal Welfare Science, Ethics and Law, Bristol University Veterinary School, Langford, Somerset UK

Preface to second edition

The aim of *The Complete Textbook of Veterinary Nursing* has always been to provide information for the whole of a veterinary nurse's working life and in this second edition this is even more true with the addition of new chapters on ethics and welfare, the art of communication, physiotherapy techniques and a new section on nursing models and reflective practice. All the chapters have been updated, additional information has been added and the contributors have included changes to legislation and current nursing techniques all of which have resulted in a comprehensive work which continues to fulfil its original aims.

When I was editing the first edition I was faced with a change in the RCVS VN syllabus for veterinary nurse training and it was essential that the book provided the range of information to cover it. Imagine my surprise, when editing this second edition, I discovered that coincidentally there was to be another change in the training process and the syllabus and I was faced with the same problem! However the changes to the syllabus have not been as great as I feared and I am confident that this book will present any student nurse with sufficient relevant, current and accurate knowledge to pass the professional exams. It is also important to remember that this book has become a significant contributor to other modes of study such as animal science and veterinary nursing degrees and to a range of animal management courses – the use of the word 'veterinary' in the title should not prevent its use by everyone interested in the study of animals at many levels.

To satisfy the requirements of a more technological age there is an updated website which provides a new added dimension. The website takes the form of extra chapters, videos illustrating many of the techniques commonly used in veterinary practices and large numbers of multiple choice questions. I recommend that you visit the website and use it to gain extra information and as a visual guide to those routine techniques. For those student nurses preparing for the professional exams, the more MCQs that you do the better. This site will give you questions written by the book's contributing authors to test your understanding of the chapters you have read and to help you get used to answering questions written by people other than your usual tutors.

As before, this book represents many hours of dedicated work by the contributing authors all of whom have regular contact with the veterinary nursing fraternity and they have my undying thanks.

Victoria Aspinall
March 2011

Acknowledgements

As ever I would like to thank my husband not only for his support and forbearance but also for the radiographs that have been used to illustrate several chapters. I would also like to thank Peter Neville for reading through the chapter on dog and cat behaviour, all the hard working contributors who have taken time to read and revise their chapters and Raystede Animal Welfare Centre, Plumpton College Sussex and the staff at Aspinall Auld and Stevenson for providing some of the new photographs. The filming of the videos on the website took up the free time of Kirsty Gwynne and Kirsty Jones for which thank you so much.

Finally as I sit looking out at rainy March fields, I ask myself the question: why do my two cats Roly and Thomasina feel that their contribution to the editing process is treading muddy paw marks all over every piece of clean paper? Perhaps the answer lies in Chapter 10?

CHAPTER 1

Ethics and animal welfare

James Yeates

Key Points

- Ethics is about how people *should* act.
- Think about the predictable problems in advance and after you have made decisions.
- Rules-based and virtue ethics schools of ethical thought are primarily concerned with the person acting, e.g. the nurse.
- Consequences-based and rights-based schools of thought are primarily concerned with who is affected, e.g. animals, owners, colleagues, the practice, the profession and the environment.
- Discussion with other people is useful and sometimes necessary, but letting other people tell you what to do is still an ethical choice.

What are ethics and morality?

Each individual, society and profession has a way of making decisions about how to act and how other people should act. An individual veterinary nurse has a personal way of making decisions, which she (or he) reveals in what she does and what she says. The veterinary nursing profession also has its way, which it describes in the Royal College of Veterinary Surgeons (RCVS) *Guide to Professional Conduct*. A society has its way, which leads to its laws.

Ethics is the study of these ways of making decisions. It can be studied by sociologists, such as a survey of whether people approve of tail docking – this is called **descriptive ethics**. It can be studied by philosophers, who try to decide the best way to make decisions in general. This is called **normative ethics** and is discussed later; however, normative ethics is not limited to philosophers. It is done whenever one considers the ethics of a person, a profession or a society. People can then decide how to make decisions in real-life cases – this is called **applied ethics**. Applied ethics is an important part of many scientific and medical professions, and recently, the veterinary profession has begun to consider applied ethics in more depth.

Ethical conflicts

For much of the time, one obvious ethical responsibility must be followed, and in these situations, a nurse may not need to think about how to act, let alone have any complicated theories about it; however, at other times, nurses have conflicting ethical responsibilities. An **ethical conflict** is a situation in which a person has two or more ethical pressures that cannot both be fulfilled.

It is worth looking out for ethical conflicts that you deal with each day. Common ones include decisions about:

- Balancing an animal's quality of life and its quantity of life
- Balancing an animal's welfare and the owner's or practice's finances
- Being asked to assist in a procedure that you think is unethical for any reason
- Situations where the 'best option' is illegal
- Possibly reporting a colleague or owner to authorities
- Being given contradictory instructions by different vets or employers.

There are several ways to solve an ethical conflict. Two common methods are asking someone else or relying on 'gut feeling'. Both are quick and easy and involve a minimum of thought, and these characteristics make them useful for situations where a nurse has to act fast. However, just as such methods might not always reach the best solution in clinical issues, so too are they likely to be ethically less accurate than decisions that are better thought out.

It is worth following a rough procedure for dealing with an ethical conflict such as the one shown in Box 1.1. It is not necessary, and sometimes impossible, to follow this order rigidly, but the scheme lists important steps describing these is more detail.

Think about the predictable problems in advance (Box 1.1)

Many conflicts can be predicted and anticipated.

- Some problems are created by the owners, e.g. some dog breeders breed bulldogs but the puppies often need to be delivered by Caesarean section. Some veterinary nurses consider it is unethical to breed bulldogs because of the health problems that they have and unethical to help to perform a Caesarean, or think that one should insist on neutering the bitch at the same time.

- Think about the predictable problems in advance
- Describe the question and your choices
- Identify the choices that you have available physically
- Identify the choices that you have available legally
- Identify the stakeholders and predict how each one might be affected
- Choose a school of thought or a framework
- Identify choices you think are ethically acceptable
- Discuss your decision with other stakeholders
- Act
- Reflect on the decision and outcomes
- Prepare for next time

Box 1.2 Common options when faced with a case of euthanasia

- Kill the animal
- Let the animal die naturally
- Try to cure the animal's disease
- Palliate any suffering
- Rehome the animal with the owner's consent
- Take the animal and rehome it against the owner's wishes
- Do nothing
- Report the owner for cruelty

- Other dilemmas are caused by the vet, e.g. when a nurse sees a vet acting unethically, there is a dilemma as to whether to 'whistle-blow'.
- Other dilemmas are caused by the law, e.g. in the UK non-native species such as grey squirrels cannot be released back into the wild after treatment.
- Many dilemmas depend on the owner, the law and the vet, e.g. nurses can expect many different cases of euthanasia. Some animals brought for euthanasia are completely healthy and might have a good life if the owner and vet did not agree to euthanize it. Others have been suffering for some time but their owner does not want them euthanized. Some do not have owners. Each case causes a different ethical dilemma.

Thinking about these issues in advance allows you time to think when you are relaxed and not pressured by other people. It gives you time to get more information and discuss matters with other people. For example, you may need to discuss with an owner whether to resuscitate an animal if it crashes under anaesthesia *before* the animal crashes, as there is no time when it does. If you have some idea in advance that you might not be happy to assist a vet with a procedure, then it is useful to say so *before* the animal is admitted because:

1. It may avoid the vet trying to do the procedure on his own because you refused to help after he had committed himself.
2. You may end up helping with the procedure to prevent him doing it on his own and then feeling inconsistent and weak.
3. Your decision might make the vet change his mind before he has committed himself.

Describe the question and your choices

You cannot make a decision without knowing what that decision concerns. It is useful to describe the question as neutrally as possible so that it does not determine your answer in advance. For example, questions such as 'Should I fail to care appropriately for this animal?' or 'Should I act uncharitably to this owner?' will be answered by 'No', even though there might actually be very good reasons not to care for the animal, e.g. because it would cause danger to your colleagues, or to act uncharitably to the owner, e.g. because it would cost the practice money.

It is useful to separate the question you have to answer from the situation. Often situations could and should have been avoided, and it is very easy to moan about the situation and fail to make a decision. For example, if an animal is aggressive because it has been poorly trained or is unsuitable for the owner, then this is a situation that should have been avoided, but you still have to make a decision now about what you are going to do.

Once you have phrased the question, you can consider the possible answers. Some options are not immediately obvious and are revealed only by reflection. Doing nothing is always a choice but often not the right one. As an example, your choices when faced with a decision about euthanasia are listed in Box 1.2. It is useful to think of all these choices at this point, however imperfect or silly they seem, because you may find that the sensible options are not possible in some cases.

Identify the choices that you have available physically

Very often you will find that some choices are physically impossible. For example:

- Treating an aggressive dog may be much more difficult than treating a nicer dog because you may be unable to get close to it.
- Some diseases may not be treatable because a cure has not yet been discovered.
- Sometimes you are limited by your own competence levels or available time.

It is psychologically important not to feel guilty for not achieving the impossible, and in some cases it may be better to be realistic.

Identify the choices that you have available legally

Legal rules and the rules in the RCVS *Guide to Professional Conduct* are based on the official ethics of your profession and of society. Following the law is generally the right thing to do and breaking the law is not usually an ethical option.

The law is discussed in more detail in Chapter 3, but here it is worth noting that the law often agrees with one's own ethics, e.g. allowing unreasonable suffering is illegal, unprofessional and unethical. Similarly, there are some ethical arguments as to why it is a good thing that owners own their pets and why informed consent is important – imagine what it would be like if other people could just decide whether your pet is killed or rehomed.

It is important in ethical decision-making to see the difference between options available to you as a nurse and options available to other people. Nurses do not have all the legal options available to the owner and the vet. If these other people will not do what is right, this limits the options open to the nurse. In these cases, the nurse must choose the best from the options she does have – which may be a less than ideal treatment or even euthanasia. She should then not feel guilty for the poor ethics of other people.

Identify the stakeholders and predict how each one might be affected by each choice

Any decision in practice will involve a 'cast' of people or animals involved, referred to as stakeholders. Common stakeholders are:

- The patient
- The owner
- The nurse's colleagues
- The practice
- The profession
- The public
- The environment
- The nurse.

The stake for each person or animal may be different and may create conflicting duties. It is useful to consider how each stakeholder may be affected by each available option.

The patient

This is probably the most important stakeholder; however, an animal cannot be asked what it wants and it cannot make veterinary decisions for itself because it does not understand medical treatment, e.g. if hospitalized, animals cannot decide when to go to the toilet outside, or whether to receive visitors. This means the nurse has to make these decisions.

A popular way to think about how animals are affected is in terms of animal welfare. You can think about animal welfare in terms of inputs and outcomes. **Inputs** are things provided for animals in terms of their environment, medical treatment, husbandry, and the animal's condition and genetics. **Outcomes** are the effects of those inputs on the animals' quality of life. This is classically defined as 'the state of the animal as it attempts to cope with its environment' (Fraser and Broom 1990), but there is disagreement about which outcomes are important.

Some argue that you should only look at **physical welfare**. You can assess how well an animal functions by looking at its biology. Biological assessments look at how well the animal is functioning as an organism. You can measure its levels of substrates such as stress hormones or urea and/or look for signs of pathology such as stomach ulcers. Clinical assessments, such as palpation, temperature, capillary refill time, biochemistry, radiography and so on are usually biological assessments.

Many argue that welfare is about the **feelings** of animals. Welfare scientists have been surprisingly resistant to such ideas, mainly because they are not measurable from the outside – no person can ever know *for sure* whether an animal is feeling pain; however, welfare science has begun to recognize that it can guess an animal's feelings from its behaviour. Firstly, it looks at what animals choose. Secondly, it looks at behaviours that show negative feelings such as pain, stress, fear, malaise, boredom and lethargy or positive feelings such as in play and company. Pain may be shown by increased sensitivity in the area local to an injury or an altered posture and also in general behavioural signs such as quietness or inappetance. Similarly, stereotypes such as feather plucking in parrots or pacing in a caged zoo animal can suggest anxiety or boredom.

Assessment of feelings can be done in practice through simple observations and empathy; however, it must be remembered that animals experience the world and illness in a very different way to a human in an equivalent situation. This means you cannot merely ask whether *you* would want to be treated in this way. You should try to imagine what it might be like to be a *dog* in the situation, knowing what you know about canine brains. For example, unlike a person, a dog is unlikely to want to survive until Christmas or worry about its diagnosis; however, like a person, it may dislike being in a strange place and without any control over its treatment.

Assessment in practice can be assisted by using a formal tool or framework. Frameworks such as the Five Freedoms, shown in Box 1.3, combines inputs and outcomes of animal welfare.

Often the best assessment is one that combines the abilities of the nurse, owner and veterinarian. Owners usually see the animal far more than you, often every day for many years, but owners might not have much experience of assessing welfare. They might have had bad previous experiences or personal feelings that may affect their judgement. The nurse and the vet can help the owners to be more objective. Owners usually do not know about the clinical facts and may also be unable to perceive future problems. The vet may have a great deal of knowledge and experience, but still only sees the animal for a few minutes and may try not to get too close to the animal in order to remain objective. The assessment of a nurse, especially one that is experienced and empathetic, is a useful addition to the assessment of the owner and veterinarian.

An animal might also be affected in other ways. Being dead does not involve suffering, but it does deprive the animal of

---

Box 1.3 The Five Freedoms (Farm Animal Welfare Council 1993)

1. Freedom from thirst, hunger and malnutrition *by ready access to fresh water and a diet to maintain full health and vigour*
2. Freedom from discomfort *by providing a suitable environment including shelter and a comfortable resting area*
3. Freedom from pain, injury and disease *by prevention or rapid diagnosis and treatment*
4. Freedom from fear and distress *by ensuring conditions that avoid mental suffering*
5. Freedom to express normal behaviour *by providing sufficient space, proper facilities and company of the animal's own kind*

good welfare and/or avoid future bad welfare. An animal may have **rights** that can be broken such as a right to life or liberty, e.g. killing a grey squirrel might breach its right to life; keeping it captive deprives it of a basic right to live as a wild animal (and causes poor welfare too).

An animal may also be affected in terms of whether its **integrity** is damaged. If an animal is mutilated, such as being declawed, this damages its integrity on top of any pain or other problems caused. The same is true if animals are deprived of living naturally. If a dog is prevented from performing certain species-specific behaviours (its 'telos'), then it loses some of its 'doggyness'. It might also be harmful to make animals live in an unnatural way. Taking a parrot from its natural environment and making it live in a house is unnatural, *as well as* possibly being bad welfare.

The owner

Owners are important stakeholders who may be seriously affected by the different outcomes. Owners may be heavily involved with the animal, sharing in its suffering and feeling grief, guilt and loss at its death. Treatment can cost the owners time or money. Owners legally prosecuted might get a criminal record.

As you may not know the owner very well, the best way to find out what is in their interests is to ask them what they want. This is important not only legally but also ethically because going against owners' wishes can be traumatic for them. It is unpleasant to be told by someone else what to do with your beloved pet, and some owners think it important that *they* fulfil their responsibility to their pet and want to be involved in all decisions. Feeling judged or bullied might even lead to owners being less keen to bring animals to your practice, or to veterinary practices at all.

Sometimes owners might not know all the choices available or the clinical facts about a decision. They may not know what happens to an animal in an operation or that there are effective treatments for conditions such as incontinence. Owners may be embarrassed or scared to say what they really want, such as if they cannot afford treatment. Owners may feel cruel for asking for euthanasia too early or for not asking early enough – and their idea of cruel can be very different from yours. Some owners find talking to nurses easier than to veterinary surgeons. In all these cases, effective communication can help owners make informed, reflective decisions.

Bereavement is an important aspect of how an owner may be affected. Research suggests that bereavement is experienced by about two in three clients and is severe in one in three (Adams et al. 2000). Grief can range from numbness to hysteria, from self-blame to anger. The well-known five stages of grief are shock and disbelief; anger and guilt; bargaining; depression; and finally, acceptance. They will vary in duration, severity and order. Sometimes stages occur before the animal is dead. These can be quite unpredictable, but still, anticipation and preparation can help in dealing with them. There is widespread recognition that appropriate grief is normal and emotionally useful, but also that every person deals with grief differently (Kubler-Ross 1969). Nurses can help with an owner's grief by letting the owner know it is acceptable and healthy to grieve and by not belittling it, e.g. by saying 'it's only a dog!' (see Chapter 2).

The nurse's colleagues

Nurses usually work under the direction of a vet. The veterinary surgeon will have an interest in the case that may be personal, academic and financial and often bears full responsibility for the animal's treatment. The vet may suffer sadness, disappointment, loss of respect and anxiety if a case does not go well and they may resent too much interference or feel in need of help or sympathy. The personality of the vet and the nurse–vet relationship will make each nurse's duties to the vet very different. A nurse will have different duties if she is a dogsbody, boss, colleague, friend or wife.

Other colleagues also count in everyday decisions, e.g. whether to do some work or just laze about is an ethical decision. It is an ethical duty not to speak badly of colleagues without good reason, or to put colleagues in difficult situations, including placing them in ethical conflicts.

One difficult ethical decision can be whether or not to pass a responsibility onto another colleague. Sometimes they are in a better position to decide than you are, or sometimes it is a decision that concerns them, e.g. it is their case. However, at other times, 'passing the buck' can actually make matters worse for the animal and should not be used as a way to avoid making a decision yourself. A nurse should generally try to avoid placing colleagues in ethically tricky situations, e.g. by booking euthanasia in for a vet in a busy consulting period or when it is another vet's case.

The practice

The practice can be considered to be a stakeholder in two ways, either as a boss who makes money or as a society who work together. A practice boss is sometimes the vet involved in the case as well, but increasingly often, the boss (e.g. practice manager or corporate owner) has no veterinary training and may not even be known personally by the nurse. Bosses can have control over various aspects of practice (e.g. by limiting options) and authority (e.g. by paying wages).

In contrast, a practice can be considered as a small society that benefits all its members and local community. Whether helping the practice is seen as helping the practice owner or all of the staff may depend on whether the boss is more concerned about making money than about the staff or patients. Nurses in family-like practices may feel loyalty and trust, whereas nurses for more money-grabbing firms may justifiably have only a business-like relationship with their employers.

In most cases, money made by the practice is money paid by the owners, and any money that the owner is 'let off' paying comes out of the practice's budget. This leads to conflicts between the interests of the practice, of the owner and of the animal. For example, if an owner cannot pay for the best treatment, then the animal may have to have a less efficacious treatment. If the owner will not pay for any treatment, the practice may have to either refuse to treat the animal or work for free.

As a society, a practice can have a societal ethic. It can be easier to make ethical decisions if all staff help each other and 'sing from the same hymn sheet'. If one nurse refuses to assist in bulldog Caesareans but another one does it unthinkingly, all that has been achieved is that the first nurse has made a stand – it could be better if all refused. Sometimes practices try to achieve a societal ethic by having standard operating procedures (SOPs) that advise nurses to make a certain type of decision in a certain way, which may be to maximize welfare or maximize profit. A nurse is still morally responsible for deciding to follow an SOP and should not follow one that she thinks is immoral.

Profession and public

Every nurse, whether a Registered Veterinary Nurse (RVN) or not, is a representative of nurses in general. This adds a further responsibility for the nurse to act well because her actions reflect on all nurses, and they may also reflect on vets too. As for a practice, 'singing from the same hymn sheet' can have benefits for all members. For these reasons, the RCVS has written down rules about what is professional conduct in its *Guide to Professional Conduct*.

The wider public might also be affected by some of the choices, e.g. humans or animals might be harmed if an animal with a notifiable disease is at large or benefitted by a free neutering clinic. In general, the public also benefit from knowing that they can rely on the nursing profession to treat their animals well, thus harming the profession may also harm the public and vice versa.

Some everyday decisions even have to consider the environment, e.g. leaving a light on in the premises overnight will have environmental effects; the cost of recycling must be balanced with the costs for the practice; and the release of non-native animals such as grey squirrels can have an effect on the native species as well as being illegal.

Nurse

On the one hand, nurses should not be too selfish and should rule out any irrational or overly selfish motivations; on the other hand, nurses should recognize their own values and biases. Contrasting these with those of the other stakeholders may help identify disagreements and resolve conflicts because you can see how your own interests and values differ from those of others.

Choose a school of thought or a framework

There are many schools of thought about the different ways to make ethical decisions, and in general terms, we can divide these into two types:

1. Those that are mainly concerned with the nurse's actions
2. Those concerned with the stakeholders.

Often people 'mix and match' but being able to roughly separate the different schools of thought can be useful in conflicts.

1. Schools of thought concerned with the nurse

These examine the rules that a nurse should follow in terms of her actions or in terms of the virtues she should have. The terms 'morality' or 'immoral' usually refer to this kind of school of thought.

Rules

A moral theory that is primarily concerned with rules that people have a duty to follow is called a **deontology**. In these theories, it is the rules that are important and not the consequences of following them, e.g. 'Do not kill' should be followed even if killing would help you or others or even if the victim would die anyway.

Many modern philosophers argue for a deontological approach based on the writings of Immanuel Kant. Kant argued that moral rules could be worked out by considering what would be acceptable if everyone did the same thing. Others have argued that duties can be worked out by imagining that everyone has to sign a contract agreeing on what morals to follow. Rules that are considered **absolute** should never be broken for any benefit. This means that no two rules could conflict (otherwise a nurse would have to break one of them). In order to prevent rules from conflicting with each other, Kant argued that absolute moral duties always say 'Do not…', which leaves the option of doing nothing.

Deontological theories could include animals, but most do not. Kant argued that only animals that appreciate moral rules can have moral status. This means that humans should never be killed or exploited but non-human animals can be exploited. In a similar way, animals cannot sign a contract. Animals (and humans who cannot reason or sign contracts) may still have an indirect moral status based on the psychological worry that being cruel to them might make one cruel to humans or because other people love them, but this is a lesser status.

Virtue ethics

The Ancient Greek teacher Aristotle argued that people should try to be virtuous and his philosophy has been revived by modern writers. Virtues might include compassion, generosity, integrity, charity, humility, loyalty and so on. A moral person is one who balances these virtues correctly in the right character.

One 'virtue' that may be important in veterinary nursing is being **caring**. Caring involves personal, committed relationships between a nurse and the animals for which she has responsibilities (Donovan and Adams 1996). One problem for care-based ethics is that it is unavoidably biased to the animals we love. It might allow us to cause a lot suffering to large numbers of battery chickens or lab rats in order to help our own dear pet a little.

Respectfulness is another virtue. One might think that dressing animals up or making them do party tricks does not respect their dignity even when it does not actually cause bad welfare. Respect for animals may require giving ethical conflicts at least some thought, whatever is decided in the end. Nurses may sometimes feel bad for thinking about a decision too little as if it was unimportant. Disrespect can also extend to treatment of animal corpses.

Another important virtue might be **moral integrity**. This involves not sacrificing one's own morality too easily just because of the situation, e.g. a nurse who believes that bulldogs should not be bred might be faced with a decision whether to help in a Caesarean on a bulldog. Looking only at the single case, it might be thought that she should help; however, if the nurse believes that bulldogs should not be bred at all, then she risks sacrificing her integrity in helping with something she thinks is wrong.

Taking **responsibility** is also a virtue. A nurse should be able to take responsibility for when she has to make a decision and act. She should also take responsibility for what she has done. This may mean 'owning up' to things she has done wrong, but it can also involve feeling legitimate self-satisfaction for having done something right (indeed feeling pleased is often worth missing out on the benefits of a more selfish option).

2. Schools of thought concerned with the stakeholders

These are concerned with how people and animals might be affected by any decision or action. They consider the effects of what people do usually in terms of harms and benefits, rights or fairness. These schools of thought can be used to formulate rules or virtues, but they are primarily concerned by the outcomes. Some of these frameworks are described below.

Animal rights

Rights theory is one of the most popular theories in modern ethics when considering humans. A person can have a positive right to have or do something, or a negative right to be left alone, e.g. a positive right to life means other people should help a person stay alive, a negative right not to be killed means only that other people should not kill them. Rights theories usually exclude non-human species from having rights, especially positive rights; however, people such as Hermann Daggett, Henry Salt and Tom Regan have argued that animals do have some negative rights.

Consequence-based theories

Some people argue that one stakeholder can be harmed if this is sufficiently useful for other stakeholders. 'Utilitarians' argue that the correct way to make ethical decisions is to add up the 'utility' or 'usefulness' of each option for all stakeholders. The right option is the one that causes 'the greatest good for the greatest number'.

This sounds very sensible but there are problems with **utilitarianism**. It misses the distinction between letting someone die and murdering them because the consequences are the same in each (ignoring indirect considerations, such as the harm of being arrested, etc.). Also, by allowing some stakeholders to be harmed to benefit others, utilitarianism could, at least in theory, allow some extreme harms for minimal benefits. It could allow exploitation of poor ethnic minorities or animals in order to benefit the rich, so long as the rich benefit more than the poor suffer. It could allow a cruel blood sport if the enjoyment it created was greater than the fear and suffering of the animals.

There are many different ways that ethicists have defined 'utility'. A founder of utilitarianism, the Reverend Jeremy Bentham, argued that morality should maximize pleasure and minimize pain. You literally add up the total pleasure and subtract the total pain that would result from each available option and the right action is the one where this number is highest. Clearly, animals should count in this equation. Bentham famously asserted that the morally relevant question is not 'Can they *reason*?' nor 'Can they *talk*?' but 'Can they *suffer*?'(Bentham 1789). Bentham's successor J.S. Mill thought that some enjoyments such as relationships and poetry were more valuable than the pleasures that animals experience, thus a human is more valuable than an animal;

however, Mill still thought animals counted and their pain should be minimized (Mill 1987).

As well as being a science, animal welfare can also be considered as a type of utilitarianism that aims to minimize animals' pain and suffering, e.g. the '**3Rs**' is an ethical framework to minimize the suffering of laboratory animals. Suffering can be decreased by *reduction* of the number of animals used, *replacement* of animals with alternatives and *refinement* of procedures to cause less suffering.

Naturalness

As previously described, some people argue that animals should be allowed to live natural lives. Animals should be allowed to have natural breeding, natural environments and natural interactions with other animals and to be free from mutilations 'as nature intended'. A related school of thought is **environmentalism**. The environment should be protected or left alone, and we should avoid exploiting it (too much). Sometimes these schools of thought disagree with animal welfare, e.g. some people think wild animals should be left to live their natural lives entirely unaffected by human interference, which means that humans should not get involved even when a wild animal is injured and in pain.

Justice

Others have argued that the outcome of any action should be just. You might be able to avoid pain for many animals by doing lots of painful experiments on just one, but this might seem unjust on that one animal. Justice can be considered in terms of legal justice, in terms of rights or in terms of fairness to all the different stakeholders – and these may disagree. For example, it might be thought unfair that the law says you have to kill a grey squirrel because it is grey, when red squirrels are not killed – it is not the squirrel's fault which colour it is.

Frameworks

Some ethicists have thought that no single theory or school of thought is correct and they have come up with ethical frameworks to help analyse a problem without having to decide on just one ethical theory. Such frameworks do not always automatically generate an answer about how to act, but they help identify the different issues to consider and the different views of the stakeholders.

The Five Freedoms (Box 1.3) can be thought of as an ethical framework that combines different theories as well as being a framework for welfare assessment. A nurse can try to act so that the animal is as free from hunger, thirst, discomfort and so on as much as possible. In many European countries, they replace the 'Freedom to Perform *Normal* Behaviour' with 'Freedom to Perform *Natural* Behaviour'.

A common framework in medical ethics is based on **four principles** shown in Table 1.1. This approach combines elements of theories on rights, utilitarianism and justice.

Food ethicist Ben Mepham devised an '**ethical matrix**' framework that applies the four principles to each stakeholder. This is a tool that helps people look at all the angles on a decision and helps different people communicate their views in the same framework. Table 1.2 is an adapted example.

Religious ethics

Religious ethics are also often a combination of ethical approaches. The Jewish, Christian and Islamic faiths have been important in forming the ethics of much of Western society. For example, Jesus laid down some specific rules, e.g. 'love thy neighbour' and also provided a role model for how to be virtuous. Western religions are often thought to be against animal welfare, e.g. in ritual slaughter, but each religion has rules against cruelty and there are many different opinions within each religion. For example, many Christians preach the importance of caring for animals. In fact, the symbol of the British Veterinary Nursing Association (BVNA) is Francis of Assisi, a Christian saint, who preached to the animals and told people to care for all life.

Other religions such as Buddhism and Jainism vary in their respect, but some forms argue for complete avoidance of even accidental killing. Hinduism and Hare Krishna afford special respect to cows. All of these can affect how people think about animals and can even lead to legal battles when parties disagree, especially when people fail to appreciate the strength or logic of others' convictions.

Identify choices you think are ethically acceptable

Using the range of ethical schools of thought, you can try to work out which of the choices is ethically the best one for you and the situation. In some cases, several options are acceptable and you can choose the best among them.

You may think that one option should not be done, because:

- It would be wrong if everyone did it (a deontological position)
- It suggests a less caring nurse (a virtue ethics position)
- It breaches someone's right (a rights position)
- It causes unnecessary pain to animals (an animal welfare position)
- The harm is not outweighed by a greater good to another stakeholder (a utilitarian position)
- It is unnatural (a naturalist or environmentalist position)
- It is unfair (a justice position)
- Or a combination of any of the above, e.g. in a framework.

Discuss your decision with other stakeholders

The different stakeholders might have different views. For example, in a decision on euthanasia, an owner might want their animal kept alive at all costs because they want to avoid grief, because they are scared to make the decision, because they think killing an animal is cruel, even if it is suffering, or because they may feel guilty for the animal's situation. Alternatively, they might want their animal killed because they cannot reasonably afford treatment, because it is aggressive or incontinent, or because they think that rehoming is less caring or less responsible than euthanasia. Some owners might want to be persuaded or given other options; others will have already made up their mind and resist challenges, such as the idea that their animal might be owned by someone else.

Talking to the other stakeholders as part of your decision making can be useful to:

Table 1.1 Four principles and what they mean

Principle (Beauchamp and Childress 1979)	Meaning	Equivalent principle in the ethical matrix
Respect for autonomy	Respecting the decisions that patients or owners make	Autonomy
Non-maleficence	Not making animals worse off	Well-being
Beneficence	Making animals better off	
Justice	Fairness and respect for rights	Fairness

Table 1.2 Generic ethical matrix

Principles* Stakeholders	Well-being	Autonomy	Fairness
THE ANIMAL	Animal welfare	Respect for *telos* (e.g. doggyness)	Intrinsic value
THE VET	Peace of mind; job satisfaction	Clinical freedom; conscientious objection	Professional and legal roles and responsibilities
THE CLIENT	Owner quality of life; money, time, convenience; enjoyment of pet	Respecting owner's wishes; informed consent	Outcome appropriate to their situation; getting the best service they can afford
THE PROFESSION	Maintain professional privileges	Maintain self-regulation	Not having overly large influence on public opinion of profession
THE PRACTICE	Public relations	Practice policies and SOPs	Need to keep business going

* as shown in Table 1.1.

- Help you test your own position by hearing it said out loud
- Give a chance for them to notice weaknesses in your argument
- Find out more information about how they would be affected
- Help you understand their position
- Help them understand your position
- Identify disagreements
- Help with resolving disagreements.

You might disagree for several different reasons. You might have different ethical principles, be less or more willing to take responsibility for the decision, or have different factual beliefs, such as a different assessment of the animal's quality of life. Identifying any or all of these can help to resolve the disagreement. Good communication is therefore essential. Being overly argumentative, judgemental or not showing understanding, compassion or flexibility can be offensive and can make people less likely to reach the best decision.

Good communication can also help a nurse recognize other people's conflicts. Often when one feels that someone has done something wrong, the person who did it may have been in an ethical conflict. They may have decided to do the harm because it was the 'lesser of two evils', e.g. a vet might have struggled with a decision whether to perform a bulldog Caesarean, and thought it is better than letting the animal suffer or killing it. Similarly, some employers make their nurses tell them if they are pregnant. This may mean the nurse telling them before they would want to, but it may be necessary to avoid the greater harm of the fetus being exposed to harmful gases and radiation.

Euthanasia

As an example, one important case in which discussion is useful is in making a choice about the use of euthanasia or of life-saving treatment. Owners and vets might be experiencing ethical dilemmas and need help to make decisions. In addition, euthanasia usually cannot be done legally without the owner's consent and veterinarian's direction.

Getting the owner to make a good decision about euthanasia can be difficult, especially with a grieving client, and an understanding of the five stages of grief, described previously, may be useful. Shock may prevent owners being able to make any decision, and disbelief may make owners question the veterinary surgeon's advice or yours. Others may resist understanding, e.g. by misunderstanding phrases like 'put to sleep' – so these should be avoided. Anger and guilt occur in at least 50% of clients (Adams et al. 2000). Both may bias their decision making, e.g. guilt for not seeking veterinary advice earlier can make owners less keen to seek it now. Anger and guilt can also strain client–nurse relationships, tempting you to blame clients when you are angry, but this can inflame their anger and/or their guilt and is usually not productive. Guilt can also prevent owners from asking for euthanasia, or make them ask in a veiled way.

Bargaining involves the owner trying to alter the facts or your decision making, or trying to get some concessions. When this stage occurs at the time of the euthanasia decision (e.g. owners bargaining to delay euthanasia), compromising with the owner can be useful (e.g. using your discretion about matters such as payment and disposal). The owner's depression should be taken into account in euthanasia decisions; however, this is quite usual whenever a pet dies, so delaying euthanasia to avoid owner depression is not necessarily beneficial except where it may help them to make a more rational decision.

Disagreements between stakeholders

It may be the case that the different people involved will think that different things should be done. A nurse may disagree with an owner, a veterinary surgeon, an employer or all three. A major part of ethical thinking involves coming up with methods to resolve or avoid these conflicts. There is a spectrum of options that a nurse can do, from doing just what she is told to doing just what she wants.

1. Do what other people want

Doing whatever the owner, vet or employer wants is, in general, a good way to keep within the law and to maintain good public and work relations. In this way, the vet's ethics becomes the nurse's (deontological) ethics. The risk is that owners, vets and bosses have no more training in ethical reasoning than nurses and may well make wrong decisions however qualified/old/experienced/wage-paying they may be. When they do makes bad choices, this may harm the animal, nurse, owner and vet (even the person making the decision), and the nurse who has carried out their wishes is still morally blameworthy for deciding to do so.

2. Make joint decisions

It is helpful to remember that your assessment may not be perfect and that you can learn from other people. Discussion can help you improve your position and help the other stakeholders reflect on theirs. Wherever possible, this is likely to be the best decision, but where stakeholders cannot agree, constructive discussion may be difficult and other methods might be sought.

3. Influence the owner or vet

A nurse might try to influence the owner or vet. Legally, the owner's decision should be informed and not unduly influenced but there is a very fine line between 'neutral' advice and undue influence.

There are legitimate and acceptable ways to influence clients. Generally, owners rely on the veterinary team to provide advice and often ask directly, 'What is the best course of action?' or 'What would you do?' Even once they have been informed by the vet, owners may still need guidance in deciding between options, and the nurse can give useful advice on the decision-making process as well as providing the information. Similarly, vets may benefit from advice on certain issues – they are not always as sure as they may appear. With effective communication and empathy, nurses can provide education and advice about both the clinical issue and the welfare concepts and their ethical implications. So long as care is taken not to *unduly* influence the owner, this can legitimately achieve the nurse's goals. There are no such legal limits on influencing the vet, beyond professionalism and common decency.

4. Direct opposition

Sometimes it may be necessary for a nurse to tell the owner or vet that they disagree with their choice. It is tricky to know when such comments are appropriate. Clearly, when nurses witness something they feel is unethical, they should not feel obliged to remain silent out of deference or out of fear of the personal consequences. On the other hand, comments may be inappropriate if the owner's or vet's decision is different from the nurse's but still perfectly reasonable or if the disagreement is too trivial to make it worth any ensuing unpleasantness. Criticisms from the benefit of hindsight are especially risky, as people can be very touchy about cases where the outcomes were not what they hoped.

Conscientious objection

In addition to a nurse stating her disagreement with a decision, she can also decide not to be involved. This is called 'conscientious objection'. Even if nurses cannot force owners or vets to do the right thing, they can maintain their integrity by refusing to be involved. As with influencing, this has its ethical limits and a nurse should not refuse to do reasonable options just because there is an even better option available. In cases where both vet and nurse may object to the owner's requests, communication between vet and nurse can help each other to check the reasonableness of their position and strengthen their resolve. In cases where the vet is compliant with the owner and where conscientious objection might harm the animal, the nurse may have to reconsider her own position bearing in mind that two other people agree; but if she feels sure she is right, then she may still wish to refuse to help.

Direct action

In some cases, a nurse might actively act without other people's consent, e.g. treating an animal without consent and refunding money against the boss's instructions. This is legally safer when the owner's/boss's wishes are unknown and the nurse acts reasonably. It is legally more risky when the nurse's actions affect other peoples' property against their wishes.

Whistle-blowing

A step further than direct action and is to actively report the owner or vet. You can report a colleague to their employer (although this will not work if the problematic person *is* your employer). You can report veterinarians and Registered Veterinary Nurse (RVN) to the RCVS professional conduct department by making a formal complaint. Employers can be reported to bodies such as the Health and Safety Executive, the Office of Fair Trading, Veterinary Medicines Directorate (VMD) or the police for contravening laws, such as fraud or misuse of drugs. Anyone who harms an animal or fails to provide for their needs – including owners, veterinarians and RVNs – can be reported to the police or Royal Society for Prevention of Cruelty to Animals (RSPCA) (Scottish Society for Prevention of Cruelty to Animals [SSPCA] in Scotland). The law governing these offences is covered in Chapter 3.

The ethical reasons to report someone can be based on avoiding certain consequences that cannot be legally achieved otherwise, e.g. preventing continued abuse, future harm to other animals or even children, where a nurse has additional concerns that a child might also be likely to be abused. They might also be based on justice, in that wrongdoers should not be allowed to get away with their misdeeds.

At the same time, there are ethical reasons *against* reporting. As well as being a legal and professional matter, respect for confidentiality has ethical bases. For example, the owner or other clients might be less keen to get their animals treated if they fear being reported. The person reported may suffer enormously. If they are found guilty, this can lead to the person being struck off from working as a vet or RVN. If not, then it is a source of embarrassment and antagonism for the nurse who reported them. So the option of reporting should not be taken lightly. One general rule might be to report only if a person has acted *unreasonably*, and the whistle-blowing is likely to have a desirable effect overall.

Act

The final act is often the hardest bit. Many philosophers have written about **weakness of will**, where people make decisions but then somehow do not quite put them into practice. Sometimes we forget to do things or wrongly assume that a colleague will do it. It can be useful to put a system such as care plans in place to help people remember and communicate better. Sometimes selfishness can stop a nurse from enacting her decision – a nurse might resolve to be more helpful or be less irritable but then feels tired or poorly and does not do it.

At other times, it is hard to complete a plan that harms one of the stakeholders. It can be very hard to kill an animal even when you think it is the right thing to do. When thinking about an imaginary animal suffering, it is easy to say 'Yes I would kill it', but with the animal and owner in front of you, it can be much harder. It is especially hard if it is your own animal. Such feelings are natural and they should not make you feel guilty or embarrassed. It can be good to remind yourself that you are doing what you think is right. Remember that owners face this problem as well, so you may need to help them carry out their decisions.

Reflect on the decision and outcomes and prepare for next time

One of the most important stages is to think back over a decision. Reflective practice is a good way to develop one's ethical reasoning skills and improve as a nurse. It also helps prepare for next time, so this step and thinking about ethical problems before they occur may be combined.

Firstly, reflective practice can help you avoid future conflicts, just as owners can learn to recognize early signs of ear or anal gland disease and avoid it flaring up, so you can get better at avoiding awkward situations. You can warn owners or vets in advance that you will not help with a bulldog Caesarean. You can tell members of the public not to bring healthy grey squirrels into the practice.

When a decision has gone well, one usually does not think to reflect on it, but reflecting on good decisions is useful. It can be a 'reward' that might help you act well next time. It can also help see ways in which a decision could be improved; so next time, it is even better. It may help identify *why* a decision was good (e.g. was it down to good communication, empathy, integrity, animal welfare assessment, fairness, etc.) so that you can make sure you do the same next time. Reflecting that you did the right thing can reduce the guilt felt at the final act. The same goes for the vet and the owner, and it can be good to remind them that they did the right thing.

When a decision has gone badly, one may not want to think about it because you feel guilty, but this only makes matters worse. It can be better to bring this guilt out into the open; indeed this is one of the main aspects of psychotherapy. Reflecting on decisions that have gone wrong can help identify why they went wrong, e.g. was it down to not enough information, bad reasoning, weakness of will, etc. in preparation for next time.

Reflection after the event is dangerous if done wrong. It is very easy to spot mistakes *after* they have been made. You forget that at that time you did not have the knowledge and experience that you do now that it is all over. This is true for clinical decisions as well. It is easy for a team or owner to think that one should, or should not, have operated once the dog is dead, but it may be that at the time, operating was, or was not, the best thing to do however it turned out. In reflecting on one's own decisions, it is wrong to feel guilt if the decision was right at the time, even if it turned out badly. Thus, you should not feel bad and you may also have a role in helping owners and vets avoid guilt for good past decisions. Conversely, in reflecting on other people's decisions, you should consider what they knew at the time. Judging people after the event can cause enormous offence and annoyance. This 'moralizing' is one danger of ethical reasoning that you should make sure you avoid: ethics should be a constructive exercise helping everyone to make better decisions and achieve desirable outcomes in practice.

Bibliography

Adams, C.L., Bonnett, B.N., Meek, A.H., 2000. Predictors of owners' response to companion animal death in 177 clients from 14 practices in Ontario. J. Am. Vet. Med. Assoc. 217, 1303–1309.

Bentham, J., 1789. Introduction to the Principles of Morals and Legislation. Clarendon Press, Oxford.

Donovan, J., Adams, C.J. (Eds.), 1996. Beyond Animal Rights: A Feminist Caring Ethic for the Treatment of Animals. Continuum, New York.

Engster, D., 2006. Care ethics and animal welfare. J. Soc. Philos. 37 (4), 521–536.

Farm Animal Welfare Council, 1993. Second Report on Priorities for Research and Development in Farm Animal Welfare. FAWC, London.

Glass, R.M., 2005. Is grief a disease? JAMA 293 (21), 2658–2660.

Kant, I., 1963. Lecture in Ethics (L. Infield, Trans.). Harper & Row, NY.

Kant, I., 1996. Metaphysics of Morals (M. Gregor, Trans.). CUP, Cambridge, pp. 192–193.

Kubler-Ross, E., 1969. On Death and Dying. Collier Books/Macmillan, NY.

Mill, J.S., 1987. In: Ryder, A. (Ed.), Utilitarianism and Other Essays. Penguin, New York, pp. 272–338.

Recommended reading

Animal Ethics Dilemma. Available from: <www.ethicaltools.com>.
A fun interactive tool that challenges you in a number of cases. It gives you an indication of your own underlying moral theories, but you should be careful not to pigeonhole yourself and then try to live up to that classification (remember it is only a tool).

Beauchamp, T., Childress, J., 1979. Principles of Biomedical Ethics. Oxford University Press, Oxford.
The original book describing the Four Principles, updated several times since. It uses medical cases, which makes it less directly relevant.

DeGrazia, D., 2002. Animal Rights: A Very Short Introduction. Oxford University Press, Oxford.
A brief and readable guide to animal ethics from a prominent philosopher. It is useful for considering the 'bigger picture' issues, rather than veterinary matters.

Fraser, A.F., Broom, D.M., 2007. Domestic Animal Behaviour and Welfare. CAB International, Oxford.
A good general review of welfare issues of different animals, this latest edition contains sections on companion animals.

Mepham, B., Kaiser, M., Thorstensen, E., Tomkins, S., Millar, K., 2006. Ethical Matrix Manual. LEI, The Hague. Available from: <http://www.ethicaltools.info>.
A brief guide to making and using ethical matrices.

Pullin, S., Gray, C., 2006. Ethics, Law and the Veterinary Nurse. Butterworth-Heinemann, Oxford.
A collection of essays on aspects of ethics and law for veterinary nurses. It is well written and focuses on nurse issues. It does have a high variation in quality of chapters, and some overlap.

Rollin, B., 2006. An Introduction to Veterinary Ethics. Wiley-Blackwell, Oxford.
This has been the main textbook on veterinary ethics. It is divided into a theoretical introductory part and a discussion of specific cases. The cases relate to real life and Rollin writes engagingly and passionately.

Sandøe P., Christiansen, S., 2008. Ethics of Animal Use. Wiley-Blackwell, Oxford.
An excellently written book that considers several approaches to ethics in a number of contexts and issues.

Stewart, M.F., 2003. Companion Animal Death. Butterworth-Heinemann/Petsavers, Oxford.
A simple and short book on bereavement in pet owners.

CHAPTER 2

The art of communication

Kirsty Jones

Key Points

- Effective communication is necessary to pass information from one person to another and is only successful when both parties have understood the same information.
- The many types of communication can be broadly divided into verbal and non-verbal forms.
- Communication can be affected by a range of factors such as culture, grief and anger.
- The efficiency of a practice and its ability to communicate effectively with its clients is based on a strict practice hierarchy and the knowledge that each person in the organization is competent to carry out all aspects of his or her job.

Introduction

Effective communication is all about conveying messages to other people clearly and unambiguously. It is also about receiving information from others with as little distortion as possible. Communication is only successful when it results in both the sender and the receiver understanding the same information.

Methods of communication

There are many forms of communication used in daily life and they can be broadly divided into two areas, verbal and non-verbal communication. According to research, it is widely accepted that there are three major factors involved in face-to-face human communication and these are:

- 55% of impact is determined by body language, e.g. postures, gestures and eye contact
- 38% by the tone of voice
- 7% by the content of the words.

Verbal communication

Verbal communication is largely concerned with words, although this does not necessarily mean that it only involves speech. Any message that is portrayed using words and the alphabet as a medium can be classed as verbal communication. The medium by which information is transported could include:

- Speaking and listening
- Telephone
- Video conference/web cam
- Letter writing
- Email
- Formal notices
- Poster.

The list is endless!

The most common methods of communication in a veterinary practice with colleagues or clients are speaking or writing by a sender and listening or reading by the receiver (Fig. 2.1).

Non-verbal communication

Methods of non-verbal communication do not directly involve spoken or written language but convey the message by such things as:

- Hand gestures
- Facial expressions such as smiling or frowning
- Posture and body movements
- Eye contact
- Touch
- Voice – speed, pitch
- Other aspects of physical appearance such as clothing or hairstyle.

These are all powerful means of transmitting messages. It is very important to realize that, at times, a person's body may be 'talking' even as he or she maintains silence (Fig. 2.2), and when people do speak, their bodies may sometimes say different things from what their words convey. A *mixed message* occurs when a person's words communicate one message, while non-verbally, he or she is communicating something else. Every verbal message comes with a non-verbal component. Receivers interpret messages by taking in meaning from everything available. When non-verbal cues are consistent with verbal messages, they act to reinforce the message; however, when these verbal and non-verbal

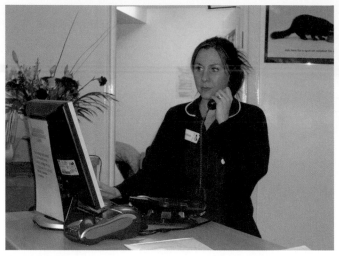

Fig. 2.1 A receptionist demonstrating the use of verbal communication by telephone. She is also receiving two forms of verbal communication via the telephone and the computer screen

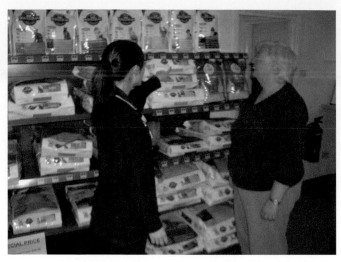

Fig. 2.3 The receptionist explaining the different types of food to a client. Face-to-face communication permits rapid transfer of ideas and also allows information to be conveyed by non-verbal means

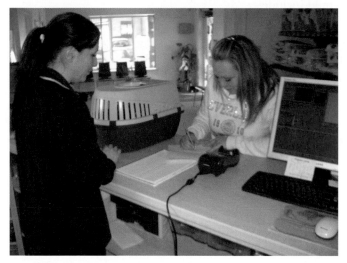

Fig. 2.2 The receptionist remains silent and relaxed, allowing the client time to read, understand and sign a consent form

messages are inconsistent, they create confusion for the receiver. It is essential to avoid inconsistency in communication with clients and colleagues.

In face-to-face interactions, a person can judge how the other party is reacting, get immediate feedback and respond accordingly. Face-to-face communication permits the exchange of words and the opportunity to see the non-verbal communication (Fig. 2.3).

Verbal styles

All speech will fall into one of the four basic communication styles shown in Table 2.1.

With reference to Table 2.1, clearly, the only healthy communication style is assertive communication, but most people use a combination of all four styles, depending on the situation. The styles chosen generally depend on what past experience has taught us will work best to meet our

needs in a specific situation. Understanding the four basic types of verbal communication will help you learn how to react effectively when confronted with a difficult person. It will also help you recognize when you are using manipulative behaviour to meet your own needs.

Written communication

Written communication has the advantage in that it provides a record for referral and follow-up, and it is a means of providing identical messages to a large number of people. Its major limitation is that the sender does not know how or if the communication is received unless a reply is required.

The following are some guidelines for effective written communication:

- Plan each message
- Draft the message with the reader(s) in mind
- Give the message a concise informative title and use sub-headings where appropriate
- Use simple words and short, clear sentences and paragraphs
- Back up opinions with facts
- Avoid 'flowery' language and euphemisms
- Summarize main points at the end and let the reader know what they must do next.

Questioning skills

Asking the correct question is at the heart of effective communication and information exchange. By using the right questions in a particular situation, it is possible to improve a whole range of communications skills, e.g. better information for use in history taking, build stronger relationships and manage clients more effectively.

a. **Closed questions** – These usually receive a single word or very short, factual answer, e.g. 'Are you thirsty?'; the answer is 'Yes' or 'No'. 'Where do you live?'; the answer is generally the name of your town or your address.

Table 2.1 Types of verbal style

Style	Quality
Aggressive communication	• Aggressive communication always involves manipulation • Attempts to make people act by inducing guilt (hurt) or by using intimidation and control tactics (anger) • Covert or overt, insistence that needs must be met (and right now!) with no regard for the other party
Passive communication	• Based on compliance and hopes to avoid confrontation at all costs • Passive communicators do not talk much, question even less and actually do very little • Do not want to 'rock the boat' • Passives have learned that it is safer not to react and easier to disappear than to stand up and be noticed
Passive-aggressive communication	• A combination of styles, passive-aggressive avoids direct confrontation, but attempts to get 'heard' through manipulation • This style of communication often leads to office politics and rumour mongering
Assertive communication	• This is natural expression when self-esteem is intact, confident communication without games and manipulation • Assertiveness leads to communication of needs clearly and forthrightly • The individual cares about the relationship and strives for a win-win situation • Limits are maintained and the individual refuses to be pushed beyond them despite the insistence of another party

Closed questions are good for:

■ Testing the understanding of yourself or the other person, e.g. 'So, if I obtain this qualification, will I get a pay rise?'

■ Concluding a discussion or making a decision, e.g. 'Now we know the facts, are we all agreed this is the right course of treatment?'

■ Frame setting, e.g. 'Are you happy with the service from your vets?'

b. **Open questions** – These require longer answers. They usually begin with what, why or how. An open question asks the respondent for his or her knowledge, opinion or feelings. 'Tell me' and 'describe' can also be used in the same way as open questions. Here are some examples:

■ What happened at the meeting?

■ What happened when you took him for a walk?

■ How was the puppy party?

■ Tell me what happened next.

■ Describe the circumstances in more detail.

Open questions are good for:

■ Developing an open conversation, e.g. 'What did you get up to at the weekend?'

■ Finding out more detail, e.g. 'What other things have you noticed that are a bit "odd" about Fluff's behaviour?'

■ Finding out the other person's opinion or problems, e.g. 'What do you think about the changes to the rota?'

c. **Funnel questions** – This technique involves starting with general questions, then homing in on a point in each answer and asking more and more detail at each level. The technique can be useful to clarify details from clients.

d. **Probing questions** – Asking probing questions is another strategy for finding out more detail. Sometimes it is as simple as asking a respondent for an example to help the understanding of a statement they have made. At other times, you need additional information for clarification e.g. 'How do you know that the new database can't be used by reception yet?'. Make sure

when questioning a client or colleague that the person is given enough time to respond. They may need to include thinking time before they answer. Do not just interpret a pause as a 'No comment' and carry on talking.

Active listening

Listening is making sense of what is heard and requires paying attention, interpreting and remembering. Some say we were born with one mouth and two ears for a reason and they must be used in that order! Effective active listeners do the following:

• Make eye contact

• Smile and nod during the conversation

• Genuinely seek information

• Avoid being emotional or attacking others

• Paraphrase the message heard, especially to clarify the speaker's intentions

• Keep silent; do not talk to fill pauses, or respond to statements in a point–counterpoint fashion.

• Ask clarifying questions

• Avoid making distracting gestures

• Schedule sufficient, uninterrupted time for meetings.

Factors affecting communication

There are many factors that affect our ability to communicate: they may make it more effective, but they may also make it more difficult and spoil the final result. They include the following:

Emotion

For many clients, a visit to the surgery is an emotional experience. Clients may be suffering with grief from the loss of their pet or anxious about bringing in their pets for surgery, tests and consultations. It may be an ordinary everyday occurrence for veterinary staff, but, to a client, it can be an extraordinary occurrence. Many clients will be emotional to some degree when they come to visit, and this can lead to a breakdown in communication.

Unsurprisingly, clients find it difficult to listen when they are focusing on their pet in a busy veterinary practice. By following the advice here about appropriate questioning and active listening, you can ensure that the breakdown in communication is minimal. Supporting any veterinary advice e.g. pre-/postoperative care, feeding, bandage care with well-written literature can reduce this further. A follow-up phone call may be useful in establishing that the client is happy and satisfied. Quite often, it is not until the client has gone home that they realize they have more questions, so the phone call can be a good way of keeping communication channels open and checking that all is well.

Terminology

The use of complicated terminology or jargon may be a hindrance in the communication process. A nurse's role can be a vital 'bridge' between a veterinary surgeon and the client. Quite often, a client will not want to ask the vet to repeat what they have said, especially if they do not understand when the vet has used a lot of specialized terminology. It is often the nurse's role to 'interpret' to the client what the vet has said. It is also important to avoid using complicated jargon yourself or, if it is necessary, take a moment to explain what the terms mean in plain English.

Culture

Cultural diversity includes differences in national origin, race, ethics, language and religion. Working with people from various cultures and subcultures can be both interesting and stimulating. However, it can also be stressful, confusing and frustrating when we do not understand what they are trying to say and vice versa. When working with clients who have English as a second language, try to be as patient as possible.

Special needs

As in any other service industry where direct communication with the public is a major component, it is important to be aware of the rights and responsibilities towards those clients and staff members who have special needs. This could range from problems with sight, hearing or mobility to learning difficulties and mental health issues. Such clients will require more time and assistance. This is an area where ongoing professional development can benefit individuals within the organization and help build the reputation of the practice for outstanding public service.

Dealing with aggressive or angry clients

Truly aggressive or violent clients are, thankfully, quite rare, but there is often no warning that they are going to be aggressive as aggression is not always accompanied by anger. However, they may have an intention to do harm to someone or something. It may be prudent to remember that some clients may be seriously ill and are therefore showing signs of aggression.

If a client has a known aggressive or violent history, ensure that:

- There is an accompanying person in the room; a 'note taker' can be a good excuse
- Panic buttons are available
- A room with an escape route is available.

In extreme cases, the practice may decide to ban the aggressor from the premises.

Case studies have shown that there can be two factors causing a potentially aggressive person to 'snap':

- **Internal factors** – they may be defensive, fearful, resistant to information or suggestions, manipulative, or grieving
- **External factors** – such as language problems, literacy problems, a busy waiting room, breaking bad news or poor environment.

Signs of anger

These are listed in the order that they occur:

1. Facial expression changes
2. Physiological changes – blood pressure and respiratory rate increase
3. Tone of voice – becomes louder and faster.

When faced with these signs of anger, it is important to remain calm and passive in your speech and facial expression. Here are a few tips that may help when dealing with an angry or emotional person:

1. Find a quiet area away from the bustle of the practice and offer them a seat and keep offering until they sit. If they do not sit, sit down yourself – a client will find it very hard to keep shouting if you are sitting down.
2. Use empathy as a tool. Overestimate their level of anger, e.g. 'I can see that you are really angry…' or 'I can see this has made you really angry'.
3. Show you want to help out, listen to them and summarize at the end to ensure you have all the facts and that they agree.
4. Acknowledge their feelings. It is normal for us all to feel frustrated at times, so acknowledge this.
5. Plan a strategy on how to deal with the problem and involve the client in this.
6. Summarize again; ensure everything is understood by both of you.
7. Ask if there is anything else you can help them with.
8. After the incident is over, take time to quietly reflect on what has taken place and how it could have been improved. If it went well, allow yourself a moment of self-congratulation.

Supporting clients through the grieving process

Grief is not an abnormality for which one should feel ashamed – it is a normal, natural and painful emotional reaction to loss. As in any relationship, when an animal companion dies or is ill, the owners are likely to feel stress, sorrow and grief. The significance of a pet dying and the consequent emotional impact on the owner is now clearly recognized within the veterinary profession, and educational materials, support groups, hotlines and counselling are available. The relatively short lifespan of dogs and cats means that clients face losing several animals during a lifetime. Most vets and nurses themselves have painful memories of losing a particular animal and understand only too well the pain that their clients feel.

An extra burden comes in having to take responsibility for the timing of death by euthanasia. Seventy per cent of animals are euthanized rather than dying naturally so this is a common problem. Some clients may feel a philosophical dilemma of balancing the relieving of pain and suffering while thinking it is wrong to kill on religious or cultural grounds, but the majority will just not want to say goodbye to a much loved friend. The difficulty of the decision overlays the loss with feelings of overwhelming guilt and the thought that there must have been some other step that could have been taken to preserve the animal's life.

How to help grieving owners

It is not only in situations of euthanasia that clients are affected by grief – traumatic accidents, sudden collapse or an unexpected diagnosis will all have a similar effect on a client. There are many stages to grief (Table 2.2), and an understanding of these stages will help you to help them

- **Shock** – Find a quiet area for the client to sit, offer them a drink, your time and empathy. Listen to the client and if they are expressing disbelief, do not contradict them; sympathize with them. Discuss all areas of what has happened to help put things in order for the client. If the client does not want to talk, do not make them. Do not let them leave the surgery, or drive, until they feel ready to do so. If needed, call a relative or a friend or a taxi to get them home.
- **Emotional release** – Let the owner cry; supply tissues and listen. Tears are the healthiest expression of grief. Show you care and empathize. You may not know how they feel, but you can understand how they feel.

- **Panic** – This is potentially more likely to happen away from the surgery. If you recognize that a client may be panicking, medical help should be sought.
- **Guilt** – Reassure owners that it is not their fault. If an animal has died from a disease, it may be helpful to sympathize with the owner and gently acknowledge that it is often easier to spot the symptoms after the diagnosis has been made. If an animal has been injured, help them recognize they could not have done any more. Do not intensify owners feelings of guilt – try to run through the events to alleviate any 'what I should have done' thoughts.
- **Hostility** – The practice may be the first target for a hostile 'attack' when a client is grieving over what has happened to their pet. This may be because the owner feels guilty and needs to attribute blame. The quality and type of treatment provided by the practice may be questioned. Meticulous record keeping by members of the practice team should remove any worries over litigation, but dealing with any complaint promptly and with empathy should be the practice's first priority.

In keeping with a practice's client communication and care policies, it is advisable to call clients a few days after a loss to see if they have any questions or unresolved issues surrounding the treatment of their pet. Many practices have a policy of sending a sympathy card to all owners whose animals have died.

Practice organization

The veterinary care we give to our clients and their animals is often quite complicated and difficult to understand by the outsider. A visit to the practice is often under stressful circumstances and can be emotionally charged. Understanding that everybody takes in information in different ways, our communication skills and professional presentation must be of a high standard to ensure that we achieve a good working relationship with our clients. As a rule, most clients cannot judge medical knowledge or surgical skills, so they judge the

Table 2.2 The stages of grief

Shock	Immediately following the death of an animal, it is difficult to accept the loss. A feeling of unreality occurs. This usually only lasts a few hours.
Emotional release	The awareness of just how dreadful the loss is accompanied by intense pangs of grief. In this stage, a grieving individual sleeps badly and weeps uncontrollably.
Panic	For some time, a grieving person may feel in the grip of mental instability. They may find themselves wandering around aimlessly, forgetting things and not being able to finish what they started. Physical symptoms may also appear, e.g. tightness in the throat, heaviness in the chest, an empty feeling in the stomach, tiredness and fatigue, headaches and migraines.
Guilt	At this stage, an individual can begin to feel guilty about failures to do 'enough' for their pet or guilt over what happened or what did not happen. They may also feel guilty that life has become much easier without the animal.
Hostility	Some individuals feel anger at what caused the loss of their pet, and there may be a tendency to blame others for what happened.
Reconciliation of grief	A balance in life returns little by little. There are no set time frames for healing – each individual is different.
Hope	Grief will lessen. Plans are made for the future. The owner is able to move forward with good feelings knowing that he or she will always have memories of their pet.

Table 2.3 Factors affecting a client's perception of a practice

Tangibles	• Appearance of building and surroundings • How professional the staff look • Delayed appointments handled well, refreshments offered
Reliability	• Ability to correctly perform what is promised • Estimates are accurate; if going to be increased, a call to inform the owner may be prudent
Assurance	• Knowledge • Competence • Credibility • Courtesy
Responsiveness	• Willingness to help when asked • Promptness with appointments • Calls to follow up appointments
Empathy	• Ease of contact • Understanding the clients needs

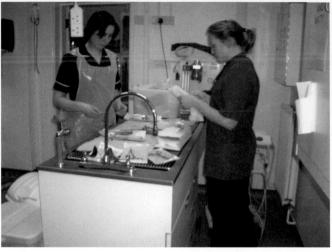

Fig. 2.4 A veterinary surgeon and a nurse wear different types of uniform, which communicates to the client and to other staff their roles in the practice hierarchy

level of service. Clients look for subtle indicators of quality to confirm that they and their pets are valued, respected and getting value for money. Think about it – does the evidence that your practice presents support this?

Every activity, person, place and document should tell the same story to every person and patient. Everything matters no matter how small or apparently insignificant – clients notice small things and staff should be sure to notice them too!

Public image is important

All practices should have a code of attitude to clients based on the findings from a study carried out in the USA. This discovered what was most important to clients and these are listed, in no particular order, in Table 2.3.

1. It is helpful to ask your clients at regular intervals how they feel that the practice is doing. Produce a client survey questionnaire and welcome any client complaints as a motivation to improve.
2. Make first impressions count. Either you or a 'hired' friend should do a complete walk-through of your waiting room and the rest of your practice using their 'client eyes'. It is useful to bring an animal and start from the time you enter the car park.
3. Look critically at the environment and the service.
   - Is it clean and tidy (car park free from weeds and faeces, etc.)?
   - Is signage and paintwork fresh and up to date?
   - Is access easy?
4. Sit in the waiting room for 20 minutes, look around you, and watch what is going on.
   - How happy is your pet to be there? Are there separate dog and cat waiting areas?
   - Is everything clean and tidy in the waiting room and around the reception desk?
   - Are the receptionists ready to help you immediately, or are they gossiping behind the desk?
   - What do clients hear as they wait? Do they hear happy and calm professional staff or a complete frenzy?

5. Go through each part of the surgery premises and detail everything.
   - Are you looked after throughout your visit?
   - Are staff roles clear and identifiable?

This list is not exhaustive and each practice should make its own judgements about how to improve. However, it is vital to make this sort of check at regular intervals because as staff change, so may the service. Always remember that 'the customer is right' even if you disagree and that they can always go elsewhere. Happy, satisfied clients mean a happy, satisfied business with lots of clients (and a pay increase!).

Practice structure

The smooth running of a busy practice depends on all staff having detailed roles and responsibilities and understanding their position in the practice hierarchy and the part they play in the running of the practice machine. The practice hierarchy should also be obvious to the clients, and this is helped by the wearing of different uniforms (Fig. 2.4) – in some cases, the veterinary surgeons wear their own clothes, which separates them from the other members of the practice.

The personnel found within a practice usually include the following:

Veterinary surgeon (MRCVS)

Veterinary surgeons work to safeguard the health and welfare of animals. In general practice, they are responsible for the diagnosis and prevention of disease and for the medical and surgical treatment of animals in homes, farms, zoos and wildlife parks. Vets are also employed in other sectors, such as education and research, government agencies, animal charities and pharmaceutical companies.

- Principal – or senior partner – he or she is usually the person who has been in the practice for the longest time and may also have a bigger financial stake in the practice.

- Partners – there may be several – they have a financial stake in the practice and are involved in the running and management of the practice.
- Assistants – veterinary surgeons employed by the partners. They are mainly involved in the clinical side of practice in seeing clients and their animals.
- Locum tenens – usually referred to as a 'locum' – employed on temporary contracts of varying length. They are often employed to cover colleagues on sick leave, study leave or maternity leave.

Veterinary surgeons practicing in the UK must be members of the Royal College of Veterinary Surgeons (RCVS). They must comply with the RCVS Guide to Professional Conduct and the Veterinary Surgeons Act 1966 and are able to use the post-nominal MRCVS accompanied by their appropriate degree.

Registered veterinary nurse (RVN)

Veterinary nurses work alongside veterinary surgeons in order to provide a high standard of care for animals. They normally work within a veterinary surgery or veterinary hospital and are involved in a wide range of care and treatment. Veterinary nurses provide skilled supportive care for sick animals as well as undertaking minor surgery, monitoring anaesthesia, medical treatments and diagnostic tests under veterinary supervision.

Qualified nurses who are registered (Listed) with the RCVS are able to use the post-nominal RVN and are entitled by law to undertake a range of veterinary treatments under the direction of a veterinary surgeon. They can also accept delegated work under Schedule 3 of the Veterinary Surgeons Act 1966 if they feel comfortable and competent in doing so. Veterinary nurses also play an important role in the education of owners about good standards of animal care.

Nurses, like vets, can also be employed in other sectors such as research establishments, laboratories, education, zoological/wildlife parks, charities, pharmaceutical companies and breeding/boarding kennels. Veterinary nurses must follow the *Guide to Professional Conduct*, which is available from the RCVS. Box 2.1 shows the main professional principles of the profession.

Equine veterinary nurse (EVN)

In the past few years, equine practice has advanced and increased, resulting in an increasing need for nurses to be skilled in the care of equine patients. In response to this need, the British Veterinary Nursing Association (BVNA), the British Equine Veterinary Association and the RCVS have developed an equine veterinary nursing qualification.

Animal nursing assistant (ANA)

The role of an ANA is to assist veterinary surgeons and veterinary nurses in the general husbandry and care of patients. ANAs may also play an active role in assisting other members of practice staff in the day-to-day running of the practice, including reception and client communication. They offer a vital supportive role in the busy practice. Upon passing an examination, ANA students may progress to veterinary nurse training.

Box 2.1 The 10 guiding principles

Those who commit animals to the care of a veterinary nurse are entitled to expect that she or he will:

1. Make animal welfare the first consideration in seeking to provide the most appropriate attention
2. Ensure that all animals in care are treated humanely and with respect
3. Maintain and continue to develop professional knowledge and skills
4. Foster and maintain a good relationship with the clients, earning their trust, respecting their views and protecting client confidentiality
5. Uphold the good reputation of the veterinary nursing profession
6. Ensure the integrity of statements signed by veterinary nurses
7. Foster and endeavour to maintain good relationships with professional colleagues
8. Understand and comply with legal obligations in relation to the supply, administration, safe-keeping and, if a suitably qualified person (SQP) working from registered premises, prescription of veterinary medicinal products
9. Be familiar with and observe the relevant legislation in relation to veterinary nurses as individual members of the profession and as employers, employees and business owners
10. Respond promptly, fully and courteously to complaints and criticism

---

Practice manager

The practice manager is responsible for some or all of the practice management tasks that are essential to the running of the business. They may be called office managers, practice administrators or practice managers. In some cases, they are partners in the practice or other senior veterinary surgeons who have a particular interest in the 'business' side of practice. The practice manager may be a veterinary nurse who has been 'promoted' into a managerial role. A growing number of practices employ individuals with a background in senior or middle management outside the veterinary profession but who have the experience, knowledge and business skills that are necessary to oversee all the non-clinical administrative and management tasks essential for success in veterinary practice.

Practice receptionist

Receptionists work alongside vets and nurses to ensure smooth and efficient running of the practice. They are principally responsible for scheduling appointments, dealing with phone calls, ensuring that emergencies are offered immediate attention and dealing with clients as they come into the practice for appointments or to buy medicines. The veterinary receptionist is usually the first person an owner may encounter over the phone or upon arriving at the surgery and so is integral to shaping the clients first impression of the practice. They must be extremely organized, have good administrative skills, be calm, positive, welcoming and be able to give reassurance to a client who may be worried about their pet. In some practices, the receptionist may also be required to process invoices and payments and manage shop stock and orders.

Governing bodies

These governing bodies and organizations play a part in the smooth running of veterinary practice in the UK.

Royal College of Veterinary Surgeons (RCVS)

The RCVS is the regulatory body for veterinary surgeons in the UK. Its role is:

- To safeguard the health and welfare of animals committed to veterinary care through the regulation of the educational, ethical and clinical standards of the veterinary profession, thereby protecting the interests of those dependent on animals and assuring public health
- To act as an impartial source of informed opinion on animal health and welfare issues and their interaction with human health.

British Veterinary Nursing Association (BVNA)

The aim of the BVNA is to promote animal health and welfare through the ongoing development of professional excellence in veterinary nursing. The BVNA undertakes to:

- Represent the veterinary nursing profession and, specifically, its members
- Develop, provide and monitor continuing professional development for veterinary nurses
- Provide education and training for associated individuals and allied professionals
- Promote the veterinary nursing profession and work proactively with other organizations and professions to shape its future development and disseminate advice and guidance to its members.

British Small Animal Veterinary Association (BSAVA)

The BSAVA exists to promote high scientific and educational standards of small animal medicine and surgery in practice, teaching and research. The association was founded as a professional body to serve veterinary surgeons that treat companion animals.

On behalf of its members, the BSAVA:

- Encourages veterinary surgeons to develop their professional skills
- Runs numerous continuing education courses and seminars throughout the UK
- Hosts the biggest annual small animal conference in the world
- Publishes books, manuals, CD-ROMs and videos on a diversity of small animal topics
- Publishes the monthly *Journal of Small Animal Practice*
- Maintains contacts with small animal practitioners through the Regional Officers, who organize local meetings
- Through its charity, Petsavers, funds clinical investigations into the diseases of companion animals
- Works with the Kennel Club on identification and control of hereditary diseases in pedigree dogs

- Provides a forum for the discussion of issues of importance to veterinary surgeons in small animal practice and submits evidence on their behalf to the British Veterinary Association (BVA) and the RCVS as well as to government departments
- Liaises with other veterinary professionals through regular meetings
- Represents member interests internationally through various European and world small animal organizations.

British Veterinary Association (BVA)

The BVA mission statement is to represent the veterinary profession and help members fulfil their professional roles. In promoting and supporting the interests of their members, and the animals under their care, they are committed to developing and maintaining channels of communication not least with government, parliamentarians and the media. Members of the BVA have the benefits of being part of a national association, with tangible services and benefits and with access to a range of highly regarded publications. The BVA is a not-for-profit organization.

Society of Practicing Veterinary Surgeons (SPVS)

SPVS was founded to promote the interests of veterinary surgeons in private practice. They are also a division of the BVA that concentrates primarily on matters of practice management and finance, providing a source of information, advice and practical guidance for both partners and assistants. They produce an annual yearbook, which gives practitioners across the country an overview of the issues of the day and is a useful source of practical information to refer to time and time again. This is sent free of charge to all UK practices.

More information can be found on the web sites of each organization. There are many more specialized organizations to support veterinary surgeons in their chosen fields, from equine and large animal to the veterinary cardiovascular society.

Practice protocols

In the day-to-day running of a veterinary practice, there are various protocols that must be used to ensure a professional, reliable and confidential service to the clients.

Client confidentiality

- The veterinary surgeon/client relationship is founded on trust and, in normal circumstances, a veterinary surgeon must not disclose to any third party any information about a client or their animal either given by the client, or revealed by clinical examination or by post-mortem examination. This duty also extends to associated support staff.

- In circumstances where the client has not given permission for disclosure and when the veterinary surgeon believes that animal welfare or public interest is compromised, the RCVS may be consulted before any information is divulged.
- Permission to pass on confidential information may be expressed or implied. Express permission may be either verbal or in writing, usually in response to a request. Permission may also be implied from circumstances, e.g. in the making of a claim under a pet insurance policy, when the insurance company becomes entitled to receive all information relevant to the claim and to seek clarification if required.
- Registration of a dog with the Kennel Club permits a veterinary surgeon who carries out surgery to alter the natural conformation of a dog to report this to the Kennel Club.

Case records

- Case records including radiographic films and similar documents are the property of, and should be retained by, veterinary surgeons in the interests of animal welfare and for their own protection. Copies with a summary of the history should be passed on request to a colleague taking over the case. (Where a client has been specifically charged and has paid for radiographs or other reports, they are legally entitled to them. The practice may however choose to make it clear that they are charging not for the radiographs, but for diagnosis or advice only. In appropriate circumstances, they may be prepared also to provide copies of the radiographs.)
- The Data Protection Act 1998 gives anyone the right to be informed about any personal data relating to themselves on payment of an administration charge.
- At the request of a client, veterinary surgeons must provide copies of any relevant clinical records. This includes relevant records that have come from other practices, if they relate to the same animal and the same client. It does not include records that relate to the same animal but a different client. Where any significant expense is involved in providing such copies, as there might be, for example, with the provision of radiographs, a charge can be made. Expense should not be a reason for declining to provide copies.
- It follows that the utmost care is essential in writing case notes or recording a client's personal details to ensure that the latter are accurate (particularly in relation to financial details) and that the notes are comprehensible and legible.

- Disclosure of records may be ordered in disciplinary or court hearings, and the RCVS may request copies of case records routinely in the course of investigating a complaint.

More information can be found on the RCVS web site (www.rcvs.org.uk).

Data Protection Act 1998

This Act of Parliament defines the legal basis for handling information in the UK. It is the main piece of legislation governing the protection of personal data in the UK. Although the Act does not mention privacy, in practice, it provides a way in which individuals can enforce the control of information about themselves. Most of the Act does not apply to domestic use such as the keeping of a personal address book. Anyone holding personal data for other purposes is legally obliged to comply with this Act.

Patient records

The medical history of an animal is obtained by careful questioning either of the owner or the carer of the patient. The aim of taking a good history is to formulate a diagnosis and to provide treatment to the patient. It is very important to realize that a diagnosis is only as good as the history – if the facts are incorrect or exaggerated, then the diagnosis and, subsequently, treatment may be inappropriate. The terms 'symptoms' and 'clinical signs' are frequently used terms and the difference is:

Symptoms – the problems reported by client.
Clinical signs – ascertained by direct examination of the patient by the veterinary surgeon.

Communication skills, particularly questioning, are vital in being able to obtain an accurate history. One of the roles of the nurse is triaging a patient over the telephone when a short history is taken and written down (e.g. name, age, sex, complaint, contact details). The nurse can then, with more open and funnel questioning, determine if the patient is an emergency or can wait until the next free appointment.

When the patient arrives at the surgery, a more detailed history can be taken by the vet or nurse. It is often the last thing a client says that is the key to the whole issue, and it may be a good idea to let a client just talk as you direct them with careful questioning.

Patient records are usually kept on a computer, but some practices still use case cards. These records are confidential and must not be made public. This is particularly relevant to veterinary nurse training where client/patient information may be used to build up case logs for the portfolio or Nurse's Progress Log (NPL) – there should be no mention of the owner's name and address.

Bibliography

Corsan, J., Mackay, A.R., 2009. The Veterinary Practice Receptionist. Essential Skills for Client Care, second ed. Elsevier Health Sciences, Oxford.

Gorman, C., 2000. Clients, Pets and Vets. Communication and Management. Pocket Practice Guide. Threshold Press Ltd, Newbury.

Gray, C.A., 2009. Dealing with Aggressive Clients. University of Liverpool, BSAVA, Gloucester.

Mehrabian, A, Ferris, SR, 1967. Inference of attitude from nonverbal communication in two channels. J. Counsel. Psychol. 31, 248–252.

Shilcock, M., Stutchfield, G., 2008. Veterinary Practice Management: A Practical Guide, second ed. Elsevier Health Sciences, Oxford.

Segal, J., Emotional Intelligence. Available from: <http://www.emotionalintelligencecentral.org>.

Recommended reading

Corsan, J., Mackay, A.R., 2009. The Veterinary Practice Receptionist. Essential Skills for Client Care, second ed. Elsevier Health Sciences, Oxford.

Written specifically for the veterinary receptionist, but well worth reading for all who have contact with clients. It gives practical advice on how to deal with many situations.

Gibbs, G., 1988. Learning by Doing: *A guide to Teaching and Learning Methods*. Further Education Unit. Oxford Polytechnic, Oxford.

For those who want to research and understand fully their learning styles and for those who teach students, to help understand how vocational learning benefits many students.

Gorman, C., 2000. Clients, Pets and Vets. Communication and Management. Pocket Practice Guide. Threshold Press Ltd, Newbury.

A practical, light-hearted guide that provides advice on 'real' client situations. Covers a wide variety of situations that occur in veterinary practice and how to deal with them. An essential read.

Honey, P., 2001. Improve Your People Skills, second ed. Chartered Institute of Personnel and Development, London.

An in-depth guide for those wanting to research and improve their people skills.

Kolb, D.A., 1984. Experiential Learning: Experience as the Source of Learning and Development. Financial Times/Prentice Hall, London.

For those who want a more in-depth guide to the reflective process and learning in a vocational field.

Shilcock, M., Stutchfield, G., 2008. Veterinary Practice Management: A Practical Guide, second ed. Elsevier Health Sciences, Oxford.

An essential guide, written for practice managers, but contains useful information for owners, vets and nurses.

CHAPTER 3

Legislation and the veterinary nurse

Suzanne May

Key Points

- Health and safety legislation is concerned with providing a safe working environment for both employers and employees.
- It comprises many different Acts of Parliament, each of which deals with a different aspect, e.g. first aid, manual handling and substances that may be hazardous to health.
- The use of radiation to produce radiographs is of particular concern to those working in veterinary practice and is controlled by the Ionizing Radiation Regulations 1999.
- Animal welfare legislation is aimed at both maintaining animal health and protecting the people working with animals.
- There are numerous pieces of animal welfare legislation, many of which concern dogs.
- It is essential that all personnel working in a veterinary practice are familiar with the legal side of their work.

An introduction to legislation

Legislation in the UK refers to both Acts of Parliament and regulations.

A law or statute is created by Parliament. The process involves a draft of legislation called a bill being first presented and debated within the House of Commons and the House of Lords. It then goes before a parliamentary committee before finally obtaining the Queen's signature to make it law. It is then placed in the Statute Book as an Act of Parliament.

Regulations detail the implications of laws. Further regulations can be added to laws as necessary with the approval of Parliament.

Where animal welfare is concerned, welfare codes are also required to have parliamentary approval. If the provisions of the code are not complied with, it is not an offence. However, this could be used in evidence if prosecution followed.

Veterinary Surgeons Act 1966

This Act of Parliament controls the work of both veterinary surgeons and veterinary nurses.

Definition of veterinary surgery: the Act defines this as 'the art and science of veterinary surgery and medicine, and

without prejudice to the generality of the foregoing, shall be taken to include:

- The diagnosis of diseases in, and injuries to animals including tests performed on animals for diagnostic purposes
- The giving of advice based upon such diagnosis
- The medical or surgical treatment of animals
- The performance of surgical operations on animals.'

The Act prohibits anyone other than a veterinary surgeon who is a Member of the Royal College of Veterinary Surgeons (MRCVS) from practising veterinary surgery. There are, however, a number of exceptions to this rule, some concerning lay persons and two concerning veterinary nurses:

- Schedule 3 of the Act allows anyone to give first aid in an emergency for the purpose of preserving life and relieving suffering. The owner of an animal or a member of the owner's household or employee of the owner may also give it minor medical treatment. There are several exceptions to this general rule, mainly relating to farm animals.

Veterinary nurses, like anyone else, may give first aid and look after animals in a way that does not involve acts of veterinary surgery. However, there are further provisions for qualified listed veterinary nurses under Schedule 3 of the Act.

- Schedule 3 of the Veterinary Surgeons Act 1966 details that qualified listed veterinary nurses can administer medical treatment and perform minor surgery (not involving entry into a body cavity) under the direction of the veterinary surgeon that is providing care for that animal (cat, dog or exotic species but NOT equine species, unless a certificate in equine nursing is also held). The veterinary surgeon must be satisfied that the nurse is competent to carry out their instructions as he/ she is ultimately responsible and accountable for their actions.

Amendment to paragraphs 6 & 7 of Schedule 3 to the Veterinary Surgeons Act 1966, as amended by the Veterinary Surgeons Act 1966 (Schedule 3 Amendment) Order 2002 clarifies the term 'veterinary nurse' within the Act as one whose name is entered on to the list of veterinary nurses maintained by the RCVS. It also makes provisions for the training of student veterinary nurses, allowing them to perform Schedule 3 procedures as detailed above, but only with direct, continuous and personal supervision from a registered veterinary surgeon, or veterinary nurse under veterinary instruction where surgery is concerned. The definition of a student veterinary nurse is one who 'has been enrolled under the RCVS bylaws for the purposes of training as a veterinary nurse and who is employed at an approved training practice'.

Occupational health

What is health and safety all about?

Health and safety laws exist to assist in the provision of a satisfactory, safe working environment, preventing people from being injured or harmed at work by taking the right precautions and knowing what action to take when things go wrong.

The Health and Safety Commission (HSC) is the body which oversees and monitors health and safety, producing reports and advising the government on health and safety matters. The Health and Safety Executive (HSE) is the enforcement body of the HSC, and at present veterinary practices come under the jurisdiction of HSE inspectors, whereas shops, offices, hotels, etc., are the responsibility of local authority environmental health officers.

HSE inspectors can visit any practice at any time to ensure that all relevant legislation is being complied with. Their job is to advise and enforce accordingly. Where they find a breach in health and safety law, there are a number of actions they can take based on how severe the problem is:

- If the breach is minor, an inspector will usually informally tell the employer what the problem is and how to correct it.
- If the breach is more serious, an **improvement notice** may be issued which identifies the situation that needs to be corrected and sets a specific date by when this should be done.
- Where an inspector believes that a breach could cause serious personal injury, a **prohibition notice** can be used to halt an activity immediately, i.e. this notice takes effect as soon as it is issued.

Failure to comply with either an improvement notice or a prohibition notice can result in fines of up to £20,000. Both types of notice can be appealed against through the Employment Tribunal.

The main Acts of Parliament affecting occupational health within veterinary practices are as follows.

Health and Safety at Work Act 1974

This applies to all businesses, however big or small, and to those who are self-employed. It generally places the responsibility for minimizing health and safety risks onto those who create them, usually the employer.

Employer responsibilities include:

- Appointing a competent person to oversee health and safety
- Carrying out risk assessments

- Supplying health and safety information to employees and visitors
- Providing health and safety training for employees.

Employee responsibilities include:

- Taking reasonable care of their own health and safety, and that of others
- Co-operating with the employer over health and safety matters
- Using equipment and substances in accordance with health and safety training
- Informing the employer of any health and safety risks or lack of protection.

A health and safety policy is required by any business that employs five or more people. This written policy contains information as to how the employer will maintain the health and safety of their employees, and usually includes the following information:

- Responsibilities for health and safety, i.e. who has overall responsibility and to whom specific responsibilities have been delegated
- The risk assessments that will be undertaken
- How the practice will organize consultation with its employees
- How the safety of equipment will be maintained and who is responsible for this
- Implementation of COSHH
- Arrangements for the provision of health and safety training
- Accident and first-aid arrangements
- Fire and emergency evacuation procedures
- How reviews of health and safety will be undertaken.

Management of Health and Safety at Work Regulations 1999

These regulations follow on from the Health and Safety at Work Act 1974, redefining and reinforcing the requirements of the Act to include the following activities:

- Planning
- Organization
- Control
- Monitoring
- Review.

Health and Safety at Work Regulations 1992

The 1992 Health and Safety at Work Regulations state that 'it shall be the duty of every employer to ensure so far as is reasonably practicable the health, safety and welfare of all their employees.' With this legislation came the requirement for employers to carry out risk assessments, and later that year the first six regulations requiring risk assessments were published:

- Manual Handling Operations Regulations
- Workplace (Health and Safety at Work)
- Personal Protective Equipment Regulations
- Provision and Use of Work Equipment Regulations
- Health and Safety (Display Screen Equipment) Regulations

- Management of Health and Safety at Work Regulations.

Leading from these, other areas have since been identified as also requiring risk assessment including:

- Fire
- First aid
- Electrical safety
- Ionizing radiation
- Young people at work
- Lone workers
- Noise
- New and expectant mothers
- Working time
- Work-related stress
- COSHH.

Risk assessments

A risk assessment involves looking at the workplace and the type of work undertaken, and identifying anything that could cause harm to people. The assessment involves identifying **hazards,** and then determining the level of **risk** each hazard is likely to have to employees.

- A *hazard* is anything that can cause harm
- A *risk* is the likelihood that someone will be harmed by the hazard.

The HSE recommends the following three actions with regards to hazards:

1. Eliminate the source of the hazard wherever possible
2. Substitute the source of the hazard if it cannot be eliminated
3. Control the source of the hazard if it cannot be substituted.

The following steps should be considered when undertaking risk assessment:

- Careful consideration of the task/situation
- Identification of the hazards
- Identification of those people who carry out the task or are exposed to the hazard
- Assess the level of risk involved
- Consider what control measures are already in place
- Identify any other control measures needed
- Record all of the findings of the assessment
- Implement control measures that have been identified as being required
- Inform all relevant staff of the risk assessment and its outcomes – development of a standard operating procedure (SOP) may be required if not already in place.
- Train staff if required
- Monitor and review on a regular basis.

An example risk assessment can be seen in Table 3.1.

Table 3.1 Example of a risk assessment

Activity	Radiography
Location	Radiography room
Potential hazards (the actual things that are likely to cause harm)	Primary beam
	Secondary radiation (scatter)
	Animal (if conscious)
Risk (the likelihood of the potential hazard causing harm)	Consider:
	Protective clothing
	Protective screening
	Persons inside the controlled area
	Any manual restraint of animal
	Any protective restraint of animal, e.g. muzzle
	Possibility of machine malfunction – continuous emission of X-rays
Who is at risk? Is anyone more at risk than others?	Any persons remaining within the controlled area are most at risk. Those more at risk but who should not be participating anyway are those who are pregnant, under 18 or who have been advised not to undertake radiography by their GPs
Control measures	Authorized personnel only
	Personal dosemeters
	Protective clothing/screens
	Extension enabling radiographer to stand out of the controlled area when exposure is taken
Training required	Health and safety training on radiography. Those involved must have read and understood the local rules and systems of work
Emergency action	Shut off power to X-ray machine from fuse box
	Inform RPS and RPA and arrange for immediate service of the machine

Standard operating procedures (SOPs)

These are written documents designed to cover the full range of work performed within the practice. They provide clear and concise information in line with the individual protocols of the practice.

Control of Substances Hazardous to Health Regulations 2002

The Control of Substances Hazardous to Health Regulations 2002 (COSHH) were introduced specifically to cover the management of risks associated with hazardous substances. This includes all pharmaceutical products and chemicals used in veterinary practice.

Risk assessments should be in place for all such substances. In assessing the level of risk involved the following should be considered:

- Who uses it?
- How is it used?
- How long are people exposed?
- By which route would the substance enter the body?
- Are there any particular people at risk (e.g. asthmatics, expectant mothers)?

Employees should be familiar with the common hazard warning symbols illustrated in Figure 3.1 when dealing with a substance and what personal protective equipment is needed.

In addition the particular hazards of a substance can be identified by using a numerical code system introduced in 1996 as a result of the Chemicals (Hazard Information and Packaging for Supply) Amendment Regulations 2002 (CHIP 96). Manufacturers should also supply COSHH data sheets to help the practice produce its risk assessments.

Standard operating procedures should be in place for substances which present a hazard and for how to deal with spillages, i.e. the cleaning-up procedure and whether any protective equipment is required (Box 3.1).

It should be noted that clinical waste also comes under COSHH regulations in terms of risk assessment, but there are also different legal requirements as to its disposal.

Box 3.1 Rules for working with chemicals

- Never eat, drink or smoke when working with chemicals
- Ensure area is adequately ventilated
- Use the appropriate protective clothing
- Ensure the chemical is correct for use in this situation
- Keep the chemicals in their original containers with the label intact and legible
- Use the correct concentration
- Read the label and the product COSHH sheet
- Store appropriately according to manufacturers instructions – out of direct sunlight, away from animals and children – in a locked cupboard if necessary
- Do not mix unless recommended by the manufacturer
- Dispose of chemical according to manufacturers' guidelines
- Wash hands after use
- Deal with accidental spillage immediately and report as necessary

---

Hazardous Waste (England and Wales) Regulations (HWR) 2005

Disposal of waste from the practice

The legal definition of clinical waste is given in the Controlled Waste Regulations 1992 as 'any waste which consists wholly or partly of human or animal tissue, blood or other bodily fluids, excretions, drugs or other pharmaceutical products, swabs or dressings, or syringes, needles or other sharp instruments, being waste which unless rendered safe may prove hazardous to any person coming into contact with it'. This includes waste from medical, nursing, dental, pharmaceutical, teaching, research and veterinary practices.

The Environmental Protection Act 1990 states that 'all establishments are responsible for their own waste' but this was amended in 1992 to include 'a duty of care for controlled waste'. This means that the responsibility for disposing of waste created by a business lies with the employer or self-employed person, which includes ensuring that waste disposed of by an outside company, e.g. collectors of clinical waste from a veterinary practice, is disposed of legally and safely. Should the outside company be found to be negligent according to law then the people who employ that company are also liable for prosecution.

Within the veterinary practice there must be a waste storage area separate from any other area, which must be secure against both humans and vermin, with access only to authorized personnel. Within the area the waste is stored in appropriate receptacles ready for disposal and collection by the designated company.

There are many different types of waste, which must be disposed of correctly. They can be classed as:

- Hazardous waste – the premises must keep a waste register, use consignment notes and keep these records for 3 years.
- Non-hazardous waste.

All waste has an EWC classification number for identification. There is also a colour code system of containers for the disposal of waste (see Table 3.2).

Hazardous waste

In 2005, the Hazardous Waste Regulations replaced the Special Waste Regulations and introduced new definitions of hazardousness for infectious and pharmaceutical wastes. This group is divided into:

1. Cytotoxic and cytostatic pharmaceuticals – includes medicinal products which are toxic, carcinogenic and/or mutagenic. Following identification, these may include glass containers, syringes and sharps, animal bedding and clinical items such as swabs and gloves.

HARMFUL   IRRITANT   CORROSIVE   TOXIC

Fig. 3.1 Some common hazard warning signs

Table 3.2 Colour coding for waste containers

Container colour	Contents
• Yellow	Infectious waste which requires disposal by incineration
• Orange	Infectious waste which requires treating to render it safe or it is incinerated
• Purple	Cytotoxic and cytostatic waste
• Yellow and black	Offensive or hygiene waste
• Black	Domestic waste which cannot be recycled

They must be disposed of by segregating into purple or yellow containers for high-temperature incineration.

2. Contaminated sharps – includes all sharps contaminated with blood or pharmaceuticals (other than cytotoxic or cytostatic as above). They must be disposed of by segregating into yellow sharps containers for high-temperature incineration. Non-contaminated sharps can be disposed of in orange lidded containers for treatment such as autoclaving.

3. Infectious waste – includes waste containing microorganisms or their toxins which are believed to have caused disease in another living organism. Following identification, these may include clinical items such as swabs and gloves, animal bedding , body parts and cadavers.

4. Photographic chemicals – includes waste fixer and developer solutions. They must be disposed of by segregating into separate containers and treated at a permitted facility which can be arranged via the practice waste contractor. There is no standard packaging.

Non-hazardous waste

This group is divided into:

1. Pharmaceuticals – does not include cytotoxic or cytostatic pharmaceuticals but it does include controlled drugs, prescription-only medicines, out-of-date drugs and contaminated bottles, syringes and packaging. It can be further divided into:
   - Disposal of controlled drugs – all controlled drugs should be denatured before disposal with other pharmaceuticals above. Schedule 2 drugs required denaturing in the presence of a person authorized by the Secretary of State, e.g. a police officer.
   - Disposal of other pharmaceuticals – should be segregated into leak-proof containers and done without mixing them together. There is no standard packaging. They should be incinerated at a permitted facility which can be arranged via the practice waste contractor.

2. Offensive waste – this is soft waste, e.g. swabs, gloves and animal bedding that is not 'clinical waste' but is unpleasant to the senses. It should not present risk of infection or hazard to another living organism. Material containing bodily fluids should not be placed in this waste unless the veterinary surgeon can demonstrate that procedures that ensure the waste does not pose a threat of infection to another living organism have been implemented The waste should be segregated into yellow and black containers for disposal into landfill.

3. Non-infectious cadaver – any pet cadavers that are not infectious can be buried at home, buried in a pet cemetery or cremated. There is no standard packaging and disposal can be arranged via the waste contractor for the practice.

4. Domestic waste – includes domestic waste such as unsoiled newspaper, food waste and other household waste not fit for recycling. This waste goes to landfill.

Further information of the disposal of waste can be found on the BVA website at <http://www.bva.co.uk> or in the BVA *Good Practice Guide to Handling Veterinary Waste* (Fig. 3.2).

Manual Handling Regulations 1992

This Act expands on the general provisions of the Health and Safety at Work Act 1974. The requirements and applications of these regulations are clearly outlined in their booklet – *Manual Handling, Guidance on Regulations.*

General provisions outlined include:

- Avoid hazardous manual handling operations so far as is reasonably practicable
- Assess any hazardous manual handling operations that cannot be avoided
- Reduce the risk of injury so far as is reasonably practicable.

The regulations do not set out any guidelines for weight limits, etc. It is expected that each individual task will be assessed according to:

- The task
- The load (an animal being carried may suddenly move, which makes it different from carrying a box)
- The working environment (moving around objects, slippery floors, etc.)
- The individual's capabilities (these vary with age, pregnancy, etc.)

The Health and Safety Executive (HSE) guidance for manual lifting and the main elements of a good lifting technique can be found in Figures 3.3 and 3.4, respectively.

The Health and Safety (First Aid) Regulations 1981

This requires employers to provide adequate and appropriate equipment, facilities and personnel to enable first aid to be given to employees if they are injured or become ill at work. The minimum first-aid provision in any workplace is:

- A suitably stocked first-aid box
- An appointed person to take charge of first-aid arrangements.

Requirements increase with the size of the workforce and the type of work being done. A veterinary practice is considered as a medium-risk environment, and as such must appoint a person responsible for first aid if there are fewer than 20

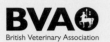 **BVA** British Veterinary Association

GOOD PRACTICE GUIDE TO HANDLING VETERINARY WASTE

All businesses have a duty of care to ensure that:

- All waste is stored and disposed of responsibly
- Waste is only handled or dealt with by those authorised to do so
- Appropriate records are kept of all waste that is transferred or received

HAZARDOUS WASTE   Register your premises, keep a Waste Register, use Consignment Notes, keep all records for at least three years.

CYTOTOXIC AND CYTOSTATIC PHARMACEUTICALS

Waste contaminated with cytotoxic and cytostatic pharmaceuticals, which are medicinal products that are toxic, carcinogenic, toxic for reproduction or mutagenic. Following a veterinary assessment waste deemed to be contaminated may include:

- Glass bottles and vials
- Clinical items (for example, swabs, masks and gloves)
- Syringes and sharps
- Animal bedding.

DISPOSAL

- Segregate into appropriate purple and yellow containers, sharps into purple-lidded sharps containers
- High temperature incineration
- European Waste Catalogue (EWC) = 18 02 07*.

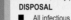

INFECTIOUS WASTE

Any veterinary waste containing viable micro-organisms or their toxins which are known or reliably believed to cause disease in man or other living organisms. Following a veterinary assessment waste deemed to be contaminated may include:

- Clinical items (for example, swabs masks and gloves)
- Animal bedding
- Blood, body parts and cadavers.

DISPOSAL

- All infectious material can be segregated into appropriate yellow containers for high temperature incineration only
- EWC = 18 02 02*.

  - Infectious clinical items can be further segregated into orange containers for suitable alternative treatment (for example, autoclaving) as best practice
  - EWC = 18 02 02*.

PHOTOGRAPHIC CHEMICALS

This may include:

- Waste fixer and developer solutions.

DISPOSAL

- Segregate into separate fixer and developer containers for treatment at an appropriately permitted facility
- There is no standard packaging so specific requirements should be discussed with your waste contractor
- EWC = 09 01 01 (developer) and 09 01 04 (fixer).

CONTAMINATED SHARPS

All sharps contaminated with animal blood or pharmaceuticals (other than cytotoxic or cytostatic). This may include:

- Partially and fully discharged sharps, hypodermic needles and other sharp instruments.

DISPOSAL

- All sharps can be segregated into yellow sharps containers for high temperature incineration only
- EWC = 18 02 02* and 18 02 08.

  - Non-pharmaceutically contaminated sharps can be further segregated into orange-lidded bins for suitable alternative treatment (for example, autoclaving) as best practice
  - EWC = 18 02 02*

NON-HAZARDOUS WASTE

PHARMACEUTICALS (NOT CYTOTOXIC OR CYTOSTATIC)

Waste contaminated with pharmaceuticals (not cytotoxic or cytostatic). This may include:

- Controlled drugs
- Prescription-only medicines
- Out-of-date drugs
- Contaminated bottles, syringe bodies and packaging.

DISPOSAL OF CONTROLLED DRUGS

- All controlled drugs should be denatured or made not readily recoverable and then be disposed of with other pharmaceuticals (not cytotoxic or cytostatic)
- Schedule 2 controlled drugs should be denatured in the presence of a person authorised by the Secretary of State (for example, a police officer).

DISPOSAL OF OTHER PHARMACEUTICALS

- Segregate into leak proof containers
- Avoid mixing
- There is no standard packaging so specific requirements should be discussed with your waste contractor
- Incineration at an appropriately permitted facility
- EWC = 18 02 08.

OFFENSIVE WASTE

Offensive waste is soft veterinary waste that is **not** 'clinical waste' (as defined on the reverse side of this poster) but which is unpleasant and may cause offence to the senses. This waste must have been subjected to a detailed item and patient specific assessment that clearly demonstrates it does not present a risk of infection or other potential hazard to any animal or person that may come into contact with it, even if mismanaged. As a result of this assessment the veterinary surgeon is declaring that the waste **is not 'clinical waste' that requires any incineration or other treatment prior to landfill.** Following a veterinary assessment waste deemed to be non-hazardous offensive waste may include:

- Clinical items (for example, swabs, masks and gloves)
- Animal bedding.

Material contaminated with body fluids (for example, blood) should not be placed in this waste stream unless a veterinary surgeon is able to demonstrate that they implemented procedures that meet the requirements set out in the accompanying web guidance (see www.bva.co.uk).

DISPOSAL

- Landfill or other suitable permitted facility
- EWC = 18 02 03.

NON-INFECTIOUS CADAVERS

Any pet carcasses that are not considered to be infectious waste after assessment in accordance with the accompanying web guidance (see www.bva.co.uk).

DISPOSAL

- Burial at home
- Burial in a pet cemetery
- Cremation

- There is no standard packaging so specific requirements should be discussed with your waste contractor
- EWC = 18 02 03.

DOMESTIC WASTE

Waste that only contains domestic rubbish. This may include:

- Unsoiled newspapers and magazines
- Sandwich wrappers
- Drink cans.

DISPOSAL

- Landfill or recycling at a suitably permitted or licensed site
- EWC = 20 03 01.

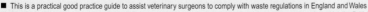

- This is a practical good practice guide to assist veterinary surgeons to comply with waste regulations in England and Wales
- The Environment Agency supports this *Good practice guide to handling veterinary waste* written and published by the British Veterinary Association (June 2008)
- Further information on handling veterinary waste is available at www.bva.co.uk and www.environment-agency.gov.uk

 BSAVA BRITISH SMALL ANIMAL VETERINARY ASSOCIATION   THE GOAT VETERINARY SOCIETY   © BVA 2008

Fig. 3.2 *Good Practice Guide to Handling Veterinary Waste (From BVA)*

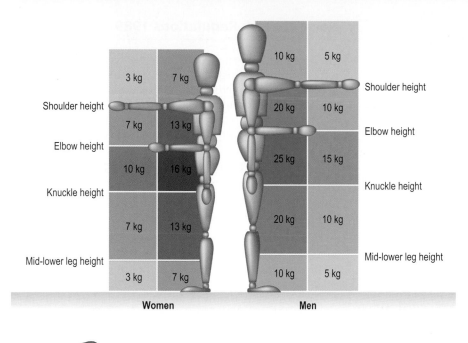

Fig. 3.3 Health and Safety Executive guidance for manual lifting *(Crown copyright material, with permission of the Controller of HMSO and the Queen's Printer for Scotland)*

	Women			
Shoulder height	3 kg	7 kg		
Elbow height	7 kg	13 kg		
Knuckle height	10 kg	16 kg		
Mid-lower leg height	7 kg	13 kg		
	3 kg	7 kg		

			Men	
Shoulder height	10 kg	5 kg		
Elbow height	20 kg	10 kg		
Knuckle height	25 kg	15 kg		
Mid-lower leg height	20 kg	10 kg		
	10 kg	5 kg		

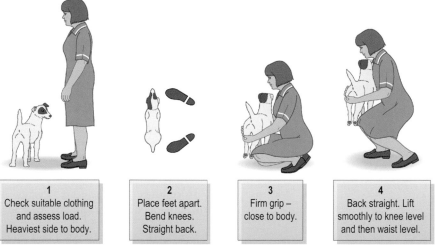

1	2	3	4	5	6
Check suitable clothing and assess load. Heaviest side to body.	Place feet apart. Bend knees. Straight back.	Firm grip – close to body.	Back straight. Lift smoothly to knee level and then waist level.	With clear visibility move forward without twisting.	Set load down at waist level or to knee level and then floor.

Fig. 3.4 The main elements of a good lifting technique

employees. If there are between 20 and 50 employees, a trained first aider must be appointed.

What is the difference between an appointed person and a first aider?

An *appointed person* is someone who is appointed by management to take charge when someone is injured or ill. This includes calling an ambulance if required. Appointed persons are also responsible for keeping the first-aid box stocked and recording any treatments given.

A *first aider* is someone who has undergone an HSE-approved training course in First Aid at Work and holds a certificate to prove this. Training should be repeated every 3 years to ensure that the certificate is kept up to date.

The *First Aid at Work: Approved Code of Practice and Guidelines* 1997 states that staff must know who the first-aid officer is and where the first-aid box is kept. First-aid boxes should be clearly marked with a white cross on a green background. There is no 'standard' list of items that should be kept in the first aid box; it depends on what the practice assess the needs to be. The HSE offers further guidance on this.

All accidents that occur within the workplace must be recorded in an Accident Book approved by the HSE (form B1 510). Details of what should be recorded in the Accident Book include:

- Full name, address and occupation of individual who had the accident
- The signature of the person who is filling in the Accident Book and the date of the occurrence

- When and where the accident took place
- Details of occurrence and record of injuries
- Indicate whether the incident needs to be reported to the HSE under RIDDOR (see below).

Reporting of Injuries, Diseases and Dangerous Occurrence Regulations 1995 (RIDDOR)

The Reporting of Injuries, Diseases and Dangerous Occurrence Regulations 1995 (RIDDOR) legislate for the reporting of certain serious events directly to the HSE. These can be broadly divided into:

- Major or fatal accidents
- Any accident or illness resulting in absence from work for more than three days because of an incident at work
- Dangerous occurrences and near-misses.

Fatal accidents include those where death occurred within one year as a result of an original accident at work.

Major accidents are defined as:

- A fracture of the skull, spine or pelvis
- A fracture of a long bone of a limb
- Amputation of a hand or foot
- Loss of sight of an eye
- Any other accident that results in an injured person being admitted to hospital as an inpatient, unless they were only kept in for observation.

Major or fatal accidents must be reported as soon as possible by telephone, followed by written confirmation within 7 days using the HSE form F2508. There is a list of dangerous occurrences that must be reported whether an injury occurs or not. These include:

- Explosion from a gas cylinder or steriliser
- Uncontrolled release of substance (including X-radiation, gases, etc.)
- Any escape of substances that might result in problems due to inhalation or lack of oxygen
- Any cases of ill health that could have resulted from exposure to pathogens in infected material
- Any unintentional ignition or explosion.

The employer must ensure that RIDDOR is enforced.

Health and Safety Display Screen Equipment Regulations 1992

Incorrect use of display equipment and poor design of work stations can result in problems like headaches, eye strain, neck and back problems. This legislation requires the way in which work stations are used to be regularly assessed.

The work station itself should be adequately lit with appropriate room and leg space with an adjustable chair and foot rest if required.

Equipment should be of a low-radiation type, have no glare and good contrast with a stable image. Monitors should be adjustable and keyboards should be legible with a wrist rest provided if needed.

Noise at Work Regulations 1989

These regulations state that the employer must assess the level of noise to which employees are exposed and take any necessary action to eliminate, control or reduce exposure. If noise levels are found to be above the 'first action noise level' of 85 decibels for continuous periods, e.g. due to barking dogs, then hearing protection **must be provided.**

The Working Time Regulations 1998

These set out entitlement for rest periods, night work and annual leave in line with the hours worked. They state that:

- The average working time is limited to 48 hours during each 7-day period
- There must be a minimum of 11 hours rest in any 24-hour period
- There must be a minimum rest period of 24 hours in each 7-day period. This increases to 48 hours for persons under 18 years of age
- There must be a minimum rest break of 20 minutes if the working day is longer than 6 hours or if the person is under 18 years of age they are entitled to 30 minutes if the working day is over 4 ½ hours.
- If an employee works at least 3 hours between 11.00pm and 6.00am, they are limited to 8 hours in every 24 hour period
- All employees are entitled to a minimum of 4 weeks paid annual leave.

Electricity at Work Regulations 1989

This governs safety procedures that should always be employed when dealing with electrical equipment (Box 3.2).

Portable appliance testing

Portable appliance testing (PAT) comes under these regulations. Appliances that have been tested will often have a label attached to the cable detailing the date and who tested

---

Box 3.2 Basic electrical safety

Remember:
- Electricity and water do not mix – never touch electrical equipment with wet hands
- Loose connections and exposed wires may short-circuit and cause fire
- Always use the correct fuse for the appliance
- Do not overload sockets
- When investigating or repairing electrical circuits SWITCH OFF THE POWER FIRST
- When using extension leads always unwind them fully, as this prevents overheating.
- Always follow the manufacturers' instructions
- Report any damaged/faulty equipment to your supervisor immediately.

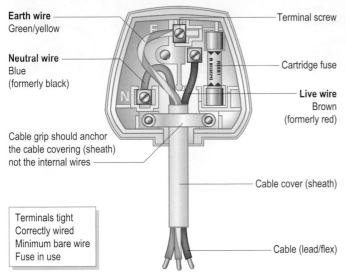

Earth wire
Green/yellow

Neutral wire
Blue
(formerly black)

Cable grip should anchor
the cable covering (sheath)
not the internal wires

Terminal screw

Cartridge fuse

Live wire
Brown
(formerly red)

Cable cover (sheath)

Cable (lead/flex)

Terminals tight
Correctly wired
Minimum bare wire
Fuse in use

Fig. 3.5 How to wire a plug

it. The frequency of testing is dependent on the type of equipment and is usually somewhere between every 6 months and every 2 years.

Electrical circuits and circuit breakers

Every electrical circuit should have a fuse in it, which is a simple safety device. A fuse is simply a thin wire through which the current of electricity flows. If a fault occurs in the circuit it usually causes an increase in the electrical current. This results in the wire melting, which breaks the circuit. It is very important to use the correct fuse within a circuit (Fig. 3.5). If a fuse that is used in a circuit has too low a value, the fuse will constantly 'blow'. However, if a fuse is used with too high a value, a fault may result in the risk of fire or electrocution.

A circuit breaker is a device used to protect against short-circuits and is found on the main fuse board. These electromagnetic devices switch off the current if a fault occurs. A trip switch or RCD (residual current device) can be plugged into a socket to give added protection for a portable appliance. Circuit breakers are reset by either pressing a button or by switching them back on.

The Regulatory Reform (Fire Safety) Order 2005

This legislation came into force in October 2006 and replaces most of the previous fire legislation. It requires the following to be undertaken:

- Risk assessment with reference not only to employees but also to clients and other visitors who may be in the practice
- Implementation of fire precautions such as fire detection systems, fire-fighting equipment and suitable escape routes.

On discovering a fire, the alarm should be raised and the fire brigade alerted immediately. A specified member of staff should be appointed as Fire Officer and it is this person's responsibility to ensure that the building is evacuated, that all occupants are accounted for and that no-one re-enters the building until the all-clear is given by the Fire Department. Local fire rules describing what to do in the event of a fire should be displayed within different areas within the building. Fire exits should be well labelled and well lit and not blocked with rubbish, etc., as should fire assembly points. There should be adequate fire-fighting equipment and staff must know the location of the equipment. Fire doors should be kept shut at all times. Care should be taken with the handling and storage of flammable and explosive materials.

Fire extinguishers

These are now all red, with a coloured strip indicating the contents and usage. There should also be a label mounted on the wall above the extinguisher, showing in green the fires that can safely be extinguished with that particular fire extinguisher and in red those that cannot (Fig. 3.6).

Ionizing Radiation Regulations 1999

Damage from radiation is cumulative, i.e. exposure to tiny amounts of radiation over a period of time can be just as serious as one exposure for a length of time. In addition to damaging cell structure, genes of reproductive cells (sperm and ova) can also be harmed, causing gene mutation. The effects of this may not be immediately obvious and may take a long while to emerge.

Harmful effects of radiation:

- Inflammation
- Blood disorders
- Death of tissue
- Death or mutation of developing fetus
- Damage to gonads
- Infertility
- The production of tumours.

The main beam that is produced when making an exposure is called the primary beam. This represents the biggest hazard to personnel. No part of the operator's body should ever be placed in the primary beam.

Secondary radiation or scatter is produced when particles of energy from the primary beam hit a surface (such as tissue or inanimate objects) and cause the production of lower-energy particles. These lower-energy particles 'bounce' of the surface at random and, like X-rays, travel in straight lines (Fig. 3.7).

Everyone who is involved with radiography must be protected from its dangers.

All practices should have written local radiation rules and a system of work, a copy of which should be displayed in the designated X-ray room. This should include a list of all personnel within the practice who are authorized to undertake radiography.

The main principles associated with radiation protection are:

- Radiography should only be undertaken if there is a definite clinical justification for the use of the procedure
- Exposure of personnel should be kept to a minimum

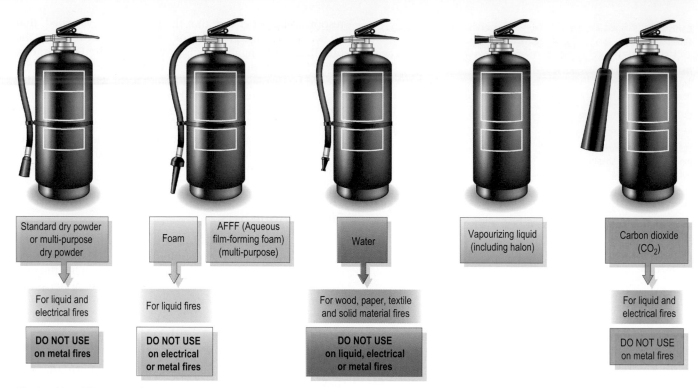

Standard dry powder or multi-purpose dry powder	Foam	AFFF (Aqueous film-forming foam) (multi-purpose)	Water	Vapourizing liquid (including halon)	Carbon dioxide (CO$_2$)
For liquid and electrical fires	For liquid fires		For wood, paper, textile and solid material fires		For liquid and electrical fires
DO NOT USE on metal fires	**DO NOT USE** on electrical or metal fires		**DO NOT USE** on liquid, electrical or metal fires		**DO NOT USE** on metal fires

Fig. 3.6 Use of fire extinguishers *(redrawn with permission from Health and Safety Executive 2004 Fire Safety: An Employer's Guide. Stationery Office, London)*

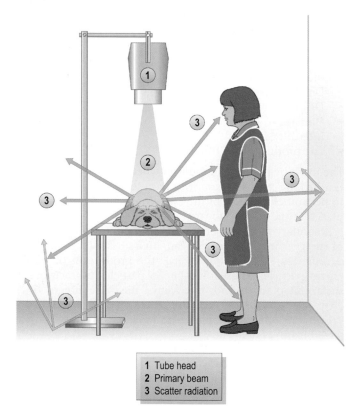

1 Tube head
2 Primary beam
3 Scatter radiation

Fig. 3.7 The hazards of radiation *(redrawn from Lane and Cooper 2003 Veterinary Nursing, third ed. Butterworth-Heinemann, Oxford)*

- There must be personal monitoring of staff involved with radiation to ensure that dose limits are not exceeded.

Under the legislation, practices must appoint:

A Radiation Protection Supervisor (RPS) – A listed veterinary nurse or veterinary surgeon employed in the practice whose responsibility it is to ensure that radiography is carried out safely and in accordance with local rules and the associated system of work

A Radiation Protection Advisor (RPA) – A suitably qualified person not employed by the practice who is responsible for periodically visiting the practice and inspecting/giving advice regarding aspects of radiation protection. The RPA is responsible for writing the local rules. They must either:

- Hold a Diploma in Veterinary Radiography (DVR) or
- Be qualified in appropriate radiation physics with an interest in veterinary radiography.

Controlled area

A specified room should be identified for small-animal radiography. It should have sufficiently thick walls and no part of the controlled area should extend beyond it (brick walls are adequate; thin walls may be reinforced with barium plaster or lead ply).

The room should be large enough to allow any people that have to remain in it during exposure to stand at least 2 metres from the primary beam. If this is not possible, a protective lead screen must be provided. Unshielded doors and windows may be acceptable if the work load is low and the room is large enough. Special recommendations are made for flooring in rare cases where there is an occupied area below the radiography room.

Technically, the controlled area is the area around the primary beam within which the average dose rate of exposure exceeds a given limit. This is usually within a radius of 2 metres (6 metres for large animal work) as laid down in the regulations.The controlled area must be clearly labelled and a red warning light should be displayed (usually by the entrance to the controlled area) when radiography is taking place, warning others not to enter.

In addition, all X-ray machines should have lights visible from the control panel indicating:

- When the machine is switched on and being supplied by electricity
- When exposure is taking place.

Once radiographic examination has been completed the machine should be disconnected from the electricity supply. All staff should be aware of what to do in an emergency, i.e. if the machine jams while emitting X-rays. This usually involves knowing where to shut down power without having to re-enter the controlled area. Any fault must be reported to the RPA.

Staff involved with radiography

Persons 16–18 years of age have restrictions on radiography work. There is a smaller dose limit for them, although if possible they should not be allowed in the controlled area as their bodies are still developing and are at a slightly greater risk.

Maximum permissible dose

The maximum permissible dose (MPD) is the amount of radiation that can be received by the body or a specific part of it without causing harm.

Personal monitoring

Designated persons (a list of whom will be displayed in the local rules) should all have a dosemeter that they wear while at work. The dosemeter should only be worn by its designated wearer. There should be no swapping and sharing. Dosemeters should be worn on the trunk beneath any lead apron.

Different types of dosemeter are available. Commonly used types include:

- Film badge (blue holder)
- Thermolucent crystal badge (bright orange holder).

They should not leave the building, nor be placed in direct sunlight or next to any other sources of radiation, e.g. a computer. Dosemeters are supplied by the National Radiation Protection Board (NRPB) and are periodically exchanged, when the old dosemeters are sent back for reading. A printout of all readings is sent to the practice so staff can see if they have registered any exposure. Records of these printouts must be kept in the practice for at least 2 years.

Persons who should not take part in radiography:

- Persons under 16 years of age
- Pregnant women
- Those advised not to by their GP.

Protective clothing

It is important to realize that any protective clothing protects against scatter and not the primary beam. Clothing available may include:

- Aprons
- Gloves
- Sleeves
- Thyroid guards.

They are made of plastic or rubber that is impregnated with lead and known as 'lead rubber'. Aprons may be single- or double-sided (double-sided giving better protection). They should be long enough to reach mid-thigh level. The aprons should be worn by any persons remaining in the controlled area while an exposure is taken, even if standing behind a lead screen. Gloves and sleeves are worn when manual restraint of an animal is necessary. Even when wearing these, the hands should not be placed in the primary beam.

Protective clothing must be checked regularly for signs of wear and tear. Visual inspection is usually enough but, where further investigation is needed, X-raying the clothing may be necessary. Aprons should never be folded; they should be hung up to prevent cracking of the lead.

X-ray records book

Every practice should have a record of exposures taken. Columns may be detailed, as shown in Figure 3.8. This is used to keep an accurate record of exposures and also enables staff to see which exposures have produced diagnostic radio-

Date	Owner Details	Animal Name	Breed	Wt (kg)	Consc Or GA	View	Plate	Grid Y/N	Exposure	Comments	Initials
1.6.01	Jones	Sam	GSD	37	GA	VD Hips	Large	Y	85 x 5	V. good	DM SKM

Fig. 3.8 Example of records kept in a radiography book

graphs, thus helping to reduce the number of unnecessary radiographs.

Manual restraint

Manual restraint while taking radiographs:

- Should only be done when there is just cause, e.g. if the patient is a severe anaesthetic or sedation risk
- Details of any persons manually restraining during X-rays should be recorded in the X-ray book so their exposure can be monitored.

Processing chemicals

Processing chemicals for use in automatic or wet processors may be supplied as powders, liquid concentrates or ready-to-use liquids. All chemicals should be handled with care in a well-ventilated room. Gloves, goggles and face mask should be worn.

When spent, waste chemicals should be placed in the original container and collected by an authorized person. Local hospitals and laboratories may provide this service. As with all potentially hazardous substances, a risk assessment

Table 3.3 Summary of laws that protect the public

Animal Health Act 1981 and Quarantine regulations	This Act gives government ministers powers to make orders to prevent and control the introduction and spread of zoonotic disease and assist in the eradication of diseases carried by animals in the UK. The orders and regulations covered include the following: • The Rabies (Control) Order 1974, now incorporated into the Animal Health Act • Quarantine for imports and exports • Points of entry into Britain • Transport method and conditions • Seizure of animals and their disposal (dogs and wildlife) • Disinfection of places and vehicles.
The Pet Travel Scheme (PETS)	PETS, introduced in 2001, allows dogs and cats coming from EU countries, certain other European countries and rabies-free islands to enter the UK without having to undergo quarantine provided they can be shown to meet the necessary criteria regarding vaccination and identification. Requirements: • Microchipped with electronic chip • Vaccinated against rabies using an inactivated vaccine • Treated for exotic diseases not present in the UK • Blood-tested at an approved laboratory to prove efficacy of vaccine • Has an official health certificate • 24–48 h before re-entry into UK the dog or cat must be treated against ticks and tapeworm • Pre-entry checks carried out by train operators, ferry companies and airlines • Random spot checks on animals arriving in the UK by the Department of the Environment, Farming and Rural Affairs (DEFRA) and official carriers.
Dangerous Dogs Act 1991, 1997	Applies to the following breeds of dog: • American pit bull terrier • Japanese tosa • Dogo argentino • Fila braziliera. The Act states that the rules for ownership of a dangerous named breed of dog are as follows: • Notifying the police of ownership • Obtaining a certificate of exemption from the police, which is issued when the dog has been neutered and identified with a microchip or other permanent method • The dog is covered by third-party liability insurance • In public places, the dog is always muzzled and on a lead • The dog is always in the company of a person over 16 years of age • It is an offence to sell, exchange or abandon the dog • It is an offence to breed from these dogs. Any dog dangerously out of control and a risk to the general public comes under the remit of this Act. Where such a dog has caused injury, the owner may be subject to prosecution and an unlimited fine
Guard Dogs Act 1975	Governs the safe use and control of dogs that guard property or sites. This must be done in a way that does not put the general public at risk. A notice must be displayed to inform the public that a dog is in use and the dog must only be off the lead if accompanied by a handler
Animals Act 1971	This Act covers liability for damage that has been caused by animals, including damage, death and injury caused to people, property and livestock. The owner of a dangerous animal must take precautions to ensure that it has no opportunity to inflict damage as defined by this law. If a dog kills or harms farm animals, farmers are entitled to protect the stock in their care. If, for example, a dog is found injuring sheep, the farmer may kill the dog but must report the incident to the police
Dog Fouling of Land Act 1996	Local authorities and councils use this Act to prevent dogs fouling where there is public access to property or pavements, but allowing the exemption of guide dogs for the blind

and standard operating procedure should be in place for use and disposal of these chemicals.

A summary of other legislation designed to protect the public is included in Table 3.3.

Animal Welfare Act 2006

The Animal Welfare Act 2006 defines an 'animal' as being any living vertebrate animal.

It imposes a 'duty of care' (a legal phrase which means that someone is obligated to do something) on those persons responsible for animals. This includes if he/she is:

- The owner of the animal
- In charge of the animal, e.g. the owner of a cattery, or looking after a neighbour's dog whilst the owner's are on holiday
- A parent or guardian of a person under 16 years of age who is responsible for an animal.

Before the Animal Welfare Act was introduced, people only had a duty to ensure that their animal did not suffer unnecessarily. This new Act builds on this, making owners and keepers responsible for ensuring that the welfare needs of their animals are met, including the need for:

- A suitable environment
- A suitable diet
- The ability to exhibit normal behaviour
- Any need the animal has to be housed with; or apart from other animals
- Protection from pain, suffering, injury and disease.

Collectively, the above are known as the 'Five Freedoms' (see also Chapter 1).

Under the Act, there are two different types of action that can be taken in the event of someone breaking the law:

Table 3.4 Current animal welfare legislation

Animal Boarding Establishments Act 1963	Boarding kennels or catteries must be licensed by their local authority in order to trade. The following conditions apply: • Records kept of animal arrivals and departures and details of owners • Provision of suitable accommodation • Adequate and appropriate supplies of food and water • Exercise facilities available • Animals protected from disease and risk of fire. In order to ensure that the conditions of the licence are met, the local authority can at any time instruct inspection by an authorized officer or veterinary surgeon. Licences are renewed annually.
Breeding of Dogs Act 1973	The law was altered in 1991, allowing authorized officers or veterinary surgeons to enter premises with a warrant if they suspect an offence under the 1973 Act has been committed. The term 'breeding establishment' refers to any premises where more than two bitches are kept for the purpose of breeding animals for selling. The 1973 Act prohibits: • Obstruction of inspection by authorized personnel • Breeding dogs for sale without a licence from the local authority • If disqualified under other Acts of Parliament, holding a licence for the breeding of dogs.
Pet Animals Act 1951, 1983	Prohibits the keeping of a pet shop without a licence. A licence is granted after inspection of the premises by an approved veterinary surgeon authorized by the local authority. An amendment in 1983 now makes it illegal to sell pets in public places. A licence is granted if the following conditions are met: • Proper care • Suitable accommodation • Housed in the correct conditions with reference to heating, lighting, etc. • Provided with appropriate food • Observed and checked at suitable intervals during the day • Sold only after weaning and after a suitable age has been reached • Prevention of spread of disease • Emergency and fire precautions for the premises are in place and operational.
Protection of Animals Acts 1911, 1988	This series of Acts forms the main statutory control on cruelty to animals by humans. These Acts are used when bringing prosecutions related to animal welfare cases. The Act makes it an offence to cause unnecessary suffering to any domestic or captive animal either deliberately or by omission (neglect). The Act lists offences such as: • Inflicting physical cruelty by beating, kicking, etc. • Inflicting mental cruelty by teasing or terrifying • Causing unnecessary suffering during transportation by failing to provide food or water at appropriate intervals • Performing surgery or operations without anaesthetic • Poisoning without reason.

(Continued)

Table 3.4 Continued

Protection of Animals (Anaesthetics) Acts 1954, 1982	It is illegal for any operation to be conducted on an animal that will cause pain unless under anaesthetic (local or general).There are, however, several exceptions to this Act. • Does not apply to birds, fish or reptiles • In emergency first-aid situations • Under permitted Home-Office-licensed procedures • Minor painless operations carried out by a veterinary surgeon or a listed veterinary nurse.
Welfare of Animals during Transport 1973, 1994 (Amendment) Order 1995	This order is designed to protect all animals during transport by road, rail, sea and air. From 1997, a standard set of regulations covering EU countries on journey times, hauliers' journey plans and routes amended the original order. The regulations cover: • Loading and unloading of animals • Housing and containers for transit • Access to food and water • Specified number of animals contained together for transit.
Abandonment of Animals Act 1960 Dangerous Wild Animals Act 1976	This Act applies to the abandonment of an animal in circumstances likely to cause it unnecessary suffering, whether temporarily or permanently. This Act was introduced following a rise in the 1960s and 1970s in the numbers of members of the public keeping animals more associated with zoos and wildlife parks. There was cause for concern over their standard of living and also about the danger posed to the general public. The legislation involves strict control and inspection by authorized veterinary surgeons, who may inspect premises in which these animals are kept. If the inspection is approved, a licence may be issued by the local authority. The Secretary of State has the power to change the list of animals at any time and any animal on the list is classified as a 'dangerous wild animal'. The Act states that anyone keeping these listed animals must: • Pay a fee to the local authority for the issue of the licence • Take out liability insurance • Provide suitable accommodation • Be over 18 years of age.
Performing Animals (Regulation) Act 1925	This Act was introduced following public concern over the treatment of animals in circuses. As a result, the local authority must be informed of anyone who trains animals for exhibition to the public or exhibits a performing animal to the public, even if it is free of charge, and any such person must be registered to that effect. The exceptions to this rule are when animals are trained for sporting purposes, military or police work and display.

Zoo Licensing Act 1981	The term 'zoo' refers to the exhibiting of wild animals to the public for educational purposes. It applies to animal collections that are open to the public for 7 days or more in any year.
	  This Act was passed after the dramatic increase of zoos and wildlife/safari parks in the 1960s. It is intended to protect the zoo animals and the general public by ensuring that measures to safeguard standards of care, the welfare of the animals and the safety of the public are in place.
	  The zoo must obtain a licence from the local authority, which is renewed initially after 4 years and then every 6 years.

The Wildlife and Countryside Acts 1981, 1985	These Acts replace several existing laws and regulations and cover the protection and conservation of wild animals and their habitats. Land, sea and airborne species of wild animals are protected. The minister can add or remove species on this list, which may not legally be injured, killed or taken from the wild. The Act protects habitat from humans and species in captivity which, if released into the wild, would seriously affect many other species. Within the Act, licences can be granted which exempt the holder from the above provisions: • Relating to the protection of farming or forestry interests • Relating to the conservation, reintroduction, photographing and identification of wildlife.
Convention of International Trade in Endangered Species of Wild Flora and Fauna (CITES) 1973	This is an international agreement in place to protect the world's endangered species. This is done through control of their export and import on a worldwide scale. Animals within this agreement fall into one of two categories: • Those that are threatened with extinction • Those likely to become so threatened.

- An improvement notice can be issued. This explains why someone is failing to meet the welfare needs of the animal, what they need to do to rectify the situation, the time in which they must comply with the notice and the action that will be taken if they fail to do so. It is not a criminal penalty, but can lead to a criminal record if there is failure to meet the welfare requirements of the notice.

- Criminal prosecution can be pursued; if found guilty a person can be fined up to £20,000, imprisoned, have the animals taken away or be banned from keeping animals in the future.

A summary of other animal welfare legislation is included in Table 3.4.

Bibliography

Dallas, S., 2002. Animal Biology and Care. Blackwell Science, Oxford.

Hotston-Moore, A., Simpson, G., 1999. Manual of Advanced Veterinary Nursing. British Small Animal Veterinary Association, Gloucester.

Hughes, P., Ferrett, E., 2003. Introduction to Health and Safety at Work. Butterworth-Heinemann, Oxford.

Lane, D., Cooper, B., Turner, C., 2007. BSAVA Textbook of Veterinary Nursing, fourth ed. BSAVA, Gloucester.

Moore, M., Simpson, G., 1999. Manual of Veterinary Nursing. British Small Animal Veterinary Association, Gloucester.

Shilcock, S., Stutchfield, G., 2003. Veterinary Practice Management; A Practical Guide, second ed. Saunders Elsevier, Oxford.

Useful websites

British Veterinary Association: <http://www.bva.co.uk>

DEFRA: <http://www.defra.co.uk>

Health and Safety Executive (HSE): <http://www.hse.gov.uk>

Royal College of Veterinary Surgeons: <http://www.rcvs.org.uk>

Recommended reading

Hotston-Moore, A., Simpson, G., 1999. Manual of Advanced Veterinary Nursing. British Small Animal Veterinary Association, Gloucester.

Lane, D., Cooper, B., Turner, C., 2007. BSAVA Textbook of Veterinary Nursing, fourth ed. BSAVA, Gloucester.

A detailed discussion about the legal responsibilities of a veterinary nurse within a practice.

Moore, M., Simpson, G., 1999. Manual of Veterinary Nursing. British Small Animal Veterinary Association, Gloucester.

Both manuals provide added information about animal welfare law and the responsibilities of a veterinary nurse.

CHAPTER 4

Canine and feline anatomy and physiology

Sue Dallas

- The cell is the basic unit of the body. All cells contain a nucleus, cell membrane and cytoplasm. They also possess other features that are specific to their type and function.
- Cells form the four basic tissues, which are arranged into organs, which form the body systems.
- The systems of the body comprise a set of organs, each of which has a function that contributes to the overall function of the system.
- Anatomy is the study of the structure of the organs; physiology is the study of how the organs function.

Introduction

Knowledge of anatomy and physiology in the dog and cat is essential as a foundation to many aspects of veterinary nursing and care. From this knowledge evolves an appreciation of how disease and injury affect normal function and how in turn treatment can be designed to alleviate the symptoms. This chapter is not written as an all-inclusive description of anatomy and physiology but merely as a reminder of the important and most relevant facts.

Cells and basic tissues

The cell is the functional unit of all tissues and each cell has the ability to perform all the essential life functions. Within the various tissues of the body, the constituent cells show a wide range of adaptations to perform a particular functional specialization. All cells conform to a basic structure (Box 4.1).

The diversity of cells

Cells are not identical and their shape and contents show variation according to their function, but wherever they are found in the body they have the same basic features. Some examples of different cells are:

- **Epithelial cells** – found lining the surface of the body, the body cavities and the organs within it.
- **Glandular cells** – responsible for producing some kind of secretion, e.g. mucus to lubricate the tissues.
- **Osteoblasts** – produce bone tissue.
- **Erythrocytes (red blood cells)** – their shape is designed to hold the red pigment haemoglobin to convey oxygen around the body; they are one of the few cells in the body that has no nucleus.
- **Nerve cells, or neurons** – have slender arm-like processes that will transmit electrical impulses through the nervous system to reach the whole body.
- **Muscle** – capable of contracting to bring about body movement.

Cells

All cells have the following features in common:

- **Cell membrane** – encloses the cytoplasm and controls the internal environment of the cell.
- **Cytoplasm** – a jelly-like material that contains all the structures and chemicals that make the cell function.
- **Nucleus** – to control all the functions of the cell and to hold the inheritable material in the form of chromosomes. (See also Chapter 16.)

Cell membrane

The cell membrane is 0.00001 mm thick and forms the outer boundary of the cell. It is here that all exchanges take place between the cell and its surrounding environment. In a manner that is not yet fully understood this membrane allows certain chemicals to pass in and out of the cell but prevents the passage of others – the cell membrane is said to be selectively permeable.

Cytoplasm

The term cytoplasm refers to all the living parts of a cell except the nucleus and is a jelly-like material containing a large number of important structures and substances, many of which are concerned with metabolism. It contains:

- Organelles – the free-living structures within the cell other than the nucleus.

- Mitochondria – some of the most important organelles in which the chemical reactions involved in cellular respiration take place; energy is released for cellular function.
- Rough endoplasmic reticulum – lined by ribosomes produced in the nucleus; protein is synthesized here and the cell may transport it for use in the manufacture of digestive enzymes and hormones.
- Smooth endoplasmic reticulum – not lined by ribosomes but is concerned with the synthesis and transport of lipids (fats) and steroids of body origin
- Ribosomes – these granules, rich in ribonucleic acid, are sites of protein synthesis.
- Centrosome – lies near the nucleus and is made up of two centrioles; it is important during cell division and the formation of the cilia and flagella, which are slender projecting hairs needed by some cells.
- Lysosomes – dark, round bodies containing enzymes (lysozymes) responsible for splitting complex chemical compounds into simpler ones. They also destroy worn-out organelles within the cell.
- Golgi body or complex – a system of flattened tubes in which lysozymes are stored.

Nucleus

A nucleus is found in the living cells of all organisms. The nucleus of a cell contains rod-shaped objects called chromosomes. These are only visible when a cell is about to divide into two during mitosis and meiosis (see Ch. 16). Chromosomes contain a complex chemical called deoxyribonucleic acid (DNA). DNA controls the development of the features that an organism inherits from its parents. In other words it contains the chemical 'instructions' for making an organism.

Basic tissue types

Muscular tissue

Brings about movement.

- Skeletal (voluntary, striated) – causes movement of the skeleton, e.g. locomotion
- Smooth (involuntary, non-striated) – concerned with movement within organs and blood vessels, e.g. vasoconstriction, peristalsis
- Cardiac – concerned with the beating of the heart.

Epithelial tissue

Forms a protective layer both inside and on the surface of the body, e.g. skin, glands and linings of the various body

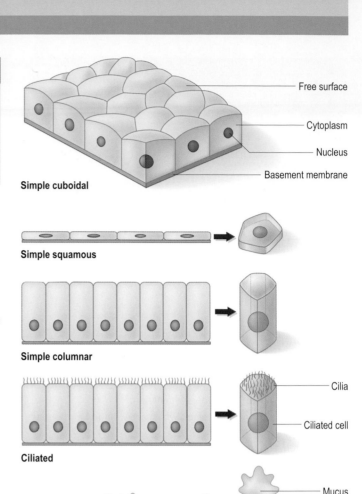

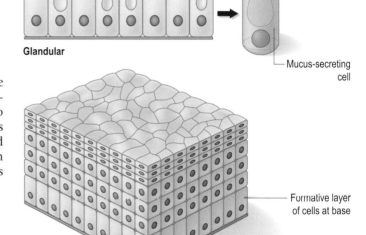

Fig. 4.1 Types of epithelial tissue

systems. Its function is to protect and, depending on its location and density, to allow absorption. Epithelial tissue may be simple or compound (Fig. 4.1). The many and varied functions of epithelium mean that it takes many different forms.

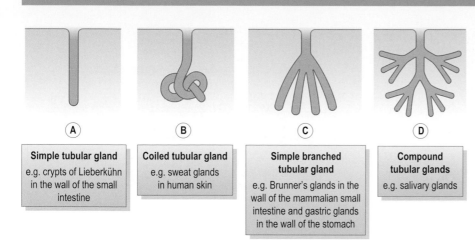

Fig. 4.2 Examples of endocrine glands

A — **Simple tubular gland**
e.g. crypts of Lieberkühn in the wall of the small intestine

B — **Coiled tubular gland**
e.g. sweat glands in human skin

C — **Simple branched tubular gland**
e.g. Brunner's glands in the wall of the mammalian small intestine and gastric glands in the wall of the stomach

D — **Compound tubular glands**
e.g. salivary glands

a. Simple

The layer of cells is one cell thick:

- Squamous – cells are flat and plate-like. Found where absorption is required, e.g. blood vessel walls and lining the renal nephrons.
- Cuboidal – cells are cube-shaped with a central spherical nucleus. Found in glands and ducts.
- Columnar – tall and rectangular; the layer of cells may contain mucus-secreting goblet cells or may be ciliated, i.e. covered in a fine covering of hairs. Found in the respiratory tract (ciliated), lining the gut with a covering of microvilli, and in secretory glands of the digestive and endocrine systems.

b. Compound

More than one layer of cells.

- Stratified – the first layers of cell are cuboidal, becoming flatter as they are moved towards the surface of the tissue by new cells forming beneath them, e.g. in skin.
- Transitional – modified, stratified, containing a combination of shapes; found where ability to stretch is required, e.g. urinary bladder.
- Glandular – consisting of either individual goblet cells with a single unbranched duct or a mass of secretory cells with a branched duct system forming a gland; there are two types:
  - **a.** Endocrine – surrounded by an extensive capillary network and are ductless, secreting hormones directly into the blood stream, e.g. thyroid gland (Fig. 4.2).
  - **b.** Exocrine – defined as simple or compound, have ducts and secrete on to an epithelial surface, e.g. sweat glands.

Connective tissue

Supports and connects tissues and acts as a transport system to move essential materials, e.g. nutrients around the body. Examples of this tissue are:

- Loose connective tissue (also called areolar tissue) – this consists of a loose network of collagen fibres and surrounds organs providing support and flexibility, e.g. under skin, around blood vessels. Adipose tissue is similar to areolar tissue but has an increased proportion of fat cells, which provide an energy reserve, insulation and protection.
- Dense connective tissue – has a large proportion of collagen fibres, which provide great strength, e.g. tendons, which connect muscle to bone, and ligaments, which connect bone to bone.
- Blood – transports essential nutrients, gases, waste products, hormones and enzymes to and from all body cells. Consists of many cell types, e.g. erythrocytes, leucocytes and thrombocytes, suspended in a liquid matrix called plasma.
- Cartilage – a mixture of collagen and elastic fibres provides shape, provides protection for organs and allows movement. It is a dense, clear, blue/white material that is tough and can be elastic or rigid. Found mainly in joints, it has no blood vessels but is covered by a membrane called the perichondrium from which it receives its blood supply. The cells of cartilage are called chondrocytes.
  There are three types of cartilage:
  - **a.** Hyaline – chondrocytes lie within a hyaline matrix with collagen fibres running through, e.g. forming the articular surfaces of the joint; C-shaped rings that keep the trachea open for air passage into the lungs
  - **b.** Fibrocartilage – stronger than hyaline cartilage and the matrix contains more fibrous collagen fibres, e.g. surrounds the articular surface of some bones, e.g. in the hip joint and the shoulder joint; also found in the stifle as pads of cartilage called menisci; intervertebral discs within the vertebral column
  - **c.** Elastic – has a hyaline matrix and many elastic fibres that gives it elastic properties, e.g. in the ear pinna; in the epiglottis.
- Bone – provides support for the body and a means of attachment for skeletal muscles. It consists of cells embedded in a comparatively hard matrix or ground substance. The cells are arranged as cylinders in layers known as Haversian systems, which give bone its strength (Fig. 4.3). Bone is made of three types of cell:
  Osteoblasts – responsible for the secretion of material which, when mineralized or calcified, will become bone

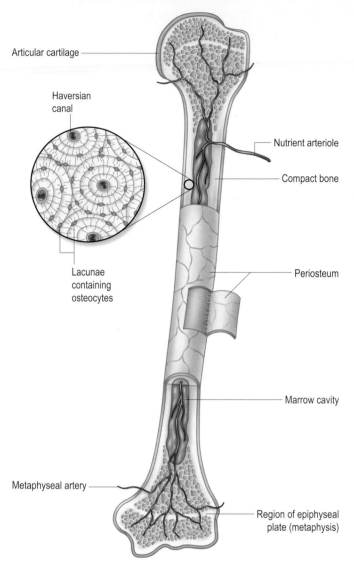

Articular cartilage

Haversian canal

Lacunae containing osteocytes

Metaphyseal artery

Nutrient arteriole

Compact bone

Periosteum

Marrow cavity

Region of epiphyseal plate (metaphysis)

Fig. 4.3 Structure of compact bone

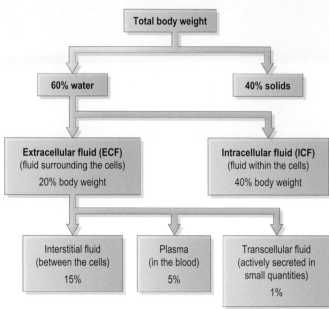

Total body weight

60% water   40% solids

Extracellular fluid (ECF) (fluid surrounding the cells) 20% body weight

Intracellular fluid (ICF) (fluid within the cells) 40% body weight

Interstitial fluid (between the cells) 15%

Plasma (in the blood) 5%

Transcellular fluid (actively secreted in small quantities) 1%

Fig. 4.4 Distribution of body fluids into compartments

surface of bone is covered by a delicate connective tissue layer called the endosteum. Both the periosteum and endosteum contain osteoclasts, which assist in the remodelling and repair of bone if it becomes damaged.

- Haemopoietic tissue – responsible for the formation of all blood cells from haemopoietic stem cells which are found in the spleen, liver, lymphoid tissue and in bone marrow. As the animal reaches maturity the bone marrow is the main site of haemopoiesis.

Nervous tissue

Conducts electrical or nerve impulses to and from the central nervous system by means of neurons. Each neuron consists of a cell body, many dendrons, which conduct impulses towards the cell body, and a single axon, which conducts impulses away from the cell body. Neurons are supported by neuroglial cells, which are a form of connective tissue (see Nervous system, below).

Body fluids

The body consists of approximately 60% fluid, which is often referred to as body water and is distributed into 'compartments' (Fig. 4.4), which are delicately balanced. The total volume of body fluids is affected by:

- Input, i.e. by drinking and eating.
- Output, i.e. major losses include:
    Respiration – within exhaled gases
    Skin – sweating
    Gastrointestinal – faeces
    Kidneys – urine.

The proportion of body fluids varies between individuals:

- Fat animals – lower percentage of fluid, as fat displaces water within the cells
- Very young animals – higher percentage of fluid, as the solid elements of the body are underdeveloped.

Osteoblasts – become trapped in the forming bone and are then called osteocytes
Osteoclasts – responsible for reabsorbing materials and for the remodelling of bone, e.g. after a fracture.

Long bones, e.g. femur, humerus (Fig 4.3), are made up of two types of bone tissue:

a. Compact bone – forming the dense walls of the bone shaft
b. Cancellous or spongy bone – forming the central medullary cavity and providing support for haemopoietic tissue.

The medullary cavity of most bones contains red marrow, which is responsible for the production of platelets or thrombocytes and red and white blood cells. The yellow, rather fatty-looking material sometimes found in the medullary cavities is inactive bone marrow. The outer surface of bone is covered with a layer of dense fibrous connective tissue called the periosteum into which are inserted tendons and ligaments for the attachment of muscles. The inner

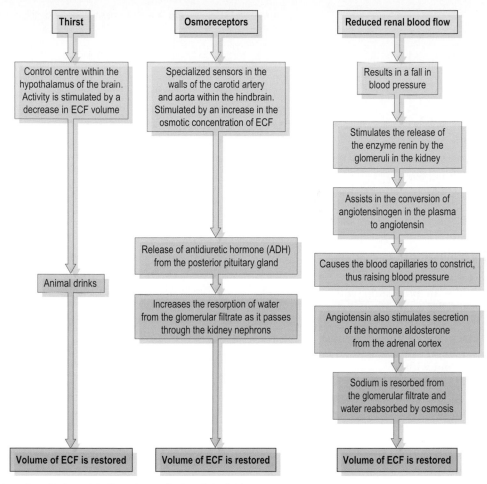

Fig. 4.5 Physiological reactions that regulate the volume of extracellular fluid

The daily fluid loss in terms of body weight is calculated as:

- 20 ml/kg body weight/day – respiration and sweating
- 10–20 ml/kg body weight/day – faeces
- 20 ml/kg body weight/day – urine.

The total loss of fluid from the body is estimated to be 50–60 ml/kg body weight/day.

The losses from the respiratory tract and the skin cannot be regulated and are described as insensible or inevitable water loss. Losses from the kidney are linked to thirst and osmoregulatory mechanisms involved in the maintenance of extracellular fluid volume (Fig. 4.5).

Within the body, fluid moves between compartments and this movement depends on the osmotic concentration within each compartment. Water crosses most cell membranes by a process of osmosis and moves rapidly to equalize the osmotic concentration between the cells and their surroundings. The osmotic concentration of plasma is vital in controlling fluid movement, and the kidneys and thirst regulate the osmotic concentration of both extracellular and intracellular fluid by affecting water taken into the body and excreted in urine (Box 4.2).

Electrolytes

An electrolyte is a substance that, when dissolved in water, breaks up into ions or charged particles, e.g. sodium chloride (NaCl) becomes Na^+ and Cl^- when dissolved in water.

Box 4.2 Movement of fluid

Osmosis – the movement of water through a semipermeable membrane from an area of low concentration to an area of high concentration (Fig. 4.6). The cell membrane is said to be semipermeable, permitting the passage of some substances but not of others. Osmosis will continue through it until the concentration is equal on either side. The pressure that must be applied to prevent this movement is called the osmotic pressure or potential

Isotonic – osmotic pressure is equal to that of the plasma and refers to solutions which cause no transfer of fluid either into or out of a cell

Hypertonic – solutions with an osmotic pressure higher than that of plasma

Hypotonic – solutions with an osmotic pressure higher than that of plasma

Diffusion – the movement of substances from an area of high concentration to one of low concentration. The substances are passing down a diffusion gradient

---

There are two types of ion:

- Cations are positively charged ions, e.g. sodium, potassium, calcium, magnesium
- Anions are negatively charged ions, e.g. chloride, bicarbonate, sulphate, phosphate.

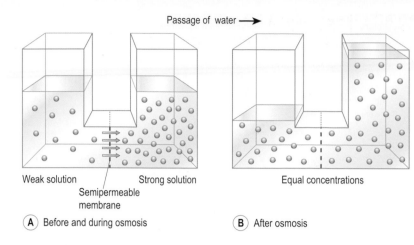

Passage of water ⟶

Fig. 4.6 Processes that occur during osmosis

Weak solution   Strong solution   Equal concentrations
        Semipermeable
        membrane

(A) Before and during osmosis   (B) After osmosis

The body fluids contain electrolytes as follows:

- The main **cations** found within:
  a. Intracellular fluid – are potassium, with sodium and magnesium in smaller quantities.
  b. Extracellular fluid – are sodium, with potassium, calcium and magnesium found in smaller quantities.
- The main **anions** found within:
  a. Intracellular fluid – are phosphate with chloride and bicarbonate in smaller quantities. There is no protein in intracelluar fluid.
  b. Extracellular fluid – are chloride with smaller quantities of phosphate. Plasma contains plasma proteins – the main ones are albumin, prothrombin, fibrinogen and globulin and their function is to maintain blood volume and blood pressure by exerting osmotic pressure. These are not present in other forms of extracellular fluid because the molecules are too large to escape through the capillary walls under normal conditions.

Knowledge of which electrolytes are found within each of the fluid compartments enables the veterinary surgeon to decide which type of fluid replacement therapy is appropriate in different disease conditions.

Body cavities

The body is divided into three main cavities:

1. **Thoracic cavity** – lies within the chest. Its boundaries are:
   - Cranial – the thoracic inlet or aperture formed by the first thoracic vertebrae, the first pair of ribs and the manubrium at the cranial end of the sternum, through which the trachea and oesophagus pass
   - Caudal – the diaphragm
   - Dorsal – the thoracic vertebrae and muscles
   - Ventral – the sternum
   - Lateral – the ribs and intercostal muscles.
2. **Abdominal cavity** – its boundaries are:
   - Cranial – the diaphragm
   - Caudal – the pelvic opening
   - Dorsal – the lumbar vertebrae and part of the diaphragm
   - Lateral and ventral – the abdominal muscles.
3. **Pelvic cavity** – often described as a separate cavity but there is no physical barrier between it and the abdominal cavity. Its boundaries are:
   - Cranial – the pelvic inlet
   - Caudal – the pelvic outlet
   - Dorsal – the pelvic girdle – the pubis, ileum and ischium
   - Lateral – the muscles or ligaments attached around the pelvic girdle.

The pericardium, not one of the major cavities of the body, contains the heart. It consists of a double layer of membrane and lies within the mediastinum in the thoracic cavity.

The cranial cavity is another small cavity, formed by the bones of the cranium, and contains the brain.

Body cavity linings

All cavities are lined with a layer of serous endothelium or serous membrane, which secretes a small amount of serous (watery) fluid that acts as a lubricating layer between two tissue surfaces. The cavity between two layers of serous membrane is a serous cavity. Serous membranes are composed of a simple squamous surface epithelium and a connective tissue groundwork or stroma. This connective tissue is composed of yellow elastic and white fibrous tissue and provides support to the delicate membrane. The layer covers all the organs within the cavity and is named according to the cavity.

- Thoracic cavity – the serous membrane is called the **pleura** and forms the pleural cavity, which is divided into right and left by a double layer of pleura known as the mediastinum. The space between the two layers contains the heart and other structures (Fig. 4.7). The pleura covering the lungs is the pulmonary or visceral pleura. The remaining pleura is the parietal pleura. Where the parietal pleura covers the ribs it is called the costal pleura and where it covers the diaphragm it is called the diaphragmatic pleura.
- Abdominal cavity – here the serous membrane is called the **peritoneum** and forms the peritoneal cavity. The visceral peritoneum closely covers the abdominal organs, forming suspensory folds or mesenteries that connect the intestines to the dorsal abdominal wall (Fig. 4.8). Each mesentery is named according to the organ it suspends; for example, the mesoduodenum

suspends the duodenum. The lining of the abdominal wall is the parietal peritoneum.

- Pelvic cavity – the peritoneum continues into the pelvic cavity and covers the cranial surfaces of the organs within the cavity, e.g. bladder and uterus. The remainder of the cavity is filled with organs, muscles and connective tissue and is not lined by a serous membrane.

Locomotor system

The function of the locomotor system is to bring about movement of the animal. It consists of two major systems:

- The skeletal system – made up of the skeleton and the joints
- The muscular system – made of the muscles attached to the skeleton.

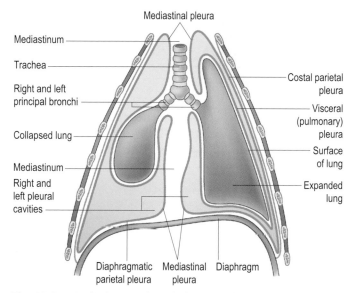

Mediastinal pleura

Mediastinum

Trachea

Right and left principal bronchi

Collapsed lung

Mediastinum

Right and left pleural cavities

Costal parietal pleura

Visceral (pulmonary) pleura

Surface of lung

Expanded lung

Diaphragmatic parietal pleura   Mediastinal pleura   Diaphragm

Fig. 4.7 Longitudinal section through the thorax showing the arrangement of the pleura

The skeletal system

The skeleton is divided into three parts:

- Axial skeleton – the skull, vertebral column, ribs and sternum
- Appendicular skeleton – the fore and hind limbs
- Splanchnic skeleton – bones that develop in soft tissues, e.g. the os penis.

The skeletal system consists of bone and cartilage whose function is to provide support for the body and a rigid but all-moving framework (see Basic Tissues Types, p. 38).

Bone growth or ossification

Bone develops within the embryo in two ways:

- Intramembranous – bone formed directly from fibrous tissue, e.g. flat bones of the skull
- Endochondral – bone formed within a preformed cartilaginous model.

The **function** of the skeletal system is to:

- Support the body
- Provide leverage for muscle contraction, which brings about movement
- Protect the organs, e.g. heart, lungs, brain
- Maintain calcium and phosphorus levels in the body.

There are over 200 bones in the skeleton, many of which are shown in Figure 4.9. For more detailed descriptions of the skeleton you are advised to look at a more specialized anatomy book (see Recommended reading).

Joints

Joints are places where two or more bones meet. There are several methods of joint classification:

Degree of movement

- Synarthrosis – joint that is immovable, e.g. joints of the skull, known as sutures

Fig. 4.8 Sagittal section through the abdominal cavity to show the arrangement of the peritoneum

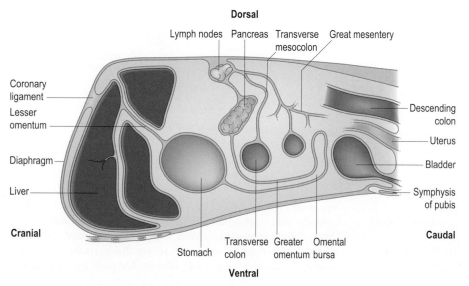

Dorsal

Lymph nodes   Pancreas   Transverse mesocolon   Great mesentery

Coronary ligament

Lesser omentum

Diaphragm

Liver

Descending colon

Uterus

Bladder

Symphysis of pubis

Cranial

Caudal

Stomach   Transverse colon   Greater omentum   Omental bursa

Ventral

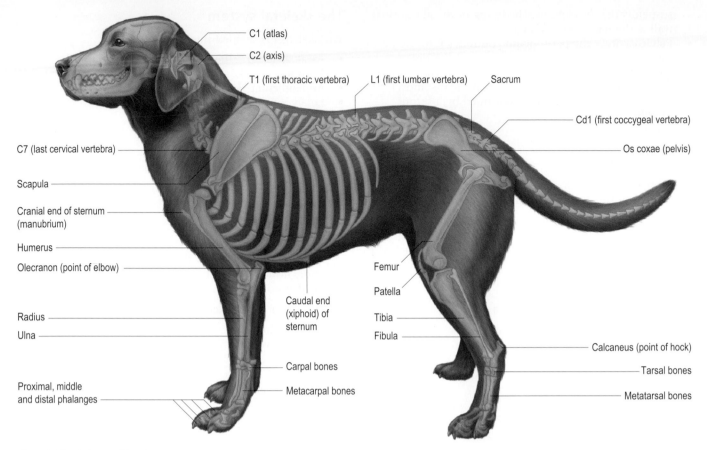

C1 (atlas)
C2 (axis)
T1 (first thoracic vertebra)
L1 (first lumbar vertebra)
Sacrum
Cd1 (first coccygeal vertebra)
Os coxae (pelvis)
C7 (last cervical vertebra)
Scapula
Cranial end of sternum (manubrium)
Humerus
Olecranon (point of elbow)
Femur
Patella
Caudal end (xiphoid) of sternum
Tibia
Fibula
Radius
Ulna
Calcaneus (point of hock)
Tarsal bones
Carpal bones
Metatarsal bones
Proximal, middle and distal phalanges
Metacarpal bones

Fig. 4.9 The skeleton of the dog

- Amphiarthrosis – joint that shares some of the characteristics of the synarthroses and diarthroses and has limited movement, e.g. between the vertebrae of the spine
- Diarthrosis – joint in which there is a great deal of movement; these are usually related to the limbs, e.g. synovial joints (Fig. 4.10)
- Syntosis – joint that becomes fused with bone as the animal ages, e.g. pubic symphysis, sutures of the skull.

Structure

- Fibrous – connected by dense fibrous connective tissue that allows very little movement, e.g. sutures of the skull
- Cartilaginous – connected by cartilage and found where the right and left sides of the body join, e.g. mandibular symphysis and pubic symphysis
- Synovial – allow plenty of movement (Fig. 4.10). Synovial joints have several anatomical features:
  - Hyaline cartilage covers the bone ends to form the articular surfaces
  - The surfaces of the joint are linked by a dense, fibrous, connective-tissue joint capsule
  - The capsule is lined by a synovial membrane which secretes synovial fluid
  - The joint cavity is filled with synovial fluid, which acts as a lubricant and a 'shock absorber'.

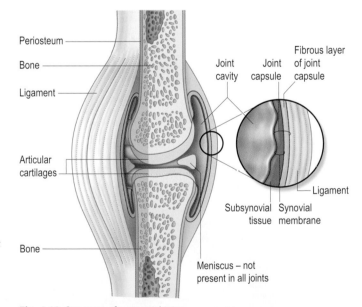

Periosteum
Bone
Ligament
Joint cavity
Joint capsule
Fibrous layer of joint capsule
Articular cartilages
Bone
Ligament
Subsynovial tissue
Synovial membrane
Meniscus – not present in all joints

Fig. 4.10 Structure of a synovial joint

Synovial joints may be called simple joints if they contain two articular surfaces, e.g. the shoulder joint formed by the glenoid cavity of the scapula and the head of the humerus. Compound joints have more than two articular surfaces, e.g. the elbow formed by the distal end of the humerus, the proximal ends of the ulna and radius.

Type of movement

- Pivot (radius/ulna or atlas/axis)
- Ball and socket (femur/acetabulum)
- Hinge (humerus/radius and ulna)
- Plane or gliding (between carpals/tarsals)
- Saddle (between phalanges)
- Condylar (stifle).

During locomotion joints undergo a great deal of stress and strain and their stability is improved by:

- Surrounding muscle and tendons
- Ligaments, which link one bone to another
- Correct bone conformation, particularly at the articular surfaces, which ensures that the weight is supported by the correct part of the bone – poor conformation leads to lameness and arthritis.

The muscular system

The main tissue of the muscular system is striated or skeletal muscle, i.e. that which is attached to the bones of the skeleton. Its contraction is controlled voluntarily.

Skeletal muscle structure

Muscle tissue consists of cells that are long, thin and thread-like and are referred to as muscle fibres. They vary in size from about 1 mm to 5 cm in length. Under the microscope the fibres of striated muscle appear striped, which gives them their name. This is due to the microscopic appearance of the two contractile proteins actin and myosin.

Skeletal muscles attached to a bone are formed from parallel muscle fibres held together in small bundles or fascicles by connective tissue. These are collected into larger groups, also enclosed in connective tissue, and ultimately form the muscle, which is surrounded by yet more connective tissue, commonly called the muscle sheath (Fig. 4.11). When muscles lie close to one another, the sheaths may thicken to form what is called an intermuscular septum. During muscle contraction the arrangement of the myofilaments, both thick and thin, remain constant in length regardless of the muscle contractions. Thick filaments remain parallel, whereas thin filaments are united in a disc-like formation; this allows the thick and thin filaments to slide over each other, altering the length of the sarcomere (Fig 4.11).

All the connective tissue within and around the muscle merges into the connective tissue of the periosteum of the bone to which the muscle is attached, forming a tendon (Fig. 4.12) or a fibrous sheet called an aponeurosis. Aponeuroses are seen attached to the abdominal muscles and within the diaphragm.

Each skeletal muscle consists of a thick central part, the belly, tapering at each end to form a head that inserts via a tendon on to a bone (Fig. 4.12). When the muscle contracts it pulls the bones closer together.

Muscle action is defined in the following terms:

- Flexion – the angle between the bones is reduced
- Extension – the angle between the bones is increased

- Abduction – the whole limb moves away from the midline of the body
- Adduction – the whole limb moves towards the midline of the body
- Protraction – the whole limb moves cranially
- Retraction – the whole limb moves caudally
- Supination – the under-surface of the paw is turned downwards
- Pronation – the under-surface of the paw is turned upwards.

There are many different skeletal muscles within the body, with varying shapes and actions that influence the name by which they are known. For example, the superficial digital flexor lies superficially on the lower limb and flexes the digits; triceps has three heads; biceps femoris has two heads and is attached to the femur. The key to learning the action of each muscle is to know at which two points on the skeleton each inserts and then imagine how the relevant bones move in relation to each other. (For more detail about the muscles look in the Recommended reading list for more specialized anatomy books.)

Nervous system

The nervous system provides a rapid means of communication and coordination for all body systems and enables the body to respond to events within its environment and thus survive.

The functions of the nervous system are to receive information from both the internal and external environment, to integrate and analyse this information and to bring about the appropriate response.

Components of a coordinated nerve pathway are:

- Stimulus – any change inside or outside the body that provokes a change in behaviour; it could be sight, pain, touch, change in blood pressure or pH
- Receptors – specialized cells which detect stimuli: some receptors are housed by the special sense organs, e.g. ear, eye, nose; others are found within blood vessel walls, joints or muscles, e.g. stretch receptors, osmoreceptors
- Coordinators – the brain and spinal cord (central nervous system, CNS) receive information in the form of nerve impulses from the receptors, coordinate the information and initiate the response
- Effectors – muscles and glands produce a response, e.g. contraction or secretion, and are controlled by the CNS.

The nervous system is divided into:

- Central nervous system (CNS) – the brain and spinal cord.
- Peripheral nervous system (PNS) – composed of all nerves given off by the CNS:
  - Cranial nerves
  - Spinal nerves
  - Autonomic nervous system – sympathetic and parasympathetic branches.

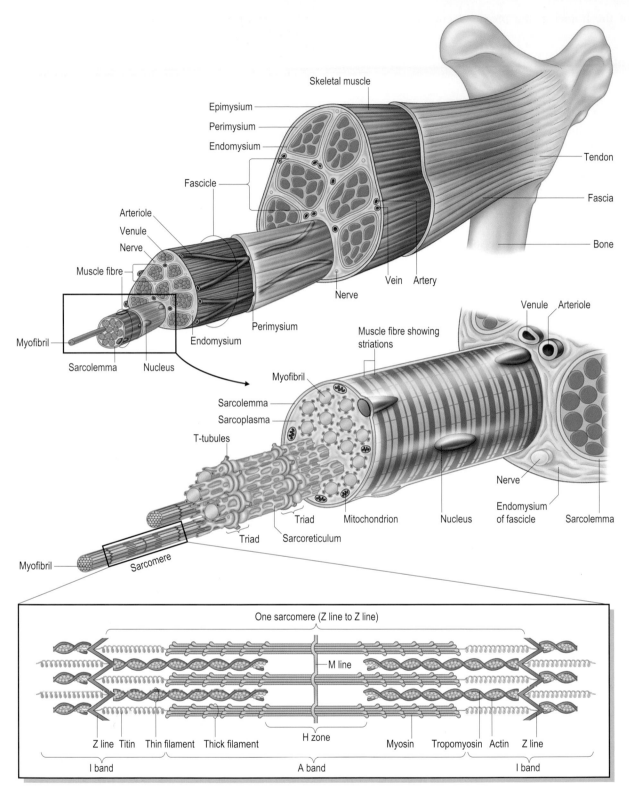

Fig. 4.11 Microscopic structure of skeletal muscle

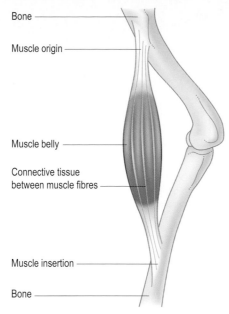

Fig. 4.12 Gross structure of a skeletal muscle

Nervous tissue

The nervous system consists of nervous tissue which connects to all parts of the body. The main cell is the **neuron** (Fig. 4.13) and nervous tissue consists of thousands of long, thin nerve fibres supported by various types of glial cell. 'Nerves', identified grossly as flattened white strands, are made up of many nerve fibres.

Neuron

All neurons have the same basic structure:

- A cell body containing the nucleus
  - An axon, which carries the nerve impulse away from the cell body
  - One or more dendrons or dendrites, which branch extensively like tiny trees and carry nerve impulses towards the cell body.

There are several shapes of neuron (Fig. 4.14) and this depends on their function:

- Multipolar neuron – have many dendrons and one axon. These are found as motor neurons in the spinal cord; Purkinje fibres in the heart are specialized multipolar neurons.
- Bipolar neuron – have one dendron and one axon and are found in the retina of the eye and in the nasal mucosa.
- Pseudo-unipolar neuron – appear to have only one fibre leaving the cell body (Fig 4.14), but in fact they have one dendron and one axon which are wound around each other giving this appearance. They are found as sensory nerves.

The majority of the axons leaving the neurons are enveloped by specialized Schwann cells, which provide both structural and metabolic support and secrete a lipoprotein material known as myelin (Fig. 4.13). Large-diameter fibres are wrapped by a variable number of concentric layers of the

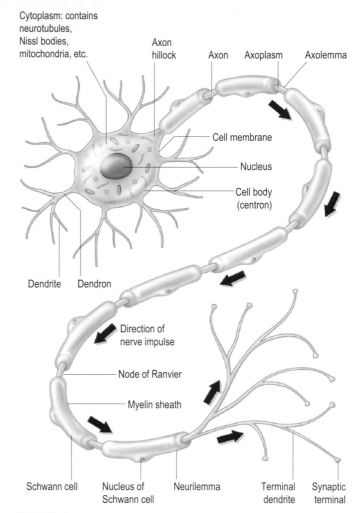

Fig. 4.13 A neuron

Schwann cell plasma membrane forming the so-called myelin sheath. These nerve fibres are said to be myelinated. Non-myelinated fibres are found within the cornea of the eye and within the grey matter of the CNS. The myelin sheath increases the rate and efficiency of electrical conduction along the axon, by allowing the impulse to jump between gaps within the myelin, called the nodes of Ranvier. At this point the axon is exposed to the external environment. The jumping from node to node is known as saltatory conduction and greatly enhances the conduction speed of axons.

Nerve impulses pass along nerve fibres in one direction only and are named accordingly:

- Sensory neurons – conduct impulses from receptors such as those in the eyes, ears and stretch receptors in the muscles and carry them **towards** the CNS
- Motor neurons – conduct impulses **away** from the CNS towards effector organs, e.g. muscles and glands.

Nerves that supply the visceral organs, i.e. those of the respiratory, digestive, urinary and reproductive systems and the heart, are known as visceral nerves. They may be visceral sensory or visceral motor nerves.

Nerves that supply all other organs, e.g. skin, joints, skeletal muscles, are known as somatic nerves. They may be somatic sensory or somatic motor nerves.

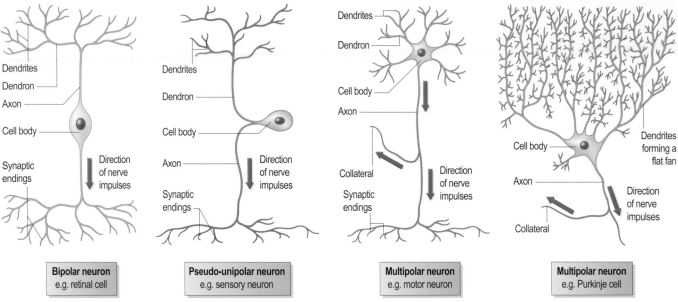

Bipolar neuron
e.g. retinal cell

Pseudo-unipolar neuron
e.g. sensory neuron

Multipolar neuron
e.g. motor neuron

Multipolar neuron
e.g. Purkinje cell

Fig. 4.14 Types of neuron

Neuroglial tissue

Neuroglial tissue provides support for the neurons and their processes and there are four types:

- Astrocytes – numerous star-shaped cells thought to provide mechanical and metabolic support for neurons. They cover the capillaries in the brain and help to form the blood–brain barrier.
- Oligodendrocytes – similar to the Schwann cell of peripheral nervous tissue and are responsible for myelination and holding nerve fibres together.
- Microglia – small phagocytic cells that are thought to be the CNS representatives of the macrophage/monocyte defence system.
- Ependymal – a simple epithelium that lines the cerebral ventricles of the brain and central canal of the spinal cord.

Nerve impulses

Nerve impulses can be considered to be a form of electrical impulse resulting from a chain reaction in the form of a wave of rearrangements of sodium and potassium ions across the cell membrane. The nerve fibre must recover before it can conduct another impulse. This recovery period, known as the refractory period, lasts for only a few thousandths of a second.

Impulses passing along a nerve fibre eventually reach the end of it, where they encounter a microscopic gap called a synapse (Fig. 4.15) lying between the tip of one fibre and the beginning of the next. Transmission of the impulse across the gap is dependent upon the presence of chemical or neurotransmitters, e.g. acetylcholine (most common), adrenaline (epinephrine) or serotonin (5-hydroxytryptamine). The chemical is released from vesicles in the axon terminal to activate (excite or inhibit) other impulses in the dendrites of the connecting neuron. The neurotransmitters mediate their effects by interacting with

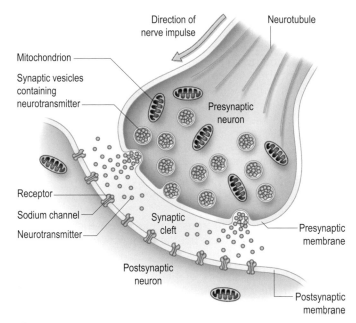

Fig. 4.15 A synapse

specific receptors in the opposing plasma membrane. Nerve fibres terminate on muscle fibres at a motor endplate or a neuromuscular junction.

Reflex action

The simplest arrangement of neurons is seen in the reflex arc (Fig. 4.16). A reflex action is a behaviour in which a stimulus results in a response that does not have to be learned and that occurs very quickly without conscious thought, e.g. withdrawal from a painful stimulus. Stimulation of pain receptors in the skin fires off impulses in sensory neurons that pass through the spinal cord along spinal nerves. They

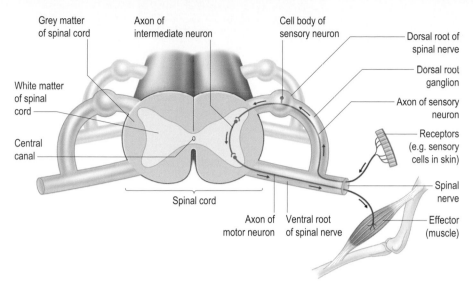

Fig. 4.16 Components of a reflex arc

enter the spinal cord via a separate dorsal root (containing the sensory nerve fibres) and leave via a ventral root (containing motor nerve fibres) (Fig. 4.16). The grey matter of the cord contains the nerve cells and bodies of the motor nerve cells whose axons run out into the ventral roots. Nerve impulses are conveyed to the appropriate muscle by motor nerves and the muscle contracts and moves the limb away from the cause of the pain.

Central nervous system

The CNS is the control area of the nervous system comprising the brain, located in the cranium, and the spinal cord, lying within the spinal cavity of the vertebral column. Both are protected by the skeletal system. It is composed entirely of neurons and neuroglia arranged as white matter and grey matter.

The brain

The brain is subdivided into three regions

Forebrain – telencephalon and diencephalon

This consists of the right and left cerebral hemispheres connected in the midline by a band of tissue known as the corpus callosum (Fig. 4.17). The cerebral hemispheres are concerned with conscious thought. The outer layer of grey matter is known as the cerebral cortex and is divided into lobes whose names correspond to the skull bone nearest to the lobe:

- Frontal lobe – the most anterior of all the lobes, is the centre of voluntary movement. It is often referred to as the motor area, containing areas for control of gross, fine and complicated muscle movements.
- Parietal lobe – collects, recognizes and organizes sensations of pain, temperature, touch, position and movement.
- Temporal lobe – contains the centres for awareness and correlation of auditory stimuli
- Occipital lobe – forms the posterior extremity of each cerebral hemisphere. It involves visual perception and visual memory with a role in eye movements.

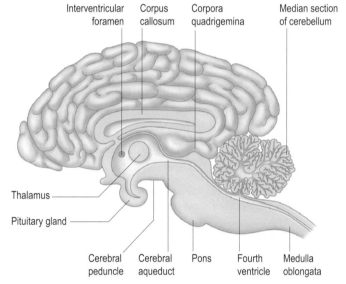

Fig. 4.17 Median section through the canine brain

On the ventral surface of the forebrain is the optic chiasma, which is a cross-shaped arrangement of nerve fibres associated with the eye and the pituitary gland, part of the endocrine system. Dorsal to the pituitary gland and lying within the brain tissue is the hypothalamus, which is the coordinating centre of the endocrine system. At the anterior point of the cerebral hemispheres are the olfactory bulbs. These paired structures lie close to the nasal chambers and are concerned with the sense of smell. The thalamus at the base of the cerebral hemispheres acts as a relay station for sensory impulses. The epithalamus holds the pineal body, which is involved in the regulation of gonad hormones. Cranial nerves I (olfactory nerve) and II (optic nerve) are attached to the forebrain. Running through the centre of the forebrain are the lateral ventricles – part of the ventricular system, which contains cerebrospinal fluid (CSF). Damage to tissue in the forebrain can cause personality change.

Midbrain – mesencephalon

Consists of a tube through which runs part of the ventricular system known as the cerebral aqueduct, carrying the CSF. It contains centres for control of muscle, sight and hearing and is involved in the positioning of the body to maintain balance. Cranial nerves III (oculomotor nerve) and IV (trochlear nerve) are attached to the midbrain. Damage to tissue in the midbrain results in coma.

Hindbrain – metencephalon and myelencephalon

Consists of the cerebellum, which has a ridged surface resembling a small cauliflower and is composed of two hemispheres joined in the midline (Fig. 4.18). Each hemisphere controls and coordinates balance and movement. Ventral to the cerebellum is the medulla oblongata, which passes through the foramen magnum of the skull and becomes the spinal cord. It contains centres that control respiration, heart rate and blood pressure. Linking the cerebrum, cerebellum and the medulla oblongata is the pons, which forms a crossover tract of white matter involved in the control of respiration. Within the hindbrain is the fourth ventricle, which is continuous with the cerebral aqueduct and the central canal within the spinal cord. Cranial nerves V (trigeminal nerve), VI (abducens nerve) and XII (hypoglossal nerve) are located on the ventral surface. Damage to the hindbrain results in rapid death.

Protection of the central nervous system

If an animal is to survive, the CNS must be protected from mechanical and chemical damage.

- Cranium – the bones of the skull form a hard outer covering to the brain.
- Vertebral column protects the spinal cord.
- Meninges – three layers of membrane composed of white, fibrous connective tissue envelope the entire CNS providing support and protection:
    - **Dura mater** – the outermost layer is tough, fibrous and lines the cranium. In the vertebral canal there is an epidural space between it and the periosteum of the vertebrae
    - **Arachnoid mater** – named for its web-like appearance. More delicate and cushions the CNS and facilitates diffusion of oxygen and nutrients into the nervous tissue beneath. CSF runs in the subarachnoid space below this layer.
    - **Pia mater** – the innermost layer. Delicate, very vascular supplying blood to the CNS tissues and closely follows the contours of the brain surface.

Cerebrospinal fluid (CSF) consists of a watery, transparent fluid, similar to plasma with less protein, which flows within the ventricular system of the brain, the central canal of the spinal cord and subarachnoid spaces (Fig. 4.19). It is secreted by networks of capillaries referred to as choroid plexuses located within each ventricle. The function of CSF is to act as a shock absorber during movement, provide an antibacterial effect and transport nutrients and waste materials from the nervous tissue.

The spinal cord

The spinal cord runs from medulla oblongata to the lumbar region terminating at the sixth or seventh lumbar vertebrae

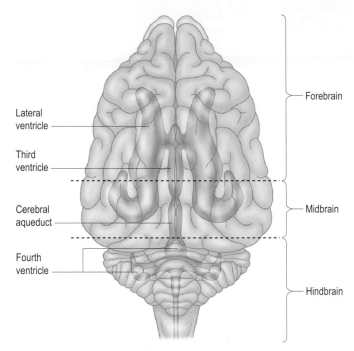

Fig. 4.18 Ventricular system of the brain

Labels: Forebrain, Lateral ventricle, Third ventricle, Cerebral aqueduct, Fourth ventricle, Midbrain, Hindbrain

as the cauda equina or 'horse's tail'. Pairs of spinal nerves leave the cord throughout its length via intervertebral spaces, linking the brain to all the organs of the body.

The spinal cord is composed of nerve fibres running in organized tracts. Its structure is similar over its entire length and the tissue is divided into outer white matter surrounding the central grey matter. It is covered by the meninges and bathed in CSF, which also flows in the central canal (Fig. 4.19).

In transverse section (Fig 4.19) the grey matter has a characteristic butterfly shape. The ventral horns are more prominent and contain the cell bodies of the large motor neurons. The dorsal horns contain the cell bodies of smaller sensory neurons. Sensory information, particularly concerning pain and temperature, is relayed to the brain via afferent neurons. Smaller lateral horns, containing the cell bodies of preganglia and sympathetic efferent neurons, are located in the upper lumbar and thoracic regions. This corresponds to the level of sympathetic outflow from the cord. More grey matter is required in the cervical and lumbar regions because of the greater activity of both sensory and motor innervation of the limbs. This in turn increases the diameter of the spinal cord in these areas.

The white matter contains a greater proportion of myelin and consists of ascending tracts of sensory fibres and descending motor tracts that increase in volume, especially in the sacral to cervical regions, as more and more fibres pass up towards the brain.

Peripheral nervous system

The peripheral nervous system is made up of the nerves which leave the central nervous system. It links the CNS to all the organs of the body.

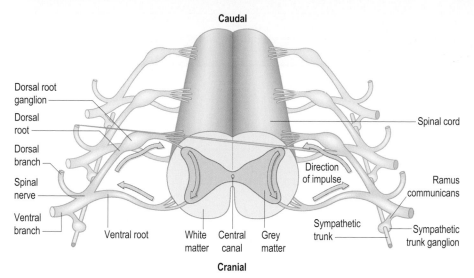

Fig. 4.19 Transverse section through the spinal cord of the dog

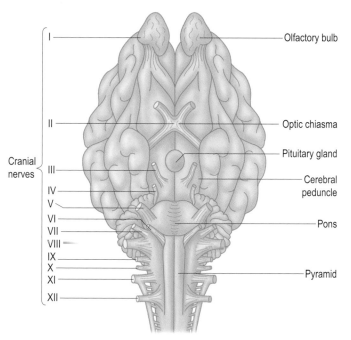

Fig. 4.20 Ventral view of brain showing cranial nerves

Cranial nerves

Cranial nerves are given off by the brain and leave the cranium via foramina in the bones (Fig. 4.20). Most supply structures on the head and are relatively short. They may carry sensory or motor nerve fibres or a mixture of the two. These nerves have specific names and are always referred to by Roman numerals (Table 4.1).

Spinal nerves

Spinal nerves are given off by the spinal cord. They contain both sensory and motor fibres and are, therefore, mixed nerves. They supply all the musculoskeletal system and are numbered according to the number of the vertebra in front of their point of exit from the cord. The exception is in the cervical region, where the first nerve leaves the cord *before* the first vertebra – there are eight cervical nerves in total.

The spinal nerves on each side of the cord are divided into two roots:

- The dorsal root carries sensory fibres into the cord and the cell bodies of the nerves are contained in the dorsal root ganglion (Fig. 4.19).
- The ventral root carries motor fibres away from the cord and their cell bodies are within the grey matter of the cord. The nerve supply to the limbs is:
  - Fore limb – spinal nerves Cervical 6 (C6) to Thoracic 2 (T2; forms the radial nerve). Together these form the brachial plexus
  - Hind limb – spinal nerves Lumbar 4 (L6) to Sacral 2 (S2; forms the sciatic nerve). Together these form the lumbo-sacral plexus.

Autonomic nervous system

The autonomic nervous system consists of spinal nerves that supply motor fibres to the viscera and may be described as the visceral motor system. It is considered to be self-governing, i.e. it is not under conscious control but will assist in the regulation of the internal body organs by means of both sympathetic and parasympathetic innervation.

Sympathetic system

The nerves for this system are located in the thoracolumbar areas of the spinal cord, i.e. T1 to L4 or L5. Short preganglionic fibres synapse within a series of ganglia on each side of the vertebral column forming a nodular cord (looking like a string of beads) known as the sympathetic chain. Long postganglionic fibres then travel to their intended organs using the routes of blood vessels. The function of the sympathetic system is to prepare the body for stressful or hazardous situations (the fight, flight or frolic reflex) and relies on noradrenaline (norepinephrine) as a transmitter at the synapses within the system (Table 4.2).

Parasympathetic system

This originates in the brain stem, sending impulses via the oculomotor (III), facial (VII), glossopharyngeal (IX) and

Table 4.1 Cranial nerves

Cranial nerve number	Name	Nerve type	Function
I	Olfactory	Sensory	Smell
II	Optic	Sensory	Vision, pupil light response
III	Oculomotor	Motor + parasympathetic	Eye movement, pupil constriction, focus
IV	Trochlear	Motor	Eye movement
V	Trigeminal	Mixed	Muscle for mastication, upper and lower jaws, face
VI	Abducens	Motor	Eye movement
VII	Facial	Mixed (motor) + parasympathetic	Salivation, facial expression, taste, ears, head
VIII	Auditory/vestibulocochlear	Sensory	Hearing, balance
IX	Glossopharyngeal	Mixed + parasympathetic	Taste, laryngeal muscles, swallowing, salivation
X	Vagus	Mixed (motor) + parasympathetic	Vocalization, swallowing, gastrointestinal tract, thoracic organs, abdominal organs
XI	Accessory	Motor	Head and shoulder movement, vocalization, swallowing
XII	Hypoglossal	Motor	Tongue movement, swallowing, vocalization

Table 4.2 Comparison between the functions of the sympathetic and parasympathetic systems

Sympathetic system	Parasympathetic system
Neurotransmitter chemical – noradrenaline (norepinephrine)	Neurotransmitter – acetylcholine
Prepares body for fight, flight or frolic, e.g dilates the pupils	Assists in the day-to-day functions of the body
Inhibits salivation and slows gut movement	Stimulates gut movement and salivation
Increases heart rate	Returns heart rate to normal
Increases respiratory rate	Decreases respiratory rate
Dilates the bronchi and bronchioles	Lacrimal secretions increase

vagus (X) cranial nerves and via the sacral nerves S1 and S2. The ganglia are embedded in the wall of the effector organ, thus requiring long preganglionic and short postganglionic nerve fibres. The function of the system is the opposite of the sympathetic system and relies on the use of acetylcholine at all the synapses (Table 4.2).

Special senses

The special senses, i.e. sight, hearing and balance, smell and taste, are detected by sophisticated sensory receptors that respond to a stimulus or change in the environment. These specific neural receptors are housed within the special sense organs, e.g. eye or ear, which enhance and refine the reception of incoming stimuli before it is passed on the CNS.

Sensory receptors are found all over the body and can be divided into:

- Proprioceptors – lie within muscle and joints and are used to detect the body's spatial position in the environment; also linked to the ear for balance
- Exteroceptors – involved in the response to external stimuli collected by the special sense organs
- Interoceptors – respond to changes in the internal environment of the body, e.g. pH or blood pressure, and stimulate homeostatic mechanisms, e.g. respiration, vasodilation.

Smell – known as olfaction

The chemoreceptors for the sense of smell are located in the nasal mucosa covering the turbinate bones in the nasal cavity. In the dog and cat the olfactory tissue is extensive and is an essential function for survival in the wild. The olfactory receptor cells are true bipolar neurons containing a single dendritic process extending from the cell body to the tissue surface and terminating as a small swelling giving rise to a number of long, modified cilia. The cilia receive information from smell chemicals dissolved in the mucus over the epithelium, passing it to receptor cells. Nerve impulses travel along the olfactory nerve (cranial nerve I) and reach the olfactory bulbs in the forebrain. The sense of smell and taste are linked, with smell being by far the more sensitive of the two.

Taste – also known as gustation

Taste buds are located in the epithelium of the papillae of the tongue and scattered in other parts of the tongue, palate,

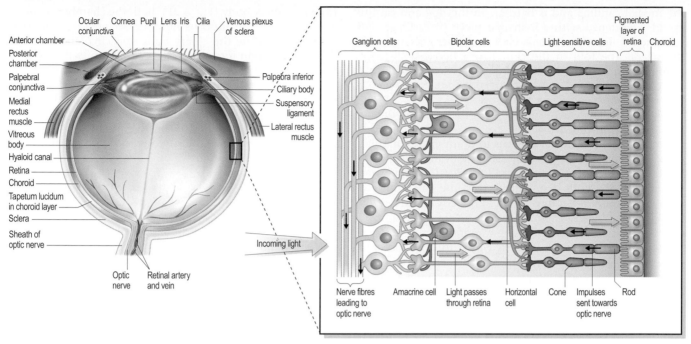

Fig. 4.21 Cross-section through the eye. Section through the retina showing the rods and cones

pharynx and epiglottis. The taste bud consists of gustatory cells which are chemoreceptors and support cells, both having long microvilli extending into the taste pore. The gustatory cells have receptor function and respond to taste chemicals dissolved in the mucus over the surface of the tongue. They pass information to the facial (VII), glossopharyngeal (IX) and vagus (X) nerves and then to the brain. Although four basic tastes – sweet, salt, sour and bitter – are recognized in man, it is not thought that animals show the same discrimination and their sense of taste is directed mainly at identifying what is good or bad for the individual.

Sight – the eye is the organ of sight

The eye is a highly specialized organ of photoreception that involves the conversion of different wavelengths of light into nerve impulses.

The eye

Perception of an image

Light radiating from an image is received by photoreceptor cells which are located in the inner layer of the eye, the retina. These cells are modified dendrites of two types of nerve cell (Fig. 4.21):

- Rods – receptive to light of differing intensity seen in black and white images and used in night vision; located outside the fovea in the more peripheral parts of the retina
- Cones – receptive to different colours, enabling a coloured image to be perceived in day light levels; located in the fovea to give high levels of visual accuracy.

The tapetum lucidum lies over the retina of the dog and cat, within the uvea. It is a reflective layer, enhancing light enter-

ing the eye and improving vision when there are low light levels by reflecting it back to the retina. The retina contains many sensory and connector neurons and processes. At an area in the back of the retina there is an optic disc where the nerve fibres from the eye meet to form the optic nerve (II). The optic nerve is joined by an artery and vein from the choroid, which together form a blind spot in which there are no rods and cones.

Light passes through the overlying retinal layers to the photoreceptor cells where an inverted image is produced. The light that misses the receptor cells on its way through the retina is reflected back to the retinal layers by the tapetum lucidum. The bipolar receptor cells then transmit the image through the optic nerve to the cerebral cortex of the brain.

Structure of the eye

The remaining structures of the eye (Fig. 4.21) support the retina and assist in the focussing of light rays on to the retina.

The eyeball comprises three layers:

- Sclera – the tough outermost layer of dense connective tissue, divided into the cornea and the sclera
- Uvea – the vascular pigmented layer, divided into the choroid, tapetum lucidum, suspensory ligament, ciliary body and iris
- Retina – the innermost layer, which contains the photoreceptor cells.

The eye (Fig. 4.21) is situated within the orbit of the skull and is cushioned in fat and connective tissue. Attached to the eyeball are the optic nerve (II), ocular musculature, other nerves and its blood supply. The eye is protected by the eyelids, covered by a thin, highly folded skin externally and by smooth conjunctival epithelium on the inner surface. The upper and lower eyelids are hairy and meet at the medial canthus close to the nose and the lateral canthus nearer to the ear. The third eyelid or nictitating membrane comes from the medial canthus and is hairless. In the dog and cat this eyelid is stiffened with a T-shaped piece of cartilage. The conjunctiva lines the inner eyelids and lines the surface of the sclera. The fold in the conjunctiva between the layer lining the eyelids and the layer lining the sclera is the fornix. The conjunctival mucous secretions contribute to the protection of the exposed surface of the eye.

Lachrymal glands are responsible for the secretion of tears and this is distributed over the eye surface by the eyelids, collecting near the medial canthus to drain via the nasolacrimal duct into the nasal cavity. The Meibomian glands lie under the lashes of the upper and lower eyelids. They are a specialized sebaceous gland attached to the hair follicle of each eyelash and open directly on to the edge of the eyelid, producing oily tears. These tears float on the surface of the watery tear film and help prevent evaporation.

The front of the eye is protected by a thick, transparent cornea behind which lies the iris, which is continuous with the ciliary body and contains circular and radial muscles. Contraction of these muscles alters the size of the aperture or pupil and controls the amount of light falling on to the retina. The transparent biconvex lens is located directly behind the iris of the eye, supported by the suspensory ligament and attached to the ciliary body, which encircles the lens. The lens focuses light rays on to the retina.

The fundus of the eye comprises the anterior and posterior chambers formed by the iris extending in front of the lens from the ciliary body (Fig. 4.21). Both the chambers contain a watery fluid, the aqueous humour, secreted into the posterior chamber by the ciliary body and circulated through the pupil to drain into the canal of Schlemm in the anterior chamber. The aqueous humour is a source of nutrients for the lens and the cornea, which are non-vascular. It also acts as a non-refractive optical medium, maintaining the shape of the cornea by the resulting intraocular pressure. The vitreous chamber at the back of the eye, behind the lens, contains a gelatinous mass called the vitreous body or humour, which also provides a non-refractive optical medium and supports the lens and retina.

Hearing and balance

Hearing is the detection of sound waves or vibrations in the air. These sound waves have differing frequencies and are detected by the ear and interpreted by the brain as differences in pitch. Balance is perceived by the semicircular canals within the inner ear.

The ear

The ear (Fig 4.22) can be divided into:

- External ear – concerned with reception of sound
- Middle ear – involved with transmission and amplification of incoming sound waves

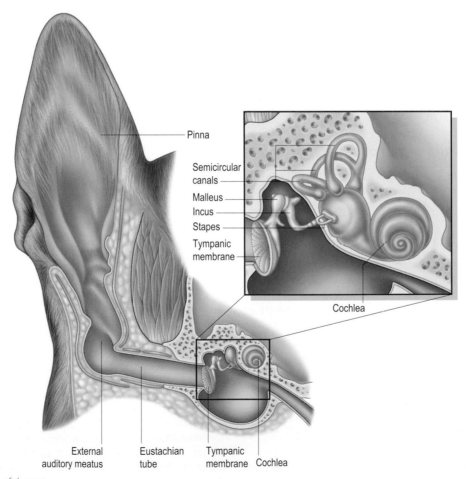

Pinna
Semicircular canals
Malleus
Incus
Stapes
Tympanic membrane
Cochlea

External auditory meatus Eustachian tube Tympanic membrane Cochlea

Fig. 4.22 The structure of the ear

- Internal ear – containing specific sensory receptors for both movement and sound.

The external ear

Receives and conducts sound waves to the ear drum or tympanic membrane. The external auditory meatus or ear canal (Fig 4.22) is lined by hairy skin containing sebaceous glands and modified apocrine sweat glands that secrete a waxy material called cerumen. The shape of the ear canal and the pinna or ear flap are maintained by elastic cartilage. The ear canal consists of a vertical and then a horizontal section.

The middle ear

The middle ear is an air-filled cavity located within the tympanic bulla of the temporal bone and separated from the external ear by the tympanic membrane. The Eustachian or auditory tube links it to the pharynx and equalizes the air pressure on either sides of the tympanic membrane. Sound waves reaching the tympanic membrane are converted into mechanical vibrations, which are then amplified by a system of levers made up of three small bones called ossicles. These are the malleus, nearest to the tympanic membrane, the incus and the stapes, next to the oval window below which is a membrane called the round window (Fig. 4.22). The ossicles articulate with each other via synovial joints and ligaments. The muscle linking the tympanic membrane and stapes reduces excessive sound vibrations that might otherwise damage the middle and inner ear. The oval window is covered by the base of the stapes to assist transmitted vibrations. The round window permits vibrations passed to the sensory receptors for sound to be dispersed.

The inner ear

The inner ear consists of an interconnected fluid-filled membranous labyrinth located within a bony labyrinth within the temporal bone. This is shaped specifically to house the membranous labyrinth.

The two are separated by fluid known as perilymph and the membranous labyrinth is filled with endolymph (Fig. 4.22).

The membranous labyrinth consists of the:

1. Vestibular apparatus
2. Cochlea.

1. Vestibular apparatus – the vestibule gives rise to three semicircular canals which lie in vertical, horizontal and transverse directions at right angles to each other. They are concerned with balance and the detection of movement. The vestibule also contains the utricle and the saccule, whose walls contain a specialized area of sensory receptor cells known as a macula. Axon fibres pass from the macula into the vestibulocochlear or auditory nerve (VIII), serving as part of the sensory input for balance.

Close to one end of each semicircular canal is a dilated area called the ampulla. In each ampulla there is a ridge called a sensory crista containing sensory receptors (hair cells) which move back and forth influenced by the movement of the head and thus the endolymph in the canals. The hair cells send nerve impulses along the vestibulocochlear nerve to the brain to record movement of the head in all directions.

2. Cochlea – this takes a spiral form similar to a snail shell with a canal divided into channels within which is the organ of Corti. This contains receptor hair cells, which respond to movement of the endolymph caused by the vibrations of the sound waves and convert it into sensory receptor information. The resulting nerve impulses are carried by the vestibulocochlear nerve to the brain where they are interpreted as sound.

Endocrine system

The endocrine glands are the sites of synthesis and secretion of substances called hormones. The hormones are disseminated throughout the body by the blood and act on specific target organs. Hormones coordinate and integrate the functions of all the body systems in conjunction with the nervous system. Both systems provide a means of communication within the body and both involve the transmission of a message, triggered by a stimulus to produce a response. The difference between the two systems concerns the nature of the message – in the endocrine system the message takes the form of a chemical substance conveyed through the blood system while in the nervous system it is a rapid nerve impulse.

Endocrine glands are ductless and are composed of secretory cells of epithelial origin supported by connective tissue that is rich in blood and lymphatic capillaries. The secretory cells discharge hormones into the interstitial spaces from which they are rapidly absorbed into the circulatory system.

Some endocrine glands form organs, e.g. pituitary, thyroid, parathyroid, adrenal, while others are associated with exocrine glands, e.g. pancreas. Some form a part of complex organs, e.g. kidney, testis and ovary.

For the full list of endocrine glands see Table 4.3, but some of the more significant endocrine glands are:

Adrenal gland

This can be considered to be two separate glands wrapped around each other:

- **The medulla** – produces the hormones **noradrenaline** (norepinephrine) and **adrenaline** (epinephrine). Their effects on body organs are identical to those produced by the stimulation of the sympathetic nervous system, i.e. they raise heart rate and systolic blood pressure and cause peripheral vasoconstriction in preparation for 'fear, flight or fight. Noradrenaline is the more potent hypertensive agent.

Adrenaline also decreases gut motility and increases:

- Cardiac output
- Glycogen breakdown in liver and muscle
- Fatty acid release
- Skeletal muscle tone.

The action of adrenaline and noradrenaline is short-lived as they are rapidly inactivated. Both are regarded as 'emergency hormones' and the adrenal medulla is not essential to life.

- **The cortex**
  Surrounds the medulla and consists of three concentric layers each of which secretes a different group of steroid hormones belonging to two groups:
  a. **Corticosteroids** – these are essential for life. Individual corticosteroids vary in their ability to produce the full glucocorticoid or mineralocorticoid

Table 4.3 The endocrine glands and their hormones

Gland	Hormone	Action
Thyroid	Thyroxine	Increases metabolic rate
	Calcitonin	Regulates calcium levels
Parathyroid	Parathormone (parathyroid hormone)	Regulates calcium and phosphorus levels
Adrenal cortex	Glucocorticoids	Protein and carbohydrate metabolism and anti-inflammatory
	Mineralocorticoids	Stress resistance, potassium and sodium levels
	Gonadocorticoids	Male/female sex hormones
Adrenal medulla	Adrenaline (epinephrine)	Sympathetic nervous system
	Noradrenaline (norepinephrine)	Sympathetic nervous system
Pituitary	Growth hormone	Stimulates growth
	Thyroid-stimulating hormone (TSH)	Stimulates thyroid gland activity
	Adrenocorticotrophic hormone (ACTH)	Stimulates adrenal cortex
	Follicle-stimulating hormone (FSH)	Stimulates growth of ovarian follicle
	Luteinizing hormone (LH)	Ovulation and development of the corpus luteum
	Interstitial cell-stimulating hormone (ICSH)	Stimulates interstitial cells of the testis
	Prolactin	Stimulates formation of milk
	Oxytocin	Milk 'let down'; uterine contraction in parturition
	Antidiuretic hormone (ADH)	Reabsorption of water from renal collecting ducts
Pancreas	Insulin	Decreases blood glucose
	Glucagon	Increases blood glucose
	Somatostatin	Smoothes out blood glucose fluctuations
Ovary	Oestrogen	Female sex characteristics and oestrus behaviour
	Progesterone	Prepares uterus and uterine horns; maintains the pregnancy
Testis	Testosterone	Male sex characteristics; spermatogenesis
Pineal	Melatonin	Coordinating circadian and diurnal rhythms

effects (Table 4.3). In the dog and the cat the two most important corticosteroids are cortisol, which has mainly glucocorticoid effects, and aldosterone, which has primarily mineralocorticoid effects.

b. **Adrenal sex hormones**, i.e. androgens, oestrogens and probably progestagens. These are produced in small quantities and may be called gonadocorticoids.

Adrenocorticotrophic hormone (ACTH), secreted by the anterior pituitary gland, controls the formation of cortisol and androgens but has little effect on the formation of aldosterone, which is controlled by the renin–angiotensin pathway in the kidney.

Thyroid gland

This lies as paired bilateral glands below the larynx near to the upper trachea. It produces:

- **Tri-iodothyronine (T3) and thyroxine (T4),** together known as thyroid hormone and based on iodine. They are vital for growth and the regulation of the metabolism. Secretion of these hormones is regulated by thyroid-stimulating hormone (TSH), secreted by the anterior pituitary (Table 4.3).
- **Thyrocalcitonin or calcitonin** regulates blood calcium levels in conjunction with parathormone. Calcitonin lowers blood calcium levels by inhibiting the rate of decalcification of bone by osteoclasts and by stimulating bone growth or osteoblast activity.

Pancreas

This is a mixed gland lying within the loop of the duodenum (see Digestive system). Hormones are secreted by discrete areas of endocrine tissue known as the islets of Langerhans lying within the exocrine tissue. The islets consist of three types of cell, each secreting a different hormone:

- α cells secrete glucagon, which increases blood glucose levels by breaking down stores of glycogen in the liver by a process of glycogenolysis
- β cells secrete insulin, which reduces blood glucose levels by enabling glucose to pass into the cells where it is used as a vital source of energy. Excess glucose is

stored as glycogen in the liver by a process of glycogenesis
- δ cells secrete somatostatin, which smooths out the daily fluctuations in blood glucose levels.

Cardiovascular system

The cardiovascular system consists of four separate components:

- Blood
- The heart
- The circulatory system
- The lymphatic system.

Blood

Blood is a highly specialized connective tissue consisting of several types of cell suspended in a fluid medium called plasma. Blood performs a wide range of functions:

1. **Transportation** – blood is responsible for carrying the following vital components around the body:
   - Oxygen – carried by haemoglobin in the red blood cells
   - Carbon dioxide – formed by the tissues and carried in solution in the plasma to the lungs
   - Nutrients – products of digestion carried from the small intestine to the liver and other tissues
   - Waste products – resulting from metabolism and transported to the point of excretion, e.g. kidney and liver
   - Hormones and enzymes – carried to their target organs.
2. **Homoeostasis** – regulation of the systems responsible for maintaining the internal equilibrium of the body:
   - Defence against disease – white blood cells and immunoglobulins protect against invasion by antigens
   - Body temperature – blood conducts heat around the body to where it is needed
   - Acid–base balance – presence of buffers in the blood maintain pH at approximately 7.4
   - Osmotic concentration and volume of body fluids – presence of plasma proteins and electrolytes controls fluid flow between compartments and maintains blood volume and pressure
   - Blood clotting – cascade mechanism controls blood loss from injuries and prevents entry of infection.

Composition of blood

Blood is a connective tissue that circulates around the body in a continuous system of blood vessels. It makes up about 7% of the body weight and has a pH of 7.35–7.45. Plasma makes up about 60% of the volume and the cells and other materials in transit make up the remaining 40%.

Plasma

Plasma is an aqueous solution containing a variety of dissolved substances, e.g. oxygen, hormones and nutrients, which are transported from one part of the body to another and constantly exchanged with the interstitial fluid of the tissues.

Plasma consists of:

- Water
- Electrolytes, e.g. sodium, chloride, potassium
- Plasma proteins, e.g. albumin, globulin, fibrinogen, prothrombin
- Nutrients, e.g. amino acids, fatty acids, glucose
- Gases, e.g. oxygen, carbon dioxide
- Waste products, e.g. urea, creatinine
- Hormones, e.g. adrenaline, insulin, thyroxine, oestrogens
- Enzymes, e.g. alanine aminotransferase (ALT), amylase, lipase
- Antibodies.

Plasma proteins

Plasma proteins are large molecules in the blood, which exert a colloidal osmotic pressure within the circulation to help regulate the exchange of fluid between the plasma and the extracellular fluid. The main plasma proteins are:

- Albumin – binds with plasma calcium, which is required for clotting, bone formation and restructuring. It maintains blood pressure by keeping fluid within the plasma by osmosis – its large molecular size means that under normal circumstances it cannot pass between the endothelial cells of the blood capillaries into the extracellular fluid
- Globulin – binds with thyroxine and bilirubin, iron, cholesterol and vitamins A, D and K, and is involved in defence against infection. They also maintain blood pressure
- Fibrinogen and prothrombin – are both involved in the clotting mechanism. Fibrinogen is converted to fibrin and used in the formation of a clot. The remaining fluid seen at the site of an injury is serum. Serum is thus plasma without fibrinogen/fibrin.

Blood cells

Haemopoiesis is the process by which mature blood cells develop from precursor or stem cells. Production takes place in the liver and spleen of the embryo and the bone marrow, mainly of the pelvis, ribs, long bones and lymph nodes in the neonate and adult animal. The exception is the lymphocyte, which is formed in lymphoid tissues in the lymph nodes and the spleen. Erythrocytes and platelets function entirely within blood vessels, while the leucocytes are able to function outside the blood vessels in the interstitial tissue spaces. They are found in circulating blood only in transit between their various sites of activity.

a. **Red blood cells – erythrocytes** – produced in the red or active bone marrow. They are non-nucleated biconcave discs filled with the protein haemoglobin and are about 7 μm in diameter – those of the cat are slightly smaller than those of the dog (Fig 4.23). Their main function is to carry oxygen, as oxyhaemoglobin, from the lungs to the tissues.

Erythropoiesis – the production of erythrocytes – takes about 1 week and is controlled by the hormone erythropoietin, secreted by the kidney and regulated by the amount of oxygen reaching the tissues.

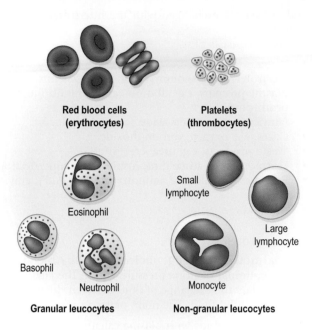

Fig. 4.23 Blood cells

Haemoglobin is synthesized from iron, folic acid and vitamin B_{12}. Immature erythrocytes are known as reticulocytes and their presence in the blood is an indication of red cell regeneration – a significant factor in some types of anaemia. Cat erythrocytes live for 58–68 days while those of the dog live for 107–120 days.

b. **White blood cells – leucocytes** – these are fewer in number and can be divided into two groups:
1. Granulocytes – have granular cytoplasm and a multilobed nucleus Also known as polymorphonuclear leucocytes (Fig. 4.23). They are:
    ■ Neutrophils – phagocytic cells which increase rapidly as juvenile or band cells in acute infections described as a neutrophilia. The granules stain purple.
    ■ Eosinophils – involved in the inflammatory reaction to tissue damage and in allergies. The granules which are released from the cytoplasm, deactivating histamine and heparin, take up acid dye and stain red.
    ■ Basophils – granules produce heparin and histamine, take up alkaline dyes and stain blue.
2. Agranulocytes – have a clear cytoplasm:
    ■ Lymphocytes – round nucleus that almost fills the cells (Fig. 4.23). They support the immune system and are classified as B lymphocytes and T lymphocytes depending on their origin.
    ■ Monocytes – are the largest of the white cells and their function is phagocytosis. They have a horseshoe-shaped nucleus and are highly motile cells, migrating into connective tissues, where they are termed histiocytes or macrophages. Macrophages play an important role in the immune defence system. Monocytes appear to have little function in circulating blood and are seen in chronic conditions, assisting in the removal of debris arising from normal turnover of cells within the tissues.
3. Thrombocytes or platelets – small, non-nucleated cells formed in the bone marrow by break-up of huge megakaryocyte cells. They participate in blood clotting in two main ways:
    ■ They clump together to plug small defects in the walls of small blood vessels
    ■ In the presence of a damaged vessels they release a substance called serotonin that reduces blood flow by constriction of the area.

The heart

The heart is a muscular pump located in the thorax and held within the mediastinum, slightly to the left of the midline and covered in a double layer of serous membrane known as the pericardium. Between the two layers is the small pericardial cavity.

The heart, whose sole function is to pump blood around the circualtory system, is a hollow, muscular, cone-shaped organ divided into four chambers – the right and left atria and the right and left ventricles (Fig. 4.24). Its size varies depending on the size of animal and it lies between the third and sixth rib. The right side of the heart receives deoxygenated blood from the systemic veins and the left side of the heart receives oxygenated blood from the lungs via the pulmonary circulation.

The heart wall consists of three layers:

*   Endocardium – a smooth inner layer of epithelium involved in the formation of valves and continuous with the endothelium of the blood vessels
*   Myocardium – the cardiac muscle layer; the left ventricle muscle is three times thicker than the right. Blood supply to this muscle is through the coronary vessels
*   Epicardium or serous pericardium – the outer layer of the heart covering the muscle wall. It produces serous fluid, which lies within the pericardial cavity and lubricates the movements of the heart.

Heart valves

These ensure that the flow of blood through the heart goes in one direction only (Fig. 4.24). There are two sets of valves:

1. Left side
    ■ Left atrioventricular valve, also known as the bicuspid or mitral valve, lying between the left atrium and ventricle. It has two cusps or flaps.
    ■ Aortic valve, which lies at the base of the aorta. This is described as being a semilunar valve because of the shape of its three cusps.
2. Right side
    ■ Right atrioventricular valve also known as the tricuspid valve, lying between the right atrium and ventricle. It has three cusps.
    ■ Pulmonary valve lies at the base of the pulmonary artery. This is also a semilunar valve and has three cusps.

Each cusp of the right and left atrioventricular valves has several tendinous attachments or chordae tendinae running

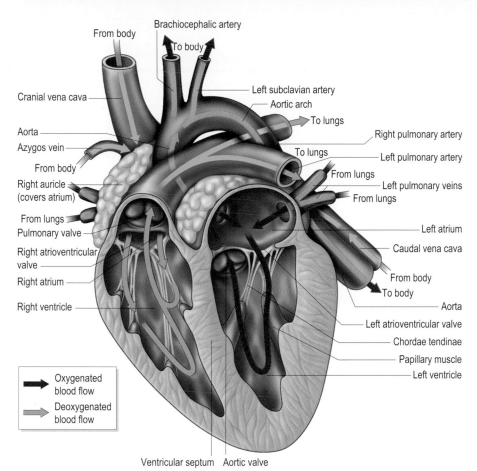

Fig. 4.24 Structure of the heart

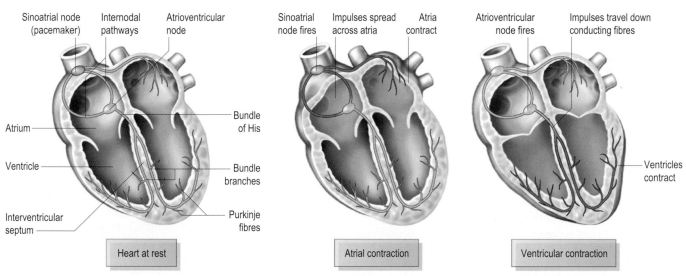

Fig. 4.25 Conduction system of the heart

from their margin to the papillary muscles on the ventricular surface of the heart. They prevent the valves everting as blood is forced out during the strong ventricular contractions.

Nervous control of the heart

Cardiac muscle has an inherent ability to contract at a set rate and contraction is coordinated by a conduction system (Fig. 4.25), which consists of:

- Sinoatrial node (SA node) – situated in the wall of the right atrium. This initiates each heart beat and is known as the pacemaker.
- Atrioventricular node (AV node) – lies at the top of the interventricular septum between the right and left sides of the heart.
- Bundle of His – specialized cells within the interventricular septum.

Table 4.4 Characteristics of the different types of blood vessel

Arteries	Veins	Capillaries
Transport blood away from the heart	Transport blood towards the heart	Link arteries to veins, and are site of exchange between blood and tissues
Tunica externa – outer fibrous layer		Consist of a single layer of squamous endothelium (epithelium)
Tunica media – middle layer of muscle and elastic fibre Tunica intima – inner layer of endothelium	Tunica media layer is thinner, with less muscle and few elastic fibres	
No semilunar valves	Semilunar valves at intervals along the length to prevent any back-flow of blood	No semilunar valves
Blood pressure high and with pulse that reflects the heart beat Blood flow rapid Low blood volume Smaller arteries are known as arterioles Main artery of the body is the aorta	Blood pressure low and no pulse Blood flow slow Increasing blood volume Smaller veins are known as venules Main vein of the body is the caudal vena cava	Blood pressure gradually falls as blood flows through the capillary bed. No pulse Blood flow slowing High blood volume

- Purkinje fibres – specialized nerve cells within the walls of the ventricles.

Nerve impulses, initiated by the SA node, travel across the atrial walls and stimulate the AV node. They then continue down the bundle of His to the Purkinje fibres at the apex of the ventricles. As a result of this electrical wave, the atria contract (atrial systole), forcing blood into the ventricles. The atria relax (atrial diastole) and the ventricles then contract (ventricular systole) and blood is forced upwards, closing the AV valves but opening the aortic and pulmonary valves and moving blood from the ventricles into the systemic and pulmonary circulations. The ventricles then relax (ventricular diastole) and the semilunar valves close.

In order to meet the changing demands of the body the heart rate must be able to alter. This is done by nerves of the autonomic nervous system, which act on the SA node – the sympathetic branch of the autonomic nervous system increases the heart rate, while the parasympathetic branch (the vagus nerve) slows the heart rate.

Pulse rate – the number of heart beats per minute

The pulse is produced by the heart pumping blood into the aorta, increasing and decreasing the expansion of the arterial vessel wall with each heart beat. The pulse is measured by palpation of a superficial vessel as it passes over a bone. The pulse quality, i.e. its rate, rhythm and character, is a reflection of the function of the heart. Normal sites for measuring the peripheral pulse in the dog and cat are the femoral, brachial, lingual and coccygeal arteries.

Circulatory system

This consists of a continuous series of blood vessels that transport the blood pumped by the heart around the body. Figure 4.26 shows the route taken by the blood around the body.

Blood vessels

Table 4.4 compares the characteristics of the different types of blood vessels:

- Arteries – carry blood *away* from the heart, except for the pulmonary artery, which carries blood towards the heart. Arteries carry oxygenated blood.
- Veins – carry blood *towards* the heart, except for the pulmonary vein, which carries blood away from the heart. Veins carry deoxygenated blood.
- Capillaries –thin-walled vessels that link arteries to veins and are the site of gaseous and nutrient exchange within the tissues.

Lymphatic system

The lymphatic system is closely linked to the circulation and is a means of returning lymph or excess interstitial tissue fluid back to the circulation via a system of lymphatic vessels and ducts.

The functions of the lymphatic system are:

- To return excess tissue fluid or lymph to the circulation.
- To produce lymphocytes to fight infection.
- To transport fatty acid molecules, produced during digestion, as chyle, which is collected by the lacteals. These are a form of lymphatic capillary found within the finger-like villi of the small intestine and they drain the chyle into the cisterna chyli in the dorsal abdomen.
- To act as a filter for lymph.

Formation of lymph takes place at the arterial end of blood capillaries, where the hydrostatic pressure exceeds the colloidal osmotic pressure exerted by plasma proteins. Fluids and electrolytes pass out of the blood capillaries into the extracellular spaces with some plasma proteins, which leak through the endothelial wall. At the venous end of the blood capillaries the pressure relationships are reversed and fluid is drawn back into the blood vascular system. In this way

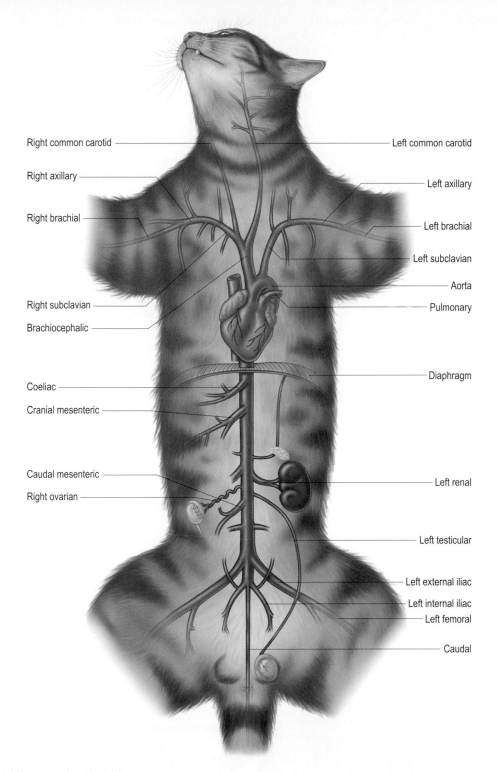

Right common carotid — ——— Left common carotid

Right axillary — ——— Left axillary

Right brachial — ——— Left brachial

——— Left subclavian

——— Aorta

Right subclavian — ——— Pulmonary

Brachiocephalic —

——— Diaphragm

Coeliac —

Cranial mesenteric —

Caudal mesenteric — ——— Left renal

Right ovarian —

——— Left testicular

——— Left external iliac

——— Left internal iliac

——— Left femoral

——— Caudal

Fig. 4.26 Major arterial blood vessels in the body

about 2% of plasma passing through the capillary bed is exchanged with the extracellular tissue fluid. The rate of tissue fluid formation at the arterial end of capillaries generally exceeds the reuptake of fluid at the venous end, leaving quantities in the interstitial spaces. The excess fluid becomes known as lymph once it drains into the system of lymphatic capillaries, which converge to form progressively larger-diameter lymphatic veins or vessels. Movement of lymph along the vessels relies on the surrounding tissues, particularly skeletal muscles, squeezing the fluid past non-return valves in the walls.

Lymph re-enters the venous circulation via the right atrium of the heart via a single duct on each side of the body:

- The right lymphatic duct and the right and left tracheal ducts drain lymph from the right forelimb and from the head and neck.
- The thoracic duct drains lymph from the whole of the rest of the body. The contents of the cisterna chyli in the abdominal cavity also empty into the thoracic duct.

Lymph nodes

Along the route of the regional lymphatic vessels are lymph nodes from which lymphocytes and antibodies enter the general circulation. Lymph nodes are small kidney-bean-shaped organs whose function is to filter lymph or bacteria or other particulate matter by the phagocytic activity of macrophages and to produce and store the T and B lymphocytes. Lymph passes through one or more nodes before re-entering the circulation.

A lymph node is an encapsulated mass of lymphoid tissue supported by dense connective tissue trabeculae between which are channels containing the flowing lymph (Fig. 4.27). Each node is supplied by many afferent lymphatic vessels and drained by a single efferent vessel, which leaves at the hilus of the node. As lymph nodes are responsible for draining lymph from specific regions of the body they monitor the health status of that area. All areas of the body

have their own nodes, e.g bronchial or mesenteric lymph nodes, but some nodes are quite superficial and can be palpated, particularly if they become enlarged or diseased (Fig. 4.28).

Lymphoid tissue is also found in other sites:

- Spleen – located in the left cranial abdomen, it is highly vascular and acts both as a lymph node and a blood reservoir
- Tonsils – three pairs located within the pharyngeal area and referred to as the palatine, lingual and pharyngeal tonsils

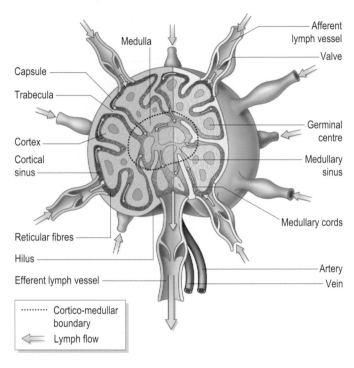

Fig. 4.27 Structure of a lymph node

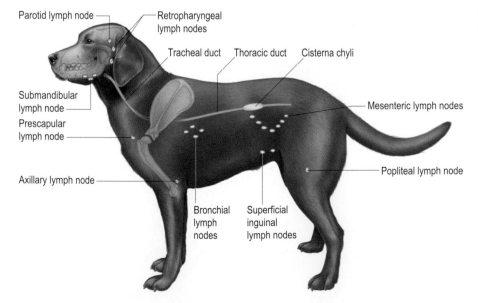

Fig. 4.28 Lateral view of a dog showing the position of palpable lymph nodes. NB. Bronchial and mesenteric lymph nodes are not palpable.

- Thymus – located in the anterior part of the thoracic cavity, its role is vital to the developing immune system in young animals.

Respiratory system

Respiration describes two interrelated processes:

- Cellular respiration – the process in which cells derive energy from the breakdown of organic molecules in the presence of oxygen
- Mechanical respiration – the process by which oxygen required for cellular respiration is absorbed from the atmosphere into the blood and the process by which carbon dioxide produced by the cells during metabolism is excreted into the atmosphere.

It is mechanical respiration that occurs in the respiratory system.

The respiratory system has two functional components:

- A conducting system or the respiratory tract, for the transport of inspired and expired gases between the atmosphere and the circulatory system
- An interface for the passive exchange of gases between the atmosphere and the blood – the pulmonary membrane.

Nasal cavity

The entrance to the cavity is via the nostrils or external nares and the exit is via the internal nares or the opening to the pharynx. The nasal cavity is divided into left and right chambers separated by a septum and filled by coiled turbinate bones. These are covered with ciliated mucous membrane to

filter out dust and other foreign matter and it also enables the air to be moistened and warmed prior to entry into the lower tract. Leading from each chamber are the air-filled frontal and maxillary sinuses which assist in this function and reduce the weight of the skull.

Pharynx

The pharynx is divided by the soft palate into the nasopharynx and the oropharynx. It has six openings into it: i.e. from the nasal chambers, the mouth, the Eustachian tube from the middle ear on each side, the oesophagus and the larynx. It acts as a crossover point between the digestive and respiratory tracts (Fig. 4.29).

Larynx

A hollow box-like structure consisting of cartilage, muscle, fibrous tissue and ciliated mucous membranes, its function is to:

- Provide the means of vocalization
- Control the flow of inspired gases during breathing
- Prevent the entry of solid particles into the trachea.

The larynx consists of a collection of cartilages, the most cranial of which is the epiglottis, which closes the glottis or the opening of the larynx. Inside the larynx, paired vocal folds form a narrow passageway for air flow. Movement of the cartilages controls the size of the glottis and regulates the flow of air through it. During normal breathing the larynx lies in its resting position with the epiglottis lying above the soft palate, making a continuous opening for the air to pass through and the glottis is open (Fig 4.33). During

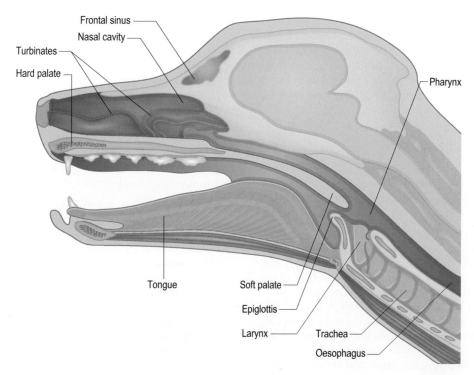

Fig. 4.29 Longitudinal section through the head of a dog to show the upper respiratory tract

swallowing the epiglottis lies over the glottis, closing it and preventing the passage of food down the trachea.

Trachea

The trachea is a non-collapsible tube extending from the larynx through the thoracic inlet to the bifurcation or point of division into the left and right bronchi. It is made up of a series of incomplete C-shaped rings of hyaline cartilage separated by fibrous connective tissue and smooth muscle and lined with ciliated epithelium. The open area of each ring is on the dorsal aspect, which enables the oesophagus, lying close to it, to expand without hindrance when a bolus of food passes through.

Bronchi, bronchioles and alveolar ducts

The bronchi are similar in structure but the cartilage rings are complete. Each bronchus enters the lung tissue at the root of the lung and continues to divide into smaller and smaller bronchi and bronchioles. Eventually the cartilage within the walls disappears altogether. The divisions continue until the smallest branches become the alveolar ducts and finally blind-ending alveoli. The arrangement of smaller and smaller air passages is referred to as the bronchial tree.

The lining epithelium of the tract is a ciliated mucous membrane. The cilia and the mucus trap particles and pass them up to the pharynx where they are either coughed out or swallowed. Deeper into the bronchial tree the alveolar ducts and alveoli are lined by a thin simple squamous epithelium known as the pulmonary membrane – it is across this that gaseous exchange takes place.

Lungs

The right and left lungs are essentially spongy organs that lie in the thorax on either side of the mediastinum (Fig. 4.30). They are divided into lobes, as shown in Table 4.5 – the right side is larger than the left. The lung tissue is covered by the pulmonary pleura and enclosed within the pleural cavity, in which there is nothing but a vacuum and a little serous fluid. These are essential to provide smooth movement between the lungs and thoracic wall during breathing and to bring about inflation of the lungs.

The mechanics of breathing

Lung tissue contains no muscle, so it cannot expand on its own. It is, however, very elastic and will return to its collapsed state when there is nothing to expand it. Breathing occurs in two phases:

- **Inspiration** – the cavity volume increases by the flattening of the diaphragm (a dome-shaped muscular partition separating the thoracic and abdominal cavities) and the lifting of the ribs by contraction of the external intercostal muscles. The lungs increase in size as they are sucked outwards by the vacuum in the pleural cavity. The pressure in the lungs reduces and air passes from the outside down into the lungs, which fill the pleural cavity.
- **Expiration** – the diaphragm relaxes and returns to its domed position and the ribs return to their natural

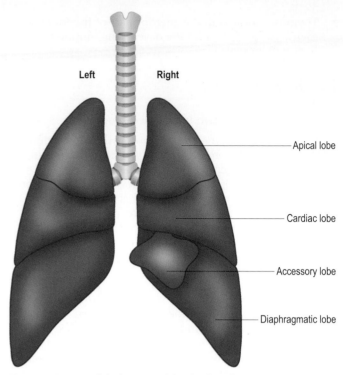

Left   Right

— Apical lobe

— Cardiac lobe

— Accessory lobe

— Diaphragmatic lobe

Fig. 4.30 Division of the lungs into lobes by deep fissures

Table 4.5 Structure of the lungs

Left side	Right side
Cranial or apical lobe	Cranial or apical lobe
Cardiac or middle lobe	Cardiac or middle lobe
Diaphragmatic or caudal lobe	Diaphragmatic or caudal lobe
	Accessory lobe

position, decreasing the volume of the cavity and increasing the pressure of the air in the lungs. Air is forced up the trachea and out of the body.

Control of respiration

Respiratory centres in the pons and medulla oblongata of the hindbrain control:

- Inspiration via the inspiratory centre.
- Expiration via the pneumotaxic and apneustic centres.
- Hering–Breuer reflex – prevention of overinflation of the lungs by stretch receptors in the bronchiole walls. When stretched by air in the bronchioles, these receptors provide information to the hindbrain and stimulate expiration.
- Blood pH – chemoreceptors in the aortic and carotid artery walls and within the medulla oblongata receive information on the changing levels of carbon dioxide and oxygen in the blood which affect the pH. They stimulate respiration to restore the correct pH by expelling the carbon dioxide.

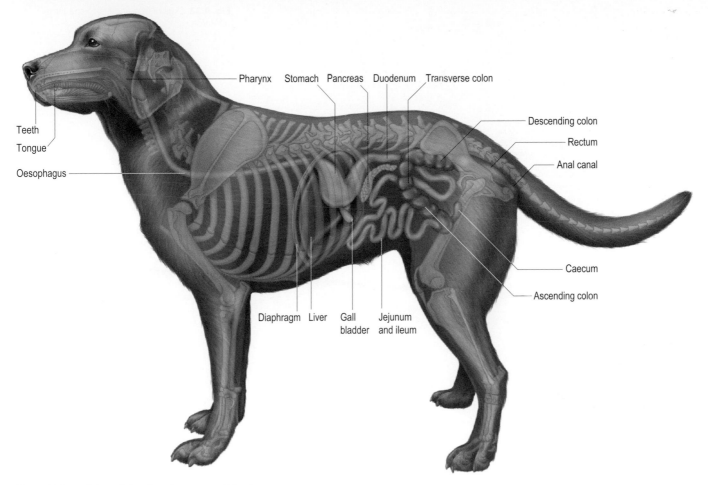

Teeth
Tongue
Oesophagus

Pharynx Stomach Pancreas Duodenum Transverse colon

Descending colon
Rectum
Anal canal

Caecum
Ascending colon

Diaphragm Liver Gall bladder Jejunum and ileum

Fig. 4.31 Lateral view of the digestive system of the dog

Respiratory terminology

- External respiration – transfer of gases between the external environment and the circulation
- Internal or tissue respiration – transfer of oxygen from the blood to the tissues and carbon dioxide from the tissues to the blood
- Tidal volume – the amount of air breathed in and out in one respiration
- Residual volume – the air left in the lungs following a forced exhalation
- Functional residual volume or capacity – the amount of air left in the lungs after normal exhalation
- Total lung capacity – the total amount of air in the lungs
- Vital capacity – the greatest volume of air that can be made to pass out of lungs following forced exhalation
- Anatomical dead space – the volume of air in the trachea, bronchi and bronchioles that never reaches the alveoli.

Digestive system

The digestive or gastrointestinal tract is a muscular tube lined by a mucous membrane which runs from the mouth to the anus. It comprises a variety of structures, reflecting the many functions of the system that work together to bring about the digestion of food in order to provide a source of energy to the body tissues (Fig 4.31).

Oral cavity

Forms the beginning of the tract and consists of the tongue, teeth, cheeks and lips. Its boundaries are (Fig. 4.32):

- Laterally, the cheeks and teeth. Each cheek holds a pad of fat, the buccal pad, which during eating prevent the cheeks from being bitten.
- Dorsally, the palate, which is divided into the hard and soft palates – the hard palate is a bony structure covered with mucous membrane, parts of which are set out in thickened ridges on its surface. The soft palate is a flap of tissue dividing the pharynx into the nasopharynx and oropahrynx.
- Ventrally, the tongue and sublingual muscles, which anchor the tongue, enabling it to assist with prehension, swallowing of food and water, grooming and licking.
- Cranially, the lips and teeth.

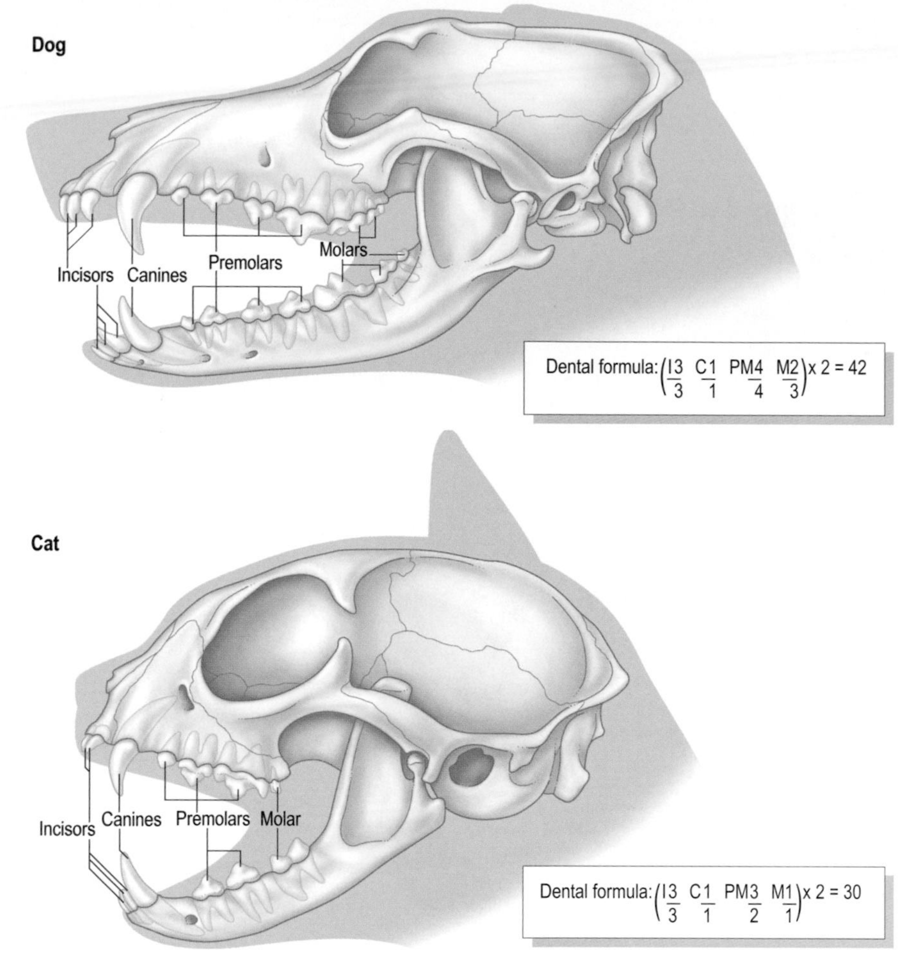

Fig. 4.32 Skull of dog and cat to show the dentition

Dog

Incisors Canines Premolars Molars

Dental formula: $\left(\dfrac{I3}{3}\ \dfrac{C1}{1}\ \dfrac{PM4}{4}\ \dfrac{M2}{3}\right) \times 2 = 42$

Cat

Incisors Canines Premolars Molar

Dental formula: $\left(\dfrac{I3}{3}\ \dfrac{C1}{1}\ \dfrac{PM3}{2}\ \dfrac{M1}{1}\right) \times 2 = 30$

Salivary glands

Paired primary salivary glands include:

- Zygomatic or dorsal buccal
- Sublingual
- Mandibular.

Minor glands also secrete saliva and include the labial, lingual and palatine glands. These glands all have ducts which pass saliva directly into the mouth when stimulated by the smell, sight or thought of food. Saliva is used for moistening food in the mouth and for the formation of a bolus which is swallowed and passed down the oesophagus.

Pharynx

The pharynx is a short muscular tube that acts as a crossover between the digestive and respiratory tracts and serves as a common passageway for air and for food. When food enters the pharynx, all other openings, including the larynx, are blocked in order to direct the food to the oesophagus (Fig 4.33). The tongue presses against the hard palate to close the oral cavity and the food bolus passes through the pharynx. The larynx, attached to the hyoid apparatus, then moves backwards, and the epiglottis falls forward, leaving the larynx open again when swallowing or deglutition is complete. The

bolus of food enters the oesophagus and moves downwards by peristalsis into the stomach.

Oesophagus

A hollow muscular tube which is capable of considerable distension during the passage of a food bolus. It has a good supply of nerves, blood vessels and mucous glands that lubricate the inner lining during the passage of food material by peristalsis. It extends from the pharynx through the thorax and diaphragm via the oesophageal hiatus to the stomach.

Stomach

Lies within the abdomen on the left side of the cavity. It is divided into sections:

- Cardia – area adjacent to the cardiac sphincter, a poorly defined ring of muscle at the junction with the oesophagus which controls the passage of food into the stomach.
- Fundus – major area of digestive glands, which secrete gastric juices and some protective mucus.
- Body – or corpus, which is a continuation of the fundus.

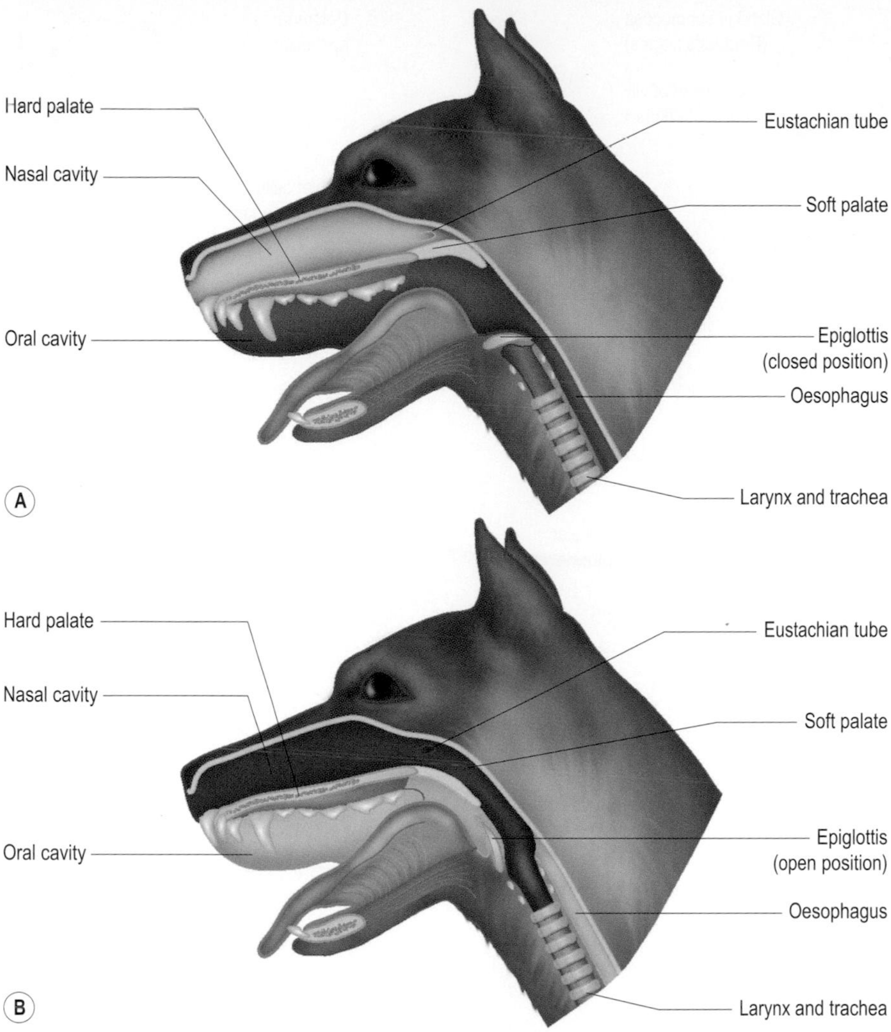

Fig. 4.33 Function of the pharynx during (**A**) swallowing and (**B**) breathing

- Pylorus – a narrowing of the body in which mucus and the hormone gastrin are secreted. It joins the duodenum at its narrowest point as the pyloric sphincter and controls the passage of liquid, partially digested food or chyme, which is squirted into the duodenum.

The stomach is composed of an inner mucous membrane supported on a submucosal layer and known as the gastric mucosa. It is arranged in numerous folds or rugae, which become flattened when the stomach is distended with food. Gastric pits or glands within the gastric mucosa produce hydrochloric acid, mucus and the enzyme pepsin. The lining of the stomach is protected from autodigestion by a thick surface covering of mucus. The middle layers of the stomach consist of smooth muscle, which is responsible for the mixing of food. The outermost layer is a layer of mesentery or visceral peritoneum forming the omentum, which suspends the stomach from the dorsal body wall.

The function of the stomach is to store and mix food with the gastric digestive enzymes. This process takes about two hours, requiring the muscular contractions of the stomach wall, and results in the formation of chyme, which passes into the duodenum.

Within the lining of the stomach wall are gastric pits that secrete gastric juices in response to the hormone gastrin, which is secreted in response to the presence of food passing through the cardiac sphincter. The gastric pits are made up of:

- Goblet cells in the fundus and body of the stomach which secrete mucus which lubricates the passage of food and protects against autodigestion
- Parietal or oxyntic cells distributed in the gastric pits of the fundus and secrete hydrochloric acid. This protects the gastrointestinal tract from harmful bacteria by creating an environment in which they cannot survive and it also denatures protein prior to its digestion
- Chief cells secrete pepsinogen and are clustered at the base of the gastric pits. Pepsinogen is converted into the active enzyme pepsin in the presence of hydrochloric acid and it digests protein.

Small intestine

Receives acidic chyme from the stomach (Fig. 4.31) via the pyloric sphincter. Here the process of digestion is completed and the digested food products are absorbed. Effective absorption depends on a large surface area and this is

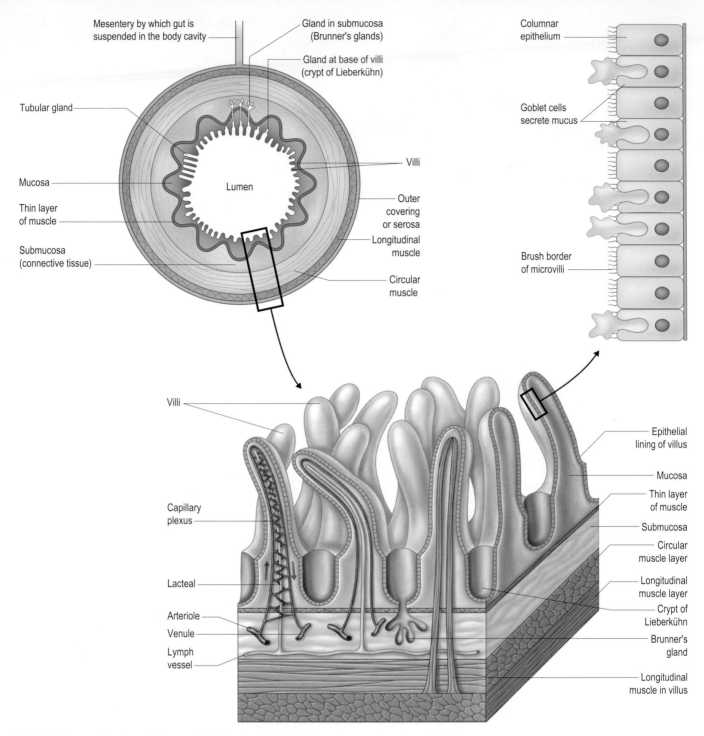

Fig. 4.34 Cross-section through the small intestine showing its structure

achieved by the development of finger-like villi within the intestinal mucosa. These are covered by a layer of epithelium within which lie the digestive glands (Fig 4.34).The small intestine is divided into three parts:

- Duodenum – lies on the right side of the abdomen, and within its U-shaped loop lies the pancreas. It is held in position by part of the visceral peritoneum known as the mesoduodenum. The duodenal mucosa has characteristic villi and Brunner's glands, which

open between the villi. The presence of chyme in the duodenum stimulates the Brunner's glands to secrete a mixture of enzymes known as succus entericus. There are ducts opening into the duodenum from the pancreas and the bile duct.

- Jejunum and ileum – it is difficult to distinguish between these two parts, which form a long mobile tube with no fixed position within the abdominal cavity. It is suspended by the mesojejunum and the mesoileum. The lining epithelium contains villi at the base of which are digestive glands known as the crypts of Lieberkühn. The ileum terminates at the ileocaecal junction.

Pancreas

Lies within the U of the duodenum and is a mixed gland, i.e. has exocrine and endocrine parts. It is an elongated gland, highly lobulated and covered by a loose connective tissue capsule.

- Endocrine tissue – consists of the islets of Langerhans, which secrete several hormones including insulin (see Endocrine system)
- Exocrine tissue – consists of closely packed secretory cells forming the major part of the gland. Pancreatic juices drain into a highly branched duct system and then into the main pancreatic duct which joins the common bile duct to drain into the duodenum. The secretions are alkaline because of a high content of bicarbonate ions, which helps to neutralize the acidic chyme. They are also rich in enzymes which digest proteins, carbohydrates and fats. Many are in an inactive form, preventing autodigestion of the pancreas and must be activated by other enzymes before they can function.

The secretion of pancreatic juices occurs in response to the sight, smell and taste of food. In addition, food entering the duodenum as chyme stimulates secretion via the gastrointestinal hormones cholecystokinin and secretin from the duodenal mucosa.

Gall bladder

Lies within the lobes of the liver and stores bile produced by the liver. Bile containing bile salts is needed for the breakdown or emulsification of fats prior to its digestion and is added to the ingesta via the common bile duct in the duodenum.

Digestion

Food eaten by an animal consists of a mixture of protein, carbohydrate and fat. These food materials are too large to be absorbed into the blood stream and must undergo the process of enzymic digestion (Boxes 4.3–4.5). A cocktail of digestive enzymes are secreted by the gastric pits, Brunner's glands within the duodenum, the crypts of Lieberkühn in the jejunum and ileum, the pancreas and the gall bladder. Enzymes are proteins that act as catalysts to increase the speed of a chemical reaction. Each enzyme is specifically adapted to act on a particular substrate: e.g. lipases act on lipids; proteases act on proteins. The result of the digestive process is the production of small molecules that can be absorbed into the blood stream and carried to the tissues and the liver where they are used for the metabolism of the body.

Absorption

The main site for absorption into the blood stream is within the small intestine.

- Amino acids resulting from protein digestion and monosaccharides and disaccharides from carbohydrate

---

Box 4.3 Protein digestion

- Protein in food as polypeptide chains
- Pepsinogen in gastric juices is converted to pepsin
- Pepsin + protein = peptides
- Enterokinase within succus entericus from Brunner's glands activates trypsinogen in pancreatic juices to form trypsin
- Trypsin converts chymotrypsinogen to chymotrypsin
- Chymotrypsin and other proteases act on peptides and produce amino acids

---

Box 4.4 Carbohydrate digestion

- Carbohydrates present in food as polysaccharides
- Carbohydrate digestion begins in the small intestine
- Enzymes are present in succus entericus, intestinal and pancreatic juices
- Amylase + starch = maltose
- Maltose + maltase = glucose
- Sucrose + sucrase = glucose and fructose
- Lactose + lactase = glucose and galactose
- Sucrose and maltose are disaccharides
- Glucose and fructose are monosaccharides

Box 4.5 Fat digestion

- Fat is present in the diet as triglycerides
- Fat is emulsified by bile salts within the duodenum
- Bile salts activate the lipase enzymes
- Fats + lipase = fatty acids and glycerol
- Fatty acids and glycerol are monoglycerides
- Monoglycerides become coated in protein to form chylomicrons

---

digestion pass through the walls of the villi into the blood capillaries and are carried by the hepatic portal vein to the liver, where they are used for metabolism.
- Fatty acids and glycerol resulting from fat digestion are converted into chylomicrons by the addition of a protein coat. These are absorbed through the walls of the villi into the lacteals and are carried as a milky liquid known as chyle to the cisterna chyli (see Lymphatic system) before entering the circulation via the heart.

Metabolism

Although metabolism also takes place in many tissues, the most significant organ is the liver.

The Liver

The liver is the largest organ in the body, occupying approximately 3–4% of total body weight in an average dog or cat. It lies just behind the diaphragm, cranial to the duodenum and the right kidney, resting against the stomach. It is attached to the abdomen wall by a fold of fibrous tissue and fat called the falciform ligament, which is the remains of the umbilical blood vessels in the fetus. Approximately 75% of the liver's blood supply comes from the hepatic portal system, which delivers blood from the small intestine carrying the products of digestion. The remaining 25% of the blood supply comes from the hepatic artery, which delivers oxygenated blood. The hepatic vein carries waste materials, including carbon dioxide, away.

The liver is thought to perform several hundred functions, all carried out by one type of cell – the hepatocyte. Hepatocytes store significant quantities of glycogen and process large quantities of lipid. The hepatocytes are arranged in hexagonal lobules with the cells arranged in rows radiating from the centre of each lobule towards the periphery. Running alongside each lobule are branches of the hepatic artery, hepatic portal vein and bile duct.

The hepatic artery and hepatic portal vein may be referred to as the interlobular blood vessels since they are located between adjacent lobules. In the centre of each lobule is a branch of the hepatic vein, referred to as the central or intralobular vein. The vessels are connected with the central vein by a system of capillary-like sinusoids that run parallel to, and come into close contact with, the chains of lower cells. The sinusoids are surrounded by fine channels called canaliculi. These connect up with the bile ducts at the edge of the lobule. The hepatocytes are located close to both sinusoids and canaliculi.

Blood reaches each lobule via the interlobular vessels, flowing along the sinusoids towards the central vein. The liver cells take up from the blood what they require and shed products into it. The only exception is bile, which is secreted not into the sinusoids but into the canaliculi to flow into the gall bladder where it is stored until it is needed.

Functions of the liver include:

- Bile production – synthesized by liver hepatocytes. Contains bile salts and the pigment bilirubin, reduced from the green pigment biliverdin, which results from erythrocyte breakdown. Stored in the gall bladder until food enters the stomach and duodenum. This stimulates contraction of the gall bladder and the bile is squirted along the common bile duct into the duodenum.
- Carbohydrate metabolism – occurs when glucose molecules arrive in the liver via the hepatic portal vein. They are polymerized to become glycogen and are stored in the liver. When energy is required by the body, glycogen is broken down to release glucose by a process known as glycogenolysis.
- Fat metabolism – lipids are synthesized to produce cholesterol and fatty acids used to produce energy or stored around the body in adipose tissue.
- Protein metabolism – needed for the following purposes:
  - Use in cells
  - Polymerized to make plasma proteins, e.g. albumin, globulin, fibrinogen and prothrombin
  - As an energy source
  - Deaminated to form urea and eliminated by the kidney.
- Heat production – from synthesis, deamination and transporting of products through the liver combined with its blood supply, the liver produces and then distributes heat around the body, especially to peripheral sites.
- Hormone elimination – after their functions have been performed, some are modified chemically, some are eliminated by the kidney, others expelled in the bile via the intestinal tract.
- Haematinic principle – assisting in the quality of the blood cell production by increasing the haemoglobin level in cells by use of iron and B vitamins.
- Storing blood – using the expansion and contraction ability of the liver veins, the total blood volume in the circulation can be altered as required by the body.
- Detoxification – of nitrogenous waste from cell metabolism prior to excretion.

Large intestine

The indigestible liquid residue from the small intestine passes through the ileocaecal junction joining the ileum and the caecum, into the large intestine. The large intestine is divided into three parts:

- Caecum – a blind-ended sac through which food residue is forced by peristalsis (Fig. 4.31). The lining changes from villi to a glandular form. The function of the caecum is not significant in carnivores.
- Colon – divided into three sections, ascending, transverse and descending according to the position in the abdomen, all attached to the dorsal body wall by the mesocolon. The main function is the absorption of water from the ingesta and the pushing forward of the increasingly solid faeces to the rectum prior to defaecation.

  The mucosa of the colon has no villi but is lined by goblet cells which secrete mucus to aid the passage of the faecal mass. The thickened mucosa is folded in appearance when not distended with faecal material. Commensal bacteria within the colon further degrade food residues, but the colon walls are protected from damage by the presence of numerous leucocytes and cells of the immune system.
- Rectum – this is a short dilated tube lying within the pelvic cavity. Its function is to store the semi-solid faeces prior to defaecation. The mucosa is lined by increased numbers of goblet cells. It terminates in the anal canal and internal and external anal sphincters which control the passage of faeces to the outside. Lying within the anal sphincters are a pair of modified cutaneous glands – the anal sacs – which produce a smelly secretion used to coat the faeces as a form of territorial marking.

Urinary system

The urinary system is primarily responsible for maintaining the balance of water and electrolytes within the body fluids, i.e. homeostasis. The kidney provides the route by which excess water and electrolytes are eliminated as urine, which is then stored within the bladder before being excreted.

The functions of the urinary system are:

- Excretion of nitrogenous waste products, e.g. urea and creatinine
- Regulation of the volume and chemical constituents of the body fluids – osmoregulation
- Secretion of the hormone erythropoietin, which initiates formation of new red blood cells within the bone marrow in response to low blood oxygen levels
- Activation of vitamin D after its synthesis within the skin
- Storage of urine in the bladder prior to micturition.

The kidney

There are two kidneys located in the dorsolumbar region of the abdominal cavity, one on each side of the midline. The left kidney is slightly caudal to the right kidney and both are retroperitoneal, i.e. lie beneath the parietal peritoneum (Fig. 4.35). Urine is produced by the kidneys and conducted to the bladder by the ureters to be stored, prior to micturition via the urethra.

Each kidney is supplied with blood by a renal artery which arises from the aorta. The total blood volume of the body circulates through the kidneys continuously and each kidney receives 20% of cardiac output at any one time. Renal blood pressure is high as the glomeruli consist of a capillary bed between arterioles (not between arterioles and venules as in other sites) and the efferent arterioles are able to constrict under the influence of renin. The high pressure forces the plasma through the perforated walls of the glomeruli into the tubules for modification. Blood is then returned via the renal vein directly to the caudal vena cava. Both the renal artery and vein are positioned in a depression on the medial side of the kidney called the hilus.

The substance of the kidney is contained within a tough, fibrous capsule and is divided into two layers:

- Cortex – outer layer containing the major part of each kidney nephron, including the glomeruli.
- Medulla – the inner area arranged in pyramid-shaped units separated by extensions of cortical tissue. Each pyramid is formed by several collecting ducts which discharge urine into the renal papillae. The calyx, into which the papillae link, forms the larger renal pelvis to conduct urine to the bladder via the ureter.

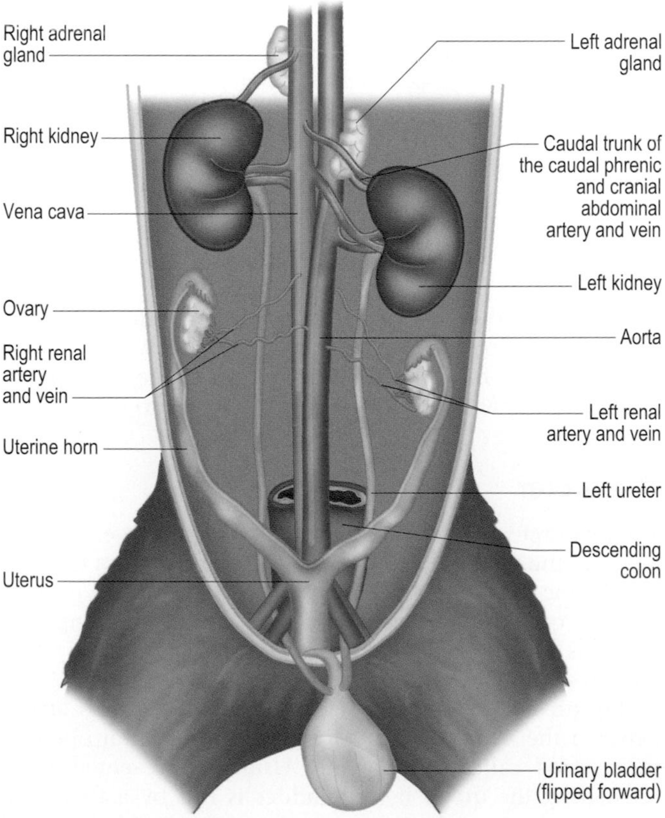

Nephron structure

The functional unit of the kidney is called a nephron (Fig. 4.36) and each healthy kidney will contain about one million nephrons. Each nephron consists of:

- The **glomerular or Bowman's capsule** – consists of a double layer of flattened cells connecting with a perforated basement membrane forming a hollow, distended, cup-shaped structure.
- The **glomerulus** – a tightly coiled network of capillaries that is closely applied to the basement membrane of the glomerular capsule. A glomerulus sitting within its glomerular capsule is known as a renal corpuscle. It is here that a process of ultrafiltration, in which plasma is forced from the glomerular capillaries into the glomerular space, takes place. The filtering action of the glomerulus holds back molecules the size of the plasma proteins or larger. It also retains substances bound to these proteins, e.g. hormones and calcium. Any molecule that is smaller and freely dissolved in plasma will appear in the ultrafiltrate or primitive urine, e.g. sugars, amino acids, small proteins such as myoglobin and haemoglobin, drugs, toxins and electrolytes. The ultrafiltrate then passes into the next section of the renal tubule.
- The highly convoluted renal **tubule** extends from the glomerular capsule to the connection with the collecting duct. The duct is lined by a single layer of epithelial cells. The function of the tubule is to selectively reabsorb water, electrolytes and other molecules from the glomerular filtrate. The renal tubule has three physiological areas:
  1. The proximal convoluted tubule is the longest section, in which 75% of water and electrolytes are reabsorbed from the filtrate.
  2. The loop of Henle descends from the cortex into the medulla and is in close association with wide capillary loops arising from the efferent arterioles. The loop is impermeable to water but electrolytes

Right adrenal gland

Right kidney

Vena cava

Ovary

Right renal artery and vein

Uterine horn

Uterus

Left adrenal gland

Caudal trunk of the caudal phrenic and cranial abdominal artery and vein

Left kidney

Aorta

Left renal artery and vein

Left ureter

Descending colon

Urinary bladder (flipped forward)

Fig. 4.35 Ventrodorsal view of the urinary tract

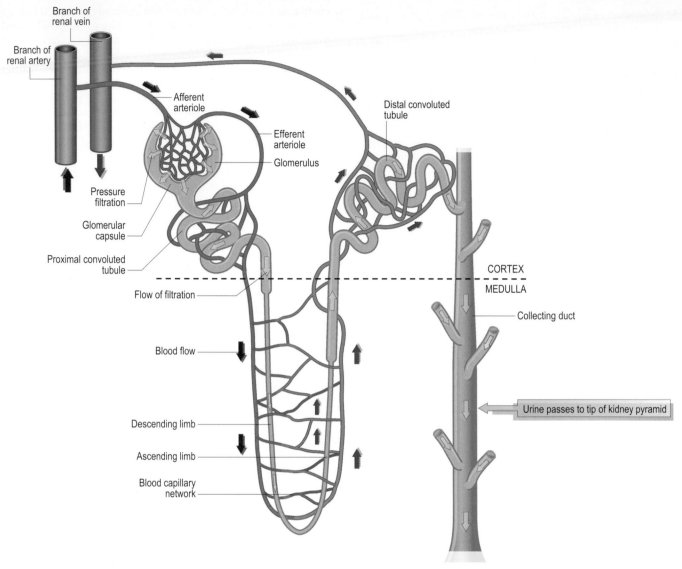

Fig. 4.36 A renal nephron

(sodium and chloride) and some urea are reabsorbed and recycled in the local capillaries (vasa recta), causing high concentrations in the surrounding medullary tissues. This leads to a high osmotic pressure in the extracellular fluid, which is the main function of this area. The outcome is fine control of sodium, chloride and water reabsorption.

3. The distal convoluted tubule is a shorter section of the tubule and is less convoluted. Here sodium electrolytes are reabsorbed along with the secretion of hydrogen or potassium. This is controlled by the release of the hormone aldosterone from the cortex of the adrenal gland.

The terminal section of the distal convoluted tubule drains the urine into the collecting ducts situated in the medulla. The collecting ducts are not permeable to water except in the presence of antidiuretic hormone (ADH) secretion from the posterior pituitary gland (see Endocrine system). Water is then drawn out by the high osmotic pres-

sure of the medullary extracellular fluid and returned to the blood circulation by the vasa recta capillaries. Urine, now formed, drains from the collecting ducts to the renal pelvis at the hilus, leaving the kidney via the ureter to the bladder (Box 4.6).

The ureter

The two ureters are thin tubes, one leading from each renal pelvis to the bladder (Fig. 4.35). They are lined with mucous membrane and have three layers of smooth muscle in their wall – required for peristalsis to move the urine along. The lumen is lined by transitional epithelium that is folded when relaxed and dilates during the passage of urine.

The ureters enter the bladder on the dorsal aspect between the neck of the bladder and the urethral opening in an area called the trigone. Urine is prevented from re-entering the ureter if the bladder is full by a flap-valve within each ureter that compresses against the bladder wall (Fig. 4.38).

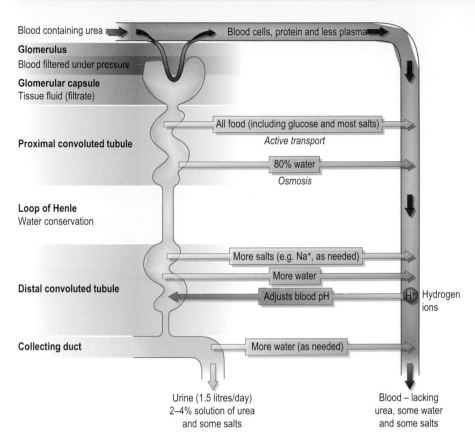

Blood containing urea → Blood cells, protein and less plasma →

Glomerulus
Blood filtered under pressure

Glomerular capsule
Tissue fluid (filtrate)

Proximal convoluted tubule

All food (including glucose and most salts)
Active transport

80% water
Osmosis

Loop of Henle
Water conservation

More salts (e.g. Na⁺, as needed)

More water

Distal convoluted tubule

Adjusts blood pH ← H⁺ Hydrogen ions

Collecting duct

More water (as needed)

Urine (1.5 litres/day)
2–4% solution of urea
and some salts

Blood – lacking
urea, some water
and some salts

Fig. 4.37 Diagrammatic representation of nephron function

Box 4.6 Physiology of filtration

- Proximal tubule function is to reabsorb about two-thirds of the primitive urine, along with the useful substances like sodium and water (Fig. 4.37).
- The loop of Henle acts if blood plasma is too concentrated and the body needs to retain water in order to dilute the fluid. It is here that the final concentration or dilution of urine is decided.
- Antidiuretic hormone (ADH) from the posterior pituitary gland acts in response to the osmotic gradient provided by the concentrated interstitial fluid surrounding the collecting ducts in the medulla.
- The distal tubule is where the final urinary loss of sodium takes place. If the body is sodium-deficient, the hormone aldosterone, secreted by the adrenal cortex, will promote sodium reabsorption back into the body.

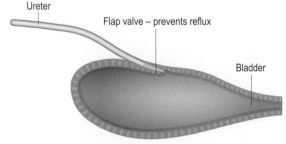

Fig. 4.38 Site of entry of the ureters into the bladder

The bladder

The bladder is a vesicle or sac used for the temporary storage of urine (Fig. 4.35). It is a pear-shaped sac with three layers of smooth muscle in its walls, which contract during micturition. The lining of transitional epithelium resembles that of the ureters. When empty the bladder lies on the pelvic cavity floor and the lining epithelium is folded; when full it may expand as far forward as the umbilicus within the ventral abdomen.

Micturition or bladder emptying occurs when stretch receptors in the bladder wall monitor the degree of filling and relay the message to the spinal cord via the pelvic nerve. Nerve impulses from the spinal cord are sent to the internal bladder sphincter at the neck of the bladder, which is made of smooth muscle and allows urine to pass down the urethra. Emptying is a reflex action but voluntary control involving the external bladder sphincter, which is made of striated muscle, can be learned using reward training.

The urethra

The urethra carries urine from the bladder to the outside. It is a tubular canal lined with transitional epithelium. There is a difference between the urethra of the male and of the female animal.

a. **Female urethra**
   - Shorter than in the male
   - Serves only the urinary system
   - Exterior opening embedded in the vaginal wall and called the urinary meatus.

b. **Male urethra** (Fig. 4.39)
- ■ Longer and narrower than in the female
- ■ Divided into three sections:
  - – Prostatic – surrounded by prostate gland, ducts from prostate open into it
  - – Membranous or pelvic – narrowest part of the urethra, passing along pelvic floor
  - – Cavernous or penile – lies within the body of the penis and opens to the outside
- ■ Urethral opening is called the urinary meatus
- ■ Serves both urinary and reproductive systems.

NB. In the tomcat, the urethra is short, the opening lies within the perineum and is directed caudally.

Urine production

Normal urine contains the following:

- • 96% water and 4% solids
- • Electrolytes
- • Urea
- • Other metabolic waste:
  - ■ Creatinine
  - ■ Phosphate
  - ■ Sulphate.

Volume: approximately 20 ml/kg bodyweight per day.
  Specific gravity: Dog – 1.016–1.060. Cat – 1.020–1.040
  pH: Dog – 7.5. Cat – 6.5.

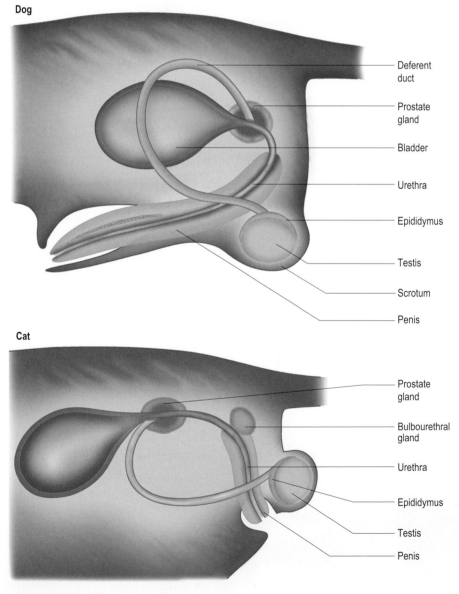

Fig. 4.39 Male urino-genital system of the dog and cat

The rate of urine production varies with ambient temperature, water intake and disease processes. Factors affecting urine composition, other than disease, include:

- Species – variation in specific gravity, which varies with the ability to concentrate urine (compare the volume produced by a cat to that produced by a horse)
- Diet – affects pH values – herbivores produce alkaline urine while carnivores produce acid urine.
- Fluid intake – affects specific gravity concentration
- Exercise – influences fluid loss from body by sweating.
- Medication – some drugs are excreted unchanged in the urine.

Reproductive system

The male tract

Testis

The testes are paired, oval in shape and develop embryonically within the abdomen close to the kidneys (Fig. 4.39). At later stages of embryonic development they migrate caudally through the abdominal cavity, taking their blood supply with them, and pass out through the inguinal canal to lie in the scrotum. This is complete by the age of 12 weeks – if the testis fails to descend the animal is described as being a cryptorchid. The scrotum consists of thin, pigmented skin supplied with sweat glands and is divided into two cavities surrounded by a double fold of peritoneum, the internal and external tunica vaginalis (Fig. 4.40). In mammals the testes are held outside the body because the normal internal body temperature is too high for sperm development. The blood vessels, nerves and ducts supplying the testes run from abdomen to scrotum in the spermatic cord. The cremaster muscle surrounds the spermatic cord and controls the position of the scrotum in relation to the body.

The testicular tissue is divided into numerous conical compartments, each containing a coiled mass of seminiferous tubules between which lie the interstitial cells or cells of Leydig, which secrete the male hormone testosterone (Table 4.3). The seminiferous tubules are lined by two types of cell:

- Spermatogenic cells to produce sperm.
- Sertoli cells, which provide support, nutrients and protection for the developing sperm. They also secrete small amounts of the hormone oestrogen.

The seminiferous tubules eventually join to form the epididymis, which runs on the dorsolateral border of the testis and leads into the deferent duct or vas deferens. This then passes through the inguinal canal and joins the urethra in the area of the prostate gland.

Sperm formed in the seminiferous tubules mature during their passage into the epididymis, where they are stored within the cauda epididymis before being propelled along the deferent duct during ejaculation.

The prostate gland surrounds the junction of the deferent ducts with the urethra close to the neck of the bladder and secretes prostatic fluid. This is alkaline, in order to protect

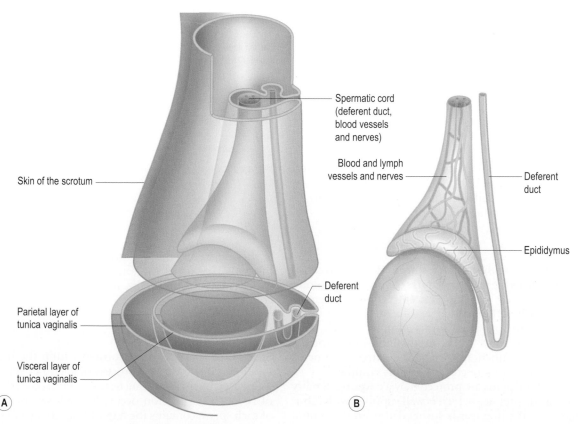

Spermatic cord (deferent duct, blood vessels and nerves)

Blood and lymph vessels and nerves

Deferent duct

Skin of the scrotum

Epididymus

Deferent duct

Parietal layer of tunica vaginalis

Visceral layer of tunica vaginalis

(A)

(B)

Fig. 4.40 The testis within the scrotum. (**A**) Testis enclosed within the internal and external tunica vaginalis. (**B**) Testicular structure

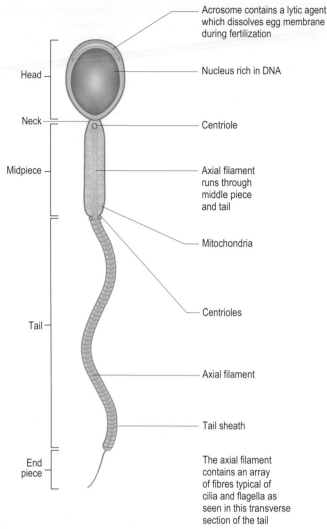

Head —

Acrosome contains a lytic agent which dissolves egg membrane during fertilization

Nucleus rich in DNA

Neck —

Centriole

Midpiece —

Axial filament runs through middle piece and tail

Mitochondria

Centrioles

Tail —

Axial filament

Tail sheath

End piece —

The axial filament contains an array of fibres typical of cilia and flagella as seen in this transverse section of the tail

Fig. 4.41 Structure of a spermatozoon

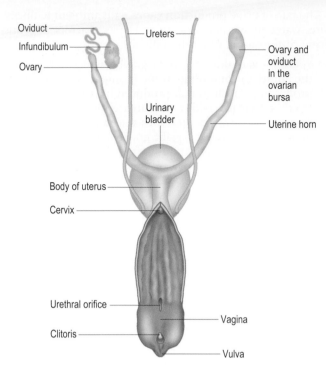

Oviduct —
Infundibulum —
Ovary —

— Ureters

Ovary and oviduct in the ovarian bursa

Urinary bladder

— Uterine horn

Body of uterus —

Cervix —

Urethral orifice —

— Vagina

Clitoris —

— Vulva

Fig. 4.42 Dorsal view of the female reproductive tract of the dog and cat

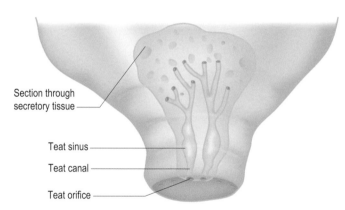

Section through secretory tissue —

Teat sinus —

Teat canal —

Teat orifice —

Fig. 4.43 Section through a mammary gland

the sperm from possible damage by the acidity of urine, and helps to increase the volume of sperm in order to wash it into the female tract. Bulbourethral glands, found only in the cat contribute to the action of the prostate gland.

Penis

The penis consists of the urethra surrounded by layers of cavernous erectile tissue which becomes engorged with blood during sexual arousal, enabling its entry into the female vagina during coitus. Embedded within the erectile tissue close to the tip is the os penis. This is a tunnel-shaped bone that in the dog lies dorsal to the urethra and in the tomcat lies ventral to it. Its function is to aid the entry of the penis into the female tract before erection is fully complete.

The tissues of the penis are protected by a covering of hairy skin known as the prepuce, which is well supplied with lubricating glands. In the dog this is suspended from the ventral abdomen and in the tomcat is much shorter, as the opening

to the urethra and the scrotum lie in the perineum ventral to the anus. The tip of the tomcat's penis is covered in barbs, which play a part in the induction of ovulation during coitus.

Spermatozoon structure

Spermatozoa or sperm are formed within the seminiferous tubules of the testes by a process of spermatogenesis. This is influenced by the hormone testosterone, secreted by the cells of Leydig. Cell division occurs by meiosis and the nucleus of each sperm contains the haploid number (half the normal number) of chromosomes (See Chapter 16).

Each sperm (Fig. 4.41) consists of the following:

- **Head** – this carries the chromosomes (DNA) within a large nucleus and accounts for more than half the dry weight of the head. The nucleus is surmounted by a thin acrosome cap, which contains the enzymes necessary for penetrating the outer membrane of the ovum.
- **Neck and midpiece** – within the midpiece, the axial core is surrounded by densely packed mitochondria rich in respiratory enzymes. This section is concerned with releasing energy for driving the sperm.
- **Tail** – a modified flagellum, which, by lashing from side to side, propels the sperm along the female tract towards the ovum.

The female tract

Ovary

There are two ovaries found in the dorsal abdomen caudal to the kidneys at the level of the third and fourth lumbar vertebrae (Fig. 4.42 and Fig. 4.35). Each is a small, round structure consisting of a central medulla and an outer cortex of connective tissue surrounded by a layer of epithelial cells continuous with the peritoneum known as the mesovarium. This forms a pouch known as the ovarian bursa, which masks the ovary and contains an opening into the peritoneal cavity.

Within the ovarian connective tissue are many primary follicles, each of which can develop into a mature or Graafian follicle. Each mature follicle contains a small amount of fluid and an ovum. The bitch and the queen are litter-bearing (multiparous) species, so they release several ova at the same time.

During ovulation, the follicle ruptures on the surface of the ovary, releasing the ovum, which passes down the uterine tube. After ovulation there may be some bleeding into the ruptured follicle. This is resorbed and replaced by a corpus luteum, which releases progesterone to maintain the pregnancy. In the bitch the corpus luteum remains even in the non-pregnant animal for several weeks and the resulting high levels of progesterone may cause a false pregnancy.

Uterine tube

The uterine tube, oviduct or Fallopian tube is a narrow tube running from the trumpet-like infundibulum, which encloses the ovary, to the uterine horn. The edges of the infundibulum are fringed with fimbriae, which aid in the capture of the newly released ova. The tube is convoluted, lined with ciliated epithelium and suspended by the mesosalpinx, which is continuous with the mesovarium. Its function is to convey the ova to the uterus. Fertilization takes place within the uterine tube.

Uterus

The function of the uterus is to contain the embryos/fetuses during pregnancy and provide nourishment for them to develop to full term. The non-pregnant uterus lies in the pelvic and abdominal cavities; when pregnant the weight of the fetuses pulls the uterus down into the abdominal cavity.

The uterus is a Y-shaped, hollow, muscular organ composed of two long uterine horns, which unite, forming the small body or fundus. This is described as being a bicornuate uterus and is characteristic of litter-bearing species. The inner layer of epithelial and glandular tissue is called the endometrium and this thickens during pregnancy to receive the placenta. The endometrium is surrounded by layers of smooth muscle that form the myometrium. It is suspended from the abdominal wall by the mesometrium or broad ligament, which forms the outermost layer.

The uterus has a dual blood supply:

- An ovarian artery arises from either side of the aorta just caudal to the kidney to supply each ovary and the uterine horn
- Each ovarian artery anastomoses with a uterine artery, which runs down the side of the uterine body and cervix, and supplies the more caudal parts of the tract.

Cervix, vagina and vulva

The cervix lies between the uterus and the vagina and is a thick-walled structure through which runs the cervical canal. It acts as a sphincter, only opening in the healthy animal during oestrus, mating and parturition. The vagina is a hollow muscular organ that extends from the cervix to the external genitalia. It is capable of great dilation and is lined by stratified epithelial cells. These cells change throughout the oestrous cycle under the influence of oestrogen and progesterone.

The vagina continues into the vestibule, a short passage that is shared by both reproductive and urinary systems – the urethra enters in the floor of the tract and marks the change from vagina to vestibule. It contains vestibular glands, which lubricate the caudal genital tract. The muscles in the wall of the vestibule constrict around the dog's penis and aid the 'tie' during coitus.

The vulva forms the external opening of the tract guarded by a pair of vertical labia. These contain striated muscle and under normal conditions are held closed to keep the vulva sealed. It is the vulval labia that become visibly engorged with blood when the bitch is in season. Lying ventrally between the labia is a knob of erectile tissue known as the clitoris.

Mammary glands

Mammary glands are highly modified sweat glands. The glandular tissue is surrounded by connective tissue and fat (Fig. 4.43). The secretion – milk – is produced by secretory epithelial cells and drains into gland sinuses and then into teat sinuses. These narrow into teat canals and link to the outside via the teat orifices. In the bitch and the queen the mammary glands lie between the musculature of the body wall and the skin, in two parallel rows along the ventral abdomen and thorax. The bitch has five pairs and the queen has four pairs.

Mammary glands enlarge during pregnancy and start to produce milk a few days before parturition. Their development is controlled by the following hormones:

- Oestrogen – causes initial development at puberty
- Progesterone – enlargement during pregnancy
- Prolactin – formation of milk during last third of pregnancy

- Oxytocin – causes contraction of smooth muscle around the glands and squeezes milk out of teats – known as milk 'let down'.

The oestrous cycle

The oestrous cycle is the regular cycle of events that occurs in the ovary and the reproductive tract of the postpubertal non-pregnant female.

Reproductive function is under the control of gonadotrophins produced by the anterior pituitary gland (Table 4.6). Gonadotrophins are hormones that stimulate the gonads, i.e. ovary or testis. The release of gonadotrophins is controlled by gonadotrophin-releasing hormone (GRH), which is produced in the hypothalamus and transported down the pituitary blood portal system. The hypothalamus is sensitive to both internal and environmental stimuli such as heat, light and particularly the daylength. It may also be stimulated by pheromones, secreted by other females and by the male animal. The oestrous cycle is controlled by a complex interplay between these stimuli, the hypothalamus and the reproductive tract.

The oestrous cycle occurs in distinct phases during which events take place within the ovary, the reproductive tract and in the female animal's behaviour. (For further details see Chapter 17.) Table 4.7 shows the details of the oestrous cycle of the bitch and the queen.

Fertilization

The ova released at ovulation from the ovaries are propelled down the uterine tubes by the ciliated epithelium and the peristaltic action of the muscles lining the tube walls. At the time of ovulation the ova contain the haploid number of chromosomes (half the normal number) and are immature

Table 4.6 Interaction between gonadotrophins and sex hormones

	Follicle-stimulating hormone (FSH)	Luteinizing hormone (LH)	Luteotrophic factors
Site of action by hormone	Developing follicle	Mature follicle and corpus luteum	1. Corpus luteum 2. Mammary glands
Effect of hormone	1. Follicular growth 2. Secretion of oestrogen	1. Ovulation and formation of the corpus luteum 2. Secretion of progesterone	1. Progesterone secretion maintained 2. Stimulates mammary gland enlargement
Action/effect on the pituitary gland	Oestrogen secretion exerts negative feedback and prevents further secretion of FSH but positive feedback stimulates secretion of LH	Progesterone exerts negative feedback on the hypothalamus and prevents further release of GRH	

Table 4.7 Phases of the oestrous cycles of the bitch and the queen

The bitch			The queen		
Notes: Spontaneous ovulator. Monoestrous. Age at puberty – approx. 6 months but breed-dependent			Notes: Induced ovulator. Seasonally polyoestrous – breeding season is between January and September. Age at puberty – approx. 5 months but depends on month of birth		
Phase	Length	Signs	Phase	Length	Signs
Pro-oestrus	9 days	Enlarged vulva, bloodstained vaginal discharge. Flirty, excitable behaviour. Will not allow mating	Oestrus	4–10 days	No external signs. Very affectionate, rubs against objects, rolls over, lordosis, loud 'calling'
Oestrus	Approx. 9 days. Ovulation occurs on Day 10 of the complete cycle	Vaginal discharge becomes straw-coloured. Vulva even more enlarged. Excitable, flirty, stands to allow mating	Dioestrus	Up to 14 days	Behaviour returns to normal
Metoestrus I	Approx. 20 days	Vulva shrinks, discharge dries up, behaviour returns to normal	Anoestrus	Up to 4 months. Occurs only in the non-breeding season.	Normal behaviour
Metoestrus II	Approx. 70 days	Behaviour and appearance is normal			
Anoestrus	Variable – 3–9 months	Behaviour and appearance is normal			

and incapable of being fertilized. They are known as primary oocytes and they mature to become secondary oocytes approximately 3 days later.

Mature spermatozoa (sperm) pass from the seminiferous tubules of the testes into the epididymis where they undergo a maturation period within the cauda epididymis. During ejaculation they are propelled up the ductus deferens into the urethra, through the penis and into the female tract. The sperm, containing the haploid number of chromosomes, use their tails to swim from the vagina through the cervix into the uterus. They then enter the uterine tubes where fertilization takes place. Sperm are able to survive within the female tract for up to 7 days waiting for mature ova to be available. Fertilization occurs when a single sperm penetrates an ovum and the nuclei coalesce (Fig. 4.44).

Each ovum released from the ovary is protected by a double layer of cells – an inner layer of glycoprotein, the zona pellucida, and the outer layer of cells, the corona radiata. Sperm come into contact with the ova by random movement. When the head of a sperm hits the zona pellucida the acrosome, the tip of the sperm head, bursts open, releasing an enzyme that softens the connecting tissue membrane of the ovum. The sperm is then able to penetrate into the cytoplasm of the ovum. Further spermatozoa are prevented from entering by a rapid chemical change known as the fertilization reaction, which causes thickening of the surface of the ovum. After penetrating the ovum, the sperm tail is discarded. The head and mid section are drawn through the cytoplasm toward the nucleus. The nuclear membrane breaks down, forming a spindle along which the chromosomes of the sperm and ovum arrange themselves as in mitosis (see Chapter 16).

Fertilization of the ovum by the sperm results in a zygote (Box 4.7). The diploid number of chromosomes is restored (haploid + haploid = diploid) and the fertilized ovum or zygote is ready for its first mitotic division (Fig. 4.44). As further divisions take place the zygote continues to move down the uterine tube towards the uterine horns.

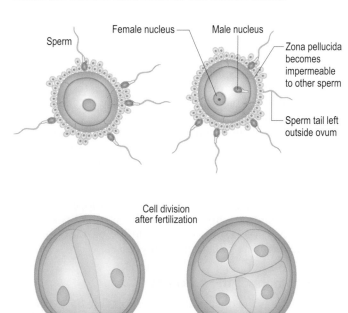

Fig. 4.44 Fertilization of the ovum

Pregnancy

After fertilization the zygote moves down the uterine tube and by the time it reaches the uterine horns it has already divided several times. At the 16–32 cell stage the structure is called a morula and is a solid mass of cells resembling a blackberry. Following a long journey down the tube during which the ball of cells floats free in the lumen of the tube it develops a fluid-filled cavity and is known as a blastocyst. By about the 19th day the blastocysts space themselves evenly along the uterine horns and implantation begins (Fig. 4.45). In order to create equal numbers within each uterine horn, thus allowing equal space for development, one or more blastocysts may cross the body of the uterus to implant in the opposite horn – this is known as transuterine migration.

During the oestrous cycle the uterus prepares to receive the fertilized ova. In the follicular phase of the cycle there is growth both of the myometrium and endometrium and an increase in the blood supply of the uterus. The endometrium thickens, new blood vessels grow and glandular structures hypertrophy. In the luteal phase of the cycle these changes continue and the endometrium becomes secretory. When the blastocysts reach the uterine horns they are bathed in the uterine secretions, which provide nutrients and create the correct environment for survival.

Embryonic development

The cells of the blastocyst become organized to form on one side of the cyst the inner cell mass and on the other side a thinner layer known as the trophoblast. The inner cell mass becomes the embryo and divides into three germ cell layers, each of which has a specific role (Box 4.8).The inner cell mass curves around to become C-shaped, enclosing the endoderm and mesoderm, which form the internal organs. Table 4.8 shows the stages and timing of puppy development. Kittens develop in a similar way but are usually slightly in advance of puppies.

Formation of the extra-embryonic membranes

The trophoblast consists of the peripheral cells of the blastocyst and is eventually responsible for attachment to the uterine wall, i.e. implantation (Fig. 4.45). It develops small,

---

Box 4.7 Reproduction

Gamete – male (spermatozoa) and female (ova) germ cells – each are formed by meiosis and contain the haploid number of chromosomes.

Zygote – the fertilized ovum which contains the diploid number of chromosomes. Undergoes cell division by mitosis.

Embryo – the stage of development in which the major organs are forming. Up to about 35 days

Fetus – the stage from which the development of the major internal organs is complete. From 35 to 63 days.

Conceptus – the embryo or fetus, the extra-embryonic membranes and the placenta.

Neonate – the newborn animal – until the animal is about 1 week old.

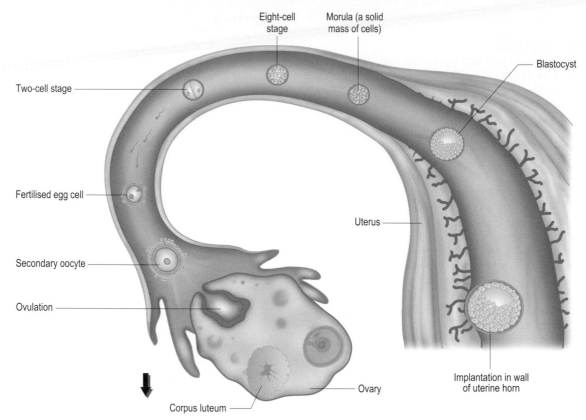

Fig. 4.45 Development and implantation of the embryo

---

finger-like outgrowths that project into the surrounding tissue of the uterine wall, contributing to the placenta and the extra-embryonic membranes and enabling absorption of nutrients across the villi.

There are four extra-embryonic membranes that surround the developing embryo. They protect the embryo and provide a means of attachment to the uterine wall (Fig 4.46).

1. Cells from the endoderm multiply and line the trophoblast, forming the **yolk sac**. This shrinks away sometime before birth.
2. Between the yolk sac and the trophoblast, mesodermal cells divide into two layers forming a cavity – the outer layer lies close to the trophoblast and forms the **chorion**, and the inner layer lies close to the yolk sac.
3. The trophoblast and mesoderm expand and push up around the embryo, forming a fluid-filled cavity – the amniotic cavity. This is entirely separate from the other cavities and it is the surrounding membrane or **amnion** in which the fetus is delivered.
4. Around the outer surface of the amnion creating a double layer is the chorion, which is now in contact with the uterine endometrium. Projections called chorionic villi grow out from its surface to connect with the maternal tissues as the placenta. Both amnion and chorion consist of ectoderm and mesoderm.
5. From the caudal end of the primitive embryonic gut endodermal cells multiply and form a diverticulum known as the **allantois**, which lies beside the yolk sac. This collects urine from the fetal kidneys via a tube or urachus that connects to the fetal bladder. During development the allantois increases in size, pushing between the amnion and the chorion, eventually surrounding the embryo. The inner layer fuses with the amnion, forming the allantoamnion, which contains lubricant fluids to assist movement towards the birth canal during parturition. The outer layer forms the **chorioallantois** with the chorionic layer and is known as the 'water bag'. This ruptures during parturition as the fetus moves toward the birth canal.

Development of the placenta

The placenta is the organ which is responsible for providing nourishment of the developing embryo and fetus. Villus structures develop from the chorioallantois and contain capillary loops derived from the umbilical artery (Fig. 4.47).

Table 4.8 The stages of puppy development

Stage of development	Time (post-fertilization)	Event
Pre-implantation		
	96 hours	Fertilized ovum divides into two cells
	20 hours	Four cells
	144 hours	Eight cells
	192 hours	Ball of cells becomes a morula
	8–9 days	Morula passes down uterine tube and then into uterine horn
Embryonic development		
	15 days	Blastocyst forms and floats free in the uterus
	17–18 days	Placenta begins to develop
	20–21 days	Embryos of less than 13 mm in diameter begin to implant at equal distances within the walls of the uterine horns. Central nervous system is forming
	21–28 days	Brain and spinal cord are developing. Embryo curls around into the 'fetal position'. All body organs, limb buds, head, eyes and face are forming
	28 days	Embryo is about 25 mm in diameter and oval in shape
	29–30 days	Eyelids are closed and eyes begin to develop beneath them. Male and female external characteristics are forming
Fetal development		
	35–44 days	Organogenesis is complete by 35 days. Body is about 100 mm long. Body hair and coloured markings are developing
	45–55 days	Calcification of the skeleton is complete and will show up on a radiograph. Fetus grows rapidly
	57 days	Further rapid growth. Fetus is about 150 mm long. Hair covering is complete; pads developed

They burrow into the endometrium of the uterus and project into the maternal blood spaces, which receive blood from the uterine artery. Only a thin endothelial layer separates the fetal and maternal systems and here nutrients and oxygen are able to pass into the fetus and waste gases and nitrogenous waste pass from the fetus into the maternal circulation.

The placenta forms a thickened band around the conceptus and is described as being a zonary placenta (Fig. 4.48). At the edges are areas of capillary degeneration and haemorrhage into the uterine endothelium caused during implantation. These are referred to as the marginal haematoma. During parturition the broken-down blood in these haematomata colours the parturient discharges. It is normal to see a green discharge in the bitch and a brown discharge in the queen – any other colour should be a cause for concern.

The placenta produces small amounts of oestrogen and progesterone, which act together to prevent further ovulation and oestrous cycles during pregnancy. Their effects are responsible for more vascular development of the uterine endometrium and glandular secretions. The uterine muscle relaxes and size increase becomes possible during the pregnancy.

Changes during pregnancy

The gestation period may be defined as the time between mating and parturition. The time is always expressed as a range as there is great individual variation and the exact timing of fertilization is difficult to determine.

- Bitch 59–72 days – average 63 days or 9 weeks. Smaller breeds whelp earlier than larger breeds.
- Queen 61–70 days – average 63 days or 9 weeks. Siamese and Persians will often go to 70 days.

Changes during pregnancy include:

- Enlargement of abdomen
- Mammary gland enlargement
- Enlargement of the teats
- Vulva remains enlarged and elastic throughout pregnancy

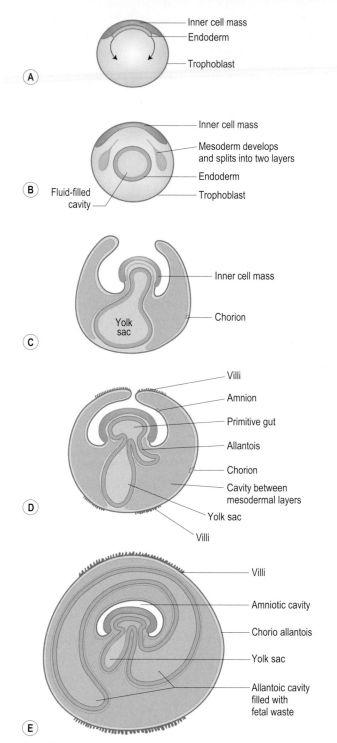

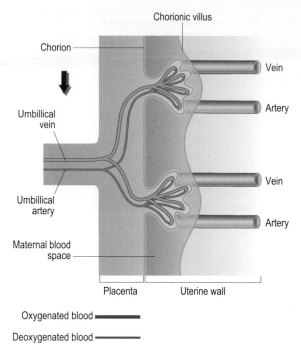

Fig. 4.47 Arrangement of blood capillaries within the placenta

Oxygenated blood ▬▬▬

Deoxygenated blood ▬▬▬

Fig. 4.47 Arrangement of blood capillaries within the placenta

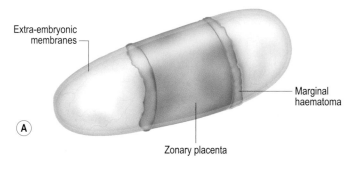

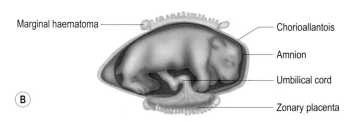

Fig. 4.46 Stages in the development of the extra-embryonic membranes. (**A**) Cells of the endoderm multiply and line the trophoblast. (**B**) Mesodermal cells divide into two layers forming a cavity between them. (**C**) The trophoderm and mesoderm expand and push up around the inner cell mass or embryo. (**D**) The amniotic cavity is formed; the yolk sac begins to shrink and the allantois develops from the primitive hindgut. (**E**) The allantois fills with waste products and extends around the embryo. Placental villi form around the outer surface and aid implantation

Fig. 4.48 The zonary placenta of the dog and cat. (**A**) Conceptus, showing zonary placenta. (**B**) Section through the conceptus

- Clear mucoid vaginal discharge may be seen in some animals.

Relaxation and loosening of the ligaments in and around the pelvic girdle area occurs a few days before actual birth. Alterations in abdominal configuration accompany such ligament relaxation. The abdomen, which earlier shows a uniform bulge, develops a 'hollow' in the flank area. This change is clearly visible both in profile and from above and is frequently referred to as a 'pear-shaped' abdomen.

Parturition

Parturition occurs in three stages:

- First stage – uterine contractions begin and cervix dilates
- Second stage – delivery of the fetuses
- Third stage – expulsion of the membranes and placenta or after-birth.

It may be referred to as whelping in the bitch and kittening in the queen. Other species also have colloquial names for parturition, e.g. calving in cows, foaling in horses and lambing in sheep (see also Chapter 17).

Hormonal changes

Parturition is the expulsion of the fetus and its membranes from the uterus. It involves interaction between the hormonal and nervous system control mechanisms. It is thought to be initiated by the fetuses within the uterus. As they grow larger they outgrow the available space, which results in distress and the secretion of cortisol from the fetal adrenal glands. Cortisol causes the corpus luteum within the ovary to degenerate and the levels of progesterone secreted by it throughout pregnancy to fall. At the same time oestrogen levels begin to rise and the uterine muscles, which were relaxed under the influence of progesterone, regain their ability to contract and are described as being 'sensitized'.

By this time the dam may feel ready to give birth, will be sensitive to external stimuli such as darkness or privacy and will search for somewhere to have her young. The presence of the external stimuli will stimulate the hypothalamus and the pituitary gland secretes two hormones:

- Prolactin – from the anterior pituitary gland stimulates the formation of milk from the mammary glands.
- Oxytocin – from the posterior pituitary gland acts on the sensitized uterine muscle and initiates strong contractions, which result in expulsion of the fetuses. It also causes the milk to be released from the mammary glands when the neonates begin to suckle.

A hormone produced by the placenta called relaxin causes relaxation and opening of the cervix and also primes the myometrium of the uterus to respond to oxytocin. Prostaglandins are produced by the uterine tissue and help to supplement uterine contractions.

Signs of imminent parturition

Subtle signs that indicate that parturition will soon occur may be seen for a few days before the event.

- Changes to the external sex organs, e.g. vulval lips swell and become softer; vulval opening enlarges
- Slight vaginal discharge may be seen as the cervix begins to dilate
- Body temperature may drop by a few degrees 6–18 hours before parturition
- Some bitches may go off their food
- Some bitches may tear up newspaper and start to prepare a nest.

These behaviour patterns vary between individuals and some bitches show no signs at all (see Chapter 17). Most queens will search for somewhere to give birth and this is usually in private where they can remain undisturbed; however, some queens seem to need human company.

First stage

Mild uterine contractions start sweeping over the uterus and gradually bring about dilation of the cervix. This stage may last for up to 48 hours but is very variable.

The dam may show evidence of mild physical discomfort, e.g. restlessness, agitation, panting, licking the vulva. Strings of mucus may hang from the vulva and the first 'water bag' or chorioallantois may rupture within the vagina. Milk may be present in the mammary glands. The fetus becomes active and moves from the curled fetal position to the extended position ready for birth and the immature cardiac and respiratory systems become ready to take over from the placental exchanges that occur in utero. The contractions push the first fetus up against the cervix as it starts to dilate. Once the cervix is fully dilated the second stage begins.

Second stage

Increased uterine contractions propel the fetus through the cervix into the vagina. Once the fetus is in the birth canal abdominal contractions help to increase the propulsive force. The fetus must rotate to meet the centre of the cervix and the surrounding bags of fluid lubricate the passage of the fetus (Fig. 4.49).

The young of litter-bearing or multiparous animals, e.g. cat and dog, are born in longitudinal presentation, i.e. with the long axis of the puppy parallel to the long axis of the bitch. They may be born in anterior presentation, i.e. head and fore limbs first or in posterior presentation, i.e. hind limbs first – either is quite normal (Fig. 4.49). Any other position may cause dystocia or difficult birth (Fig. 4.50). A breech birth is abnormal and occurs when the rump of the puppy is presented with the hind limbs pointing cranially.

After the birth of each puppy the bitch will break the amniotic sac over the head and lick the puppy to stimulate respiration. She will also break the umbilical cord to separate it from the placenta. A healthy puppy will then make its way around to the teats and begin to suckle.

The time between the onset of straining and birth varies from 10 to 30 minutes – any longer may indicate a problem.

Third stage

Delivery of the fetus is usually followed by expulsion of the placenta within about 30 minutes. During this stage the uterus involutes or contracts and a green/brown discharge is passed – this lochia may continue for several days but may be licked away by the bitch or queen.

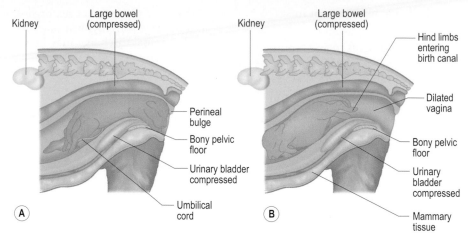

Fig. 4.49 Position of puppy during normal birth. (**A**) Anterior presentation. (**B**) Posterior presentation

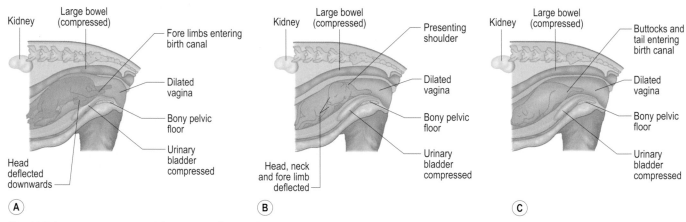

Fig. 4.50 Incorrect presentation. (**A**) Downward flexion of the head. (**B**) Sideways deviation of the head. (**C**) Breech presentation

In reality, in multiparous animals, the second stage often alternates with the third stage so the placenta may follow the delivery of the puppy and then another puppy and placenta may follow.

The integument

The integument refers to the outer covering of the body and includes the skin, hair, claws and footpads.

The skin

The coat of a dog or cat is often its most striking feature but it is the skin beneath which is the more complex structure. The skin forms an unbroken layer over the body and is continuous with the mucous membranes of the mouth, nose and genital openings. It is the largest organ of the body and has a number of vital roles.

Structure

Some features of skin vary depending on the area of the body but the basic structure is always the same. It is tough, stretchable and of varying thickness, e.g. thickest where it is most exposed such as the footpads of the dog. It is also thicker over the dorsal and lateral surfaces of the body but at its thinnest over the ear flap, thorax, ventral surface of the abdomen and inner surface of the legs.

The skin (Fig. 4.51) is composed of three main layers:

1. **Epidermis** – layer of non-vascular stratified epithelium of varying thickness. The epidermis is composed of four layers of cells:
   - **Stratum basale or germinativum** – lowest layer in which cells divide rapidly by mitosis. Melanocytes (pigment cells) are found in this layer and are responsible for skin colour.
   - **Stratum granulosum** – cells contain granules in the cytoplasm and begin to die as they gradually move to the surface. Keratin, a fibrous protein, develops and gives a hardened texture to the cells.
   - **Stratum lucidum** – cells lose their nuclei and develop a clearer appearance. This layer develops in areas of harder wear.
   - **Stratum corneum** – flat, cornified cells, overlapping each other as dry scales. If these scales remain intact, this top layer prevents the entry of harmful materials. Keratinization is completed here and gives the modified epidermal structures, e.g. hooves, beaks and hair, their strength. Dead cells or squames from

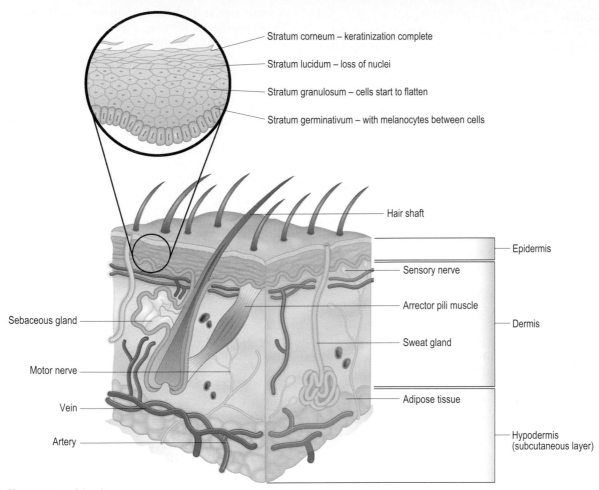

Stratum corneum – keratinization complete

Stratum lucidum – loss of nuclei

Stratum granulosum – cells start to flatten

Stratum germinativum – with melanocytes between cells

Hair shaft

Epidermis

Sensory nerve

Arrector pili muscle

Sebaceous gland

Sweat gland

Dermis

Motor nerve

Vein

Adipose tissue

Artery

Hypodermis
(subcutaneous layer)

Fig. 4.51 The structure of the skin

this layer are continuously sloughed off as dandruff, scurf or dander and replaced by new cells growing up from the base layer.

2. **Dermis or corium** – made up of dense, fibrous, elastic connective tissue, which contains blood vessels and nerves. Bundles of smooth muscle called the arrector pili muscles are attached to hair follicles and when contracted cause hairs to become erect. The effect of this action increases the animal's ability to keep warm in cold weather and, if used in the 'fight or flight' reaction when the animal raises its hackles along the back and neck, increases the animal's apparent size. This layer also contains sebaceous glands, sweat glands, sensory nerves and blood capillaries.

3. **Hypodermis or subcutaneous layer** – contains connective tissue and adipose tissue, allowing the skin to move over deeper structures without tearing or damage.

Function

The many functions of skin include:

- **Protection**
  - Acts as a barrier between the internal structures and the external environment.
  - Prevents entry of microorganisms.
  - Protects underlying structures from injury.
  - Protects against damage from water loss, mechanical trauma and ultraviolet light.
  - Prevents absorption of toxic or harmful substances.
- **Production**
  - Vitamin D, required for the absorption of calcium from the intestines, is synthesized from dihydrocholesterol in sebum by the action of ultraviolet light.
  - Sebum from sebaceous glands forms a water-repellent layer over the skin and helps control bacterial growth.
  - Sweat, which assists in the removal of some waste products.
  - Pheromones, produced in special scent glands, are used for communication with other animals for reproductive or territorial purposes.
  - Milk, released from the mammary glands.

- **Sensation**
  - Sense organ with receptor nerves throughout the skin's surface needed to perceive touch, temperature, pressure and pain.
- **Storage**
  - Fat, as adipose tissue, is an energy store and acts as an insulation layer to help maintain the body temperature in cold weather. It also helps to protect some organs such as the kidney.
- **Thermoregulation**
  - Heat loss – dilation of surface blood vessel walls and sweating from the skin glands assists in the loss of water and salts that evaporate and cool the skin surface.
  - Heat gain – constriction of surface blood vessel walls conserves heat in the body.
  - Insulation – adipose tissue under the skin insulates the body. Erection of hairs traps a layer of warm air.
- **Communication**
  - Pheromones – scents produced by special skin glands and used for communication with other animals of the same species. The production of pheromones is used mainly for reproductive purposes.
  - Visual communication or camouflage involving coat colour or pattern.
  - Response to threat or attack, the animal will raise its 'hackles' in order to appear larger.

Skin glands

Glands in the skin produce a variety of secretions:

- Sebaceous glands opening into the hair follicles secrete sebum whose function is to form a thin, oily, water-repellent layer over the skin surface. It gives the coat hair a shiny appearance and encourages the growth of bacteria that produce an acid pH. This acidity protects the skin from growth of other bacterial species.
- Sweat glands or sudoriferous glands open on to the skin surface. Sweat evaporates and causes cooling of the body and also contains some waste from the body.
- Anal glands or anal sacs – lie on either side of the anal sphincter. Their secretion has an unpleasant smell and is thought to be used as a pheromone for territorial marking. These sacs are intermittently emptied by the passage of faeces.
- Mammary glands – their function is to produce milk. They are the characteristic feature of mammals and are present in both male and female animals.

Modified epidermal structures

Hair

Individual hairs develop from pegs of epidermal cells which project downwards into the dermis and form a hair follicle.

A small area at the base invaginates and fills with a knot of blood capillaries forming the hair papilla. Cells above the follicle divide to produce the keratinized hair shaft, which pushes up through the centre of the follicle and on to the centre. Each follicle develops an arrector pili muscle and a sebaceous gland.

There are three main types of hair:

- **Guard hairs** – longer and coarser than the other hairs; prevent water soaking into the coat and protect against mechanical damage.
- **Wool hairs** – softer and wavier than other hairs; lie close to the body surface forming an insulating layer.
- **Sinus hairs** (includes the vibrissae or whiskers) – long coarse hairs that protrude beyond the outline of the body. The base of each hair is in contact with a blood-filled sinus with a good nerve supply. Movement of the hair 'tweaks' the nerve fibres and a nerve impulse is sent to the brain, where it is interpreted.

Claws

These are beak-shaped structures forming the protective outer covering of the distal phalanges of each digit. Each claw consist of two sheets of epidermis which form the claw walls. The sole lies between them, facing the ground surface, and is filled with a soft, flaky horn. At the base of the claw, where it attaches to the skin covering the digit, is a fold of skin called the claw fold. In the centre of the claw between the last bone of the toe and the horn of the claw is the dermis, which contains blood capillaries and nerve fibres – often referred to as the 'quick'

The functions of a claw include:

- Assisting in locomotion by providing grip
- Used for obtaining food
- Fighting, especially in cats.

Each of the five digits of the foot has a claw. The first digit or dew claw is small and bears no weight so the claw is not worn down and may cause problems with overgrowth. The claws of the cat are narrower than those of dogs and are usually retracted into the claw fold by ligaments. The claws can be quickly unsheathed by muscular action when required.

Footpads

These are the weight-bearing surface of the animal's foot. The footpad is hairless and covered in specialized epidermis that is thick, roughened and normally pigmented. Sweat glands are present in the dermis and beneath this is the toe or digital cushion, made of fatty or adipose tissue with a good blood supply. The pads are oval, or heart-shaped depending on their location in the dog and are more rounded in the cat. The pads provide protection against wear, provide grip when walking and act as shock absorbers when running or jumping.

Bibliography

Allen, W.E., 1992. Fertility and Obstetrics in the Dog. Blackwell Scientific Publications, Oxford.

Aspinall, V., Capello, M., 2009. Introduction to Veterinary Anatomy and Physiology, second ed. Butterworth-Heinemann, Oxford.

Lane, D.R., Cooper, B., 2007. Veterinary Nursing, fourth ed. BSAVA, Gloucester.

McBride, D., 1996. Learning Veterinary Terminology. C V Mosby, St Louis, MO.

Tighe, M., Brown, M., 1998. Mosby's Comprehensive Review for Veterinary Technicians. C V Mosby, St Louis, MO.

Recommended reading

Aspinall, V., 2005. Essentials of Veterinary Anatomy and Physiology. Butterworth-Heinemann, Oxford.

Quick reference guide to all the important facts – useful for revision.

Aspinall, V., Capello, M., 2009. Introduction to Veterinary Anatomy and Physiology, second ed. Butterworth-Heinemann, Oxford.

This book is designed to cover the veterinary nursing syllabus and provides the correct depth of knowledge for student veterinary nurses.

Aspinall, V., Bowden, S., Capello, M., 2009. Introduction to Veterinary Anatomy and Physiology Flashcards/Anatomy and Physiology Workbook. Butterworth-Heinemann, Oxford.

The fun way to revise anatomy and physiology! Provides a series of games and exercises to test your knowledge.

Tartaglia, L., Waugh, A., 2002. Veterinary Physiology and Applied Anatomy. Butterworth-Heinemann, Oxford.

Provides in-depth coverage of the subject at a more advanced level. Recommended for those who wish to take the subject further.

CHAPTER 5

Comparative anatomy and physiology of the exotic species

Victoria Aspinall

Introduction

It is no longer rare to be presented in the surgery, with an animal that is classed as an exotic species, i.e. one that is neither a cat nor a dog. In order to understand their care within the practice it is necessary to have some knowledge of their individual anatomy and physiology. This chapter will take the basic plan of the mammal as exemplified by dogs and cats and highlight the differences.

Small mammals

The rabbit

Rabbits are warm-blooded mammals and members of the class Lagomorpha, which also includes the hare and a guinea-pig-like creature known as the pika. The feature that distinguishes them from members of the rodent family is that they possess two pairs of upper incisor teeth while the class Rodentia has only one pair. In the wild rabbits are subject to constant predation by carnivorous species and much of their anatomy and physiology is adapted to sensing danger and making a rapid escape.

Morphology

The wild rabbit is covered in brown ticked fur, which camouflages it. The average rabbit weighs about 2.5 kg but selective breeding has led to the development of at least 50 different breeds, which vary in colour and size. The head is rounded, with protuberant eyes set laterally, providing a wide field of monocular vision that enables the individual to detect predators. The ears are long and black-tipped and can be moved independently to pick up sound. They represent about 12% of the body surface and are extremely vascular, making them a useful means of thermoregulation. The lips are soft and the upper lip is divided by a deep philtrum, which allows the rabbit to nibble grass very short.

The skin of the rabbit is well supplied with scent glands, particularly under the chin, around the anus and in the inguinal region. The rabbit is strongly territorial and the development of these glands which are affected by the reproductive hormones reflects the degree of sexual activity. As the female rabbit matures she develops a large flap of skin or the dewlap under her chin from which fur is pulled to line the nest prior to giving birth.

The forelimbs are relatively short and used for digging while the hind limbs are long and powerful. They provide the main force needed for the hopping motion that is a characteristic of the rabbit. There are no footpads and the undersurface of the foot is covered in coarse fur. There are five toes on each forepaw and four on each hind paw, each of which ends in a sharp claw. The tail is short and fluffy and its white underside 'flashes' as the animal runs, acting as a warning to other members of the group.

Musculoskeletal system

The skeleton represents only 7–8% of the body weight and the bones are thinner and much more fragile than those of

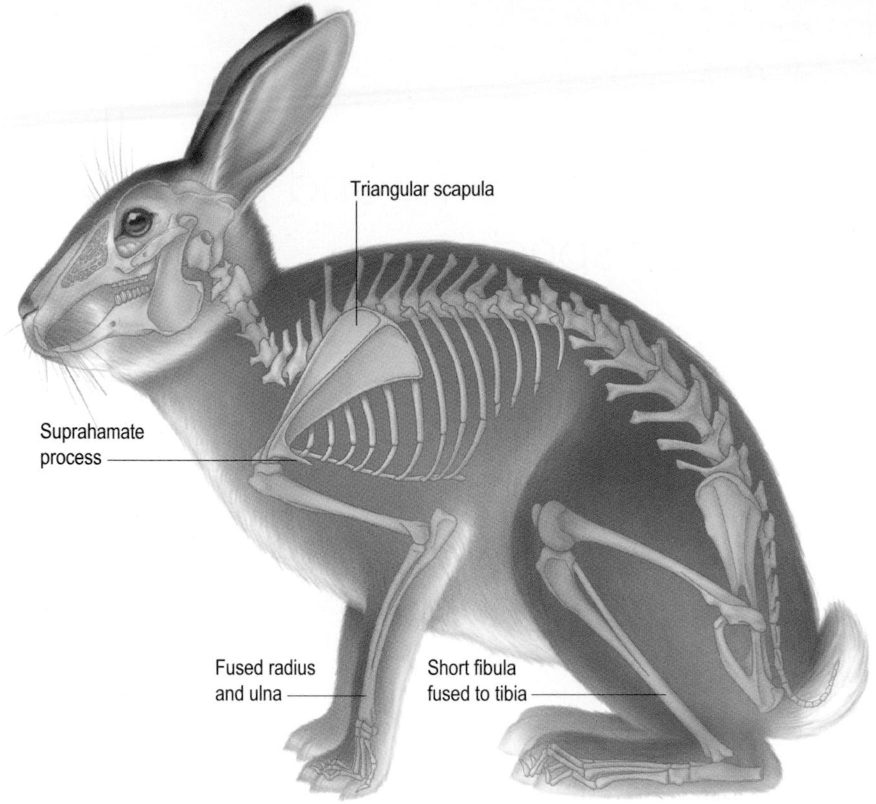

Fig. 5.1 Skeleton of the rabbit

Triangular scapula

Suprahamate process

Fused radius and ulna

Short fibula fused to tibia

the cat, whose skeleton occupies 12–14% of the body weight. Incorrect or clumsy handling of the animal may cause fractured limbs or spine. In addition, older rabbits, those that are overweight or those not given sufficient exercise, may develop osteoporosis or thinning of the cortex.

Apart from obvious differences in conformation (Fig. 5.1), the skeleton is largely similar to that of the cat. The number of vertebrae in the vertebral column is C7, T12–13, L7, S4, Cd16.

Digestive system

The rabbit is a herbivore and thrives on coarse plant material with a high fibre content. The oral cavity is long and narrow and the tongue is fleshy. The teeth are all open-rooted, which enables them to grow continuously throughout life. Dental problems are the most common reason for visiting the veterinary surgery. The dental formula is shown in Table 5.1. The incisor teeth are chisel-shaped for nibbling food, while the premolars and molars are flatter and ridged for grinding fibrous grass and hay. There are no canine teeth (Fig. 5.2). The gap between the incisors and the premolars is known as the diastema.

The digestive tract is long compared to that of the dog and cat as plant material is relatively difficult to digest. The stomach is simple and thin-walled and acts as a reservoir for food and ingested faeces. Both the cardiac and pyloric sphincters are well developed and rabbits are unable to vomit, making starvation prior to anaesthesia unnecessary. The duodenum, jejunum and ileum are long, with a small lumen. The ileum terminates at the caecum in a rounded structure known as the sacculus rotundus or the ileo-caecal

Table 5.1 Dental formulae of the commonly kept small mammals

Species	Latin name	Dental formula
Rabbit	*Oryctolagus cuniculus*	[I 2/1 C 0/0 PM 3/2 M 3/3] × 2 = 28
Mouse	*Mus musculus*	[I 1/1 C 0/0 PM 0/0 M 3/3] × 2 = 16
Rat	*Rattus norvegicus*	[I 1/1 C 0/0 PM 0/0 M 3/3] × 2 = 16
Syrian or golden hamster	*Mesocricetus auratus*	[I 1/1 C 0/0 PM 0/0 M 3/3] × 2 = 16
Gerbil	*Meriones unguiculatus*	[I 1/1 C 0/0 PM 0/0 M 3/3] × 2 = 16
Chipmunk	*Tamias sibiricus*	[I 1/1 C 0/0 PM 0/0 M 3/3] × 2 = 16
Guinea pig	*Cavia porcellus*	[I 1/1 C 0/0 PM 1/1 M 3/3] × 2 = 20
Chinchilla	*Chinchilla lanigera*	[I 1/1 C 0/0 PM 1/1 M 3/3] × 2 = 20
Ferret	*Mustela putorius furo*	[I 3/3 C 1/1 PM 3/3 M 1/2] × 2 = 34

tonsil (Fig. 5.3) inside which is a network of lymphoid follicles.

The caecum is the largest organ in the abdominal cavity, occupying most of the right side. It is thin-walled, sacculated and coils in on itself, ending in a vermiform appendix,

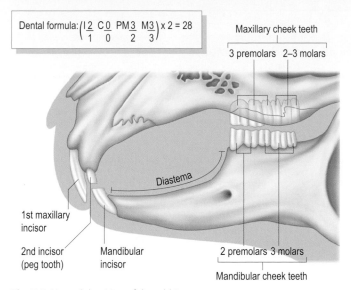

Dental formula: $\left(I\frac{2}{1} \; C\frac{0}{0} \; PM\frac{3}{2} \; M\frac{3}{3}\right) \times 2 = 28$

Maxillary cheek teeth

3 premolars 2–3 molars

1st maxillary incisor

2nd incisor (peg tooth)

Mandibular incisor

Diastema

2 premolars 3 molars

Mandibular cheek teeth

Fig. 5.2 Normal dentition of the rabbit

which also contains lymphoid material. The colon is also sacculated and leads into the rectum.

Digestion

The rabbit is a herbivorous, monogastric hindgut fermenter. Plant material is masticated within the oral cavity with the aid of the flattened surfaces of the molars and premolars. After swallowing, the food undergoes monogastric digestion within the stomach in a similar way to that seen in the dog and cat. The ingesta passes into the small intestine and then into the caecum. When it enters the colon, muscular contractions separate the fibrous from the non-fibrous components. The fibrous material travels on down the digestive tract and is passed out as hard pellets within about 4 hours of eating. The remaining softer and more fluid material passes back into the caecum where it undergoes fermentation by colonies of microbes that are able to produce the enzyme cellulase for the breakdown of the cellulose plant cell walls. At intervals the now digested material is squeezed into the colon by peristalsis and leaves the anus as softer pellets or caecotrophs which are eaten by the rabbit – a process known as coprophagia or caecotrophy. These are produced within 3–8 hours of ingestion of the original food material, often at night, and are covered in mucus, which protects them from the stomach acid. Food ingested by the rabbit passes through the digestive tract twice in 24 hours and in this way nutrients produced by microbial fermentation are made available to the rabbit. Although fibre has very little nutritional value it is an essential component of a rabbit's diet to wear the teeth down and to stimulate peristalsis and digestive function.

Urinary system

The kidneys are unipapillate in contrast to the multipapillate kidneys of the dog and cat. The structure of the kidney varies with the species of rabbit and its associated environment. Desert-living rabbits have large kidneys with an extremely well-developed ability to concentrate urine, and thus con-

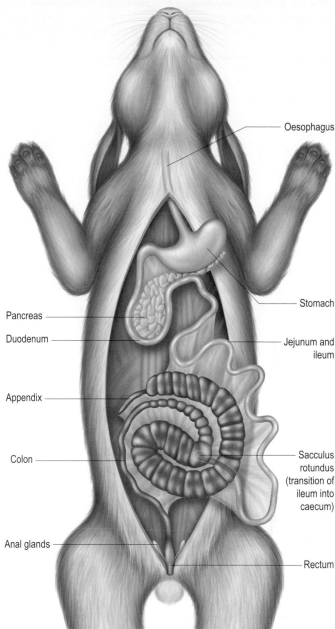

Oesophagus

Pancreas

Duodenum

Appendix

Colon

Anal glands

Stomach

Jejunum and ileum

Sacculus rotundus (transition of ileum into caecum)

Rectum

Fig. 5.3 Digestive system of the rabbit

serve water, while those of alpine rabbits are small and produce more dilute urine.

The urine of the rabbit is the main method of calcium excretion and the urine, depending on the intake of calcium in the diet, is often thick and creamy because of its high calcium carbonate content. The colour also varies from white to yellow or even red. These changes are normal and are due to certain pigments excreted by the kidney.

Reproductive system

Male or buck

The almost hairless scrotum contains two testes and lies cranial to the penis. This position is unlike that of any other

Table 5.2 Biological data relating to rabbits and small mammals

	Chinchilla	Gerbil	Guinea pig	Golden hamster	Mouse	Rat	Rabbit
Life span (years)	10–12	3–4	4–8	2–3	2–3	3–4	5–12
Adult weight	400–600 g	50–60 g	750–1000 g	80–120 g	20–40 g	400–800 g	1–8 kg
Body temperature (°C)	38–39	37.4–39	38.6	36.2–37.5	37.5	38.0	38.3–39.4
Respiratory rate (breaths/min)	40–80	90–140	90–150	70–80	100–250	70–150	35–60
Pulse rate (beats/min)	100–150	250–500	130–190	280–412	500–600	260–450	130–325
Oestrus cycle (days)	41; seasonally polyoestrous	4–6	15–17	4	4–5	4–5	No regular cycle; induced ovulator
Age at puberty	8 months	10 weeks	M 8–10 weeks; F 4–5 weeks	6–10 weeks	6–7 weeks	8–10 weeks	4–6 months
Gestation period (days)	111	24–26	63	16	19–21	20–22	28–32
Development of young at birth	Precocial	Altricial	Precocial	Altricial	Altricial	Altricial	Altricial
Weaning age	6–8 weeks	24–27 days	2–3 weeks	3–4 weeks	3–4 weeks	3–4 weeks	4–6 weeks
Type of diet	Herbivorous; coprophagic	Omnivorous; coprophagic.	Herbivorous; need vitamin C	Omnivorous; coprophagic	Omnivorous; coprophagic	Omnivorous; coprophagic	Herbivorous; coprophagic
Natural behaviour	Nocturnal; social	Nocturnal; monogamous	Diurnal; social	Nocturnal; solitary	Nocturnal; social	Nocturnal; social	Crepuscular; social

Source: Adapted from Aspinall V 2003 Clinical procedures in veterinary nursing. Butterworth-Heinemann, Edinburgh

placental mammal, where the scrotum lies caudal to the penis. The testes descend at about 12 weeks of age and the inguinal canal remains open. There is no os penis. The buck has no nipples.

Female or doe

The bicornuate uterine tract has evolved to produce large litters of young and consists of two long uterine horns, each of which enters the vagina via its own cervix. There is no uterine body. The mesometrium that suspends the tract within the peritoneal cavity contains abundant amounts of fat and is a major fat storage area.

The doe is an induced ovulator and does not have a well-defined oestrous cycle. Periods of sexual receptivity occur in domestic rabbits at 4–6-day intervals. Ovulation takes place within 10 hours of coitus. (For further details of reproduction see Table 5.2.) The doe has four or five pairs of nipples. The young are altricial, i.e. blind, deaf and bald, and entirely dependent on their mother until they are weaned.

Small rodents

Members of the order Rodentia – the rodents – make up 40% of all mammals but only a few species are kept as pets. Those that are kept in captivity include mice, rats, gerbils, hamsters, chipmunks, guinea pigs and chinchillas. Their common characteristic is that they have incisor teeth with a persistent pulp cavity, i.e. the cavity remains open, unlike the pulp cavity of the incisors of the cat and dog, which shrinks once the tooth is fully developed. As a result the teeth continue to grow and the animal must gnaw on hard food, wood or stone to keep the incisors at a normal length.

Rodents can be subdivided into three groups. These are:

- The myomorphs – the mouse-like rodents. They are all omnivores and include rats, mice, gerbils and hamsters. The young are altricial.
- The sciuromorphs – the squirrel-like rodents. They are all omnivores and include the chipmunks. The young are altricial.
- The histricomorphs – relates to their reproductive patterns. They are all herbivores and include guinea pigs and chinchillas. The young are precocial, i.e. born fully furred with their eyes open and capable of eating solid food within the first 24 hours of life.

Rodents are warm-blooded mammals and as such they have many similarities with the dog and cat. However the most notable difference is in the anatomy of the digestive system, which has evolved to deal with a range of diets.

Digestive system

Omnivores, e.g. mouse, rat, gerbil, hamster and chipmunk

These species eat a wide variety of different foodstuffs, including leaves, seeds, roots, fruit, insects such as crickets and locusts, cheese, hard-boiled egg and cooked meat. Their dentition consists of one pair of chisel-shaped incisors designed to gnaw and bite the food and flattened premolars and molars or cheek teeth for grinding and breaking up the plant material. Dental formulae are shown in Table 5.1. The incisors retain an open pulp cavity and grow throughout life, while the cheek teeth stop growing once they have reached full size. The gap in the jaw between the incisors and the cheek teeth is known as the diastema. Malocclusion or difficulty in closing or bringing the teeth together caused by abnormal growth is the most common problem seen in pet rodents.

Both the hamster and the chipmunk have cheek pouches, which are diverticula from the oral cavity lined with mucous membrane and used to carry food long distances back to the food storage chambers within their nest complexes. The pouches can become impacted, particularly in newly weaned animals.

The stomach is simple and digestion within it is monogastric. In the rat, mouse and gerbil the lining epithelium is mostly non-glandular. Lying between the oesophagus and the cardiac region is a ridge that prevents regurgitation and makes vomiting impossible. The intestine is relatively longer than that seen in the carnivorous dog and cat but shorter than that seen in the herbivores. As plant material makes up only part of the diet there is no organ specifically adapted for microbial fermentation and breakdown of cellulose; however, the hamster has a distinct forestomach which is adapted for this purpose. The rat has no gall bladder but it is present in the other omnivores.

All omnivores show a degree of caecotrophy or coprophagia and the faecal pellets are thought to contain a significant amount of vitamin B produced by the microbial flora living in the colon.

Herbivores, e.g. guinea pig and chinchilla

These species live mainly on the leafy parts of plants and in the guinea pig in particular it is essential that it receives fresh green food daily. The liver of the guinea pig is unable to manufacture vitamin C and if deprived of green food containing the vitamin it will begin to show symptoms and will eventually die.

The dentition consists of chisel-shaped incisor teeth and flattened premolars and molars, all of which retain an open pulp cavity and grow throughout the animal's life. The dental formulae are shown in Table 5.1. As with the other species, malocclusion is a common problem. The stomach is simple and lined with a glandular epithelium, and digestion is monogastric. The small intestine is moderately long and lies mainly on the right of the side of the peritoneal cavity.

The much longer large intestine fills the left and central parts of the cavity. The most significant part of the large intestine is the caecum, which is large and thin-walled and has many lateral pouches created by bands of smooth muscle in the walls (Fig. 5.4). Inside the caecum are large numbers of microorganisms, which are responsible for the fermentation and breakdown of cellulose within the plant cell walls. They also contribute extra nutrients such as vitamin B to the digested food mixture. Both guinea pigs and chinchillas exhibit caecotrophy. Animals deprived of the opportunity to eat their own faeces may suffer from malnutrition.

The ferret

The domestic ferret is a member of the family Mustelidae and is therefore related to other members of the family such as the polecat, weasel, stoat and badger. These species are noted for their pungent smell, which comes from sebaceous glands distributed within the skin and also the anal glands. They are carnivorous mammals and as such show many similarities to the cat. Working ferrets are used to kill rats

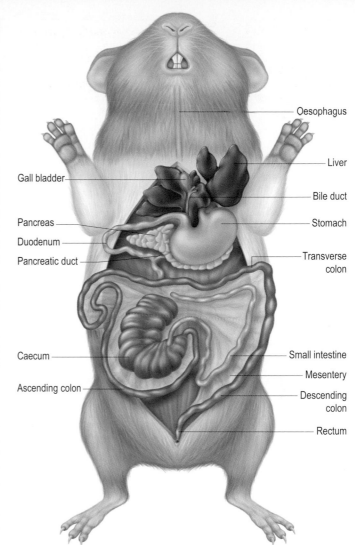

Fig. 5.4 Digestive system of the guinea pig

and rabbits but they are also becoming popular as domestic pets.

Morphology

The tubular body is long and very flexible and is designed to go down holes in pursuit of prey. The neck is long and muscular with a similar diameter to that of the rest of the body. The head is small, with small ears set on the crown of the head and eyes that point forwards. These provide binocular three-dimensional vision, which enables the ferret to locate its prey accurately. Their eyesight is poor and is adapted to the low light levels found within tunnels.

The legs of the ferret are short and are used mainly for digging. Ferrets are excellent climbers and if the surface is rough enough to grip they may reach great heights. There are five toes on each foot, each ending in a non-retractable claw. The skin is thick to provide protection from bites and the fur is very dense. The natural colour is cream, with black guard hairs, black feet and tail and a black mask on the face. This is the colour of the closely related polecat and in the

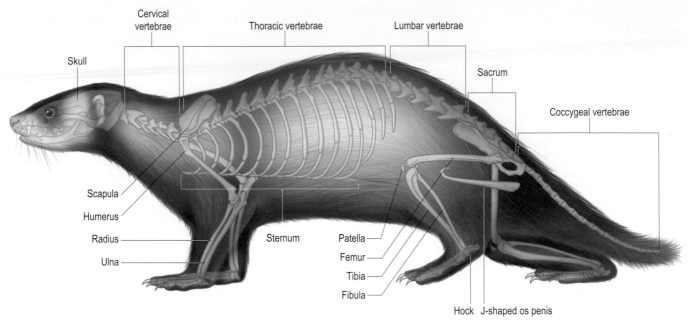

Fig. 5.5 Skeleton of the ferret

ferret is described as 'fitch'. Other colours that may also occur naturally include albino, sandy or cinnamon.

Musculoskeletal system

The pattern of the skeleton is similar to that of the cat (Fig. 5.5). The spine is extremely flexible and allows the ferret to bend at an angle of at least 180°. The arrangement of the vertebral column is C7, T15, L5–6, S3, Cd18. The thoracic inlet is small and may quite easily be blocked by an abnormal mass, which will interfere with breathing and swallowing.

Digestive system

The ferret is a true carnivore and this is reflected in its dentition and the anatomy of the digestive tract. The teeth are extremely sharp and are adapted for killing prey and tearing flesh off the bone. The incisors are prominent; the canines are large and may be visible when the mouth is closed. The premolars and molars are similar to those of the cat. The third upper premolars are the largest of the cheek teeth and are known as the carnassials. The dental formula is shown in Table 5.1.

As in all carnivores the digestive tract is quite short as meat is easily digested and therefore takes less time. The stomach is simple and small but capable of enormous distension with food. The small and large intestines follow a similar pattern to that seen in the cat. There is no caecum or ileocaecal valve. The ferret has a six-lobed liver, a gall bladder and a pancreas that has two parts, which open into the duodenum close to the pylorus.

Reproductive system
Male or hob

The two testes lie externally within the scrotum and once the testes have descended the inguinal ring closes. During the breeding season the testes become noticeably enlarged as spermatogenic activity increases. There is a J-shaped os penis lying within the caudal section of the penis and dorsal to the urethra (Fig. 5.5). The opening of the prepuce is on the ventral abdomen in a similar position to that of the dog. The male ferret has teats. Further reproductive details are shown in Table 5.3.

Female or jill

The bicornuate uterus consists of two long uterine horns with no uterine body. This adaptation is essential to produce the litters of 8–10 young commonly seen in the ferret. The small slit-like vulva lies ventral to the anus and becomes enlarged during the oestrous cycle. The jill is seasonally polyoestrous and an induced ovulator. Coitus may last for 1–3 hours and can be a violent procedure. Ovulation takes place within 30–40 hours of coitus. The young, known as kits, are altricial. (For further details see Table 5.3.)

Birds

Birds are members of the class Aves and as such have an outer covering of feathers. There are about 8500 species of bird but only a relatively few species are commonly kept as cage and aviary birds; examples of these are shown in Table 5.4. Most species of bird are able to fly although there are some species, e.g. penguin, ostrich, kiwi, which remain land-bound. The ability to fly has contributed to their great ecological success and they are distributed within most habitats in the world. Their anatomy and physiology is very different to that seen in the mammal and adaptations to the metabolically demanding ability to fly are shown in almost every body system and affect such factors as metabolism, body weight, stability and wind resistance.

Table 5.3 Biological data relating to the ferret

Parameter	Measurement	Comment
Life span	5–11 years	
Adult weight	Jill: 600–900 g Hob: 1–2 kg	Weight fluctuates with the time of year – heavier in the winter
Body temperature	37.8–40°C	Rises to 40°C when excited
Respiratory rate	30–40 breaths/min	
Pulse rate	200–400 beats/min	
Oestrous cycle	Seasonally polyoestrous. Induced ovulator	Season starts in March and continues until September. Female remains in oestrus until mated. Ovulation occurs 30–40 h after mating
Age at puberty	Jill: 7–10 months Hob: 5–14 months	Puberty occurs in the spring after birth, so age varies
Gestation period	38–44 days	Young are altricial. May be eaten by the jill if disturbed
Litter size	2–6	
Weaning age	6–8 weeks	
Diet	Carnivorous	Require 30% protein, 30% fat. Can be fed on tinned or dry cat food

Source: Adapted from Aspinall V 2003 Clinical procedures in veterinary nursing. Butterworth-Heinemann, Edinburgh

Table 5.4 Commonly kept species of cage and aviary birds

Order	Species	Common name
Psittaciformes – noted for their bright plumage and ability to mimic sounds	*Psittacus erithacus*	African grey parrot
	Amazona species	Amazon parrots
	Ara species	Macaws
	Eclectus species	Eclectus parrots
	Nymphicus hollandicus	Cockatiel
	Melopsittacus undulatus	Budgerigar
	Trichoglossus species	Lories and lorikeets
	Cacatua sulphurea	Lesser sulphur crested cockatoo
Passeriformes – so-called perching birds; contains over half the living species of bird	*Serinus canaria*	Canary
	Poephila quattata	Zebra finch
	Chloebia gouldiae	Gouldian finch
	Gracula religiosa	Mynah bird
Columbiformes	*Columbia livia*	Pigeons and doves
	Coturnix species	Quail

The skeleton

The skeleton of the bird (Fig. 5.6) is adapted to support both walking and flying and has many specialized features, which result in a strong but light framework. These include:

- A reduction in the total number of bones
- Fusion of some joints to form strengthening plates of bone
- A reduction in the density of bone – many bones have a thin cortex which is strengthened by the addition of a network of bony struts
- Loss of the internal components – many bones are hollow and filled with air sacs.

Axial skeleton

- The skull shows many adaptations, which contribute to the overall reduction in weight. A lightweight beak covers the mandible and replaces the teeth. The upper beak articulates with the rest of the skull by means of the craniofacial hinge, which increases the mobility of the beak during feeding. The lower beak hinges on the quadrate bone, which enables the beak to open wide and makes dislocation of the beak very unlikely. The large eyes are housed within a pair of thin-walled orbits. Each orbit is surrounded by a ring of bony plates, known as the sclerotic ring, which protects and supports the structure of the eyeball.

- The vertebral column is divided into the different regions as in other animals; however, there are fewer vertebrae in the central regions and more in the cervical and coccygeal regions, which allows greater flexibility. The neck may contain as many as 25 vertebrae, depending on the species. Birds have 12 caudal or coccygeal vertebrae, the first few of which are mobile to enable movement of the tail and the remaining ones are fused to form the pygostyle, which carries the tail feathers. The thoracic, lumbar and sacral vertebrae are fused to form a rigid frame to support the rib cage and the legs.

- The sternum is extended into a large concave keel, which provides an increased surface area for the attachment of the flight muscles. Flightless birds do not have a keel.

Appendicular skeleton

- The pectoral girdle is formed from three pairs of bones – the coracoids, scapulae and clavicles. On each side the glenoid cavity is formed by the junction of the coracoid and the scapula and the humerus of the upper wing inserts into this cavity, forming the shoulder joint. The pair of clavicles, often referred to as the wishbone, keep the shoulders separated.

- The wings (Fig. 5.7) attach to the body at the shoulder joint, which allows rotation in several planes. The bones of the wing are reduced to the humerus, a separate radius and ulna, fused carpal and metacarpal bones and two digits. Digit 3 is fused to the metacarpal bones and is the main digit. It carries the primary feathers. Digit 1 forms the alula or bastard wing and carries a few feathers for controlling takeoff and

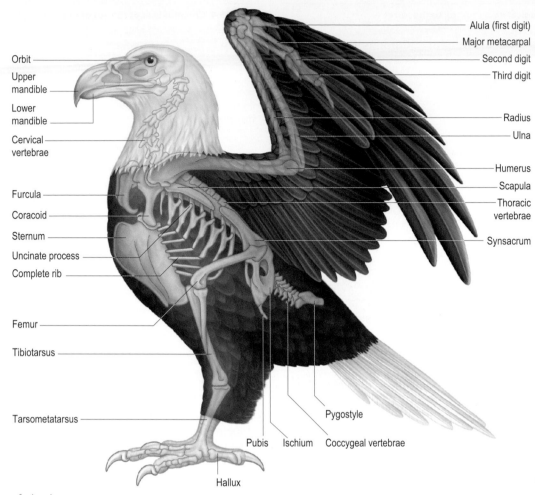

Orbit
Upper mandible
Lower mandible
Cervical vertebrae
Furcula
Coracoid
Sternum
Uncinate process
Complete rib
Femur
Tibiotarsus
Tarsometatarsus
Hallux
Pubis
Ischium
Coccygeal vertebrae
Pygostyle
Synsacrum
Thoracic vertebrae
Scapula
Humerus
Ulna
Radius
Third digit
Second digit
Major metacarpal
Alula (first digit)

Fig. 5.6 Skeleton of a hawk

landing. The shape of the wing, which varies with the species and affects the type and speed of flight, is slightly curved from front to back, forming an aerofoil shape that creates lift as the bird flaps its wings.

- The pelvic girdle is formed by three pairs of bones – the ilium, ischium and pubis – which join to form the joint into which the femur of the leg inserts. The distal ends of the three bones are not fused, leaving the lower part of the pelvis open to allow the passage of eggs out of the body cavity.
- The upper leg is formed by a short, wide femur which ends at the stifle joint. This is directed forward so that the lower leg is under the bird's centre of gravity. The middle of the leg consists of a fused tibia and fibula known as the tibiotarsus, which ends at the hock joint, consisting of a single fused tarsometatarsus. Most species of bird possess four toes, with three pointing forwards and one pointing back. However, the members of the parrot family and the woodpeckers have two toes pointing forwards and two pointing backwards. Owls and ospreys have a fourth toe that is opposable and can face backwards or forwards, which enables them to use their feet to pick up their prey.

Muscular system

The average bird has between 175 and 200 muscles, many of which are placed on the ventral surface of the body close to the centre of gravity.

Wing muscles

The most prominent are the pectorals, which are large and superficial and responsible for the powerful down beat of the wing, and the supracoracoids, which lie deep to the pectorals and are responsible for the up beat of the wing. Both pairs originate on the keel, with the pectoral inserting on the underside of the humerus and the supracoracoid inserting on the upper surface of the humerus. In strong, long-distance fliers these muscles make up about 25% of the body weight and in the pigeon they make up 40% of body weight.

Leg muscles

Most of the muscles lie high up the leg or on the body itself and they control movements by means of long tendons that run down the leg. Extensor tendons run down the front of the tibiotarsus and the tarsometatarsus while the flexor

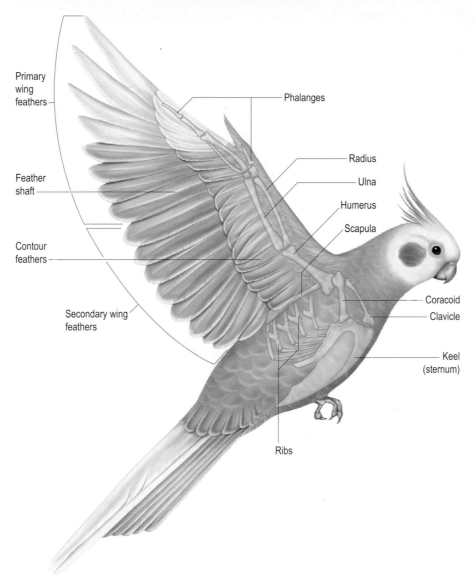

Fig. 5.7 Bird in flight showing the structure of the wing. Thrust is provided by outer primaries; lift is provided by inner primaries and secondaries

tendons run down the back of the leg. The digital flexor tendon runs in a groove at the top of the tarsometatarsus and supplies each of the digits. As the bird bends its leg to perch the tendon is pulled taut and the toes flex and tighten the hold on the branch. This is the perching reflex and is the reason why birds can sleep on a branch without falling off.

Integument

The integument of the bird consists of skin and its derivatives – the claws, beak and feathers. The structure of the skin and its associated glands is similar to that of the dog and cat and the claws and the beak are made of a tough horn that grows throughout the bird's life. However, it is the feathers that are the distinctive characteristic of the bird family.

Feathers derive from epidermal cells in a similar way to the hairs of mammals. They are made of keratin and have several functions. They:

- Form a waterproof covering that protects the thin skin from physical and chemical damage
- Create a smooth outer covering to the wing that cannot be penetrated by air, enabling the downward force of the wing to bring about lift
- Provide insulation of the body
- Provide camouflage
- Are involved in communication between birds of the same species.

All feathers have a similar structure, consisting of a central shaft or rachis that is filled with blood capillaries during growth but later becomes hollow (Fig. 5.8). The shaft gives off the flattened vane, which consists of barbs and interlocking barbules that hook together to produce a wind-resistant surface. It is essential that the feathers are kept in good condition and a healthy bird will constantly preen itself and apply sebum obtained from the preen gland at the base of

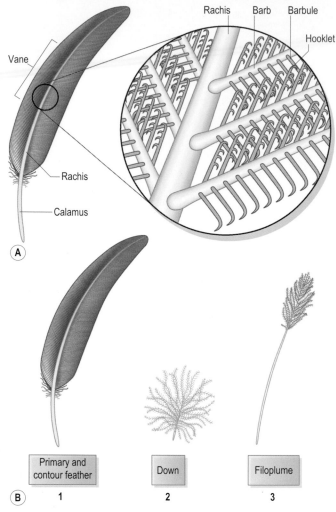

Fig. 5.8 (**A**) Feather structure and (**B**) types of feather

the tail to the feathers. This helps to 'zip up' the barbules and makes the feathers waterproof.

There are four main types of feather (Fig. 5.8):

- **Flight** – long rigid feathers attached to the wing and tail. The primaries are attached to digit 3 and to the fused metacarpals bones. The major thrust of the down beat is provided by the outer primaries. The shorter secondaries are attached to the ulna and, in combination with the inner primaries, provide lift during flight.
- **Contour** – cover the rest of the wing and may be known as coverts. They create a smooth cover over the body. They are shorter and more flexible than the flight feathers and the lowest part closest to the body may be fluffier.
- **Down** – lie close to the body underneath the contour feathers, forming an insulating layer.
- **Filoplume** – also lie close to the body. Designed to break up and form feather dust, which absorbs dirt and moisture, helping to keep the bird clean. Both down and filoplume feathers are barbless, so they look fluffy (Fig. 5.8).

Respiratory system

The metabolic rate and the energy level of the bird are high so the body has a high demand for oxygen and for the removal of carbon dioxide. To satisfy this, the respiratory system is adapted to supply oxygen as the bird flies both at speed and at high altitudes.

There are three main differences between the respiratory system of the bird and that of the mammal:

- There is no diaphragm dividing the body cavity into thorax and abdomen
- The lungs are more rigid and do not expand as they fill with air
- Air sacs extend from the lung tissue and fill every spare space within the body cavity and in the medullary cavity of bones such as the femur and humerus.

Respiratory tract

Air enters the body via the nostrils and the beak and passes into the glottis on the floor of the oral cavity. Air entering via the nostrils passes from the nasal chambers into the oral cavity via a cleft in the hard palate known as the choana. The glottis is surrounded by a complex larynx, which controls the passage of air down the trachea but plays no part in the production of sound.

The trachea consisting of cartilaginous rings linked by muscle and connective tissue runs down the neck to a point above the sternum where it enlarges to form the syrinx. This contains muscles, air sacs and vibrating membranes and is the 'voice box' of the bird. The enormous variation in birdsong depends upon the number of muscles within the syrinx, which is dependent on the species. Just distal to the syrinx the trachea bifurcates into two bronchi, which pass along the ventral side of each lung, ending in the posterior air sacs. Within the lung tissue the bronchi lose their cartilaginous rings and are known as mesobronchi. These give rise to four to six ventrobronchi which further divide to form parabronchi. The parabronchi are connected to air capillaries, which are surrounded by pulmonary blood capillaries, and it is here that gaseous exchange takes place. Gaseous exchange is a similar process to that seen in mammals.

Leading from the various bronchi are thin-walled air sacs. These are covered in minute capillaries and account for 80% of the respiratory volume. Most birds have nine pairs of air sacs (Fig. 5.9), which fill the spaces within the body cavity and penetrate into the insides of many bones. They are not involved in gaseous exchange but act as a reservoir for air and have a bellows-like effect that helps to push the air back through the lungs. They also reduce the weight of the skeleton, so aiding flight and the buoyancy of water birds.

The lungs containing the different bronchi are bright red, vascular and quite rigid and are attached to the thoracic vertebrae and ribs in the dorsal part of the body cavity. The volume of the lungs is only 2% of the total body volume.

Respiration

Air flows through the lungs and air sacs via the following route:

1. The bird inspires by muscular expansion of the body cavity, which reduces the pressure within the respiratory

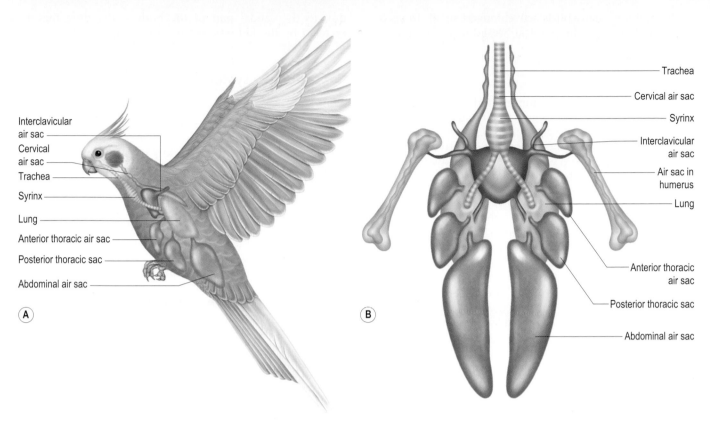

Interclavicular air sac
Cervical air sac
Trachea
Syrinx
Lung
Anterior thoracic air sac
Posterior thoracic sac
Abdominal air sac

(A)

Trachea
Cervical air sac
Syrinx
Interclavicular air sac
Air sac in humerus
Lung
Anterior thoracic air sac
Posterior thoracic sac
Abdominal air sac

(B)

Fig. 5.9 Respiratory system of a bird

tract and air is drawn in; most of the air is drawn into the posterior air sacs where it is warmed and moistened.

2. The bird expires and the air is pushed from the posterior air sacs into the lung tissue where gaseous exchange takes place.

3. The bird inspires again and the air moves out of the lungs into the anterior air sacs.

4. The bird expires again and the air leaves the anterior air sacs and exits the body via the trachea.

In order to make use of one 'unit' of air the bird has two inspirations and two expirations. Fresh air follows a one-way path and does not get mixed with the air containing carbon dioxide. This allows almost all the oxygen within the inspired atmospheric air (21%) to reach the capillaries and it is thought that the respiratory system of the bird is about 10 times more efficient than that of the mammal.

Digestive system

The digestive system is very efficient and enables the energy in food to be used rapidly to satisfy the high metabolic rate of the bird.

The basic plan of the digestive tract is similar to that in other groups of animal but there are certain modifications.

Oral cavity

A lightweight beak replaces the lips and teeth. Its shape varies with the species and is adapted to the type of diet. In most species the tongue is not very mobile but in members of the parrot family it is large and fleshy and is used to move food around for easy swallowing. Most birds have salivary glands, which secrete saliva consisting of mucus and a starch-digesting enzyme. Those species eating dry food such as seeds have many glands while those eating a wetter diet such as fish have very few.

Oesophagus and crop

Food passes down the muscular oesophagus on the right side of the neck into a diverticulum known as the crop. This lies outside the body cavity and is mainly used for food storage. Its size varies according to the species – granivorous birds have large, bilobular crops while species such as the insectivores and the owls have no crop. Some species, particularly members of the pigeon family, secrete 'crop milk' from the lining to feed their young. This is rich in proteins and fat and is stimulated by the hormone prolactin.

Stomach

This is divided into two parts:

• Proventriculus – lined by an epithelium, which secretes mucus, hydrochloric acid and pepsin; here food is stored, mixed with these digestive juices and protein digestion begins.

• Gizzard – the walls are lined with bands of muscle that contract and expand to grind up the harder components of the diet such as seeds, bones and scales;

in addition, many birds actively ingest small stones or grit to help with the physical breakdown of food in the gizzard.

Small intestine

Consists of a duodenum, jejunum and ileum that are not clearly delineated. The duodenum is the major site of digestion and absorption. The pancreas is relatively large and lies in the loop of the duodenum, pouring its secretions into the lumen of the duodenum via three ducts. The liver is bilobed; the right lobe is usually larger than the left.

Large intestine

Consists of a pair of blind-ending caeca, which lie at the junction of the small and large intestines. Their function seems to be associated with the bacterial fermentation of cellulose and the reabsorption of water, and their presence varies with the diet of the species. The rest of the large intestine, whose main role is concerned with water and mineral reabsorption, is the relatively short length between the small intestine and the cloaca.

Cloaca

This is the common exit from the body shared by the digestive, urinary and reproductive systems. It is divided into three parts:

- Coprodeum – anterior part, which receives faeces from the intestine.
- Urodeum – middle part, which collects the discharge from the kidney and the reproductive system.
- Proctodeum – posterior part, which collects and stores the discharges from all three systems. It is closed by a muscular anus, which controls the passage of 'bird droppings' or mutes and, in the case of the hen bird, the passage of eggs out of the body. In the wall of the cloaca is an area of lymphoid tissue known as the bursa of Fabricius.

Urinary system

The function of the urinary system, which consists of a pair of kidneys and a pair of ureters but no bladder, is the same as that in the mammal. However, birds excrete nitrogenous waste in the form of uric acid and urates rather than the familiar mammalian urea. The waste materials are suspended in urinary water rather than being dissolved and the resulting semi-solid urine leaves the kidneys via the ureters. It enters the urodeum of the cloaca and then passes by retroperistalsis into the large intestine, where more water is reabsorbed. The resulting mutes consist of white urates, greeny-brown faeces surrounded by clear urine.

Birds, like reptiles, possess a renal portal system. This consists of a valve at the junction of the common iliac vein with the renal portal vein that enters the kidney. The valve consists of a muscular sphincter that opens and closes in response to nervous stimulation – when it is closed blood flows into the kidney and when it is open blood bypasses the kidney and flows into the caudal vena cava. This may be of significance when administering medication by injection to the caudal part of the body – the drug may be excreted by the kidneys without reaching the cranial parts of the body.

Reproductive system

Male

The two bean-shaped testes lie within the body cavity and are connected to the urodeum of the cloaca by the vas deferens. In many species the left testis is much larger than the right and in the non-breeding season both may be relatively small. The anatomy and physiology of the system is similar to that of mammals except that the seminal fluid needed to wash the sperm along the tract is produced by the testes rather than by accessory glands. At the distal end of each vas deferens is a seminal vesicle, which acts as a storage organ for the sperm prior to their use.

Sperm is transferred into the female vagina either by means of the grooved erectile penis attached to the wall of the cloaca in species such as geese, ducks, storks and flamingos or, as in most other species, by the male and female simply bringing their cloacae close together.

Female

The tract consists of a pair of ovaries and oviducts, which lead to the cloaca. In most species the right side is rudimentary and in the non-breeding season the left ovary may be quite small. The ovum is released by the ovary and begins to pass down the tubular oviduct, which is divided into several different parts:

- Infundibulum – funnel-shaped opening, which engulfs the ovum, preventing it falling into the body cavity; fertilization takes place here and the first layer of albumen is added
- Magnum – glandular part, which adds the remaining albumen
- Isthmus – walls are lined by layers of thick circular muscle; inner and outer shell membranes are added
- Uterus or shell gland – walls are lined by thick layers of longitudinal muscle lined with goblet cells; the egg spends as much as 15 hours in this part while the shell and any pigmentation is added
- Vagina – mucus is secreted to aid egg laying and sperm from the male may also be stored for several days.

The female bird lays her eggs in a clutch and then begins incubation. The number within the clutch and the number of clutches per year varies with the species of bird. Many species lay one egg per day while others, such as ducks and geese, lay every other day. During incubation the eggs must be kept warm and damp – the average temperature is 35°C. The bird will also turn the eggs at regular intervals using her feet. This prevents the embryo from sticking to the side of the shell, which may impair the development of the chick. Incubation times vary with the species. Smaller birds have short incubation times: for example, many passerines hatch their eggs within 14–21 days, while larger birds such as hawks have an incubation time of around 30 days. The young may be described as being:

- **Nidicolous**, i.e. they are featherless and blind and dependent on the parent birds until fledged; for

example, young pigeons (known as squabs), robins and sparrows
- **Nidifugous**, i.e. they are covered in down feathers, eat adult food and are capable of surviving away from their mother; for example, ducklings, goslings and chicks.

Reptiles

Reptiles are members of the class Reptilia and as such are cold-blooded vertebrates that breed on land. They are dependent on the external environment to raise their internal body temperature and increase their metabolic rate. To do this they alter their behaviour patterns and will seek out warm spots or flatten themselves on the ground in order to increase the surface area exposed to the sun.

There are about 6500 species, which can be classified into four separate orders:

- Rhynchocephalia – includes the tuatara, which is rare and unlikely to be encountered as a captive pet
- Crocodilia – crocodiles and alligators – rarely kept as pets
- Squamata – further divided into suborder Sauria (lizards), suborder Serpentes (snakes) and suborder Amphisbaenia, members of which are not kept in captivity
- Chelonia – shelled reptiles, which includes the tortoises, terrapins and turtles.

All the orders of reptiles have a common evolutionary pathway so they share many anatomical features. For the purposes of this book the common features will be described and followed by the notable characteristics of each group.

General anatomy

Skeletal system

Reptiles are vertebrates and have an internal skeleton that in most cases follows a similar pattern to that of the mammal.

Integument

Reptilian skin is covered in thick, keratinized protective scales. They grow by moulting or shedding this covering of scales in a process known as ecdysis. The underlying new skin is soft and enables the body to expand rapidly until the replacement scales harden. Snakes usually shed their skin in one piece, wriggling backwards out of it, while lizards shed their skin in several pieces, many of which may then be eaten. The integument of the chelonians is modified into a tough outer shell.

Cardiovascular system

All reptiles have a heart that comprises two atria and one ventricle. This is functionally divided into three subchambers and receives blood from both atria. Reptiles also possess a renal portal system that is similar to that seen in the bird. Blood from the hind legs and tail may drain directly into the kidneys, so any drug injected into the hind end may be excreted via the kidneys without circulating around the fore end.

Respiratory system

Reptiles use oxygen taken from atmospheric air. They possess lungs but they do not have a diaphragm so the body cavity is not divided into two. Gaseous exchange takes place in the same way that it does in the mammal.

Digestive tract

The anatomy of the digestive tract varies with the species and with the type of diet on which the animal depends. Many species possess a specialized olfactory organ in the roof of the oral cavity that is known as Jacobsen's organ. This is used in conjunction with the tongue, which 'tastes' the environment by flicking in and out of the mouth and is then drawn across the organ. Information is then conveyed to the brain via branches of the olfactory nerve. In all species the tract ends in a cloaca. As in the bird this is divided into the coprodeum to collect faeces, the urodeum to collect urinary waste and the proctodeum, which is the final collecting chamber before elimination of the combined waste.

Urinary system

The paired kidneys do not have loops of Henle, which means that the excreted urine is very dilute. Snakes do not possess a bladder but this is present in lizards and chelonians.

Reproductive system

All reptiles lay eggs, i.e. they are oviparous, and the yolk within the egg provides nourishment for the developing embryo. Some species of reptile are ovoviviparous, which means that they appear to give birth to live young. In fact the egg is retained within the oviduct and hatches to release the young. Nutrition is still supplied to the young via the yolk and not via a placenta, as happens in mammals.

Lizards

Most lizards (Fig. 5.10) have four legs, which are attached to the body at right angles and allow the body to be raised off the ground. The tail is well defined and some species are able to shed their tail as a defence against predators. This process, known as autotomy, means that once the tail has been shed it continues to squirm, diverting the predator's attention while the lizard escapes.

The skin is thick and scaly and its texture varies according to the species. Some lizards, such as the skinks, have scales that fit tightly together, creating a smooth outline, while others are covered in much thicker and more protective scales. Species such as the chameleons have cells known as chromatophores within the skin that are able to alter the colour of the skin and thus camouflage the lizard. The gecko family has layers of overlapping scales on the underside of their feet which enable them to grip on to apparently smooth surfaces such as glass.

Digestive system

Most species have teeth that are fused to the sides of the mandible and are shed and replaced at intervals. The shape

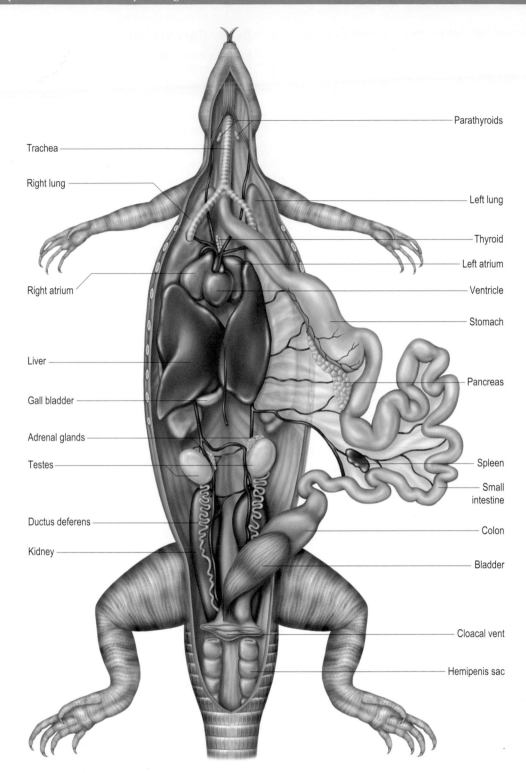

Fig. 5.10 Internal anatomy of the male lizard

of the tongue varies with the species and is used in conjunction with Jacobsen's organ. The diet may be herbivorous, insectivorous, carnivorous or omnivorous depending on the species. The stomach is simple (Fig. 5.10) and in herbivorous species the caecum is enlarged to facilitate plant digestion.

Urinogenital system

Males possess paired copulatory organs known as hemipenes, each of which lies invaginated within the base of the tail posterior to the cloaca. Only one hemipenis is used during mating, when it is erected by filling with blood and inserted into the cloaca of the female. Females have a pair

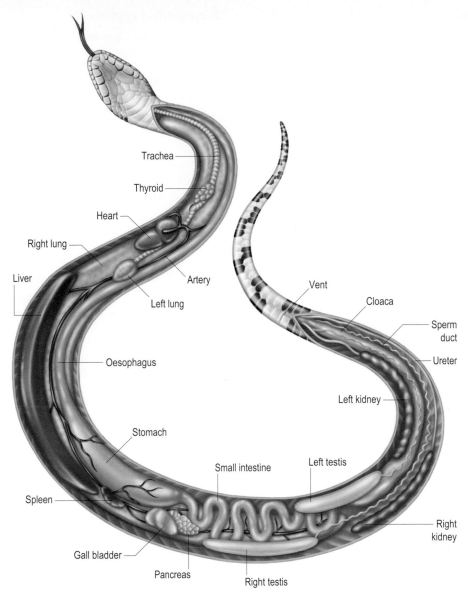

Fig. 5.11 Internal anatomy of the snake

of ovaries, which produce the ova, which are transported out of the body via the paired oviducts and the cloaca. Most species of lizard have a bladder.

Snakes

Snakes have long bodies that taper into their tails, the start of which is in the area of the vent. They have no legs, although some species such as the boas and the pythons possess vestigial pelvic limbs, which are manifested as spurs on the external surface. The skeleton consists of as many as 400 similar-shaped vertebrae, each one giving off a pair of ribs. There is no sternum, so the ribs are not joined in the midline.

Integument

This is covered in scales, which vary in shape according to the area of the body. The ventral scales are larger and thicker, while those in the dorsal and lateral parts are much smaller. The scales on the ventral surface project outwards and, as the muscles of the body wall contract and expand, the scales exert pressure on the surface and pull the snake forwards with an undulating movement. The eyelids of the snake are transparent and fused together to form the spectacle. During ecdysis when the outer layer of scales lifts off and is discarded, the spectacle also lifts off the surface of the eye and comes away as part of the shed skin.

Respiratory system

In order to fit inside the long, thin body, the left lung of most snakes is reduced or absent (Fig. 5.11). Gaseous exchange takes place in the anterior part of the right lung; the remainder is avascular and acts as an air sac and a reservoir of air, which may be needed during periods of apnoea.

Digestive system

All snakes are carnivorous. There are six rows of teeth, which are fused to the mandibles and replaced continuously. Some species have modified fangs connected to poison glands above the oral cavity and used to inject venom into the prey. The forked tongue is used to 'taste' the environment and is used in conjunction with Jacobsen's organ. The stomach is elongated and the intestines are relatively short. The organs are arranged in an elongated fashion to fit into the thin body (Fig. 5.11).

Urinogenital system

Male snakes have hemipenes, which are folded into the base of the tail. During mating the hemipenis evaginates and is inserted into the cloaca of the female. The females of slender species have only one ovary and oviduct.

Tortoises, terrapins and turtles

This group of chelonians, which is characterized by the presence of a horny outer shell, encompasses the land-living tortoises, the fresh-water terrapins and the marine turtles. In the USA they are all referred to as turtles. Tortoises have limbs that enable them to walk on land while terrapins and turtles have limbs that are primarily adapted for swimming. The shell forms a box to protect the internal organs and consists of a domed upper part, known as the carapace, and a flattened ventral part, known as the plastron. The shell develops from keratinized epidermal cells, forming a series of horny plates or scutes (Fig. 5.12), which are named according to their most adjacent organ. Growth is not brought about by shedding of the horny epidermis, as it is in other reptiles, but occurs by the deposition of epidermal cells around the perimeter of each scute, forming annual rings that can be counted to assess the age of the animal.

Skeletal system

This follows the pattern of all vertebrates except that the pectoral and pelvic girdles are within the rib cage and are directed vertically to support the shell (Fig. 5.12). The vertebral column, comprising ten vertebrae, forms the undersurface of the carapace.

Respiratory system

The lungs lie in the dorsal part of the body cavity and aid buoyancy in aquatic species. As the shell is rigid, the body is unable to expand during respiration. This is brought about by movements of the head and limbs, which move in and out, changing the internal pressure of the body cavity, thus drawing air in or pushing it out.

Digestive system

All chelonians possess a horny beak instead of teeth. The tongue is large and fleshy. The oesophagus lies on the left side of the neck, entering a simple stomach that lies across the body cavity (Fig. 5.12).

Urinogenital system

A pair of kidneys produce relatively unconcentrated urine, which is transported by a pair of ureters into a thin-walled bladder. Males have a single large penis, which is able to protrude from the floor of the cloaca.

Fish

Fish are cold blooded vertebrates that are adapted to live in water, from which they extract the oxygen needed for their metabolism. There are approximately 30 000 species of fish, which can be divided into two main groups:

- Cartilaginous fish – comprising the rays and sharks.
- Bony fish – comprising all other species. These can be further subdivided into:
  - Lower teleosts, e.g. carp and salmon
  - Higher teleosts, e.g. perch and mackerel.

Although these bony fish show an enormous range of external shapes and sizes, they all have a similar basic anatomy.

External anatomy

Most species of fish have a typical fusiform shape that enables them to pass through the water with a minimum of energy expenditure. Most fish are covered in flexible, overlapping plates known as scales. Each scale is formed by and is embedded within the dermis, with the free edge covered in a thin layer of epidermis. The scales are covered in a layer of mucus called the glycocalyx, which reduces frictional drag as the fish swims and also has a fungicidal and bactericidal action. The scales contain pigment cells that give the fish its colour and many species are able to change their colour to blend into the background.

The fish is able to swim, manoeuvre and maintain its balance in the water by the presence of flexible fins, which consist of a web of skin supported by bony or cartilaginous rays. Each fin is attached to muscle, enabling the fin to make rapid precise movements. Most fish have seven fins. These are the:

- Caudal fin or tail – shape indicates the swimming pattern
- Dorsal fin – set vertically along the back
- Anal fin – on the underside close to the tail. In some species this is adapted to form the gonopodium, which assists in internal fertilization of the female
- A pair of pectoral fins – set on either side just behind the head
- A pair of pelvic fins – set just below and behind the pectoral fins.

Fish have the range of special senses seen in mammals but in addition they have a lateral line system. This is used to detect vibrations in the water caused by the presence of other fish, which might be prey or predators. It consists of a series of shallow channels running over the surface of the body along the lateral midline. Along the line, arranged at intervals, are groups of hair cells embedded within a cup or cupula. Vibrations cause movement of the hairs, which stimulate nerve impulses, which reach the brain and the appropriate nerve impulse is initiated.

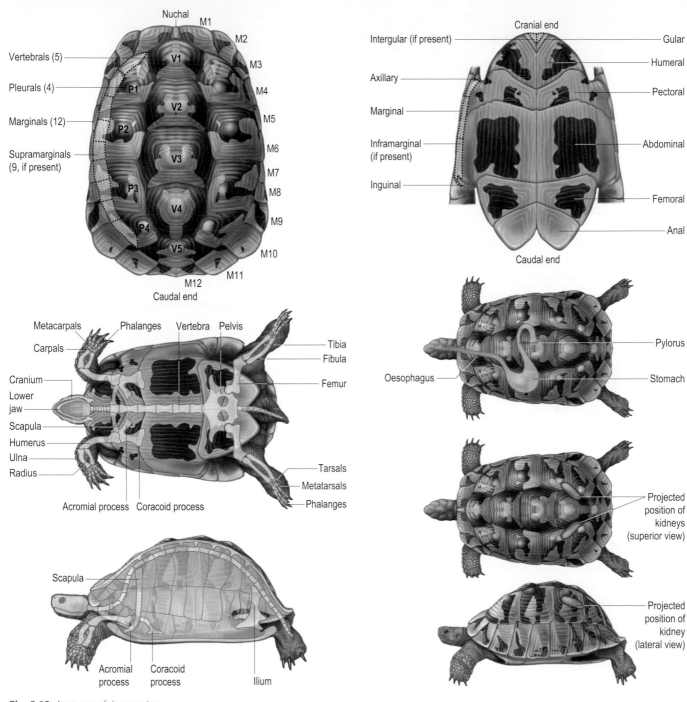

Fig. 5.12 Anatomy of the tortoise

Internal anatomy

Musculoskeletal system

Although the skeleton (Fig. 5.13) appears to be completely different from that of the mammal, it has similar components. The pectoral and pelvic girdles comprise the remnants of the pentadactyl limb (five digits) seen in mammals, birds and reptiles and provide a key to the evolutionary pathway of the fish. The muscles of the body are arranged in blocks or myomeres attached on either side of the axial skeleton. They enable the body to flex laterally, providing the propulsive force to move forward. The number of vertebrae varies with the species. The ribs in the thoracic region articulate with the vertebrae and support the walls of the body cavity.

In order to maintain buoyancy in the water most bony fish possess a swim bladder, which lies just below the vertebral column within the body cavity. The specific gravity of the fish is greater than that of the surrounding water, so it sinks if it stops swimming. This is overcome by altering the volume of gas within the swim bladder and the fish is able to rise or fall according to its needs. The structure of the swim bladder depends on the species of fish:

- Lower teleosts – the swim bladder is said to be physostomous and is a diverticulum of the foregut

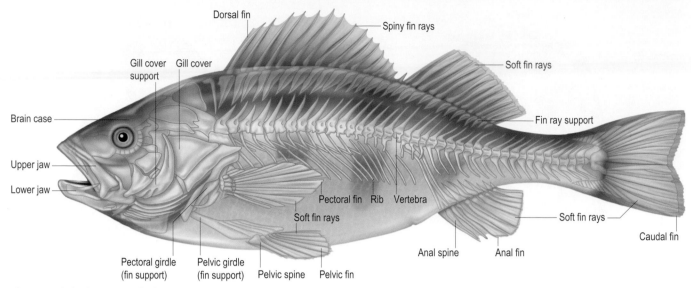

Dorsal fin — Spiny fin rays

Soft fin rays

Gill cover Gill cover
support

Brain case — Fin ray support

Upper jaw —

Lower jaw —

Pectoral fin   Rib   Vertebra

Soft fin rays

Soft fin rays —

Caudal fin

Anal spine   Anal fin

Pectoral girdle   Pelvic girdle
(fin support)   (fin support)   Pelvic spine   Pelvic fin

Fig. 5.13 Skeletal structure of a fish

linked by a pneumatic duct. The swim bladder is refilled by the fish rising to the surface and taking a mouthful of air and is mainly seen in shallow water species.

- Higher teleosts – the swim bladder is said to be physoclistous. There is no connection between the swim bladder and the foregut and depending on the species it is either filled during larval development, when there may be a temporary connection, or it may be filled by specialized cells forming a gas gland within the sac. The secreted gas is mainly carbon dioxide and it is kept in the bladder by an impermeable lining.

In addition to its function as a buoyancy aid the swim bladder acts as resonator for sound, giving the fish a more acute sense of hearing than is provided by its inner ear.

Cardiovascular system

The heart is a long, folded organ consisting of a single atrium and a single ventricle. The circulation is described as being single because blood passes once through the heart in a complete circuit. This is compared to the double circulation of the mammal. Oxygenated blood leaves the ventricle and is pumped to the tissues, where it gives up its oxygen. The blood picks up carbon dioxide from the tissues and is carried to the gills, where it is excreted into the water. At the same time the blood picks up oxygen and is carried to the atrium of the heart.

Respiratory system

Fish breathe using a system of gills (Fig. 5.14). Each gill consists of a bony gill arch supporting the gill filaments. Projecting from these are delicate secondary filaments or lamellae, which contain the blood vessels through which gaseous exchange occurs. On each side of the pharynx are five lateral gill slits through which water drawn in through the mouth passes. The entrance to each gill slit is 'guarded' by stiff projections known as gill rakers, which act as a screen

to filter out food particles which could damage the delicate gills. On the external surface of the head the gills are covered by cartilaginous protective flaps or opercula (sing. operculum). Water is drawn in through the mouth by constant opening and closing, forced into the pharynx, over the gills and out through the opercula. Because of the difference in concentration between the gases in the blood and the water, oxygen dissolved in the water diffuses into the blood and carbon dioxide in the blood is released into the water.

Digestive system

This varies according to the diet of the species. Predatory species have teeth on the front and the roof of the mouth and they may also have throat teeth just in front of the oesophagus. These are mainly used to hold the prey and position it ready for swallowing head first. Some species have teeth for biting; others have teeth to rasp food from rocks; while others have no teeth at all. Ingested food travels down the oesophagus into a tube-like stomach and then into an intestine of uniform diameter. The length depends on the type of diet, herbivorous species having the longest intestine. Faeces are evacuated from the body via the rectum and anus.

Urinary system

The kidneys lie below the vertebral column and in some species may sit like a saddle over the swim bladder. They have several functions, e.g. haemopoiesis, excretion, osmoregulation and secretion of hormones. Nitrogenous waste is excreted in the form of ammonia, which is extremely toxic and is only excreted by organisms that live in a watery environment where it can flow away. The main site for excretion is the gills, not the kidneys as occurs in mammals.

Reproductive system

Among the huge number of fish species there are examples of a range of reproductive patterns, including parthenogen-

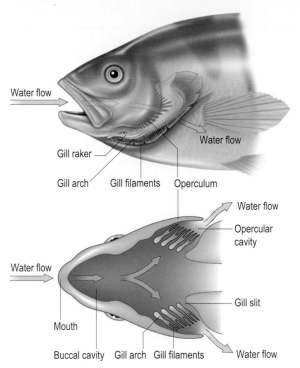

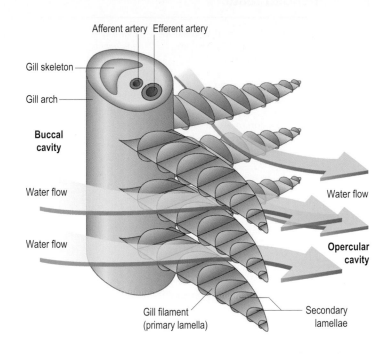

Fig. 5.14 The gill system of the fish

esis and hermaphroditism. However, the majority of teleosts have separate sexes. Fertilization may be:

- Internal – the male introduces the sperm into the female. She retains the fertilized eggs in her body until they hatch to produce live young.
- External – the female lays her eggs in the water and the male adds his sperm or milt in a process known as

spawning. Many of these eggs and sperm are lost so millions are produced. The eggs may then be scattered or deposited in a nest or in the mud on the river bed. Some species are mouth brooders and incubate the eggs in the mouth. This is often done by the male and once the young are hatched they may continue to use the mouth as a refuge from predators.

Bibliography

Aspinall, V., O'Reilly, M., 2003. Introduction to Veterinary Anatomy and Physiology. Butterworth-Heinemann, Oxford.

Beynon, P. (Ed.), 1996. Manual of Psittacine Birds. British Small Animal Veterinary Association, Cheltenham.

Beynon, P.H., Lawton, M.P.C., Cooper, J.E., 1992. Manual of Reptiles. British Small Animal Veterinary Association, Cheltenham.

Bowden, C., Masters, J. (Eds.), 2001. Pre-veterinary Nursing Textbook. Butterworth-Heinemann, Oxford.

Butcher, R.L. (Ed.), 2001. Manual of Ornamental Fish. British Small Animal Veterinary Association, Gloucester.

Colville, T., Bassett, J.M., 2002. Clinical Anatomy and Physiology for Veterinary Technicians. Mosby, St Louis, MO.

Cooper, J.E., 2002. Birds of Prey – Health and Disease. Blackwell Scientific Publications, Oxford.

Cooper, B., Lane, D.R. (Eds.), 1999. Veterinary Nursing, second ed. Butterworth-Heinemann, Oxford.

Dyce, K.M., Sack, W.O., Wensing, C.J.G., 1996. Textbook of Veterinary Anatomy, second ed. W B Saunders, Philadelphia.

Flecknell, P. (Ed.), 2000. Manual of Rabbit Medicine and Surgery. British Small Animal Veterinary Association, Quedgeley.

Harvey Pough, F., Heiser, J.B., McFarland, W.N., 1993. Vertebrate Life, third ed. Macmillan, Basingstoke.

Hillyer, E.V., Quesenberry, K.E., 1997. Ferrets, Rabbits and Rodents – Clinical Medicine and Surgery. W B Saunders, Philadelphia, PA.

King, A.S., McClelland, J., 1984. Birds – Their Structure and Function. Baillière Tindall, London.

Laber-Laird, K., Swindle, M.M., Flecknell, P. (Eds.), 1996. Handbook of Rodent and Rabbit Medicine. Pergamon, Oxford.

McArthur, S., 1996. Veterinary Management of Tortoises and Turtles. Blackwell Science, Oxford.

Mader, D.R., 1996. Reptile Medicine and Surgery. W B Saunders, Philadelphia, PA.

Meredith, A., Redrobe, S. (Eds.), 2002. Manual of Exotic Pets, fourth ed. British Small Animal Veterinary Association, Quedgeley.

Okerman, L., 1994. Diseases of Domestic Rabbits. Blackwell Scientific, Oxford.

Phillips, W.D., Chilton, T.J., 1989. A-level Biology. Oxford University Press, Oxford.

Roberts, R.J. (Ed.), 2001. Fish Pathology, third ed. W B Saunders, Philadelphia, PA.

Sturkie, P.D. (Ed.), 1976. Avian Physiology. Springer Verlag, New York.

Warren Dean, M., 1995. Small Animal Care and Management. Delmar, New York.

Recommended reading

Aspinall, V., Capello, M., 2009. Introduction to Veterinary Anatomy and Physiology, second ed. Butterworth-Heinemann, Oxford.

This book provides three chapters on exotic animal anatomy and physiology.

Aspinall, V., Bowden, S., Capello, M., 2009. Introduction to Veterinary Anatomy and Physiology – Flashcards and Workbook. Butterworth-Heinemann, Oxford.

Fun way to revise your knowledge of exotic anatomy using flashcards and a wide variety of games and tests.

Colville, T., Bassert, J.M., 2002. Clinical Anatomy and Physiology for Veterinary Technicians. Mosby, London.

Very detailed coverage of the anatomy of the bird.

Cooper, B., Lane, D.R. (Eds.), 2007. Veterinary Nursing, fourth ed. BSAVA, Gloucester.

New chapter on exotic anatomy.

Hillyer, E.V., Quesenberry, K.E., 1997. Ferrets, Rabbits and Rodents – Clinical Medicine and Surgery. W B Saunders, Philadelphia, PA.

Each section begins with detailed descriptions of the relevant anatomy and physiology.

CHAPTER 6

Equine anatomy and physiology

Catherine Phillips

Key Points

- All species of horse belong to the class Mammalia and as such they have much in common with other mammals, e.g. respiratory system, urinary system, structure of the integument, etc.
- The horse has evolved the ability to run fast for long distances and this is reflected in the anatomy and physiology of its skeleton and muscular system.
- Horses are adapted to eating relatively poor-quality roughage over long periods of the day and this is reflected in the anatomy and physiology of their digestive tract.

Introduction

In Chapter 4 we looked at the anatomy and physiology of the dog and cat, which, as they are mammals, show many similarities to those of the horse so in this chapter we will only look at the systems in which there are differences.

The horse has evolved from a small multitoed animal, *Eohippus,* into the creature that we know today with a specialized digestive tract to allow the consumption of grass and grains and a single-digit elongated limb which enables the horse to make a rapid escape from predators. Knowledge and understanding of these complex anatomical and physiological structures are essential to allow us to plan the management and nursing of this species.

The skeletal system

The skeleton (Fig. 6.1) can be divided into two main sections:

- The axial skeleton – made up of the skull, the vertebral column, ribcage and pelvis
- The appendicular skeleton – made up of the bones of the limbs.

The skeleton is a framework of hard structures creating strength and rigidity that will support and protect the soft tissues, facilitate movement and allow locomotion. Note that there is no splanchnic skeleton in the horse as there is in the dog and cat.

The axial skeleton

The skull

The skull is constructed of a large number of bones joined by fibrous joints or sutures that allow little movement between them (Fig. 6.2). The main function of the skull is to protect the brain, inner ear, parts of the eye and nasal passages.

The major part of this structure comprises the following bones:

- The mandible (the lower jaw)
- The maxilla, incisive and palatine bones (the upper jaw, hard palate and base of the nasal cavity)
- The nasal bone (completing the nasal cavity)
- The frontal bone (forming the rostral section of the cranium)
- The supraorbital process (supporting and protecting the eye)
- The temporal bone (containing and protecting the middle ear)
- The occipital bone (forming the back of the skull)
- The hyoid bones (constitutes the apparatus that supports the guttural pouches, pharynx, larynx and base of the tongue).

The nasal septum divides the nasal cavity into two nasal chambers and a bony, membranous septum divides the maxillary sinus into rostral and caudal compartments. The maxillary sinus communicates with the nasal cavity through an opening into the middle nasal meatus.

Teeth

Dental formula:

Deciduous teeth – (I3/3 PM3/3) × 2 = 24

Permanent teeth – (I3/3 C1/1 PM3/3 or 4/3 M3/3) × 2 = 40 or 42

The roots of premolar teeth 4 and molar 1 extend into the rostral maxillary sinus and the last two cheek teeth, i.e.

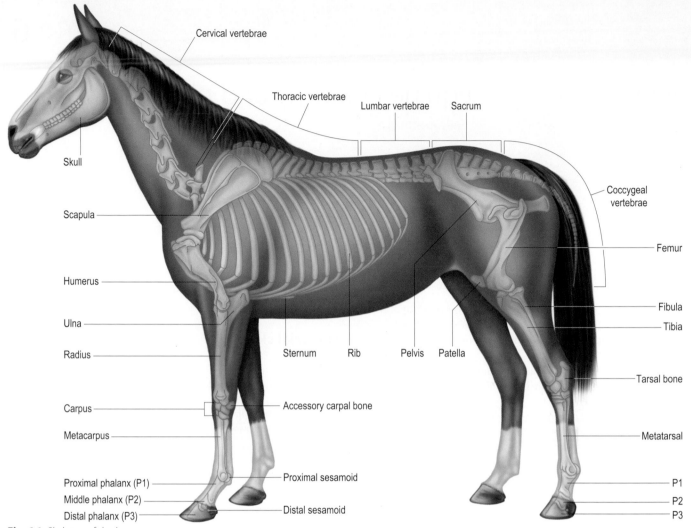

Fig. 6.1 Skeleton of the horse

molars 2 and 3, communicate with the floor of the caudal maxillary sinus. If these teeth suffer injury or infection, then infection of the sinus may also occur.

The horse has hypsodontic teeth, i.e. they do not have a surface covering of enamel and they are all of the same height (Fig. 6.4). This creates an abrasive surface necessary for the grinding up of plant material and includes vast reserve crowns that allow the teeth to continually grow for some years, ensuring a long working life. As the horse chews, the occlusal surfaces are worn down by about 2–3 mm a year. The extent of wear and the appearance of the occlusal surface of the tooth can be used to identify the approximate age of the horse (Fig. 6.3).

Canine teeth may not be present or may be vestigial in the mare. The wolf tooth is a small upper premolar that is often extracted to prevent interference with the bit during training.

The vertebral column

The vertebral column (Fig. 6.1) is made up of groups of vertebra as seen in the dog and cat. The functions of the vertebra are to house the spinal cord, support the skull and thorax and provide attachment for the pelvis and insertion of many of the muscles.

There are five different types of vertebra (Fig. 6.5), making up the column as follows:

- Cervical vertebrae – 7 bones, the first 2 being the atlas and axis
- Thoracic vertebrae – 18 bones
- Lumbar vertebrae – 6 bones, occasionally 5 or 7 are found in some Arabs
- Sacral vertebrae – 5 bones, fused to form a triangular sacrum
- Coccygeal vertebrae – 15–20 (average 18 bones), sometimes called caudal vertebra.

The vertebral formula may be quoted as follows: C7 T18 L6 S5 Cd15–20

The ribs

The horse has eighteen pairs of ribs – the first eight pairs are described as being true, as they articulate directly with the

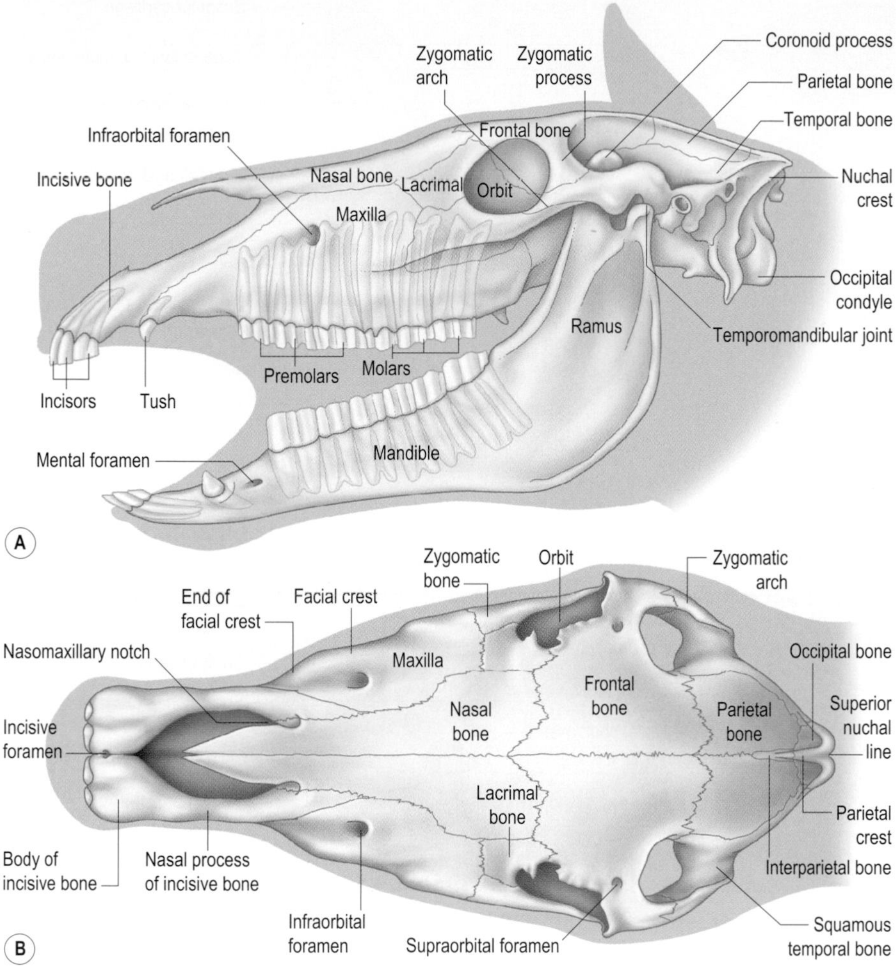

Fig. 6.2 The equine skull. (**A**) Lateral view. (**B**) Dorsal view

Coronoid process

Zygomatic arch

Zygomatic process

Parietal bone

Frontal bone

Temporal bone

Infraorbital foramen

Incisive bone

Nasal bone

Lacrimal

Orbit

Nuchal crest

Maxilla

Occipital condyle

Ramus

Temporomandibular joint

Premolars

Molars

Incisors

Tush

Mental foramen

Mandible

(A)

Zygomatic bone

Orbit

Zygomatic arch

End of facial crest

Facial crest

Nasomaxillary notch

Maxilla

Occipital bone

Nasal bone

Frontal bone

Parietal bone

Superior nuchal line

Incisive foramen

Lacrimal bone

Parietal crest

Body of incisive bone

Nasal process of incisive bone

Interparietal bone

Infraorbital foramen

Supraorbital foramen

Squamous temporal bone

(B)

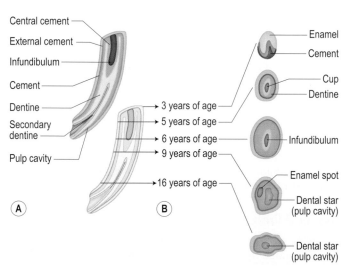

Central cement

External cement

Infundibulum

Cement

Dentine

Secondary dentine

Pulp cavity

Enamel

Cement

Cup

Dentine

3 years of age

5 years of age

6 years of age

9 years of age

16 years of age

Infundibulum

Enamel spot

Dental star (pulp cavity)

Dental star (pulp cavity)

(A)

(B)

Fig. 6.3 (**A**) Longitudinal section through an incisor tooth. (**B**) Cross-sections indicating the appearance of the occlusal surface as the tooth wears down

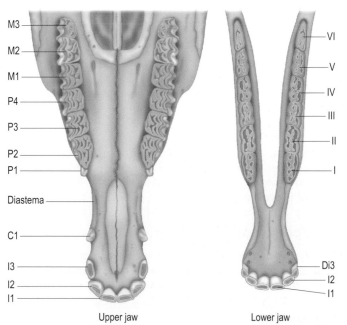

M3

M2

M1

P4

P3

P2

P1

Diastema

C1

I3

I2

I1

VI

V

IV

III

II

I

Di3

I2

I1

Upper jaw

Lower jaw

Fig. 6.4 Teeth in the jaw of a 4 1/2-year-old horse

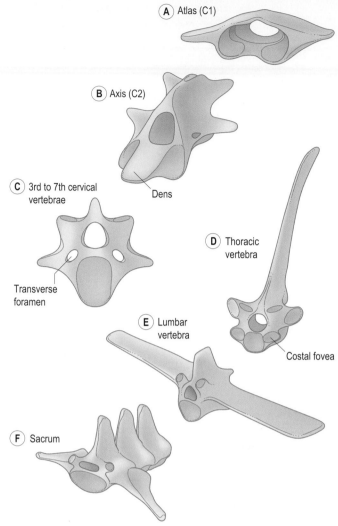

(A) Atlas (C1)

(B) Axis (C2)

(C) 3rd to 7th cervical vertebrae

Dens

Transverse foramen

(D) Thoracic vertebra

(E) Lumbar vertebra

Costal fovea

(F) Sacrum

Fig. 6.5 The shape of each vertebral type – from Aspinall, V., Capello, M., 2009. Introduction to Veterinary Anatomy and Physiology, second ed., page 192. Elsevier, Oxford.

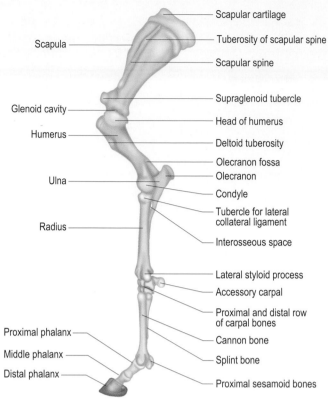

Scapular cartilage

Scapula

Tuberosity of scapular spine

Scapular spine

Glenoid cavity

Supraglenoid tubercle

Head of humerus

Humerus

Deltoid tuberosity

Olecranon fossa

Ulna

Olecranon

Condyle

Tubercle for lateral collateral ligament

Radius

Interosseous space

Lateral styloid process

Accessory carpal

Proximal and distal row of carpal bones

Proximal phalanx

Cannon bone

Middle phalanx

Splint bone

Distal phalanx

Proximal sesamoid bones

Fig. 6.6 Forelimb of the horse

sternum. The remaining ribs are false or asternal, as they articulate with the rib in front to form the costal arch.

The sternum

The sternum forming the ventral surface of the thorax is composed of seven sternebrae. The first sternebra is called the manubrium and the terminal segment is called the xiphoid process or xiphisternum.

The appendicular skeleton

This comprises the limbs, which have been adapted to allow great leverage for the application of speed, and the bony girdles that attach them to the body.

The forelimb

This is attached to the trunk by means of the scapula (Fig. 6.1), which in turn is attached by strong muscles.

The forelimb (Fig. 6.6) comprises the following bones running from proximal to distal:

- The scapula (shoulder blade).
- The humerus.
- The ulna and radius.
- The proximal row of carpal bones (medial to lateral) – radial carpal bone, intermediate carpal bone, ulnar carpal bone, accessory carpal bone (Fig. 6.7).
- The distal row of carpal bones (medial to lateral) – first carpal bone (may be absent), second carpal bone, third carpal bone, fourth carpal bone.
- The metacarpal bones (medial to lateral) – second metacarpal bone, third metacarpal bone, fourth metacarpal bone. The second and fourth metacarpal bones are also called medial and lateral splint bones, respectively.
- The medial and lateral proximal sesamoid bones.
- Proximal phalanx (P1, long pastern).
- Middle phalanx (P2, short pastern).
- Distal sesamoid bone (navicular bone).
- Distal phalanx (P3, pedal bone).

The hind limb

This is attached to the body by means of the pelvic girdle, which is made up of three fused bones:

- Ilium
- Ischium
- Pubis.

The hind limb (Fig. 6.8) comprises the following bones, running from proximal to distal:

- The femur
- The patella

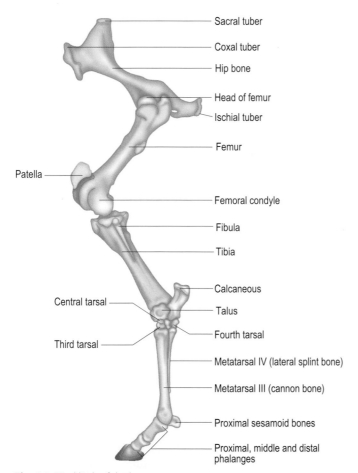

Fig. 6.7 Left carpus of the horse. (**A**) Lateral view. (**B**) Dorsal view

A

Radius

Intermediate carpal bone

Accessory carpal bone

Ulnar carpal bone

III carpal bone

IV carpal bone

III metacarpal bone

IV metacarpal bone

B

Radius

Intermediate carpal bone

Radial carpal bone

Ulnar carpal bone

III carpal bone

IV carpal bone

III metacarpal bone (cannon)

II metacarpal bone (medial splint)

IV metacarpal bone (lateral splint)

Sacral tuber

Coxal tuber

Hip bone

Head of femur

Ischial tuber

Femur

Patella

Femoral condyle

Fibula

Tibia

Calcaneous

Central tarsal

Talus

Fourth tarsal

Third tarsal

Metatarsal IV (lateral splint bone)

Metatarsal III (cannon bone)

Proximal sesamoid bones

Proximal, middle and distal phalanges

Fig. 6.8 Hind limb of the horse

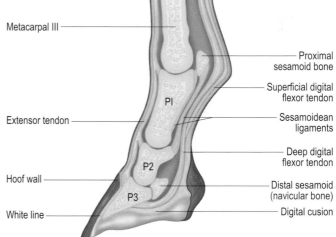

Metacarpal III

Extensor tendon

Hoof wall

White line

PI

P2

P3

Proximal sesamoid bone

Superficial digital flexor tendon

Sesamoidean ligaments

Deep digital flexor tendon

Distal sesamoid (navicular bone)

Digital cusion

Fig. 6.9 Lateral view of the distal part of the forelimb

- The tibia and fibula
- The calcaneus
- The talus
- The central tarsal bone
- The first and second tarsal bones – fused
- The third tarsal bone
- The fourth tarsal bone
- The second metatarsal bone – also known as the medial splint bone
- The third metatarsal bone
- The fourth metatarsal bone – also known as the lateral splint bone
- The medial and lateral proximal sesamoid bones – found on the plantar surface
- Proximal phalanx (P1, long pastern)
- Middle phalanx (P2, short pastern)
- Distal sesamoid bone (navicular bone)
- Distal phalanx (P3, pedal bone).

The foot

The equine foot has a bony base that consists of the distal half of the middle phalanx (short pastern), the complete distal phalanx (pedal bone) and the distal sesamoid (navicular bone) (Fig. 6.9). Several important soft-tissue structures are also housed within the foot, including the digital cushion and the navicular bursa. Covering this is a highly vascular modified dermis called the corium, which is named according to the insensitive structures that it underlies, i.e. perioplic corium, corium of the frog, corium of the sole, etc. (Fig. 6.10). The hoof is the insensitive cornified layer of epidermis

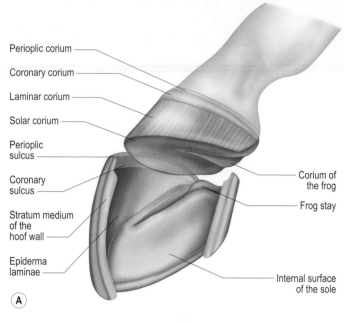

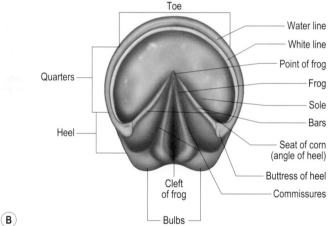

Fig. 6.10 The hoof. (**A**) Dissected view of the relationships of the hoof to the underlying regions of the corium. (**B**) Weight-bearing surface

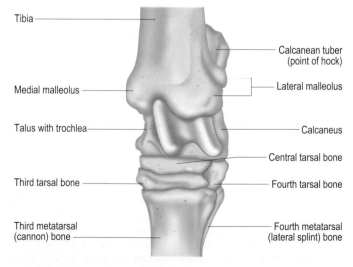

Fig. 6.11 Dorsal view of the left hock

that covers the distal end of the digit. The insensitive structures of the hoof include the periople, wall, bars, laminae, sole and frog. These are all produced by the germinative layer of the epidermis, which lies close to the corium of the same name, which is well supplied with blood capillaries and nerve fibres (Fig. 6.10).

Joints of the fore and hind limbs

The joints of the limbs are extremely important if the horse is going to be able to move fast. Table 6.1 summarizes the anatomy of the major joints of both limbs.

The muscular system

The muscular system brings about movement of the horse. Muscles are often found in pairs, working together with opposite actions, e.g. flexion and extension, which creates coordinated movement and balance (Table 6.2).

The suspensory apparatus

The suspensory apparatus consists of a collection of ligaments connected with the proximal sesamoid bones in both the fore and hind limb, as follows:

- Suspensory ligament
- Intersesamoidean ligament
- Collateral sesamoidean ligament
- Distal sesamoidean ligaments.

This apparatus acts to suspend and support the fetlock joints and prevent overextension and collapsing of the limb. The suspensory apparatus also forms part of the stay apparatus (Fig. 6.12).

The stay apparatus

The stay apparatus consists of an arrangement of muscles, tendons and ligaments in both the fore and hind limbs that allows the horse to stand and sleep while using minimum muscular effort (Fig. 6.12). The apparatus locks the joints in position so that they can bear the weight of the body for long periods. The flexor tendons allow extension to a certain point, in combination with the check ligament to take the work of standing upright away from the muscles. The suspensory ligament will also support weight with minimum effort. In the hind limb the peroneus tertius, flexor tendons and medial patellar ligament, which hooks over the end of the distal femur, lock the limb in a secure position, preventing flexing of the distal limb and stifle.

For more detail of these vital ligamentous structures refer to a more detailed equine anatomy text.

The digestive tract

The physiology of the digestive tract and the process of digestion are covered in more detail in Chapter 9. In this section we will consider the anatomy of the tract. The parts of the tract are the same as those of the dog and cat but as the horse is a herbivore, some of them have different functions (Fig. 6.13, Table 6.3).

Table 6.1 Joints of the fore and hind limbs of the horse

	Fore limb	Hind limb
Shoulder joint	Consists of the glenoid cavity of the scapula and head of the humerus	
Elbow joint	Consists of the condyles of the humerus, radius and ulna	
Carpal joints (knee)	1. Radiocarpal joint – radius and proximal row of carpal bones 2. Midcarpal joint – proximal and distal row of carpal bones 3. Carpometacarpal joint – distal row carpal bones and metacarpal bones 2–4	
Metacarpophalangeal joint (fetlock) or metatarsophalangeal joint	Metacarpal bone III or metatarsal bone III, proximal phalanx P1, medial and lateral proximal sesamoid bones	
Proximal interphalangeal joint (pastern)	Proximal phalanx P1 and middle phalanx P2	
Distal interphalangeal joint (coffin)	Middle phalanx P2, distal phalanx P3 and distal sesamoid bone (navicular)	
Hip joint		Ilium, pubis, ischium all combine to form the acetabulum, head of femur
Stifle joint		1. Femorotibial joint – femur and the medial and lateral condyles of the tibia 2. Femoropatellar joint – femoral trochlea with the patella
Tarsal joint (hock; Fig. 6.11)		1. Tarsocrural joint – cochlea of tibia with trochlea of talus 2. Proximal intertarsal joint – talus and calcaneus with central and fourth tarsal bones 3. Distal intertarsal joint – central tarsal with I–III tarsals 4. Tarsometatarsal joint – I-IV tarsals with II–IV metatarsals

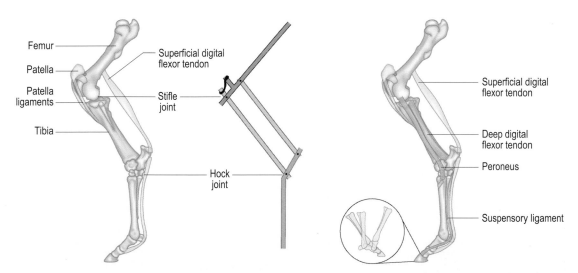

Fig. 6.12 Diagram to show the stay apparatus and the suspensory apparatus of the hind limb. There is a similar mechanism in the forelimb

Oral cavity

The mouth is small but the cavity itself is very deep and is bounded by soft, flexible and sensitive lips. It is formed by the maxilla, incisive and mandibular bones and the hard palate, which is broad and ridged, forms the roof of the mouth. The soft palate extends from the hard palate and is exceptionally long – at rest it hangs down in front of the epiglottis, making mouth breathing difficult and normal vomiting impossible. The tongue is long and broadens out towards its apex. Its upper surface is covered in delicate papillae, which give it a velvety texture. Taste buds are distributed over the tongue and soft palate but their gustatory

Table 6.2 Important muscles, ligaments and tendons of the equine muscular system

Muscle/ligament/tendon	Origin	Insertion	Action
Rhomboideus	Nuchal ligament	Medial scapula	Lifts head and pulls scapula forward and up
Brachiocephalicus	Cranial cervical vertebra	Shoulder to humerus	Protraction of limb, extends shoulder, bending of head and neck
Sternocephalicus	Sternum	Mandible	Moves the head and neck
Splenius	Base of skull	Beginning of trapezius muscle	Lifts head and bends neck
Trapezius	Occipital bone and vertebra C7–T10	Spine of the scapula	Pulls shoulder forward and backward in addition to upward movement
Latissimus dorsi	Lower thoracic and lumbar vertebrae	Caudal humerus	Flexes the shoulder and retracts the forelimb
Longissimus dorsi	Ilium, sacrum and thoracic spine	Cervical spine 4–7, lumbar and thoracic vertebrae, ribs	Raises and supports head lateroflexion and extension of the back
Nuchal ligament	Skull	Cranial thoracic spine	Aids muscles of the neck support the head
Deltoid	Scapula	Proximal humerus	Flexes and abducts shoulder
Supraspinatus	Below the trapezius	Point of the shoulder	Maintains shoulder extension
Pectoral	Sternum and ribs 1–4	Humerus and scapula	Protracts, retracts and adducts limb
Triceps brachii	Scapula and humerus	Olecranon	Extends the elbow
Biceps brachii	Distal scapula	Radius	Flexes the elbow
Extensor carpi radialis	Humerus	Metacarpals	Extends carpus and flexes elbow
Flexor carpi radialis	Humerus	Metacarpal III	Flexes carpus and extends elbow
Common digital extensor tendon	Distal humerus	P1–P3	Extension of P1–P3, carpus and flexion of elbow
Lateral digital extensor tendon (forelimb)	Lateral aspect of the elbow	P1	Extension P1–P3 and carpus
Superficial digital flexor tendon (forelimb)	Medial humerus and posterior radius	Distal P1 and proximal P2	Flexion of P1–P3 and carpus, extension of the elbow
Deep digital flexor tendon (forelimb)	Medial humerus and olecranon	Palmar aspect of P3	Flexion of P1–P3 and carpus and extension of the elbow
Long digital extensor tendon	Distal femur	Dorsal proximal aspects of P1–P3	Extension of distal P1–P3 and flexion of hock
Lateral digital extensor tendon (hindlimb)	Lateral stifle and proximal tibia	Long extensor tendon mid metacarpal III	Extension of distal limb and flexion of hock
Superficial digital flexor tendon (hindlimb)	Distal femur	Tuber calcis, proximal and distal P2	Flexion of distal limb and extension of hock
Deep digital flexor tendon (hindlimb)	Proximal tibia	Palmar aspect P3	Flexion of distal limb and extension of hock
Intercostal muscles	Between ribs	Between ribs	Aids breathing
External and internal abdominal oblique	Ribs	Pelvic bones	Supports internal organs and aids breathing
Superficial gluteal	Tuber coxae	Proximal femur	Hip flexion
Biceps femoris	Sacroiliac ligament, and tuber ischii	Distal femur, patella, tibia crest and tuber calcis	Extension of hip, stifle and hock
Semitendinosus	Tuber ischii and tail base	Proximal tibia	Extends hip and hock

Table 6.2 Continued

Muscle/ligament/tendon	Origin	Insertion	Action
Semimembranosus	Tuber ischii and sacrosciatic ligament	Distal femur	Extends hip and adducts limb
Gastrocnemius	Caudal femur	Point of hock	Maintains hip extension
Peroneus tertius	Femur	Metatarsal III	Flexion of hock when stifle in flexion
Achilles tendon	Distal gastrocnemius	Point of the hock	See Gastrocnemius
Radial check ligament	Distal radius	Proximal superficial flexor tendon	See Superficial digital flexor tendon
Carpal check ligament	Distal carpus	Proximal deep digital flexor tendon	See Deep digital flexor tendon
Tarsal check ligament	Distal tarsus	Proximal deep digital flexor tendon	See Deep digital flexor tendon
Suspensory ligament	Proximal palmar metacarpus	Dorsal extensor tendon at the level of distal P2	Suspends and supports fetlock joint

Table 6.3 Size and function of the parts of the equine digestive tract

Structure	Approximate length or capacity	Function
Oesophagus	1.5 m	Passage of food from mouth to stomach at approximately 35–40 cm per second
Stomach	18 l	Mixing of food with acids, enzymes and mucus; protein digestion
Small intestine	22 m, 64 l	Absorption of nutrients, breakdown of non-fibrous material and addition of pancreatic juices and bile
Caecum	1 m, 30 l	Microbial fibre breakdown into fatty acids and absorption of water
Large colon	3.5 m	Continuation of microbial breakdown of fibre, absorption of water and nutrients
Small colon	2.5 m	Absorption of water and nutrients
Rectum	0.5 m	Transfer of faeces through anus as excreta

function is less efficient than those of the dog and cat. Teeth have been covered within the skeletal system.

Pharynx

The pharynx lies entirely within the skull. Part of the roof and the lateral walls are enveloped by the guttural pouches, which are found only in the horse. They are large caudoventral diverticula of the auditory tube that connect the nasopharynx to the middle ear. Several large and vital blood vessels, e.g. internal carotid artery, and cranial nerves, e.g. glossopharyngeal (IX) and vagus (X), run over their surface. They are lined with mucous membrane and mucus drains from them into the pharynx – the normal downwards position of the head during grazing promotes drainage.

The pharynx is divided into the upper nasopharynx and lower oropharynx by the soft palate. The walls of the oropharynx contain diffuse areas of lymphoid tissue. The function of the pharynx, which acts as a crossover point between the digestive and respiratory systems, is similar to that of the cat and the dog. During swallowing, the back of the tongue raises and pushes the food material against the hard palate while the laryngeal entrance to the respiratory tract is covered with the epiglottis. The movement of these structures creates pressure within the pharynx and the food is forced into the oesophagus. Peristalsis pushes the food material towards the stomach.

Oesophagus

The oesophagus is located close to the trachea on the ventral surface of the neck and slightly to the left of the trachea. The structure passes through the mediastinum and oesophageal hiatus into the stomach.

Stomach

The stomach is a small, J-shaped organ and food enters from the oesophagus via the cardiac sphincter. The oesophageal region of the stomach is similar to the oesophagus in that it does not contain secretory glands. The cardiac and pyloric gland regions contain digestive and mucus glands to initiate the process of protein digestion. The exit of the stomach is

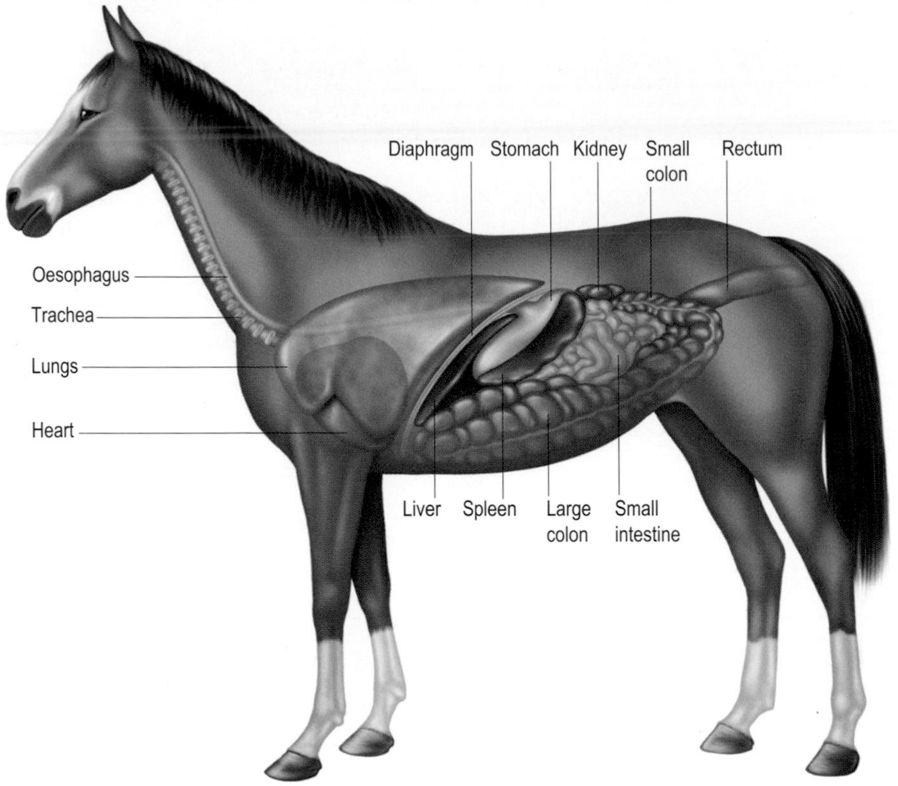

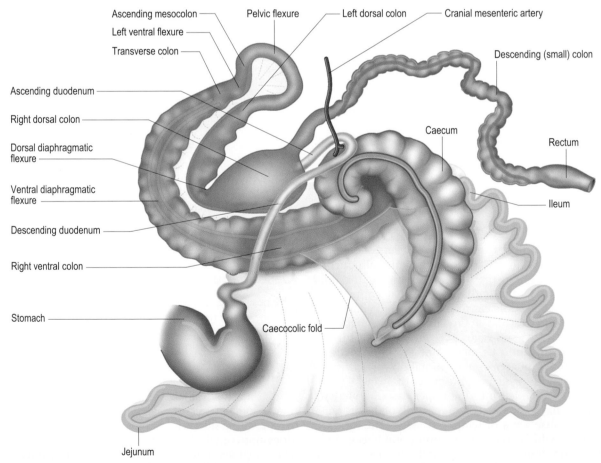

Fig. 6.13 Left lateral view of the equine digestive tract

Diaphragm Stomach Kidney Small colon Rectum

Oesophagus

Trachea

Lungs

Heart

Liver Spleen Large colon Small intestine

Ascending mesocolon Pelvic flexure Left dorsal colon Cranial mesenteric artery

Left ventral flexure

Transverse colon

Descending (small) colon

Ascending duodenum

Right dorsal colon

Dorsal diaphragmatic flexure

Ventral diaphragmatic flexure

Descending duodenum

Right ventral colon

Caecum

Rectum

Ileum

Stomach

Caecocolic fold

Jejunum

Fig. 6.14 Diagrammatic representation of the equine digestive tract

via the pyloric sphincter, which controls the flow of stomach contents into the small intestine.

Small intestine

The small intestine (Fig. 6.13) is a tube which is approximately 22 m in length divided into three regions:

- Duodenum
- Jejunum
- Ileum.

The bile and pancreatic ducts empty into the duodenum close to the pyloric sphincter. The ileum is the terminal section of the small intestine, joining with the caecum of the large intestine at the ileocaecal junction.

Large intestine

The horse has the largest and most complex large intestine of all domestic animals (Fig. 6.14). It has an enormous capacity and consists of:

- Caecum
- Colon
- Rectum.

The walls of the caecum and colon are characteristically sacculated by the presence of bands of muscle and elastic fibres. In order that the large intestine can fit into the relatively small abdominal cavity of the horse it is folded many times and this predisposes to various types of obstruction and displacement, which lead to the group of conditions known as colic. The caecum is a blind-ending, comma-shaped organ that extends from the right side of the pelvic inlet to the abdominal cavity floor just behind the xiphoid cartilage of the sternum (Fig. 6.14). It has a capacity of about 30 litres. It leads into the ascending colon at the caecocolic orifice. The colon is divided into the ascending and transverse colon, which are often referred to as the large colon because of their diameter, and then the descending colon, which is long and arranged in coils and often referred to as the small colon. The descending colon terminates at the rectum.

Bibliography

Budras, K.-D., Sack, W.O., Röck, S., et al., 2003. Anatomy of the Horse, fourth ed. Schlütersche, Hanover.

Budras, K.-D., Sack, W.O., Röck, S., Bragulla, H., Pellmann, R., Reese, S., Coumbe, K., 2001. The Equine Veterinary Nursing Manual. Blackwell Science, Oxford.

Dyce, K.M., Sack, W.O., Wensing, C.J.G., 2002. Textbook of Veterinary Anatomy and Physiology, third ed. W B Saunders, Philadelphia, PA.

Frandson, R.D., Spurgeon, T.L., 1992. Anatomy and Physiology of Farm Animals, fifth ed. Lea & Febiger, Philadelphia, PA.

Sisson, S., Grossman, J.D., 1969. Anatomy of the Domestic Animals, fourth ed. W B Saunders, Philadelphia, PA.

Recommended reading

Aspinall, V., Capello, M., 2009. Introduction to Veterinary Anatomy and Physiology, second ed. Elsevier, Oxford.

This new edition includes a chapter on equine anatomy and physiology.

Aspinall, V., Capello, M., Bowden, S., 2009. Introduction to Veterinary Anatomy and Physiology Revision Aid (Flashcard and Workbook). Elsevier, Oxford.

This provides a fun way of revising anatomy and physiology.

Dyce, K.M., Sack, W.O., Wensing, C.J.G., 2002, Textbook of Veterinary Anatomy and Physiology, third ed. W B Saunders, Philadelphia, PA.

Provides an excellent detailed section on the horse.

Sisson, S., Grossman, J.D., 1969. Anatomy of the Domestic Animals, fourth ed. W B Saunders, Philadelphia, PA.

Old-fashioned but very detailed text and photographs.

Canine and feline nutrition

Alison Jones

Introduction

The correct diet is vital in maintaining health and in the management of disease. Understanding nutrition and its role in both health and disease is an important skill for all qualified veterinary nurses and your advice will frequently be sought by your clients.

Traditionally the breeder, neighbours, friends, relatives, the pet shop owner and even the local supermarket have been a source of advice on feeding. Recently there has been a great increase in public awareness about the relationship between diet and disease, thanks to media interest and to marketing tactics by major manufacturing companies. Few people will not have heard about the alleged health benefits of 'high fibre', 'low fat' and 'low cholesterol' diets.

Breeders have always actively debated the 'best way' to feed dogs and cats. Most owners are aware of the importance of good bone development and the role of nutrition in achieving optimal skeletal characteristics. However, as a veterinary surgeon in practice, I am constantly amazed and bewildered at the menus given by breeders to new puppy owners. These all too frequently consist of complex home-made recipes, usually based on large amounts of fresh meat, goat's milk and a vast array of mineral supplements. These diets are often very unbalanced and could easily result in skeletal and other growth abnormalities.

Domesticated dogs have little opportunity to select their own diet so it is important to realize that they are solely dependent upon their owners to provide all the nourishment they need. Pet cats are less reliant on their owners' dietary selection as they are able, through hunting, to supplement their diet. This chapter will explain the principal components of healthy nutrition to allow you to recommend a balanced diet which avoids both nutritional excess and deficiency. It will look at the practical feeding of dogs and cats of all ages, while giving you an insight into the key nutritional differences between dogs and cats as well as the different types of pet food available commercially.

Essential nutrition

Dogs have a common ancestry with, and are still often classified as, carnivores, although from a nutritional point of view they are actually omnivores. This means that dogs can obtain all the essential nutrients that they need from dietary sources consisting of either animal or plant material. As far as we know, dogs can survive on food derived solely from plants. The same is not true for domesticated cats, which are still obligate carnivores (see Chapter 4).

A nutrient is any food component that helps support life. Any nutrient required by the animal that cannot be synthesized in the body is called an essential nutrient. It must be present in the diet. If any essential nutrient is missing or present in too low a level then the diet as a whole is inadequate.

Nutrients are divided into six basic classes:

- Protein
- Fat
- Carbohydrates
- Minerals
- Vitamins
- Water.

Water

Water is the most important nutrient of all. Animals can lose almost all their fat and half their protein and still survive. A 15% loss of body water would mean death. Good-quality water should always be available except when an animal is persistently vomiting, when temporarily withholding oral fluid intake may be advised. Water intake increases with habit, with increased salt intake and with anything that increases water losses – bleeding, diarrhoea, polyuria, lactation, increased body temperature, etc. The amount of water animals should consume per day in millilitres is roughly equivalent to their daily energy intake in kilocalories.

Energy

In addition to providing specific nutrients, food also provides energy. The energy content of the diet is derived solely from the fats, proteins and carbohydrates, and the proportion of these energy-producing nutrients in the diet will determine its energy content (also referred to as the energy density).

All living cells require energy and the more active they are the more energy they use. Individual animals have unique energy needs, which can vary, even between members of the same breed, age, sex and activity level. Breeders will recognize the scenario in which some littermates develop differently, one tending towards obesity, another on the lean side, even when they are fed exactly the same amount of food. If your clients are feeding a commercially prepared food, you should be aware that the feeding guide recommended by the manufacturer is also based on average energy needs, and therefore you may need to increase or decrease the amount you recommend to meet the individual pet's requirements. In some countries (such as those within the European Union) legislation may not allow the energy content to appear on the label of a prepared pet food; however, reputable manufacturing companies can and will provide this information upon request.

When considering different foods it is important to compare the metabolizable energy (ME), which is the amount of energy in the food that is available to a pet. Some companies will provide you with figures for the gross energy, which is not as useful because some of that energy (sometimes a substantial amount) will not be digested, absorbed and utilized.

Dietary fat supplies 2.25 times as much energy per gram as protein or carbohydrate. Water has no energy value and so a diet with a high moisture content will contain a low energy density and therefore fewer calories. It is important that energy intake is carefully controlled to allow the animal to reach and maintain optimum body condition. Excess energy can lead to obesity and growth abnormalities. Inadequate energy intake leads to poor growth and weight loss. Both conditions are potentially damaging to health and should be avoided by careful dietary management.

Animals eat to satisfy their energy requirements unless a diet is excessively palatable, when overeating may occur. In a balanced diet when an animal has consumed the amount of diet to meet its energy needs then the requirements for all other nutrients should also have been met. If the energy density of the diet is low, nutrient deficiencies may occur

since the animal will stop eating when the gut is full but before all the nutritional requirements have been met. The diet is said to be bulk-limited. Examples of bulk-limited diets are:

- Puppies and kittens on a poor-quality maintenance diet
- Weight loss in lactating bitches fed on a maintenance not a growth diet
- Some weight-control foods are bulk-limited for the energy-producing nutrients but not for the non-energy-producing nutrients – this is deliberate to achieve weight loss.

Energy requirements vary from individual to individual according to an animal's:

- Age
- Breed
- Sex
- Activity level
- Reproductive status
- Environment
- Health status.

This should be borne in mind when advising your clients on the most appropriate diet for the pet and when calculating the daily feeding amount.

Owners may think that protein is the source of energy needed for exercise and performance but this is not true. Protein is a relatively poor source of energy because a large amount of the energy theoretically available from it is lost in meal-induced heat. Meal-induced heat is the metabolic heat 'wasted' in the digestion, absorption and utilization of the protein. Fat and carbohydrates are better sources of energy for performance.

For obese or obesity-prone dogs a low energy intake is indicated, and there are now specially prepared diets that have a very low energy density; those that are most effective have a high fibre content.

Energy requirements

The basal energy requirement (BER) is the amount of energy expended while asleep, 12–18 hours after feeding in a thermoneutral environment.

The maintenance energy requirement (MER) is the amount of energy required by a moderately active animal in its daily search for and utilization of food (Table 7.1). It does not

Table 7.1 Daily maintenance energy requirements

Weight in kg	Energy in kcal/kg
Dogs	
3	110
6	85
10	75
>25	65
Cats	
2.5–5.5	65–70

include the energy required for growth, repair, pregnancy, lactation or work.

- MER in dogs is approximately 2 × BER
- MER in cats is approximately 1.4 × BER.

Most of the energy used by the body is given off as heat through radiation and convection from the body surface. Energy expenditure is related to body surface area. Small animals have a larger surface area related to body weight and therefore have greater heat loss and so a greater BER. Surface area can be determined from conversion tables using the animal's body weight but this can be complex and time-consuming.

In order to determine BER without the need to convert body weight to surface area, a simpler equation has been formulated, which seems to be accurate:

$$BER = (30 \times wt \text{ in kg}) + 70$$
$$MER = 2(30 \times wt \text{ in kg}) + 70 \text{ for dogs over 2 kg}$$
$$MER = 1.4(30 \times wt \text{ in kg}) + 70 \text{ for cats over 2 kg}$$

If the animal is very small, i.e. under 2 kg, use 70 × wt in kg.

In sickness the energy requirement varies considerably. Pets are often less active, sleep more and lie in a warm environment. The BER is therefore lower. However, if the animal has suffered from trauma, surgery or sepsis, the BER rises sharply. The precise rise will depend upon the illness factor involved. In pregnancy, lactation, growth and the control of obesity, the energy needs vary (Table 7.2).

The gross energy of nutrients (Table 7.3) varies but only a proportion of these nutrients are actually digested by the animal. The figures must therefore be adjusted to provide accurate values of the metabolizable energy obtained from the nutrient. The figures shown in Table 7.4 allow for digestibility. If a diet is highly digestible the energy content is higher; if a diet is poorly digestible because of lower-quality ingredients, the energy content is lower.

The only way to accurately determine the nutrient content of a diet as shown in Table 7.5 is by laboratory analysis. Many manufacturers give some information on the label. This is called the guaranteed analysis. This tells you that the diet contains at least x amount or has a maximum y amount of each nutrient. The true value could be much higher or much lower.

- If the guaranteed analysis is used to calculate the energy density of a food, a more accurate figure can be obtained by multiplying the calculated amount by 1.2 for canned diets and 1.1 for dry diets.
- The carbohydrate content may not be stated on the label but can be calculated by subtracting the total amount of all other nutrients from 100.
- The water content may not be given for all dry diets. Assume a figure of 10% if none is stated.
- This diet therefore contains 333.8 kcal/100 g of food, i.e. 3.338 kcal/g.

Using the above information, the energy provided by each nutrient can be calculated as a percentage of the total energy:

Percentage protein calories = 77/333.8 × 100 = 21%
Percentage fat calories = 78.3/333.8 × 100 = 21.3%
Percentage carbohydrate calories = 178.5/333.8 × 100 = 48.6%

Protein

Proteins are complex molecules composed of chains of amino acids. There are only 23 amino acids and all animals need all 23 of them. These 23 amino acids can be arranged in any combination, giving an almost infinite variety of

Table 7.2 Daily energy requirements for cats and dogs

One full day's work	1.5 × MER
Gestation post 3 weeks	1.3 × MER
Peak lactation	2–4 × MER
Birth to 3 months	2.0 × MER
Sub-freezing temperatures	1.7 × MER
Tropical heat	2.5 × MER
Resting	0.8 × MER
Obesity	0.6 × MER
Geriatric	0.6 × MER

Table 7.3 Gross energy content of nutrients

Nutrient	kcal/g
Protein	5.64
Fat	9.40
Carbohydrate	4.15

Table 7.4 ME content of nutrients

Nutrient	kcal/g
Protein	3.5
Fat	8.7
Carbohydrate	3.5

Table 7.5 Nutrient content of a typical diet

Nutrient	Amount (%)	kcal/g nutrient	kcal/100 g diet
Protein	22	× 3.5	77.0
Fat	9	× 8.7	78.3
Fibre	3	0	0
Water	10	0	0
Ash	5	0	0
Carbohydrate	51	× 3.5	178.5
Total	333.8		

naturally occurring proteins, each with its own characteristic properties, e.g. hair, skin, muscle, hormones, antibodies.

Many amino acids can be synthesized within the animal's body and so do not have to be provided in the diet. However, there are some that cannot be synthesized and so must be included in the diet. These are termed the essential amino acids. There are 10 amino acids essential in the diets of dogs and 11 amino acids essential in the diets of cats. These are:

- Phenylalanine
- Valine
- Tryptophan
- Threonine
- Isoleucine
- Methionine
- Histidine
- Arginine
- Leucine
- Lysine.

The 11th amino acid that is essential for cats only is called **taurine**. Inadequate taurine in the diet of cats can cause irreversible blindness and heart problems. Plant proteins do not contain taurine. The only source of taurine is animal protein, providing evidence that the cat is an obligate carnivore.

Proteins are essential components of all living cells, in which they have several functions including regulation of metabolism, a structural role in cell walls and muscle fibres. They are an important requirement for tissue growth and repair. Proteins may also be used as a source of energy in the diet. Animals cannot synthesize new amino acids so they require a dietary protein source to prevent a loss of body function or an inability to produce new tissue.

The quality of a protein varies with the number and amount of essential amino acids it contains. The quality of a protein is referred to as its **biological value**. This will depend on how:

- Acceptable
- Digestible
- Utilizable

the protein is: e.g. leather is not edible and so has 0% acceptability and therefore 0% biological value; chicken is edible, is 80% digestible and is 70% utilizable – the biological value is 87%.

Dietary protein in **excess** of the animal's requirements cannot be laid down as muscle but is broken down in the liver by a process of deamination. The amino part is converted to urea, which is excreted by the kidneys. The acid part of the amino acid is converted to glycogen or fat and is stored. Excess dietary protein can therefore be damaging to animals with liver and kidney problems and so control of dietary protein is prudent in the ageing pet.

Protein **deficiency** can result from insufficient dietary protein or from a deficiency of a particular amino acid. Signs of protein deficiency include:

- Poor growth or weight loss
- Dull hair coat
- Muscle wasting
- Increased susceptibility to disease
- Oedema
- Death.

Fat

Dietary fat may be referred to as oils, lipids or fats and consists of mainly triglycerides, which are composed of one molecule of glycerol and three molecules of fatty acids.

The specific fatty acids present determine the physical and nutritional characteristics of the fat. Fats are required in the diet:

- To provide energy
- To aid absorption of the fat-soluble vitamins (A, D, E, K)
- To enhance palatability
- As a source of essential fatty acids.

Inadequate dietary fat may lead to fatty acid deficiency and/or energy deficiency. Fats containing a high percentage of unsaturated fatty acids are liquid at room temperature and are called oils. Those with a low percentage of unsaturated fatty acids are solid at room temperature and are called fats.

Just as some amino acids cannot be synthesized by the body and must be provided in the diet, some fatty acids are also termed 'essential'. The three essential fatty acids are:

- Linoleic acid
- Linolenic acid
- Arachidonic acid.

Linoleic acid is an essential fatty acid required in the diet of all animals. It is common in vegetable oil and makes up 15–25% of poultry and pork fat but only 5% of beef tallow. Arachidonic acid is synthesized from linoleic acid in dogs but not in cats and so it must be present in the diet of the cat. Arachidonic acid is only found in fats of animal origin. Linolenic acid is synthesized from linoleic acid by both dogs and cats. Therefore neither species requires linolenic acid in dietary fat.

Fatty acids are needed as constituents of cell membranes, for the synthesis of prostaglandins and in controlling water loss through the skin. Essential fatty acid **deficiency** may result in impaired reproductive performance, impaired wound healing, a dry coat and scaly skin. This can predispose the skin to bacterial infection and eczema 'hot spots'. Essential fatty acid deficiency occurs most commonly in dogs receiving low-fat dry dog foods containing beef tallow or dry food that has been stored too long, especially under warm or humid conditions. Fatty acids become rancid due to the oxidation of their double bonds. Once rancid they lose their nutritional value. This oxidation is hastened by high temperatures and humidity. Oxidation of fats is prevented by the inclusion of substances called antioxidants such as vitamin E and ethoxyquin.

Certain fatty acids (such as docosahexaenoic acid or DHA) have been shown to play an important role in neural development in puppies and kittens. DHA is one of the 'building blocks' of brain tissue during growth. Eggs, meat and fish, such as salmon, sardines and tuna, are rich in DHA. Bitch and queen milk is also rich in DHA but once weaned puppies and kittens suffer a drop in DHA intake. Some super-premium pet growth foods are now supplemented with higher levels of DHA and these foods have been shown to improve trainability and vision development of puppies and kittens.

Excess dietary fat can lead to pansteatitis or 'yellow fat disease'. Signs include cutaneous pain, anorexia, pyrexia and nodular fat deposits within the skin. This can occur in cats eating a diet chiefly composed of red meat or tuna. Treatment involves correction of the diet and vitamin E therapy. Excess dietary fat may also lead to obesity, a serious condition that has many lifelong health consequences, including diabetes, heart disease, increased risk of joint disease and skin disorders. More than 50% of British pets are considered to be overweight and so educating clients as to the dangers of obesity and helping them choose the most appropriate diet for their pet are valuable skills for all veterinary nurses to learn.

Carbohydrates

There are three main groups of carbohydrates:

- Monosaccharides – glucose, fructose
- Disaccharides – maltose, sucrose, lactose
- Polysaccharides – starch, glycogen and fibre.

Carbohydrates provide the body with energy and may be converted to body fat. All animals have a metabolic requirement for glucose but, provided the diet contains sufficient glucose precursors (amino acids and glycerol), most animals can synthesize enough glucose to meet their metabolic needs without dietary carbohydrate. However, sugars and cooked starches are an economical and easily digested energy source. Sugars increase palatability to dogs but cats do not respond to the taste of sugar.

The value of certain carbohydrates is limited by the animal's ability to digest them. Digestion of disaccharides such as sucrose and lactose is controlled by the activity of the intestinal enzymes, i.e. disaccharidases sucrase and lactase. The activity of lactase decreases with age and so an excessive consumption of lactose-containing products in older animals can lead to diarrhoea.

Dietary fibre

Dietary fibre, or roughage, consists of a group of indigestible polysaccharides such as cellulose, lignin and pectin. They are the main constituents of plant cell walls and are relatively indigestible within the gut of dogs and cats. In these species the role of fibre in the diet is to provide bulk to the faeces, regularizing bowel movements and helping to prevent constipation and diarrhoea. Fibre also has therapeutic uses in the treatment of fibre-responsive diseases. Since fibre is largely indigestible, it decreases the energy content of the diet and so has a role in the correction and prevention of obesity.

Minerals

The term mineral is used to denote all inorganic elements in a food. Minerals are sometimes referred to on pet food labels as ash.

More than 18 minerals are believed to be essential for mammals. They are divided into macrominerals, which are needed in larger amounts, and trace elements, which are required in smaller amounts. Electrolytes are minerals in their salt form and are found in body tissues and fluids.

Minerals have many varied functions in the body. They are required for the maintenance of:

- Skeletal structure (especially calcium, phosphorus and magnesium)
- Acid–base and fluid balance (especially potassium, sodium and chloride)
- Cellular function
- Nerve conduction (especially potassium and magnesium)
- Muscle contraction (especially magnesium and calcium).

The absorption of different minerals is often linked, so that an excess intake of one mineral can lead to a deficiency of another. This is important since supplementation of one mineral can cause deficiency of another.

There are seven macrominerals. These are:

- Calcium
- Phosphorus
- Magnesium
- Sodium
- Potassium
- Chloride
- Sulphur.

1. **Calcium and phosphorus** are the major minerals involved in maintaining structural rigidity as components of the bones and teeth. The level of calcium and phosphorus in the blood is controlled by a complex series of reactions involving parathormone, calcitonin and vitamin D. It is the absolute concentrations of these minerals that are of most importance, but the ratio of calcium to phosphorus is also significant. The correct ratio for growth is 1 : 1. Imbalance in this ratio with either in excess leads to skeletal deformities. Meat meals are a rich source of calcium because of their bone content but most cereals are low in calcium. Calcium deficiency occurs most commonly in diets that are high in phosphorus (high meat and offal diets) and in lactating bitches it can cause eclampsia. Calcium excess occurs when high-calcium diets are fed, especially to large-breed puppies. It most commonly occurs when calcium supplementation is given in addition to a growth type diet. Many skeletal abnormalities have been attributed in part to excess calcium, including osteochondritis dissecans (OCD), canine hip dysplasia (CHD) and wobbler syndrome.

2. **Magnesium** is required for the normal function of heart and skeletal muscle. Foodstuffs containing bone, grains and fibre are rich in magnesium. Magnesium deficiency can cause muscular weakness but is very unlikely to be due to a lack of magnesium in the diet. Very high intakes of magnesium have been associated with feline lower urinary tract disease (FLUTD) and the formation of struvite crystalluria.

3. **Sodium and chloride** are the major electrolytes in the body water. They are needed for acid–base balance and for the regulation of the concentration of the body fluids. Chloride is a component of bile and hydrochloric acid. Fish, eggs, whey and poultry meal are rich in both sodium and chloride. A deficiency of these minerals can arise from excessive fluid loss, such as occurs in vomiting and diarrhoea. Signs include exhaustion, inability to control water balance, dry skin and hair loss. An excess will cause a greater than normal fluid intake and may predispose animals to hypertension and therefore heart and kidney problems.

4. **Potassium** is plentiful within cells and has an important role in maintaining both acid–base and osmotic balance. Potassium is also needed to facilitate the transfer of nerve impulses and muscle contractility. Potassium is present in a wide variety of foods, including soya, rice bran, grains and wheat bran. A deficiency of potassium is termed hypokalaemia and will cause anorexia, lethargy and muscle weakness. An excess of potassium is rare but may occur when potassium excretion is impaired; it leads to bradycardia.

There are at least 11 trace elements, the most important of which are as follows:

1. **Iron** is an essential component of haemoglobin, the oxygen-carrying pigment of the blood, and myoglobin, the oxygen-carrying pigment found within muscle. Most meat ingredients are high in iron and primary dietary deficiency is rare. It may arise as a consequence of chronic blood loss causing anaemia and fatigue, or occur in young puppies and kittens if milk is fed for too long a period, as milk has a low iron content.

2. **Copper** is needed for the formation of red blood cells and in the normal pigmentation of the skin and hair. Most meat ingredients, especially ruminant livers, contain plentiful copper. Copper deficiency may occur when zinc and iron excess arise and causes poor reproductive performance, early fetal loss and hair depigmentation. Copper toxicity is very rare in dogs and cats with normal metabolisms and occurs mainly in Bedlington terriers, West Highland White terriers and Doberman Pinschers – these breeds are all prone to an inherited metabolic defect that causes liver cirrhosis.

3. **Zinc** is required by all animals for maintaining a healthy skin and coat. Very high calcium diets can increase the animal's need for zinc. Zinc is relatively non-toxic and signs of dietary excess are rarely encountered in animals consuming normal commercial pet food but have been reported as a result of pica, following the consumption of large numbers of pennies. Signs of zinc deficiency have been reported in dogs fed cereal-based foods because of the presence of phytates that bind the zinc and prevent its absorption. The most common presentation of zinc deficiency is poor skin, hyperkeratosis and a sparse hair coat.

4. **Manganese** is of little practical relevance in the dietary management of cats and dogs but is an essential component in the diet of all birds. Manganese is required for the activation of many enzymes and is thus involved in a wide variety of important metabolic processes. Fibre sources and fish meal are rich in manganese.

5. **Iodine** is a major constituent of thyroid hormones, which are required for thermoregulation, reproduction, growth and metabolism. An animal's iodine requirement is influenced by its physiological state and diet. Lactating animals have a greater need for dietary iodine since about 10% of intake is excreted in the milk. Fish, eggs and poultry by-products are rich sources of iodine.

6. **Selenium** is an important constituent of the body's antioxidant protective system, in which it functions in combination with vitamin E. Selenium deficiency will cause muscular dystrophy and reproductive failure in ruminants but has not been reported in dogs and cats.

Vitamins

In order to be classified as a vitamin a substance must have five basic characteristics:

- It must be an organic compound different from fat, protein and carbohydrate
- It must be a component of the diet
- It must be essential in minute amounts
- Its absence must cause a deficiency syndrome
- It must not be synthesized in sufficient quantities to support normal physiological function.

Not all vitamins are essential for all species: e.g. guinea pigs and primates must have a dietary source of vitamin C, whereas other species can synthesize it themselves.

Vitamins can be divided into two main groups, depending on whether they are soluble in fat or water:

- Water-soluble – B complex and C
- Fat-soluble – A, D, E, K.

Vitamins assist in regulating energy metabolism and are involved in many biochemical reactions. Most vitamins cannot be synthesized in the body and so must be present in the diet. Since the water-soluble vitamins are readily lost via the urine and are poorly stored in the body, a daily supply must be available. Fat-soluble vitamins are more readily stored and so a daily intake is not so important. However, toxicity arising from excessive intake is much more common. There is no daily dietary requirement for vitamin C (ascorbic acid) in dogs and cats, since they can synthesize all they require from glucose.

Many factors influence an animal's individual requirement for vitamins. During growth and reproduction animals are making new tissues and so require higher levels of all nutrients, including vitamins. Various disease conditions also affect vitamin status through a reduced intake, e.g. following prolonged anorexia, or due to increased losses or decreased production, e.g. reduced synthesis of vitamin D during renal failure.

All commercial pet foods contain added vitamins both from synthetic and natural sources. It is therefore unnecessary and indeed contraindicated to supplement the diet of healthy dogs and cats with additional multipurpose vitamin formulations.

Water-soluble vitamins

1. **Vitamin B complex** – this includes thiamine, riboflavin, niacin, biotin, folic acid and cyanocobalamin. The water-soluble B vitamins are generally considered to be non-toxic. Since commercial pet foods contain plentiful supplies of B vitamins, deficiency states in pets fed such foods are very unlikely.

   Deficiencies can occur as a result of overconsumption of certain foods that contain specific antivitamins: e.g. avidin in egg white binds biotin; thiaminases in raw fish can lead to thiamine deficiency in cats. Water-soluble vitamin deficiencies can also be demonstrated in pets fed unusual home-prepared diets. Dogs fed exclusively on cereals such as porridge have been reported to develop niacin deficiency (termed pellagra), which presents as dermatitis, diarrhoea, dementia and death.

2. **Vitamin C** – this is not technically a vitamin for healthy dogs and cats because all that is required can be synthesized by the animal. Vitamin C mainly functions in the body as an antioxidant and free radical scavenger and is needed for the synthesis of collagen. It was postulated that huge doses of vitamin C could be beneficial in preventing hip dysplasia but this has not been proved. Recent research has focused on the use of supplemental vitamin C in the prevention of some types of cancer.

3. **L-carnitine** – this is a vitamin-like substance found in red meat and dairy products. It is needed in the metabolism of fat to produce energy. Although L-carnitine can be synthesized by both the liver and kidneys, certain animals may benefit from additional dietary supplementation, especially during weight loss programmes using a calorie-controlled diet food. It has been shown that a higher level of dietary L-carnitine can improve the rate of weight loss and can help to preserve lean body tissue during the weight-reduction phase.

Fat-soluble vitamins

1. **Vitamin A** – also called retinol, is the most nutritionally important vitamin. It is required for normal vision and for healthy coat, skin, mucous membranes and teeth. Naturally rich sources of vitamin A include fish oil, liver, eggs and dairy products. Plants do not contain active vitamin A but instead are rich in provitamins called carotenoids.

   Deficiencies are uncommon but cats require a source of preformed vitamin A, which is only found in animal tissue, and thus theoretically could become deficient if fed a vegetarian diet. Vitamin A toxicity is fairly common in cats receiving a diet high in liver or following oversupplementation with cod liver oil, since these foodstuffs contain abundant amounts of preformed vitamin A. Clinical signs of vitamin A toxicity include liver damage and painful bone disease, especially of the cervical vertebrae and long bones of the forelimb.

2. **Vitamin D** – this is required for the intestinal absorption of calcium and for the mobilization and bone deposition of both calcium and phosphorus. It can be absorbed from the diet in the small intestine and also can be synthesized in the skin following exposure to sunlight. Marine fish and fish oils are the richest natural sources of vitamin D and can potentially be a source of toxicity. Vitamin D deficiency is very rare but can cause rickets in young animals and severe bone disorders in adults. Toxicity can occur due to oversupplementation and causes hypercalcaemia, soft-tissue calcification and ultimately death.

3. **Vitamin E** – this is an important antioxidant and the requirement for vitamin E increases with the dietary levels of polyunsaturated fatty acids (PUFA). Vitamin E is only synthesized by plants and the richest natural sources are vegetable oils, seeds and cereal grains. The clinical manifestations of vitamin E deficiency vary markedly between species. In dogs the main clinical signs are degenerative skeletal disease with muscular weakness and gestational failure. In cats deficiency can arise when diets that are high in PUFA, such as oily fish, are fed. The clinical signs associated with vitamin E toxicity in cats include the occurrence of painful subcutaneous nodules, termed steatitis, as well as myocarditis and myositis.

4. **Vitamin K** – this regulates the formation of several blood-clotting factors and can be found in green leafy vegetables. The daily requirement for both dogs and cats is easily met in the healthy animal by synthesis from bacteria and so a deficiency is unlikely. However, the poison warfarin is a potent vitamin K antagonist and causes haemorrhage.

Neutraceuticals

Neutraceuticals are substances that are required for normal body structure and function and when given orally in a purified form improve the health and well-being of the animal.

The most common neutraceuticals in relation to pet food are:

- L-carnitine
- Glucosamine
- Chondroitin sulphate.

1. **L-carnitine** – this is a water-soluble vitamin-like substance found naturally in red meat and dairy products:
   - Most prepared pet foods are low in natural L-carnitine because they do not contain much red meat.
   - L-carnitine is needed in the body to help in the oxidation of body fat to form energy.
   - In normal animals all the L-carnitine needed can be synthesized in the liver and so animals do not rely on a dietary source of this vitamin.
   - Dogs and cats that are overweight and put on a lower-calorie diet have a higher requirement for L-carnitine, since they are using up more fat.
   - 'Light' diets for overweight dogs and cats should be supplemented with L-carnitine.

2. **Glucosamine and chondroitin sulphate** – these are called chondroprotectives. This means they help maintain the health of cartilage.
   - Chondroprotectives are produced naturally by the body but, as pets get older or as stress on the joints increases, this production decreases.
   - The addition of extra glucosamine and chondroitin sulphate has been shown to help maintain joint mobility and health.
   - Large-breed dogs by their very size have greater stresses on their joints.
   - The addition of extra chondroprotectives in the diet of large-breed dogs may be beneficial.

Table 7.6 The potential sources of free radicals

Internal sources	External sources
Mitochondria	Smoke
Phagocytes	Pollution
Reactions involving iron	Radiation
Exercise	UV light
Inflammation	Drugs
Ischaemia	Ozone
	Pesticides

Antioxidants

The role of antioxidants in preserving fat in pet food is well known and understood; however, there is now a considerable body of evidence to suggest that dietary antioxidants can have a positive effect on health and disease prevention through preventing cellular damage by free radicals. Oxidation of dietary fat causes the food to go rancid, whereas oxidation of endogenous fat causes tissue damage termed lipid peroxidation and the production of a continuous supply of free radicals.

Free radicals are reactive, unstable molecules that cause cellular damage to proteins, nucleic acids (DNA) and membrane lipids. Free radicals are unstable because they have a single unpaired electron in an outer orbit. Unpaired electrons attempt to regain stability by attacking and modifying other molecules. Free radicals can propagate damaging chain reactions within the body in an attempt to produce more stable atoms and molecules. This process of transferring electrons from one atom or molecule to another is called oxidation.

Free radicals are produced in the body by everyday metabolism and following exposure to adverse environmental conditions. Potential causes of increased free radical production are shown in the Table 7.6.

Cell damage due to free radicals has been implicated as a causative factor in many disease processes, including:

- Cancer
- Diabetes mellitus
- Cardiovascular disease
- Kidney disease
- Arthritis
- Cataracts
- Inflammatory bowel disease
- Pancreatitis
- Accumulated injury (wear and tear)
- Ageing changes.

An antioxidant is a substance that has the ability to scavenge free radicals (in reactive oxygen species) and reduce the overall number of oxidants in the system. The body has a complex antioxidant defence system that limits the effect of free radicals on tissues. This includes:

- Enzymes (catalase, superoxide dismutase)
- Free radical scavengers (vitamins A, C, E)
- Flavenoids.

Some antioxidants are made in the body and others are supplied by the diet. The main dietary antioxidants are:

- Vitamin E
- Vitamin C
- Carotenoids.

The role of vitamin E in preventing the oxidation of polyunsaturated fatty acids (PUFA) is well documented. Antioxidant defences are therefore highly dependent on adequate nutrition; indeed, inadequate ingestion of vitamins C and E mimics the effects of radiation exposure. Cells of the immune system are sensitive to changes in levels of antioxidants due to the very high percentage of PUFA in their cell membranes.

The best food sources of dietary antioxidants are fruit and vegetables. They are especially high in vitamin C and carotenoids and also contribute a significant amount of vitamin E and non-nutrient antioxidants to the diet. It is a well-held belief that people should try to consume at least 5 daily portions of fresh fruits and vegetables in an attempt to reduce their risk of degenerative diseases and cancer. Unfortunately the typical diet for the majority of the population in the Western world falls far short of this goal.

Pet dogs and cats very rarely consume this type of diet. Many commercially available pet foods now contain added dietary antioxidants designed to protect dogs and cats against the risk of disease. These products have added levels of vitamin C, vitamin E and selenium to provide antioxidant protection.

Types of pet food

Home-made diets

Some owners like to feed home-cooked diets to their pets. Most home-made diets are unbalanced and they are not recommended. The main problems encountered with home-made diets for pets are that they are:

- Often very high in calories and can encourage overeating and weight gain
- Usually unbalanced and so do not provide the best nutrition
- Often high in salt and may be addictive
- Not consistent and so can cause upset stomachs and diarrhoea.

Although it might appear dull to us, it is better to advise clients to feed their dogs and cats the same amount of the same food every day.

Commercial diets

Commercially available diets have undergone extensive research by vets and nutritionists at the pet food companies. They provide the best balance of nutrients combined with convenience and excellent value. There are three main types of dog and cat foods available: canned foods, dry foods and semi-moist foods.

Canned foods

Most canned foods are complete foods, i.e. they can be fed on their own with just water to drink and the dog or cat will be getting everything they need. Canned foods contain about 80% water (you may see this written as 'moisture' on the label). Canned foods come in many different flavours. Many cat owners like to give their cats a different taste each day, although this has been shown to increase the chances of the cat getting fat.

Some canned foods are complementary foods, i.e. they must be fed with something else (usually mixer biscuits) to give a proper diet and it is not recommended to feed just the canned food. It should be clearly stated on the packet or can if the food is complete or complementary.

Dry foods

Most dry foods are complete, although some are complementary. Dry foods contain about 10% water, although legally the label does not have to state the water content if it is less than 14%.

Semi-moist foods

These foods are usually complete and contain about 25% moisture. They are usually sealed in foil pouches or small plastic bags to retain their freshness. One pouch is often equivalent to one can of food. Semi-moist foods tend to be preserved using sugars and so should be avoided in all pets with diabetes.

Premium foods

Premium pet foods are highly sophisticated foods that have been developed by veterinary surgeons and specialist nutritionists. They are usually available in both canned and dry forms. Premium foods contain higher-quality ingredients than regular pet foods and this makes them much more digestible. Premium foods may at first glance seem more expensive than economy brands, but they have several advantages:

- They are fed in smaller amounts so the cost compares favourably with other foods.
- The pet produces smaller firmer faeces, as the food is more digestible; this makes toilet training easier and less messy.
- The high-quality ingredients often lead to improved skin condition.
- They are complete and so no extra supplements are needed.
- They are always made to the same consistent recipe; this is called fixed formulation and reduces the likelihood of digestive upsets.
- They tend to be lower in potentially harmful nutrients such as salt.
- They are available in different life stages to suit both the pet's age and its lifestyle.

Treats

Most pet owners like to buy treats for their pets but if the pet is receiving a complete balanced diet then this is not necessary. However, providing that the total number of calories eaten each day in treats is no more than 10% of the pet's daily intake, they can be safely fed. It is best to get owners to reduce the daily feeding amount by about 10% to compensate for the additional calories from the treats.

Some treats, such as rawhide chews, are very poorly digestible and so provide very few calories. These can be fed more freely but it is good advice to stop people giving treats at family mealtimes, as this can lead to begging. Most new puppy owners will use treats as a reward when they are training their puppies – the main meal should be reduced to compensate for this.

Feeding puppies and kittens

Puppies

Puppies should be weaned at 3–4 weeks of age. Many puppies will start to eat solid food before this by exploring their surroundings and coming into contact with their mother's food. If the mother is fed a good-quality balanced growth food during the latter stages of pregnancy and throughout lactation, then this is a suitable weaning ration for the puppies too. In the first few days the kibble can be soaked to allow smaller puppies to chew them more easily, but very soon puppies will learn to accept dry kibble. If a commercial balanced food is chosen then no supplements should be needed and in fact adding other nutrients will only cause dietary imbalances.

The musculoskeletal system changes constantly throughout life but these changes are most rapid during the first few months of life. The exact point of maturity varies between breeds but is usually between 12 and 18 months of life. The skeletal system is most susceptible to physical and metabolic insult during the first 12 months because metabolic activity is heightened during this time. If damage occurs at this stage of development the structural soundness of the adult dog can be affected, leading to lameness or growth defects.

Optimum growth, including skeletal development, is dependent upon a combination of good genetics, the correct environment and balanced nutrition. Breeders put considerable effort into selecting the best breeding animals to maximize genetic potential, avoiding those with overt conformational defects. The environmental influences include litter size, and thus space available within the womb for development, activity level in the first few weeks of life and housing conditions. Rearing puppies on a non-slippery floor can help reduce stress damage to developing joints, including the hips.

Nutrition is certainly one of the most important factors in optimal growth and many scientific studies have shown that development can be adversely affected by both under- and overnutrition. With the advent of modern commercial pet food, nutrient deficiency as a cause of developmental skeletal disease has virtually been eliminated. Today we see far more cases where the plane of nutrition has been too high because of overfeeding or oversupplementation. The main nutritional risk factors for puppies are:

- Obesity in smaller breeds, due to an excessive intake of energy
- Skeletal disease in larger breeds, due to a combination of excessive energy intake and high intake of specific nutrients.

About one-third of all dogs fall into the category of 'large-breed'. These puppies will weigh more than 25 kg when adult and as the group includes some of the nation's favourite breeds, they will be very frequent visitors to your clinics.

Excessive nutrient intake has been shown to be a factor in the main developmental skeletal disorders of larger-breed puppies, including hip dysplasia, osteochondrosis, wobbler syndrome, un-united anconeal process and panosteitis. The key nutritional influences on skeletal development are the:

- Energy content of the food
- Feeding method employed
- Specific nutrient content, including calcium, phosphorus, protein, vitamin D and vitamin A.

Most dog owners are aware that puppies need relatively more energy, protein, calcium and phosphorus than adult dogs, i.e. in relation to their body weight, but many do not realize that too much of any one of these nutrients can be harmful. When it comes to nutrition, more is not better!

The intake of too much calcium is more common than the intake of too little. This is because of the tendency of owners to overfeed and to supplement the diet with additional minerals and vitamins in the form of powders, tablets and capsules, as well as by adding high-calcium foods, e.g. milk, bonemeal, treats and titbits, to the growth ration. This high intake of calcium has the effect of inhibiting the natural remodelling process of bone that has to occur during development in response to changing stresses on the skeleton. The consequences of this overnutrition are proportionately greater in puppies that grow more rapidly, i.e. the larger breeds, and this explains why the majority of the developmental skeletal conditions are diagnosed in breeds weighing 25 kg or more when adult.

New puppy owners have to digest a huge amount of information during their first few visits to the surgery. This information includes vaccination policies, worming regimes, flea treatments, neutering, insurance, training as well as the correct way to feed their new family member. When speaking to new puppy owners it is very useful to use diagrams, graphs and charts to help illustrate the different growth rates in the different breeds. Encourage owners to come back regularly to have their puppies weighed and their growth rate checked. By offering puppy growth checks every 2 weeks for the first 6 months of life, you can offer a valuable preventative health care service.

To assess a growth food for optimum development in growing puppies we must consider a number of factors:

Energy content

Growing puppies need twice as much dietary energy on a per-kilogram basis as adults. This need is greatest just after birth and then decreases as the dog grows and matures. Excessive dietary energy may support a growth rate that is too fast for proper skeletal development, which results in increased frequency of skeletal disorders in large and giant breeds. As fat has twice the calorific density of protein or carbohydrate it follows that dietary fat is the primary contributor to excess energy intake. Not only does excess energy result in rapid growth but also dietary energy in excess of the

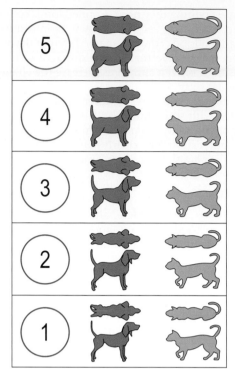

Fig. 7.1 Estimation of body condition score

puppy's needs will be stored as fat and hence predispose to juvenile obesity. Puppies that are allowed to get fat will increase the number of fat cells they have (called fat cell hyperplasia) and are then predisposed to obesity for the rest of their lives.

Body condition scoring (BCS) evaluates body fat stores and therefore confirms if the energy intake is suitable (Fig. 7.1). Maintaining a proper BCS during growth not only avoids juvenile obesity but also helps control excessive growth rates and is a valuable practical step you can take to improve the long-term health of your clients' puppies. Limiting food intake (while avoiding deficiencies) to maintain lean body condition will not impede a dog's ultimate genetic potential; however, it will reduce food intake, faecal output and obesity and also lessen the risk of skeletal disease.

Protein content

Excess protein intake has not been shown negatively to affect the developing skeleton. However, any protein in excess of what is needed for growth may be converted to energy and so may increase growth rate. Protein deficiency has been shown to be harmful. The minimum adequate level of dietary protein will depend upon the protein's:

- Digestibility
- Amino acid profile
- Ratio of essential amino acids
- Bioavailability – the amount actually utilizable by the body.

A growth food should contain at least 22% protein (on a dry matter basis DMB) of high biological value. Once the puppy reaches maturity this level may be reduced.

Calcium content

It is the absolute level of calcium and the calcium:phosphorus (Ca:P) ratio that influences skeletal development. One study showed that young giant-breed puppies fed a food containing excess calcium (3.3% dry matter basis, DMB) with a phosphorus level that was either normal (0.9% DMB) or high (3.3% DMB to maintain the correct Ca:P ratio) had a significantly increased incidence of developmental bone disease. Thus we cannot just increase the phosphorus to make up for the fact that the calcium is too high.

It was postulated that switching from a growth to an adult food earlier than normally advised might help protect puppies from excess calcium intake, since the adult food would contain a lower level of calcium and should therefore lead to a reduced calcium intake. However, the puppy must consume a greater volume of the lower-energy adult food in order to meet its higher calorie needs. This means that ultimately the puppy consumes a greater amount of calcium when eating the adult food. This reinforces the fact that puppies are not small versions of adult dogs but have unique nutritional needs that can only be satisfied by feeding a balanced growth food.

Feeding treats or giving supplements that contain calcium will further increase calcium intake. Two level teaspoons of a typical calcium supplement added to a growth food for a 15-week-old, 15 kg puppy would more than double the daily calcium intake. This would take the total calcium intake to a level much higher than has been shown to significantly increase the risk of developmental skeletal disease.

Studies demonstrate the safety and adequacy of 1.1% calcium (DMB) in the food. The Association of American Feed Control Officials (AAFCO) minimum recommended level of calcium is 1% DMB and this should be with no supplementation, especially for at-risk puppies.

Other nutrients

- **Vitamin C** has been recommended in the prevention and treatment of several skeletal diseases; however, the relationship between vitamin C and disorders such as OCD and CHD has not been proved. Vitamin C (L-ascorbic acid) is required for the biosynthesis of collagen, a major component of ligaments and bones, but a study found that feeding puppies growth diets totally devoid of vitamin C caused no skeletal problems and did not affect growth. There are no known requirements for dietary vitamin C in the dog.
- **Vitamin D** metabolites regulate calcium metabolism and therefore the skeletal development of growing animals. These metabolites aid in the absorption of calcium and phosphorus from the gut, increase bone cell activity, influence endochondral ossification and alter calcium excretion via the kidney. Unlike other omnivores, the dog seems to be dependent on a dietary source of vitamin D as well as that produced endogenously by the action of ultraviolet light on the skin. Commercial pet foods contain ample vitamin D, making vitamin D deficiency (rickets) very rare. Excess vitamin D can cause hypercalcaemia, hyperphosphataemia, anorexia, polydipsia, polyuria, vomiting, muscle weakness, soft tissue mineralization and lameness. Vitamin D supplementation should be avoided in growing dogs since it may disturb normal skeletal development because of increased calcium and phosphorus absorption.
- The **trace minerals copper and zinc** are involved in normal skeletal development. In dogs, bone copper levels are not influenced by dietary supplementation. Long-term studies of the effects of dietary zinc on canine growth have shown no significant clinical influence on skeletal development. So, even though these minerals are required for normal skeletal development, their exact role in the dog has yet to be determined.

Feeding techniques for use in growing puppies

There are three basic methods:

1. **Free-choice feeding** – this is an effortless way to feed growing puppies. Frequent trips to the always-full food bowl may help to limit boredom. Timid or unthrifty animals have less competition when eating, as they can choose to feed at quieter times. However, free-choice feeding has been shown to encourage overeating, which increases the risk of developmental bone diseases. Therefore free-choice feeding methods are contraindicated for all 'at-risk' breeds until they have reached skeletal maturity (12–18 months of age, or at least 80% of their adult weight and height).

2. **Time-limited feeding** – this can be used for most breeds. The food is only available for a set period two or three times daily, leading to a reduced intake in most breeds. This slightly reduced intake results in slower growth rates but does not diminish the adult size achieved. Close attention should still be paid to the total amount of food consumed, since certain individuals (very greedy feeders) are still able to consume large amounts of food during this limited time period. If this method is chosen, it is recommended to allow three 5–10 minute feeding periods for the first month after weaning, reducing to two per day after that.

3. **Food-limited feeding** – this is the method of choice for feeding puppies to maintain optimum growth rate and body condition. Food-limited feeding involves giving a measured amount of food based on calculated energy requirements. This will have been done by the manufacturer and is indicated by the feeding guide. Clinical monitoring of growth and adjustment of feeding amount are critical. Large and giant-breed dogs grow rapidly and thus have steep growth curves. Their intake should be monitored closely and will have to be adjusted more frequently than for dogs of smaller breeds. These 'at risk' breeds should be weighed, evaluated and have their feeding amount adjusted every 2 weeks. This is still an uncommon approach to feeding many puppies but a trained veterinary nurse can, through education and support, explain the benefits of this method to their clients.

Regardless of a food's nutrient profile and how it is fed, the ultimate measurement of appropriate intake is the physical condition of the puppy. The only way to reduce potentially harmful nutritional risk factors that can affect skeletal development is to assess body condition and adjust the amount fed to ensure lean, healthy growth. The ideal BCS of a growing puppy is represented by a score of 3 (Fig. 7.1). The ribs are palpable with a thin layer of fat between the skin and the bone. The bony prominences are easily felt, with a slight amount of overlying fat. Animals over six months of age should have a pronounced abdominal tuck when viewed from the side and a well-proportioned lumbar waist when viewed from above.

Nutritional management alone will not completely control developmental diseases. However, skeletal diseases can be influenced during growth by feeding technique and nutrient profile. Dietary deficiencies are of minimal concern now that most dogs consume commercial foods specifically prepared for young, growing dogs. The potential harm is in overnutrition from excess consumption and oversupplementation.

Kittens

Growth problems in kittens resulting from unsuitable nutrition are very rare. Veterinary surgeons will sometimes see kittens with growth problems that have been fed on very unusual diets. These kittens have usually been fed home-made diets, especially 'all-meat' diets and diets high in liver.

All-meat diets are very high in phosphorus and very low in calcium. This mineral imbalance can upset the development of the skeleton and cause very thin, weak bones. The kittens may develop bone fractures after very minimal trauma, e.g. being dropped. Alteration of the diet to a more suitable balanced growth food can reverse the problem if caught early enough. Diets that are very high in liver are also very high in vitamin A. An excessive intake of vitamin A can cause abnormal bone development, leading to fusing of the bones in the neck, spine or joints. This condition is very painful and difficult to reverse even after the feeding is corrected.

Optimum growth in kittens is achieved by feeding a high-quality, complete, balanced kitten food. Supplementation with vitamin or mineral tablets and powders is unnecessary and could be harmful. Home-prepared diets for kittens are often unbalanced, containing very high levels of fat, protein and salt. They are best avoided.

The following points should be taken into consideration when recommending a growth food for kittens:

- The product chosen should be complete and balanced for growth. All-purpose foods that claim to be suitable for pregnant and lactating queens, kittens, adult cats and senior cats should be avoided, since these different life stages have differing nutritional requirements.
- A fixed-formula product will reduce the incidence of gut upsets, including diarrhoea; this will make litter training the kitten much easier.
- A highly digestible product (made from high-quality ingredients) will result in smaller, firmer stools with less smell, again aiding litter training – since many cat owners keep the litter tray in the kitchen, any advice you can give to help reduce unpleasant smells will be appreciated.
- The product should contain an increased level of protein, since more protein is needed during growth.

- The product should be high in energy (fat), since this means that the kitten can consume all the calories needed in a smaller amount of food – remember, a kitten's stomach is very small and so large-volume foods should be avoided.
- The product should produce naturally acidic urine; this has been shown to help reduce the incidence of bladder problems in cats. The natural urine pH for cats is 6.2–6.4.
- Milk should be avoided. Kittens do not need cow's milk and in fact lack the enzyme needed to digest the milk sugar (lactose). Giving milk to a kitten can cause diarrhoea and will also upset the balance of the diet, since the milk also contains protein, fat and calcium. Kittens should be provided with an ample supply of fresh, clean drinking water.

Feeding during pregnancy and lactation

The aims of a good feeding programme during pregnancy and lactation are to reduce the number of matings needed to achieve pregnancy, i.e. to maximize conception rate and produce the very largest numbers of healthy puppies or kittens per litter. Good nutrition is also needed to maximize the growth rate of the newly born puppies and kittens and to ensure a healthy immune system in the early days of life.

Many of your clients seeking advice will be breeding from their pet dogs for the first time. These inexperienced hobby breeders will benefit from time spent giving sound nutritional advice and help with product selection. Serious breeders often hold very strong opinions regarding feeding programmes for breeding dogs and raising puppies and so it may be a challenge to alter their preconceptions.

As a general rule, only healthy adult dogs and cats in a good nutritional state, i.e. neither too fat nor too thin, should be considered for breeding. This is an important point, since often poor nutritional status prior to mating is only noticed once the puppies are born. Breeding from overweight bitches should be avoided since it has been shown that these dogs are at a greater risk of insufficient milk production as well as having an increased risk of difficulties giving birth. Breeding from thin animals should not be encouraged either as the strains of pregnancy and lactation can cause health problems for the already weak dog or cat. Bitches tend to have a reduced appetite around the time they are in oestrus and it is advisable to feed small frequent meals at this time or even to withhold food for the time immediately before and after mating.

The pregnant and lactating bitch

Gestation in the bitch lasts on average for 63 days and is typically divided into three 21-day 'trimesters'. Adequately fed bitches will gain about 15–25% additional body weight between mating and whelping. After whelping the bitch should weigh no more about 5–10% more than the pre-breeding weight. This weight gain can be explained mainly by the development of the mammary tissue. In the first 40 days of pregnancy the fetuses only gain about 5% of their final birthweight. This means that during the first two-thirds

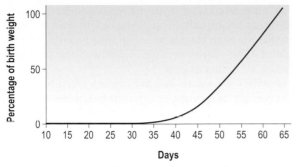

Fig. 7.2 Increase in weight of fetal puppies with time during gestation

Table 7.7 Target nutritional profile for pregnancy and lactation

Nutrient	Recommended level	
	First 6 weeks of pregnancy	**Last 3 weeks of pregnancy and during lactation***
Energy (kcal/g)	3.5–4.5	4–5
Protein (%)	22–32	25–35
Fat (%)	10–25	> 18
Carbohydrate (%)	> 23	> 23
Phosphorus (%)	0.6–1.3	0.7–1.3
Calcium (%)	0.75–1.5	1.0–1.7

*Large-breed bitches may need this type of diet throughout pregnancy and lactation.

of pregnancy the energy requirements of the pregnant bitch are no different from those of the non-pregnant bitch. However, after day 40 the weight of the fetuses increases dramatically and energy intake should increase correspondingly during week 5 to reach a peak between weeks 6 and 8 (Fig. 7.2).

The following nutritional parameters are important during pregnancy:

Energy intake

This reaches about 30% above adult maintenance for bitches with small litters but may reach as high as 60% above maintenance if the litter size is large (Table 7.7). It may be physically difficult for the bitch to eat sufficient calories in the final days since the abdomen will be filled with the large uterus containing the puppies. This means it is vital to slowly change the diet for a pregnant bitch so that by the last third of pregnancy, i.e. the last 3 weeks, she is eating a growth ration. It is important to remember that large-breed puppy foods are not suitable for pregnant and lactating bitches since they are restricted in both fat (energy) and calcium. These two nutrients are needed in higher amounts in the pregnant bitch, regardless of breed size. Giant breeds may sometimes need a higher-energy food throughout pregnancy and not just in the last 3 weeks. Food intake often decreases just prior to whelping and many bitches become totally anorexic. This may be a sign that whelping is imminent.

Protein intake

Just as the energy requirement of the pregnant bitch increases with the developing fetuses, so does the protein requirement (Table 7.7). Foods for dogs in late gestation should contain increased levels of protein and reduced levels of fibre. This can be achieved by switching to a ration formulated for growth. A food containing 20–25% crude protein on a dry matter basis has been recommended. Protein deficiency during pregnancy may decrease the birthweight of the puppies and decrease their ability to survive.

Carbohydrate intake

Studies have shown that feeding a carbohydrate-free diet to pregnant bitches dramatically decreases the rate of survival of the puppies, as well as causing weight loss in the bitch. This is because the developing fetus obtains more than 50%

of its energy from glucose. Bitches should have at least 20% of the energy provided by carbohydrate. This is important, since many commercial canned dog foods contain almost no carbohydrate. Inexperienced owners may choose to feed these foods, since their labels often indicate that they are suitable for growth, pregnancy and lactation.

Calcium and phosphorus intake

In the last 35 days of pregnancy the requirement for calcium and phosphorus increases by 60%. This is because the skeletons of the puppies are developing and need calcium and phosphorus to form properly. Excessive intake of calcium at this time can, however, be detrimental since it may upset the delicate balance that controls calcium and phosphorus levels. It is recommended that the calcium intake during pregnancy is between 0.75% and 1.5% on a dry matter basis.

Lactation

Optimum milk production depends on several key factors, including:

- Breeding only from bitches in good physical condition
- Good nutrition during pregnancy
- Good nutrition during lactation.

During lactation the nutritional requirements are directly related to the amount of milk the bitch has to produce, which in turn depends on the number of puppies in the litter (Table 7.7). Lactation puts the bitch under tremendous nutritional strain, more so than at any other stage of her life. The bitch must produce a huge amount of milk, since her puppies have to double their birthweight in the first 9 days of life. A German shepherd bitch with six puppies can produce up to 2 litres of milk per day. At peak lactation the bitch produces milk at a rate similar to that of a dairy cow. Bitch's milk is very rich, containing more than twice the fat and protein of cow's milk. This very nutrient-dense milk is needed to support such rapid growth rate in the puppies.

Water must be provided in large quantities. Always remind owners of lactating bitches to provide clean, fresh drinking water at all times – a 35 kg bitch at peak lactation may need up to 6 litres of water per day.

A summary of the dietary recommendation for pregnant and lactating bitches is:

- Complete adult food for the first 6 weeks of pregnancy
- Complete puppy food for the final 3 weeks of pregnancy and throughout lactation
- Complete puppy food may be required by giant-breed bitches, e.g. Great Danes, during the entire pregnancy and lactation
- Puppy large-breed foods should not be fed to pregnant or lactating bitches since they are too low in both energy and calcium.

Feeding adult dogs and cats

Obesity-prone dogs and cats

Obesity is the most common nutritional disease in the Western world in both pets and their owners. A staggering 50% of dogs and cats in the UK are considered to be above their ideal weight. This means that every other dog and cat owner you speak to in your practice will have a pet that might benefit from a weight-management product. When discussing weight control it should be remembered that many owners might feel guilty that their pet has become overweight. You are as much counselling them as giving nutritional advice for their pet.

True obesity, where the pet is more than 15% over the ideal body weight, is considered to be a clinical condition and requires careful weight reduction under the guidance of a veterinary surgeon. This is important, since severe obesity can contribute to many other clinical conditions that would require veterinary attention. Also, in a few rare cases the weight gain may be due not to the accumulation of fat but to pregnancy, fluid retention, the growth of a tumour or other serious health problems, which are best dealt with by a veterinary surgeon.

The causes and risks of excessive weight gain

The cause of weight gain is essentially very simple – a pet is given more calories to eat on a daily basis than it requires. Overeating results in the extra calories being converted to fat and then the fat is laid down in the body tissues. These extra calories can be from treats and titbits given by the owner or simply by giving too much of the pet's usual food.

The way in which the pet is fed also has an influence on whether or not it gains weight. It has been shown that regular flavour rotation can increase the risk of obesity in cats. Pets that are fed on an 'ad lib' basis are also at a greater risk of weight gain.

Other factors that increase the risk of a pet becoming overweight include:

- **Breed** – certain pure-bred dogs seem to be more prone to becoming overweight than crossbreed dogs (Box 7.1); however, pedigree cats are less likely to develop obesity than crossbreed 'moggie' cats.
- **Age** – older dogs tend to be less active and if their feeding level is maintained, they will gain weight.

- **Sex** – neutered dogs and cats require fewer calories than entire animals. To prevent weight gain the energy intake for both dogs and cat should be reduced by about 15% after neutering; 'light' products should be fed to all neutered pets.
- **Lifestyle** – pets with inactive owners often become overweight as a result of physical inactivity. Many cats are kept indoors, never going out, so may gain weight, especially if fed on an 'ad lib' basis.
- **Body condition during growth** – it has been shown that puppies and kittens that are allowed to become overweight during growth are always more prone to becoming overweight adults. This is because, when an immature animal overeats, the additional calories not only cause an increase in the size of the fat cells but also an increase in their number – fat cell hyperplasia. This means that the pet now has more fat cells that when it was born, resulting in a greater risk of becoming overweight.

You may also find that clients seeking nutritional advice for overweight pets have a similar problem themselves. This requires tactful handling and careful choice of words. It is best to avoid the word 'obese', since many people find this offensive and unkind. Try discussing 'weight management' or call the pet 'heavy' or 'over the ideal body weight' instead.

Excessive deposition of body fat is damaging to both the quality and length of the pet's life. Overweight dogs and cats are at a greater risk of developing many conditions (Box 7.2).

To determine how overweight a dog or cat actually is requires careful observation or questioning of the owner. Ideally, all pet owners should know what their pet's ideal weight is and be encouraged to weigh their pets at least every month and record it. Unfortunately, very few actually do.

Box 7.1 Dog breeds that are commonly prone to obesity

- Labrador retriever
- Cairn terrier
- Cocker spaniel
- Shetland sheepdog
- Beagle
- King Charles spaniel
- Basset hound
- Long-haired dachshund

Box 7.2 Common disorders in overweight dogs and cats

- Heart disease
- High blood pressure
- Constipation
- Joint disease
- Diabetes
- Liver disease (cats)
- Breathing problems
- Exercise intolerance
- Feline lower urinary tract disease (FLUTD)

You should encourage all your clients to keep a regular check on their pet's weight and it is very helpful if you offer a free pet weight-check service.

Once you have determined the pet's weight, you can then assess the degree of obesity. Breed weight charts are available that show the ideal weight ranges for all the popular breeds of both dog and cat. Sometimes, despite being within the ideal breed range, you may feel that the pet is in fact overweight. This is due to individual variation in shape and size. Other methods should then be used to determine if a weight-management product is required. These include:

- Feeling along the pet's ribs – you should be able to feel (but not see) the ribs with light fingertip pressure; if you cannot feel the ribs then they are covered by a layer of fat and the pet is overweight.
- Looking down on the pet from above – dogs should have a definite waist (an hourglass shape) when viewed from above. If, instead, the dog resembles a coffee table, then there is too much fat laid down over the lumbar region.
- Cats often lay down excess fat in their inguinal region (between the back legs) rather than over their backs; the customer may say that their cat 'waddles' rather than walks.
- You may notice that the dog's collar has recently been let out a notch or two. This is often a telltale sign of weight gain.
- Keep a regular record of the pet's waist or chest measurement – this is especially useful if a calorie-controlled diet is needed since it is an easy way for the owner to check their pet's progress.

Feeding regime

Once you have convinced a client that their pet requires a weight-management product, you will need to explain the key features of an ideal 'low-calorie' pet food. Essentially, the concept is very simple: providing fewer calories on a daily basis than the pet requires leads to utilization of the stored body fat to provide the additional energy needed, and consequently weight loss. Pet owners facing the challenge of getting their pet to lose weight will often ask you if simply feeding less of the pet's usual food will produce the desired weight loss. This approach is usually unsuccessful because:

- Most commercial pet foods contain high levels of fat; fat is very easily digested and so high-fat foods tend to support weight retention, even if fewer calories are fed.
- The pet will be getting a much lower volume of food than it has been used to, which often leads to it seeking out food or begging; many owners will give up if they think their pet is suffering hunger.
- Remember, if you feed half the usual amount of food, then not only is the pet getting half the calories but also half the protein, vitamins and minerals too; this may lead to deficiencies if a reduced amount is fed for a long period of time.

Pet food manufacturers decrease the calorie content of a pet food by reducing the fat content of the food. The fat needs to be replaced by another, less energy-dense nutrient (remember that fat provides more than twice the calories per gram than either protein or carbohydrate). There is much debate among pet food manufacturers as to the best method of reducing the energy content of the food. There are several different methods widely used. The fat can be replaced with:

- **Air** – used to fill out the kibble of food and so make the volume of food appear larger. The owner thinks that a large meal is given and that the pet will not therefore feel hungry. However, this air is quickly removed once the food is eaten and so does not maintain a feeling of fullness. Many dogs on this type of reduced calorie food show signs of hunger and begin begging.
- **Water** – has a similar short-acting effect to fill the pet up and make the meal size appear larger; again, the gut quickly absorbs the water and so little satiety is achieved.
- **Fibre** – research scientists have proved the value of fibre as a replacement for fat in reduced-calorie pet foods. Fibre provides bulk and so a satisfying feeling of fullness, while contributing few calories (since the fibre remains within the gut and is not digested or absorbed). Fibre has an added benefit in that its presence within the gut limits the absorption of other nutrients, including protein, fat and carbohydrate. The concept of high-fibre weight-loss diets for people too is well known and so many customers will understand this principle.

Many pet foods claim to be higher in fibre and lower in calories. It should be noted that, to achieve weight loss or adequate prevention of weight gain, the fibre levels need to be significantly higher than is usual in commercial pet foods. Most commercial pet foods contain around 1–2% crude fibre. It should be noted that adult dogs and cats that simply need to lose weight should not be fed a low-protein food. They still have the same protein requirement as other adult dogs and cats. It is simply their energy (fat) intake that needs to be controlled. Recent research has shown the benefit of supplementing lower-calorie foods with the vitamin-like substance L-carnitine. The key features of an ideal controlled-calorie food are shown in Table 7.8.

Feeding senior dogs and cats

You will often be asked for dietary advice regarding the optimum nutrition of the seemingly healthy older dog and cat. If at any stage you feel that the pet may have an illness, it is best to suggest that the client consults the veterinary surgeon, rather than attempting to make a feeding recommendation.

Table 7.8 Nutrient profile of the ideal controlled-calorie pet food

Nutrient	Level
Energy	Reduced
Fat	Reduced
Fibre	Increased
Protein	As adult maintenance
L-carnitine	Supplemented

- Cancer
- Heart disease
- Kidney disease
- Liver disease
- Constipation
- Joint disease
- Obesity
- Impaired hearing
- Impaired vision
- Dental disease
- Behavioural changes

Senior individuals represent a significant, and increasing, proportion of both the canine and feline populations. Improvements in health care and nutrition have extended the average lifespan for pets as they have for humans. Approximately one-third of all dogs and cats owned by your clients will fall into the senior life stage, which is defined as being older than 7 years of age. These individuals are at a much greater risk of developing many disorders (Box 7.3) but, with appropriate dietary management and veterinary health care, the onset of such disorders can be delayed or even prevented. Most pet owners pay particular attention to quality as well as quantity of life for their pets and all you can do to help them in this will be much appreciated.

Feeding the healthy older dog

We have increasing evidence that small-breed dogs live significantly longer than large- and giant-breed dogs. One survey revealed a 12 : 1 ratio of small- to large-breed dogs at the age of 17 years or more. We can consider a dog as being older when it reaches half its life expectancy. A change of diet would thus be considered around the age of 5 for large- and giant-breed dogs and around 7 years for small dogs.

Nutritional assessment

In view of the wide variation among the older dog population, nutritional management should be tailored to the individual dog. A good evaluation of the animal must be obtained to rule out possible risk factors such as obesity, malnutrition and underlying or hidden diseases. The nutritional status of a dog can be evaluated through a dietary history and assessment of body condition. This is best done by the veterinary surgeon, but a few simple questions regarding the type of food currently being fed will help in choosing the most suitable product for the pet.

A good diet history should include:

- Brand name of the food
- Quantity fed
- Information about the giving of treats and titbits, including home-made foods.

Body condition scoring (Fig. 7.1) can be very useful in certain individuals that, although within the breed standard for weight, are actually overweight because of their particular body conformation. Many of your clients will try to tell you

that their dog is 'big-boned'! If you run your hand down the side of the chest and cannot feel the ribs or if, when viewed from above, the dog does not have an obvious waist, then the dog is overweight. Any pet that is obese, i.e. more than 15% over the optimum weight for the breed, should be referred to a veterinary surgeon for a gradual weight-reduction programme. If the dog is just a little overweight you may recommend a reduced-calorie food until optimum body weight is achieved and then switch to a senior food.

Nutritional choices for the older dog

It is important to remember that we cannot make a single dietary recommendation for the aged dog. It is good advice to carefully monitor food intake in very old dogs, since in very old people it is known that low food intake increases the risk of vitamin and mineral deficiencies. Feeding an older dog smaller meals more frequently increases nutrient utilization and may improve food intake.

Canned or dry?

Most dogs in the UK are fed a combination of canned and dry food (meat and mixer). Many dog owners may think that older dogs should have softer foods but this can add to the problem of dental disease. Because of the increased incidence of dental disease in older dogs, a complete dry food is recommended, together with regular home care, e.g. toothbrushing. If the dog is used to a canned-only diet, gradual introduction of the dry product can usually be achieved by using it as if it were a mixer and slowly reducing the amount of canned food offered.

Fixed formulation

The incidence of gut upsets increases with age, since dogs become more susceptible to changes in nutrient intake. A fixed-formula food can help reduce the occurrence of gut upsets including vomiting, diarrhoea and loose stools.

Protein requirements

Numerous factors may affect the choice of the percentage of protein required in the diet and those such as protein digestibility, amino acid profile, caloric density of the food and health status of the dog have to be considered. The protein requirements of elderly dogs are controversial, and the same debate goes on in humans.

Protein given in excess of that required on a daily basis must be broken down and removed from the body. Animals cannot store this extra protein for later use. The process of breaking down this extra protein occurs in the liver, and urea is produced. Urea is toxic and must be removed from the body via the kidneys. Since many older dogs may have kidney or liver disease, it is beneficial to help reduce the load on these organs by reducing the amount of protein the dog has to deal with each day. This does not mean that older dogs should be fed a low-protein diet, just one containing controlled levels of high-quality protein.

Protein is also a source of the mineral phosphorus. It has been discovered that, in dogs with kidney disease, a reduced intake of phosphorus can help slow down the rate at which kidney function gets worse. Therefore, a controlled protein intake is beneficial. A diet containing 18–20% protein (DMB) of good quality and digestibility will provide sufficient protein (Table 7.9).

Table 7.9 Recommended levels of key nutrients for healthy senior dogs

Nutrient	Recommended amount (% DMB)
Protein	18–20
Fat	10–20
Fibre	3–7
Calcium	0.6
Phosphorus	0.5
Sodium	0.2–0.35

Fat

Fat improves palatability, enhances the absorption of fat-soluble vitamins and provides essential fatty acids. A relatively low fat content would be beneficial to prevent obesity in middle-aged dogs. Later in life, however, old dogs show a tendency to lose weight so a balance should be maintained between prevention of obesity and providing enough calories. As a general guide, the diet for an older dog should contain a minimum of 10% (DMB) fat, with a maximum of 20% DMB.

Recently, the question of how essential omega-3 fatty acids are in dogs has received more attention. Omega-3 fatty acids have proven beneficial effects on the body's immune response. The absolute fat content and also the omega-6 to omega-3 fatty acid ratio seem to be important to obtain adequate levels in the tissues. The debate about the best level of these fatty acids continues and currently we have no proven 'best' level. However, the diet for a healthy older dog should contain a high level of essential fatty acids to help improve and maintain good skin and coat condition.

Fibre

Constipation is probably the most common digestive abnormality seen in older dogs. This may be partly due to a reduction in the amount of exercise given to older dogs, since exercise stimulates the gut. Increasing the fibre content of the diet can help to correct this, so a higher-fibre diet (3–7% DMB) may be preferred in older dogs.

Calcium and phosphorus

Osteoporosis (thinning bones) similar to that seen in older people is not common in dogs. Most fractures in dogs are due to trauma and are not age-related. Many people think that, because older people are recommended to take additional calcium to help prevent thinning of the bones, the same must be true for dogs. In fact there is no special need for extra calcium or vitamin D_3 in older dogs provided a balanced diet is fed. However, because of possibly decreased kidney function and the high chance of kidney disease, older dogs should be fed a food containing a low level of phosphorus (around 0.5%) (Table 7.9).

Sodium

A dog's requirement for sodium is not well understood. It is widely assumed that animals fed a generous (often excessive) amount of dietary sodium can be regarded as having a 'normal intake'. When switched to a low-sodium diet, healthy dogs are able to maintain normal blood sodium levels by decreasing faecal and urinary sodium losses accordingly. There is no nutritional need for the levels of sodium found in some pet foods today and the reasons for using salt in canine diets are badly founded, i.e. it is added as a cheap palatability enhancer and not to serve any true nutritional need.

The incidence of heart disease is relatively high in older dogs. Hypertension in dogs may be more common than would be expected and it becomes particularly important in dogs with obesity and kidney disease. Dogs with high blood pressure and heart disease may benefit from a food with a controlled sodium content. An older dog should not receive more than 0.2–0.35% sodium DMB.

Vitamin requirements

Dogs receiving a complete and balanced commercial pet food are unlikely to become deficient in any vitamin. Home-made diets may be low in vitamins if not supplemented. Since many older dogs drink more water (because of poor kidney function) they will lose more of the water-soluble vitamins in their urine. The diet for a healthy older dog should therefore be supplemented with B vitamins.

Zinc

Zinc is an essential part of many substances in the body and zinc supplementation has been associated with enhanced immune response. One study showed that levels of zinc and copper start decreasing in dogs over 7.5 years of age. This may indicate a decrease in the availability of zinc or an increase in losses, resulting in higher nutritional needs. Low levels of zinc have been shown to affect the condition of the skin and coat as well as the body's ability to fight infection and heal wounds. Additional zinc is therefore beneficial in the food for all ageing dogs.

Water

Many older dogs need to drink more because of kidney or liver disease. A plentiful supply of fresh, clean drinking water should always be available. This is especially important in the summer and during long car journeys.

Feeding the healthy older cat

A change of diet should be considered around the age of 7 for all breeds of cat. As with older dogs, we must treat each older cat as an individual. A dietary history and body condition score are also useful aids to determine the cat's current physical condition. In contrast to the situation in older dogs, obesity is much less common in older cats. Many older cats, in fact, become thinner because cats are less well able to digest their food as they age. A highly digestible diet is therefore recommended and this can be achieved by feeding a diet with high-quality ingredients.

Nutritional choices in the older cat

Canned or dry?

Most cats in the UK are fed canned cat food. Many of your clients may think that older cats would be reluctant to eat dry food because of dental disease, which is very common in old cats – many old cats have no teeth left at all. Surprisingly, cats tolerate dry food very well, even when they have no teeth left, and many older cats prefer dry food. Some commercial senior cat foods have been developed with a softer kibble to make chewing easier. Another benefit of dry food is that, because of the higher calorie content, smaller meals are needed. This is of benefit to older cats who do not like to eat very large meals.

Protein requirements

Unlike dogs, cats are obligate carnivores. This means that they must obtain some of their dietary protein from animal sources. A cat's normal protein requirement is much higher than a dog's because cats must also use some of this protein for the production of energy. As cats get older this conversion of protein to energy becomes much less efficient and often leads to weight loss and muscle wastage. It is not possible to reduce the protein intake for healthy older cats to the same degree as we can with dogs. A diet containing 30–40% protein (DMB) of good quality and digestibility will provide sufficient protein.

Fibre

Constipation is very common in older cats because of a reduction in general activity with increasing age. Older dogs can have their activity level increased with relative ease by the owner taking the dog for more frequent walks. However, it is very difficult to persuade an older cat to exercise more. A higher fibre level can help to reduce the risk of constipation developing. Fibre also binds with calcium to reduce the absorption of this mineral. This is beneficial in older cats, which are at a greater risk of developing calcium oxalate bladder disease.

Calcium and phosphorus

Calcium intake should be controlled to help reduce the occurrence of bladder problems caused by calcium oxalate crystals and stones. A reduced intake of phosphorus is also very important in the diet of older cats because of the very high incidence of kidney disease. For older cats, a food with relatively low levels of phosphorus (around 0.7%) and correct calcium to phosphorus ratio is recommended.

Feline lower urinary tract disease (FLUTD)

FLUTD is characterized by an increased frequency of urination, pain on attempting to pass urine and blood in the urine (cystitis). All cats may be affected but it is more common in overweight, inactive cats, especially those living entirely indoors.

FLUTD has many causes but the formation of irritant crystals and stones in the bladder is one major cause. Cats under the age of 7 are more at risk from developing the condition due to the formation of struvite crystals (magnesium ammonium phosphate, also called triple phosphate). Struvite crystals form best in alkaline urine and so all foods for cats under the age of 7 years should be designed to help prevent the disease by producing fairly acidic urine (pH 6.2–6.4). The incidence of struvite bladder disease decreases with increasing age and cats over the age of 7 years are at a greater risk of FLUTD due to calcium oxalate crystals and stones. These oxalate crystals form better in more acidic urine and so senior cat foods should be designed to produce less acidic urine (pH 6.4–6.6).

Water

Many older cats need to drink more because of the likelihood of kidney or liver disease. A plentiful supply of fresh, clean drinking water should always be available. Since many older cats spend long periods of time asleep, often upstairs, it can be useful to suggest that your clients provide at least one source of drinking water for their cats upstairs.

Bibliography

Hand, M.S., Thatcher, C.D., Remillard, R.L., Roudebush, P., 2000. Small Animal Clinical Nutrition, fourth ed. Mark Morris Institute, Topeka, KA.

Recommended reading

Agar, S., 2001. Small Animal Nutrition. Butterworth-Heinemann, Oxford.
Text written especially for veterinary nurses and covers all aspects of the syllabus as well as providing information for work in practice.

Burger, I. (Ed.), 1993. The Waltham Book of Companion Animal Nutrition. Pergamon Press, Oxford.
Deals with the needs of companion animals in depth.

Cooper, B., Lane, D.R., 2006. Veterinary Nursing, fourth ed. BSAVA, Gloucester.
One chapter designed to cover the normal nutritional requirements of a range of companion animals.

CHAPTER 8

Clinical nutrition

Alison Jones

Key Points

- Certain disease conditions change the animal's nutrient requirement and are described as nutrient-sensitive diseases.
- Part of the treatment of these diseases involves dietary management or clinical nutrition.
- The diet for each of these disease conditions must still provide the correct balance of the essential nutrients.

Introduction

Many disease conditions may result in an alteration in the patient's nutrient requirement and they are described as nutrient-sensitive diseases. Their treatment may be facilitated by dietary management and the use of these specialized diets is known as clinical nutrition, which has gained increasing importance in recent years. Clinical nutrition is an area in which veterinary nurses are becoming more involved and a thorough understanding of how diet can influence the patient's recovery is invaluable in modern veterinary practices. Dietary management is important in the conditions described below.

Gastrointestinal disease

There are many different types of gastrointestinal disease and the clinical signs depend on which part of the gastrointestinal tract is primarily affected.

Gastritis

The term gastritis refers to inflammation of the stomach. Dogs vomit readily as a protective mechanism due to their natural scavenging nature. If they eat spoiled or rancid food they are able to vomit and so prevent illness. Conversely, cats are naturally hunters and will kill and eat fresh food. They are therefore much less likely to eat spoiled food and so vomiting is a much more unusual occurrence in the cat.

Gastritis patients should have a short period of gut rest, with or without parenteral fluids, depending on the frequency and severity of the vomiting. When enteral feeding recommences the chosen diet should be bland, low fat and highly digestible, i.e. low in fibre. Low-fat foods are recommended because high-fat diets delay gastric emptying and so remain for longer in the stomach, increasing the chances of the vomiting persisting.

Bloat

Bloat is an acute-onset condition of the stomach and is often fatal. It is also called gastric dilatation and volvulus (GDV). It commonly affects large, deep-chested breeds, especially Great Dane, Weimaraner, St Bernard, Gordon setter, Irish setter and standard poodle.

The cause is unknown but risk factors include:

- Increasing age – dogs over 7 are twice as likely to succumb
- Obesity
- Body conformation, e.g. a narrow, deep chest in Irish setters and a narrow, deep abdomen in Great Danes
- Diet has been implicated, especially high-cereal diets
- Stress
- Aerophagia, i.e. swallowing air during eating
- Lax gastric ligaments – large-volume, bulky, cereal-based diets may predispose to this
- Overdrinking – may stretch the stomach ligaments
- Postprandial exercise, i.e. exercise just after eating.

Dilatation precedes volvulus (twisting of the stomach). Following dilatation the stomach wall and muscle undergo potentially irreversible damage due to lack of blood supply. Treatment of GDV involves immediate decompression and shock therapy. This situation is a true veterinary emergency.

It is controversial as to whether diet affects the incidence of recurrence. Most experts recommend feeding a meat-based, canned, highly digestible diet at least three times daily. Avoidance of postprandial exercise and competitive feeding may also help reduce aerophagia. At-risk dogs should not be competitively fed, as this may increase the ingestion of air. Very greedy dogs should have a large stone placed in the feeding dish to slow down the feeding rate and some people also advocate soaking dry food prior to feeding.

Enteritis

Enteritis means inflammation of the small intestine and the most common clinical sign is diarrhoea. Gut rest is the classic treatment for diarrhoea, i.e. a short (24–48 hours) period of starvation, during which fluids are given either orally or intravenously, is followed by small, low-fat, highly digestible meals. As the diarrhoea improves the animal can be slowly put back on to the normal diet (over a 5–7-day period).

Colitis

Colitis means inflammation of the large intestine and the most common clinical signs are watery diarrhoea, often containing blood and mucus (jelly), with excessive straining and often a dramatic increase in the number of motions passed each day. The affected animal may be constantly trying to pass faeces, only achieving a small amount of blood-stained mucus. Animals with colitis often benefit from diets containing an increased amount of fibre. Some cases of colitis have been linked to food allergy so a strict elimination diet trial with a single novel protein source is recommended in cases that fail to respond to higher fibre levels alone.

Constipation

Animals are said to be constipated when too slow a passage of faeces through the large bowel causes difficulty in passing hard, dry stools. This may be more common in older dogs and cats partly due to decreased physical activity. Since fibre increases the rate of passage of stools through the large intestine, diets that contain higher levels of fibre have proven beneficial in constipation. Many senior pet foods contain a higher level of insoluble fibre in an attempt to help prevent constipation.

Obesity

Obesity is the most common form of malnutrition in pet animals and occurs when there is an increase in body weight that is 15% over the optimum weight for the animal's breed, age and sex. Recent surveys suggest that as many as 40% of dogs and 15% of cats may be clinically obese and most owners are totally unaware of their pet's problem.

The diagnosis of obesity is simple, requiring no specialist equipment. To diagnose obesity simply weigh the pet and compare with breed average, then palpate the area over the ribs – you should be able to feel ribs but not see them. The presence of fat pads over the hips and tail and a pendulous abdomen (especially in cats) are also common signs of obesity.

It is important to remember, when embarking on a weight-reduction programme for a pet, that you are treating the owner as well as the pet. You should always consider a planned exercise programme as well, but any increase in exercise should be undertaken with caution, especially if the pet has joint or heart disease.

The aim of dietary management for obesity is to produce safe, effective weight loss, at the same time maintaining healthy levels of protein, vitamins and minerals. Many commercial low-calorie foods are available but the best effects are achieved using balanced high-fibre, low-fat foods. The fibre provides bulk, which improves satiety while at the same time reducing the energy density of the food and in some way controlling the absorption of the other energy-containing nutrients. It is important that owners are made aware that a planned weight-loss programme is not a crash diet and that gradual weight loss is safer and more effective. A large dog should lose no more than 3% of its body weight per week and a cat no more than 2% each week. To achieve safe weight loss you should aim to provide 60% of the metabolizable energy requirement (MER) needed to maintain optimum body weight in dogs and 70% of MER in cats.

Osteoarthritis

Wear and tear on joints over the life of a pet can lead to oseteoarthritis. Acute injuries such as a ruptured cruciate ligament or joint infection can also damage cartilage and cause arthritis in both dogs and cats. Osteoarthritis (OA) is a common condition that affects up to 1 in 5 dogs over the age of 5 years old and as many as 70% of cats over 12 years old.

The clinical signs associated with OA are due to degeneration of articular cartilage, loss of proteoglycans and collagen, proliferation of new bone and inflammation. This leads to pain and disability; owners will recognize lameness, stiffness and reluctance to exercise as well as a reduced ability to jump, play and use the stairs. Many cats with OA go unnoticed, since owners believe the lack of mobility is just associated with 'old age'. However a lack of grooming and relutance to jump up are good indicators of OA in cats.

Recent studies have shown that supplementing pet food with certain omega-3 fatty acids such as eicosapentaenoic acid (EPA) in dogs and docosahexaenoic acid (DHA) in cats can lead to a reduction in the clinical signs associated with OA by diminishing joint inflammation (and so controlling pain) and by a reduction in the activity of proteoglycan-degrading enzymes such as aggrecanase. Such diets offer a valuable additional therapy for many dogs and cats with OA.

Skin disease

To achieve a healthy-looking coat requires good overall health and nutrition throughout the year. A period of poor skin and hair condition may take several weeks or months to completely recover. For hair to regrow after shaving may take 3–4 months in a short-haired dog and up to 18 months in a long-haired breed.

The skin and coat can influence nutrient requirements. Hair length, thickness and density affect temperature regulation in cold environments. The hair cycle is influenced by general health status, genetics, seasons, temperature, hormones and nutrition as well as poorly understood intrinsic factors. Hair does not grow continuously, but in cycles. Each cycle consists of a growing period (anagen) during which the follicle is actively producing hair, and a resting period (telogen). During telogen, hair is retained in the follicle as dead hair, which is subsequently lost. Hair growth is maximal in summer and minimal in winter when up to 90% may be telogen. Illness, malnutrition and stress from reproduction may shorten anagen considerably and force many hair follicles to enter into telogen at the same time. Since telogen hair is shed easily, malnutrition can result in a visible thinning of the hair coat and cause a dull, lustreless hair coat through nutrient deficiency.

The skin and coat account for about 30–35% of the daily protein requirements of the healthy adult small-breed dog with a long coat. Nutrition is important in achieving and maintaining good skin and coat condition. Important nutrients include:

- Protein (especially sulphur-containing amino acids)
- Energy
- Fat
- Fatty acids
- Vitamin A
- Vitamin B
- Vitamin D
- Vitamin E
- Zinc
- Copper.

Irrespective of the nutritional cause of the disease, the skin usually only responds to nutritional imbalance in a limited number of ways. Skin changes that often indicate nutritional abnormality include:

- A sparse, dry, dull, brittle coat with hairs that epilate easily
- Slow hair growth or regrowth following clipping
- Abnormal scale (seborrhoea sicca)
- Loss of hair, crusting and erythema
- Decubitus ulcers
- Poor wound healing
- Loss of normal hair colour.

In healthy pets eating high-quality commercial pet foods, deficiencies of protein, fat, carbohydrate, vitamins and minerals causing skin disease are very rare. However, nutritional deficiencies may be noted when animals have been anorexic for a period of time. Concurrent disease may reduce the ability of the animal to digest, absorb or metabolize nutrients. Animals fed home-made diets are more likely to develop nutritionally related skin and coat disease, since many of these diets are not balanced.

Nutritional imbalance may occur when owners overfeed a single food type. This is most commonly seen in cats fed on a liver-only diet which contains very high levels of vitamin A. Imbalances may also occur from the improper use of mineral supplementation. This can cause skin disease when the oversupplementation of one nutrient affects the levels of another nutrient that is important in maintaining skin and coat health. This is most commonly seen where oversupplementation of calcium gives rise to zinc deficiency.

Genetic factors may mean that the animal is unable to absorb or utilize a particular nutrient, causing skin or coat disease, e.g. zinc deficiency in Alaskan malamutes.

The common clinical signs of skin and coat disease are:

- Pruritus
- Seborrhoea
- Alopecia
- Hyperkeratosis
- Pyoderma
- Otitis externa
- Slow hair regrowth after clipping.

Animals with non-specific skin disorders should be fed a high-quality, complete, balanced diet containing adequate levels of fat and essential fatty acids plus good-quality, highly digestible protein.

Food-allergic skin disease

In rare cases the animal may actually be allergic to the protein within the diet. This is true food allergy, but the term food allergy is often misused. Many pet owners refer to the reaction their pet had to a particular food as an 'allergic' reaction when it may have just been food intolerance. A true food allergy must involve the pet's immune system and takes many months or even years to develop. A dog or cat that reacts to a new food the first time it is exposed to it probably has food intolerance.

Food allergy or hypersensitivity is an immunological response to one or more dietary proteins. It is considered the third most common skin hypersensitivity disease in dogs and the second most common in cats, accounting for up to 5% of all canine dermatoses and 6% of feline. The prevalence and severity of food hypersensitivity reactions is greatest in younger animals.

Clinical signs are predominantly associated with the skin and/or gastrointestinal tract. A high proportion of food allergies produce skin signs, primarily non-seasonal pruritus; the other skin signs mostly result from self-trauma. Cutaneous signs of food allergy include:

- Pruritus, generalized or localized – including pedal, perineal and facial areas
- Otitis externa
- Miliary dermatitis in cats
- Crusting/scaling
- Secondary pyoderma.

Studies have shown that in more than 65% of all the reported cases dogs were allergic to one of three main foods, i.e. beef, dairy products or wheat (or, more accurately, wheat gluten). Similar studies in cats have found that more than 80% of reported cases could be attributed to beef, dairy products or fish.

An elimination diet trial, for up to 10 weeks, is considered the only certain method of confirming food allergy and without it food allergy may remain undiagnosed. However, diet trials can present difficulties and they have been eliminated by the use of protein hydrolysate technology. Major food allergens are proteins with molecular weights between 10 000 and 70 000 daltons. Hydrolysate technology uses digestive enzymes to break down these proteins to their components (peptides and amino acids), reducing their antigenicity up to 66 times. Hydrolysed protein components have an average molecular weight less than 6000 daltons, too small to trigger an immune reaction.

Essential fatty acid deficiency

The epidermis depends on a supply of essential fatty acids (EFAs) derived either directly from the diet or via synthesis in the liver and transported to the skin in the blood. EFAs have a structural function in the lipoproteins of cell membranes. One of the most important functions of EFAs in the skin is to provide an essential barrier to prevent the loss of water and other nutrients through the epidermis. Linoleic acid must be provided in the diet of dogs and linoleic and arachidonic acids in the diet of cats.

Clinically, EFA deficiency can occur in animals fed low-fat dry or semi-moist commercial foods, or patients fed special low-fat therapeutic diets. Inexpensive or poorly stored foods and those with inadequate antioxidants are more likely to cause an EFA deficiency.

Skin changes have been described in dogs and cats with EFA deficiency. Skin abnormalities include:

- Scaliness (seborrhoea sicca)
- Matting of hair
- Loss of skin elasticity
- Alopecia
- Dry, dull coat
- Hyperkeratosis
- Interdigital exudation
- Otitis externa
- Lack of hair regrowth
- Extensive hair loss.

Fatty acid deficiency is rapidly reversible if the diet is supplemented with EFAs. Although the deficiency may take up to 6 months to develop, clinical signs often start to resolve within a few days of EFA supplementation and the skin is usually healthy within 6–8 weeks. Cats with EFA deficiency must be given pork or poultry fat as well as vegetable oils, since arachidonic acid is only found in fat of animal origin.

Diabetes mellitus

The diet chosen for the diabetic patient should:

- Be balanced to support long-term maintenance
- Help achieve and maintain normal serum glucose levels – this is important since it has been shown that good glycaemic control is important in preventing vascular and neurological complications that are often associated with uncontrolled diabetes
- Decrease postprandial glucose peaks
- Achieve as normal as possible metabolism of carbohydrates, fats and proteins
- Normalize body weight
- Be suitable for the senior life stage, since most cases of diabetes in dogs and cats are diagnosed in pets over the age of 7 years.

The key nutritional factors in diabetes are energy, protein, fat and carbohydrate, both soluble and insoluble.

Protein

The chosen diet should contain sufficient protein to ensure normal development and maintenance of body functions. Diabetic dogs and cats have increased urinary losses of amino acids and this should be remembered when considering the optimum protein intake for the diabetic patient. A balance must be achieved between providing sufficient protein to meet daily needs and replace urinary losses whilst preventing an excess intake that may enhance renal damage or contribute to increased insulin secretion.

Protein levels for diabetic dogs should be approximately 15–25% on a dry matter basis (DMB) and more than 28% DMB for cats. Recent advances in the management of feline diabetes have involved feeding high-protein (50% DMB), low-carbohydrate foods. These have been shown to increase tissue sensitivity to insulin and reduce cholesterol, leading to improved glycaemic control.

Fat

Dogs and cats with diabetes have abnormal fat metabolism. Many diabetic pets have increased serum levels of cholesterol and concurrent pancreatitis is a common finding. High-fat diets cause insulin resistance and decrease the number of insulin receptors. Therefore, high-fat diets should be avoided in dogs and cats with diabetes mellitus.

The supplementation of the diet with omega-3 fatty acids is controversial and in human diabetics there is conflicting evidence that these are beneficial. Omega-3 fatty acid supplementation has been shown to reduce the incidence of atherosclerosis, but not without other complications to glycaemic control. Since the risk of vascular damage is less in pets than in humans, the inclusion of omega-3 fatty acids does not seem to be desirable. The fat content of the diet should be restricted to less than 20% on a DMB.

Soluble carbohydrate

The composition and quantity of dietary carbohydrates for the management of diabetes mellitus in humans is controversial and has also been an area of recent research in small-animal clinical nutrition; however, as yet, absolute recommendations have not been made.

Diabetic cats should not be fed diets containing fructose. Fructose is often found in commercial semi-moist foods as a humectant and as high-fructose corn syrup. Cats do not metabolize fructose, causing fructose intolerance, polyuria and potential renal damage. Some nutritionists believe that high carbohydrate diets may be partly responsible for the onset of diabetes mellitus in cats. As a rule, soluble carbohydrates should make up no more than 30% of the total dietary carbohydrate level.

Insoluble carbohydrate

Dietary fibre is one of the most important nutrients to consider in the management of diabetes mellitus in both dogs and cats.

Food type

The physical presentation of the diet for dogs and cats with diabetes mellitus warrants some consideration. It has been shown that soft, moist foods (those marketed as individual meal-sized portions, usually in foil packets) have a hyperglycaemic effect compared to dry foods because they contain increased levels of simple carbohydrates (sugars) and the ingredients used as humectants (such as propylene glycol). These diets are unsuitable for diabetic pets and should be avoided. Providing the nutritional profile of the chosen food is within the desirable range, there is no advantage or disadvantage in using either canned or dry foods.

Dental disease

Dental disease is the most common disease affecting pet dogs and cats. It is so widespread that it could be thought of as an epidemic. Pet owners can easily identify the signs associated with dental disease, especially bad breath, but often do not link these signs with dental disease. Prevention is an important step in helping to keep pet dogs and cats healthy, since the presence of dental disease has been linked with an increased incidence of systemic diseases, including heart disease, kidney disease and respiratory disorders.

Dental disease begins with the accumulation of an invisible substance, called pellicle, on the surface of the tooth. Pellicle forms within a few minutes of tooth-brushing and is formed from proteins found within saliva (Fig. 8.1).The natural development of pellicle encourages the deposition of plaque, which in turn becomes mineralized to form tartar (dental calculus) and also gives rise to halitosis (oral malodour). Tartar formation, by providing a rough surface, encourages further plaque deposition. The toxins from the bacteria in plaque, aided by the irritation caused by tartar, result in gingivitis (sore, red, inflamed gums that bleed). This is the beginning of periodontal disease and if this disease progresses, periodontitis results. Periodontitis causes the supporting structure of the tooth (the periodontal ligament) to become damaged and ultimately destroyed, leading to loosening, and finally loss, of the teeth.

The best way to keep teeth and gums healthy is to encourage your clients to brush their pets' teeth daily. However, despite awareness that tooth-brushing is how we keep our own teeth clean, most pets never have their teeth brushed. This may be due to the temperament of the pet or simply due to lack of time or motivation on the part of the owner.

Life-stage diets are now available that help to avoid the occurrence or recurrence of periodontal disease, by wiping away accumulated plaque and tartar when the pet animal chews. These foods are designed to allow a tooth to penetrate each piece of food (kibble) before the kibble splits. The fibres in the kibble are non-randomly aligned to clean the surface of the tooth as they come into contact with it and they wipe the accumulation of plaque, stain and tartar from

the tooth's surface. By reducing plaque accumulation these dental foods may help to control bad breath.

Dogs and cats with severe periodontal disease require appropriate veterinary treatment to control bacterial spread and promote healing. The advanced nature of the condition, with severe inflammation and pain, means that they cannot chew effectively on affected teeth. Attempts at chewing might force food particles into exposed tooth sockets, causing bleeding and local irritation. If a pet has had extensive treatment for severe periodontal disease the veterinary surgeon and the client will need to monitor the healing and postoperative oral pain to determine when the feeding of an appropriate dental food can begin.

Cancer

Few diseases evoke as much emotion as cancer. A diagnosis of cancer is traumatic for both the owner and sometimes the veterinary practice team. Many owners already have some personal experience of cancer and they may approach cancer in their pets with some preconceived ideas, especially with regard to the use of chemotherapy. They may need considerable support and assistance during the initial weeks following the diagnosis.

Common forms of cancer in dogs include mammary cancer, ovarian cancer, lymphoma, skin tumours (certain breeds such as boxers are more prone to these types of cancer) and tumours of the spleen (haemangiosarcoma or haemangioma). Lymphoma (also called lymphosarcoma) is a cancer of the lymphatic system and in the most common form of lymphoma; you may notice that the dog's lymph nodes become enlarged and can be easily palpated.

Cancer cachexia may occur in dogs with seemingly good nutritional intake because the composition of the food is inappropriate for the canine cancer patient. The general metabolism of patients with cancer is forced to compete with the tumour for glucose and amino acids which are used for energy. The dog must therefore rely on fat as a source of calories since the tumour has a limited ability to use fat as an energy source. The following nutrients have been found to be vital in the management of cancer.

Carbohydrate

Dogs do not have an essential requirement for carbohydrate in the diet. However, most dogs have a remarkable ability to utilize carbohydrates for energy so they are often used by pet food manufacturers as a primary source of dietary energy. Dogs with cancer develop high levels of insulin and lactate, as the tumour uses glucose and produces lactate. High-carbohydrate foods should be avoided in dogs with cancer since they would add to this hyperinsulinaemia and hyperlactataemia. Carbohydrates should comprise less than 25% of the food's dry matter.

Fat

Dogs use fat as a source of energy and to aid in the absorption of the fat-soluble vitamins. Canine cancer patients must rely on fat as a source of calories, so to facilitate this and to reduce the loss of body fat stores, the ideal food should be

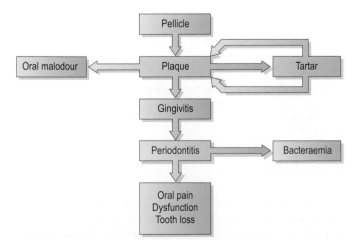

Fig. 8.1 Significance of the development of pellicle on the signs of periodontal disease (*Adapted from Hill's Pet Nutrition*)

high in fat. Dietary fat should make up 25–40% of the food's dry matter.

Omega-3 fatty acids

Dietary levels should be in excess of 5% of the food's dry matter and research has shown that a food high in omega-3 fatty acids is beneficial to the cancer patient by:

- Inhibiting tumour growth and cancer spread
- Reducing cachexia by decreasing protein breakdown
- Enhancing immune function
- Reducing radiation damage to healthy cells.

Protein

Normal healthy dogs use protein and amino acids to build muscles and organ tissue and to maintain immune status. In the dog with cancer the tumour is competing for these same amino acids. The ideal food for the canine cancer patient should therefore be higher in protein than a normal adult maintenance food. This is a very unusual profile for a canine senior food (many canine cancer patients will be in the senior stage of life), which would normally have controlled levels of protein. Dietary levels should be between 30% and 45% of the food's dry matter.

Arginine

Arginine has been found to be essential in dogs with malignant tumours and high levels improve both immune function and anabolism. Dietary levels should be in excess of 2% of the food's dry matter.

Chronic renal failure

Chronic renal failure (CRF) is a progressive deterioration of renal function that occurs throughout an animal's lifetime as part of the normal ageing process. In renal failure the kidney is unable to excrete metabolites at normal plasma levels under normal fluid loading or to retain electrolytes when the intake is normal. In the majority of adult dogs and cats, some degree of renal disease exists.

Clinical signs of renal failure include:

- Polyuria/polydipsia
- Weight loss
- Inappetance
- Uraemia/azotaemia
- Ulceration of oral/gastric mucosa
- Vomiting
- Dehydration
- Unkempt appearance.

The main problem facing the clinician is that changes do not occur in the blood of affected animals until 75% of nephrons have ceased functioning, i.e. the animal has lost the equivalent of one whole kidney and half of the other and these nephrons can never be repaired.

Early diagnosis of kidney disease can be made by considering urine specific gravity, daily water intake and urine chemistry. The animal with early renal problems will lose the ability to produce the most concentrated urine when about 66% of nephrons have ceased functioning. This stage is termed renal insufficiency and it is now that dietary intervention should begin rather than leave it until the animal is uraemic and in renal failure.

The aim of dietary management in renal disease is to ameliorate clinical signs and slow down progression of the disease. Correct diet for an animal with renal compromise is critical. The animal still needs a nutritionally balanced diet that provides all the nutrients required for maintenance. However, it has been shown that, by reducing the daily intake of phosphorus, renal deterioration can be slowed down. Moderate protein restriction can help to reduce the clinical signs caused by uraemia but adequate protein must be included in the diet to prevent the breakdown of lean body mass to provide essential amino acids. It is best if the protein source for animals with chronic renal failure is of very high biological value.

Dietary management is the cornerstone of the management of CRF in both the dog and the cat; however, other medical therapies can be beneficial to the overall well-being of the pet. Renal failure causes imbalances in minerals and electrolytes that can make the animal feel unwell:

- Hypokalaemia is common in cats with CRF. This causes muscle weakness, inappetance, anaemia and lethargy. Dietary supplementation is best but clinical cases can be treated with oral potassium gluconate and then maintained on a diet with adequate levels of potassium.
- Hyperphosphataemia can occur in CRF as a result of decreased ability of the damaged kidney to excrete phosphorus and reduced renal production of active vitamin D. This high circulating level of phosphorus stimulates the parathyroid glands to increase secretion of parathormone (PTH), leading to the development of renal secondary hyperparathyroidism. Excess levels of PTH have a deleterious effect on bone metabolism and result in pain and osteomalacia (termed 'rubber jaw', or renal rickets). Control of blood phosphorus levels is best attempted by dietary restriction of intake; however, some cases may benefit from oral phosphate binders if dietary restriction alone fails to correct hyperphosphataemia within 2–4 weeks. Intestinal phosphate binders can be administered with food at a dose rate of 60 mg/kg/day, increasing to 150 mg/kg/day if tolerated.

The ideal nutrient profile for the management of renal failure is:

- Controlled protein
- Controlled sodium to help prevent hypertension
- Controlled phosphorus
- Buffered
- High fat.

Liver disease

Liver disease is common in both dogs and cats. The liver has an enormous capacity to regenerate, so liver disease is not often diagnosed until the later stages of the disease process. In recent years significant new information has emerged concerning the metabolic changes that occur in patients with liver disease. These studies have also found that the correct nutrition is a vital step in helping to reverse these metabolic changes and facilitate recovery.

There is a vast array of supportive therapy for the liver patient in order to optimize regeneration; however, nutritional support is the cornerstone of therapy. A fine balance must be achieved between providing sufficient high-quality nutrients to allow regeneration, without overwhelming the metabolic capacity of the diseased liver, which may lead to the accumulation of toxic metabolites. The key objectives of dietary management are to:

- Maintain homeostasis
- Correct electrolyte disturbances
- Avoid accumulation of toxic by-products
- Support liver repair and regeneration
- Support storage and synthesis within the liver
- Prevent or reduce encephalopathy
- Improve the overall nutritional status of the animal.

The key nutrients of concern for the dog and cat with liver disease are as follows.

Protein

Hyperammonaemia is a common finding in dogs and cats with liver disease because of the development of portosystemic shunts and the impaired activity of the urea cycle. This is the key metabolic abnormality that leads to hepatic encephalopathy. The clinical presentation of animals with hepatic encephalopathy can vary from mild lethargy to the severe classic central nervous system disturbances. Finding the correct level of protein in the diet for the liver patient presents a nutritional dilemma. A balance must be found between reducing the level of protein to control hepatic encephalopathy and at the same time providing sufficient protein to allow for adequate production of plasma proteins and for hepatic regeneration and repair.

The current recommendation is to provide a moderate level of high-quality protein containing a low level of aromatic amino acids. This will allow regeneration but limit the development of metabolic neurotoxins. Arginine is an essential amino acid for both dogs and cats. It is needed for the synthesis of protein and amino acids and is essential in the optimal function of the urea cycle. In patients with liver disease a high intake of arginine has been found to be beneficial by reducing blood ammonia levels and improving nitrogen balance.

Energy

Patients with liver disease have decreased glycogen stores and develop insulin resistance through increased glucagon levels. These metabolic abnormalities lead to the early onset of gluconeogenesis. This protein catabolism can be reduced by providing frequent small meals and by ensuring that sufficient calories are provided in the form of carbohydrate and fat.

Carbohydrate

A very high carbohydrate intake must be avoided because insulin resistance commonly occurs in liver disease and can lead to glucose intolerance. This can be avoided by providing sufficient calories in the form of fat.

Fat

This is the most energy-dense nutrient, providing over twice as many calories per gram as either carbohydrate or protein. The provision of calories from fat supports protein synthesis and prevents gluconeogenesis. Fat also improves the palatability of the diet, an important fact in the liver patient where inappetance is very common. Fat also provides fatty acids, the major fuel for the liver, heart and skeletal muscles. The intestinal assimilation of fat is not compromised in dogs and cats with liver disease unless there is severe extrahepatic biliary obstruction, which is rare. This means there is no need to routinely restrict dietary fat in the liver patient; in fact, studies have shown a correlation between high-fat diets and increased survival in dogs with hepatic insufficiency.

L-carnitine

The final step in the synthesis of L-carnitine occurs in the liver and consequently it may be deficient in cases of liver disease. This deficiency may lead to the accumulation of free fatty acids in the cytoplasm and failure of the mitochondria, with impairment of the citric acid cycle, fatty acid oxidation and the urea cycle. This combines to cause an increase in blood ammonia levels. By supplementing the diet with additional L-carnitine this deficiency is avoided and thus the fatty acids provided from the dietary fat can be utilized as an energy source. Additional L-carnitine also decreases the risk of hepatic lipidosis, which is of particular concern in cats.

Soluble fibre

This is fermented in the gastrointestinal tract to produce short-chain fatty acids, which provide an alternative energy source for enterocytes, stimulate intestinal motility and encourage bacterial proliferation and epithelial cell growth. These all combine to result in a significant reduction in the production and absorption of ammonia, which helps to reduce the degree of hepatic encephalopathy.

Copper and zinc

Copper toxicosis is a well-recognized syndrome in Bedlington terriers, West Highland white terriers, Dobermans and Skye terriers. However, copper accumulates in the liver of all breeds in most forms of hepatobiliary disease, especially when a degree of cholestasis is present. The ideal diet for liver patients should be low in copper. Increased zinc intake decreases the intestinal uptake of copper and may also have a local protective effect against copper toxicity. Adequate zinc also helps to limit hepatic encephalopathy and may have an antifibrotic effect.

Critical care of the anorexic patient

Anorexia is defined as a loss of appetite. It is important to differentiate between an animal that is unable to prehend, masticate and swallow food (dysphagia) from an animal that is anorexic because of secondary systemic disease.

Many conditions cause a patient to become anorexic and these include:

- Alteration in taste or smell, due to profuse nasal discharge, old age, etc.
- Pain due to ulcers or foreign bodies, e.g. bones, needles
- Systemic disease, e.g. renal failure
- Trauma, e.g. head injury, jaw fracture
- Gastrointestinal tract dysfunction, e.g. intestinal obstruction, tumour
- Neoplasia.

When treating an anorexic patient consideration should be given to fluid and electrolyte balance as well as the calorie and protein content of the food. Water is the most important nutrient, since two-thirds of an animal's lean body mass consists of water and a 15% loss of body water would be fatal. An animal's water needs are met by drinking, by water in food and by water produced from energy metabolism in the body, but severe water loss may occur through vomiting, diarrhoea, salivation and burns. During periods of reduced water intake or increased water loss the kidneys attempt to conserve body water by producing more concentrated urine. If water loss exceeds water intake, dehydration occurs. All dehydrated critical care patients should have their fluid deficit measured and replaced as a matter of urgency via intravenous fluid therapy.

As well as fluid therapy, additional nutritional support is indicated if there has been recent weight loss of more than 10% or a history of anorexia for more than 3–5 days. The food chosen for the critical patient should be high in both protein and fat. As a general rule, if the gut works, then use it. This means that, apart from those patients with severe acute vomiting, acute pancreatitis or in some cases, post-surgery removal of a foreign body, oral feeding is recommended and desirable.

Protein makes up 15–20% of body weight. Initially an anorexic animal will use up all body glucose and then stored glycogen. After the first 4 days of food deprivation, muscle protein is catabolized. If this anorexic animal has malignant disease or burns, further protein losses will be occurring, leading to basal protein requirements increasing by up to 2–3 times depending upon the severity of the disease.

Animals will need extra protein as a source of calories and to support wound healing, maintain the immune system and reverse the hypermetabolic processes. When feeding a critically ill or anorexic patient you should aim to supply at least 4 g protein/100 kcal for the dog and at least 6 g protein/100 kcal for the cat. The total amount of both protein and calories needed will vary with the severity of the illness, e.g. a patient with a major burn will need 2 × basal energy requirement (BER), while immediately post-surgery the additional calorie needs will only be around 1.25 × BER (see Ch. 7). Animals with severe fluid loss may require supplemental water-soluble vitamins, especially B vitamins.

Some patients will refuse to eat voluntarily or may be too severely ill or injured to accept oral feeding. The enteral route is still preferred, since it is the most efficient and allows nutrition of the enterocytes. Failure to supply the enterocytes with their preferred fuel (glutamine) can result in defects in the intestinal mucosa and bacterial translocation from the gut into the blood stream. If a patient refuses voluntary nutrition, tube feeding should be considered. Many different types of feeding tube are available, including:

- Naso-oesophageal tubes – simple to place and tolerated in most animals, although problems may arise if an animal sneezes or gags the tube out.
- Pharyngostomy tubes – may also be associated with gagging and local infection, but in most patients they are well tolerated.
- Gastrostomy tubes – becoming more popular and percutaneous endoscopic gastrostomy (PEG) tubes may be placed using an endoscope. There is also a piece of equipment called an ELD applicator that allows a gastrostomy tube to be placed without the need for an endoscope. The main advantage of a tube placed directly into the stomach is that it can be left in situ for considerably longer periods and it allows the use of larger quantities of food. When feeding through a tube, care should be taken not to exceed the maximum stomach capacity for the patient. This is 90 ml/kg/feed for an adult dog and 45 ml/kg/feed for a cat.

The diet used for tube feeding should be balanced, easily digested, easily assimilated and easily utilized. It should be in a form that does not block the tube. Powders that have to be mixed with water are best avoided, especially if very small-bore tubes are used.

Canine urolithiasis

Common forms of canine bladder stones and crystals include:

- Struvite – composed of magnesium ammonium phosphate (also known as triple phosphate). These crystals and stones are common in puppies, bitches and any dog with bacterial infection in the urine. Most cases of bladder stones and crystals in puppies are due to struvite formation. Bacterial infection is present in 95% of all cases and causes an increase in urinary pH, facilitating the formation of struvite, which forms in alkaline urine. One of the most important factors in preventing struvite crystals and stones is maintaining a normal, i.e. acidic, urine with a pH of 6.2–6.4. This can be achieved by dietary management.
- Calcium oxalate – tend to form in more acidic urine. They are more common in male dogs over the age of 8 years and in certain breeds, especially the Lhasa Apso, Shih Tzu and Yorkshire terrier. Calcium oxalate stones are more likely to also occur within the kidney. Dogs that consume high amounts of oxalate in their diets, e.g. vegetables, tea, nuts and chocolate, are at a greater risk of developing these stones. One of the most important factors in preventing their occurrence is reducing the calcium content of the urine and maintaining slightly alkaline urine. This means that the dog's urine should have a pH in the range 7.1–7.7, which can be achieved by dietary management.
- Ammonium urate – tend to form in more acidic urine. They are more common in certain breeds of dog, especially the dalmatian and Yorkshire terrier. Dogs with liver disease are also more prone to the development of ammonium urate bladder crystals and stones.

- Cystine – tend to form in acidic urine. Most individuals affected with cystine urolithiasis are male bulldogs. It is assumed that they form as a consequence of a genetic defect in kidney function.

Dietary control is vitally important in the management of canine urolithiasis. Dietary management is useful both in the short-term treatment and in the long-term prevention of recurrence of the problem.

Struvite can be dissolved using a combination of drugs, including antibiotics if a bacterial infection is present, and diet. This is achieved by reducing the intake of the 'building blocks' of the stone. Struvite stones are composed of magnesium, ammonium and phosphate. Dissolution diets should therefore contain a controlled level of the minerals magnesium and phosphorus, plus an increased level of sodium. This increased sodium level encourages the dog to drink more water and produce a greater volume of urine, and so flushes the bladder out more frequently. The special dietary formulation also causes the formation of acidic urine, with a pH of about 6.0. At this level the formation of further struvite crystals is inhibited and those already present dissolve in the urine.

Disease caused by calcium oxalate uroliths can only be treated surgically, as these stones do not dissolve once formed. To prevent recurrence, provide a diet that contains a controlled level of the 'building blocks' of this stone type, plus one that produces more alkaline urine. The diet should contain controlled levels of both calcium and oxalate and produce a urinary pH of 7.1–7.7.

Feline lower urinary tract disease

Feline lower urinary tract disease (FLUTD) is not a single disease but a group of conditions, many of which cause inflammation of the lower urinary tract. The most common presenting signs of FLUTD are:

- Difficulty passing urine – dysuria
- Altered frequency of urination
- Incontinence
- Haematuria.

Dietary control is vitally important in the management of FLUTD, especially in those cases caused by urolithiasis (most commonly struvite and calcium oxalate in the cat) and is useful both in the short-term treatment of FLUTD and in the long term to prevent recurrence of the problem.

Struvite can be dissolved using a combination of drugs, including antibiotics if a bacterial infection is present, and dietary management. This is achieved by reducing the cat's intake of the 'building blocks' of the stone. Since struvite stones are composed of magnesium, ammonium and phosphate a diet that contains a controlled level of the minerals magnesium and phosphorus, plus an increased level of sodium (as salt) should be fed. This increased sodium level encourages the cat to drink more water and produce a greater volume of urine and so flushes the bladder out more frequently. The special dietary formulation also causes the formation of acidic urine, with a pH of about 6.0. At this level the formation of further struvite crystals is inhibited and those present dissolve into the urine.

Dietary management is also important in the prevention of recurrence of FLUTD. In cases of struvite urolithiasis the diet should contain a controlled level of the 'building blocks' of the stone plus it should produce a naturally acidic urine (pH 6.2–6.4). This prevention of recurrence food should not be high in sodium, as long-term high intake of salt may be detrimental to health. Since obesity is a major predisposing factor in the development of FLUTD, calorie intake should be controlled in all overweight cats.

In cases of calcium oxalate urolithiasis, feed a diet containing controlled levels of both calcium and oxalate that produces a urinary pH of 6.6–6.9. This helps to inhibit the formation of calcium oxalate crystals. A dietary source of soluble fibre is also helpful, since the fibre will bind with calcium in the gut to further reduce the amount of renally excreted calcium. Every effort should be made to ensure that cats affected with FLUTD drink more water. Reducing the urine specific gravity will reduce the chance of recurrence.

Bibliography

Hand, M.S., Thatcher, C.D., Remillard, R.L., Roudebush, P., 2000. Small Animal Clinical Nutrition, fourth ed. Mark Morris Institute, Topeka, KA.

Recommended reading

Agar, S., 2001. Small Animal Nutrition. Butterworth-Heinemann, Oxford.
Written especially for veterinary nurses and covers all aspects of the syllabus as well as providing information for work in practice.

Hand, M.S., Thatcher, C.D., Remillard, R.L., Roudebush, P., 2000. Small Animal Clinical Nutrition, fourth ed. Mark Morris Institute, Topeka, KA.
Very detailed coverage of the subject. Good reference text.

Kelly, N., Wills, J., 1996. Manual of Companion Animal Nutrition and Feeding. British Small Animal Veterinary Association, Cheltenham.
Good reference book that covers all aspects of nutrition in health and disease. Includes feeding of small pets and exotic species.

Markwell, P.J., 1992. Applied Clinical Nutrition of the Dog and Cat. Waltham, Melton Mowbray.
Excellent coverage of clinical nutrition.

CHAPTER 9

Equine nutrition

Corinna Pippard

Key Points

- The anatomy and physiology of the equine digestive system is designed to deal with poor-quality food that is eaten throughout the day and digested slowly.
- A healthy horse must be provided with a similar range of essential nutrients to any other mammal, but the relative proportions of each depend on the type of horse and the 'work' it is undertaking.
- All food must be stored in such a way as to prevent deterioration and supplied to the horse using appropriate equipment.

Introduction

The genus *Equus* has evolved to roam large areas in search of its main food ingredient, grass. As a prey species, it has to be constantly aware of its surroundings and ready to flee instantaneously. As a result, the digestive system has evolved to deal with a poor-quality diet eaten over a long period of time and undergoing a slow but constant digestive process.

There are generally considered to be six species within the genus *Equus*, and a number of subspecies: *Equus przewalskii*, the wild horse; *Equus asinus*, the African ass; *Equus hermionus*, the Asian ass; and *Equus burchelli*, *Equus zebra* and *Equus grevyi*, the zebras. The origin of *Equus caballus*, the domestic horse, is something of a mystery, since it does not occur in the wild. The nearest relative of *E. caballus*, *E. przewalskii*, has one extra pair of chromosomes, 33 pairs compared with the 32 pairs of the domestic horse.

With domestication, many horses have to cope with being confined for large periods of time and fed three or four meals a day, a situation that is good for neither the mental nor physical health of the horse. The original purpose and design of the digestive system should always be considered when feeding horses and care should be taken to try and ensure that a feeding system as close to nature as possible is chosen.

The digestive system

(See also Ch. 6.)

The digestive system of the horse can be divided into two parts:

- The foregut – comprises the mouth, oesophagus, stomach and small intestine; function is similar to these parts of the digestive system of other monogastric animals, e.g. dog and cat
- The hindgut – comprises the caecum, colon and rectum; the caecum and colon fulfil a function analogous to the reticulo-rumen in ruminants, providing a region where extensive microbial fermentation of food can take place.

Precaecal digestion

In this, the first part of the horse's digestive system, physical and chemical digestion take place as they would in humans, cats or dogs. Food is ingested and ground by the teeth before being swallowed and entering the stomach, where enzymatic digestion starts. Enzymatic digestion, followed by absorption, continues in the small intestine.

Mouth

Teeth

Adult dentition in the horse consists of a total of 40–44 teeth in the male (stallion or gelding) and 36–40 teeth in the mare. All horses have three upper and lower incisors on each side of the jaw, three upper and lower premolars, and three upper and lower molars. In the male, and occasionally the female, canine teeth known as tushes are found and many horses have extra premolar teeth, known as wolf teeth, which are frequently removed to aid placing of the bit. There is a large gap between incisor and premolar teeth, known as the diastema, which aids the separation of newly ingested and partly masticated food (Fig. 9.1A).

Foals are normally born without teeth, and the central incisors erupt during the first week of life, followed, at about 4–6 weeks and 6–9 months, by the lateral and

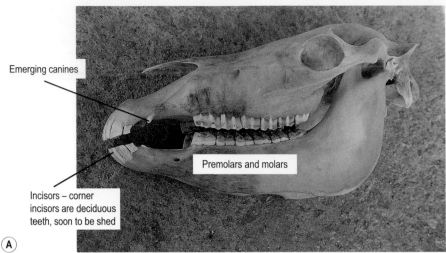

Emerging canines

Premolars and molars

Incisors – corner incisors are deciduous teeth, soon to be shed

(A)

Fig. 9.1 (**A**) Dentition of a 4-year-old male horse. (**B**) The same horse, showing the ridges on the teeth that enable a rough surface to be applied to the food

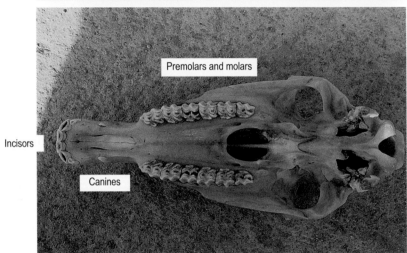

Premolars and molars

Incisors

Canines

(B)

corner incisors, respectively; premolar teeth also erupt at this time. Deciduous teeth are replaced by permanent teeth in the same order between the ages of about 2.5 and 4.5 years.

All the permanent teeth in the horse are constantly erupting and the grinding surface is made up of ridges of enamel and dentine (Fig. 9.1B). Since enamel wears more slowly than dentine and the horse subjects its food to a shearing and grinding movement, the surfaces of the teeth maintain a rough profile. They may develop sharp edges, which must be removed for efficient mastication of food. There is evidence that feeding from the ground leads to a more natural pattern of wear than feeding from a height (e.g haynets).

The eruption of the deciduous and permanent teeth and the pattern of wear may be used as a means of determining the age of a horse; however, as the horse gets older this becomes less accurate.

Tongue

The tongue of the horse feels very soft because of the presence of shorter and softer filiform papillae than in other animals. Fungiform, foliate and circumvallate papillae are also present. Taste buds are present, and the horse can detect sweet, sour, bitter and salt flavours.

Lips

Lips are prehensile and very sensitive and are used by the horse to aid food selection and prevent the ingestion of potentially harmful material. A horse is capable of selecting individual ingredients out of a coarse mix or eating the last blades of grass from around a poisonous plant without touching it.

Salivary glands

Horses secrete a large quantity of saliva (10–15 litres per day), the main purpose of which is to lubricate food. A small amount of salivary amylase is secreted but is probably of little importance. Bicarbonate is also secreted which has some buffering capacity.

Oesophagus

A muscular tube, similar to that found in other domestic animals, the oesophagus passes down the left side of the neck. The passage of food and water may easily be observed.

Stomach

The stomach of the horse is simple and digestion is monogastric as in the dog and cat. The stomach is small

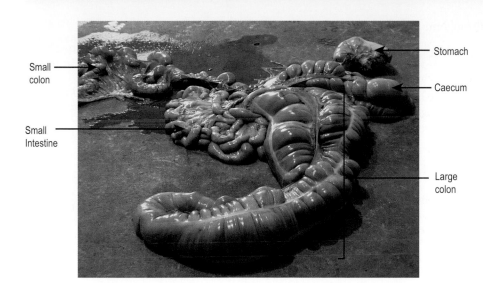

Fig. 9.2 Gastrointestinal tract of the horse

Small colon

Small Intestine

Stomach

Caecum

Large colon

(7–14 litres) compared with the size of the animal and accounts for only about 7.5% of the total digestive tract. Living in natural circumstances the horse would normally graze for a large proportion of the day and food would continually enter and leave the stomach with little actual digestion occurring apart from the initial breakdown of protein. The horse is unable to regurgitate food. In the stabled horse the stomach fills rapidly when a concentrate meal is fed and then acts as a storage organ, enabling food to enter the small intestine in small quantities for maximum digestion. The buffering capacity of the saliva may enable a limited amount of fermentation to take place in the first part of the stomach.

Small intestine

The small intestine is responsible, as in other animals, for the majority of enzymatic digestion of food and its subsequent absorption. In the horse the tract is long (about 16 m) and accounts for around 75% of the length of the gastrointestinal tract, but only 27% of its volume. As in other animals, it is divided into three parts, the duodenum, jejunum and ileum, and the ileum ends at the ileocaecal junction (Fig. 9.2). Digesta moves rapidly along the small intestine but, despite this, under normal circumstances digestion and absorption of soluble material are usually complete by the time it reaches the ileocaecal junction.

Large intestine

It is in the large intestine or hindgut that fibre digestion takes place, undergoing a microbial fermentation similar to that seen in ruminants and rabbits. The main areas involved in this process are the caecum and colon (Fig. 9.2). The size and complexity of the hindgut in the horse are what makes its digestive system so different from that of other monogastric animals; the hindgut accounts for around 65% of the volume of the digestive tract.

Caecum

The caecum is a large (25–35 litres), blind-ending sac about 0.8 m long, running forwards along the base of the abdomen,

and it is here that food entering from the ileum starts to undergo microbial fermentation. The digesta contains around 90% water but by the time defecation occurs the water content has fallen to about 60%, the largest proportion of water being reabsorbed in the caecum.

Colon

This can be divided into two parts: the large colon, mainly concerned with the digestion of fibre, and the small colon, where further water reabsorption takes place. Both are about 3–3.5 m long; however, parts of the large colon are up to 50 cm in diameter, while the small colon is only about 7.5 cm in diameter.

The large colon houses a considerable number of microorganisms, similar to the rumen in cattle and the caecum and colon of rabbits. It runs from the ileocaecal junction cranially towards the sternum – the right ventral colon, where it makes a turn – sternal flexure, back towards the pelvis – left ventral colon, then a sharp turn – the pelvic flexure, forwards again towards the diaphragm – left dorsal colon, and then backwards again – diaphragmatic flexure and right dorsal colon. Finally, the large colon makes another turn and crosses from one side to the other – transverse colon – before becoming the small colon. An important point to note, and a potential problem area, is the pelvic flexure, where the colon narrows from a diameter of about 25 cm to around 2 cm while undergoing a 180° turn. In the grass-fed horse this serves to slow down the passage of food, allowing ample time for microbial digestion; however, in the stabled horse fed a much drier diet and unable to move around freely, it can sometimes be the site of an impaction.

The small colon is approximately the same length as the large colon but of a smaller diameter (Fig. 9.2). Microbial fermentation does not stop here; however, it is of less importance and the main function of the small colon is to slow the passage of digesta and reabsorb water to enable relatively dry faeces to be voided.

Rectum and anus

The rectum acts as a storage area for faeces, as in other mammals. Horses will defecate frequently throughout the day and night, maintaining a constant throughput of material through the gastrointestinal tract.

Microbial activity in the hindgut

Unlike many other monogastric species, the horse is capable of living on a diet solely composed of fibrous roughage and a large population of microorganisms is housed in the enlarged hindgut. These microorganisms consist of about $0.5–5 \times 10^9$ bacteria per gram of contents and $0.5–1.5 \times 10^5$ protozoa. Fungi are also present, but in much smaller numbers.

Microbial enzymes are capable of breaking the β-1,4 linkages found in cellulose, unlike mammalian enzymes, and produce end-products of volatile fatty acids (largely acetic, propionic and butyric acids) and lactic acid, which can be absorbed directly from the hindgut. Other products of microbial fermentation of potential use to the horse are amino acids and a number of vitamins.

The microorganisms in the hindgut are very specific to the type of food eaten by the horse and also to the pattern of meals eaten when the horse is fed concentrates. Changing the diet suddenly can result in the death of large numbers of microorganisms that were digesting the old foodstuff and an insufficient number capable of digesting the new foodstuff. Such changes in diet can result in impaction, colic, laminitis and swollen legs.

Unlike some other hindgut fermenters, such as the rabbit, the horse does not normally practice coprophagia, although foals may be observed eating the faeces of adult horses, usually their mother's. This may be done in an attempt to populate the hindgut with suitable microorganisms. As they do not generally eat their own faeces, horses probably make little use of the amino acids synthesized by their microorganisms, although some may be absorbed.

Dietary management

Essential nutrients

The basic nutrients required by the horse are the same as for most other domestic animals. However, the form in which they are offered differs.

Water

An adult horse will drink about 25 litres of water a day, more in hot weather, after strenuous exercise or in the case of a lactating mare. For the horse at grass much of or the entire water requirement may be obtained from its food. Although it is usually advocated that water should be available at all times, it is likely that, under wild conditions, horses only drink at dawn and dusk, thus increasing the distance that can be travelled in search of food during the intervening time. However, unless all food is fed damp it is advisable to make sure that water is regularly available. All water supplies should be clean and easy to reach. Dehydration in the horse will reduce performance, since the horse relies extensively on sweating as a cooling method and severe dehydration (loss of 10–12% bodyweight) can be fatal. Donkeys are much more resistant to water deprivation than horses.

Energy

This can be obtained from carbohydrate, fat or protein. In the horse, the largest proportion normally comes from carbohydrate. Energy deficiency in the diet will result in a thin and probably lethargic horse; too much energy will result in either an unmanageable horse or one that is overweight, which can lead to a variety of other problems.

Carbohydrate

The majority of the natural diet of the horse consists of carbohydrate and this can be divided into soluble and insoluble carbohydrate. Unlike many monogastric animals, the horse has evolved to make good use of insoluble carbohydrate by utilizing microbial action in the hindgut. The gross energy (GE) content of carbohydrates is about 17.5 MJ/kg.

- **Soluble carbohydrate** – consists of sugars and starches. Grass, especially young grass, contains large amounts of sugars which are readily digested in the small intestine and will produce abundant energy quickly. Starch is found less in the natural diet but is a major component of commercial concentrate diets. It must always be remembered that the horse does not digest starch particularly effectively, although some starches are more easily digested than others with cooked starches being the most readily digested. Any soluble carbohydrates undigested in the small intestine will enter the large intestine where they may upset the balance of the microbial population and cause serious problems.
- **Insoluble carbohydrate** – like the ruminants, the horse is capable of digesting a large proportion of the fibre in its diet. The structural parts of plants are made up of a variety of celluloses, hemicelluloses, lignins and other materials. None of these are digestible by mammalian enzymes but, with the exception of lignin, can be digested by microorganisms. In the hindgut, these are broken down to volatile fatty acids and lactic acid, which are used by the horse for energy and produce a large amount of gas, which is either absorbed into the bloodstream or released via the anus. Unlike the digestion of soluble sugars, the process is a slow one and also produces a considerable amount of heat.

Since the horse relies only partly on **glucose** absorbed from the gastrointestinal tract for energy, and obtains a large proportion of its energy from volatile fatty acids, the glucose concentration of a horse's blood is lower than that seen in other monogastric animals. The only volatile fatty acid that can be metabolized to glucose is propionic acid.

Lack of **fibre** in the diet is detrimental to the horse's health, both physical and mental. Various physical problems result from the lack of activity in the gastrointestinal tract, and boredom, with the possible development of stereotypic behaviour, may also occur in the stabled horse fed too little fibre.

Fat

Despite the fact that fat is present in relatively small quantities in the horse's natural diet, it is very well digested and utilized. Since fat contains about 2.3 times the GE (39 MJ/kg) of a similar weight of carbohydrate, it is an excellent energy source, especially where bulk intake or heat production must be restricted, e.g. in the endurance horse. The metabolism of fat also releases a considerable quantity of water, which the horse can utilize.

Protein

Like most animals, the horse has a requirement for amino acids, rather than protein, and 10 of these amino acids are believed to be essential (arginine, histidine, isoleucine, leucine, lysine, methionine, phenylalanine, threonine, tryptophan and valine). A high-quality protein will contain a good balance of these amino acids such that the horse can build its own proteins without a large wastage of unnecessary amino acids.

Protein cannot be stored in the body and any excess will be broken down in the liver. The carbon skeletons are then used for energy (protein contains about 24 MJ/kg GE), and the nitrogen is excreted as urea. Feeding excess protein is detrimental to horses since the deamination process requires energy and gives rise to considerable heat production. The urea produced requires water for its excretion, thus increasing water requirements, and in the case of the stabled horse, the urea breaks down to ammonia in the bedding and contaminates the stable air.

Protein deficiency gives rise to reduced protein and amino acids in the blood, resulting in reduced tissue synthesis. This is obviously of greatest importance in growing or reproducing animals but will also limit performance in the working animal.

Vitamins

Under normal conditions, the horse requires very few actual vitamins in its diet as it is capable of synthesizing most of them itself. Vitamin A can be formed from β-carotene, which is abundant in grass. Vitamin A, along with vitamin D, is stored in the liver and a horse kept at grass during the summer can synthesize enough of both vitamins to avoid any deficiency during the winter. Vitamin D can be formed by the action of sunlight on the skin in a similar fashion to that seen in other animals. Vitamin E is found in many plants and, although not so readily stored, is rarely deficient in the horse's diet. Vitamin K is formed in the large intestine as in other mammals. Of the water-soluble vitamins, most of the B complex are formed by the microbes in the hindgut and a horse fed plenty of bulk is unlikely to suffer from any deficiencies of these. Vitamin C can be formed by the horse from glucose.

Minerals

The minerals required by the horse are similar to those required by other mammals, and are divided into macrominerals and microminerals, or trace elements. Since horses are often involved in heavy work that results in considerable sweating, electrolyte needs may be greatly increased at these times.

Common foodstuffs

Roughage

Grass

Grass is the most natural form of food for horses and the foodstuff around which the gastrointestinal tract has evolved.

Grass has a natural cycle of growth according to the seasons and as a result its feeding value varies. Growth starts in the spring when the ground warms up sufficiently and at this time the grass is low in dry matter but what dry matter there is is high in sugars and proteins. As the season progresses growth rate increases, as does dry matter and fibre content, and, as a result, protein and sugar levels fall.

During a very dry summer, and in the autumn as the soil cools, growth slows down and may cease altogether and what grass is available is very high in fibre and low in protein and sugar. Left to its own devices, a horse will put on weight over the spring and summer when grass growth and quality are at their maximum and use the stored fat to carry it through the winter when there is little high-quality grass around. Foals are born in the late spring and early summer, allowing the mares to make best use of available foodstuffs at the end of pregnancy and during early lactation.

Domesticated horses, expected to perform throughout the year, will need their diets supplemented during the winter months to avoid the loss of too much weight. They are also generally confined to much smaller areas than their wild counterparts would have been and thus cannot rove in search of better pasture. Conversely, many animals, especially 'good doers' such as native ponies, need to have their intake restricted in the spring and summer to prevent them becoming overweight and possibly developing other problems such as laminitis.

All pastures for horses should be securely fenced, have a good water supply and be free of toxic weeds, especially ragwort. Many garden plants are toxic to horses and if a field borders a garden it is best double-fenced (this will also keep the owners of the garden happy).

Conserved grass

Since it is necessary to continue feeding throughout the winter despite the poor quality of grass, a number of methods of conserving excess spring and summer growth for feeding throughout the colder months have been developed.

Table 9.1 shows the nutrient contents of some forms of roughage that may be fed as replacements for grass.

Hay

Hay is the most common form of conserved grass fed to horses. Like the grass from which it is made, hay varies in quality according to the time of cutting and the care spent making it. It is always of lower quality than the grass from which it is made because of the inevitable losses which occur during the process of haymaking (Table 9.1). The majority of hay used for horses is cured in the field and thus cannot be made until day length is sufficiently long and the weather sufficiently settled for the drying process to be carried out without fear of rain. As a result, much hay is made late in the season, when the grass is well past its best. The increased

Table 9.1 Approximate nutrient contents of some roughages

Roughage	Dry matter (g/kg)	Crude protein (g/kgDM)	Fibre (g/kgDM)	Soluble carbohydrate (g/kgDM)
Grass	180–300	80–170	130–270	5–460
Hay	850–880	45–110	300–380	20–50
Haylage	500–650	80–100		50–90
Silage	200–350	100–190	230–340	10–100
Lucerne	230–240	170–220	240–300	60–80
Swedes	120	108	100	590
Carrots	115–130	100	95	
Sugar beet pulp (molassed)	876	90–120	130	300
Sugar beet pulp (unmolassed)	900	100	175–200	80
Oat straw	860	34	394	
Barley straw	860	30–40	390–410	

Roughages vary widely in their nutrient contents; these figures are a guide only.
g/kgDM, grams per kilogram of dry matter.

volume available is also a factor, and farmers may delay making hay in order to achieve more bales per hectare.

Hay can also be barn-dried and here the weather ceases to be a major factor, allowing hay to be cut much earlier. However, the cost of drying and the reduced quantity mean that the cost is prohibitive for most horse owners, although the resulting hay is generally of very high quality.

The dry matter content of hay is high (around 850 g/kg), but during the process of hay making there is some loss of protein and sugar and a corresponding increase in the amount of fibre. Vitamin D increases, because of the action of sunlight on the cut grass, but carotene decreases dramatically. Contrary to popular opinion, the quality of hay cannot be assessed by its smell and appearance and analysis is needed. A good overall guess can be made if the source is known, together with the time of cutting, length of drying, weather conditions, etc., but these are no substitute for chemical analysis.

Two types of hay are generally available to the horse owner:

- Seeds hay – cut from specially sown grass leys. This tends to contain fewer species of grass, sometimes only one, and few other plants.
- Meadow hay – cut from permanent pasture. This will contain whatever was growing at the time, often a wide variety of grasses and broad-leaved plants, some of which may be toxic.

Opinion varies as to which is better for horses, but meadow hay has more variety and if hay forms the main bulk of an animal's diet throughout the winter it is more likely to fulfil nutritional requirements than hay made from a single grass species. Meadow hay is generally leafier and may have a higher nutritional value than late-cut seeds hay, which is sometimes little better than straw.

Hay is generally relatively cheap. Small bales are easy to handle (although still quite heavy, especially directly off the field) and easy to store in a watertight barn. Large bales, although otherwise satisfactory, require mechanical assistance to move them.

Hay can be fed off the floor, in a rack or in a net. Many horses prefer to eat off the floor, as this is a natural position for them; however, this can lead to wastage, as some hay is trampled on. Nets and racks both raise the hay off the ground. Generally, nets are better, and can be filled in the barn and carried to the horse with little loss. A net with small holes will slow down the rate of consumption, which may be advantageous for the stabled horse.

One major disadvantage of hay is its potential dustiness and mould content. Hay that is obviously very dusty or mouldy should never be fed to horses, as the mould spores can be dangerous to both the horse and its owner. Low dust levels can be dealt with by damping the hay, either by steaming it in a bin or by immersing it briefly in water. Long soaking washes out nutrients and is not recommended. The quality of hay decreases during storage and hay should not be kept from year to year.

Haylage/silage

The popularity of haylage and silage for feeding to horses has greatly increased in the last few years. Neither is as dependent as hay on the weather for its satisfactory conservation, although better products will be made in good weather.

Silage is made by cutting a crop (generally grass, maize or cereals grown especially for cutting), packing it into a clamp or wrapping large bales in polythene and leaving it to ferment in an anaerobic environment. Once the fermentation process is complete the silage will keep indefinitely provided no air is allowed in. The dry matter content of silage is relatively low, although it is very variable and generally a silage with a high dry matter content will be better than one with low dry matter. Silage for horses should always be made with great care, avoiding soil contamination, which can lead to detrimental fermentation and possible toxicity.

The use of additives is generally not recommended. Little loss need take place during the process of silage making, so the conserved product will have the same feeding value as the grass from which it was made provided the process was carried out well.

Haylage combines the qualities of hay and silage and is made by allowing the cut grass to dry to a certain extent and then packing it into polythene, where a limited fermentation takes place. The resulting product combines the characteristics of hay and silage, having a dry matter content higher than silage but lower than hay. There will be small losses of protein and sugar, with an increase in fibre, but these are much less than in hay. Well-made haylage has a very sweet smell, and is extremely palatable to horses.

Both haylage and silage deteriorate on contact with air so, unless they can be obtained in small bales, are not really satisfactory for the one-horse owner. The bales, because of their water content, are much heavier than hay bales and will probably require mechanical handling. Recently there has been a large increase in feeding of haylage to horses, with the result that many contractors have started to produce it. Small bales are much more readily available and, as they are easy to handle, they suit the one-horse owner; however, they are relatively expensive.

Despite some problems, both silage and haylage are suitable feeds for horses and do not have the dust and mould problems associated with hay (although mould patches will sometimes be found in haylage if a bale has been damaged and these should be disposed of). Silage, because of its high water content, is probably best left to horses not expected to perform very strenuous work but haylage, with its higher energy content, is an ideal roughage food for the performance horse.

When fed by weight, more haylage or silage is needed than hay because a larger proportion of the weight is water, and it will usually be possible to cut down on concentrates because of the higher energy content. The horse owner should not be misled into feeding less because of the higher energy content – this may result in diarrhoea due to a reduced fibre intake.

Legumes

Legumes are plants that fix nitrogen by means of bacteria located in nodules in their roots. As a result they contain higher levels of crude protein than grasses. Several varieties of clover are frequently found in pasture and they have the capacity to increase the overall feeding value of that pasture, in terms both of its protein and mineral levels and the length of time the pasture is of high quality. This is because the nutrient content of legumes falls more slowly during the growing season than that of grasses.

Lucerne (also known as alfalfa) is a legume often used in horse feeds both as a source of roughage and to increase the protein content of the diet. In many countries lucerne is fed as hay; however, in the UK it is usually fed either as chaff or as pellets. Feeding lucerne will increase the protein content of the diet and also the calcium content, since it has a very high ratio of calcium to phosphorus. Lucerne also has a higher energy level than grass so, if fed dried by weight, it should be possible to decrease the concentrate intake.

Roots

Roots may also be fed to horses – mangolds, swedes, turnips, carrots and sugar beet, for example, are all suitable. Roots contain a high proportion of water and sugar as well as containing roughage. They are therefore succulent and a useful addition to the diet of the stabled horse. Sugar beet pulp is also available in dried form, both molassed and unmolassed, and after soaking makes a palatable addition to the diet as well as supplying a useful amount of energy and roughage. Since it absorbs three or four times its own weight in water, the amount to be fed should be weighed out before soaking!

Straw

Straw can be fed to horses. Wheat straw is best avoided, since it is very hard, although many horses bedded on wheat straw will happily eat it. Both barley and oat straw are suitable and may be particularly useful for adding bulk to the diet of animals that would otherwise get too fat. Some straw, fed at night to the stabled horse along with its hay and concentrate feeds, will keep it occupied once the higher-quality foods have been consumed.

Concentrates

When a horse is expected to perform more than the lightest of work, a diet composed purely of roughage foodstuffs rarely provides sufficient energy, since the horse is restricted in the amount of food that can be consumed. In order to overcome this, concentrate foodstuffs in the form of a variety of grain-based diets are fed. Grains, although containing a higher energy level than grass and other roughage, contain poor-quality protein and thus if they are added to the diet it is usually necessary to add an extra protein source as well. Concentrate foodstuffs can be given either in the form of straights (single foodstuffs) or compounds (mixtures of two or more foodstuffs).

Straights

Any single foodstuff such as oats, lucerne or soya beans can be classed as a straight foodstuff. The addition of grain to the ration increases the starch content and care needs to be taken that the capacity of the horse's small intestine to digest and absorb starch is not exceeded. Excess starch reaching the large intestine is likely to give rise to rapid fermentation with a subsequent lowering of pH and possible serious results. Grains tend to be low in protein and have a poor balance of amino acids, being generally short of lysine and one or more other essential amino acids. They also tend to have a poor calcium : phosphorus ratio, which can lead to bone disorders.

These deficiencies in grain can be counteracted by adding other straight foodstuffs. For example, lucerne has an excellent calcium : phosphorus ratio, and contains a high level of good-quality protein. As it is a roughage, much of it is digested in the hindgut, which makes it an excellent foodstuff. Another good protein source is soya bean, which has the best level of lysine of any of the vegetable protein sources generally fed to horses. Table 9.2 shows the nutrient contents of some straight foodstuffs.

Table 9.2 Approximate nutrient contents of some straight foodstuffs

Foodstuff	Energy (DE) (MJ/kgDM)	Crude protein (g/kgDM)	Fibre (g/kgDM)	Ca (g/kgDM)
Oats	10.9–13.4	100–140	100–125	0.5–1.1
Barley	12.8–15.4	100–130	50–65	0.5–0.6
Maize	14.2–16.1	90–105	24–25	0.2–0.5
Linseed	11.5–18.5	220–380	66–100	2.3–4.3
Soyabean meal	13.3–14.7	500–540	40–70	3.0–4.0
Sunflower meal	9.5–11.7	280–490	130–320	2.9–4.5
Field beans	13.1	275	75–80	1.0
Dried lucerne	9.2–10.0	156–220	240–290	11.3–15.1

DE, digestible energy; g/kgDM, grams per kilogram of dry matter; MJ/kgDM, megajoules per kilogram of dry matter.

Oats

In the UK, oats have been the traditional foodstuff for horses and of all the cereal grains they are still probably the best for this purpose. Oats have a higher fibre content than other cereals, which, while lowering the energy content, also improves the texture of the grain in the stomach and aids digestion. Naked oats without the husk are also available. They have considerably higher energy levels than other oats and should be fed with great care. Oats are normally fed crushed, since, if a horse does not chew its food properly and the husk is not damaged, the oat grain can pass through the gastrointestinal tract undigested. However, whole oats can be fed to a horse that chews its food properly.

Barley

Barley may be fed in the form of extruded rings. It can also be fed as a grain but it is best rolled, as it is very hard. Barley has a higher energy content than oats and is also more dense, so care must be taken to feed by weight not by volume. Extruded barley is lighter and the cooking process makes the starch more digestible, so it is probably preferable to the uncooked grain.

Maize

Maize is fed extensively to horses in America and the UK. It is usually in a flaked form, although other forms are available, and the cooking process improves digestibility. Maize has the highest energy content of all the cereals and should be fed with caution to all but the hardest-working horses.

Compounds

Feeding a horse on straight foodstuffs is possible but these days the majority of horses are fed on compounds produced by animal feed companies. Although this is more expensive than feeding straights, compounds are usually more satisfactory because they are produced to suit all types of horse and pony and are nutritionally balanced, taking the onus off the owner to get the balance correct. They are available as cubes and mixes. Both consist of a range of grains with protein sources and usually some vitamin and mineral additives. Their palatability is usually high, not least because molasses

Table 9.3 Approximate nutrient contents for different types of compound foodstuff

Foodstuff	Energy (MJ/kgDM)	Crude protein (g/kgDM)	Fibre (g/gkDM)
Maintenance and light work	8.5–10.5	85–105	135–200
Hard work	11.5–13.0	120–140	60–140
Showing	10.0–12.5	100–150	95–190
Stud	11.5–12.0	140–160	65–100
Fibre replacer	8.0–8.5	100	200

g/kgDM, grams per kilogram of dry matter; MJ/kgDM, megajoules per kilogram of dry matter.

is used in their manufacture. Table 9.3 shows the nutrient contents of some typical types of compound foodstuff.

Cubes

The cubes fed to horses vary slightly in size but are usually fairly small with a diameter of about 5–6 mm. The ingredients used are generally the same as in coarse mixes but are ground up, mixed with molasses and forced through a die before being bagged up and sold. Although it is not possible to see the individual ingredients, if bought from a reputable firm there should be no reason to doubt them.

Coarse mixes

Many owners prefer coarse mixes largely because they look more appetizing and it is also possible to see what has gone into making them. One possible disadvantage lies in the ability of some horses to sort through foodstuff and they may become very adept at leaving certain ingredients, thus unbalancing the ration.

Additives

Where a reputable brand of compound is fed at the level recommended by the manufacturer it is not generally necessary to give the horse any additives. Many horses, however, are given less than the stipulated amount or may have a particular problem such as poor hoof quality. These horses may benefit from certain additions to their diets. All additives should be fed with care: unnecessary additives are at best expensive and at worst toxic.

Molasses

Molasses is a by-product of the sugar industry used widely in the animal foodstuffs industry. For horses it can be obtained in liquid form and poured on to a feed to encourage a shy feeder. Most compound foodstuffs contain quite a high proportion of molasses, e.g. to bind cubes together and to reduce the dust in coarse mixes.

Herbs

Herbs are a popular addition to both human and equine diets. A large number of herbal supplements are produced to suit a variety of situations, e.g. oestrus problems, skin conditions and stiff joints. In its natural state the horse would have access to a wide variety of plants and would seek out for itself those required.

Vitamin and mineral supplements

A large number of vitamin and mineral supplements are produced for the equine industry. For many horses these are a waste of money, but some situations require them.

Prohibited substances

As with human athletes, equine athletes are subject to restrictions regarding diet and supplementation. Foodstuffs produced for the competition horse should be sold with a guarantee that they contain no prohibited substances. The owner must also make sure that the horse does not consume any of these substances in the form of titbits, topically applied substances or from the pasture.

Nutritional requirements

The nutritional requirements of the individual horse depend on a number of factors, e.g. age, workload, health. Although some horses are kept at maintenance levels, many are kept either for reproduction or to carry out some physical task. Requirements have generally been split into a requirement for maintenance and an additional amount that can be considered as production, in the form of either growth or work.

Whatever activity the horse is required for, it must be borne in mind that there is a physical restriction on intake, generally believed to be around 2–2.5% of bodyweight. In practical terms a horse of around 15.2 hands high (hh) (155 cm) weighing 500 kg can eat about 10–12.5 kg of dry matter a day, or the equivalent of approximately half a bale of hay. Hay alone may be sufficient for maintenance and, for a 'good doer' fed good hay, even this amount may be too much. For the horse in hard work there is a limit to the amount of concentrates that can be substituted for hay, since a certain amount of roughage must always be fed and this limits the potential energy intake.

Maintenance

Maintenance requirements are considered to be the amount required by an animal to maintain its current weight and condition, with the addition of an allowance for essential movement such as foraging. Maintenance requirements allow the body to function, without any additional activity.

Production

- **Working** – many horses are kept for work, which can vary from light hacking at weekends to the strenuous demands made by 3-day eventing or endurance riding. Depending on the level of work required, the energy requirements are considered to be maintenance plus an additional fraction of maintenance energy. NRC (1989) considers that a horse in:
  - Light work, e.g. gentle hacking, requires 1.25 × maintenance energy
  - Medium work, e.g. show jumping, requires 1.50 × maintenance energy
  - Hard work, e.g. eventing or endurance riding, requires 2 × maintenance energy.

However, opinions vary as to what can be termed light/medium/heavy work, and the condition of the horse in question must always be carefully monitored and feeding adjusted accordingly. Little extra protein is required for work and any extra is normally supplied by the increased rations fed without any further additions.

Horses in strenuous work (Fig. 9.3) sweat copiously and the fluid and electrolytes lost must be replaced if the horse is not to suffer from dehydration. There are a number of ways of doing this but probably the most satisfactory is to administer an electrolyte paste via a syringe into the horse's mouth and then allow access to fresh water. Because the fluid lost in sweat is isotonic with blood, many horses will not feel significant thirst in spite of the water loss and will refuse to drink unless the electrolytes are first replaced.

Because the digestive system of a horse is designed for a poor-quality roughage ration, it does not take kindly to a high intake of concentrate foods with a consequent lowering of roughage intake. Stabled horses may suffer from a number of physical and mental problems that are partly due to the nature of their feeding, and it should be possible to alleviate these with more turnout and adequate provision of roughage. The problem arises with the horse in hard work, which has a high energy requirement that cannot be met unless a large proportion of the roughage part of the diet is replaced by concentrates. This is further exacerbated by many horses in hard work being shy feeders, possibly because of the high-concentrate nature of the diet. Energy levels can be satisfactorily increased by the addition of oil to the diet, but care must be taken that sufficient protein is also fed since oil contains none.

Reproduction

Reproduction or breeding is not an unnatural process for the horse and in fact the working situation is far more unnatural. Thus feeding the breeding horse should be easier than feeding the working horse. Problems arise when an

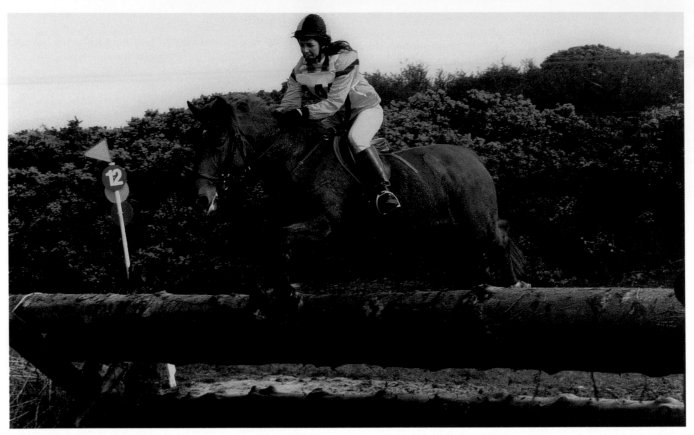

Fig. 9.3 Horse in work – eventing

exceptionally high growth rate is required of foals, to prepare them either for the show ring or for sale.

Stallions

Stallions during the covering season need a good all-round diet and their general condition and temperament should always be considered. Many stallions today are also used for work, especially for competition, where their natural presence gives them an edge over other horses, and these will normally be fed as any other working horse. For the stallion covering large numbers of mares, some increase in nutritional content of the diet is required and the condition and mental attitude of the stallion should be a good indication of how much extra to give.

Pregnant mares

Pregnancy in the mare lasts for 11 months and for the first 8 the developing fetus is relatively small and makes few demands on the mare. A good all-round diet is recommended, and many mares continue to work during this period of their pregnancy.

During the last 3 months the fetus grows very fast and the mare needs some extra energy and quite a lot of extra protein. Feed manufacturers produce special diets for pregnant and lactating mares, usually with a protein level of about 16% (160 g/kg). These diets, combined with good hay, should be ideal, although if a mare is foaling late in the season a good grass paddock should supply all her needs. During the last month of pregnancy (Fig. 9.4), when the

fetus is taking up a considerable amount of space in the abdomen, some mares will decrease their intake and may need a higher proportion of concentrates than would normally be the case.

Lactating mares

Like heavily pregnant mares, lactating mares have a high requirement for protein but energy needs are also greatly increased. A good stud diet should be fed unless ample high-quality pasture is available. Mares vary in their ability to produce milk. Some provide large quantities and sometimes lose their own condition in order to do so; others will produce less and use the extra food to build up their own fat stores. Figure 9.5 shows a 13-year-old mare with her first foal, both doing well on summer grass alone, an indicator of the feeding quality of grass at this time of year!

Youngstock

Most foals will start to investigate solid food within 1 week of birth. For a mare at grass, no extra feeding of the foal should be necessary at this stage. Where a mare is fed a compound food the foal will usually start to nibble it.

In the young foal, the hindgut is relatively small and undeveloped. As the foal starts to eat more solid food, especially roughage, the hindgut develops to cope with the new demands placed on it.

Many foals are weaned at 6 months old and it is important that by this time the foal has a good intake of solid food to compensate for the loss of its mother's milk. Creep feeding

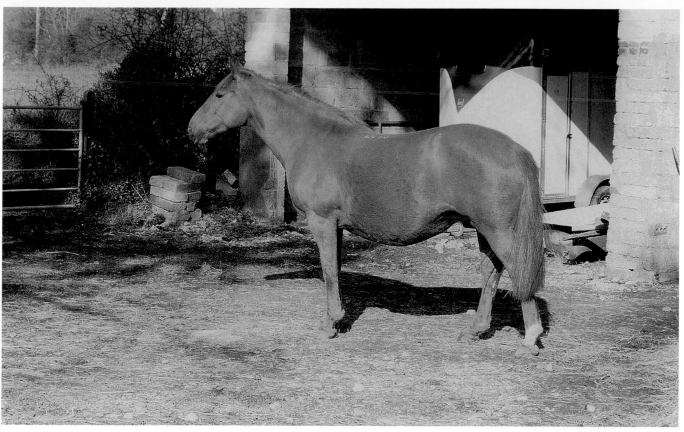

Fig. 9.4 Mare 1 week prior to foaling

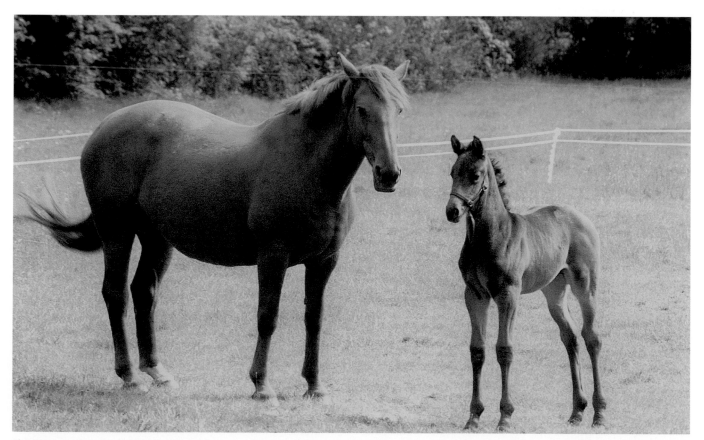

Fig. 9.5 Lactating mare with healthy foal at foot

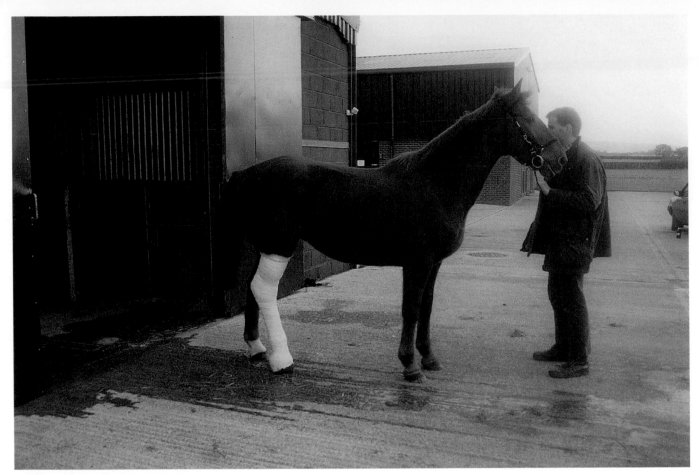

Fig. 9.6 A candidate for box rest!

is often carried out, in which food is placed in such a way that the foal can reach it but the mare cannot. Generally, foals that have been creep-fed suffer less stress during weaning, since the gastrointestinal tract is accustomed to this type of food. Although foals have a higher need for concentrate foods than adult horses, good-quality roughage must always be fed to them alongside the concentrates. It is very important at this stage not to overfeed, since a variety of limb abnormalities can occur if this is the case. Foals do, however, have a considerably greater requirement than adults for both energy and protein in order to sustain growth, which can be at a rate in excess of 1 kg per day in the first months.

As the young horse grows, its requirement for high levels of protein falls, as does its need for higher levels of concentrate food. By the age of 3 years its diet will be the same as that of an adult horse. Most young horses are left to themselves during the spring and summer and fed extra food during the autumn and winter when grass growth is insufficient.

Sickness and convalescence

The horse on box rest does not have to move around in order to seek food and its energy requirements are therefore less than maintenance. Hay alone will generally suffice for these horses but some supplementation may be necessary if the hay is not of good quality or the horse is under a particular stress, e.g. from surgery (Fig. 9.6).

Donkeys and exotic equids

Donkeys and zebras originated in the tropics. They are therefore not well suited to the British climate and may have nutritional requirements as yet unknown. It is often believed that donkeys digest fibre better than horses but this is not proven. Donkeys do conserve water better than horses and are able to withstand water deprivation for much longer, coming second only to camels in their ability to do this. Little is known about the requirements of zebras and until further research has been carried out on these species it is probably best to treat them like horses at maintenance, remembering that a tropical diet, consisting as it does of tropical plants, may contain different constituents from those manufactured in this country and that unexpected problems may arise.

Practical feeding

Water

It is generally recommended that water is available at all times, and there are a number of ways in which it may be provided:

- In the field, a self-filling trough is ideal. It should be situated away from trees and where it can be inspected regularly. It is worth bearing in mind that the ground around a trough usually gets very cut up, especially in wet weather, so having it too close to a gate is inadvisable.

- In the stable, water can be provided by self-filling drinkers. There is some evidence that horses drink less from self-filling drinkers and many people dislike them, since it is harder to tell how much a horse is consuming. The saving of labour is considerable, however, and the water is always fresh.
- Buckets allow the horse's consumption to be measured, but water in a bucket becomes stale and will absorb ammonia from the atmosphere. It is also liable to be kicked over or occasionally used as a foot bath. When a horse is stabled overnight and fed dry hay, it will usually drink the contents of two 15-litre buckets.

Roughage

The digestive system of the horse is designed to cope with a diet consisting of large quantities of low-quality roughage and all diets must be based on roughage. This can be difficult to achieve if the horse is performing hard work and has a greatly increased requirement for energy, since intake is limited and, as concentrate foods increase, so the roughage portion of the diet must necessarily decrease. This effect can be reduced by increasing the quality of the roughage fed, and generally at least one-third of the diet should be roughage.

Hay is the traditional conserved roughage feed for horses but recent years have seen a considerable increase in the use of other types of forage-based roughage: haylage being the most popular. Other roughage suitable for feeding to horses includes barley or oat straw for horses needing lower energy levels; silage or lucerne (alfalfa) for those needing higher energy levels; and roots, of which dried sugar beet pulp is the commonest and most convenient.

Roughage can be fed in a number of different physical forms:

- Long, e.g. hay, straw, and haylage; often given in a net which has the added advantage of keeping the horse occupied.
- Chaff, e.g. lucerne, hay and straw, chopped up into short lengths and mixed with the concentrate ration. Feeding chaff helps to slow down the rate at which concentrates are eaten and leads to better digestion, both through the slowing down the process and by making the food less dense in the stomach and so more readily available for enzyme activity.
- Pellets or shreds, e.g. sugar beet pulp. This must be soaked before use and it absorbs up to four times its own volume of water. It should never be fed before this water has been absorbed, otherwise it will swell within the horse's stomach and, as the horse is unable to regurgitate its food, this could in extreme circumstances lead to rupture of the stomach. In hot weather, soaked sugar beet can start to ferment if left too long and it will then become unsuitable for feeding.

Concentrates

Concentrates are fed as a concentrated source of energy and can either be in the form of straight, single foodstuffs, such as oats, or as a compound from a feed company made up of a number of different ingredients. Most horses today are fed manufactured compounds, either cubes or coarse mixes, which have the advantage of being nutritionally balanced for the different types of horse. For example, a low-energy cube can be obtained for a child's pony and a power mix for an event horse. Compounds are also produced for elderly horses, breeding animals, youngstock and invalid horses.

Frequency and timing of feeding

When feeding a horse, remember that in nature it eats for about 16 hours a day and as far as possible this should be mimicked in the stable. It is rarely possible to give a horse constant access to food but a good supply of roughage should keep it occupied for some time. Concentrate feeds are usually given separately (although some feed companies are developing complete feeds) and, unfortunately, are rarely given more often than two or three times a day because of the owner's other commitments. An ideal feeding regime would probably enable the horse to be fed a complete ration at hourly intervals throughout the day and night; however, without the development of sophisticated automatic feeding this is unlikely to be possible!

Stabled horses

The stabled horse is usually fed a concentrate food three times a day and hay two or three times daily depending on the working schedule, etc. It is possible with horses at maintenance or in low work to give large amounts of forage, possibly including oat or barley straw, thus occupying them for long periods of time. Horses in more strenuous work need more concentrate food, with a consequent reduction in roughage – this can lead to boredom and the development of stereotypical behaviour.

Horses at grass

Horses kept at grass are under the most natural conditions for the domesticated animal. The pasture should be well fenced and free from toxic plants, although a variety of plants other than grass are beneficial to the horse's health. Horses have a tendency to graze some areas of a paddock very closely and leave other areas rough and untouched. They will tend to defecate in the rough areas. Since horses are naturally herd animals it is best to keep them in consistent groups if at all possible – introduction of new animals to a group will cause some transitory disruption as the pecking order is re-established to accommodate the newcomer.

Combined system

This system allows for the animals to be at grass for part of the day or night and stabled for the rest of the time. During periods of stabling, horses are fed a roughage and concentrate ration suitable to their work and physiological condition but the quality and quantity of grass available to them should be taken into account and the ration varied accordingly.

Food storage and preparation

Storage of foodstuffs should be considered as poor storage may have an effect on the efficacy of the contents and in particular the labile, readily oxidized pigments, unsaturated fats and fat-soluble substances are destroyed. Fat-soluble vitamins are all reduced during storage, as are unsaturated fatty acids, and rancidity of fats reduces acceptance. The synthetic forms of vitamins A and E are more stable than their natural forms but have little antioxidant capacity (see Ch. 7). B vitamins are relatively resistant to breakdown during storage, but riboflavin will be lost when exposed to light. Compound feeds may have permitted antioxidants added to them to guard against various forms of deterioration but these will not stop all forms of deterioration for ever. Acceptability of all foods is reduced on deterioration.

Fungi may grow during storage and may produce toxins as well as causing decay and lack of acceptability and nutritional value will decline. Insects also cause deterioration and may carry fungal spores – some of these insects are visible to the naked eye while others are not. Rodent infestation leads to food loss and their droppings are dangerous to both man and animals.

Hay and straw are frequently bought off the field and stored throughout the winter to be used as required. This system is entirely satisfactory as long as the hay in particular has cooled down after making. Hay stored too early will heat in the stack, with a subsequent loss of nutrients. Both hay and straw can be obtained either in small or large bales. Large bales require mechanical handling, so unless they can be delivered direct to the barn small bales will be easier to deal with. Hay should not be fed before it has cooled down, since fermentation continues. Last year's hay should not be fed, as hay deteriorates gradually with time and by the following year will have little feeding value left. Hay must be stored in a dry place with plenty of air circulation, ideally in the dark to reduce the loss of carotene from the bales. Storing on pallets will prevent upwards seepage of damp, which can render the lowest layer of bales unusable.

Haylage, which is purchased in sealed bags, can either be bought in early in the season and used as required, or bought in as required. As long as the bags remain airtight there should be no loss of quality and the same is true of silage bought in big bales. Both silage and haylage can be stored outside, since the wrapping is also watertight, but bird damage can be a problem.

Concentrate foodstuffs and sugar beet pulp are usually purchased in sacks. They should be bought in as required, as the contents deteriorate with time. The purchase of a few weeks' supply at a time is generally satisfactory.

All foodstuffs should be stored at a low and uniform temperature, with low humidity, good ventilation and a dry environment. Metal bins are generally advised for concentrates as these prevent access by vermin, which not only eat the food but also contaminate it with their urine and faeces. The food should not be stored in direct sunlight as this can destroy some vitamins. If possible, rodents, birds and insects should be kept out. Opinion varies as to whether cats should be allowed in the food store – they will keep down vermin but may themselves cause some damage.

Alteration to normal feeding patterns

Hospitalized or box rest

It is important to remember when feeding the horse on box rest that such circumstances are foreign to the horse's natural habitat. The inability to move around freely can in itself be detrimental to the digestive system, as movement aids the expulsion of the considerable quantities of gases produced in the hindgut (Fig. 9.6). Provided that good-quality hay is available it may be best to cut out concentrate foods altogether. The requirement for energy is obviously diminished to below a normal maintenance level and some horses will actually refuse concentrates if they are offered. If the hay is not of sufficient quality to feed alone, a diet specially produced for the invalid horse should be used. This will have a low energy level but still contain adequate quantities of vitamins and minerals, etc. Succulent foodstuffs such as roots, apples or cut grass will be much appreciated by the horse on box rest.

In some cases it may be necessary to provide specific supplements such as B vitamins (B_{12} may be given by injection). If digestive function is impaired, partial or total parenteral nutrition may be necessary.

Overweight or obesity

Many horses are overfed and this can put a strain on the limbs, especially in young animals. Manufacturers' recommendations tend to err on the side of overfeeding and it should be remembered that feed companies, as well as providing foodstuffs, are in the business of making money! The showing world is notorious for its liking for overweight horses.

One common problem is an overestimation of the amount of work a horse is doing. NRC (1989) considers that light work consists of Western and English pleasure riding, bridle-path hacking and equitation; medium work consists of ranch work, roping, cutting, barrel racing and jumping; heavy work includes horses in race training. The recommendation is to increase the energy content of the daily ration by 1.25, 1.50 and 2.00 times the maintenance requirement as appropriate. The horse doing a few hours hacking a week can probably be considered to be at little more than maintenance, especially if stabled and not requiring any energy for foraging food in a field. Horses cannot be considered to be in medium or hard work until they are doing considerable amounts of fast work, such as regular hunting, endurance work or 3-day eventing. It is always better to err on the side of safety and keep the rations below what appears to be recommended. If the horse starts to lose weight, additional food can then be given.

The overweight horse should never be starved, as this will disrupt the digestive system and may cause problems such as hyperlipidaemia. Rather they should be fed a restricted diet in such a manner that it takes them as long as possible to eat it.

Underweight or too thin

Underfeeding is most likely to occur during the winter when animals live out, or in the case of older horses whose digestion is not as efficient as that of younger horses. The thick winter coat of horses overwintered outside can hide lack of condition very effectively. It must be remembered that, during the late autumn and winter, what grass there is will be very fibrous and contain little energy or protein. Horses and ponies neglected during these months with little or no supplementary feeding are likely to be underweight.

Older horses do not generally digest their food as efficiently as younger ones and as they get older may require extra food, especially protein. Horses, like people, vary widely in the age that they are considered old and some animals in their twenties may appear younger than those in their teens. Like dogs, larger animals tend to age faster and ponies living well into their thirties are common. Another problem encountered with the older horse can be loss of teeth, which will make the consumption of long roughages difficult. There are now many substitutes on the market and it should be possible to feed the rather toothless old horse without too much of a problem!

Should a horse be suffering from starvation, food should be introduced in small quantities at first, gradually building up the amounts given as the digestive system becomes more active.

Bibliography

Bishop, R., 2003. The Horse Nutrition Bible. David & Charles, Newton Abbot.

Bone, J.F., 1988. Animal Anatomy and Physiology, third ed. Prentice Hall, Englewood Cliffs, NJ.

Frame, J., 2000. Improved Grassland Management. Farming Press, Tonbridge, Kent.

Frape, D., 2004. Equine Nutrition and Feeding, third ed. Blackwell Science, Oxford.

Kerrigan, R.H., 1994. Practical Horse Nutrition, third ed. R H Kerrigan, Maitland, NSW.

McDonald, P., Edwards, R.A., Greenhalgh, J.F.D., Morgan, C.A., 2002. Animal Nutrition, sixth ed. Prentice Hall, Englewood Cliffs, NJ.

National Research Council, 1989. Nutrient Requirements of Horses, fifth ed. National Academy Press, Washington, DC.

Pagan, J.D. (Ed.), 1998. Advances in Equine Nutrition. Nottingham University Press, Nottingham.

Pagan, J D, Geor, R.J., 2001. Advances in Equine Nutrition II. Nottingham University Press, Nottingham.

Recommended reading

Frape, D., 2004. Equine Nutrition and Feeding, third ed. Blackwell Science, Oxford.

This is the best all-round book on equine nutrition currently available, fairly expensive but worth the cost for anyone involved in equine nutrition.

CHAPTER 10

Behaviour and handling of the dog and cat

Jocelyn Lander and Jane Williams

Key Points
• A thorough understanding of the behaviour of animals is essential for the safety of anyone working with them.
• Modern theories of the domestication of the dog now consider that small dog-like creatures were attracted to living with man by the presence of food on waste dumps and that these individuals then became tame as a result of continuous proximity to man.
• Dispelling the myth of development from wolves, the concept of alpha wolves and the dominance hierarchy changes the way we think about our dogs and the methods of training them.
• The socialization period is important in the behavioural development of both puppies and kittens but the behaviour of any animal is subject to a multitude of factors and understanding these factors is vital in dealing with behavioural problems.

Introduction

Handling dogs and cats is an integral component of the veterinary nurses' role. To ensure safety in the working environment it is essential to have an understanding of the behaviour and body language of your patients. This chapter aims to explore the history of domestication of the canine and feline species and how this relates to their behaviour. The concept of behavioural therapy is introduced and includes discussion of potential approaches to common problems encountered in these species in veterinary practice.

Handling dogs and cats

It is essential that the veterinary nurse knows how to assess and interpret the body language of dogs and cats to ensure a safe approach can be made. In turn your own body language, tone and pitch of your voice and self-assurance can influence how an animal reacts to you. Generally a reassuring voice with a low tone will put animals at ease. Never put yourself in a situation where you feel uncomfortable – it is always preferable to request assistance from a more experienced member of staff than to injure yourself or your patient.

Animals require handling to allow:

- Grooming/bathing
- Examination of an injury, for vaccination, or when ill
- Administration of first aid
- Administration of drugs
- Health checks.

Dogs

All dogs are potentially aggressive so it is unwise to make assumptions about their nature.

Initial approach and restraint

It is advisable to talk to the owner prior to handling and to use the owner as much possible. Owners know their animal and their presence should reassure the dog. Owners can be particularly useful to fit muzzles without causing stress to their pets (Table 10.1). Aggressive behaviour can be the result of possessiveness over their owner or kennel, fear or pain, maternal behaviour, environmental factors (e.g. other barking dogs), same-sex aggression or due to a pathophysiological factor (e.g. the dog was bred to fight).

Animals which are overtly protective of people or kennels should be examined in the absence of their owner and often the aggression will immediately be resolved. Kennel guarding can be reduced by leaving a form of restraint on the animal to allow ease of handling. Record cards should always be clearly marked with a warning for other staff members that animals may be aggressive.

- Approach the dog in a quiet but confident manner using the dog's name for reassurance.
- Lower yourself to the animal's level whilst maintaining your own safety.
- Offer your hand for the dog to smell using a sideways movement so as not to alarm the animal.
- Avoid handling animals in confined spaces as this can lead to anxiety and aggression if the dog perceives itself to be trapped.

In situations where the animal cannot be handled safely, the use of restraint equipment or drug therapy can be an invaluable tool.

Table 10.1 Restraint techniques in dogs

Method of restraint	Procedure
Muzzling	Ensure correct size muzzle is selected and straps are adjusted to fit the dog
	Approach from the side or behind the patient
	Prevent the head from moving from side to side by holding the scruff
	Pass the muzzle over the dog's nose and pass straps behind the head and fasten, tighten to required length
Applying a tape muzzle	Select an appropriate length of non-conforming bandage to fit around muzzle, the head of dog and allow tying
	Form a loop with a square knot
	Use an assistant to restrain the dog
	Approach from the side and place the loop of the bandage over the dog's nose with the knot at the top
	Tighten and cross the free ends under the lower jaw of the dog, then pass back under the ears
	Tie the ends in a quick release bow around the back of the head

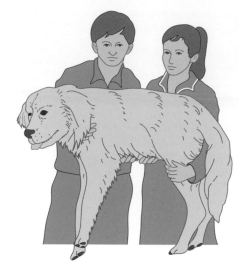

Fig. 10.1 Correct method of lifting a dog over 20 kg

All dogs should have a lead and collar fitted whilst handling occurs. Additional control can be obtained by using the following:

- Slip leads
- Haltis© or Gentle Leader©
- Muzzles
  - Wire or Baskerville© muzzles
  - Nylon or Mikki© muzzles
  - Tape muzzles
  - Box muzzles
- Dog catcher
- Chemical restraint
  - Pharmaceutical restraint includes acetylpromazine, medetomidine, Torbugesic and diazepam and should only be administered under veterinary supervision.

All restraint equipment should be fitted correctly and to avoid discomfort to the animal. Take care to avoid rubbing of the eyes or excessive tightening, and never leave a muzzled animal unattended. Never muzzle an animal which is dyspnoeic or suffering from emesis.

Lifting

- Perform a quick survey to ascertain if any injuries – if there are avoid them.
- Grasp the animal around the front and hind legs, pressing it into your own body to prevent struggling.
- Lift with your knees bent and your back straight;
- For animals over 20 kg it is a Health and Safety requirement that another member of staff assists.
- Smaller animals can be tucked under one arm to support the thorax with your body used to support the hind limbs.

- Larger dogs will require two people to lift – the first should support the front of the dog whilst restraining the head in an arm lock and the second supports the hind quarters and the abdomen (Fig. 10.1).
- Always ensure the head is safely positioned away from your face to prevent biting.

Restraint for examination – standing

Use a non-slip examination table in an area which is escape-proof. Ensure that all potentially necessary restraint equipment and examination equipment is close to hand.

- Lift the animal on to the examination table.
- Restrain by standing to one side of the animal, placing the near side hand around the animal's neck, and hold the head in a secure lock.
- The other arm is used to hold the animal's abdomen against the body or apply downward pressure on the dorsal neck region to prevent backwards movement.

This is a suitable position for administration of subcutaneous injections into the scruff or intramuscular injections.

Restraint for examination – lateral recumbency

Use a non-slip examination table in an area which is escape-proof. Putting a blanket on the table will sometimes make the animal feel more at ease. Ensure that all potentially necessary restraint equipment and examination equipment is close to hand.

- Stand beside the animal as it stands on the table.
- Place your arms across the back of the animal and grasp the off side front and rear legs at the level of the tibia and radius (Fig. 10.2).
- Gently pull the legs upwards and away from you using your chest to support the animal's body.
- The dog's body should gently roll down on to the table where it is restrained by applying downwards pressure to the limbs and using the elbows and forearms to hold down the head and body.

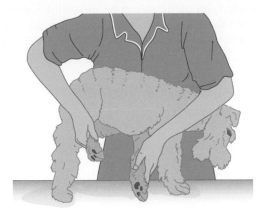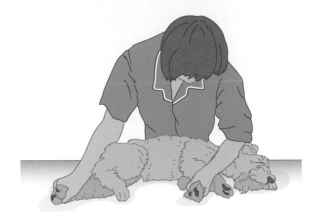

Fig. 10.2 Restraining a dog on its side

Lateral recumbency examinations may also be performed on the examination room floor, in which case you should lower yourself to the floor and support the body against your chest, restraining in a similar way.

Venepuncture

Cephalic vein

This is the most common site for both intravenous injections and for the collection of blood samples. The cephalic vein runs down the dorsal aspect of the lower forelimb.

- Restrain the dog in a sitting position. In active patients another assistant may be required to secure the rump, preventing backwards movement.
- Stand behind the animal and use the corresponding arm to the foreleg being sampled to raise and extend the leg.
- Cup the elbow in the palm of your hand, bringing the thumb across the crook of the elbow to apply gentle downwards pressure.
- Rotate the hand slightly outwards and maintain the pressure while the veterinary surgeon inserts the needle.
- If an intravenous injection is being given, the pressure can be released as the fluid is injected; if blood is being collected, maintain the pressure while the blood flows into the syringe.
- As the needle is withdrawn, apply pressure to the injection site for approximately 30 seconds to prevent subcutaneous haemorrhage.

Jugular vein

This is a less common site but is useful for the collection of larger samples. The jugular vein runs down either side of the neck in the jugular furrow.

- Restrain the patient in a sitting position or in sternal recumbency using an assistant to secure the rump.
- Hold the head upright, extending the neck. It may be necessary to apply a tape muzzle in some dogs.
- Prevent the front legs from being raised by placing your free hand across them.
- The veterinary surgeon applies pressure to the base of the jugular furrow to raise the vein and collect a sample.

Many of these procedures are illustrated on the website.

Cats

In general cats respond better to light handling and as little restraint as is practically possible.

One problem that can be encountered in cats within the veterinary practice is removing them from their kennels. Often cats are housed with or nearby other animals, especially dogs, which can cause stress or fear, resulting in aggression when the veterinary nurse attempts to remove the cat from its kennel. In this situation a towel can be used to cover the cat's head and body and then the cat can be scooped gently out. In extreme cases a cat grasper can be effective. Another method is to use a crush cage by placing it against the kennel entrance with the wire door removed effectively trapping the cat between the kennel and crush cage. A towel over the cage will make it more welcoming to the cat and hopefully they will enter it, if not then gentle persuasion can be employed. Once the cat is in the cage quickly replace the wire door and secure the animal.

There is a variety of specialist restraint equipment available for cat restraint, including:

- Cat muzzles
- Cat bags
- Crush cages
- Chemical restraint
- Towels
- Cat graspers.

Restraint for examination

As cats are small animals usually one person can safely restrain a cat for examination. This can be achieved by placing one hand over the animal's thorax and scruff with the hand securing the head and neck, whilst the other arm supports the rear of the cat and holds the body into the handler's chest. If more secure restraint is required hold the cat to your body using one arm while your hand holds the animal's forelegs, securing them between your fingers to prevent scratching. The other arm and hand is used to restrain the animal's head by placing the thumb upon the caudal skull region, the fore-finger on the bridge of the nose and the remaining three fingers are placed under the chin to keep the mouth shut. Do not scruff the cat unless it is absolutely necessary.

This position can be used for the administration of subcutaneous injections into the scruff or intramuscular injections into the quadriceps femoris muscle of the hind limb.

Lifting

There are very few cats which weigh over 20 kg so one person can safely lift them! Place one hand over the animal's thorax to support the sternum and use the other arm to support the abdomen by placing it around the side of the cat and holding the animal into the handler's chest.

Venepuncture

Cephalic vein

A very similar method is used to that in the dog (Fig. 10.3).

- The cat is restrained in sternal recumbency or in a sitting position.
- Use the other arm to hold the body close to your side and using your hand extend the forelimb towards the veterinary surgeon.
- Support the forelimb in the palm of your hand, placing your thumb across the crook of the cat's elbow.
- Apply gentle pressure with your thumb to raise the vein and rotate your hand slightly outwards.
- Maintain the pressure while the veterinary surgeon inserts the needle into the vein.

Jugular vein

There are a number of methods used for jugular vein sampling in cats:

A. Hold the animal close to the handler's body using one arm to lightly restrain the thorax and grasp the forelegs in the fingers. The other arm holds the head in extension with the hand grasping the mouth shut at the base of the jaws.

B. The handler seated holds the cat in dorsal recumbency often enclosed in a towel. The head is extended with one hand whilst the other keeps the body secure (Fig. 10.4).

C. Whilst both methods can be successful it should be noted that often just raising the cat's head with minimal restraint applied is the most successful of all.

Many of these procedures are illustrated on the website.

Evolution of the domestic dog (*Canis familiaris*)

It is thought that dogs and man first began to have a relationship in the Mesolithic period about 10 000 to 15 000 years ago. Until the start of the twentieth century the dog was largely unchanged but in the last 100 years the need for dogs to have a specific function such as hunting, herding and guarding has declined and appearance has become more important (Fig. 10.5). It may be this shift in emphasis that lies at the root of physical and behavioural problems in our modern dog breeds (COAPE course notes 2005).

Wolf to dog? Maybe not!

The process of domestication must have been very subtle and not just a case of a man hand rearing an orphaned wolf puppy and, from this, breeding generations of domesticated wolves. The animal in question was likely to have been a smaller, more dog-like kind of animal and what led to its domestication was the food source that man left behind in the form of waste dumps outside villages. Once man adapted from a hunter-gatherer lifestyle to a more sedentary one, these dumps would be a more permanent fixture, providing a rich source of food for canine scavengers. Something to keep in mind is that these dog-like creatures were not pack animals hunting down large prey but mainly scavengers which sometimes hunted smaller prey such as rats and rabbits. Once the waste dumps were more common, the dogs would have bred with others around them, rather than as thought in the past, with dogs met on their travels following the human hunter-gatherers.

In this way the animals with the least developed flight response to man naturally selected themselves and so the domestication process began. These dogs would have toler-

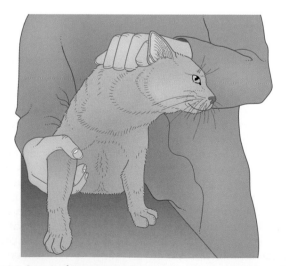

Fig. 10.3 Restraint for venepuncture using the cephalic vein in the cat

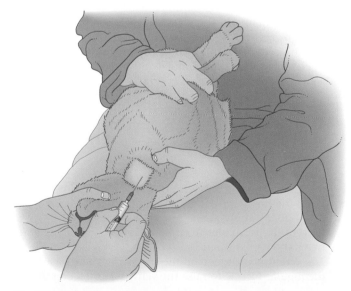

Fig. 10.4 Restraint for venepuncture using the jugular vein in the cat

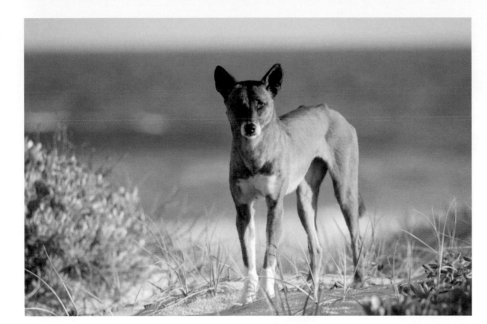

Fig. 10.5 A wild dingo

ated man and, over successive generations, they may have started living within the villages. Man would have seen the benefit of having these animals around when they alerted him to danger and may even have used them as a protein source. The dog has undergone huge physiological changes during its time with man and to compare a dog's behaviour to a wolf's is unfair and dangerous. Ray Coppinger is an eminent scientist who writes that 'The popular dog press seems to feel that if dogs descended from wolves, they would have wolf qualities, but the natural selection model points out that the wolf qualities are severely modified. Dogs do not think like wolves, nor do they behave like them.' (Coppinger and Coppinger 2001)

Dispelling the myth of dominance

Most of us have grown up assuming that dogs are descended from wolves and therefore follow the same set of rules as a pack of wolves and adhere to a strict dominance hierarchy to keep the peace. For many years, behaviourists and scientists have questioned this unproven theory and even those scientists studying wolf behaviour cannot agree. Most of our knowledge of dog behaviour has been based on the study of captive wolves – a completely unnatural situation, much like a study on human behaviour being done in a prison!

Scientists have now realized that the way wolves live and organize their social structure is different to what was originally thought. David Mech is the leading authority on wolves and has been studying them for 50 years. He has found that a wolf pack consists of a male and female and their offspring – essentially a family group. Adolescents reaching 2–3 years of age leave the pack to form their own family packs and there is no fight for top dog, no linear hierarchy. Much like a father and mother are in charge of their children, the wolf parents are in charge of theirs. This does not constitute a dominance hierarchy.

After spending time with a wild wolf pack in the 1990s Mech felt compelled to dispel the myth of the alpha wolf and this idea is very important in changing the way we view

our dogs, how we train them and how we live with them. Education on the subject is vital, as most people who are using rank reduction techniques are merely following advice found in books and, unfortunately, on television. We are doing our dogs no favours by treating them like wolves and, in fact, we are creating more problems. Dogs are a fantastic example of adaptability and opportunism and they deserve to be treated as individuals and as a species in their own right. The more people we can educate, the brighter the future for the domestic dog.

(Further information can be obtained from the Recommended reading at the end of this chapter)

Canine behaviour patterns

1. Communicative behaviour

Domestic dog populations show many of their wild relatives' social behaviour patterns although selective breeding by man has had an influence. Methods of communication tend to be via smell, facial expression and body posture, sound and physical contact.

Body posture

This is an important means of communication and it is vital that anyone dealing with a dog understands what the dog is 'saying':

- **Assertive postures** include standing tall with the tail held high, the ears erect and making direct eye contact (Fig. 10.6C). In extreme cases the dog may snarl and raise the fur along its back – the hackles. Beware of this!
- **Appeasement postures** include keeping the body low and, in extreme cases, lying on the back and presenting the inguinal region often in conjunction with urination, extreme tail wagging, nuzzling, licking, ears back and drooped and often showing an appeasement grin (Fig. 10.6B). Animals in pain or that are fearful often show extreme appeasement but care must be shown as they can still display aggression.

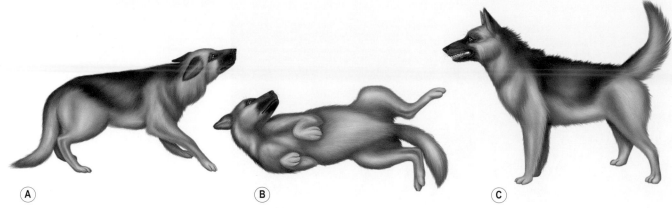

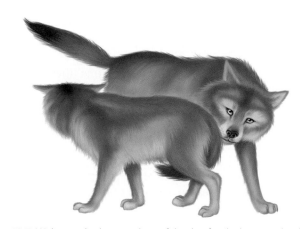

Fig. 10.6 Canine visual communication. (**A**) Fearful behaviour. (**B**) Appeasement. (**C**) Assertive posture

- **Fearful behaviour** is exhibited by the dog crouching low with its ears back, its tail held downwards and avoiding eye contact. The dog is uncertain whether to be friendly or to bite and is consequently unpredictable (Fig. 10.6A).

Olfaction – a solitary life within a household rather than in a pack may have resulted in domestic dogs relying more on olfaction than visual communication. Olfaction or the interpretation of scents is an important communication tool as scent remains in the environment, providing a long-lasting territorial marker and means of communication with other individuals of the same species.

The most frequently used olfactory sources are:

- **Faeces** – used to mark the territory and the frequency of defecation increases if alien faecal matter is encountered within the territory. Domestic dogs tend to defecate at an increased frequency when off the lead with no owner present, perhaps indicating that humans have interfered with inherent communication methods.
- **Urine** – this is the bane of many dog owners' lives! Urine marking is a common behavioural problem observed in entire male dogs. Cocking the leg or raised leg urination (RLU) is displayed by the majority of male animals. The volume of urine passed can determine if the act is for elimination or for scent marking. Male dogs will often show the raised leg display without actually urinating, suggesting a communication role. Many males and some females will scratch and kick their back legs after urination or defecation, which is thought to spread scent. Another theory is that it is to leave scent from the sebaceous glands or interdigital glands in the feet, or it could also it be a visual means of communication.

In wild dogs, double marking of male on female urine cements pair formation and improves courtship success and this is another behaviour that can be observed in their domestic cousins. Over-marking is common practice in packs but not in lone animals, suggesting territory marking. Raised leg display is often repeated after urination and is thought to affirm dominance.

Fig. 10.7 Wolves and other members of the dog family detect each other's status by sniffing the anal scents.

Urine is also an important medium for communicating the readiness of a bitch to mate and the frequency of urination increases during the oestrus period.

- **Anal glands** – these are present in all species of *Canidae*. Analysis of the glandular secretions shows differences between groups and individuals. The glandular secretions are secreted on to the faeces as they pass through the anal sphincter.
- **Other glandular secretions** – these are used by all species of *Canidae*. Glands in the facial, tail, perineum and anal regions secrete social odours. There are two types of gland – the sebaceous glands, which produce oily secretions and the suderiferous or sweat glands, which produce watery secretions and are used more commonly in social communication.

The anal region in dogs is used for postural communication – one dog will sniff the base of another's tail (Fig. 10.7). The most confident dog will present the anus to a subordinate individual and then it will check the other animal's anus. In very unconfident animals the anal region will be withdrawn, i.e. the tail clamped to prevent examination. This is more commonly seen in male animals but females do exhibit the behaviour during oestrus. Domestic dogs exhibit a similar behaviour between unfamiliar individuals and always follow

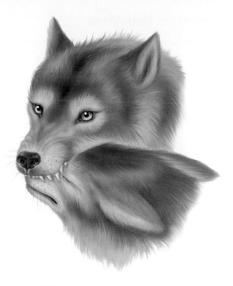

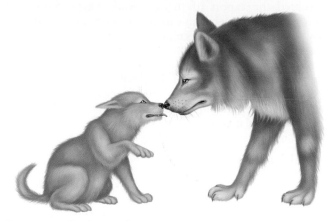

Fig. 10.9 A wolf cub using the paw raising and licking behaviours to solicit affection

Fig. 10.8 Snout grabbing is part of precopulatory play

the same sequence of behaviour or a 'fixed action' behaviour pattern: e.g. in the park dogs will

- Inspect head and anal region
- Females tend to approach the head and males the bottom
- Both try to reduce inspection by clamping.

Vocalization – this method is useful as a means of long-distance communication and in circumstances where visibility may be impaired, e.g. in dense cover or darkness. It also allows an individual's location to be identified. This behaviour is more common in the domestic dog than its ancestors and a broad repertoire of sounds have developed. Wolves howl when seeking company or trying to contact or to recall the pack after hunting. Dogs have developed numerous sounds, e.g. a growl can be defensive, a warning or a threat, and this may be the result of selective breeding.

2. Reproductive behaviour

Domestic dogs are capable of mating at any time during the year whilst their wild relatives only produce sperm within a breeding season. The bitch (in domestic and wild species) is seasonally monoestrous. During the oestrus period the bitch displays visual signs of her season including a swollen vulva and gives off olfactory signals via vaginal discharges and an increased frequency of urination. Bitches may develop a preference for specific mating partners and appear to prefer animals with whom they are already familiar. Mating behaviour includes precopulatory play such as sniffing, snout grabbing (Fig. 10.8), nipping and chasing, all particularly seen in inexperienced pairings. This is followed by exploratory sniffing and licking by the male, mounting and the resultant tie, which is unique to the canine family (see Chapter 14).

3. Maternal behaviour

When near to term the bitch will be restless and may roam. She may tear up bedding to create a nest and some otherwise affectionate animals can become aloof. She will try and find a secluded area to nest mirroring the wild situation in which the wild bitch will leave the pack and look for an abandoned hole to form her den. It is advisable to provide the bitch with a whelping box prior to her due date to allow her to acclimatize before the first stages of labour commence (see Chapter 14).

4. Care-soliciting behaviour

In wild dogs care-soliciting behaviour is particularly seen when the pack return from the hunt to the pups within the den. The pups lick around the lips of their dam, trying to place their tongue in her mouth, which stimulates a reflex regurgitation of the food in her stomach that is then eaten by the pups. The domestic dog may also do this to its owner on his or her return to the house. Wild dogs will lift a paw when asking for affection or mutual grooming and this is often accompanied by a high-pitched whining noise (Fig. 10.9). The domestic dog will also lift a paw in a similar situation with the owner and this is often converted into an apparently learned 'trick' for the amusement of others.

The evolution of the domestic cat *(Felis catus)*

The domestic cat is most likely to have descended from the African Wild Cat (*F. libyca*) and not the European Wild Cat (*F. sylvestris*) as was originally thought. This is mainly due to the fact that the African cat is more easily tameable whilst his European cousin is not and studies have also shown that the domestic cat is genetically almost identical to the African Wild Cat (Turner and Bateson 2000).

The earliest known records of the cat's relationship with man come from Egypt. Paintings on tombs dating back to 2300 BCE depict cats catching rats, indicating that they were living with humans around this time. It would seem likely that cats were initially encouraged into dwellings and villages to help control vermin and those cats that were best at their jobs or more tameable were probably selected for breeding and so the process of domestication began. Cats soon began to exert their influence over the Egyptians and their position was raised from ratters to creatures with a god-like status who were revered as symbols of fertility and strength. The Egyptians were very protective of their cats and prevented the export of them outside Egypt. Some did, however, slip through and cats made their way to Europe – Italy and Greece in particular – and they appear to have reached China around 200 BCE. With the beginnings of Christianity cats began to lose their exalted status and were seen as demons or agents of the devil and were horrifically persecuted. Modern attitudes are somewhat better, the cat having overtaken the dog as man's 'best friend' and it is now the most popular companion animal.

Social structure

Cats are social creatures, not the solitary hunters we once thought they were. Most domestic cats seek out attention and enjoy interactions with humans and other species. In a feral colony, the females are the core of the colony and make up family groups with related females and their off-spring. The size of the colony will depend on factors such as food sources and shelter – the greater the food supply, the larger the colony; when food is more scarce the colony tends to become fragmented. Females also help to raise each other's young and siblings can form strong bonds which even persist to the juvenile stage. Young male cats tend to leave the colony and live on the periphery, waiting for the chance to reproduce! They often form their own social groups or coalitions of litter mates. Hunting is largely done alone and females will bring dead and live prey back to their kittens.

A cat's sociability is largely dependent on its individual temperament, genetics and its critical socialization during the sensitive period. Cats that like to live by themselves and hate all other cats are most likely to be the product of poor socialization. This is why it is so important that cat breeders are educated with regards to correct handling and socialization, ensuring that all our pet cats can enjoy a happy, social life!

Feline behaviour patterns

Generally it has been observed that two broad types of social structure exist in feline populations and they are dependent upon food supplies:

a. **Solitary cats:**
   - Ranges overlap
   - Female ranges will be overlapped by larger male ranges
   - Thought to be food dependent
   - Male territories are bigger than females – need more food.

b. **Female social groups:**
   - Occur where there is sufficient food to sustain all
   - Males are usually loosely attached to group
   - Comprise adult females and their kittens
   - Cooperative kitten rearing/nursing
   - Structure is maintained by antagonism – strange females ousted and progeny recruited (akin to lion behaviour).

Pet cats are often forced to live in a group which is usually well-tolerated. They still have territories and ranges and those of the male cat are often 10 times larger than those of the female.

1. Communicative behaviour

Cats use many methods of communication, several of which are able to transmit information over the long distances of the home range.

Visual – this relies mainly on body posture and facial expression:

- **Body posture** – a relaxed cat will walk around with its tail down but when greeting other cats or humans to whom it is friendly it will approach with its tail raised (Fig. 10.10). An aggressive cat will hold its tail close to its body while a frightened cat will arch its back and raise its tail. The hairs along the back and covering the tail will be erected to make the animal look larger and more formidable.
- **Facial expression** – the cat has a larger range of facial expressions than the dog (Fig. 10.11) and they rely on the position of the ears and whiskers and the pupil size. A relaxed cat carries its ears upright, whiskers on the side and the pupils of the eyes are moderately dilated. When alert the pupils dilate and the whiskers are tensed; an aggressive cat has erect ears turned back, and the pupils are constricted; if frightened the ears are held flat against the head, whiskers held stiffly out to the side and pupils are dilated while a cat in conflict will alternate the ear position between flattened and turned backwards.
- **Clawing and scratching** – cats will scratch trees, fence posts and furniture and this may have two functions. Firstly it is a visual sign of territorial boundaries and the scratches may be tainted with the odour of sweat glands present around the foot pads of the cat and it may also be used to maintain claw condition.

Vocalization – sounds range from miaows which change according to their demands – some owners will claim their cats talk to them, to loud carrying yowls particularly those associated with the queen in season. Purring usually associated with contentment may also be a sign of low-grade pain. Cats also use growling and snarling to accompany their threatening body posture and facial expression.

Olfactory signs – the skin has many small glands, particularly on the cheeks, which deposit secretions when the cat rubs itself against objects in the environment, other cats or against its owner. The olfactory signals declare ownership of their territory. Cats also mark their territories using urine, which is sprayed backwards by the ventrally directed penis at the height of the next cat's nose. Urine also plays a role in reproduction, with males exhibiting the raised upper lip sniffing behaviour known as flehmen when they smell the urine of a queen in oestrus. Faeces is another significant territorial marker. Housed cats with an established territory will bury their faeces within the territory but may leave it on the surface at the boundaries – feral cats and wild cats, e.g. lions, do not bury their faeces.

2. Reproductive behaviour

Females or queens are seasonally polyoestrous and the beginning of the breeding season is determined by day length. Toms show increased activity during spring months, which then declines as the daylight hours decrease. A queen

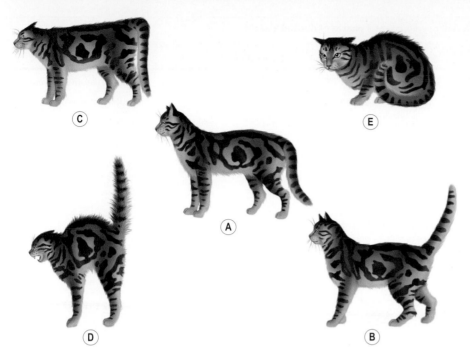

Fig. 10.10 Body postures used by the domestic cat. (**A**) Relaxed posture. (**B**) Greeting posture. (**C**) Aggression. (**D**) Fear. (**E**) Conflict

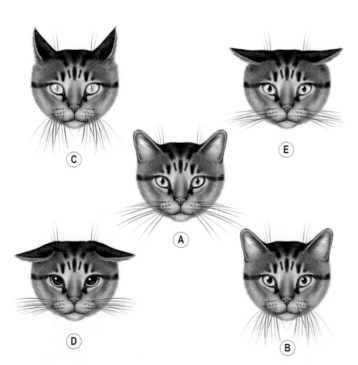

Fig. 10.11 Range of facial expression used by the domestic cat. (**A**) Friendly and relaxed. (**B**) Alert and inquisitive. (**C**) Threatening attack. (**D**) Frightened. (**E**) Conflict – cat may attack if cornered

in oestrus will roll, rub herself over objects, yowl loudly (known as calling), and exhibit lordosis, i.e. crouching low with her backside raised and her tail to one side, all of which tell the male that she is sexually receptive.

3. Maternal behaviour

Queens make use of an improvised nest and many prefer solitude while others crave attention. Infanticide may be stimulated by disturbing the queen during kittening or during early neonatal life and may also be carried out by any male cat who is not the father of the litter (mirror of lion behaviour) and in feral colonies. Communal denning and nursing among related females has been observed.

4. Social interactions

Normal meeting behaviour begins with cats nose to nose with no touching. Then the head and neck are extended with the body slightly crouched to enable a quick retreat. The cat will attempt to sniff along the neck of the other to the flank and on to the anus whilst preventing the other cat from examining its own anal region. Cats also respond to 'model' cats in the same way and humans can trigger the greeting behaviour by using an outstretched finger to substitute for the nose. In social colonies individuals indulge in a great deal of social contact and aggression is rarely seen except between strange females and young males.

Behavioural development

Developmental stages of the dog and cat

It is widely recognized that there are five phases of development in puppies and kittens as shown in Table 10.2.

The developing puppy

During the **neonatal** and **transitional** phases the puppy is completely dependent on its mother and at this time it is very important that puppies are handled, assuming that the mother is happy to allow this. Handled puppies have increased nervous system maturation, more rapid hair growth and weight gain, earlier opening of the eyes and enhanced motor development (Landsberg, Hunthausen and

Table 10.2 The characteristics seen in the different developmental phases of the dog and cat

Neonatal	Transitional	Socialization	Juvenile	Adult
1–2 weeks	2–3 weeks	3–16 weeks	10 weeks to sexual maturity	Sexual maturity onwards
Born deaf and blind	Ears open and eyes respond to light	Critical learning period	Learning continues	Behaviours fully developed
Dependent	Can move around more easily	Teeth appear	Discovers sexual behaviour!	
Reflex actions	More explorative	Exploring behaviour increases	Critical time to learn what is dangerous and what is not	
Can vocalize distress	Onset of weaning	Weaning occurs		
No hazard avoidance behaviour	No hazard avoidance behaviour	Hazard avoidance behaviour develops (respond to perceived danger)	Shows fear to unknown stimuli	

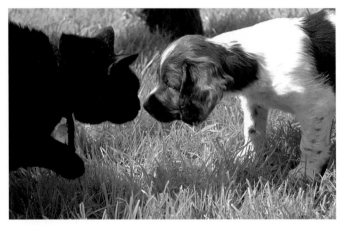

Fig. 10.12 During the socialization period puppies begin to explore new situations

Ackerman 1999). Such puppies tend to grow up more confident, have improved learning ability and are emotionally more stable.

The **socialization** period is critical up to the age of 10 weeks. It is a period of rapid social behavioural development during which the puppies begin to explore more and respond to stimuli (Fig. 10.12). Most importantly, it is during this phase that puppies begin to show fearful behaviour to new objects and stimuli. They have to get used to these things and learn that they are not dangerous – a process called **habituation.** Whatever happens during this period will set the pattern for the puppy's behaviour in later life. Behaviours and responses learned now will be difficult to change. Positive social interactions with other animals and humans are paramount to ensure the puppy develops a balanced outlook on life. 'This appears to be period of extreme sensitivity to psychological stress. The sensitivity necessary to facilitate the formation of social relationships also seems to make the puppy vulnerable to psychological trauma' (Landsberg, Hunthausen and Ackerman 1999). It is around this time that an unsocialized puppy will become increasingly fearful of anything new and will overreact to sounds and stimuli. During socialization, puppies play with each other, learning important communication skills and

what is appropriate behaviour and what is not. One of the most important things to learn during this time is bite inhibition.

Your role as an advisor to a new puppy owner is vital at this time. Stressing the importance of socialization and habituation within the correct time frame (up to 16 weeks) can mean the difference between a happy, confident puppy and a nervous, fearful puppy that could develop into an unhappy adult with a tendency towards aggression. The way in which this period is handled is very important. (see later notes on Puppy Parties).

Basic behaviours and learning capabilities have fully developed by the **juvenile period**. Although exploration during this time increases, it is also a time of increasing avoidance of social interactions, so fewer interactions occur. Learning starts to slow down by 16 weeks: 'This is likely because previous learning begins to interfere with new learning' (Landsberg, Hunthausen and Ackerman 1999) The **adult phase** begins around 6–7 months of age and most dogs are seen to be fully mature by 18 months of age.

The developing kitten

Kittens follow the same developmental phases as puppies but the phases tend to be shorter in length. The critical period during **socialization** is from two to seven weeks of age during which what they see, hear and experience will influence their behaviour in later life. Just as with dogs, sensitive handling will encourage more rapid development and reduce future fearfulness. Kittens removed from their mothers at two weeks of age or hand-raised kittens may show increased tendencies towards nervousness and aggression, although this also depends on inherited temperament and socialization by the foster mother.

During the **socialization** period the mother will start to wean the kittens and bring live prey back to the nest. At this stage, their teeth are fully developed and kittens may even begin to hunt and kill their own prey by 5 weeks of age. They will also have full control over their elimination and will cover up urine and faeces. Most kittens will be fully weaned by seven weeks of age. Social play also begins during this time and any interactions they have will influence their behaviour in the future. Kittens benefit from an environment that is full of different stimuli and objects to aid the habituation process. Too often we see cat breeders keeping kittens in an outdoor cattery until they are 9–10 weeks of age, resulting in a kitten that has not been socialized properly, only knows one environment and is often nervous and fearful in its new home.

By six months of age, most cats have reached sexual maturity and can begin to breed. They will now be self-sufficient hunters and able to care for themselves if need be.

Nature vs nurture

It is often debated whether behaviour in dogs and cats is the result of upbringing or is genetically based: i.e. 'nature or nurture.' Certain behavioural traits must be genetic or we would not have specialized groups such as pointers or collies; however, it is now apparent that behavioural development depends on two main factors:

- **Inherited or genetic factors** – these include temperament of the parents and certain innate behaviours specific to a breed of cat or dog.
- **Non-inherited factors or primary environmental influences** – these are very diverse and the list is long and includes the mother's health, nutrition, habitat and climate.

The significant thing to understand is that behavioural development is under the influence of a vast array of factors and they must all be taken into account when addressing any type of behavioural problem.

Behavioural therapy

Introduction

The science of animal behaviour is complicated with many differing opinions on the subject. We must try to understand how animals think and learn in order to interpret their behaviour as accurately as possible and by doing this we can help resolve behavioural issues professionally and with the best interests of the animal at heart.

Behavioural problems are a very common occurrence in veterinary practice ranging from aggression and fear, to clients complaining of training issues or general unruliness. Many of these problems lead to pets being rehomed or even euthanized and as veterinary professionals we are in a unique position to provide valuable assistance in resolving these issues. It is our job to identify these problems and try and help the client find a solution which will help maintain the pet/owner bond. Too often, behavioural problems can spiral into the client becoming resentful and frustrated, blaming the pet and not being able to rationalize the behaviour. Having the correct knowledge and skills can save this relationship and improve the lives of both the pet and the owner.

Veterinary surgeons are very busy people and behavioural problems are often complex and can take a great deal of time to solve or manage. This provides an ideal opportunity for a veterinary nurse to develop new skills and to take over this role. An enthusiastic, motivated and knowledgeable nurse will be a huge asset to the practice, the animals and their owners.

Learning theory

The basic principles of learning

It is important to understand the basic concepts of how animals learn in order to give the best possible advice. Further details about learning theory are included in the Recommended reading list at the end of the chapter.

The basic principles behind animal learning can be divided into four different sections:

- **Reinforcement** – what animals are prepared to work for and what they want to avoid! Reinforcement occurs when a behaviour followed by a consequent stimulus is strengthened or becomes more likely to occur again. It can be divided into **positive** and **negative** reinforcement.
- **Extinction** – ignore it and it will go away! Extinction occurs when a previously reinforced behaviour is no longer reinforced, resulting in the behaviour decreasing and eventually becoming extinct.
- **Punishment** – no! Punishment provides a consequence for a behaviour with the result that the behaviour is less likely to occur again.
- **Stimulus control** – this develops when a behaviour is only reinforced by the presence of a particular stimulus.

NB. An animal will only repeat a behaviour if it finds it rewarding in some way – if it is not rewarding it is unlikely to want to repeat the behaviour.

Reinforcement

1. **Positive reinforcement (PR)** – most of us know that we should give treats to reward a behaviour that we want. It is important to find out what motivates the animal in order to be able to reward correctly: e.g. a Labrador will always find food rewarding but a ball-obsessed Collie may not try quite so hard for a piece of liver as he will for a tennis ball!
   Timing is also crucial – for a reward to be effective, it must come within three seconds of the behaviour for the animal to make the association.
   Using PR increases the likelihood of the behaviour occurring again: e.g. trainer holds treat in front of dog's nose > dog sits > dog is immediately rewarded with treat.
   Clicker training is a very powerful PR training technique and one that has been around for a long time and has developed from the way in which marine trainers teach dolphins. Dolphins have to be trained from a distance so the trainers needed a way to let the dolphin know when they have correctly performed a behaviour. You cannot force a dolphin to do anything but, put simply, trainers use a whistle to which the dolphin has already been conditioned to understand that food is coming. When the dolphin performs a behaviour correctly, the trainer blows the whistle and the dolphin is rewarded with a fish. This technique ensures that the dolphin stays motivated and *wants* to perform. In dog training the whistle is replaced by the use of a clicker. More information on clicker training is included in the Recommended reading list.
2. **Negative reinforcement (NR)** – we use this more often than we care to admit! Most people equate NR with

punishment but these conditioning principles are very different. Put simply, a NR is more frequently used to get the animal to do a behaviour by *removing* a negative stimulus, whilst punishment is to get the animal to stop doing something by applying a punisher. An example of a NR is if a gundog refuses to release a dumbell – trainer pinches lip (NR) – dog drops dumbell – pinch is released as soon as dog drops dumbell.

Extinction

The technique involves ignoring a previously reinforced behaviour until it becomes extinct. This is often used incorrectly as humans find it hard to stay disciplined. A classic example of extinction is shown by the dog that persistently sits begging at the dinner table. The behaviour has previously been reinforced by the children dropping food onto the floor for him. If he was then not given any more food ever again, he would eventually stop begging and the behaviour would become extinct. Something to note is that animals will show an **extinction burst** during which the behaviour will become worse or more extreme before it eventually expires. It is during this extinction burst that most humans feel the technique is not working and give up. This will only serve to reinforce the behaviour more and make it stronger! It is important when using this technique, to make sure that the animal is rewarded for showing an alternative behaviour: e.g. if the begging dog goes and lies down in his bed. This behaviour must be rewarded to help develop a new more appropriate behaviour.

Punishment

'Punishment involves the application of an aversive stimulus during or immediately following a behaviour to decrease the likelihood that the behaviour will be repeated' (Landsberg Hunthausen and Ackerman 1999). Punishment is often associated with physical abuse or retribution, which gives it a negative connotation with respect to behavioural therapy and training. Its use is not recommended as the timing and the choice of the aversive stimulus must be precise and definite for it to be effective and for the punishment to be humane, it must be used correctly and only need to be used once. This very rarely happens and can result in systematic abuse of the animal. Problems that may occur are that the pet does not associate the behaviour with the punishment and so learns nothing or that the pet learns to continue the behaviour in the owner's absence. It can also lead to an increase in the behaviour, or to an increase in fear or anxiety, compromising the bond with its owner. Punishment is not motivational and does not allow for new learning. It is the lazy trainer's technique in order to get a temporary quick fix. An example of punishment is dog chases deer > trainer uses electric shock collar > dog stops behaviour temporarily.

In the end, the only reinforcement in the learning of a particular behaviour is an emotional change. The rewards and punishments discussed are how those changes are induced. Techniques and stimuli have no learning value in themselves without a consideration of how each individual feels about them.

Stimulus control

A behaviour is said to be under stimulus control when there is an increased possibility that the behaviour will occur as a result of a specific stimulus: e.g. if we see a red light, we will automatically stop; if the light changes to green, we will automatically start to move off.

Counter conditioning and desensitization

It is important to understand these concepts when dealing with and trying to solve specific anxiety- or fear-based behavioural problems.

Counter conditioning is used to counter or oppose an earlier negative experience: e.g. a young puppy becomes scared of a bicycle because his tail was once run over by one. He associates pain with the bicycle. Counter conditioning involves changing this association from bad to good for example, by feeding him his favourite treats every time he sees a bicycle and gradually getting him close enough to touch it. Eventually the puppy will see a bicycle and immediately think 'treat!'

Desensitization will occur when the dog eventually becomes non-reactive to the bicycle. Desensitization works best when done slowly and within the limits of the animal's capabilities: e.g. starting some distance away from the object that evokes fear, rewarding relaxed behaviour and then slowly working closer to the object over an extended period of time.

Flooding is the process in which the animal is exposed to the stimulus all at once and is the direct opposite of systematic desensitization. Flooding can result in overwhelming anxiety and fear and is not generally recommended to overcome fears. Animals can become aggressive and dangerous when put under such pressure – systematic desensitization is a far more humane method.

Neurochemistry – in a nutshell

Animals, like humans, respond to stimuli in the environment. We have physiological systems in place to enable us to interact with and respond to all of these stimuli. The two most important systems are the nervous system, which affects the endocrine system, which coordinates all the chemical reactions in the body. These two systems are integrated and completely reliant on each other and in order to maintain homeostasis it is vital that these systems are functioning efficiently.

'Stress' is a word we use frequently in behavioural therapy but it is often misinterpreted. It is more than just a feeling of anxiety; 'stress is fundamental to almost all behaviours as it is about the demand for adaptation and the physiological response to that demand' (O'Heare 2003). What this means is that whatever stressor causes stress in the animal is causing it to make a change or adaptation to relieve the stress. Stress is at the core of most behavioural problems, e.g. aggression, fear, anxiety. Understanding the concept of stress and how it affects an animal is fundamental to recognizing the signs and dealing with it in a scientific way.

The mammalian brain is a complex organ (see Ch. 4) but for the purposes of this chapter I have tried to simplify it. There are two major components involved in responding to our environment:

- **The amygdala** – this area deep within the cerebral hemispheres is responsible for the survival responses of fear, flight and fight. It helps the animal to 'act on instinct' to escape perceived danger. It is the most primitive part of the brain.

- **The cerebral cortex** – the more rational part of the brain responsible for cognitive function. 'Information is decoded and the brain analyzes the significance of the information based on previous learning and experience and then it goes to the frontal lobe where it is used to formulate a plan of action' (Strong).

Whilst the amygdala is active, the cerebral cortex cannot function properly. This is why most behavioural therapy is aimed at teaching animals or people to develop almost automatic coping strategies in anxious situations which enable them to gain control of their emotions and start rationalizing their fear using the cerebral cortex.

Information is conveyed from one part of the nervous system to another by **neurotransmitters**, which are chemical secretions produced at the synapses between nerve cells (see Ch. 4) and which ultimately affect the behaviour of the animal. It is important to have a basic understanding of how the brain works on a chemical level to understand why an animal behaves the way it does. Sometimes the behaviour is a result of a chemical imbalance and not the fault of the animal. This is where behavioural modification drugs can be useful but they must always be used with extreme care. Most behaviour modification therapy can help to correct any imbalances.

The main neurotransmitters are:

- **Dopamine** – this has an effect on the pleasure centre of the brain. Too much of it can promote agitation, impulsivity and over-reactivity; depleted levels can cause a lack of capacity to enjoy life. Dopamine is released after an 'adrenaline high' and is responsible for that sense of relief.
- **Adrenaline** – this is released as a result of a stressful event and prepares the body to respond to danger. Part of the 'fear, flight, fight' response.
- **Noradrenaline** – this is chemically related to adrenaline and is linked to an animal's energy levels. Trauma and chronic stress can deplete the levels of noradrenaline. High levels can result in aggression, over-arousal and impulsive behaviour, while decreased levels can cause lethargy and depression.

The effect of both dopamine and noradrenaline are regulated by an enzyme called monoamine oxidase, which deactivates them (O'Heare 2003).

- **Serotonin** – this regulates mood, controls sleep and arousal, regulates pain and controls eating. Decreased levels can lead to impulsive aggressive behaviour, impaired learning, anxiety and obsessive behaviour.
- **GABBA (gamma-aminobutyric acid)** – this is widely distributed throughout the brain and is the principal inhibitory transmitter. GABBA is complex and has receptors that have three different binding sites – one for GABBA, one for benzodiazepine drugs and the third for barbiturates and alcohol. When one of these binds to a GABBA receptor it will amplify the effects of GABBA and therefore increase neural inhibition.

Understanding emotions and their role in behaviour problems

(Centre of Applied Pet Ethology (COAPE) using the EMRA approach (emotional assessment; mood state assessment; reinforcement assessment)
'It was long thought that animals do not have emotions but merely behaved in an instinctive, automatic manner'. Recent scientific studies have shown that animals do in fact have an emotional brain and are able to experience a wide range of emotions. This has transformed the way we look at animal behaviour and more importantly, how we treat behavioural problems.

When investigating a behavioural problem, it is important to consider and try and understand the surge of feelings (*emotions*) the animal is feeling at that particular time, and also its baseline or average feelings (*mood state*) during the rest of the day.

A human example might be as follows:

Imagine your 10-year-old son is playing football outside the kitchen window and you have already asked him, to no avail, to go and play in the garden so as not to kick the ball through the window. Sometime later, the ball smashes through the window. Your initial emotion might be one of anger at your son for not doing as he was asked. Now consider the same scenario, but this time you have flu, with a grumbling headache and feel irritable. The ball comes crashing through the window. 'What is your emotion to this event this time? Explosive anger, probably, or resignation because you are too tired to bother.' (COAPE course notes)

As individuals, we all have our own mood state that fluctuates during the day. This depends entirely on what sort of day we're having, what stresses we are under, whether we are suffering from an illness or depression. Someone who is carefree and positive will have a totally different emotional reaction to an event compared to someone with chronic depression or high stress levels. This same principle applies to our pets – a nervous cat that is stressed because there is a new baby in the house is likely to have a lower mood state than a confident cat that has 24-hour access to his own three-acre garden!

When assessing any behavioural problem it is important to assess the animal as an individual and take into consideration its personality, emotional state and circumstance.

First you should base an opinion on how the animal feels from two different perspectives:

1. **Emotional assessment** – this is a measure of the surge of feelings or emotions (good or bad) experienced before, during and after the problem behaviour.
2. **Mood state assessment** – this is the average, day-to-day feelings of well-being.

Then take into account:

a. **The hedonic budget** – this is an investigation into what the animal finds rewarding or pleasurable or what things are important to the animal. It also takes into consideration what things are missing from the animal's life that may be important to it.
b. **Reinforcement assessment** – an investigation of exactly what factors, external or internal, are maintaining the problem behaviour.

Emotional assessment

An animal can feel a range of emotions from anger and frustration through to fear and anxiety, from pleasure to extreme happiness and even depression. It is important to understand what range of emotions the animal is feeling at the time of the behaviour.

Case scenario: A young dog left alone at home, barks intermittently and chews up the sofa.

a. The dog could be **bored and frustrated** as it is left at home alone all day. Barking and chewing are innately rewarding behaviours that raise the dog's mood state. They help the dog to feel better and bring him relief from the boredom and frustration.

b. The dog could be **worried and upset** to be on his own as he has never been left before. He barks to try and make contact with his owners. The longer he is left, the higher his anxiety levels rise and he starts to panic. He turns to chewing as it brings him some relief from the stress of being home alone (raises his mood state whilst he is chewing).

In both cases, if the owner comes home whilst the dog is barking, the barking will be reinforced. In the dog's mind, the barking worked and brought the owner back. Punishment would not work as the joy/relief/excitement of having the owner home would far outweigh any punishment. The treatment of each of these cases would be different as the behaviours are driven by different emotional states.

Mood state assessment

This type of assessment measures the animal's mood state on a day-to-day basis. We know that our bodies and those of animals are regulated by complex homeostatic systems to maintain physiological equilibrium, e.g. pH and body temperature. In addition, both humans and animals experience a range of negative and positive emotions during the day and it is the feeling left after the ups and downs of the day have passed that we must assess. The emotional brain tries to maintain emotional homeostasis known as the Hedonic Set Point (HSP), which aims to maintain the emotions at a 'normal' level.

Figure 10.13 demonstrates the relationship between mood state and HSP. Resting contentment (RC) is defined as having no particular emotion or feeling, such as just before you fall asleep. We would all love to be just above resting contentment everyday (Line A); however, to maintain this HSP we pursue normal everyday behaviours that are pleasurable and rewarding. If an animal is below the RC line (point B), it will partake in behaviours that help to raise its mood state, e.g. if a dog is tied up all day and very bored, he may bark a lot and run up and down on his chain. This behaviour is innately rewarding to him and will help to bring him some relief. If we can help animals to feel more contented we can overcome (i.e to raise their HSP towards RC) a multitude of behavioural issues.

The hedonic budget

Animals have many different needs that must be met for them to feel contented. They need an outlet for instinctive

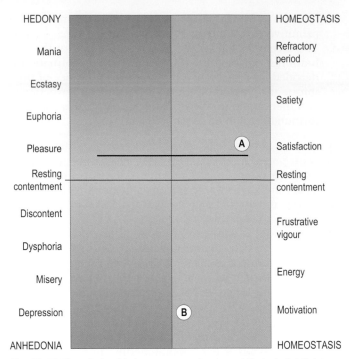

Fig. 10.13 The relationship between mood state and Hedonic Set Point (HSP)

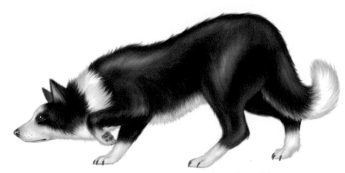

Fig. 10.14 Typical herding behaviour – a Border collie exhibiting eye stalking

and innately rewarding behaviours. Wild animals do not generally develop behavioural disorders as they are able to hunt, chase, mate and form social bonds in their natural environment. Our domesticated animals have been genetically manipulated and placed in unnatural environments and they often have no outlet for instinctive behaviour. Dogs, in particular, have been bred for many different disciplines and they all have different needs. They are descended from a predator but after much evolution and genetic manipulation, few breeds still have a full predatory motor pattern.

Example 1 – the hunting wild dog will orientate → eye → stalk → chase → grab-bite → kill-bite. During domestication we selected certain characteristics to suit our needs and culled any dogs that did not meet those criteria.

Example 2 – herding dogs would naturally orientate → eye → stalk → chase. We have removed the grab and kill part of the sequence by selective breeding as this is not a desirable trait. This is seen in breeds such as Border collies or German shepherds (Fig. 10.14).

Example 3 – dogs who guard livestock such as Anatolian shepherd dogs and Pyrenean mountain dogs would naturally eye → bark. These dogs have no tendency to chase or bite the animals they are guarding. All they are meant to do is bark when a potential predator is sighted.

Example 4 – dogs who hunt, such as spaniels, retrievers and pointers, will naturally orientate → eye → stalk → chase → grab-bite. This sequence represents the ideal hunting/retrieving characteristic as the dog holds onto its prey but does not tear it up and eat it (Fig. 10.15).

It is important to understand the different breed characteristics in order to manage any behavioural problems. Certain breeds, like the gun dogs, have a tendency to carry things around in their mouths and thus can also be more likely to guard things as they have an innate instinct to hang onto anything they grab. Herding dogs are likely to try and round things up, including children, and may be obsessive in their behaviour. They may be more orientated towards toys than food. Would it be that unusual if a herding breed nipped at a runner's heels in the park? You should always remain objective and try to see the situation from the dog's point of view. Such behaviour may be unacceptable to us, but it is completely normal for that breed of dog. We have to develop the skills to channel these behaviours into more rewarding, more appropriate behaviours. These behaviour sequences are 'hard-wired' in the dog's brain and performing them is innately rewarding and may be important in helping them to maintain a Hedonic Set Point.

When doing a hedonic budget assessment we need to first identify the behaviours that are typical or important for this breed or type of animal, then decide how well represented these behaviours are in the individual being assessed. After identifying which of the animal's behaviours are innately rewarding these can then be used in a behaviour modification programme. Using the behaviours that the animal is already programmed to do is a most effective method of dealing with the problem.

What dogs want!

In any behaviour modification programme it is important that we not only stop the undesirable behaviour but also provide an alternative, more rewarding behaviour for the animal. There are many dog toys on the market that are designed to help to do this and they include:

- Interactive food toys – these include Kong®, Busy Buddies®, Buster Cubes® and other food dispensing balls and food puzzle toys. These are important tools in helping dogs to feel contented and to ease frustration or boredom.
- Rawhide chews.
- Lots of exercise – this is by far the cheapest method and is both good for the dog and the owner.
- Training and stimulation – agility classes, clicker training, etc.

Reinforcement assessment

Reinforcement of behaviour can be both internal and external. Internal factors include problems with the animal's hedonic budget; external factors are less obvious but can be as simple as owners inadvertently reinforcing behaviours by paying attention to them: e.g. shouting at the Labrador that has chewed its owner's shoes. These reinforcers must be identified to help solve behavioural problems.

The EMRA approach is a concept used specifically by all COAPE practitioners. For more information regarding this approach please look at the Recommended reading list.

Running successful puppy parties

A well-run puppy party can be very rewarding for both the individual puppy and for the practice. It bonds clients to the practice and is important in helping dogs to become less stressed when visiting the vet. It is also a huge responsibility because behaviours learnt at a puppy party can be carried through the rest of a dog's life. It is therefore vitally important that we take them seriously and ensure that we are equipped to give the best possible advice. A puppy party should be about educating the owner as to the importance of early socialization and training using sympathetic, positive reward-based methods.

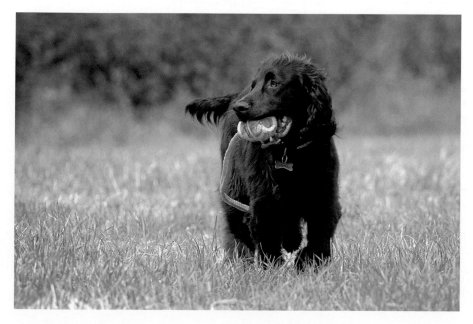

Fig. 10.15 A spaniel showing its retrieving instincts

Top tips

- Limit your class to a maximum of six puppies with two people per puppy.
- Puppies should be no older than 16 weeks. After this they start to lose their puppy teeth and social interactions are no longer on a par for the younger puppies.
- Match suitable breeds and sizes together if possible.
- Have plenty of interactive food toys and soft toys available to keep the puppies occupied whilst you talk to the owners.
- Keep your talk short and to the point. It is very difficult to keep the attention of an owner attached to a 9-week-old puppy that wants to do anything but sit still. As situations arise, this gives you the ideal opportunity to advise the owner on how to deal with the situation.
- Do not force puppies into interactions with other dogs. Allow them to sit somewhere safe to observe from a distance if that is what makes them feel comfortable. Make sure the owner does not overprotect them and reinforce fearful behaviour.
- Never let all six puppies off lead at the same time! This is a recipe for disaster and many puppies have been scarred for life after a frightening interaction at a badly run puppy party.
- Mix and match two puppies at a time that you think may interact well.
- Discuss the body language and behaviours you see with the client and help them to recognize signs of stress and anxiety and when to intervene. Be on the lookout for a puppy that is simply not coping. Remove it from the puppy party to a quieter area and see if you can get the owner to do some training/playing with it.
- Beware the overconfident puppy that tears around, trying to jump on and grab everything it sees! These puppies are best kept on a lead initially but allowed to interact with suitable puppies that can tolerate them. Letting this dog loose may cause him to learn how to be a bully and may frighten a less confident dog. This could result in a fear-based behaviour later on. Some people may not understand why they cannot all be off lead and it is important that the client understands that, just like children, puppies need to learn appropriate social skills.
- Start with a short training session to ascertain how well the owners are doing and what are their levels of skills. Demonstrate the basic principles of training. It can also be a good idea for owners to swop puppies at this point to see if they can get someone else's dog to sit!
- No puppy should be without a Kong® toy. These hollow rubber toys are ideal for teaching a puppy to be on his own, as playing with them is a rewarding experience. They are ideal for crate training and learning to be in the car. Stuff one with some tasty good-quality wet food and it will keep him occupied for a long time!
- Remember to have fun: e.g. teaching them to run through a children's play tunnel can be great fun for puppies and owners alike.

Common behavioural problems in young puppies

The first few nights

We must remember this is a very traumatic experience for the puppy. The puppy suddenly finds that it has been taken from a secure environment with the comfort of its mother and siblings and put into an entirely new environment in which it is alone. Advise the owner to make sure they take time off work to devote to the first week of the puppy's new life.

- Plug in a dog appeasing pheromone (DAP) diffuser or apply a DAP collar.
- Place the puppy in a bed or crate next to your bed so that if he cries in the night you can put your hand out to comfort him. Do not talk to the puppy. Just let him know you are there. This method is less traumatic than being left alone in the kitchen for example. If it has to be that way, it is very important you do not go downstairs when the puppy is crying, as you will reinforce this behaviour. Gradually you can move the bed/crate further away until it is outside the room.
- A hot water bottle can be comforting.
- Have a play session before bed to tire puppy out.
- Put up baby gates so that puppy gets used to being on his own in a room without closing the door. Always give him something to do when you leave him – a Kong® stuffed with something tasty would be ideal or a new toy or chew.

Crate training

Teaching your puppy to feel safe and comfortable in a crate is very important. This can become his safe haven and will make leaving him alone much easier. It will also help with house training.

Do:

- feed him in the crate
- give him a tasty chew in the crate
- keep the door open initially
- make it comfortable with snuggly blankets
- spray the blanket with DAP.

Don't:

- use the crate for punishment
- close the door until the puppy accepts the crate
- let the puppy become stressed and anxious in the crate.

Toilet training

Toilet training is entirely up to the dedication of the owner. Ideally do not encourage owners to put paper or puppy training pads down, as this sets a precedent for urinating indoors.

- Take the puppy out after every meal and have a play session. Reward the behaviour with a treat. Start putting a command to the behaviour such as 'Do your business'.
- Take the puppy out every hour if possible, thus reducing the chances of an accident happening indoors. By doing this you are setting the puppy up to succeed.
- Never punish toileting behaviour – the puppy will assume you are punishing him for toileting, not the

toileting *indoors*. It will then start to toilet on the quiet to avoid the wrath of the unpredictable human. If an accident happens indoors the owner must be even more vigilant.

Mouthing

Dogs investigate with their mouths just as we do with our hands. By mouthing they learn how hard they can bite before there are negative consequences – this is very important for learning bite inhibition. If a puppy bites too hard, squeal in a high-pitched voice and end the game for a minute or two. Encourage the mouthing behaviour onto a toy instead of hands. Make sure that any child understands this rule too.

Food guarding

Certain breeds such as terriers and gundogs may guard their food. If a puppy starts to display this behaviour advise the owner to feed food by hand initially so the puppy sees the human as the giver not the taker. Do not under any circumstances take the food away and then give it back. By taking the food away, you are reinforcing exactly what the dog is afraid of and may make him even more wary (see section on Resource Guarding, p. 182).

Coprophagia

Copraphagia or eating faeces is relatively normal behaviour in dogs although obviously it is not recommended as it can lead to the puppy picking up worms or other pathogenic organisms. If the puppy is eating his own faeces recommend the following:

- Review the diet – the puppy may not be digesting his food correctly due to an underlying medical condition or to the type of diet. His own faeces will be palatable to him as they are relatively undigested.
- Always watch the puppy and clear the faeces up before he can get to it. Teach him a recall and reward him for coming away from it. If necessary have the puppy on a long line so that you have more control of the situation initially.
- Do not punish the behaviour – he won't understand and it may encourage him to eat it quicker!

Fearful or nervous behaviour in puppies

SOCIALIZE, SOCIALIZE, SOCIALIZE using counter conditioning and desensitization techniques. Do not flood. Seek the advice of a good behaviour therapist. This will not go away as the puppy gets older and is likely to get worse if not dealt with correctly.

Common behavioural problems in adult dogs

For the purposes of this chapter I have selected the most common complaints from owners that you may come across as a nurse in practice.

Jumping up

Jumping up to greet is a common problem and one which is not acceptable to humans.

Reasons:

- This is normal greeting behaviour for dogs and for this reason, it is advisable not to punish this behaviour as you may teach the dog that people will hurt it if it approaches them, changing a sociable dog to a fearful or anxious one
- Reinforced with attention by owner, possibly encouraged.

Solution:

- Do not reinforce the jumping up with attention or touch
- Reward all four feet on the ground
- Make sure **everyone** the dog meets obeys these rules.
- Advise the owner goes to a reputable trainer.

Pulling on the lead

Reasons:

- This is simply a training issue and has nothing to do with social hierarchy or dominance
- The owner is probably reinforcing the behaviour or does not have the skills needed to retrain the dog.

Solution:

- Advise the owner to go to a reputable trainer.
- A Gentle Leader® when fitted and used correctly will help with the training process. It is not advisable to use pain or force: e.g. choke chain or jerking on the lead to get a dog to walk next to you. You would rather have a dog that walks next to you because it is more rewarding than pulling!

Inappropriate elimination

1. Indoors

Reasons:

- Insufficient house training
- Cognitive dysfunction – loss of previously learned behaviours
- The owner may be using harsh techniques causing the dog to try and eliminate out of sight of the owner – he equates owner + elimination with punishment.

Solution:

- Go back to basics with house training
- Ensure owners are using the correct techniques
- A full health check is recommended to ensure that there are no medical conditions that may be causing the problem.

2. Excitement

Reason:

- Young dogs often urinate when excited or anxious and it is normally related to fear or insecurity. It is thought that the smell of the urine may appease another dog by conveying certain messages regarding the dog's age, sex, etc.

Solution:

- Keep all greetings calm and try to distract the dog using training commands and treats to teach an alternative behaviour
- Increase the dog's confidence.

3. Marking

Both male and female dogs exhibit this behaviour but it is more likely to be prominent in uncastrated males. The incidence will be reduced if castrated but it depends on the age of the dog and the learned component of the behaviour.

Separation-related problems

Reasons:

- Being left alone does not come naturally to our social dogs. It is important that puppies are taught from a young age that being left alone can be rewarding.
- Boredom/frustration.
- Fear/anxiety.
- Cognitive dysfunction.

Solution:

- Identify the underlying emotional behaviour using the EMRA approach as previously discussed.
- If the dog is genuinely anxious and shows severe signs of stress, such as panting, salivating, sweating from pads and destruction of doors, etc., refer to a behaviourist immediately. The longer the behaviour is unresolved the worse it will become.
- If the dog appears to be barking or chewing due to boredom or frustration, advise the owner to assess his hedonic budget discussed earlier.

Food or object guarding behaviour (Resource guarding)

This behaviour can be easily avoided if the right steps are taken as a puppy.
Reasons:

- Owner insists on 'being the boss' and takes the highly prized article off the dog. This is the very thing it was worried about. This behaviour has nothing to do with being dominant – it is natural for a dog to hold onto a prized possession. It is our job to make him. understand that we are not a threat.
- Breed disposition to guarding resources – particularly in the gun dogs.
- Being punished for guarding things.

Solution:

- If a dog is showing signs of resource guarding, first identify its emotional state and review its hedonic budget
- If the dog is very anxious or fearful because it has been punished for this behaviour before, refer immediately to a behaviourist.

Guarding behaviour may be seen:

1. When feeding:
   - Do not feed from a bowl.
   - Feed bit by bit – this way you are giving the food and the dog will eagerly anticipate you being near

him during feeding time. Do this until the dog is more relaxed with you nearby and start to introduce a bowl.
   - Always put small amounts of food out so that the dog does not have a lot to guard.
   - Use this opportunity for training.
   - Start teaching that a hand on the bowl means a treat.
   - Never allow children near these dogs whilst feeding. No dog is ever 100% safe.
2. When playing with toys:
   - Whilst playing, always have another more desirable toy on hand that you can barter with. In this way you can teach the dog to relinquish the one toy and gain a better one! Teaching the dog to relinquish is the way to correct toy guarding behaviour. Don't leave desirable objects lying around.
3. Place guarding such as sofas or beds:
   - These are highly desirable areas for some dogs. Make them less desirable by making the floor or other areas of the house more desirable. Use food or toys to lure them off and reward them when they come to you.
   - Never physically try to remove them from the place they are guarding as you will force the dog to make an irrational decision.
   - Be consistent with your training and make sure everyone in the house follows the same training principles to avoid confusion.

Aggression to people or other animals

This behaviour has serious ramifications for the dog and needs to be handled professionally and quickly. Refer to a reputable behaviourist immediately. The correct advice at this time may prevent a serious injury and a euthanized dog.

Common behavioural problems in cats

Inappropriate elimination

Reasons:

- Unneutered male tom cats marking their territory
- Medical conditions such as cystitis which may cause pain and negative association with the litter tray
- Not enough litter trays per cat in the household (you should provide one tray per cat plus one extra)
- Fear, anxiety and insecurity, e.g. an aggressive cat outside, stressful multicat household. Cats will urinate in the house to create a sense of security
- Poor litter training
- Cognitive dysfunction.

Solution:

- Rule out any medical conditions
- Identify the root cause of the problem using the EMRA philosophy
- Use pheromone diffusers (Feliway®) to create a less stressful environment
- Make sure there are an adequate number of litter trays
- Refer to a knowledgeable cat behaviourist
- Advise client not to use punishment as this will increase anxiety and possibly cause the urination/defecation to increase.

Scratching furniture

Reasons:

- Natural behaviour
- Absence of a scratching post
- Boredom
- Applying scent to objects to increase the feeling of security.

Solution:

- Provide cat gyms and a sisal scratching post
- Ensure cat is stimulated and played with often
- Apply pheromone spray/diffuser to increase sense of security.

Anxiety or fearful behaviour

Reasons:

- Poor socialization
- Inherited temperament
- Punishment applied for certain behaviours
- Inappropriate environment for the cat.

Solution:

- Seek advice of behaviourist
- Use EMRA approach to make the cat's environment better and more secure
- Avoid using punishment
- Use counter conditioning and reinforcement techniques.

Aggression

Reasons:

- Poor socialization
- Inherited temperament
- Hand-raised kitten
- Reinforcement from owner, e.g. playing roughly
- Fear and anxiety.

Solution:

- Seek advice of behaviourist.
- Determine the root of the problem using the EMRA approach.
- Advise owners not to reinforce aggressive play. Use toys and NOT hands to play with kittens.
- Use counter conditioning and desensitization techniques.

What cats want!

Cats are predators and there is no getting away from this. The first time our cute little ball of fluff brings in a half-mutilated bunny or bird, we are shocked and try and save the poor creature from further trauma. Some people punish their cats for this behaviour but it is so important to educate owners that this is innate behaviour. It does not matter how much a cat is fed, he is not hunting because he is hungry; he is hunting because it provides him with an outlet for his instinctive, predatory behaviour. It is when cats are denied this opportunity to hunt, that we start to see the emergence of behaviour problems. Cats find stalking, chasing, catching and plucking of feathers or fur very rewarding and will continue to do so if

they can. Indoor cats are particularly susceptible to the build up of frustration in the absence of a predatory behaviour outlet. These cats can become cantankerous, aggressive, reclusive, bored or depressed. Help your clients enrich the lives of their indoor cats by providing them with the following:

- Surfaces at various levels to sleep on (sisal cat gyms are ideal).
- Regular play sessions simulating hunting and stalking behaviour.
- Large paper bags or cardboard boxes to hide in.
- Catnip which can encourage a feeling of well-being.
- Another feline friend to bond with and have a social interaction.
- Make eating more challenging by hiding biscuits under objects such as cushions.

Cognitive dysfunction

In older dogs and cats, it is important to recognize behavioural changes that result from ageing of the brain. Clients should be educated to recognize these changes and seek advice and treatment.

Signs to look out for are:

- Confusion and decreased awareness
- Change in social relationships
- Change in activity levels – restlessness, repetitive behaviours, apathy, decreased responsiveness
- Anxiety
- Altered sleep cycles
- Loss of learned behaviours, e.g. house soiling, remembering commands
- Change in appetite
- Irritability.

Empathizing with patients in practice

It is vital that you as a vet or veterinary nurse are able to empathize with your patients and understand something of what they might be feeling. Put yourself into a dog or cats' 'shoes' as they come through the door of the practice or the consulting room. Many animals are ill or in pain and as such are on the defensive. Treat them according to their temperament and individual needs. Learn to read their body language and adjust to each situation. This will make your job safer and the animal's stay with you less stressful. A bad experience in practice can make a normally amenable dog or cat difficult to handle which can develop into a behavioural issue.

Look for the following signs of stress:

Dogs

- Yawning
- All-over body shake as if they have just come out of water
- Panting
- Sweating paws
- Dilated pupils
- Puppy-like, appeasing behaviour
- Barking.

Give fearful patients space and time to get used to their environments. Try not to approach them immediately and drop treats on the floor.

Cats

- Hiding in the back of the cage or carrier
- Dilated pupils
- Open mouth breathing
- Sweaty paws.

Handle these cats gently and take time with them. Do not scruff as this will make a fearful cat very defensive. Use your thumb and forefinger together to create a greeting.

Bibliography

Aspinall, V., 2008. Clinical Procedures in Veterinary Nursing, second ed. Butterworth-Heinemann, Oxford.

Burch, M.R., Bailey, J.S., 1999. How Dogs Learn. Howell Book House, Hoboken, USA.

Coppinger, R., Coppinger, L., 2001. Dogs – A Startling New Understanding. Scribner, New York.

Eaton, B., Falconer-Taylor, R.F., Neville, P.F., 2007. EMRA: dominance and the alpha dog: challenging traditional thinking. Veterinary Times 37 (5), 16–19.

Falconer-Taylor, R.F., Neville, P.F., 2004. EMRA: the brain reward system and therapy induced frustration. Veterinary Times 34 (38).

Landsberg, G., Hunthausen, W., Ackerman, L., 1999. Handbook of Behavioural Problems of the Dog and Cat. Butterworth-Heineman, Oxford.

Lyon, H., Neville, P.F., Falconer-Taylor, R.F., 2006. Assessment and treatment of canine aggression problems using the EMRA approach. Veterinary Times 36 (3), 22–24.

Machell, B., Falconer-Taylor, R.F., Neville, P.F., 2006. Assessment and treatment of separation disorders in dogs using the EMRA approach. Veterinary Times 36 (16).

Mech, D., 2008. Whatever Happened to the Term Alpha Wolf? <http://www.wolf.org>.

Neville, P.F., Falconer-Taylor, R.F., 2004. EMRA: inappropriate elimination and impact of mood state assessment in a female long haired dachshund. Veterinary Times 34 (44).

O'Heare, J., 2003. Canine Neuropsychology, third ed. Behave Tech Publishing ebook.

Turner, D.C., Bateson, P., 2000. The Domestic Cat: The Biology of Its Behaviour, second ed. Cambridge University Press.

Recommended reading

Aspinall, V., 2008. Clinical Procedures in Veterinary Nursing, second ed. Butterworth-Heinemann, Oxford.

Chapter One provides all details of cat and dog handling.

Bailey, G., 2002. The Perfect Puppy. Hamlyn, London.

Ideal for first-time puppy owners.

Beaver, B.V., 1980. Feline Behaviour: A Guide for Veterinarians. Saunders, Philadelphia.

Detailed description of cat behaviour.

Donaldson, J., 1996. The Culture Clash. James and Kenneth Publishers, USA.

Goleman, D., 2004. Emotional Intelligence. Bloomsbury, London.

This book will have a huge impact on how you view your own interactions and relationships in life.

Neville, P.F., Falconer-Taylor, R.F., 2004. EMRA: the new perspective in approaching companion animal behaviour problems (1). Veterinary Times 34 (29), 28–30.

Neville, P.F., Falconer-Taylor, R.F., 2004. EMRA: the new perspective in approaching companion animal behaviour problems (2). Veterinary Times 34 (31), 14–16.

Pryor, K., 1999. Don't Shoot the Dog. Bantam Books, London.

A detailed discussion on learning theory.

Semyonova, A., 2009. The 100 Silliest Things People Say About Dogs. Hastings Press, Hastings. <http://www.non-lineardogs.com>.

An enlightened new approach to understanding your dog.

Yin, S., 2009. Low Stress Handling, Restraint and Behaviour Modifications of Dogs and Cats. Cattledog Publishing, USA.

I would recommend every veterinary practice to have a copy of this book.

For more information regarding COAPE behaviourists and on behaviour education courses available: <http://www.capbt.org> for details of local COAPE qualified, modern, fair and effective trainers and referral behaviourists.

<http://www.coape.org> for education courses in companion animal behaviour and training from basic to Diploma level.

CHAPTER 11

Equine behaviour and handling

Nicola Ackerman

- The wild horse is a sociable animal that lives in herds on open plains and most of its behaviour patterns are based on the need to survive, eat, reproduce and socialize with others of its own species.
- It is important for your own safety when handling a horse in any situation that you understand the biology and the basic behaviour of the animal so that you can predict what it may do next.
- Transportation of horses may be unavoidable but can be distressing for the horse. Correct design of the vehicle, provision of correct travel clothing for the horse and adherence to the guidelines for welfare of the horse during the journey will all help to lower the stress levels.
- Effective training of horses, particularly foals and young stock, makes use of several different methods and is based on the horse's natural behaviour and the way in which it learns.

Introduction

The horse has evolved from the small, forest-dwelling *Eohippus* into the incomparable athlete that is today's domestic horse *Equus caballus*. Wild horses are herbivorous prey animals that naturally live in herds on open plains. In these surroundings there is nowhere to hide and many of their behaviour patterns have evolved to aid their survival, mainly by rapid flight from a predator. They have also evolved to survive on a relatively poor-quality diet that is eaten over a long period. During the process of domestication the modern horse has proved to be extremely adaptable but when observing their behaviour the link back to the wild horse must not be forgotten.

Equine behaviour

The horse possesses instincts or innate behaviour patterns that revolve around four basic needs:

- Self-preservation and survival
- Food and water
- Reproduction
- Socialization and the company of others of the same species.

Self-preservation and survival

The horse has evolved over many centuries into what we now accept as the modern horse. As a prey species the horse has developed its use of eyesight and its 'flight or fight' instinct and it is important to remember these characteristics when approaching the horse and to appreciate why sudden movements in and out of the blind spot may precipitate a strong reaction. The horse's eyesight is not developed to cope with rapid changes in light intensity, e.g. going from bright outdoors to dark indoors, which explains why some horses may be reluctant to go into or falter when entering a dark stable.

The eyes of a horse lie on either side of the head high up above the mouth. This position means that the horse can graze while still keeping a look out for predators and the view from each provides a monocular panoramic view. The area in front of the head where the two monocular areas overlap, providing binocular vision in which depth can be judged, is small (Fig. 11.1). This is why a horse may refuse a fence when turned sharply to jump – it has not had time to adjust and gauge the distance to the jump. Horses will nearly always turn towards a movement in order to judge distance.

Another adaptation is that the horse is able to sleep while standing, allowing a quick response to approaching predators. Horses only lie down to sleep when in a relaxed, safe environment or when extremely tired. The stay apparatus in the limbs enables the main limb joints to lock and support the weight of the body. The system of muscles and ligaments is mainly based on the suspensory ligament running down the plantar aspect of the large metacarpal. This ligament divides into two branches inserted into the proximal sesamoid bones. Supplementing the suspensory ligament is the superficial and deep flexor tendon (see Ch. 6).

The horse will adapt its body language in order to warn off potential predators (Fig. 11.2). An unwelcome presence in a horse's field, e.g. a dog or human, can result in the horse turning its hindquarters as a threat or even charging with its head down at the object. Horses that do not want to be

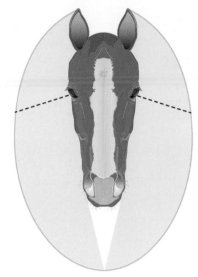

Fig. 11.1 The field of vision of the horse

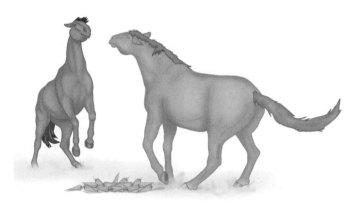

Fig. 11.2 Horses competing for food while out in the field

caught when out in a field can exhibit very distinctive body language expressing their feelings.

Food and water

The horse digests its food through hindgut fermentation in the caecum by means of colonies of symbiotic microorganisms (see Ch. 9). The horse is designed to eat low-grade forage – hay and grasses – at a constant rate. Horses do not posses a gall bladder as there is no need for the storage of bile. As horses are designed to graze for a large proportion of the day, if they is stabled and fed a concentrated diet they become bored and stereotypical behaviour, e.g. weaving and crib-biting, may develop.

Reproduction

The reproductive urge is the most fundamental of all instincts. Horses have short and seasonal reproductive periods that occur in the spring and early summer. In the natural environment a stallion will have to compete for his harem of mares and spend time interacting with them, although the mare will initiate many of these interactions. The stallion will decide who is in oestrus and will 'court' these mares for a

long time during this period. This behaviour is somewhat lost under managed breeding programmes. The horse has lost its choice of partner and may be inexperienced in communication with others.

The most frequent behavioural problems experienced are low libido. This is characterized by a lack of sexual interest and arousal when the stallion is presented to a mare in oestrus. A detailed examination of the stallion should be performed. Pain is a common cause of low libido and can become a negative reinforcement if repeatedly required to mount while in pain; for example, musculoskeletal pain, especially back pain. Low libido can also be due to low levels of hormones such as testosterone. Stallions that have been kept stabled have been reported to have lower testosterone levels than those who run with their own harem. When all other differential diagnoses have been ruled out, hormonal pharmacological agents can be used; for example, human chorionic gonadotrophin (hCG) can be used initially, administered intravenously two hours prior to mating. For stallions with low circulating testosterone levels, treatment may be with gonadotrophin-releasing hormone (GnRH).

Excessive libido also occurs in a very small proportion of stallions and is physically dangerous to both handlers and mares. Most cases result from poor handling and stallion management. Evidence has shown that this behaviour may also be inherited. Other reproductive abnormalities such as ejaculatory failure can also cause behavioural problems. Frustration can lead to aggressive behaviour towards mare and handlers. Poor semen collection technique may result in a bad experience for the stallion and may affect future behaviour.

Geldings may also exhibit sexual behaviour, although not as dramatic as in stallions. Testosterone is not always necessary for male sexual behaviour in animals – castrated dogs may still show sexual behaviour. These behaviours continue in the castrated male as their brains are thought to be 'masculinized' before birth. Geldings may herd 'their mares' away from either other geldings or humans. Aggression can also be shown either towards other geldings or towards humans, even when mares are not present. Masturbation can occur in both stallions and geldings (at a lower rate). Most owners do not normally notice this behaviour as it is associated with rest and sleep periods and therefore occurs in the early hours of the morning. This behaviour does not normally cause a problem but when a horse is shod he may be stimulated by the smell of previously shod mares on the farrier's clothing.

Socialization and the company of other horses

Horses are gregarious by nature and move around in herds. Social contact with other horses is very important and, when isolated, horses are susceptible to stress, symptoms of which can present as stereotypical behaviour or vices. The need for company is so great that it can mould the animal's personality and behaviour. Treatment of these vices is to attempt to modify the environment, returning it to a natural state.

Grooming is an important part of social interaction. When a horse is groomed the groom is essentially asking the horse to initiate a mutual grooming session and many horses respond by nibbling the person in return. If the horse does do this it is better to offer an alternative medium, e.g. coconut matting, rather than punish it.

Extrinsic factors

All the factors described above are instinctive or intrinsic factors that influence behaviour. There are, however, other extrinsic influences on behaviour and temperament that are environmental and are out of the horse's control. Most extrinsic factors experienced by the modern horse are man-made:

- **Breed or type** – a hot-blooded horse, e.g. a thoroughbred, has different characteristics from a cold-blooded horse, e.g. a draught horse. A thoroughbred is more likely to become excited at the prospect of speed, which may be a genetic influence due to the metabolic processes associated with the transfer of energy into movement. This is a generalization, and each animal should be considered as an individual – some hot-blooded horses can be extremely laid back!
- **Experience and learning** – the memory of good or bad experiences will affect the horse dramatically. Whether the intelligence of the horse influences the behaviour is questionable. Learning by exposure is essential to training and horses have shown that they will respond to this form of training. This type of learning often complements instinctive behaviour.
- **Gender** – whether this affects the behaviour and learning ability of the horse is debatable. It has been shown that the sex of a horse doesn't affect its learning ability but the temperament of the horse does. Geldings are reputed to be more consistent in their temperament than mares and stallions because fluctuating hormone levels play a part in behaviour. The health and management of the horse will also affect its behaviour.

Communication behaviour

Olfactory signals

Olfactory communication or communication by smell is the only means of communication that horses have that is capable of lasting beyond the immediate moment. Smell plays a significant role within the social context of the horse and it helps to identify individuals, their degree of dominance and the location of other potential rivals.

The odour resulting from defecation is important in olfactory communication. Stallions will defecate on existing faecal piles in order to leave distinct olfactory messages for other stallions. Mares and geldings tend to first smell the faeces of others and then defecate nearby, producing an enlarged area of faeces in the field. Most horses will not graze in this area, and particularly lush green areas may be seen in an otherwise well-grazed field. One theory of this behaviour is that it keeps grazing zones free from contamination by intestinal parasites and that there is also a slight reduction in the number of flies away from the faeces.

Stallions also use smell in order to detect when a mare is in oestrus. The horse possesses an odour-sensitive organ known as Jacobson's organ in the roof of the mouth. This consists of two parallel ducts that open into the mouth just behind the upper incisors, passing through the hard palate and communicating with the nasal passage. The ducts are lined with specialized olfactory cells that sample the air and pass the information on to the brain. The horse draws the smell-filled air through the nose and mouth over the organ and this action is characterized by the upper lip curling while the mouth is open (Fig. 11.3). As the air moves into the ducts the tongue presses against the hard palate, sealing off the duct openings and trapping the sampled air. This behaviour is called the flehmen response and all horses respond to unusual smells with it. Pheromones also play a large role in communication and our understanding of their role is increasing.

Vocalization

Horses have a limited vocal range in comparison to other mammals as they have evolved on open landscapes where they are rarely out of sight of each other. Vocalization can be used for a number of different reasons, e.g. a foal trying to find its dam, a horse warning others of impending danger. The horse's ear pinna is highly mobile to locate the source of a sound, although horses are not as accurate at pinpointing the sound as dogs, which is an important difference between the behaviour of a prey species and a predatory species.

Tactile communication

Mutual grooming provides a means of maintaining the social structure of the herd. Friendship bonds are firmly formed through grooming. These friendship bonds tend to form between horses of a similar age and social rank. Preferred grooming sites are concentrated near the autonomic nervous system's longest nerve, i.e. vagus X. Stimulation of this nerve has shown to decrease the heart rate and relax the recipient (Fig. 11.4).

Visual communication

In order to understand what the horse is 'saying' to us it is important to know and recognize normal behaviour. The horse can express its feelings through eye position, nostrils and ear position. Neighing and snorting also have a wider range of expression than is generally thought. The ears of the horse can show alertness, willingness, unwillingness or even menace. Other means of expression include the mouth (e.g. baring of teeth), the fore feet (e.g. stamping, pawing), the hind feet and carriage of the tail.

Stereotypical behaviour

Stereotypical behaviour is classed as behaviour that has been modified because of stress in the animal. It may also be described as a series of repetitive actions for no obvious reason. Stress may result from a number of different causes, e.g. change in routine, being stabled with loss of social contact, in fact anything that upsets the natural balance of the horse. It is difficult to establish whether some horses of a particular bloodline are more predisposed to stereotypical behaviour than others. However, as certain bloodlines are

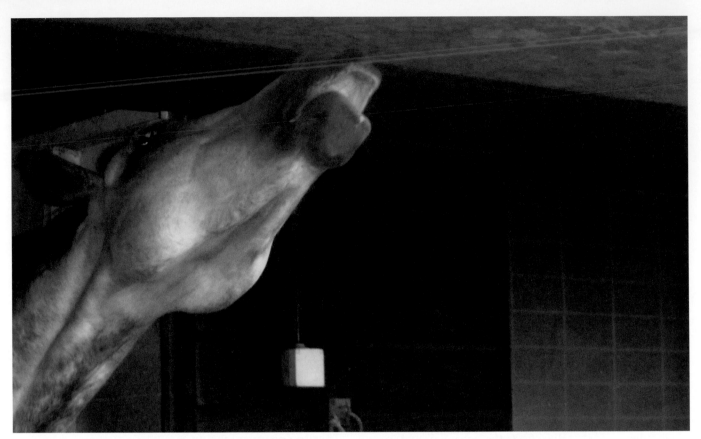

Fig. 11.3 Horse showing the flehmen response

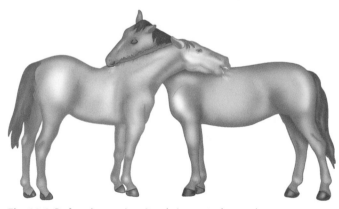

Fig. 11.4 Preferred grooming sites during mutual grooming

subjected to different management regimes, this could be the causal factor.

1. Crib-biting

Crib-biting or wood-chewing may be associated with being fed an unbalanced diet – most commonly diets low in fibre, e.g. highly concentrated pelleted foods. Boredom is also a factor and this vice tends to be highly infectious and will be copied by other horses. Pasture-kept horses will normally chew or consume trees, fences and shrubs in order to increase the fibre content of their diet. Treatment for this vice is to increase the fibre content of the diet by increasing the quantity of hay and grass. The use of hay nets with a small mesh increases the time taken to consume the food and may help the problem. Other precautions such as removing wooden edges are not always possible, but providing toys or companions may also help.

2. Cribbing

This occurs when the horse grasps an object, usually the stable door or fence, with the incisor teeth and sucks in air through its mouth. Cribbing, also called wind-sucking or aerophagia, is traditionally cited as a cause of recurrent colic and cribbers will also show excessive wear on the incisors. Some horses do not need to grasp anything and are able to swallow air just by flexing the neck. If the habit is severe, hypertrophy of the ventral muscles (sternocephalicus, omo-hyoideus and sternothyroideus) of the neck can occur.

This behaviour is a common form of self-stimulation that triggers the release of endorphins, natural opioids produced within the body, which produce a calming effect and helps to reinforce the causal behaviour. Other signs may include increased intake of water, weight loss, poor appetite and gastric ulceration. Treatment includes increasing the horse's fibre intake, use of a cribbing strap, prevention of boredom and increasing the time turned out to pasture. The use of surgery to combat this behaviour is well documented, but the efficacy of these surgical techniques has not been published. Surgical treatments include neurectomy of the glossopharyngeal nerve (cranial nerve XI) and surgical resection of the ventral neck muscles. There are also reports that in some horses where surgery was successful initially the behaviour has been relearned. The presence of scars on the neck may be an unwanted side effect, especially in show horses.

3. Weaving

Weaving is a common sign of boredom or anxiety and can be exacerbated by stress. During weaving the weight is transferred from one foreleg to the other and the head and neck sway from side to side. This process can cause undue wear and tear on the joints and tendons of the limbs and excessive wear on the shoes. Horses that weave are also more likely to show 'impulse' aggression to passers-by over the stable door, which may reflect the frustration that these animals are experiencing. It is important, however, to rule out other conditions such as forelimb lameness and neck pain.

Methods of treatment include turning the horse out to pasture, providing a more stimulating environment by siting the stable in an area in which activity is taking place or by the use of a V-shaped grill on the stable door that stops the sideways movements of the head. Studies have shown that by increasing visual stimulation weaving is significantly reduced. This factor was more successful when the horse was given the opportunity to interact with or view neighbouring horses.

4. Self-mutilation

Self-mutilation usually affects young stallions. It is thought that this behaviour occurs more in stallions than in mares as they groom themselves more often. Self-mutilation is usually initiated by a stressful event such as moving to a different yard or major changes within a breeding or exercise programme. Most self-mutilating horses bite a specific area of their bodies, often the forelimbs, the pectoral area, stifle, flanks or thighs. Some horses will grunt, stall walk and stare at the specific area prior to the act of self-mutilation. Other presenting signs include licking, alopecia and leukotrichia in one localized area.

It is important to rule out all other potential causes, e.g. seizures, skin complaints or abdominal pain. A number of stereotypical behaviour patterns are associated with abnormally high levels of opium-like compounds such as encephalins and endorphins, which are released in response to stressful stimuli. These compounds have an effect of increasing the release of dopamine in the brain and can also make the receptors more sensitive to its presence. The stress of being stabled, changes in daily routine, etc., tend to activate the stereotypical motor patterns, which in turn stimulates the release of endorphins, which further stimulates the stereotypical behaviour. Endorphins also have an analgesic effect, which may enable the horse to mutilate itself without feeling pain.

Aggression

Aggression has different evolutionary functions in the horse, which include maintaining and establishing social hierarchy within the herd, and in some circumstances aggression can be a normal behaviour pattern, e.g. maternal aggression. Horses would rather avoid aggression than attack without warning and their signals escalate gradually, ranging from flattening the ears through to lunging. Humans may put themselves at risk if they ignore the initial, more subtle visual signals. Such situations often escalate, as the human unconsciously trains the horse to believe that all the initial warning signals are unnecessary, and eventually the horse attacks without apparent warning. It is therefore vital that anyone handling horses in any way learns to read and understand their visual and vocal signals.

In most cases abnormal aggression is due to hormonal imbalances, often caused by hypertrophy of an endocrine organ. The prognosis for these abnormal aggression patterns can be good if the initiating cause can be removed.

Assessment of pain

Pain is an aversive stimulus and may be an indicator of something that could decrease the chances of survival in the wild. The horse will quickly learn to avoid anything that has been a cause of pain in the past, e.g. a horse with back pain may become saddle-shy even though the original pain has subsided long ago. Both pain and fear can produce similar behavioural responses and elicit physiological and behavioural responses that are aimed at either minimizing or avoiding the specific conditions that produced them. It is therefore important when diagnosing behavioural problems to determine whether the response is due primarily to a painful stimulus or a conditioned fear response.

It is vital that the veterinary nurse is able to recognize and assess the signs of pain in the horse. This is achieved by:

- **Observing body language** – a horse in pain, depending on severity of the pain, may be restless, sweating, kick, stamp or bite at certain body areas, kick bedding around, grind their teeth and be vocal. Horses can also become depressed, lose interest in their surroundings, hang their heads low and lose their appetite
- **Measurement of clinical parameters** such as temperature pulse and respiration.
- **Measurement of humoral factors** such as epinephrine (adrenaline), norepinephrine (noradrenaline), cortisol and endorphins in the blood can give an indication of the level of pain.

The use of a pain scoring system may help to assess the level of pain objectively. For example, a normal horse has a score of 0; a horse that is grinding its teeth has a score of 3; a horse that is rolling on the ground has a score of 5 – the higher the score the more need there is for analgesia. Such a method is non-quantitative and relies on the same person assessing the level of pain that they feel the animal is experiencing – different people may have different pain criteria. It also depends on how experienced the observer is in detecting the subtler behavioural changes in that particular animal.

Handling and restraint

The key to handling horses is to be able to anticipate through their body language and facial expression what they are likely to do. They are strong animals whose behaviour can sometimes be violent and unpredictable and an awareness of their natural behaviour will help to prevent accidents. The handler should always wear stout boots, preferably with steel toecaps, and in some cases it may be necessary to wear a safety helmet to protect the head. The majority of horses will behave better if handled with firmness and kindness and a horse will always be able to detect if you lack confidence. Always stand close to the horse near to its head and away from the hind legs – the closer you are, the less the force of any movement or kick. Make sure you know what you are going to do, have the correct equipment ready to hand and organize help if you think you may need it.

Approach and catching

- Approach from slightly to one side of the head, remembering that a horse is unable to see either directly in front or directly behind itself
- Speak to it gently using a low tone as you get near
- Place your hand on the lower neck or shoulder and put a rope around the neck
- Most horses will now accept that they have been caught and allow you to put a head collar or halter on them
- If a horse is difficult to catch it should wear a head collar in the field
- Most horses can be caught by offering them a bribe in the form of food, e.g. an apple or Polo mint, but keep it hidden until you have caught the horse
- There are many suggestions for catching difficult horses and the handler will soon invent methods suited to their own individual horse.

Tying up

All horses should be trained at an early age to stand quietly while tied up:

- Select a suitable ring, post or rail – this should be firmly attached and should not be part of anything that will bang, rattle or fall over if the horse pulls away.
- Always use a quick release knot (Fig. 11.5). A piece of string can also be incorporated into the lead rope to

allow easy breaking or untying if the horse falls over or pulls backwards. This will prevent head injuries but may develop into persistent halter breaking and escape.
- Never leave the horse unattended.

Leading

- Horses are traditionally led from the left or near side but they should learn to accept leading from both sides – use of the right or off side may be necessary when walking on the road towards oncoming traffic.
- Hold the lead rope close to the horse's head and the remaining rope loosely in the other hand – never wind it around your hand in case the horse suddenly pulls away.
- Difficult or unpredictable horses should wear a bridle with the reins taken over the head, which provides extra control.
- When you are ready to move give the command 'walk on', take a step forward and the horse should follow.
- If the horse does not move tap it on the side with a small stick held in your hand.
- Do not tug at it or stare it in the face.
- If the horse refuses to move ask someone to go behind with a broom or long whip to urge the horse forward – they should of course stay out of range of a kick.
- If 'trotting up' to show a horse's paces or for the investigation of lameness, lead the horse away from the observer in a straight line for about 25 metres. Turn the horse around away from the handler, to reduce the risk of being trodden on, and walk past the observer. Repeat at a trot.
- The lead rope should be held in an open hand to allow free movement of the head but you must be ready to grasp the rope if the horse plays up.
- When you are ready to stop, give the command 'halt' or 'stand' and stop walking – the horse should then stop.
- Young foals should be trained to these commands from an early age.

Picking up the feet

A horse should be trained to allow its feet to be picked up for daily cleaning, regular inspection and shoeing:

- Speak to the horse as you approach its shoulder.
- To lift a fore foot, stand facing the tail and run the hand closest to the body down over the elbow, back of knee and tendons until you reach the fetlock.
- Tug at the fetlock giving the command 'up'.
- As the horse lifts its foot up, catch the toe of the hoof and support it with your other hand. The horse should be encouraged to stand square, otherwise it may lean on you.
- Do not allow the horse to snatch its foot away, as it may stamp it down on your toe.
- To lift a hind foot (Fig. 11.6) run the same hand over the horse's back down the rump and back leg to the point of the hock.

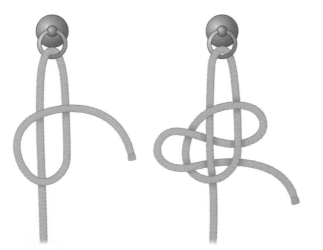

Fig. 11.5 A quick release knot

- Move your hand over the anterior part of the cannon bone to the medial part of the fetlock.
- Tug at the fetlock using the command 'up' and the horse will lift its foot up.
- Foals should be trained early to get used to this procedure. Obliging horses will soon learn to lift their feet ready for you once they know what is required.

Examination of the mouth

This may be necessary for examination of the teeth, for treatments such as tooth rasping and for determining a horse's age:

- Steady the nose with one hand and insert the other, palm downwards, into the diastema (space between the corner incisors and the first premolars)
- Grasp the tongue and gently pull it out sideways so that it is out of the way
- In this position an oral medicine can be given; for tooth rasping it may be necessary to use a gag, which keeps the mouth open and leaves the hands free.

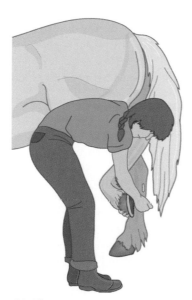

Fig. 11.6 Lifting a hind foot

Use of the twitch

Additional restraint may be needed for some individuals, particularly if you need to carry out treatment or examination on a frightened or injured animal. In most cases a twitch provides sufficient restraint. This consists of a short pole with a loop of 6–7 mm thick rope at the end:

- Using your finger and thumb, grasp the horse's upper lip and draw it through the loop of the twitch
- Twist it up firmly, having removed your hand and maintain the position for several minutes until instructed to release it (Fig. 11.7)
- Leave the twitch in place for a minimum amount of time and never for longer than 5 min
- Never apply to the ears, as permanent damage can be inflicted.

It was originally thought that the twitch provided a certain degree of pain that distracted the horse's attention from what was being done to it. However, research now shows that the natural endorphins released by the brain may have an analgesic/anaesthetic effect and the horse appears sedated after a few minutes – enough time for minor procedures to be performed.

Personal protective equipment

It is important that personal protective equipment (PPE) is worn when handling horses. Those horses that are in discomfort or in unfamiliar surroundings can behave in an abnormal and unpredictable manner. PPE include helmet (ASTM/SEI approved), correct safety shoes and body protection when riding. Gloves should be worn at all times when leading and handling horses. Difficult-to-handle horses can also be led out with a bridle rather than a head collar.

Identification and the use of horse passports

The Horse Passports (England) Regulations 2004 requires all owners to obtain a passport for each horse they own. This includes ponies, donkeys, and other Equidae. Owners cannot sell, export, slaughter for human consumption, use

Fig. 11.7 Application of a twitch

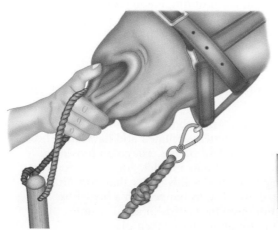

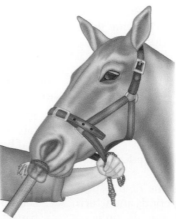

for the purposes of competition or breeding, a horse which does not have a passport. Owners of foals must obtain a passport for it on or before 31 December of the year of its birth, or by six months after its birth, whichever is later. Passports can be issued from organizations authorized by DEFRA. Some organizations will issue passports for specific breeds of horses, while others will do it for any breed. Each horse is issued a Unique Equine Life Number (UELN) which will appear on the horse's passport and identifies it. The silhouette of the horse, used as a means of identification, must be completed by a veterinary surgeon or an approved representative of the Passport Issuing Organisation (PIO) approved by DEFRA. This is completed by the use of colour, breed and distinguishing features such as whorls, stars, leg markings, etc. Freeze marks can be noted on the silhouette.

Any medicines administered to the horse should be recorded in section IX of the passport for those animals intended for human consumption. Details of the medicines concerned are contained in the consolidated Version of the Annexes I to IV of Council Regulation 2377/90. If the declaration that the horse is ultimately intended for human consumption is signed, the date when any medicines are administered that have substances not included in annexes I–IV of 2377/90 must be recorded on the section IX pages of the passport. This is to comply with the legislation relating to the withdrawal period of drugs within which a food-producing animal must not be slaughtered. Note: Annex IV drugs must never be administered to a food-producing animal.

Other forms of identification are possible and these include freeze marking, microchipping and tattooing. In all cases the owner's details are held on a database and it is important that these details are kept update. Freeze brands and tattoos can be easily altered and can fade over time, so microchipping is strongly recommended by veterinary surgeons. The microchip should adhere to the protocol set out by the International Organisation of Standards (ISO) so that the microchip can be read by all microchip readers.

Transportation of horses

Transportation can cause distress, leading to a loss of condition and even metabolic upset. Correct preparation of the animal prior to transportation is vital and can reduce stress levels. In the UK the Horserace Betting Levy Board issue guidlines on the transportation of horses. There are three legislative orders that govern the transportation:

- The Horse (Sea Transport) Order 1952 (amended in 1958)
- Transit of Animals (Road and Rail) Order 1975 (amended in 1979 and 1988)
- The Welfare of Animal Transit Order 1997; Transport of Horses came into force in July 1998.

Transportation out of the country is also included in the Horse Passports Regulations 2004.

These orders set out details of dimensions of transport vehicles, lengths of time in transport, rest periods and which animals can and cannot be transported, e.g. ill, unfit or

pregnant mares may suffer unnecessary stress or harm. Transportation of pregnant mares should be avoided during the 20–45-day stage of gestation as during this stage there is a transfer from the yolk sac to chorioallantoic placentation and the risk of abortion increases.

When transporting horses over long distances it is important to seek veterinary advice and to have the horse's health checked prior to movement. Horses with respiratory disease should not be transported if possible. Clinical examination with the emphasis on subclinical respiratory problems should be done prior to lengthy trips. Horses transported in close proximity with little ventilation and dusty hay all predispose to respiratory problems such as 'shipping fever', the name given to respiratory disease linked to transportation. This manifests itself as depression and inappetence with the presence of a soft cough, shallow frequent respiration and a febrile response. Appropriate treatment can be effective but the condition may be life-threatening. The condition may be prevented by the use of dust- and mould-extracted hay and good ventilation. Horses should not to be tied up with their heads in an abnormally high position, as this can lead to commensal bacteria spreading to the lower respiratory tract.

Stress is an important factor in respiratory disease and in the welfare of the horse during transportation. There are several factors that should be taken into consideration to reduce stress while travelling:

- The number of animals being transported in one vehicle
- Provision of food and water
- Ambient temperature
- Ventilation
- Degree of movement, which is determined by the length of rope on the head collar; the horse must be able to balance itself without undue effort and have enough room to urinate and defecate
- The presence of a stable mate or other companion
- Habituation to travelling.

Horses are sensitive to movement underfoot and are aware of the stability of the ground beneath them. This may help to explain why some horses are reluctant to cross bridges or traverse ramps and which may lead to an unwillingness to load for travelling. This may reflect genuine apprehension, stubbornness or, as is often more likely, may result from a previous bad experience, e.g. travelling too fast, poor balance or falling off the ramp during loading or unloading. If the horse is difficult to load it is important that plenty of time and patience is given to the procedure.

Travel by road

The method of transportation can have an effect on the horse:

- **Type of vehicle** – horseboxes, i.e. those with an integral cab, tend to be better ventilated and have more head and body room than trailers. They also provide a smoother journey than a trailer. Some horses prefer travelling facing backwards rather than forwards, or standing diagonally, as happens in a horsebox. Horses should not travel backwards in a trailer unless the correct modifications have taken place.

- **Ramps** – the incline of the ramp into the vehicle should be no greater than 25° and should provide secure footing.
- **Journey times** – may vary from an hour to a few days. The usual practice is for the horse to rest overnight in stables after every 24 hours of transportation. Long journeys create long periods when the horse is standing in one position. This can create muscle fatigue and associated myositis.
- **Ventilation** – poor ventilation can have a detrimental effect on the health of the horse. Exhaust fumes and fumes from excreta can affect the respiratory system, as can mouldy hay. It is advised that dust and mould particles are removed from hay prior to travelling. Exhaust fumes such as ammonia, carbon monoxide and nitrogen dioxide may disrupt the epithelial barrier between capillaries and alveoli in the lungs, which increases their permeability to bacteria. Also an altered rate of pulmonary aerosol clearance after travelling increases the bacterial numbers in the lower respiratory tract.

Travel by air

Transportation by air is becoming more common and utilizes either an enclosed 'air stable' or an open-stall system. There are strict regulations concerning air travel. The ratio of personnel to horses should be one groom to every three horses but this is not always possible because of the number of seats available on some aircraft. Most bloodstock shipping agencies arrange for an equine clinician to travel on long-haul flights. Air travel is expensive, so few horses are transported in this way. When travelling by air the horse should wear the same protective clothing as when travelling by road.

Clothing for travel

The choice of travel clothing depends on the time of year and the weather on the day of travel, and no matter what the length of journey the protective clothing must always be of the same standard (Fig. 11.8). Protective leg bandages should always be worn. They may be either stable bandages with plenty of Gamgee padding or specially designed travelling boots, which must fit correctly and be non-slip. If the bandages do not cover or protect the knees and hocks, additional hock and knee boots must be worn. Over-reach boots can also add extra protection. A poll guard should also be worn to protect the head. The low headroom of the trailer or horsebox puts a head-shy or nervous horse at risk of injury. A tail bandage and tail guard will help protect the soft tissue in the tail and stops unsightly rubbing. It should be remembered that the horse will cool more quickly if it is moving and in a draughty environment and the horse that sweats while being transported may be anxious rather than hot. A combination of a sweat sheet and a warmer rug may be necessary.

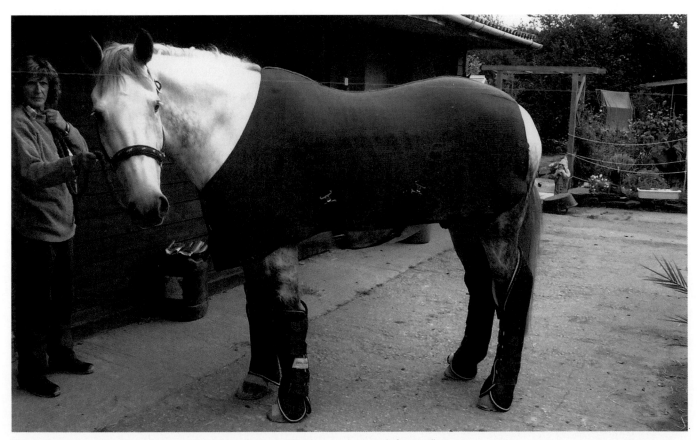

Fig. 11.8 Horse wearing protective leg wear, tail bandage, guard and sweat sheet ready for travelling

Transportation of sick or injured horses

Sick and injured horses should not be transported unless authorized by a veterinary surgeon. If such a horse has to be transported it is still vital to provide protective clothing while it is travelling. Secondary injuries to any part of the body can be detrimental to the horse – if there is already an injury to one leg, a secondary injury to one of the supporting limbs may be disastrous. Additional stress to the animal should be prevented and care should be taken not to unbalance the horse.

In some cases transportation is unavoidable, e.g. disorders such as exertional rhabdomyolysis (tying up) require that the horse is not made to walk any distance at all as this exacerbates the condition, the degree of pain and muscle damage.

The transport should always be taken to the location of the horse; not the horse to the vehicle. If the ramp of the horsebox or trailer is steep, parking on a slope or in a loading bay can reduce the angle and benefit the horse. If support is required, straw bales can be used unless a modified ambulance is available.

All fractures should be immobilized and supported prior to transportation. If the horse has a fractured forelimb, travelling the horse backwards reduces the risk of it inadvertently putting weight on the fractured limb if the vehicle stops suddenly. If a hind limb is fractured, face the horse forwards. The head and neck should be left free to move and act as a counterbalance. There is great debate on the use of painkillers before moving and transporting horses that have fractures and there is a belief that pain relief should not be given in order to discourage the horse from bearing weight on the fractured limb. A means of communication within the vehicle is important so that the handler can inform the driver of any problems. If an injured foal needs to be transported, two people can carry it or support it – one with hands around the neck and thorax and the other with hands around the abdomen and hindquarters. The mare should be allowed to remain close by.

Sedation for travelling should be avoided in all animals because the sedative creates problems with balance and thermoregulation, and when sedated the horse may over-react to certain stimuli, causing panic.

Use of equine ambulances

Equine ambulances attend most equine events and have been specially designed to cope with the types of emergencies that might happen there. The low ramp entrance is long to reduce the angle of incline into the ambulance. Internal partitions are easily positioned and moved around to allow access to different areas of the horse. Support can be provided from slings, and winches are available to drag unconscious patients into the ambulance.

Training the horse

Horses are extremely adaptable and their learning capability encourages approaches to training that work with, rather than against, their natural behavioural traits. Horses learn by four different methods and each training regime uses one or more of these. They are:

- **Habituation** – the horse becomes used to a stimulus and overcomes its initial response, e.g. fear
- **Sensitization** – the horse may be conditioned to respond to a stimulus by previous training using another stimulus
- **Observation** – the horse watches another horse performing a particular behaviour pattern and then repeats the pattern when given the opportunity
- **Association** – the horse connects a response with a particular stimulus.

Training methods

The methods used to train horses can be related to their natural behaviour patterns and can be divided into:

- **Classical or respondent conditioning** – another name is pavlovian conditioning, as the phenomenon was originally identified by Pavlov. An unconditioned stimulus produces a reflex type of response, e.g. salivation in response to the smell of food. If a neutral stimulus is then paired with the original stimulus – for example, Pavlov rang a bell when he fed his dogs – eventually the use of the neutral stimulus will produce the response and the response is said to have been conditioned.
- **Operant or instrumental conditioning** – best described as trial-and-error learning, using negative or positive reinforcement to 'reward' the behaviour that was performed. For example, the horse hears the sound of food being shaken in a bucket, it approaches and receives the food as reward. A negative reinforcement is not a punishment but a process in which the stimulus is removed. For example, pressure from the bit increases the probability of a behaviour recurring, e.g. the horse working on the bit. Unfortunately, punishment is widely overused, and there is a danger that the horse might associate the punishment, usually the whip, with the wrong aspect of the situation. A prime example of this is when a horse refuses a jump and the rider then uses the whip. Some horses may then become anxious about the situation and start rushing at the fences.

Once the goal has been reached it is important that the learning is reinforced through occasional exposure to what were previously problem elements so that the learning is not forgotten. Each training session should begin with a stimulus of a lower level than that achieved in the previous session, then worked up to the more complex stimuli and beyond if necessary.

Counter conditioning

Counter conditioning is the process whereby an animal is trained to respond in a way that is incompatible with the response that is to be eliminated, when presented with a problem-evoking stimulus.

- **Classical or respondent counter conditioning** – this uses an unconditioned response as the desired behaviour: e.g. the sound of a whistle being blown before the horse gets its food. The sound now predicts eating its favourite food. Once the response has become established the sound can be used to gain the animal's attention when a potential problem is approaching, e.g. a dog in the yard. The behaviour that the horse normally performs, i.e. eating its food, is an unconditioned response, as the horse would do this naturally.

- **Operant counter conditioning** – there are many names for operant counter conditioning. These include counter commanding, response substitution and competing response training. It uses a conditioned response such as 'lie down' in the dog, to control the undesired behaviour. For example, a dog with a history of attacking other dogs is told to lie down until the other dog has passed. A good example of this in the horse is a method of dealing with horses that barge when leaving the stable or horsebox. Standing the horse in a neutral environment while being tied up is then reinforced with food. The handler uses a keyword for example 'stand' and the horse will soon learn to associate this word with the behaviour – this behaviour is a conditioned response of standing still.

Habituation

Habituation is another aspect of learning and is seen in most animals. A great deal is known about socialization and habituation of puppies (see Ch. 10) and horses learn in the same way. Habituation occurs when the stimulus response is repeated with no reward until the response no longer occurs and is important because an animal that reacts to every stimulus in its environment is as ill-equipped as one that does not react at all. The animal learns that there is no resulting action from the stimulus and learns to ignore it.

Horse trainers use this learning capability to full effect. When exposing the horse to a new experience it is important that the trainer acts as calmly as possible and takes very little notice of what caused the response as this may reinforce the initial reaction. For example, if a horse shies at an imaginary object, ignore this behaviour; punishment of the shying will only focus the horse's attention on the incorrect response, thus reinforcing it.

Desensitization

This method is used to help overcome phobias and other anxiety-based problems and is commonly used alongside counter conditioning. It is used to raise the threshold at which an animal responds to a given object or stimulus. The horse should be shielded from the natural stimuli while the desensitization process is going on. It is important when beginning this technique that the horse is relaxed and it is then gradually introduced to representations of the feared response, e.g. if the horse is frightened of clippers use a recording of the clippers. The recording is then played at increasing volume until the horse slowly becomes desensitized to the stimulus. Progression on to each stage should not occur until full desensitization for each step has taken place. Once this has been achieved the clippers can then be introduced nearby while the horse is given food (positive reinforcement) and then progression can be made until you

are able to clip the animal. This method is time-consuming but beneficial.

Training foals

The most important time for a horse to learn is as a neonate. The correct procedures at the right time will produce dramatic results. The neonatal foal will be able to stand up and then learn to follow its mother within a couple of hours of parturition – this is known as the following response. It is known that the foal is born with a capacity for automatic limb control, a characteristic possessed by all four-limbed animals, enabling them to balance and move in a coordinated fashion within hours of birth.

Coprophagy, i.e. ingestion of faeces, is common in foals and this behaviour enables the foal to acquire the hindgut bacteria needed for fermentation of cellulose (see Ch. 9). It is also thought that this behaviour imprints on the foal the smell and taste of various plants in the faeces of its dam so that it learns to recognize what can be eaten and what cannot. Foals do not exhibit normal adult grazing behaviour until 6 weeks of age, but do exhibit play or exploratory grazing, in which they learn to select suitable grazing material through trial and error.

Imprint training

Imprinting is an adaptive form of learning and occurs very early on in a foal's life. It is especially important in prey species as newborn animals do not have time to learn through associative learning who their mother is before they have to be able to run with the herd. The process of imprinting creates a mental template that helps the foal to form an image of what a horse should look like and helps to create a special bond between the foal and its dam. It is thought that this might explain why some stallions in adult life tend to prefer mares of a particular colour.

Imprint training provides a singular opportunity to make handling easier, reduce injuries and enhance later training. It should begin immediately postpartum and requires that the mare is stabled for foaling. It also helps if the brood mare has a good temperament to allow the handler to start the imprint training.

Once the umbilical cord has been broken the foal should be rubbed down. This process has a habituating effect on the foal. Once the mare has returned to her feet, allow her to smell and clean the foal with the handler present, enabling the foal to simultaneously bond with the mare and the handler. The rubbing down of the foal is also a method of desensitization, i.e. it makes the foal less sensitive to the act. Touching and handling of the animal's ears, nose, mouth, feet, tail and other body parts will aid in desensitization and habitualization. Other activities can include placing electric clippers on the foal and rubbing the foal with crackling plastic. The foal can also be desensitized to loud noises, police whistles, loud music and gunfire. When performing imprint training it is impossible to overdo a stimulus, but it can be underdone. Most foals will habituate to 30–50 stimuli so use more than is necessary, e.g. if desensitizing the foal to having its foot picked up pick up the hoof and tap it 50–100 times.

When imprint training foals it is important to conduct all activities from both sides of the foal, as horses can become one-sided. There are many thoughts as to why this may occur, one being that most foals suckle from one side of the dam, showing a left- or right-sided preference and another is that like human infants the foals are simply born one way or the other.

Training aids

There are many commonly used training aids – bits, reins, head collars, lunge reins, cavessons, etc., and it is important to select the appropriate type for the job in hand.

Bits

There are several types of bit available and when choosing one it is important to remember that it must be:

- Of the correct size in length and thickness
- Properly fitted
- In good condition
- As mild as possible while still allowing the rider good communication and control
- Permitted within the level or discipline at which you are competing.

Bits can be placed into 'families':

- **Snaffle** – considered to be one of the mildest bits but there are several different types and some can be very severe. A simple jointed snaffle has the action of flexing the poll and lower jaw and encourages the horse to raise its head. The bit acts on the tongue, on the outside of the bars of the mouth and on the lips or the corners of the mouth. The snaffle produces a nutcracker action on the tongue. The use of rings or keys can help stimulate saliva production, which may help to relax the jaw.
- **Double bridle** – combines a snaffle (Bradoon) with a curb bit (Weymouth) and chain (Fig. 11.9) and, in order to fit both bits into the mouth, both are finer and lighter than usual. The effect of the combination of bits is to add the action of the Weymouth, which has a lever action on the lower jaw. This leverage is dependent on the length of the cheeks of the bit and the curb chain. The curb bit should not be used without the Bradoon, since the constant pressure on the lower jaw will numb the mouth.
- **Pelham** – a single bit used with a curb chain (Fig. 11.9). The bit is a combination of the curb and Bradoon in one mouthpiece. Two reins should be used so that the rider can facilitate the curb or snaffle action when required. Pelhams usually have an unjointed mouthpiece, which some horses prefer. It is commonplace to use leather rounders so that only one rein may be used. This can be an advantage for young riders but may act as a source of confusion to the horse.
- **Bitless bridle or Hackamore** – this bridle acts by exerting pressure on the nose and poll, which is achieved by the use of a single rein attached to long cheek pieces that create the required leverage. The Hackamore can be a useful means of regaining

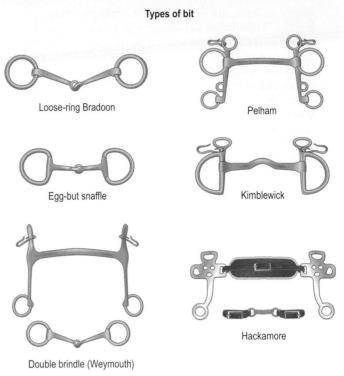

Types of bit

Loose-ring Bradoon

Pelham

Egg-but snaffle

Kimblewick

Double brindle (Weymouth)

Hackamore

Fig. 11.9 Types of bit

confidence in a horse that has suffered mouth injuries or biting problems in the past; however, it is severe and can cause a great deal of damage in the wrong hands.

All bits work as a negative reinforcement. Application of pressure on the horse's mouth from the rider makes the horse give way, relaxing the jaw. Acknowledgement from the rider by instantly relaxing the rein as soon as the horse responds is the reward. Other training aids, such as martingales, that have direct or indirect contact with the bit work as the same negative reinforcement. With indirect contact, e.g. a running martingale, pressure is applied to the reins at a different angle from that of the rider's hands. Thus, when the horse raises its head, pressure is applied by the martingale. When the horse then lowers its head in response the pressure stops, which acts as a negative reinforcement.

Reins

The reins are a direct means of contact between the horse and its rider. If the rider is tense, this is directly transferred to the horse via the bit. Rubber-covered reins are not advisable for schooling or dressage as they 'deaden' the feel and vibration to and from the horse.

Head collars

The head collar is one of the most common ways of restraining the horse. The head collar should fit well and be made of substantial materials. The use of head collars with tightening throat lashes or nosebands can increase control of the horse. The lead rein is also a point of communication with the horse and the horse will be able to detect if the handler is tense.

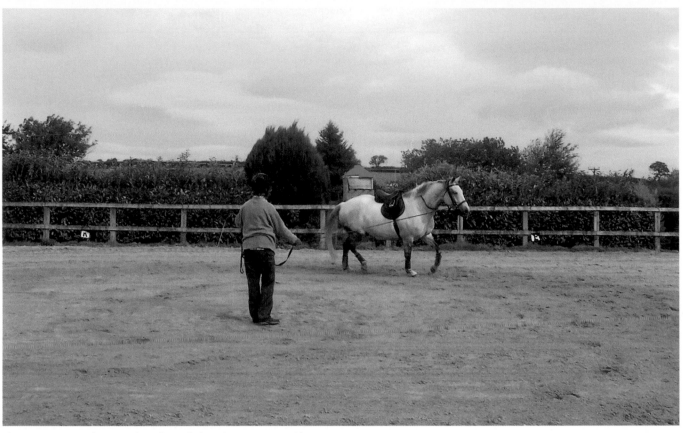

Fig. 11.10 Lunging has many benefits, including the assessment of lameness

Lunging and long-reining

Work from the ground includes lunging and long-reining and these training methods can be beneficial in the following situations:

- In the initial stages of training/breaking a young horse
- When the rider is injured and unable to ride
- When the horse cannot wear its normal tack, e.g. if it has a girth gall or a sore mouth
- In order to assess a problem that can be more easily seen from the ground, e.g. lameness
- To help improve the horse's obedience to the voice.

When **lunging** the horse, the handler is positioned in the centre of the circle slightly behind the level of the horse's shoulder (Fig. 11.10). This helps to encourage the horse to move forward. The lunging cavesson should be worn with adequate padding to the noseband, providing protection to the delicate turbinate bones of the nose. Training aids can be used when lunging, e.g. side reins, which provide an even pressure on the bit to encourage the horse to work on the bit.

Long-reining provides an alternative to lunging and provides training for horses in the initial stages of breaking a horse to harness. Instead of a single rein, two reins are used and the handler is positioned behind the horse. The pressure of the reins against the side of the horse encourages the horse to move forwards.

Bibliography

Anderson, R.S., Edney, A.T.B. 1991. Practical Animal Handling. Pergamon Press, Oxford.

Budiansky, S., 1997. The Nature of Horses: Their Evolution, Intelligence and Behaviour. Weidenfeld & Nicholson, London.

Harris, P.A., Gomarsall, G.M., Davidson, H.P.B., Green, R.E., 1999. Proceedings of the BEVA Specialist Days on Behaviour and Nutrition. BEVA, London.

Hastie, S., Sharples, J., 1999. Horselopaedia. Ringpress Books, Cheltenham.

Higgins, A.J., Wright, I.M., 1995. The Equine Manual. W B Saunders, Philadelphia, PA.

Hodgson, D.R., Rose, R.J., 1994. The Athletic Horse. W B Saunders, Philadelphia, PA.

Smythe, R.H., Goody, P.C., Gray, P., 1993. Horse Structure and Movement. J A Allen, London.

Vetstream Equis CD-ROM. Vetstream Ltd, Cambridge.

Recommended reading

McGreevy, P., 2004. Equine Behaviour. A Guide for Veterinarians and Equine Scientists. Elsevier, Oxford.
Comprehensive guide to the behaviour of the horse.

Walrond, S., 1989. Breaking a Horse to Harness: a Step-by-step Guide. J A Allen, London.
Easy-to-follow instructions for breaking a horse.

Williams, M., 1995. Horse Psychology. J A Allen, London.
Interesting subject that helps you to understand why horses behave as they do.

CHAPTER 12

Restraint, handling and administration of medicines to exotic species

Sharon Reid

Key Points

- The exotic species commonly kept as companion animals do not appreciate excessive human contact or being handled and in many cases this may be a distressing experience that may affect their health. Handling should be avoided unless it is strictly necessary.
- For the welfare of the animal and the safety of the handler it is important that anyone dealing with these species is aware of the correct methods of handling and restraint.
- It is often important to determine the sex of an animal, e.g. to prevent or to encourage reproduction, prevent fighting, increase the value of the animal or simply to give the animal an appropriate name. There are different methods of sex determination that vary according to the species in question.
- An exotic animal under veterinary treatment is likely to need medicine. There are many routes of administration and the most appropriate methods depend on the species in care.

Introduction

In many practices it is no longer rare to be presented with an exotic animal requiring some form of veterinary care and nursing. The word 'exotic' may be taken to mean any animal that is 'out of the ordinary' and neither a cat nor a dog. The needs of these species vary widely and are certainly different from most of the patients in the kennels. It is therefore important for the welfare of the animal and your own safety that you understand a little about their biology (see Ch. 5), how they should be handled and how to give them the medicines prescribed by the veterinary surgeon.

Small mammals

Before handling any small mammal you must consider whether it is really necessary to handle the animal and, if you must do it, whether it is safe to do so. Ask yourself the following questions:

- Do you know how to handle this animal safely without doing harm to yourself or to the patient?

- Is the animal a well-handled, friendly pet or an aggressive one? Some ferrets can bite severely; chipmunks are fast and can harm themselves and you as they try to make a run for freedom.
- Is the animal debilitated in any way and is there any indication of respiratory distress? For example, in rats a nasal discharge may be shown by the presence of dried discharge on the forearms; rabbits with pneumonia may have a nasal discharge and dyspnoea. Always observe the patient quietly before handling and if you are in any doubt it is best not to handle it. Any excessive or rough handling could be fatal.
- Is there any reason to suspect metabolic bone disease? Has the animal got any fractures or a past history of having had one? Are their any signs of poor growth? What is the animal being fed? Is the diet lacking in calcium or vitamin D? This mainly occurs in young animals – often rabbits and sometimes guinea pigs.

Once you have decided that the animal must be handled you must consider the method of restraint – manual restraint is preferable but chemical restraint is occasionally necessary. Before removing any animal from its cage select a room that contains few objects behind which the animal can hide if it escapes and ensure that all doors and windows are closed.

Rats and mice

Rats and mice only have one means of defence and that is their teeth. Most of them are easily handled and not very aggressive but they can give nasty nips if handled roughly or incorrectly:

- Mice tend to bite if worried, stressed or handled by an unfamiliar person. The best way of handling a mouse is to grasp it firmly by the base of the tail, lift it up carefully and then place it on to a non-slip table (Fig. 12.1). Once it is on the table you should grasp the scruff at the back of the neck firmly between the thumb and forefinger. You now have the mouse securely restrained for examination or for administration of any medication.
- Rats tend not to bite unless roughly handled. The easiest way to pick up a tame rat is by picking it up

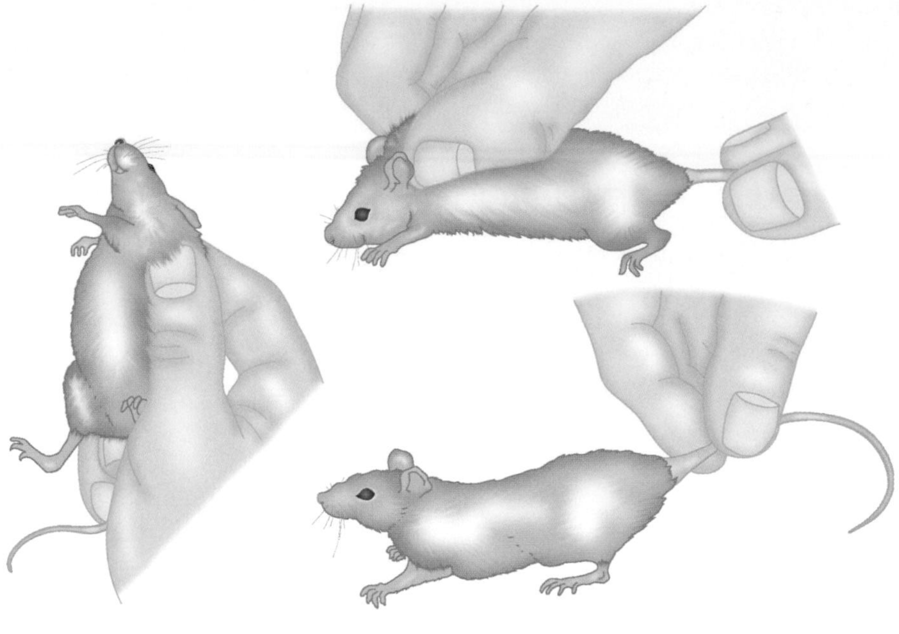

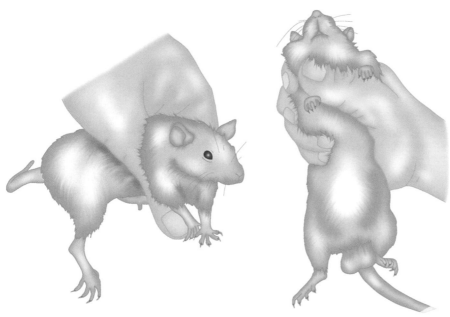

Fig. 12.1 Restraining a mouse

Fig. 12.2 Restraining a rat

around the middle with one hand just behind the front legs and putting the other hand underneath its bottom to support its weight (Fig. 12.2). If you have an unfriendly or aggressive rat then the safest way to handle it is in much the same way as the mouse. Grasp it by the base of the tail, lift it on to a non-slip table and then scruff it by the back of the neck with your thumb and forefinger.

A very important point to remember is that you should never grasp any mouse or rat by the end of the tail as the skin will slough off and cause severe damage, resulting in amputation of the tail.

Sex determination

The most common method of determining the sex of all small mammals is by measuring the anogenital distance,

i.e. the distance between the anus and the tip of the penis in the male and between the anus and the vulva in the female (Fig. 12.3). There may also be other methods (Table 12.1).

Hamsters

Hamsters only have one means of defence and that is their teeth – they can give a very nasty nip.

The larger Syrian hamsters tend to be less aggressive than the smaller Russian and Chinese dwarf hamsters, who are known for having short tempers. These animals are nocturnal and do not take kindly to be woken up and handled during the day, especially by a stranger. For minor examinations or to move a friendly hamster, simply cup your hands around the animal and lift it up. For a more detailed examination or for an aggressive hamster firmly scruff it at

Table 12.1 Methods of sexing small mammals

Species	Method of sexing
Rat	Examine the anogenital distance – it is longer in the male than in the female. Testes are large and obvious in adult males. Teats present only in the female
Mice	Examine the anogenital distance – it is longer in the male than in the female. Testes are large and obvious in adult males. Teats present only in the female
Hamster	Examine the anogenital distance – it is longer in the male than in the female. Large testes in the adult male make the hind end cone-shaped; in the female the hind end is rounded. Adult males have a pigmented scent gland on the point of each hip. Teats present only in the female
Gerbil	Examine the anogenital distance – it is longer in the male than in the female. Adult males have a scent gland on the ventral abdomen. Teats present only in the female
Chipmunk	Examine the anogenital distance – it is longer in the male than in the female. Testes are retracted during the non-breeding season and descend into the scrotum and enlarge at the start of the breeding season in February/March. Penis is visible and points caudally. Teats present only in the female
Guinea pig	Anogenital distance is less easy to measure. Gentle pressure placed on either side of the prepuce of the male will cause the penis to elongate. Testes are large. Female has a Y-shaped genital opening and a pale-coloured clitoris. Both sexes have a pair of elongated teats in the inguinal region
Chinchilla	Female has a large urinary papilla, which you may mistake for the male's penis. She also has separate exits to the urinary and reproductive tracts, unlike most other small mammals. The male's penis resembles the female's urinary papilla, although it is larger and tends to point cranially. Pressure applied on either side of the prepuce may cause it to elongate. Both males and females have teats – one inguinal pair and two pairs of lateral thoracic teats
Rabbit	Apply pressure on either side of the anal area to pop out the vulva or penis. The vulva is round, has a small slit in the middle and tends to point cranially. The penis is more cone-shaped and tends to point caudally. Adult males have large, obvious testes
Ferret	The male has a very obvious prepuce on the ventral abdomen and large testes in the scrotum unless he has been castrated. The female has a vulval opening situated ventral to the anus

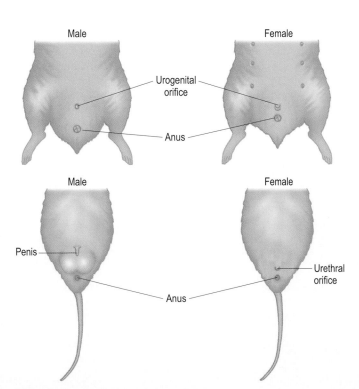

Fig. 12.3 General method of sexing small rodents

the back of the neck, ensuring that you grasp a lot of scruff between your thumb and forefinger – if you do not take enough scruff the hamster will still be able to turn around and bite you. Make sure the scruff is pulled cranially to avoid pulling it too tight around the eyes as hamsters are prone to prolapse if roughly handled. If you have an extremely aggressive hamster that you just cannot get a hold of then scoop it up into a clear plastic box, which will enable you to see if there is anything obviously wrong. If a more detailed examination is required then a gaseous anaesthetic via an induction chamber may be necessary.

Gerbils

Gerbils are fairly docile animals, easy to handle if socialized well and will only bite if frightened or stressed by rough handling. They move fast and are very good jumpers – if they get worried they will escape by jumping away. To transport gerbils from one place to another, cup them in both hands underneath their bodies and gently lift them up. If a detailed examination is required or you have an aggressive animal then firmly but gently grasp the scruff between your thumb and forefinger, lift the animal up and support it underneath with your other hand and place it on a non-slip table for examination.

Never pick up a gerbil by the tail as it will slough the skin very easily, leaving only the vertebrae showing – known as a degloving injury. This will never regrow and would have to be amputated.

Chipmunks

Chipmunks are very highly strung, fast-moving creatures that can leap extremely high to escape, so great care must be taken when handling them. Unless the chipmunk is correctly handled you are likely to be bitten. If you are lucky you may be able to grasp the scruff between the thumb and forefinger. If really well handled you may be able to cup a chipmunk in both hands and lift it out of the cage and then gently scruff it. If the chipmunk is in a large enclosure then the best way to catch it is by using a fine net. This is the safest way and will allow you to transfer it to a towel or restrain it on a non-slip table for examination. If manual restraint is not possible, gaseous anaesthesia via an induction chamber may be necessary. This is sometimes better for your safety and for that of your patient.

It is very important to remember that you should never approach a small mammal from above. To the animal your hands are like a bird of prey swooping down on them, which can make them very frightened, especially as they will already be worried by the strange environment. Always try to approach them from the side and at a low level.

Guinea pigs

Guinea pigs are very sensitive creatures and do not like being away from their natural surroundings or from their companions. To reduce their stress it is helpful to dim the light and reduce the noise. To aid in their capture it is less stressful to catch them in a small box rather than chasing them around a large enclosure. The easiest method of restraint is to gently grasp them from behind under the front legs with one hand and with the other hand support the weight of the animal (Fig. 12.4). It is very important to support the guinea pig's weight as it has a rather large abdomen and a slender spine and surrounding bones and if there is not enough support spinal damage can occur.

Chinchillas

Chinchillas are very timid and sensitive creatures that rarely bite. They are also easily stressed, so dimming the lights and reducing the noise is helpful when handling them. You must be very careful not to scruff or roughly handle them as a condition known as fur slip can occur in which clumps of fur fall out around the area being held, leaving a bald patch, which takes a few weeks to regrow. If a chinchilla is very stressed it will stand on its back legs and squirt urine at you – they have a very good aim! The best and safest way to handle a chinchilla is by quickly and gently picking it up, putting one hand around the body just under the front legs and the other hand to support the body weight. For young chinchillas, which are more wriggly than well-handled adults, it is sometimes easier to restrain them by using your fore and middle finger around either side of the head and your thumb and fourth finger under the front legs and then with your other hand support the body. You should also remember that they have powerful back legs, so you should always make sure you have a good grip of them.

Rabbits

Most domestic rabbits are very easy to handle and rarely cause injuries unless stressed or roughly handled. They are capable of using their teeth and claws, with which they can inflict deep scratches, and their back legs, which are very powerful. Some rabbits can be aggressive, especially males around the breeding season in the spring. Reducing the light and noise can help to reduce stress.

To handle a friendly rabbit it is best to pick the rabbit up by placing one hand under the thorax and using the first three fingers to gently grip the front legs by placing one finger either side and one in the middle. Using your other hand, you support the rabbit's weight. If you need to move the rabbit from one place to another, you can support the rabbit on one arm and place the rabbit's head under your arm (Fig. 12.5). With the other hand gently hold the scruff and place your arm along on its back. Being in the dark under your arm or even covered in a towel or blanket will calm the animal. Ensure that you have a good grip, as a sudden noise can spook the rabbit and it may try and escape. To restrain an aggressive rabbit you should grasp it firmly by the scruff and gently lift it up and then with your other hand

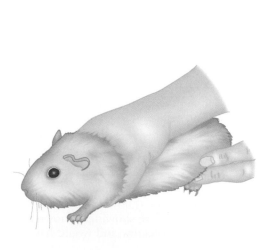

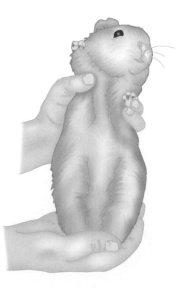

Fig. 12.4 Restraining a guinea pig

you should support its weight (Fig. 12.6). You should quickly move it onto a non-slip table, as it may struggle. Never pick a rabbit up by the ears.

For examination it is sometimes useful to reduce the stress of examination by wrapping the animal up in a towel with the head sticking out (Fig. 12.7). It is important to remember that a struggling anxious rabbit may harm you and also harm itself. Rabbits have very powerful back legs and if not properly restrained they can kick out and twist to get away, which can fracture or dislocate their spines. Another thing to remember is that severe stress can cause a cardiac arrest.

Ferrets

Some well-handled pet ferrets can be very friendly but others can be aggressive and fast, especially if not handled regularly. Working ferrets used for rabbit hunting and ratting are often not handled very much and can be aggressive. Ferrets have claws and teeth as sharp as those of a cat.

The easiest way to handle tame ferrets is to hold them from behind with one hand around the body under the front legs and support the body's weight with the other hand. The best way to restrain more aggressive ferrets is to firmly grasp the scruff behind the neck and pull them upwards. Then with the other hand, support the body by putting it around the pelvic area. It is sometimes useful to wear gauntlets for handling very aggressive ferrets.

Birds

Before handling any type of bird you must consider whether it is really necessary. Birds do not appreciate being handled

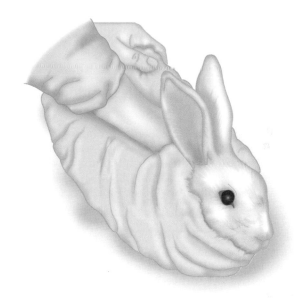

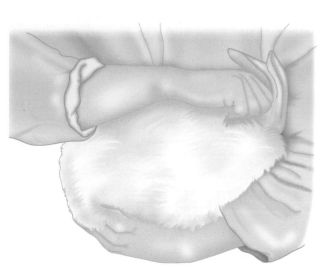

Fig. 12.5 Carrying a rabbit with the head tucked under your arm

Fig. 12.7 Restraining a rabbit using a towel

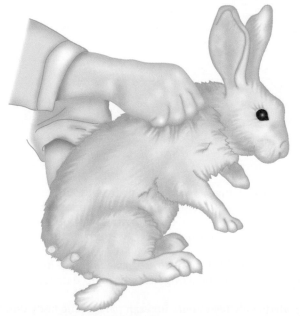

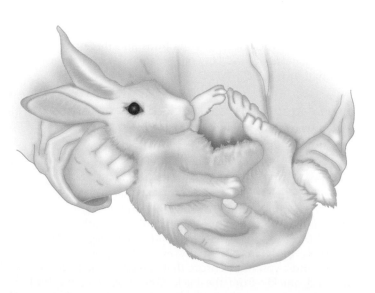

Fig. 12.6 Restraining a rabbit

in the way that dogs and cats do and some species may hurt you if handled incorrectly. Ask yourself the following:

- Is the bird a well-handled pet or is it a wild bird of prey or water fowl?
- Do you know how to handle this bird safely without causing harm to you or the bird?
- Does the bird have any signs of respiratory distress that could be made much worse by restraint?
- Do you really need to handle the bird or can you just look at it through the cage to make decisions about its condition and its treatment?
- Does the bird require oral or injectable medication or could this be given in food or drinking water?

To perform a physical examination or to administer treatment the bird will have to be restrained in some way. Before catching a bird always make sure all windows and doors are closed and that there is a warning sign on the door in case someone enters the room, allowing the bird to escape. There is nothing worse than having to tell an owner that you have lost their pet.

Small caged birds, e.g. canaries, budgerigars and finches

These small birds cannot do much harm but they do have sharp little beaks and sharp claws, which you will need to avoid when examining them. Small birds may become stressed even if they are used to handling; to reduce this, dim the lights and reduce the noise. If the bird comes in its own cage with all its toys, remove them before trying to capture the bird – there is nothing worse than trying to avoid obstacles while chasing it around the cage.

To catch the bird, use a small facecloth or something similar to provide a greater surface area than your hand. It is also a protective layer between you and the bird to prevent you from being bitten. Once you have captured the bird, hold it very gently. Birds have no diaphragm and they rely on the outward movement of their ribcage for inspiration. If you grip too tight it can be fatal, especially if they are suffering from a respiratory disease. To examine the bird, hold it in the palm of your hand wrapped loosely in a cloth with its head out, placing your thumb under its beak to prevent it pecking you. It may help to allow the bird to grip your little finger, as these are perching birds and this may make them feel more secure. Unwrap small parts at a time for examination (Fig. 12.8).

Large caged birds, e.g. cockatiels, cockatoos and parrots

The larger caged birds have powerful hooked beaks and can give a very nasty bite. They can become distressed, so dimming the light and reducing the noise will reduce this. Remove any toys or accessories from the cage to allow easier and less stressful capture. The use of a towel or small blanket will enable you to catch the larger birds, remembering not to hold them too tightly, as this can be fatal (Fig. 12.9).

As these birds are potentially more dangerous than the smaller birds, you must ensure that you grasp the bird carefully and quickly from the back. Once you have the bird out of the cage, restrain the head as this is the part that can

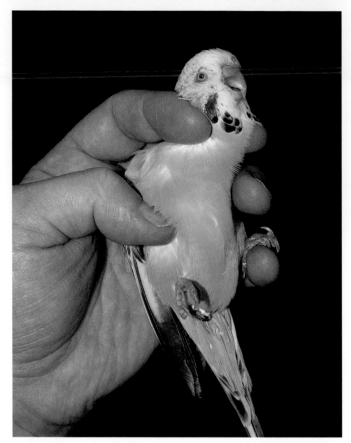

Fig. 12.8 Restraining a budgerigar

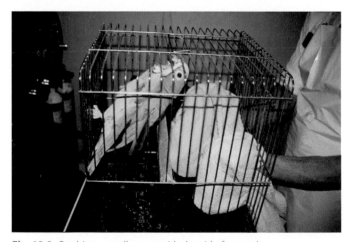

Fig. 12.9 Catching a small parrot with the aid of a towel

cause you most damage. Wrap the bird gently in the towel with your thumb and forefinger positioned under the lower beak. This will enable you to push the beak upwards to prevent the bird from biting you. Once you have the bird in this position, ensure that the wings are securely restrained in the towel. If the bird is able to struggle and flap its wings there is a risk of it breaking its wings or damaging its plumage.

Once adequately restrained, unwrap parts of the body one at a time for examination. Handling aggressive parrots and cockatoos may require extra protection – leather gauntlets come in very handy. However, it is often difficult to feel much through them so you must be careful not to squeeze the bird too tightly. Once you have the bird restrained satisfactorily, remove the gloves to prevent any harm to the bird.

Birds of prey

Birds of prey can be broadly divided into the nocturnal species, i.e. owls, and the diurnal species, e.g. falcons, hawks and eagles. These birds have extremely sharp talons and powerful beaks, both of which can be very dangerous when handling them. The method of handling differs with each type.

Diurnal species, e.g. falcons

Most handled falcons will come in wearing a leather cap or hood, which fits over the bird's head (Fig. 12.10) covering the bird's eyes but leaving its beak exposed. This calms the bird and helps to reduce stress. These birds also have a very good sense of hearing, so reducing the noise in the room reduces the stress. Most falcons will also be presented wearing leather straps or jesses around their ankles, which enable them to be restrained while on their owner's arm (Fig. 12.10). When restraining these birds, wear a leather gauntlet because it is extremely painful if they grip your arm without one.

If the bird has been transported in a box there are several ways to remove it:

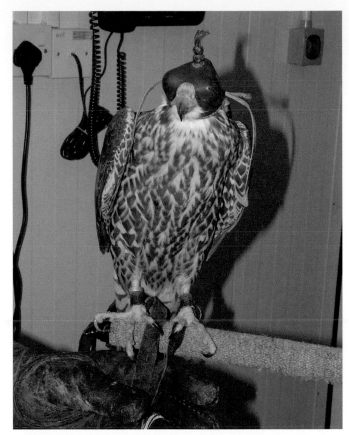

Fig. 12.10 A falcon wearing a hood and jesses – note the handler's leather gauntlets

- Ask the owner to remove the bird from the box, as it will respond to them better.
- If you are removing the bird yourself, place your gauntleted hand into the box beside the perch if it has one or beside the bird, grasp the leather straps with your thumb and forefinger and encourage the bird to step on to the glove. You must keep hold of the strap at all times. You can now remove the bird from the box and put the hood on if it is not already on. You should now be able to examine the bird safely. You must make sure that you always keep your arm up above the elbow, as otherwise the bird will attempt to climb up towards your shoulder, which can be painful.
- If the bird has no leg straps or hood and is not well-handled then you must take a different approach. Dim the lights and reduce the noise before you start. Some birds may be trained to perch on your hand and you may be able to encourage it to do this. If not you will have to grasp the bird from behind with a thick towel or blanket. Always make sure you know where the bird's head is. You must then grasp the bird over the shoulder area facing towards you and place your thumbs under its beak to push it up out of the way. You can then place a hood on the bird's head if you have one. It is best to put the bird on your gauntleted arm, as gripping on to something makes it feel more secure.

When examining these birds it is sometimes necessary to hold their feet out of the way as they may try to grasp one foot, with the other causing puncture wounds and leading to serious infections (Fig. 12.11). This method really requires

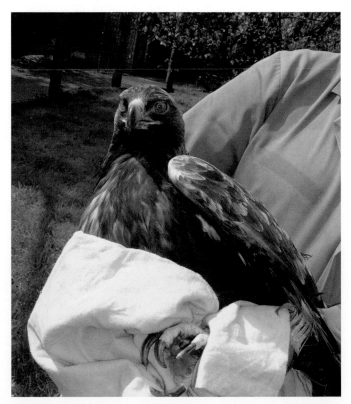

Fig. 12.11 A golden eagle with its talons wrapped in a towel to prevent damage to the handler

two people – one to hold the bird from behind, restraining the wings and body, and one to hold the legs from behind and away from the examiner.

Nocturnal species – owls

The overall technique is much the same but, as they are nocturnal, dimming the lights and wearing a hood has no real effect. Reducing noise will help reduce the stress. Owls have sharp talons but their beaks are not as large as those of falcons; however, they can still inflict a serious bite.

Waterfowl

Most waterfowl are wild but you may encounter a few 'tame' ones that are kept on ponds in farms or parks. Most waterfowl are rarely handled.

Small waterfowl, e.g. various species of duck

Restraining these birds is fairly easy as they are moderately small and have blunt-ended beaks. Grasp the duck from behind by the neck, ensuring that your thumb is securing the back of the neck while your other fingers are gently curled around the front of its neck. Make sure that you support the neck, as there is a weak area at the atlantooccipital joint. Control the wings as soon as you can by wrapping the bird in a towel and then tucking it under your arm, holding it close to your body. This position allows you to carry the bird safely. Examine one side at a time, keeping the other side restrained in the towel.

Large waterfowl, e.g. geese and swans

These species have large, powerful wings and can also be quite vicious with their beaks. The method of restraint is similar to that used for smaller birds. Restrain the head first, making sure that you support the neck, which may be difficult as they have long strong necks. The use of a swan hook or something similar may be useful. This is a pole with a smooth round hook that enables you to hook the neck of the swan or goose under the beak and gently pull it towards you to a point from which you can grasp its neck. Two people may be needed to restrain the bigger birds – one to control the head and one to control the large, powerful wings. Swan bags are available for restraining swans.

If any type of bird breaks free and tries to escape, dim the lights (unless it's an owl) and ensure that all exits are covered to prevent anyone from opening a door:

- Larger birds – throw a towel or blanket over it and wrap the bird up
- Very small birds – use a soft net, a small cloth or a light towel.

Always remember to be as gentle as possible and avoid restricting the bird's breathing whatever its size.

Sex determination

Sexing birds can be difficult and there are several ways in which it can be done:

- **Sexual dimorphism** – the male's appearance is different from that of the female. Males tend to have much more colourful feathers; for example, in the mallard duck the male is a wonderful green colour and the female is a plain brown. In most budgies the adult male has a blue cere over the beak and the female has a brown one. Male cockatiels have bright orange cheek patches and have a solid colour underneath their tails. Females have paler orange cheek patches and horizontal dark stripes under their tails. Most female birds of prey are slightly larger than the males and are less coloured.
  - **Examination of the pelvis** – requires experience. The pelvic bones of the female are wider than those of the male to allow eggs to pass through.
  - **Endoscopic examination of the gonads** – the gonads, i.e. ovary and testis, of the bird are internal (see Ch. 5). Under a general anaesthetic a rigid endoscope is passed through a small incision into the body cavity to examine the gonads and thus identify the sex. This can be a dangerous and invasive procedure.
- **DNA sexing** – used for parrots and cockatoos, as, in many species it is impossible to determine the sex externally. A blood sample or pulp from a freshly plucked feather is collected and sent to a laboratory where the DNA from the tissue is used to examine the chromosomes of the bird.

Reptiles

Before handling any reptile you must ask yourself whether it is necessary to handle this reptile, whether it is safe to do so and whether you know what to do. Consider the following:

- Is the reptile a well-handled pet or is it aggressive, or even poisonous? For example, rock pythons, Tokay geckos and some green iguanas are aggressive; adders, cobras and Gila monsters are poisonous. If you are working with reptiles it is important to be able to recognize the poisonous species.
- Do you know how to handle this animal safely to prevent harm to you or your patient?
- Is the animal in any kind of respiratory distress? Is the animal mouth-breathing or is there mucus around the mouth, which may indicate that there is a problem?
- Is the reptile very delicate? Some of the members of the gecko family are very small and fragile and if stressed or handled roughly can shed their tails. Some of them are so small that handling is really not advised.
- Is the animal suffering from metabolic bone disease? Many lizards have this as a result of incorrect husbandry and if you are in any doubt, assume that they do have problems. Their bones can be very fragile and fracture easily, so care must be taken when handling them.

If the reptile must be examined or treated, then some form of restraint will be necessary.

Reptiles can be divided into:

- Lizards
- Snakes
- Tortoises and terrapins.

Lizards

The risk involved in handling lizards varies according to their species:

- Small lizards use their teeth for defence and can give a nasty nip if stressed or roughly handled.
- Larger lizards have teeth and claws and some of them have long powerful tails, which they use like a whip and which can be very painful. Some species, e.g. the green iguana, can be very aggressive: they have sharp claws, a long tail and sharp teeth, which can all cause damage. Male iguanas are more aggressive to women during certain phases of the menstrual cycle because they can detect human female pheromones, which are similar to the ones secreted by female iguanas during the breeding season.

Even if you are very experienced, handling any species of lizard can be difficult:

- **Tiny lizards**, e.g. anoles or some geckos, are not recommended for handling as they are very fast and very delicate; it is easier to place them in a clear plastic box and examine them by observation.
- **Small lizards**, e.g. leopard gecko. Grasp them from behind around the shoulder area with the thumb and forefinger and the other three fingers around the body. If the lizard is larger than your hand, gently support the back legs with your other hand to prevent them from wriggling.
- **Large lizards**, e.g. green iguana, water dragon. Restrain by grasping the lizard from behind the shoulders (Fig. 12.12). With your thumb and forefinger, control one leg and use the middle and fourth finger to control the other leg. Using the other hand, grasp around the pelvic girdle from behind and use your thumb and forefinger to control one leg and your middle and fourth finger to control the other leg. Avoid holding the lizard too tight, as if it wriggles, this can cause spinal damage. If you have to move the animal, wrap it in a towel with its legs lying down by its sides. Then restrain the head and tuck the body and tail under your arm to prevent damage from the tail.
- **Spiky lizards**, e.g. bearded dragons (Fig. 12.13). If you restrain spiky lizards as described above you will only injure yourself. Hold the lizard's back against your body with your hand held flat against the underside and under the front legs and gently restrain the head. The other hand restrains the tail and hind legs. Another method is to wrap the lizard in a towel, but this does not allow easy access for examination. It may be possible to get your fingers behind the spiky area on the head where there is a soft fleshy part and then restrain the lizard on its back – this may not be easy to do if the patient is wriggly or aggressive (Fig. 12.14).

The vasovagal reflex is useful for putting any lizard into a form of trance and may be used as a means of restraint for

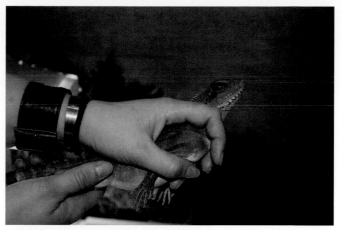

Fig. 12.12 Restraint of a water dragon

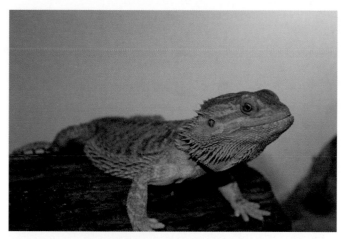

Fig. 12.13 A bearded dragon showing its spiky skin

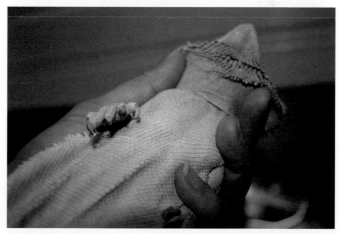

Fig. 12.14 Restraint of a bearded dragon

procedures such as radiography. This is done by putting firm but gentle digital pressure on both eyeballs, which stimulates the parasympathetic branch of the autonomic nervous system, resulting in a drop in heart rate, respiratory rate and blood pressure. This effect can last for 1–2 min if everything is quiet. The only problem is that any sudden noise will wake the lizard up and it will run off the table and escape. A useful tip is using two cotton wool balls and, placing them over the eyelids, bandage them firmly but gently in place. This is used instead of your fingers and keeps a constant pressure over the eyes for a prolonged effect. Sometimes putting lizards gently on to their backs will calm them and make restraint for examinations much easier (Fig. 12.15).

Another means of restraint for radiography is to bandage the front legs of the lizard gently along the body and the back legs along the tail. This enables you to get a clear image and keeps your patient still without you having to restrain it. This should not be done if you suspect any limb or rib fractures.

When restraining lizards it is very important not to grasp them by the tail as they can shed their tails – a process known as autotomy. Some species will also do this if they are really distressed or roughly handled. In most cases the tail will grow back but it will never look as good as the original and there are some species of lizard whose tail will not grow back, so you must be careful. Iguanas will not regrow their tails after the age of 3–4 years.

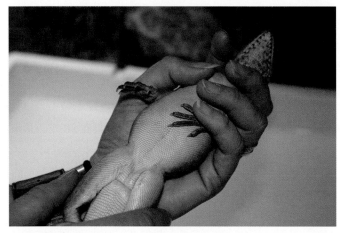

Fig. 12.15 Restraining a water dragon on its back

Sex determination

This is reasonably easy to do in a sexually mature adult but cannot easily be done in a younger reptile. Look for evidence of pores in the inguinal area of the lizard (Fig. 12.16):

- Male – obvious pores, i.e. anal, preanal and femoral pores, that vary according to the species. In some species there may also be hemipenal bulges below the entrance to the cloaca. For example, the green iguana has femoral pores and hemipenal bulges; the leopard gecko has preanal pores and hemipenal bulges. Males are often slightly larger and have more body appendages, e.g. the male chameleon has horns.
- Female – very faint pores but no hemipenal bulges.

Snakes

Most snakes are fairly docile if regularly handled but there are some species that are naturally aggressive, e.g. the rock python and the anaconda. Their main means of defence are their teeth and the larger snakes can give a nasty bite. The teeth are curved and embed themselves in your skin – if you pull away you are likely to pull a large piece of skin off your finger or thumb! The best way to remove the teeth from your skin is by using a wooden spatula or credit card and pushing it between your skin and the teeth. Do not put the snake's head under water to make it let go – snakes can hold their breath for a very long time because they have air sacs at the end of their lungs that act as reservoirs. Some of the larger boas and pythons kill by constriction, and this may be a potential danger to the handler.

Pick up a snake from behind, supporting its whole body. Snakes do not have very good eyesight and if you approach a snake quickly from the front you will frighten it and even the best-natured snake may bite. To restrain the snake for examination, use your last three fingers to grasp the snake gently around the top of the neck just below the head. Place your thumb and forefinger on either side of the head. If the snake is potentially aggressive, place a finger on the top of the head (Fig. 12.17). Use your other hand to support the rest of the body.

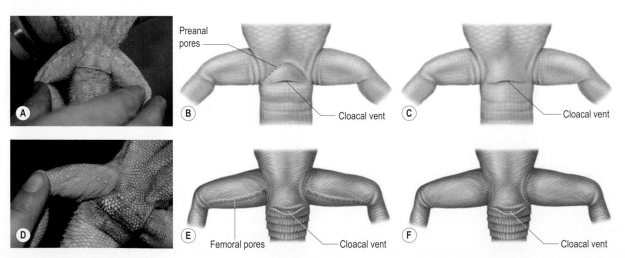

Fig. 12.16 Sexual differentiation in the lizard. (**A, B, E**) Male bearded dragon showing femoral pores. (**D, C, F**) Female bearded dragon showing lack of pores

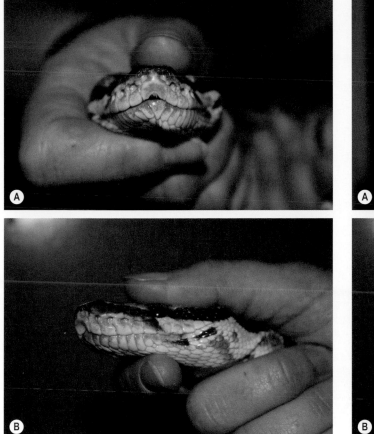

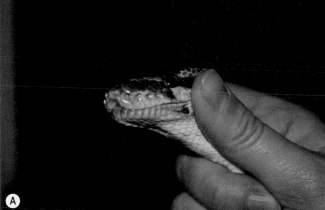

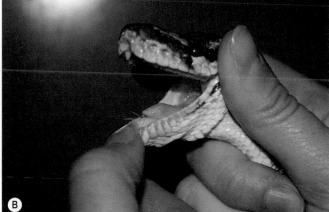

Fig. 12.17 (**A, B**) Restraining the head of the snake

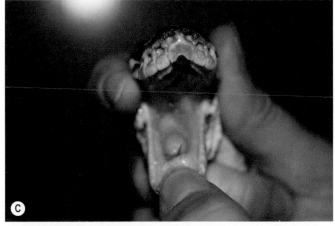

Fig. 12.18 (**A–C**) Opening the mouth of the snake

To examine the mouth (Fig. 12.18), place your thumb and forefinger on either side of the snake's head, allowing you to open its mouth using a wooden spatula. Care must be taken when controlling snakes' heads, as they have a weak point at the atlantooccipital joint that can easily be dislocated if roughly handled.

If the snake is longer than 4 ft make sure that there are two people to handle it. Most snakes that are not poisonous are constrictors and they could squeeze a limb or even asphyxiate you. If you have an aggressive snake that you are unable to pick up, you can use a snake hook, which is a smooth metal hook. Approach the snake from the side or behind and press the head gently to the ground, allowing you to grasp the snake carefully by the back of the head.

Sex determination

It is not easy to determine the sex of snake, but there are several ways to do it:

- In very young snakes you can sometimes pop out the hemipenis by applying gentle pressure from the tail to the cloaca. In a male the hemipenis should pop out but not in the female. This method requires experience.
- Measure the tail length by counting the scales between the cloaca and the end of the tail. In a male the

distance from the cloaca to the tip of the tail is greater than in a female.
- Use of a snake-sexing probe – this is the most accurate method (Fig. 12.19). Lift the cloacal scale and insert the small, round-ended probe down inside the tail into the hemipenis of the male or the vaginal sac of the female. If you do not have a probe you can use a Jackson's urinary cat catheter (always remove the metal insert). In the male the probe will go down a distance of about 8–16 subcaudal scales and in the female it will only go down about 2–5 subcaudal scales. Make sure that you lubricate the probe well before use and

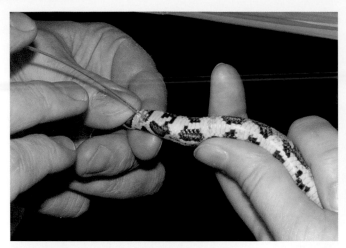

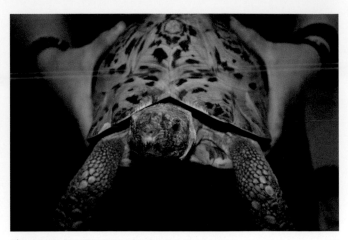

Fig. 12.19 Use of a probe to determine the sex of a snake

Fig. 12.20 Restraining a tortoise

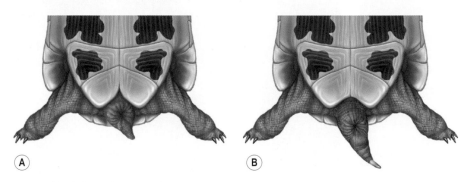

(A)

(B)

Fig. 12.21 Determining the sex of a tortoise. (**A**) Male. (**B**) Female

that you do not push the probe too hard, as you can perforate the vaginal sac.

Tortoises and terrapins

Most tortoises are harmless but some of the terrapins and turtles can be aggressive and give a nasty nip with their sharp beak, e.g. snapping turtles, soft-shelled turtles and even red-eared terrapins. Terrapins also have sharp claws.

Restraint is usually fairly easy and is achieved by holding the shell on either side just behind the front legs (Fig. 12.20) which prevents the head and claws from causing damage. If a more detailed examination is required the animal is likely to withdraw its head and legs into its shell. In some of the smaller species of mediterranean tortoise you may be able to pull the head and legs out gently. In larger species, especially the leopard tortoise, it is virtually impossible to get the head and legs to come out if the tortoise does not want to do it. Sedation may be necessary for a proper examination. If the animal is one of the more aggressive species, e.g. the snapping and soft-shelled turtles, holding any part of the shell is likely to result in you being bitten because these species have very long necks and they can reach right round to the back of their shell. You may be able to get them to snap at a piece of wood or cloth and then grasp the head, which is the dangerous part.

Note: You must wash your hands after handling reptiles, as they can carry zoonotic *Salmonella*, which occur naturally in their gut flora but are also found all over the reptile's body.

Sex determination

Sexing tortoises and terrapins is quite easy (Fig. 12.21):

- Males – have a longer tail, which is wider at the base, and the cloaca is further away from the plastron
- Females – have a short tail and the cloaca is closer to the plastron
- Some species of male terrapin, e.g. red-eared terrapin, have longer front claws than are seen in the female
- In some species of tortoise, e.g. leopard tortoise, the male has a concave plastron and the female has a flat plastron.

Administration of medication

The available routes and methods of administration of medication to most animals are as follows:

- Oral dosing
- Intramuscular injection
- Subcutaneous injection
- Intravenous injection
- Intraperitoneal injection
- Intraosseous injection – used for the introduction of fluids into the medullary cavity of the bone.

Small mammals

Oral

This method is used most often in small animals as medication can be given by this route at home by the owners, reducing the stress to the animal. Medication for small animals mainly comes in a liquid form, which makes it easier to administer. Most small mammals will take the medication if you syringe it into the side of the mouth slowly. If the medication has a particularly nasty taste, mix it into some baby food and syringe it down. Rodents are able to close off the back of the mouth with the cheek folds, which may make oral administration difficult but is quite normal, as it allows them to gnaw at wood without ingesting it.

If oral administration is difficult, a feeding tube or straight crop tube can be used. Keep the patient firmly scruffed to prevent it from wriggling and keep the head and oesophagus in a straight line to allow the tube to pass down easily. The animal may become distressed by this procedure and it should only be used for feeding and medication – not just for medication. The use of naso-oesophageal or gastric tubes can be used in the larger animals like guinea pigs, chinchillas, rabbits and ferrets but rats and mice are too small.

Intramuscular injection

This route is not often used as the muscles of most small mammals are so small. Use the quadriceps femoris muscle in the hind leg or the muscle over the spine. Use 25-gauge needles or an even smaller gauge.

Subcutaneous injection

The scruff area is the most useful but the skin over the lateral thorax can be used in the larger animals. The use of a 25-gauge needle is recommended. Use this route with care in chinchillas because if it causes pain it may cause fur slip.

Intraperitoneal injection

Used for administering fluids, not medication, it is a relatively easy procedure. Place the animal in dorsal recumbency with the head tilting downwards to help the abdominal contents to move cranially, leaving the area where you are injecting clear of organs. Select the lower right quadrant of the ventral abdomen. Insert the needle and withdraw the plunger first to ensure you have not punctured any organs; then complete the injection. The best size of needle is a 23–25-gauge 5/8-inch needle.

Intravenous injection

Only satisfactorily used in rabbits, as the other species are too small.

- The lateral tail vein of rats and mice can sometimes be used, warming the tail first and applying local anaesthetic cream to help dilate the vein – use a 25–27-gauge 5/8-inch needle.
- The cephalic and saphenous veins may be used in guinea pigs, chinchillas and ferrets but they are quite difficult to locate and the procedure is not

tolerated well, especially if a catheter is to be left in place.
- Cephalic and saphenous veins may be used in the rabbit and the lateral ear vein can also be used. The use of a 25–27-gauge needle or butterfly catheter is best for administration.

Intraosseous injection

This site is used for the administration of fluids rather than medication. It cannot be done in the small rodents as they have very fine bones with a small medullary cavity and there is no needle safe enough for the procedure.

In some larger rats, chinchillas, guinea pigs, rabbits, etc., the best site is the proximal femur in the fossa between the hip joint and the greater trochanter. The area must be surgically prepared as the needle would track bacteria straight into the medullary cavity, resulting in severe osteomyelitis. A 20–21-gauge needle or a spinal needle is screwed into the bone. Apply antibiotic cream around the needle to prevent infection. Cap the needle and bandage in place. This procedure is very painful and so requires heavy sedation or a general anaesthetic. The procedure should never be attempted if there is any sign of metabolic bone disease. A radiograph should be taken after the needle is placed to ensure that it is in the correct position.

Birds

Oral

This route is a useful method for administering medication, as many drugs can be added to food or drinking water for self-medication. It is an easy and less stressful method but you cannot be sure how much of the medication the bird has actually ingested.

A more accurate method is to use a crop tube (Fig. 12.22). Restrain the bird, maintaining its head tilted upwards to keep the head and oesophagus straight. Using a feeding tube or straight crop tube, carefully introduce it into the oesophagus until you reach the crop just below the base of the neck.

Medication may be given by simply syringing the medication straight into the mouth but the bird may choke. If the bird tolerates this method well you may demonstrate it to owners, who may not feel able to use the crop tubing method.

Intramuscular injection

This is probably the easiest and quickest method of administration of medication. Select the pectoral muscle in the breast area. Restrain the bird and inject into the ventral part of the muscle using a 23–25-gauge 5/8-inch needle. This route is relatively painless and as it is quick it reduces the stress of handling to the bird.

Subcutaneous injection

Several sites may be used:

- Inguinal skin fold cranial to each leg – useful in small birds.
- Axillary area under each wing.

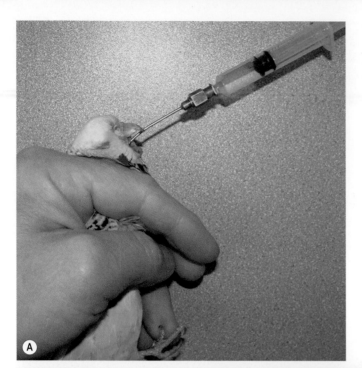

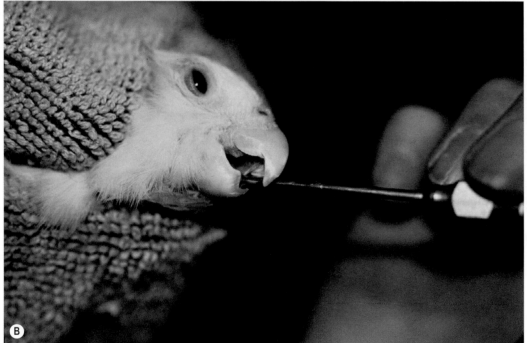

Fig. 12.22 Use of a crop tube. (**A**) In a budgerigar. (**B**) In a parrot

- Dorsal inner wing area – not the best site to use. A 23–25-gauge 5/8-inch needle is best.

Intravenous injection

Mainly used for blood sampling and the administration of fluids:

- This is not easily done in smaller birds – use the right jugular vein and a 23–25-gauge 5/8-inch needle.
- In larger birds the basilic (or brachial) vein, which runs along the ventral part of the wing just caudal to the

humerus, can be used, but it ruptures easily, causing large haematomata (Fig. 12.23).
- The ulnar vein, which runs along the ventral part of the wing just caudal to the ulnar bone, can sometimes be used but is very narrow and mobile. This vein can only be used in the larger raptors and waterfowl and it also ruptures easily.
- In larger geese and swans use the medial metatarsal vein on the leg.

Larger birds tend to tolerate repeated injections fairly well but many small birds will not and the use of a catheter is

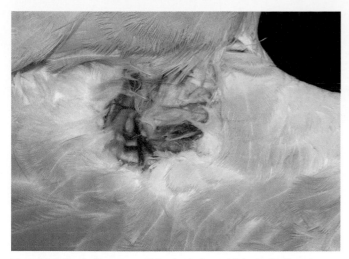

Fig. 12.23 Site for intravenous injection in larger birds: the basilic vein runs caudal to the humerus

recommended. Sedation or a general anaesthetic may be required for this procedure: 23-, 25- or 27-gauge 5/8-inch needles or butterfly catheters are best for this procedure.

Intraperitoneal injection

This route should *never* be used in birds as their body cavity is full of air sacs, which are a vital part of the respiratory system. If a needle is introduced it may rupture the air sacs.

Intraosseous injection

Only used for the administration of fluids and can be performed in both small and larger birds. In small birds the best site is the proximal tibiotarsal bone below the stifle joint; in the larger birds the distal and proximal ulna can also be used (Fig. 12.24). The procedure is painful and the use of sedation or a general anaesthetic is advised.

The area must be surgically prepared before the needle is screwed in place to prevent osteomyelitis. After the needle is placed apply an antibiotic cream around the site before bandaging the needle in place. For the smaller birds use a 25–27-gauge needle or spinal needle and for larger birds a 20–23-gauge needle or spinal needle. It is useful to radiograph the site to ensure that the needle is in the correct position.

Reptiles

Oral

This is a good route to use as the glottis is clearly visible and can be avoided. It lies at the front of the oral cavity in snakes (Fig. 12.25) and at the base of the tongue in lizards, tortoises and terrapins. Some reptiles will tolerate medication by direct syringing into the mouth but there is a risk of inhalation and it is also inaccurate.

The most efficient method makes use of a feeding tube or a straight crop tube and with practice can be carried out by owners at home and is well tolerated by most reptiles. If prolonged medication and feeding is required then the

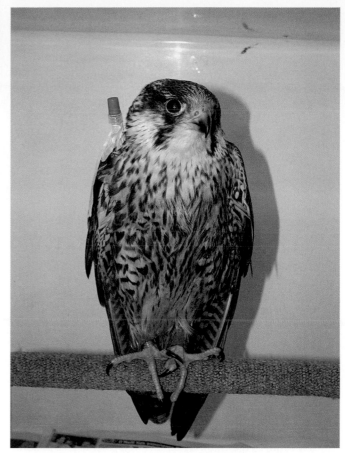

Fig. 12.24 Falcon with an intraosseous catheter placed in the ulna of the wing

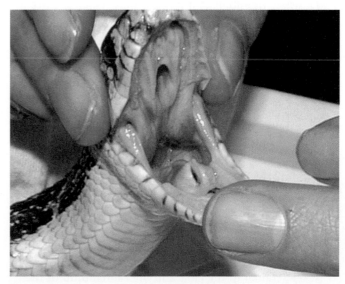

Fig. 12.25 Oral cavity of the snake showing the position of the glottis

placement of a pharyngostomy tube is advised as this will reduce the stress of repeated tubing.

To locate the stomach you should always measure the tube against the outside of the body before placing it to ensure you really are in the stomach, preventing regurgitation. In snakes the stomach is located about one-third of the way down the body; in lizards the stomach is located about half way down the body; in tortoises and terrapins you measure from the nose to the line where the pectoral and abdominal scutes meet (see Ch. 5). Mark the position of the mouth on the tube using a biro – this is the point that the tube will reach when the end is in the stomach. Open the mouth with a wooden spatula. Introduce a well-lubricated tube up towards the roof of the mouth and down the oesophagus, avoiding the glottis. Advance the tube until your marked point.

Intramuscular injection

Fairly well tolerated and easy to do:

- Snakes – inject into the caudal third of the snake, using the muscles that run parallel to the spine.
- Lizards, tortoises and terrapins – inject into the proximal part of the forearm. The hind limbs can also be used but be aware of the renal portal system. Tortoises and terrapins may withdraw their limbs into their shells, so you may have to use the pectoral muscles at the junction of the neck/forelimb with the body.

Use a 23–25-gauge 5/8-inch needle. Always clean the skin before injecting, as reptiles have very dirty skin. Always inject under the scales, never through them.

Subcutaneous injection

An easy route to use but may be less well tolerated with some drugs, as they can be painful:

- Snakes – use the first third of the body in the lateral dorsal area.
- Lizards – use the lateral thoracic area. There is a risk of the skin around the injection site becoming darkened – especially common in the chameleon family. The owner should be advised of this,
- Tortoises and terrapins – use the area cranial to the forelimbs and hind limbs. Strong tortoises tend to pull their legs in, making it very hard to inject. The use of a 23–25-gauge 5/8-inch needle is recommended. The area must be cleaned and you must inject under the scales, not through them.

Intracoelomic injection

Reptiles do not have a diaphragm and the entire body cavity is known as the coelom. The intracoelomic route is mainly used for fluid administration:

- Snakes – enter the body cavity within an area on the lateral part of the body just dorsal to the ventral scales, cranial to the cloaca in the caudal third of the body.
- Lizards – place the lizard in dorsal recumbency with the head tilted downwards to encourage the organs to move cranially away from the injection site. Select a site in the lower right quadrant of the body cavity.
- Tortoises and terrapins – this is not the easiest route as it is difficult to reach an area cranial to the hind limbs. The bladder lies in this area and can be punctured very easily.

The injection site should be cleaned before injection is performed. Inject under the scales not through them. The plunger should always be drawn back before injection to ensure you have not punctured an organ. Use a 23–25-gauge needle.

Intravenous injection

This route is more difficult than the others as you cannot easily 'raise' the vein or see it through the thick skin:

- Snakes – use the ventral tail vein. Insert the needle in the midline about one-third of the tail length from the cloaca at a 75° angle. Advance it slowly until you hit the vertebrae. Pull out slightly while drawing back on the plunger until you get blood back. Administer your medication. The palatine vein, which runs along the roof of the mouth, may be used in larger snakes when they are anaesthetized.
- Lizards – use the ventral tail vein. Insert the needle at a 75° angle about one-third of the way down the tail from the cloaca to ensure you avoid the male hemipenes in the caudal third of the body. Advance the needle until you hit the vertebrae. Pull out the needle while drawing on the plunger. When you get blood back, stop and inject the medication. You must be careful with some species of lizard as they are able to spontaneously shed their tails – this may occur if they are injected on a regular basis.
- Tortoises and terrapins – two routes are used:
  a. Jugular vein – this is the recommended route. Extend the head, tilt the body away and pull the neck towards you. Raise the vein on the right side by applying pressure at the base of the neck. The vein runs from the eardrum down the neck and can sometimes be seen when it is raised.
  b. Dorsal tail vein – more difficult. The vein lies midline on the dorsal aspect of the tail. Insert the needle at a 90° angle and advance it until you hit the vertebrae. Gently pull back while drawing back on the plunger. When blood comes back into the syringe, stop and administer the medication. Use a 23–25-gauge 1-inch needle.

Ensure that the area is cleaned well and go under the scales not through them.

Intraosseous injection

This route is mainly used for fluid administration. This route is impossible in snakes as they do not have any legs:

- Lizards – use the proximal femur, distal femur and the proximal tibia. As this procedure is painful, the use of sedation or a general anaesthetic is required. The area must be cleaned well, as the needle could introduce an infection straight into the bone and cause osteomyelitis. Use a 23–25-gauge needle or spinal needle depending on the size of the lizard. The proximal femur is entered at the fossa between the hip joint and the greater trochanter. This is not an easy route to use as it is at a difficult angle. The distal femur is a bit easier to access as you enter at the stifle joint but it does restrict the movement of the leg. The proximal tibia is really only used in the larger lizards and is entered at the tibial crest.

- Tortoises and terrapins – there are two main sites:
  a. The area at which the plastron and carapace meet just cranial to the hind legs – this is easily accessed but can be very tough, especially in older tortoises. A 21–23-gauge spinal needle is screwed into the shell, ensuring that it is kept parallel to the side of the shell.

  b. The proximal tibia – this is accessed via the tibial crest.

After the needle has been capped, apply an antiseptic cream around the site to help prevent an infection. A radiograph should be taken of the area to ensure it is in the correct place. If you suspect that the reptile may be suffering from a metabolic bone disease you should never use this route and to check this you should always radiograph the animal prior to this procedure.

Bibliography

Anderson, R.S., Edney, A.T.D. (Eds.), 1991. Practical Animal Handling. Pergamon Press, Oxford.

Aspinall, V., 2008. Clinical Procedures in Veterinary Nursing, second ed. Butterworth-Heinemann, Oxford.

Cooper, B., Lane, D.R., 2007. Veterinary Nursing, fourth ed. BSAVA, Gloucester.

Hotston Moore, A. (Ed.), 1999. Manual of Advanced Veterinary Nursing. British Small Animal Veterinary Association, Cheltenham.

Recommended reading

Aspinall, V., 2008. Clinical Procedures in Veterinary Nursing, second ed. Butterworth-Heinemann, Oxford.
Step-by-step guide to handling the more common species of exotic pet.

Hotston Moore, A. (Ed.), 1999. Manual of Advanced Veterinary Nursing. British Small Animal Veterinary Association, Cheltenham.

Detailed chapter describes all aspects of exotic animal care, including nutrition, anaesthesia and patient care.

CHAPTER 13

Introduction to genetics

Dorothy Stables

Key Points

- Every living cell contains a set of chromosomes in the nucleus – a cell containing the normal two sets of chromosomes is called diploid. Gametes (ovum or sperm) have only one of each chromosome pair present and are haploid.
- There are two mechanisms necessary for cell division, mitosis or the division of somatic cells and meiosis, the production of gametes. During meiosis the chromosome complement is halved.
- Genes are arranged in a specific order, each in the same locus on the chromosomes in every member of a species. Alleles are alternative versions of genes at a locus. If an animal has two alleles alike at a locus, it is homozygous. If the alleles differ, the animal is heterozygous.
- DNA molecules consist of a double helix made up of two complementary chains of nucleotides composed of phosphoric acid, deoxyribose and four nitrogenous bases, two purines – adenine and guanine – and two pyrimidines – thymine and cytosine.
- The full complement of DNA is called the genome. The genetic makeup inherited by an individual animal is called the genotype. The outward appearance of an animal, or the phenotype, results from gene–environment interactions.
- Congenital defects are present at birth. Not all congenital defects are inherited and may occur because of genetic/chromosomal abnormalities, the action of environmental teratogens, multifactorial disorders caused by the interaction of environment and genes or idiopathic defects with no known cause.

Introduction

Genes are special molecules within cell nuclei that spell out the blueprint for the development, structure, function and maintenance of living organisms, e.g. the control of hair colour. However, like words in a book, genes can sometimes be 'spelled' wrongly, leading to abnormal development or to diseases. As genes are involved in cell division and in the manufacturing of antibodies, cancers and some immune disorders have a genetic basis. The actions of genes may also be influenced by environmental features, leading to disorders such as hip dysplasia in dogs. It is important to understand a little of basic cell physiology to understand both normal and abnormal gene function.

Characteristics of mammalian cells

Cells are the basic structural and functional units of living organisms (see Ch. 4) and are membrane–bound units filled with an aqueous solution of chemicals and organelles (Fig. 13.1). Cells must extract raw materials necessary for their function and expel waste products. Their structure and functions are governed by genetic information. Cells create copies of themselves.

Cellular organization

A typical cell includes a single **nucleus, cytoplasm** and a cellular boundary known as the **plasma membrane**. The nucleus contains the genetic material and the cytoplasm is composed mainly of cytosol containing water, electrolytes, proteins, lipids and carbohydrates, and the organelles. The cell membrane or plasma membrane encloses the cellular contents and maintains the boundary between the cytoplasm and the extracellular environment. This chapter is concerned with the functions of the cell nucleus.

The nucleus

The nucleus is the largest structure of the cell and is its control centre. It is surrounded by a double nuclear membrane, one bilayer inside the other. The outer one is continuous with the endoplasmic reticulum of the cell cytoplasm. The nuclear membrane is penetrated by several thousand nuclear pores to allow molecules to pass through. Most cells have only one nucleus, although skeletal muscle cells are multinucleated. Nuclei contain large quantities of deoxyribonucleic acid (DNA), made up of **genes**. Several other structures are essential to the normal functioning of the nucleus, such as the **nucleoli** where ribosomal subunits are synthesized. DNA is found in a thread-like mass known as chromatin. Prior to cellular reproduction chromatin

Fig. 13.1 Diagram of the ultrastructure of a cell

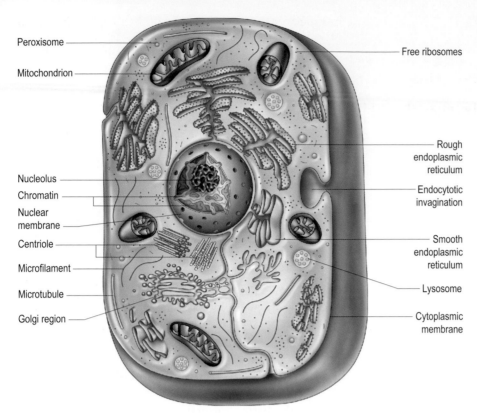

Peroxisome

Mitochondrion

Free ribosomes

Rough endoplasmic reticulum

Endocytotic invagination

Nucleolus

Chromatin

Nuclear membrane

Smooth endoplasmic reticulum

Centriole

Microfilament

Lysosome

Microtubule

Golgi region

Cytoplasmic membrane

shortens and coils into rod-like bodies, forming recognizable **chromosomes**, the number of which varies between species.

Chromosomes

When dividing cells are observed under a light microscope, the chromosomes are clearly visible. During cell division the chromosomes become condensed. At this time DNA replication results in an X-shaped structure consisting of two identical strands called **chromatids** joined by a constricted area called the **centromere.** If the DNA of a single cell was stretched out it would be several metres long yet the total length of the condensed chromosomes of an average cell placed end to end is less than 0.5 mm!

In **somatic** (body) cells chromosomes are arranged in pairs. One chromosome of each pair originates within the maternal ovum and the other chromosome within the paternal sperm. A cell containing two sets of chromosomes is called **diploid**. **Gametes** (sex cells) are haploid, i.e. there is only one of each pair. In all but one of the pairs the chromosomes are identical and these pairs are called **autosomes.** The pairs that are alike are called **homologues.** The other pair is the **sex chromosomes,** two X chromosomes in females and an X and a Y chromosome in males.

Identifying chromosomes

Circulating lymphocytes from peripheral blood are commonly used to study chromosomes. The cell samples are encouraged to divide. The process is stopped during mitosis (see below) by adding colchicine. The two chromatids have been formed from one chromosome and, if cell division had continued, the centromere would have split and each

chromatid would have become a separate chromosome in a new cell.

A photograph is taken and the chromosomes are cut out and arranged in a standard fashion and then photographed again to produce **a karyotype** (Fig. 13.2). Chromosomes are usually referred to as pairs and the total number is called the $2n$ number, where n is the number of pairs. Chromosomes are identified by their size, light and dark banding patterns and position of the centromere. A chromosome is divided by its centromere into short and long arms. The short arm is referred to as 'p' and the long arm as 'q'. Chromosomes can be classified by the position of their centromeres. If located centrally the chromosome is **metacentric**, if intermediate it is **submetacentric** and if found at one end the chromosome is **acrocentric**. It is common to use the term metacentric to cover metacentric and submetacentric (Nicholas 2003), as shown in Table 13.1.

Cell division – mitosis and meiosis

There are two mechanisms necessary for cell division. **Somatic cells** must be able to replicate themselves with minimal mistakes. During mitosis each daughter cell receives a copy of all the chromosomes. Multicellular species replace cells damaged by wear and tear or lost during programmed cell death (apoptosis) by the cycle of somatic cell division. Where ill health, trauma or surgery occurs, loss and replacement of cells will increase. Where natural cell division is halted, for example, in exposure to a large dose of ionizing radiation, the animal is likely to die within a few days because of rapid cell destruction. However, something special is required in sexual reproduction, where mother and father must contribute one of each pair of chromosomes to

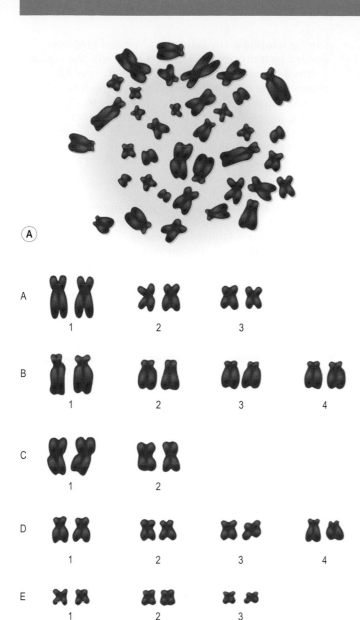

Fig. 13.2 (A, B) The chromosomes of a male cat

their offspring. During **meiosis** only one of each pair of chromosomes enters each **gamete** (sperm or ovum).

Replication of DNA

In order to produce a pair of genetically identical daughter cells, nuclear DNA must be precisely replicated and the replicated chromosomes separated into two identical cells. At the same time most cells double their mass and duplicate all their cytoplasmic organelles. Cells must not enter mitosis or meiosis until the chromosomes have been replicated, otherwise they may lack a particular chromosome, which may give rise to cancer at a later stage.

The duration of the **cell cycle** (Fig. 13.3) varies greatly from one cell type to another but always consists of three distinct phases, interphase, mitosis and cytokinesis. The standard cell cycle is fairly long, extending to 12 hours or more. In most cells the mitotic phase takes about 1 hour, a small fraction of the total cell cycle. The time between one mitotic phase and the next is taken up by interphase, which itself consists of three distinctive phases, G1 (gap1), S (synthesis) and G2 (gap2). During G1 phase the cell becomes committed to DNA replication, which occurs during S phase.

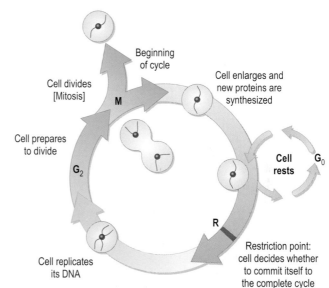

Fig. 13.3 The cell cycle

Table 13.1 Karyotypes of some domestic species (adapted from Nicholas 2003)

Species	Total (diploid 2n)	Metacentric pairs	Acrocentric pairs
Cat, *Felis catus*	38	16	2
Dog, *Canis familiaris*	78	0	39
Goat, *Capra hircus*	60	0	29
Sheep, *Ovis aries*	54	3	23
Cattle, *Bos taurus*	60	0	29
Horse, *Equus caballus*	64	13	18
Rabbit, *Oryctolagus cuniculus*	44	19	2

The subsequent G2 phase appears to provide a safety gap, allowing DNA replication to be complete before mitosis.

Mitosis

During mitosis (Fig. 13.4) the nuclear membrane breaks down and the nuclear contents condense, forming visible chromosomes. The stages of mitosis are prophase, metaphase, anaphase and telophase:

- During **prophase**, the cell's microtubules establish the mitotic spindle, which will eventually separate the chromosomes.
- In **metaphase** the duplicated chromosomes align on the mitotic spindle, in preparation for segregation (Fig. 13.4).
- During **anaphase** the chromosomes move to the pole of the spindle, where they decondense and establish new nuclei.

- During **telophase** the cell is pinched and gradually divided by a process known as **cytokinesis**, the critical point of mitosis that terminates the cell cycle. All phases of the cell cycle are variable in length but the greatest variation occurs in the G1 phase. If cells in G1 are not committed to DNA replication, they can enter a resting state known as the G0 phase for days, weeks or years before resuming proliferation.

Meiosis

During meiosis (diminution), the chromosome complement is halved. Meiosis involves two nuclear divisions rather than one. A mature haploid gamete produced by the divisions of a diploid cell during meiosis must contain half the original number of chromosomes. Only one chromosome from each homologous pair is present, ensuring that either the maternal or the paternal copy of each gene but not both

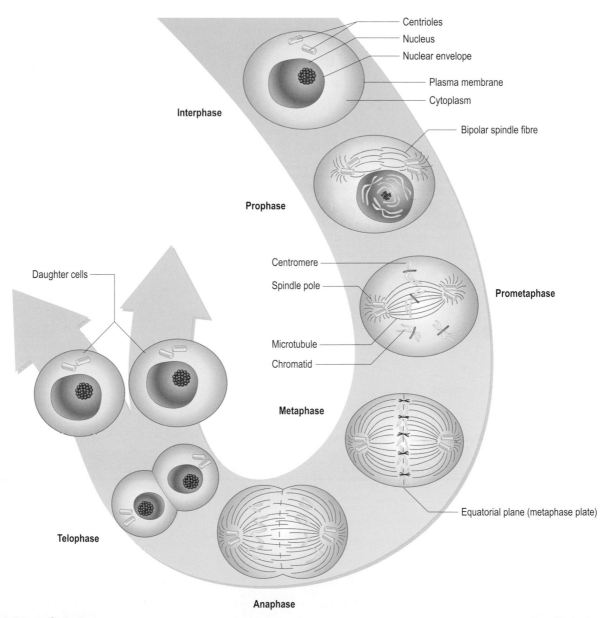

Fig. 13.4 Stages of mitosis

is present. The homologues recognize each other and become physically paired prior to lining up on the mitotic spindle.

Meiosis consists of two stages (Fig. 13.5):

- **Meiosis 1** begins with each chromosome duplicating itself, giving rise to two identical chromatids joined at the centromere. The duplicated homologous pairs form a structure containing four chromatids. This close proximity allows recombination (crossing over of genetic material) to occur. Fragments of maternal chromatids are exchanged for corresponding fragments of homologous paternal chromatids. Next, the two centromeres are pulled to opposite sides of the cell, a process called **dysjunction**. The cell now divides into two new cells, one containing a recombined maternal chromosome and one containing a recombined paternal chromosome.

- In **meiosis 2** two chromatids in each new cell are formed and move apart and these cells divide into two, each containing one chromatid or new chromosome. The result is four haploid spermatozoa but only one functional ovum because of the loss of a set of chromosomes in meiosis 1 into a dark body called the first polar body and the loss again in meiosis 2 of one set of chromosomes into a second polar body. The union of a sperm and ovum at fertilization results in a **zygote** with the normal diploid number of chromosomes.

Feline and canine chromosomes

Genes are arranged in a specific order, each in the same place or **locus** on the chromosomes, in every species such as the

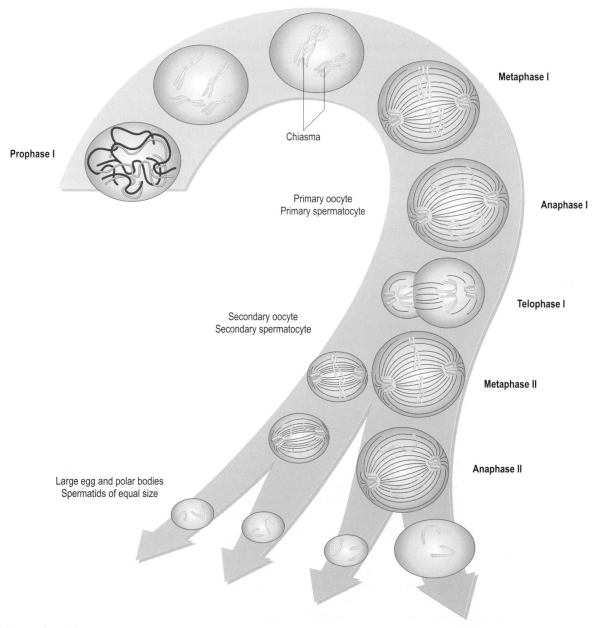

Fig. 13.5 Stages of meiosis

domestic cat (*Felis catus*). This ensures that any male cat can mate successfully with any female cat and is the defining feature of a species. Cats have 19 pairs of chromosomes carrying their genes. All domestic dogs (*Canis familiaris*) have 39 pairs of chromosomes (Table 13.1).

Development of modern genetics

In 1865 a monk called Gregor Mendel presented a paper on his experiments on garden peas. He had studied varieties of pea that differed in a single characteristic, such as tall and short plants or wrinkled and smooth seeds. He found that one of two characteristics, for example, tall plants, seemed to dominate the next generation, the first filial (F1) generation, and these were called **dominant factors**. The opposite characteristic – e.g. short plants – disappeared, only to reappear in the second or F2 generation. These were called **recessive factors.**

Mendel proposed that each pair of characteristics was controlled by a pair of factors, one arising from each parent plant. Pure-bred pea plants were **homozygous,** inheriting two identical genes from their parents. The F1 generation that resulted from the breeding of a tall plant with a short plant were all tall plants. However, they inherited two different genes from their parents and were **heterozygous**. These factors were called genes by a Danish botanist, Johannsen who shortened the term pangenia that Charles Darwin had coined for his unknown hereditary factors (Gould 2007). The alternative versions of genes at a locus are called **allelomorphs**, usually shortened to **alleles.**

For other useful definitions see box 13.1.

Mendel's laws

Three main principles developed from Mendel's work:

- **The law of uniformity** – when two homozygotes with different alleles are crossed, all the offspring of the F1 generation are identical and heterozygous. Characteristics do not blend and can reappear in subsequent generations.
- **The law of segregation** – each individual possesses two genes for a particular characteristic, only one of which can be passed on in the ovum or sperm to the next generation.
- **The law of independent assortment** – members of different gene pairs segregate to offspring independently of one another. This third law is not strictly true, because, if two genes are situated closely together on the same chromosome, they may be linked and inherited together during meiosis.

Mendel's findings were ignored until 1900, when thread-like structures were seen in cell nuclei. These were the chromosomes and in 1903 two people independently proposed that they carried the hereditary factors known as genes. However, it was only in 1952 that DNA was identified as the universal genetic material. In 1953 the structure of DNA was discovered by James D. Watson and Francis H. C. Crick. Without Rosalind Franklin, who developed the skills of X-ray crystallography, their discovery might not have occurred. The correct number of 46 human chromosomes was identified in 1956 (Jorde et al 2006).

Box 13.1 Useful definitions

- Chromosome – thread-like mass of DNA found within the nucleus of the cell
- Gene – unit of inheritance; genes consist of short pieces of DNA which, when joined together in a sequence, make up specific chromosomes
- Locus – the position of a gene on a chromosome
- Allele – a gene on the same locus of a pair of homologous chromosomes
- Homologous chromosomes – identical in size and shape
- Homozygous genes – identical genes on the same locus of a pair of chromosomes
- Heterozygous genes – non-identical genes on the same locus of a pair of chromosomes
- Phenotype – outward or visible appearance of the animal; may be affected by the environment
- Genotype – the genetic makeup of an animal

Composition of DNA

The double helix

DNA molecules consist of a double helix made up of two complementary chains of nucleotides. These are composed of several simple chemical compounds bound together in a regular pattern. The building blocks of each molecule are phosphoric acid, a pentose sugar called deoxyribose, and four nitrogenous bases, two purines – **adenine and guanine**, and two pyrimidines – **thymine and cytosine**, identified by the single letters A, G, T and C. A second form of nucleic acid is ribonucleic acid (RNA). In RNA thymine is replaced by uracil (U). Two sugar-phosphate strands wind around each other and the base pairs are stacked between these strands, pointing inwards to the centre of the double helix. The two strands run in opposite directions and are complementary to each other. A purine always pairs with a pyrimidine and the pairs stack one above the other. The complementary chains are held together by hydrogen bonds, which are easily broken, a feature necessary for DNA replication (Fig. 13.6).

Genes

The full complement of DNA is called the **genome** and the study of it is called **genomics**. DNA is arranged in segments called **genes**. Genes code for proteins, which may act as hormones, receptors, structural and regulatory proteins. Two alternative alleles of any gene are present at a specific locus, one on each of a pair of chromosomes. If both parents contribute an identical allele for a locus, the individual is **homozygous**. If the two alleles differ, the individual is **heterozygous.**

Many mammals, including humans and mice have between 20 000 to 25 000 discrete genes but these form only a small section of the DNA in the genome They are separated from each other by long runs of inactive, repetitive DNA sequences. Some of it is turning out to be organizing genes that switch on and off structural genes but most of it appears to be 'junk' (Carroll 2006). Also any gene is not a continuous stretch of DNA coding for a protein. There are non-coding intervening

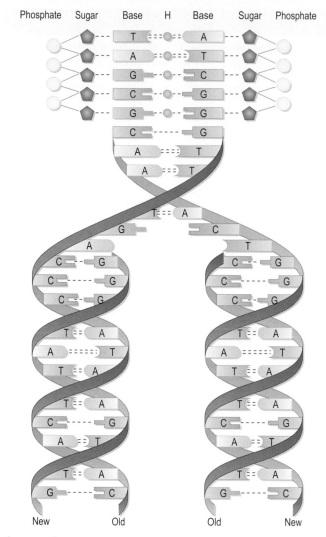

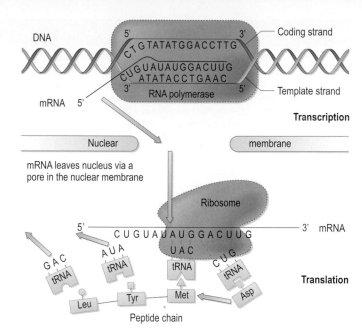

Phosphate Sugar Base H Base Sugar Phosphate

New Old Old New

Fig. 13.6 The replication of DNA, showing the unwinding of the double helix and the formation of new strands with complementary base pairs

Fig. 13.7 Synthesis of polypeptides in a eukaryote by means of transcription and translation

sequences called **introns** (intervening sequences) separating the coding sequences which are called **exons** (expressed sequences) (Turnpenny & Ellard 2007). The introns are excised by enzymes during transcription (see below) and do not form part of the coding for the gene product.

The role of the environment

Genes act in response to environmental changes. These may be internal, such as a response to fluctuations in hormone level, or external, such as the response to a meal. The full complement of genes inherited by an individual animal is called the genotype. The outward appearance of an animal, i.e. its physical, biochemical and physiological nature, is known as the phenotype and results from gene/environment interactions. For example genes may specify the adult size of an animal but the amount and type of food may alter this potential.

From DNA to RNA to protein

Proteins are the working components of the cell. DNA stores the information. RNA carries out instructions encoded in

DNA and synthesizes the proteins involved in cellular function.

The genetic code

Twenty different organic compounds called amino acids are found in proteins, so it became obvious to Watson and Crick that, as there were only four bases – ATGC – more than one base must be necessary to specify a particular amino acid. Even two bases wouldn't be enough, as 4^2 gives only 16 possibilities. However, 3^2 bases give 64 possibilities, more than enough to code for the 20 amino acids. A group of three nucleotides called a triplet codon spells out each amino acid and the sequence of amino acids shapes a particular protein. There are also codons at the ends of genes that signify 'start' and 'stop' so that a correct version of a protein is made.

Reading the genetic code

Making a functional protein from a stretch of DNA involves two processes, transcription and translation.

Transcription

In a gene only one of the two DNA strands forming the helix acts as a template for a polypeptide. It must be copied by messenger RNA (mRNA) before it can be read. This is called transcription (Fig. 13.7). Every base in the single-stranded mRNA is complementary to the DNA but uracil replaces thymine.

Translation

Following transcription, mature mRNA is transported to the ribosomes for translation into a specific protein (Fig. 13.7). In the cytoplasm a particular amino acid is bound to its transfer RNA (tRNA) for transporting to a ribosome where it is linked up with others to form a polypeptide chain to build the protein.

Box 13.2 Inheritance of coat colours in Labrador dogs

The working of single genes can be illustrated by the inheritance of coat colour in Labrador dogs. Coat colour in mammals is brought about by the presence of pigment granules called melanins in a protein framework. Two varieties of melanin are converted from the amino acid tyrosine. One is called eumelanin and gives rise to dark coat colour and the other is phaeomelanin, which produces light colour – various shades of yellow from pale to red (Nicholas 2003).

Punnett square 1

		Paternal genes	
		B	B
Maternal genes	B	BB black	BB black
	B	BB black	BB black

Labradors come in three basic colours – black, chocolate and yellow. Chocolates can vary from light to dark in colour. Two alleles of the same gene are responsible for the black and chocolate colours. Black is dominant and is represented by the upper case letter B and chocolate is recessive to black and is represented by the lower case letter b. Therefore a dog with a black coat (phenotype) may be genetically either homozygous BB or heterozygous Bb. If a dog and bitch are both homozygous all their puppies will be black BB, as shown in Punnett square 1.

Punnett square 2

		Paternal genes	
		B	b
Maternal genes	B	BB black	Bb black
	b	Bb black	bb brown

If a dog and bitch are both heterozygous Bb, three of their puppies will be black and only one chocolate, as shown in Punnett square 2. One of the black puppies will be homozygous BB, two will be heterozygous Bb. The chocolate puppy will be homozygous for the recessive gene bb.

Punnett square 3

		Paternal genes	
		BBE	BBe
Maternal genes	BBE	BBEE black	BBEe black
	BBe	BBee black	BBee yellow

The yellow colour is brought about by a second recessive gene, E, which functions to mask the dark colour by producing phaeomelanin instead of eumelanin. If the animal is homozygous for the dominant allele, i.e. EE or heterozygous Ee, there is no effect on the basic coat colour. Eumelanin will be produced and the coat colour will be black or brown. If the animal is homozygous for the recessive version ee, phaeomelanin will be produced and the coat colour will be yellow as shown in Punnett square 3. For simplicity of cell numbers in the Punnett square both dog and bitch are shown as homozygous BB.

Patterns of Mendelian inheritance

There are four basic types of single-gene Mendelian inheritance – autosomal dominant, autosomal recessive, X-linked dominant and X-linked recessive. Recessive X-linked disorders are rare and will not be discussed.

Dominant genes

- Only one copy is needed to affect the phenotype and manifests its effects in heterozygotes.
- The effect does not miss a generation.
- Every affected offspring with that particular phenotype has at least one affected parent.
- Where one parent is affected, offspring have a one in two chance of being affected.
- Normal offspring of an affected parent only produce normal offspring.

Recessive genes

- A recessive allele only affects the phenotype in homozygotes.
- Animals with one copy of the allele are carriers.
- The progeny of two carriers have a one in four chance of being affected or normal and a one in two chance of carrying the disorder.
- Matings between a homozygous affected animal and a normal homozygous animal produce normal offspring.
- The effect may be to skip generations until two carriers reproduce.
- An example of recessive inheritance is illustrated in Box 13.2.

Dominant X-linked genes

- The X chromosome carries a large number of genes involved in development and function.
- Males only have one X chromosome and are hemizygous for X chromosome genes.
- If there is an abnormal X chromosome gene, males will be affected by an X-linked disorder.
- Females are usually heterozygous for the X chromosome and will not be affected because of the opposing normal allele. They will be asymptomatic carriers.

Mitochondrial DNA

- Each mitochondrion has its own circular double-stranded DNA called mitochondrial DNA (mDNA) inherited only from mothers because sperm mitochondria rarely enter the ovum and do not contribute to the embryo.
- mDNA codes for genes that are important in cellular respiration.
- mDNA disorders affect males and females but are transmitted only through their mothers. The disorders combine muscular and neurological features, affecting cells with high energy needs.

Inactivation of the X chromosome in females

In females only one X chromosome is functional in each cell and the other is inactivated in the early embryo. This phenomenon is called lyonization (Box 13.3) (Vella et al 1999). Laura Gould has written an interesting and informative book about her male calico (tortoiseshell and white) cat George, updated 2007. It is called 'Cats are not Peas' and she discusses how George came to be – he carried two X chromosomes (XXY) instead of one and therefore half his cells carried black and half red.

Congenital defects

Congenital defects are present at birth. Some may be visible or they may be hidden, such as changes in protein molecules, e.g. haemoglobin. Not all congenital defects are inherited. Some result from environmental influences on the embryo. Congenital defects may occur because of the following factors:

- Genetic/chromosomal abnormalities may cause abnormality. Some genes (pleiotropic) support multiple functions and an abnormality may affect multiple systems. Some disorders may involve the interactions of many genes and these are referred to as polygenic.
- Teratogens reach the fetus by crossing the placenta and cause DNA mutations. During organogenesis, the embryo is vulnerable to developmental disruption.

Box 13.3 Inactivation of the X chromosome

In females one or other of the X chromosomes is randomly inactivated in cells early in embryonic life. Half the cells of a female will contain one activated X chromosome and half the other. All daughter cells of a particular cell line contain the same inactivated X chromosome. This effect is called lyonization, after its discoverer, Dr Mary Lyon. Each female is a mosaic of half paternal and half maternal X chromosomes.

The tortoiseshell cat – in cats the orange gene (O) is responsible for the colour of the ginger cat. It is carried on the X chromosome. The O gene eliminates all black or brown pigment from the hairs. A tortoiseshell cat is a female heterozygote Oo. In any cell only one X chromosome functions. Two cell lines develop at random – one with O producing hair with orange pigment and the other with o, allowing normal pigment to colour the hair with whatever the animal has inherited (Fig. 13.8).

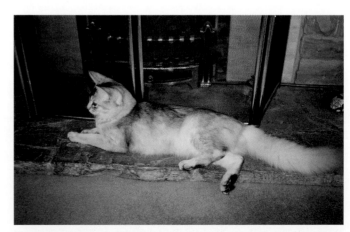

Fig. 13.8 A tortoiseshell silver Somali cat showing patches of red and black on a silver base

Examples of teratogens are infectious agents such as feline panleukopenia virus, drugs such as griseofulvin, and radiation.

- Multifactorial disorders are caused by the interaction of environment and genes, e.g. canine hip dysplasia.
- Idiopathic defects have no known cause; at present they are the largest group.

Mutations

Genes usually produce their product faithfully but occasionally a mutation or alteration in the genetic material in a cell arises either naturally or because of the effects of environmental challenges called mutagens. These include radiation, chemical or physical stressors. Mutations can be minor changes in DNA or macromutations involving alterations of large amounts of a chromosome. Mutations often result in harmful or lethal defects. A few examples include:

- Point mutations of a single base cause amino acid substitutions resulting in faulty protein products, which may cause functional defects.
- Nonsense mutations involve the creation of a stop codon in the middle of a gene; the broken gene does not code for a protein product.
- In frameshift mutations additions or deletions of a nucleotide alter the reading frame of the DNA to the left or right so that triplet codons do not code for amino acids.

Genetic defects

Slight differences in a protein brought about by a genetic mutation may cause devastating metabolic diseases such as phosphofructokinase deficiency in cocker and springer spaniels. However, not all diseases are due to alterations in metabolic pathways. Some proteins have cellular structural roles while others control embryological development. Many feline and canine disorders have their similarities to human diseases. Dogs share 85% of their genetic code with humans and over half their genetic disorders mirror a human genetic disease (Guynup 2000), e.g. severe combined immunodeficiency disease (SCID) in basset hounds and Welsh corgis. The boy in the bubble mentioned in a song by Paul Simon suffered from this disorder.

Incidence

Research has identified over 250 inherited genetic defects in the cat. Many also afflict humans, including muscular dystrophy, polycystic kidney disease and retinal degeneration (Budiansky 2002). Many genetic diseases have been identified in the dog and Donald Patterson, professor of medical genetics at Pennsylvania University, runs a 'canine genetic disease information system'. By 2007, over 500 genetic diseases had been recorded in dogs, with the poodle breed top of the list at 145 diseases (Dog Health Problems 2009). This knowledge was highlighted by the BBC in its programme 'Pedigree Dogs Exposed' (2008). Most inherited diseases are due to recessive genes (Ruvinsky & Sampson 2001). The loss of genetic diversity in pure-bred animals means that most of these disorders have been found among specific breeds of animal rather than among the outbred mongrel or moggy.

It is difficult to identify carriers of recessive disorders until affected offspring have been born from two apparently normal parents.

Chromosomal defects

Occasionally, whole chromosomes may be involved but such defects often result in stillbirth or spontaneous abortion. Numerical or structural changes may affect the autosomes or sex chromosomes.

Numerical chromosomal defects

Many of these numerical defects arise during failure of dysjunction, when sister chromatids fail to separate. This may result in too many or too few chromosomes:

- Polyploidy means the presence of multiples of the haploid number of chromosomes, i.e. three or more.
- Triploidy is the presence of three copies of each chromosome.
- Monosomy is when one of a chromosome pair is missing.
- Trisomy is the presence of an extra chromosome. Trisomy of the sex chromosomes is quite common and XXX females (triple X) or XXY males occur. This can lead to the unusual occurrence of a male tortoiseshell cat with the genotype 18XXY (18 pairs + X and Y and an extra X).
- Mosaicism results when the zygote develops into an individual with two genotypes or cell lines. The condition arises as a result of non-dysjunction during early mitosis.

Structural chromosomal defects

Pollution or radiation may induce breaks in chromosomes, resulting in macromutations. Two of these, inversion and translocation, may be transmitted from parent to offspring.

- Translocation is the transfer of a piece of one chromosome to another non-homologous chromosome. If the translocation is balanced, the normal complement of chromosomal material is received. There will be no abnormality. If the translocation results in extra chromosomal material, abnormality will occur.
- Deletion is the loss of part of a chromosome.
- Duplication is where a section of a chromosome is repeated; this is less harmful as there is no loss of chromosome material.
- Inversion occurs if a segment of a chromosome breaks free and becomes reattached in the reverse position.

Application to practice

The genome projects

Over the last few decades identification of genes through the use of molecular genetics using DNA/RNA-based technologies has given rise to a new science of genomics or the study of the genome. Fragments of known DNA can be used as a probe to identify genes on the chromosomes (Nicholas 2003). The technology has led to disease-causing gene discovery, genetic engineering, paternity testing and criminal identification (Padgett & Duffendack 2004).

The Human Genome Project, completed in 2003, involved mapping all the human genes to their chromosomes. Work has proceeded on various animal genomes, including feline and canine. Obtaining samples of DNA for study requires only a blood or saliva sample. Recent developments have greatly increased the speed at which DNA can be sequenced.

Researchers at Cornell University began sequencing the dog genome in 1990 and the genome of a female boxer dog called Tasha led the way. Similarly, Professor Stephen J. O'Brien began to study the genetics of the house cat in the 1970s. A low-resolution map of the feline genome was announced in 2005 when the DNA of an Abyssinian cat called Cinnamon was sequenced (Little 2008). As mentioned above, the domestic cat is known to have at least 250 genetic diseases, many of them having similarities to human diseases. Therefore genome research is of importance not only to our cats and dogs but also to ourselves. Once an inherited trait has been identified to a specific location a DNA test can be created for it. However, the ethics of using the new technologies have to be considered and Meyers-Wallen (2003) discusses the problems clearly.

Diagnosis of disorders

Although molecular genetics has provided sophisticated tests for identifying disorders there are other, more traditional ways of identifying risks for breeding animals and selecting against an inherited single gene problem. These are clinical screening, pedigree analysis and test matings. The technical methods include biochemical screening and DNA markers (Nicholas 2003).

Clinical screening

Although single-gene disorders give rise to serious problems such as inherited eye disorders in dogs and polycystic kidney disease in cats, they may not prevent animals from reproducing. Some disorders, especially dominant gene disorders such as feline polycystic kidney disease, can be identified by clinical examination and any affected animal prevented from breeding. The simplest way is to neuter them and sell them as pets.

Pedigree analysis

Breeders of pedigree animals are expected to keep meticulous pedigrees containing at least four generations. Studying the pedigree can help to estimate the probability that a prospective parent may be homozygous for a particular gene. There is also a retrospective use of pedigrees. When an animal has been born with a genetic disease, closely related parents who may be carriers can be identified and test matings may be carried out. Specific symbols are used to make interpretation of pedigrees universal (Fig. 13.9).

Test matings

These are time-consuming and may be expensive but allow the breeder to identify the source of an abnormal allele. The concept will be discussed more fully in Chapter 14.

Biochemical screening

Some diseases are caused by the lack of a specific protein that acts as a catalyst or an enzyme in a metabolic process. If the disease process leaves a biochemical marker in blood or other readily obtainable tissue, a biochemical screening test can be developed. Sometimes the heterozygote carrier of the gene has reduced manufacture of the particular protein and can be identified by the test.

DNA technologies

DNA technologies are being increasingly used to identify genes associated with defects. The techniques include the use of restriction enzymes, polymerase chain reaction (PCR) and Southern blotting. Nicholas (2003) gives a good account of these techniques in Chapter 2 of his book.

Restriction enzymes

In 1970 scientists discovered that bacteria produce enzymes that can break down any foreign DNA that enters their cells. These enzymes restrict viruses from damaging the bacterium, hence the name restriction enzymes. They cut the foreign DNA at specific sites and into pieces of varying lengths and these fragments can be isolated and cloned (making multiple identical copies). If a fragment is inserted into a suitable vector, such as the small circular DNA found in some bacteria called plasmids, the resulting DNA is called recombinant DNA (rDNA).

Polymerase chain reaction (PCR)

Cloning can produce many copies of a particular fragment to use in gene sequencing. Another use for cloning is the manufacture of a genomic library which could contain most of the DNA for that species. These libraries are then used to track down specific genes, including those causing inherited disease. PCR, developed in 1985, is widely used in the detection of particular genes. PCR rapidly produces more than a million copies of DNA. The original DNA can be from a cell or from any source: from a living cell, a museum specimen, a single sperm or a hair follicle.

Southern blotting

The technique is named after Ed Southern, who developed the method in 1975. Depending on their length, fragments of DNA will travel different distances through a gel when an electric current is passed through it. This is called gel electrophoresis. The fragments are denatured into single strands, separated by size and blotted onto either a nitrocellulose or nylon membrane. The membrane is baked in an oven to fix the DNA and then bathed in a solution containing labelled (with a substance that fluoresces), denatured DNA probes. The strands will combine with any complementary strand in the solution. The unattached probes are washed off, leaving the matched DNA.

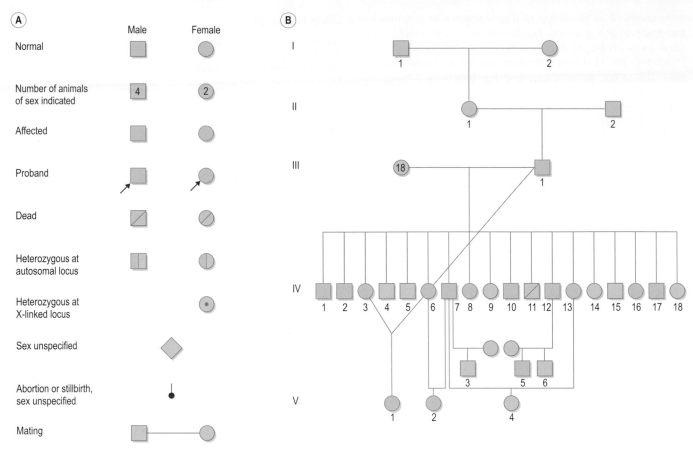

Fig. 13.9 (A) Symbols used in writing and interpreting pedigrees; a proband is an affected individual through whom the family came to the notice of an investigator. (B) BOA pedigree, showing the pattern of inheritance of multiple exostoses in horses. Reproduced with permission from Nicholas, F.W., 2003. Introduction to Veterinary Genetics, second ed. Blackwell, Oxford

Examples of screening for specific canine and feline defects

Kennel Club and British Veterinary Association

In the UK the Kennel Club (KC), together with the British Veterinary Association (BVA), currently have three screening schemes for inherited conditions. These are inherited eye conditions including peripheral retinal atrophy, hip dysplasia and elbow dysplasia.

Generalized progressive retinal atrophy

Although there are different types of generalized progressive retinal atrophy (PRA) most forms are inherited as an autosomal recessive trait (Dekomien & Epplen 2003). The genetic cause varies between breeds, making a single diagnostic DNA test difficult. Homozygous animals develop degeneration of the peripheral retina, leading to night blindness and loss of visual fields. Typically the disease progresses to complete blindness. Genetic testing is available under the eye scheme for the Irish setter but the BVA maintain a list of other breeds indicating the approximate age at which the deterioration can be diagnosed by ophthalmoscope.

Canine hip dysplasia – a multifactorial problem

Unfortunately, some serious disorders are not caused by a single gene or even a combination of genetic effects (polygenic). There may also be an environmental factor predisposing animals to a disease, i.e. the disease is multifactorial. One of these diseases is canine hip dysplasia. Others include epilepsy, autoimmune diseases, heart disease and some forms of cancer.

Hip dysplasia is a major congenital canine health problem. Large pedigree dogs such as labradors are more prone to it but smaller dogs and mongrels may also suffer. There is abnormal formation of the 'ball and socket' hip joint. Normally the ball, which is the head of the femur, fits snugly into the socket. Dogs with a genetic disposition are born with normal hips but as the dog grows the structure of the joint becomes deformed so that the head does not fit into the socket and the joint does not rotate smoothly. The dog becomes lame, may be unwilling to run around and may have difficulty climbing stairs. It may walk with a waddle. The ultimate result is arthritis and a painful, crippling disease.

Many factors work together to cause this disease. The dog must be genetically at risk, but environmental factors, especially nutrition and exercise, bring about the symptoms. There may be excess calcium in puppy food, obesity and high-protein and high-calorie diets. Incorrect levels of exercise (too much or too little) also produce symptoms but the continued breeding of dogs with hip dysplasia is a major contributor.

Total elimination of the disease may be unrealistic but selective breeding of dogs with good hips can reduce the incidence. The BVA and the KC run a scheme to test for hip dysplasia, which helps the breeder to choose good breeding stock. Radiographs from dogs more than 1 year old are submitted to ensure that skeletal maturity is sufficient. An overall hip score based on examination of specific sites for malformation in both joints is calculated. A list of breed mean scores (BMS) is published and breeders are recommended to ensure that their breeding stock has scores well below the BMS for their breed of dog. There is an excellent seven-page article called Hip Dysplasia in Dogs: Diagnosis, Treatment and Prevention online at <http://www.peteducation.com/article.cfm?c=2+1569& aid=444>.

Elbow dysplasia

Elbow dysplasia is a degenerative polygenic inherited disease of the elbow joint. The causes, diagnosis and management are similar to hip dysplasia. The Orthopaedic Foundation for Animals maintains an elbow registry and elbows can be graded from normal through grades 1, 2 and 3 as the severity of the radiographic appearance increases. Three main disorders may occur singly or in combination:

- Fragmented medial coronoid process
- Osteochondritis of the medial humeral condyle
- Ununited anconeal process.

Elbow dysplasia occurs mainly in larger dogs and is breed-related. The incidence ranges from 0% in Border collies to 47.8% in chow chows. Male dogs are more likely to be affected than females and in 20–35% of cases both elbows are affected. Affected dogs should probably be removed from the breeding programme, although the severity of symptoms is only loosely related to the radiographic signs.

The Feline Advisory Bureau

The Feline Advisory Bureau (FAB) currently organize a screening programme for the autosomal dominant problem – polycystic kidney disorder (PKD).

Feline polycystic kidney disorder (PKD)

In PKD a large number of fluid-filled cysts form within the kidneys (Feline Advisory Bureau 2004). The cysts are present from birth but increase in size until they damage the surrounding kidney tissue and cause kidney failure (Fig. 13.10). The cat will eventually die, despite supportive treatment. The disease is peculiar to Persian cats and any breed of cat where Persian genes have been included, such as the Tiffany.

The problem has become widespread in these breeds because the disease is an unfortunate combination of an autosomal dominant gene, so that only one parent needs to be affected by PKD and one in two of any offspring will be affected, and a condition whose symptoms may not be obvious until the age of 7 or 8, by which time the cat may have produced several litters of kittens, 50% of whom would be affected.

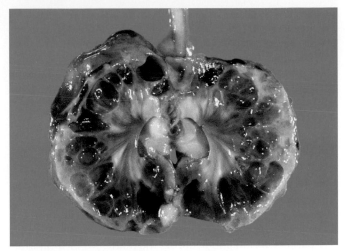

Fig. 13.10 Cross-section of a severely affected kidney showing cysts throughout. Reproduced with permission of the Feline Advisory Bureau

The Feline Advisory Bureau has developed a PKD screening scheme that relies on ultrasonography of the kidneys, looking for the presence of cysts. This is best done when the cat is more than 10 months old. An FAB-approved certificate is issued, stating the result of the scan for that cat. This enables breeders to make informed decisions about which cats to use for future breeding. Tim Gruffydd-Jones MRCVS (personal communication) believes that the disorder could be eradicated quickly if all breeders were responsible about testing their cats.

Feline erythrocyte pyruvate kinase deficiency (PKDef)

Enzymes are proteins which speed up metabolic reactions. Genetic mutations may alter enzymes so that normal metabolism cannot occur. Pyruvate kinase (PK) is an enzyme involved in breaking down glucose to release energy inside intracellular mitochondria. During this glucose cycle, PK converts phosphoenol pyruvate (PEP) to pyruvic acid.

Mature erythrocytes (red blood cells) lose their mitochondria but can still produce enough adenosine triphosphate (ATP) to cope with wear and repair. PK deficiency, especially common in Somali and Abyssinian cats, prevents energy production, resulting in irreversible cell membrane injury and premature haemolysis that leads to anaemia. PKDef is recessively inherited and an affected cat inherits an abnormal gene from each parent. To summarize:

- Animals with one copy of the abnormal gene are carriers and will show no signs of disease.
- The progeny of two carriers will have 1 in 4 chance of being affected or normal, and a 1 in 2 chance of carrying the disorder.

There is now a diagnostic test available from Bristol University for detecting both carriers and sufferers. Obtaining samples of DNA for study requires only a blood or saliva sample.

PK deficiency can also affect various breeds of dog and is a very severe disease. Affected dogs die mainly before they are 4 years old. Cats do not generally develop severe problems and may have a normal life span; however, they may develop intermittent anaemia with variable symptoms. Some develop severe lethargy, weakness, anorexia and lose weight and they may have pale mucous membranes. Damaged red cells are removed from the blood by the spleen, resulting in an enlarged spleen, and the destruction of red cells results in the release of bilirubin, causing jaundice. However, the body is good at making new red blood cells so anaemia is often mild or occurs gradually. Occasionally a severe, life-threatening anaemia may develop.

Feline blood grouping

Incompatible blood groups between the stud tomcat and the queen can lead to the devastating loss of whole litters of kittens. This problem can be solved by screening the prospective parents' blood and avoiding the mating of incompatible animals. One scheme for the identification of feline blood groups by screening is offered at the University of Glasgow by Dr Diane Addie, who also maintains a register of blood-typed stud toms and queens (Addie 2004). This problem is discussed further in Chapter 14.

Future trends in biotechnology

Cloning of animals

Genetically identical animals are produced naturally every time an early embryo splits into two or more to produce identical twins, triplets, etc. From the 1970s embryos have been split in the laboratory and each of the resulting embryos inserted into a different mother. This form of cloning has been widespread in livestock breeding (Nicholas 2003). Cloning by transferring the nucleus of a somatic cell into an unfertilized ovum was introduced in the 1980s, culminating in the birth of Dolly the sheep in February 1997. Since then many animals have been cloned in this way but the technology has major problems:

- The success rate is very low – only 1–2% of cloned embryos survive

- Many die soon after birth
- Survivors suffer from abnormalities, including abnormal enzyme expression and poor immunity.

If the technique can be perfected, gene replacement will be more effective, replacement organs and tissues could be grown and it could be used in the conservation of rare species.

Transgenesis

Transgenesis involves the insertion of genes from one species to another, e.g. a human gene into a pig. As the genetic code is universal the transferred gene will work in its new environment. The new animal is described as transgenic. The first transgenic animals were mice produced in 1980. Pigs and sheep were produced to manufacture human growth hormone in 1985. The technique is mainly used in disease research. Another use is in the production of human polypeptides for use in pharmaceuticals. Financial and ethical considerations may limit the use of this technique.

Gene therapy

Therapeutic uses of recombinant DNA techniques include gene therapy, i.e. 'the deliberate introduction of genetic material into human somatic cells for therapeutic, prophylactic or diagnostic purposes' (UK Gene Therapy Advisory Committee definition quoted in Turnpenny & Ellard 2007). When the gene enters the new cell it may change the way the cell works or the chemicals that the cell secretes. The identification of many abnormal genes and their products has led to possibilities of treatments for some important diseases, both human and animal. It overcomes the major problem of transplantation, as genes work within the cell and are not affected by immune rejection. However, it is unlikely to be of use in animal therapy, where best practice would prevent breeding from any abnormal animals by carrier detection.

Bibliography

Addie, D., 2004. What Are Feline Blood Groups? Available online at: <http://www.dr-addie.com>.

BBC programme, 2008. 'Pedigree Dogs Exposed'. <http://news.bbc.co.uk/1/hi/uk/7569064.stm>.

Budiansky, S., 2002. Happening Cats. Available online at: <http://www.smithsonianmag.si.edu.smithsonian/issues02/sept02/phenomenas.html>.

Carroll, S.B., 2006, The Making of the Fittest. Quercus, London.

Dekomien, G., Epplen, J.T., 2003. Evaluation of the canine RPE65 gene in affected dogs with generalized progressive retinal atrophy. Mol. Vis. 9, 601–605.

Dog Genetic Disease, 2009. RUF Dog Health Problems. <http://doghealthproblems.

co.uk/dog-genetic-disease/weeeee>.

Feline Advisory Bureau, 2004. Information Sheet Number 32. Polycystic Kidney Disease (PKD) in Cats. Feline Advisory Bureau, Tisbury, Wiltshire. Available online at: <http://www.fabcats.org/pkd.html>.

Gould, L.L., 2007. Cats Are Not Peas, second ed. A K Peters, Copernicus, New York.

Guynup, S., 2000, Genetic Testing for Dogs. Genome News Network, Rockville, MD. Available online at: <http://www.genomenewsnetwork.org/articles/07_00/genetic_testing_dogs.shtml>.

Jorde, L., Carey, J., Bamshad, M.J., White, R., 2006. Medical Genetics, third ed. (updated) Mosby, St Louis, MO.

Little, S., 2008. Feline Genetics: What Technicians Need to Know (proceedings). <http://veterinarycalenfdar.dvm360.com/avhc/Veterinary+technicians/Feline-genetics>.

Meyers-Wallen, V.N., 2003. Ethics and genetic selection in purebred dogs. Reprod. Domest. Anim. 38 (1), 73–76.

Nicholas, F.W., 2003 (update due October 2009). Introduction to Veterinary Genetics, second ed. Blackwell, Oxford.

Padgett, G.A., Duffendack, J.C., 2004. Canine molecular diseases. Compend. Contin. Educ. Dent. 22, 480–489. Available online at: <http://www.med.umich.edu/hg/RESEARCH/FACULTY/Brewer/compendium.htm>.

Peteducation.com. Hip Dysplasia in Dogs: Diagnosis, Treatment and Prevention <http://www.peteducation.com/article.cfm?c=2+1569&aid=444> (accessed 11.5.2009).

Ruvinsky, A., Sampson, J., 2001. The Genetics of the Dog. Kennel Club, London.

Turnpenny, P., Ellard, S., 2007. Emery's Elements of Medical Genetics, thirteenth ed. Churchill Livingstone, Elsevier.

Vella, C.M., Shelton, L.M., McGonagle, J.J., Stanglein, T.W., 1999. Robinson's Genetics for Cat Breeders and Veterinarians, fourth ed. Butterworth-Heinemann, Oxford.

Recommended reading

Jorde, L., Carey, J., Bamshad, M.J., White, R., 2006. Medical Genetics, third ed. Mosby, St Louis, MO.

This textbook on medical genetics presents its subject matter clearly and is illustrated by good diagrams. Although it is aimed at those interested in human genetics, the basic science is presented in a sensible progression to maximize understanding.

Nicholas, F.W., 2003 (to be updated late 2009). Introduction to Veterinary Genetics, second ed. Blackwell, Oxford.

This is an excellent textbook on veterinary genetics. The detailed contents pages make it easy to follow and it progresses information from the basic sciences to application to future developments.

Pet Education.com. Hip Dysplasia in Dogs: Diagnosis, Treatment and Prevention. Available at: <http://www.peteducation.com/article.cfm?c=2+1569&aid=444> (accessed 11.5.2009).

This paper is included because of its comprehensive and up-to-date data about hip dysplasia.

Vella, C.M., Shelton, L.M., McGonagle, J.J., Stanglein, T.W., 1999. Robinson's Genetics for Cat Breeders and Veterinarians, fourth ed. Butterworth-Heinemann, Oxford.

This is a long-established textbook on genetics aimed at cat breeders and vets. Although the subject is dealt with in depth, as it is written with breeders as well as professionals in mind, it is easily understood.

CHAPTER 14

Practical animal breeding

Dorothy Stables and Gareth Lawler

Key Points

- Pedigree animals are the result of selective breeding. Inbreeding, line breeding and outbreeding are strategies used by breeders to select for traits such as hair colour, body type and behaviour.
- Breeding stock, i.e. the stud male and the breeding bitch or queen, must be selected with care using criteria based on health, temperament and adherence to the breed standard.
- The mating process usually takes place on the stud male's territory and must be carefully monitored to avoid injury to either individual.
- The dam must be cared for during pregnancy and consideration must be given to nutrition, exercise, vaccination and preventative worming treatment.
- Parturition takes place in three stages and knowledge of these will ensure the delivery of healthy offspring.
- In some cases the dam may need assistance or the neonate may need extra care in order to survive.
- Colostrum ingested within the first 24 hours of life provides protective antibodies for the neonate.
- All kittens and puppies must be treated for roundworms and vaccinated.
- All pedigree animals should be registered with the appropriate organization.

Introduction

The aim of this chapter is to provide an insight into breeding pedigree animals from a breeder's point of view. The two authors, Dorothy Stables and Gareth Lawler, are both experienced breeders and in the following two sections they explain how they produce healthy kittens and puppies.

Breeding pedigree cats

Dorothy Stables

About 200 million years ago, mammals arose. They coexisted with the huge dinosaurs and were small, warm-blooded, covered in fur and fed their babies with milk but probably also laid eggs. By 65 million years ago there were many species but suddenly all the dinosaurs disappeared, as did the majority of birds and fishes. Something cataclysmic happened, possibly the arrival of an immense asteroid that landed in the Caribbean Sea. Clouds of dust cut out the light from the sun. The small, warm-blooded mammals could control their own body temperatures and were at an advantage, so most survived. By 45 million years ago all the major groups of mammals alive today had evolved. True cats are found in the fossil records from about 25 million years ago. Feline domestication may have begun in Egypt (see also Ch. 10). The African wild cat (*Felis libyca*) began to live around the grain stores, catching small rodents. Gradually the more tame amongst them allowed humans to play with their kittens. Domestication led to selective breeding for favoured features such as hair colour and length.

Selective breeding

Pedigree animals are the result of selective breeding, where specific favourable traits are chosen to be perpetuated by the breeder. In the latter half of the 19th century people started to breed specific types of cat and over the last century about 30 recognized breeds have been developed (Fig. 14.1). Alterations in features occur because natural mutations are already present in wild cats. Generally, one of the two alleles for a characteristic such as coat colour mutates but is recessive. When two cats both carrying the mutated gene mate a new characteristic appears (see Ch. 13).

Breeding strategies

'The good and bad points of the individual cats (or dogs) should be assessed and weighed against each other before mating' (Vella et al 1999):

- **Inbreeding** is the mating of closely related individuals such as father and daughter or siblings. How closely these animals are related can be calculated using the mathematical concept of the inbreeding coefficient, which can be defined as 'the probability that the two genes present at a locus in an individual are identical by descent'.

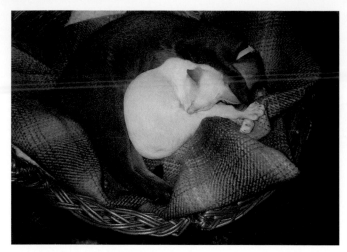

Fig. 14.1 Two short-haired breeds; a Usual Abyssinian neuter male cuddling a red point Siamese male kitten

- **Line breeding** is the mating of animals with shared ancestors but not as closely related as in inbreeding. The word 'line' is probably related to the term 'blood line'. Both strategies are used by breeders to select for desired traits, but there is a risk with mating related animals that they may both carry a harmful recessive gene and this would be expressed in the homozygous individual – a condition known as **inbreeding depression**. Advances in genetics should help breeders to identify and eliminate many harmful genes over the next few years.
- **Outbreeding** or the mating of two unrelated individuals is a method of reducing inbreeding depression. Crossbreeds, mongrels or simply 'moggies', are the extreme form of outbreeding. However, Vella et al (1999) quote Joan Miller, then vice president of the Winn Feline Foundation as saying that 'In the majority of breeds it is now impossible to find two cats unrelated to each other because every pedigree is based on a few early founding cats'.
- **Gene linkage** is another problem associated with selecting closely related animals and is a situation where a desired trait may carry with it an abnormality – if the two genes lie close together on a chromosome they may be inherited together (see Ch. 13); for example, blue eyes are often associated with white coat colour and deafness.

Two inheritable feline characteristics, coat colour and behaviour, are briefly discussed to show why an understanding of genetics is important for cat breeders.

Coat colour

Pigment production – genes in the melanocytes at the base of the hair follicles influence the production of hair pigments. As discussed in Chapter 13 (Box 13.2), eumelanin is a black pigment and phaeomelanin produces a yellowish ground colour. The dominant gene that controls the colour deposition known as agouti (A) produces agouti protein 'A', which gives a hair that is black at the tip and yellow at the base. Its recessive partner, which codes for non-agouti, is

designated 'a'. When the amount of agouti protein within the melanocytes reaches a certain level, production of eumelanin stops and that of phaeomelanin begins.

All cats have a second system of pigmentation superimposing a pattern of dark markings on the agouti coat. Some areas of skin have a poor response to agouti protein and then the hairs are coloured from base to tip by eumelanin and are black. Alternating bands of agouti and black produce the tabby pattern. In cats who are homozygous for the recessive mutation called non-agouti 'a/a', a defective agouti protein is produced that does not affect eumelanin production. The phenotype of these cats is the self black cat.

Coat colour genes – the three basic colours, black, chocolate and cinnamon, are coded for by the gene TYRP1 or tyrosine-related protein or mutants of that gene. This gene is called the B locus. The enzyme produced by TYRP1 is located in melanocytes, which produce the melanin that gives animal skin, hair and eyes their colour. TYRP1 may stabilize the enzyme tyranosinase, which is responsible for the first step in melanin production . Two different mutations of this gene give the two shades of brown known as chocolate (b-) and cinnamon (b^1/b^1 recessive) (Lyons et al 2005). Testing for these changes in the TYRP1 gene is now available at different laboratories and can determine which gene is present and therefore the colour of the cat if, as in the Somali cat, it may not be clear to the eye.

The three basic colours can be modified by the presence of other genes:

- The dominant inhibitor gene (I) suppresses the amount of pigment fed into the hair, resulting in the presence of white hairs with coloured tips.
- The recessive dilute gene (dd) causes pigment granules to be enlarged and deposited unevenly along the hair: the hair may be very lightly pigmented.
- The sex-linked orange (O) gene causes the production of phaeomelanin, resulting in a male ginger cat or female tortoiseshell.

Behaviour

Behaviour is partly instinctive (inherited) and partly learned. However, instinctive behaviour is fine-tuned by learning. Fogle (1991) believes that we can attribute human mental characteristics to cats because their brains are wired up like ours. Cats learn quickly and anticipate events such as feeding. My cat Filly remembers that she is fed separately from the other cats so she does not run into the kitchen with the rest, but goes to where her food is served.

Learning requires input from parents, litter mates and humans (Turner and Bateson 2000). Socialization is the breeder's responsibility (see Ch. 10). There is a sensitive period from 2 to 7 weeks when kittens need handling for at least 40 min a day if they are to interact with humans. Petting, playing with and talking to them (Fig. 14.2) is more important than feeding for their social development (Karsh 1983; Halls 2007). Behaviour must be considered when choosing a kitten for breeding or showing.

Breeding practices

Rice (1997) suggests that professional cat breeders take cat breeding seriously, with 'carefully planned agendas and

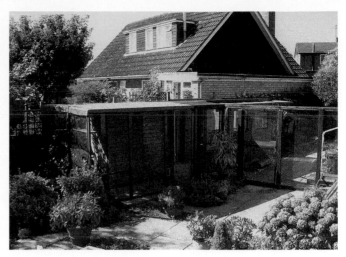

Fig. 14.3 Typical stud quarters

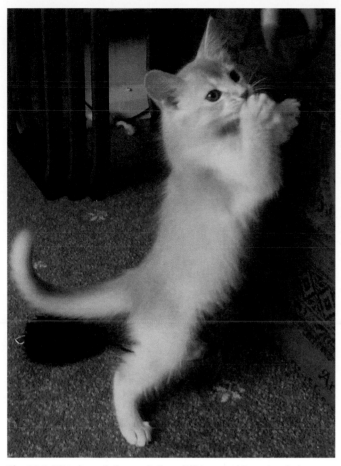

Fig. 14.2 Mistral, a red silver male Somali kitten aged 8 weeks, playing with an unseen human

well-defined motives'. They may wish to develop a particular breed to enhance certain desirable features such as coat colour or head shape, or they may wish to breed for showing.

Buying a breeding queen

Before buying a breeding queen, consider the following:

- Is the home suitable for rearing kittens? Ornaments scattered around a house may not survive a healthy litter of kittens and trailing wires may be dangerous.
- Is the expense prohibitive?
- It is better to buy a kitten rather than an older queen so that there is time to develop a bond before the first litter of kittens comes along. The potential queen should be visited in her home and her siblings and mother should be observed for type and behaviour. If the stud is owned by the breeder he should also be looked at. The pedigrees of the animal should be checked to exclude potential problems:
  - Is there a suitable stud cat in the vicinity? Some of the rarer breeds of cat may be scattered around the country, requiring a lengthy journey with a howling queen!
  - Although all kittens will have had a health check when they were vaccinated, new owners may wish their own vet to examine the kitten before purchasing it.

- The new owner should receive a receipt of purchase, a four-generation pedigree, a certificate of kitten registration and transfer of ownership with a suitable body such as the Governing Council of the Cat Fancy (GCCF), certificate of vaccination and advice on caring for the kitten.

The stud cat

Most breeders will not sell a stud tom to someone until they have been breeding for 4 or 5 years and own two or three queens. During that time they will have had experience of how other people manage their stud cat. He will need his own quarters (Fig. 14.3) near to the house because of urine spraying. They will need to be airy in summer and heated in winter, with a run attached so that he can exercise. The owner should be able to sit in with the stud and play with him.

If he is to have visiting queens there should be suitable quarters where the queen can be kept near to him but can be separated if the need arrives. He should be introduced to his stud quarters at about 16 weeks old so that by the time he matures he is happy and familiar with his own territory. A stud tom should be chosen with as much care as a breeding queen. His pedigree should be studied and discussed so that any relationships between the queens and the stud are recognized.

The mating process

The queen

Sexual maturity in a queen occurs between 5 and 12 months. However, she may not be physically or psychologically ready to have kittens and should be at least 1 year old before mating (Rice 1997). She could be allowed a breeding life of about 5 years during which she should have no more than two litters every 18 months.

Queens show few obvious physical signs of the oestrous cycle or being 'in heat' although some develop pinkness and a slight swelling of the tissue around their vaginal orifice. However, their behaviour can be quite dramatic, with vocalization (calling) and posturing. Owners have taken a queen to the vet because she was crying so loudly they thought she was in pain! Because a queen may be ready to mate without showing signs, no entire female should be allowed to go outside. The local tomcats from miles around will know she is ready!

Oestrus often begins with the queen rolling around on the floor and purring. She then shows lordosis, which involves lowering her chest, lifting up her bottom and placing her tail to one side while treading with her back legs. Oestrus can last from 3–10 days but is shortened if the queen is mated. During oestrus the female will allow the male to mount and copulate.

Cats are induced ovulators, which maximizes the chance of fertilization. Copulation releases luteinizing hormone (LH), which stimulates ovulation (see Ch. 4). The level of LH increases with each copulation so that fertilization and pregnancy are more likely to occur. Breeders allow mating over 3 days. As the penis is withdrawn from the queen's vagina the scratching of the papillae or spines covering the glans penis may stimulate a rise in LH levels.

The stud cat

A tom shows signs of sexual activity at about 7–8 months of age and may mate with a receptive queen. From about 10 months old a stud is capable of fathering kittens but this does not mean he is ready to work. The owner must allow time for him to mature.

Boy meets girl

It is usual to take the queen to the stud's home for mating. Some males prefer their own territory, as it gives them confidence. A receptive queen should be introduced to the stud cat carefully. She may be left in her carrying basket to see how the two cats react. The journey may affect the queen and it may be 24 hours before she returns to being receptive. A maiden queen should be taken to an experienced tom and a young tom should be allowed a mature, experienced queen for his first mating. If all seems well they should be allowed to have physical contact with each other. She may show her willingness by calling, rolling and flirting. The tom will respond by making a low, throaty noise. He watches for signs of acceptance and, at an opportune moment, runs in and grabs the queen by the neck. He has to be quick as she may attack him. The queen responds to the neck grasp as a kitten does, by remaining still while he mounts her (Morris 1996). With a few thrusts, he deposits his semen before withdrawing his penis. At this point the queen often screams loudly and turns to attack him. Each act of copulation takes only about 10 seconds.

Experienced studs have their escape route planned and will only let go when they can safely run. Both cats now settle down apart and vigorously wash their genital regions. Cats will mate several times in a day. Matings rarely require human intervention but it is wise to be nearby. Occasionally a tom may be too rough or a queen attack too harshly and the cats may need to be separated for a while.

Aftercare of the queen

After mating the queen may continue to call for a few days, so other entire males should not have access to her. After this, her appetite, reduced during calling, and her behaviour will return to normal. Her neck should be examined for tooth marks and any damage should be treated. Puncture wounds extending through the skin should always be examined by a veterinarian.

Pregnancy

The average length of pregnancy in the domestic cat is 63 days or 9 weeks, but a range of 58–70 days is accepted. If parturition occurs earlier than this the kittens may not be viable and if later, size problems may occur, requiring urgent intervention. There is no accepted blood or urine test available for diagnosing feline pregnancy. A vet may be able to palpate the fetuses at 15–20 days of gestation, but this is dangerous if done by inexperienced people as too much pressure may cause the loss of the kittens. Ultrasound imaging can be used from 15 days.

Breeders become experts in diagnosing pregnancy. At 21 days the queen's nipples become more vascular and turn a rosy pink. Later the nipples grow larger and a discrete area of hair loss occurs around them, often aided by the queen plucking hairs. By 35 days there should be a noticeable increase in abdominal girth and by 49 days the individual kittens may be observed and felt to move.

A queen who fails to conceive may call again any time between 28 days and towards the end of the anticipated pregnancy. Some develop a phantom pregnancy (pseudocyesis), during which their abdomens increase in girth and they do not return to oestrus. Rice (1997) believes this usually follows attempts to stimulate the vagina, produce ovulation and end oestrus artificially.

Care of the pregnant queen

Nutrition

As pregnancy progresses beyond the second week the queen requires more calories. Her daily calorie intake should increase by 70% and her body weight will steadily increase due to the rapid growth of the fetuses and the storage of fat for lactation (Rice 1997). This can be achieved by increasing the number of times a day she is fed from two to four and by giving her free access to whatever dried food she enjoys.

Nesting behaviour

As pregnancy progresses the queen seeks out a secluded place in which to have her kittens. She can be provided with two or three alternative places, which she will inspect and rearrange. If this is not done she will choose her own place, which could well be the sofa! A cardboard box that can be disposed of after the event makes an excellent nest. There are commercial boxes available (Fig. 14.4) but a queen may not like them! Any box should be large enough to allow her to stretch out and accommodate mother and kittens for at least 5 weeks. It should be enclosed, with an opening big enough for the mother to go in and out but high enough to keep the kittens confined. Bedding should be smooth and flat at first so that the kittens cannot find their way beneath the layers. A piece of synthetic fleece (Vetbed) over which a piece of sheeting can be placed is ideal. Material such as towels and blankets with loops should be avoided, as they may trap the kittens' claws and damage their feet.

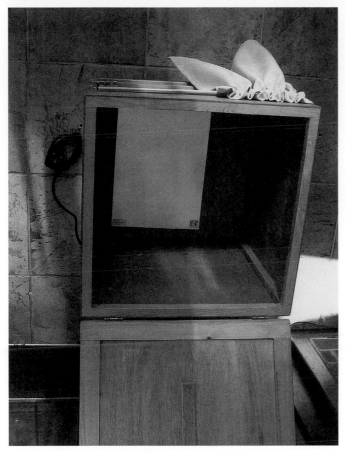

Fig. 14.4 A commercially-made kittening box

Parturition

Cats usually give birth without human interference and queens who have been given too much attention during delivery have been known to abandon their kittens (Rice 1997). However, breeding for different body shapes has increased birth problems in the modern Siamese cat and the Persian cat (Feline Advisory Bureau 2008).

A breeder should be ready to give assistance if necessary. Equipment likely to be needed includes:

- Haemostat forceps, dental floss and blunt-ended scissors for dealing with the umbilical cords
- An antiseptic solution in a shallow dish for sterilizing the instruments
- Warm, disposable cloths for receiving the kittens
- Cotton swabs
- A 2 ml syringe without needle for neonatal resuscitation
- Bags for disposing of bloodstained articles.

Signs of parturition

The onset of parturition or labour can be predicted by taking the queen's rectal temperature every 8 hours for a day or two before the expected date of delivery (EDD). There will be a drop from the normal 38.5°C to 37°C about 12 hours before labour begins. Behavioural signs are also good indicators and include reduced appetite, restlessness, pacing, making frequent visits to the nesting place, licking the genitalia and discomfort. My queens come for me when they are in early labour and insist on taking me to the delivery place! One young queen likes to get into a sleeping basket and cuddle up to her mother, an old neutered female.

During the first stage of labour, uterine contractions dilate the cervix and move the kittens towards the body of the uterus. There is usually a clear, odourless discharge of mucus, which may become tinged with blood just before delivery. Cats, though uncomfortable, rarely cry out but, in the presence of their owners, may purr loudly which is thought to indicate low-grade pain. It is difficult to pinpoint the onset of the first stage but it probably isn't necessary as long as the cat is not distressed. Normal progress is more important than length of time (Rice 1997).

The second stage is the delivery of the kittens and the third stage, which usually follows immediately for each kitten, is the delivery of placenta and membranes. If the queen has been walking about she will now lie down in her kittening box. The uterine contractions become stronger and she will actively push. A bubble of amniotic fluid may appear at the vulva but this usually bursts and slightly bloodstained amniotic fluid escapes. It is not normal to see quantities of fresh blood.

Kittens may be born head first (anterior presentation) or tail and hind legs first (posterior presentation) but as long as progress is made it does not matter. This stage may take up to 1 hour for the first kitten and the length is best related to progress and frequency of contractions rather than time. It is shortened to about 5 min or less for subsequent kittens. Once the kitten is born the mother clears the membranes from its nose and mouth, chews and separates the umbilical cord and eats the placenta.

Following the birth of the first kitten there is usually a short delay of 10 min to 1 hour before the birth of the next kitten. This gives the mother time to clean the first kitten and for it to find a nipple and commence suckling. Occasionally labour is interrupted for a time and the mother rests happily with the kittens already born.

Assisted delivery

This is usually only necessary during the late second stage where a kitten has partially emerged but progress does not continue. Most queens will deliver themselves if time is allowed, as demonstrated by my own cat Scampy, who is small but progressed in labour very well until the time came to push. An hour went by and Scampy valiantly pushed with no obvious progress. I was about to call my vet when she suddenly leapt out of her box and wedged herself upright in the angle of a corner in a 'defecating position'. Two minutes later the first kitten popped out bottom first and the other three kittens followed quickly.

Normally, if the kitten is halfway out, gentle traction should be attempted. A dry cloth should be wrapped around the kitten and, taking care to avoid compressing internal organs, traction should be applied to complete the delivery. The direction of traction is important: it should follow the shape of the feline birth canal downwards towards the mother's feet and backwards away from her body.

Resuscitating a kitten

Newborn kittens soon establish regular respirations. If a kitten continues gasping or if bubbles of fluid are coming down its nose and out of its mouth, help is needed. The mouth and nostrils should be wiped and suction using a small syringe can be used to extract mucus. A vigorous drying with a warm towel may stimulate respiration.

If the kitten is still in difficulty, some suggest holding the kitten belly down wrapped in a cloth so it is not slippery. With its head away from you but supported, swing the kitten in an arc from your waist to near the floor. This manoeuvre creates a centrifugal force that extrudes fluid from its lungs and trachea. After two swings, massage its chest. If there is still no response, hold its mouth open and blow very gently into its mouth from a distance of several inches (remember how small its lungs are). If after half an hour there is no response, stop the procedure.

Completion of parturition

Ensure that all the placentas are delivered and that there is no heavy bleeding. The kittens should be warm, dry and vigorous and have found a nipple to suckle (Fig. 14.5). Following the birth the queen will clean herself and may even take a little food and water. She may not pass urine for 24 hours and will then pass a large quantity. She should resume normal defecation at the same time.

Caring for the family

The kittens should only be checked to ensure that their condition is satisfactory. The family should be given a peaceful and quiet environment to ensure that the queen accepts and cares for them (Fig. 14.6). After 3 days a confident queen will allow handling of her kittens.

The queen's milk provides all necessary nutrients. Colostrum provides all the antibodies the kittens need. The hair from around the nipples could be trimmed before birth if the queen has long hair. The first 6 weeks put a great strain on the queen's nutritional status: she may lose 25% of her body weight and will need extra food. Once the kittens begin to eat solid food the queen's food intake will decrease, although she will continue to suckle them until they go to their new homes. Her mammary glands should be inspected frequently for signs of sore nipples or mastitis and her milk will gradually reduce as the kittens eat more.

Most queens spend 90% of their time with their kittens during the first two weeks (Rice 1997). She will lick their urogenital area to stimulate them to pass urine and faeces and consume their excretions until they are weaned. If the queen is disturbed or if the bedding becomes soiled she may move her kittens.

Neonatal examination

Each kitten should be carefully examined for any abnormality such as extra digits or cleft palate. The sex and weight of each kitten are recorded. If the litter are all the same colour some breeders identify them early by marking up a specific claw with nail polish. A spot of the same colour or notification of which toe is coloured is made in their records.

Ongoing development

Development proceeds in a craniocaudal manner, with control of the head, forelegs and hind legs developing in that order. Eyes should open between days 8 and 10 and cords usually fall off between the 3rd and 6th day. By 3 weeks the kittens wobble unsteadily around the inside of their box and a few days later they climb out and begin to explore. Specialized kitten food can now be fed to them. The aim is to wean them by about 6 weeks. As soon as the kittens begin to eat solid food they should be provided with a litter tray. They will play in this at first, digging holes. Shortly afterwards they will use it for its intended purpose.

Hand-rearing kittens

There are times when the mother is incapable of feeding her kittens or has so many she cannot cope. The young kittens must be kept warm, dry and clean and will need to be fed every 2 hours day and night for three weeks. It is important to obtain special kitten milk, as cow's milk is not suitable. It is possible to buy miniature bottles and teats but an eye dropper can be equally useful. Care must be taken to avoid inhalation of milk, which could lead to pneumonia and death. As much care should be taken over sterilizing the

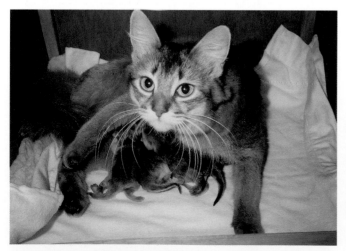

Fig. 14.5 Molly, a chocolate Somali, feeding her newborn kittens

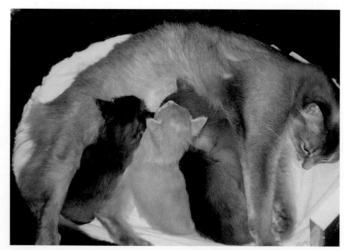

Fig. 14.6 Scampy, a tortoiseshell Somali queen, and her sex-linked kittens – a red male, a cream male and two tortie females

feeding equipment as would be used for a human baby, as infection is a great killer of young animals. If the queen is not caring for the kittens at all, their anal and vulval regions must be stimulated gently with damp, warm cotton wool to enable them to urinate and defecate.

Aftercare of the litter

Vaccination

Cats are subject to some dangerous pathogenic organisms and may become seriously ill or die, so all kittens should be vaccinated. In the UK the first vaccinations are given at 9 weeks, followed by a repeated dose at 12 weeks. Typically a kitten is vaccinated against feline panleucopenia (feline infectious enteritis), feline respiratory viruses (cat flu) and leukaemia (FAB 2008). Show cats may also be vaccinated against *Chlamydia*.

Worming

All kittens should be treated for the roundworm *Toxocara cati*. Although the lifecycle (see Ch. 27) of this worm means that the larvae do not cross the placenta into the fetal kittens, they do pass into the mammary glands so the kittens become infected when taking their first drink. Kittens should be routinely treated from 1 month old, repeated at monthly intervals until the kitten is 6 months of age and then every 3 months throughout life.

Registering and selling kittens

All pedigree kittens have to be registered with a formal organization if they are to be sold as pedigree cats, used in a breeding programme or shown. In the UK the Governing Council of the Cat Fancy (GCCF) is the main organization. Details of the kittens' parents and grandparents, their sex, colour and birth date are recorded.

It is essential to find a good home for the kittens and most breeders wish to meet the prospective purchasers before a sale is agreed. Some will deliver the kitten to its new home as a final check on suitability. The breeder must provide the purchaser with:

* A four-generation signed pedigree
* The vaccination certificate
* A certificate of transfer of ownership
* A receipt of payment.

Also recommended are:

* An advice sheet on caring for their kitten
* Insurance to cover the first 6 weeks following transfer
* Contact readily provided to discuss problems.

Showing cats

The first major cat show in the world was held at the Crystal Palace on 23 July 1871, organized by Harrison Weir. The shows are run by the official bodies such as the GCCF and certificates and titles are awarded. Kittens can be shown from 14 weeks and queens can be shown 12 weeks after they have given birth. Any cat that attends a show is 'vetted in' and may be excluded from the show if it appears ill, is pregnant, has dirty ears, fleas or other parasites or has a skin lesion of any kind. If a cat is taken ill during the show there is a duty vet

to see to it and a room is set aside as a hospital. Cat breeding is challenging, exciting and rewarding as long as the breeder follows the rules.

Breeding pedigree dogs

Gareth Lawler

Selective breeding

The artificial evolution of dogs into many different types with morphological diversity and variation in size, which is seen in few other species, is a direct consequence of years of selective breeding by man. This has resulted in the creation of a range of purebreds with individual traits and characteristics. Modern day breeds are a standardization of the desirable traits of some of the older breeds, especially those characteristics that have been useful over long periods of time. It is, or at least should be, the aim of dog breeders today to attempt to perpetuate those traits while simultaneously paying great heed to the maintenance of a friendly disposition, a characteristic so essential for a family pet.

Breeding strategies

For definitions of inbreeding and line breeding return to the section on cat breeding.

The brood bitch

The most valuable asset for anyone striving to breed good stock is a good brood bitch. There is more to breeding dogs than just producing pretty-looking specimens and the aim is to produce puppies that are sound both mentally and physically.

Consider the following factors:

* Health – avoid a bitch that has a history of ill health.
* Temperament and disposition – until the puppies go to their new homes, the pups continually learn from and even mimic the mother. Do not even consider a bitch as a breeding prospect if she panics easily.
* Freedom from hereditary diseases – there is increasing awareness of breed-specific hereditary traits and many breeds now require certain health checks before breeding. By the time a breeder reaches this stage, he/she should be fully aware of the problems the respective breed may have and which tests are required prior to breeding.
* Breed standard – as well as exhibiting special traits of the lines concerned, she should descend from very good specimens of the breed and should not depart by any significant degree from the breed standard.
* Inheritability – the ability of the bitch to pass on desirable features to her offspring.

No expense should be spared in the acquisition of a suitable bitch for breeding, as she will prove her worth time and time again. The brood bitch is the key to the immediate future because she has much more influence on her puppies than just her contribution to their genetic make-up. You should never be tempted to breed from an immature bitch.

Age of maturity differs between breeds and some breed clubs have introduced 'codes of ethics' pertaining to the minimum age for breeding from your bitch. It is essential that she is allowed to mature both physically and mentally so that she will have the confidence to cope with her own litter.

The bitch should be kept in the peak of condition, during her pregnancy and also prior to mating. She should be up-to-date with her vaccinations before mating, and she must also have been wormed regularly.

Some stud dog owners require all visiting bitches to have a vaginal swab tested as a precaution against any foreign bacteria or infections before they will use their dog. The veterinary surgeon will prescribe appropriate medication to clear any infection prior to mating, as long as the bitch is swabbed as early as possible during her season.

The stud dog

In a similar way to the brood bitch, whatever the breed, quality or even pedigree, the stud dog should satisfy some basic criteria before he is deemed suitable to pass his genes to the next generation. He must be sexually mature, entire and in good health, both physically and mentally, and, ideally, he should be mature in growth and development. It is unwise to use a young male before he has developed his adult characteristics, as he may depart from the breed standard as he matures. Some hereditary conditions, e.g. hip dysplasia and progressive retinal atrophy, are not always obvious until the dog is well into middle or old age. The older a dog is, and the more bitches he has covered, the smaller the chance of him producing an 'affected' puppy if he has not already done so.

The choice of stud dog should result from exhaustive research and breeders should be aware that no dog is suitable for every bitch – such a dog has still to be born (Fig. 14.7)!

The mating game

The bitch will normally come into season every 6 months, although some bitches, particularly in the larger breeds, cycle every 8–10 months. It is not uncommon for some bitches to go as long as 12 months between seasons. The period of oestrus or 'heat' usually lasts about 3 weeks, and the most notable sign is vaginal bleeding. Bitches vary as to the stage of the heat when they start to bleed, many starting almost at day 1 and others not until the end of the first week. Vaginal swelling is another sign of oestrus.

The optimum time to mate should be at the time the bitch ovulates. Bitches are spontaneous ovulators and textbooks indicate that the bitch ovulates on day 10 of the cycle; however, this can be variable and may be difficult to assess in some bitches. It is a fact that some bitches will ovulate as early as day 3 or as late as day 23. There are several tests available now to determine the exact time of ovulation and thus the optimum time for mating. These involve monitoring vaginal cytology and a hormonal assay. If the bitch has had a history of unsuccessful matings, it is advisable to seek veterinary advice and have, if necessary, daily or twice daily blood samples taken to determine an accurate ovulation time. There is also an ovulation detector available on the

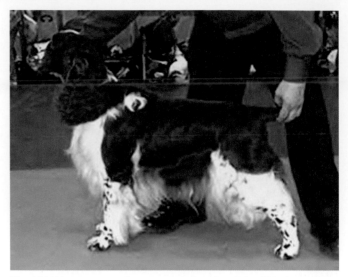

Fig. 14.7 Never compromise on your choice of stud dog. This dog was the UK's top winning English springer spaniel at the time

market that detects changes in the electrical conductivity of the lining of the uterus. This method, although available to everyone with only an initial cost in purchase of the equipment, has received a mixed reception in the dog world, some breeders proclaiming exceptional results, while others have had no improvement in their results at all. It is as well to remember that, whatever the chosen method, conception and pregnancy, even when all eventualities have seemingly been covered, can never be guaranteed!

The process of mating involves mounting by the dog and then the 'tie' during which the penis is locked into the bitch's vagina by the contraction of her vaginal muscles. The actual mechanics of mating are another potential pitfall. Some matings may take a matter of seconds before a 'tie' results, while others take rather longer. Some bitches will develop an exceptionally strong liking for a particular male, so strong that all other males may be rejected. Very often males will mount and dismount the bitch for a period of time before thrusting forward and penetrating the bitch. If the dog seems to be in position, and yet fails to get a mating, there is a possibility that the bitch has a stricture, something that will need veterinary intervention.

Once penetration occurs, there should follow a stage where the male lies on the female's back, and after a short time he will try and lift one leg over the bitch to stand rear to rear in a classic 'tie' position. It is thought by some that the purpose of the 'tie' is to prolong the mating time, as the ejaculate in a dog is dispensed in three fractions, but it would probably be rather more truthful to admit that nobody really knows why they do it – we just accept the fact that they do! The 'tie' position can last from just a few minutes to over 1 hour, and it is important to understand that it is a mutual action by the dog and the bitch, with the swelling of the bulb at the end of a dog's penis coinciding with constriction of the vaginal muscles of the bitch. It is still possible to get puppies produced in the absence of a 'tie' but most breeders feel more comfortable if a 'tie' has occurred. It is also worth noting that some dogs of certain breeds, e.g. West Highland white terriers, are well known for not 'tying' and yet are still able to produce normal litters.

Pregnancy

Pregnancy lasts for about 63 days on average but the length of gestation depends not only on the bitch and when she was mated but also on the breed – some breeds have a tendency for a longer or shorter gestation period. The normal range is considered to be 57–68 days.

It is possible to determine pregnancy from as early as 28 days by careful palpation of the abdomen. At this stage, golf-ball-like structures can sometimes be felt. From 35 days, these structures will become less palpable as their weight pulls them down into the abdomen and after this time it may not be possible for another 2–3 weeks to determine whether the bitch is pregnant.

The growth rate of the embryo is very slow for the first 35 days and this is when organogenesis takes place, but after this stage the growth of the fetus should become increasingly rapid. This should enable the owner to tell if the bitch is pregnant, but again it has been known for bitches not to 'show' until a week before they are due, when they seem to 'blow up' overnight. Ultrasound is an accurate way to determine whether a bitch is pregnant but, although it is possible to see the puppies from about 3 weeks, partial reabsorption of the litter may occur and you may not get as many puppies as you thought you would.

Antenatal care

The bitch should be treated as normal for the first 6 weeks. After this time the amount of food should be gradually increased, so she is having about 1.5 times as much as normal by the time of whelping. It is also advisable to split the food into several smaller meals throughout the day.

During pregnancy or prior to mating the bitch should be given a booster vaccination. This will raise the levels of maternal antibodies that she will pass to her puppies in the colostrum or first milk. She should also be treated for roundworms (*Toxocara canis*) to prevent the transmission of roundworm larvae across the placenta into the developing fetuses.

It is essential that the bitch is given gentle exercise right up until the time of whelping so that she can retain the muscle tone necessary for a straightforward birth. From about 6 weeks onwards, our bitches have raspberry leaf supplement morning and night, and from week 8 they receive *Caulophyllum thalictroides* twice daily. Both of these supplements are claimed to promote a more straightforward whelping as the *Caulophyllum* acts as a form of oxytocin. Table 14.1 shows the developmental stages of the puppy during pregnancy (see also Ch. 4).

Parturition or whelping

Preparation

About 1 week before the whelping is expected, it is important that the bitch is moved to her whelping quarters. She should be allowed time to become used to her whelping box and surroundings, giving her time to adjust to the new routine and the new smells. Traditionally, the whelping box was wooden, with rails inside, about 10 cm above the base, so that the bitch was not able to 'crush' the puppies against the side. The more modern whelping boxes are made of

Table 14.1 The development of the puppies during pregnancy

Weeks of developmental stage gestation	
1	Fertilization occurs; two-cell embryos are in the oviduct; the embryo is fairly resistant to external interference in development
2	Embryo increases from four cells to 64 cells. Embryo enters the uterus
3	Embryo becomes implanted in the uterus on day 19
4	Development of eyes and spinal cord; faces take shape; fetuses grow from 5–10 mm to 14–15 mm. Organogenesis begins – fetuses are most susceptible to developing defects. Days 26–32 are the best to palpate for puppies
5	Development of toes, whisker buds and claws. Fetuses look like dogs and the sex can be determined. Eyes are closed. Fetuses grow from 18 mm to 30 mm. Organogenesis complete. Puppies are now resistant to external interference in development
6	Development of skin pigment. Fetal heartbeat can be heard with a stethoscope
7	Growth and development continues
8	Detection of fetal movement when bitch is at rest. Puppies may be safely born at 8 weeks
9	Growth continues until parturition at around 63 days

uPVC, for hygiene purposes, or even disposable cardboard whelping boxes. Some breeders prefer a child's inflatable paddling pool – which obviates the necessity for rails and provides soft, cushioned sides.

Early signs

Many bitches will display nesting behaviour in the days leading up to the birth. Signs will include scratching up of the bedding and an attempt at burrowing. They may also become very restless and be rather 'clingy' to one or more people. A sudden drop in rectal temperature within 24 hours of birth may be a sign that the birth is imminent. Minor fluctuations in temperature are quite normal but when the temperature suddenly drops from about 39°C to around 37°C you may be sure that whelping is about to start. The majority of bitches may prefer to give birth at night and veterinary surgeons are usually resigned to the possibilities of a midnight call-out!

Parturition in the bitch, as in other mammals is split into three distinct stages of labour:

Stage 1

The cervix starts to dilate. During this time it is quite normal for the bitch to refuse food, become restless, start to pant and even vomit. You may also see external signs of very weak contractions. This stage can last from 1 hour to more than 1 day and it is often difficult to be certain when it started.

Stage 2

The cervix dilates fully, contractions become more obvious and the stage ends with the delivery of the puppy. As the urge to push becomes stronger the bitch's straining is very noticeable. It is quite normal for the bitch to shiver at this time. Before the first pup is born there is very often a greenish-black discharge or lochia, which results from the placenta separating from the uterus. It is important that the timing of this discharge is noted, as in an uncomplicated whelping the first pup should be born within the next 2 hours. Puppies may be born in anterior presentation, i.e. with the nose and front paws first, or in posterior presentation, i.e. with tail and hind feet first – either is quite normal (see Ch. 4). In the uterus each pup is surrounded by two sacs – the outer one, the allantochorion, tends to rupture as the pup enters the birth canal. The second sac, the amnion, may or may not rupture during birth. If it does not the bitch will break the sac to release the puppy, enabling it to begin breathing. She will also bite the umbilical cord and lick the puppy vigorously, stimulating it to breathe and to dry off.

The breeder may need to intervene at this stage to open the sac so the pup can start to breath normally. If the breeder needs to break the umbilical cord it is essential that the cord is not cut too short and that it is torn with the fingernails rather than cut with a sharp blade, as this will cause haemorrhaging. The puppy must be rubbed quite vigorously with a towel, which will mimic the bitch's licking actions. Sometimes a maiden bitch is reluctant to start licking the pups – I have found a good method is to put some butter on the pups to encourage the mother to lick them. The bitch will normally suckle pups between births. This is something I always allow as the nursing will stimulate the release of oxytocin, increasing milk let-down and causing further contractions of the uterus.

Stage 3

The fetal membranes and placenta are passed. As the bitch is a litter-bearing (multiparous) animal, stages 2 and 3 very often alternate. There is a difference of opinion as to whether a bitch should be allowed to eat the placentas but I am of the firm belief that we should only interfere when necessary. In other words, if she chooses to do so, I have no objection; after all, in the wild, there would be no-one there to remove them!

Timing

There is no definite timescale between the second and third stages of parturition as some puppies are born within minutes of the previous one, and yet it is not unknown for a bitch to go several hours between puppies. The main criterion is whether or not the process is progressing and it is important to observe the bitch during this time. Although there is no need for alarm if there are extended periods between pups, it is very dangerous to allow the bitch to have continual contractions for a prolonged period without producing a pup. This is the time to request veterinary assistance. Sometimes a car journey to the vets will stimulate another birth and it is not unknown for people to arrive at the surgery with more pups than when they left home!

Dystocia

A prolonged or difficult whelping, referred to as dystocia, is the main cause of puppies appearing rather weak at birth. An overlarge puppy, a puppy in the incorrect position or a small or abnormal birth canal through which the puppy must pass are the most common causes of dystocia. A bitch that is not in the best physical condition, through lack of exercise and corresponding poor muscle tone or through being overweight, may also result in prolonged labour due to inertia.

Inertia can be divided into:

- **Primary inertia** – can result when the uterus is so full of puppies and therefore so distended that there is little chance of strong contractions starting. Conversely, primary inertia may also be caused by the 'single puppy syndrome', when there is so little distension of the uterine muscle that there is no apparent stimulus to initiate contractions. It is imperative that bitches are kept fit and with good muscle tone, as an unfit bitch is more likely to develop primary inertia.

- **Secondary inertia** – may develop after the bitch has given birth to some of the puppies but contractions then stop. The bitch appears to be too tired to carry on and contractions stop. The veterinary surgeon may give an oxytocin injection, which should stimulate further contractions. In some cases it may be necessary to give the bitch intravenous calcium as well as giving her oxytocin.

Assisted delivery

Assisted delivery may be necessary when a puppy is lodged in the birth canal during delivery. The use of gloved fingers is the most reliable and safe way to pull a puppy through the birth canal. It should be noted, however, that in the smaller breeds this is very difficult and potentially dangerous. If it should be needed, it is better to enlist the services of a veterinary surgeon. Under no circumstances should the breeder attempt to use any instruments to assist delivery as they can do great harm to the puppy and the bitch.

In larger breeds when assisted delivery is needed it is important to locate the puppy by firm but gentle palpation of the lower abdomen. Once the puppy has been located, the breeder should apply gentle pressure to this area to prevent the puppy slipping back up the vagina (Fig. 14.8). Insertion of a clean lubricated finger into the vulva then allows the breeder to ascertain whether the puppy is presented head first or tail first.

When the presentation position of the puppy is known, it is possible, after the removal of any obstruction, to gently ease the puppy down the birth canal (Fig. 14.9). It is imperative that the puppy is pulled gently in unison with

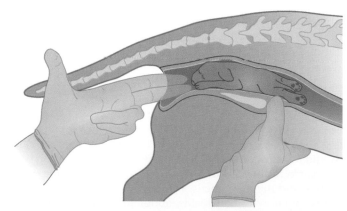

Fig. 14.8 Applying gentle pressure to the abdomen to prevent the puppy slipping back

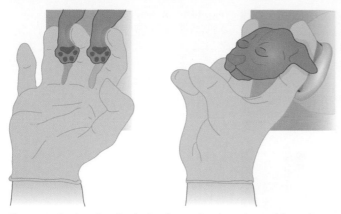

Fig. 14.9 Gentle pulling by the hindlegs or head – only possible in a large breed

the bitch's contractions. It should be noted that a breech birth is not when a puppy comes hind feet first – this is normal posterior presentation – but when the puppy is presented tail first with the hind legs curved underneath it (see Ch. 4).

Resuscitating a puppy

The most common cause of death in newly delivered puppies is hypoxia (low oxygen levels). It is essential when resuscitating a puppy that you complete the following steps:

- The puppy's airway should be cleared immediately and freed of any membranes, fluid and meconium (a puppy's first faeces).
- Excess fluid should be swabbed from the mouth and opening of the throat using a lint-free swab or the corner of a towel.
- If fluid still remains it should be expelled by gently swinging the puppy in a downward path headfirst while supporting its head and body securely in a towel. Be careful with this procedure as there have been cases of cervical dislocation.
- If breathing does not begin, it may be necessary to massage the face and chest of the puppy.

'Never give up' is a phrase that has no greater relevance than when in this situation, and even after a couple of minutes when you may feel all is lost it is not unusual for a puppy to start breathing. For a while the puppy may appear to be gasping but usually this will cease after a short period. It has been known for breeders to give up after a seemingly endless period of massage, to put the puppy to one side – possibly on a cold floor – only to find that the puppy seems to revive a short while after. Whether it is the shock of the cold surroundings that initiates the breathing is unknown but as useful as a textbook is, nature does, from time to time, throw up these little oddities!

Once the puppy is breathing satisfactorily it must be kept warm, either with the bitch or in a box warmed by dry towels placed over a lukewarm hot water bottle or heat pad – hypothermia is a killer!

Completion of parturition

The bitch will usually indicate when she has finished whelping and will appear to be more settled with her litter (Fig. 14.10). At this stage, I always give the bitch a thorough examination and palpate her abdomen to be sure there are no more pups inside. Do not be too alarmed if you can feel a hard lump inside, as very often this will be the uterus, which has yet to involute to its former state.

Once a puppy is born it will crawl around to find a teat and then begin to suckle. This may happen while others in the litter are still being born, or the breeder may remove the puppies to a warm box and return them to the bitch when parturition is over. It is vital that the puppies receive the first milk or colostrum within the first 24 hours of life. Colostrum is rich in maternal antibodies, which will provide protection against disease for about the first 12 weeks.

After whelping is complete the bitch will need to go out to go to the toilet, although you may find you have to put a lead on her to get her to leave the pups for the first few times. She will be tired and thirsty and probably hungry too. For her first meal she should be offered something appetizing but not too heavy, e.g. cooked chicken and boiled rice and a drink of some beaten eggs and milk with added glucose. She should be allowed to rest at this point and apart from keeping an eye on the proceedings there should be as little interference as possible.

For a few days after whelping, there will be a vaginal discharge known as the lochia, which is greenish-black to start with, changing to a watery red/brown discharge as the days go by. It is important to check the bitch's teats for signs of inflammation or mastitis. If you are in any way concerned about this, veterinary advice should be sought immediately.

Care of the newborn

Examination of the puppies

As soon as the puppy is breathing normally and is clean it should be carefully examined and you should check for any obvious defects, e.g. cleft palate, umbilical hernia, absence of an anus. If an abnormality is found you should inform the veterinary surgeon and the puppy may be euthanased, depending upon the significance of the problem. In some congenital conditions there is virtually no hope of the puppy surviving, and it is irresponsible to prolong the inevitable.

It is very important that the temperature in the whelping quarters is kept constant at about 23.8°C for the first few days, as puppies cannot regulate their own body temperature. By the time they reach 10 days old their sensory systems are developing rapidly and they are able to withstand temperatures of as low as 15.5°C, although this is not recommended.

Unless there are obvious problems, keep interference with the bitch and her litter to a minimum but keep a close eye on the family at the same time. At this age, up until about 3 weeks, the bitch should be able to supply all the puppies' needs and as long as she is quite settled I tend to leave her do the job that nature intended. The one time I do interfere is when the bitch returns to the puppies after going outside to relieve herself. I tend to lie the bitch on her side and place the puppies where they can get on to the teats. This is because sometimes, particularly with a younger or inexperienced bitch, an act of clumsiness at this stage can lead to the bitch unintentionally squashing a puppy.

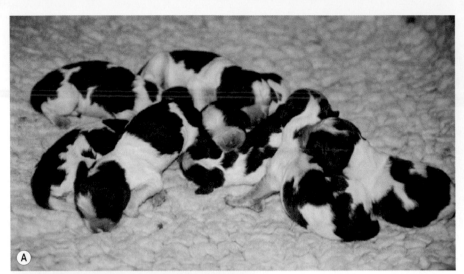

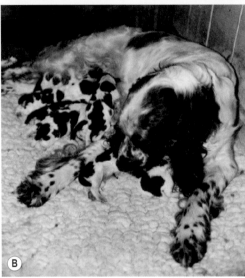

Puppy development

The development of the puppies is very rapid and, compared to humans, the growth rate is exceptionally high. This gives us some indication of the nutritional demands of the puppies. In the early stages, the nutritional requirements of the bitch to be able to sustain the constant demand by the suckling litter is therefore also very high (see Ch. 7). It is quite usual for the puppies to be constantly 'twitching', especially when they are sleeping. This is known as 'activated sleep' and is thought to be the external symptoms of the full development of the nervous system. Puppies are born deaf and blind, and these senses, among others, are fully developed within the first 2 weeks of the puppy's life. Puppies are expected to open their eyes on the 10th day, although I have yet to have a litter that does! Generally I find the 14th day a better guide but have had them as late as 20 days before the eyes are open. However, it is also quite common in some breeds for the eyes to be open as early as the 7th or 8th day.

Hand-rearing puppies

If the bitch produces no milk and is unable to feed her own puppies, or if she dies, then it may be necessary to hand-rear them. There are special formulas available for feeding puppies, which have their own guides as to how much to feed. This depends on the age of the puppies, e.g. puppies under 2 weeks must be fed every 2–3 hours; by 3– 4 weeks the pups can go up to 6 hours between feeds. Various bottle and teat designs are available, depending on the size or age of the puppies, and these must be sterilized between uses.

The bitch will normally lick the area under the tail to stimulate the puppy to urinate and defecate. In her absence, you will need to clean this area with damp cotton wool or tissues after each feed to ensure regular toileting.

Diarrhoea is a common problem in hand-reared puppies and can lead to rapid dehydration and death. It is often caused by poor hygiene, so all equipment used when dealing with the puppies must be kept rigorously cleaned. Feed the affected puppies with milk diluted with cooled boiled water, but if the diarrhoea does not reduce within 24 hours or the puppy shows other signs of illness, consult your veterinary surgeon as soon as possible.

All puppies should be:

- Wormed against roundworms from 2 weeks of age at fortnightly intervals until 12 weeks of age. They should then continue to be treated every month until they are

6 months old. The dosage depends on their weight. Timing may vary according to your veterinary surgeon's practice protocols.

- Vaccinated at 8 weeks of age with a second vaccination given at around 12 weeks – timing varies according to which vaccine is used. Some breeds in some areas require extra parvovirus injections and some litters need earlier vaccinations if they have not received the important colostrum. Contact your veterinarian for advice on the appropriate vaccination programme for your puppies.

Registering and selling puppies

If you are the breeder of a pedigree litter, you will undoubtedly want to register the puppies with the Kennel Club (KC). The KC have a code of ethics and each person who registers puppies with them must undertake to abide by this general code. It covers the general daily care of dogs in registered ownership, the responsibilities of the owner of a bitch who is going to be bred from, and the responsibility that the breeder has to new puppy owners.

Showing dogs

The first recorded dog show was held in 1859 and, since that time, showing has become the most popular canine hobby in the country. Nowadays dog shows are held almost every weekend and have become large social as well as competitive events. All dog shows are licensed by the KC and held under their rules and regulations. At early dog shows all breeds of dog were judged together. At later dog shows the dogs were divided into sporting and non-sporting breeds.

Today's championship dog shows are organized into many more groups: i.e. hounds, terriers, gundogs, toy dogs, utility dogs, working and pastoral dogs. These distinct groups have developed throughout the history of the dog. In this way dogs are judged against dogs of similar characteristics before the best dogs of each group are judged. Finally, the best of each group compete against each other for the position of overall Best in Show.

If you want to compete:

- Your dog must be registered with the KC on the Breed Register.
- Your dog must be at least 6 months old.
- You will need to train your dog to stand still while a stranger (the judge) examines him. Then he must be able move at a steady trot so that his movement can be assessed.
- When your dog is ready you will need to find out when and where shows are taking place.
- You must have trimmed or tidied up your dog as appropriate for the breed.
- You must bath your dog – if appropriate for the breed.

Commonsense tips for dog showing:

- If you want to show your dog, arrange to take your dog or bitch back to see their breeder and ask him/her for an honest opinion of its show potential before you invest time and money in entering shows
- Spend some time at shows watching how things are organized and how experienced exhibitors behave
- Don't be afraid to ask for help and advice – the advantage of being a novice is that you can ask for help without feeling foolish – remember everyone there was once a novice
- Do prepare your dog in advance, e.g. English springer and cocker spaniels will need trimming if they are not to look out of place and even Border collies need their feet tidied up – the show is not the place to start preparing your dog.

Bibliography

Abrantes, R., 1997. Dog Language. Wakan Tanka, Naperville, IL.

Caddy, J., 1995. Cocker Spaniels Today. Ringpress Books, Cheltenham.

Coppinger, R., Coppinger, L., 2001. Dogs – a New Understanding of Canine Origin, Behaviour and Evolution. University of Chicago Press, Chicago, IL.

Craige, P.V., 1997. Born to Win, Breed to Succeed. Doral Publishing, Sun City, AZ.

Evans, J.M., White, K., 2002. The Book of the Bitch. Ringpress Books, Cheltenham.

Feline Advisory Bureau, 2008. Feline Parturition When to Wait and When to Worry. Available online at: &lt: http://web.ukonline.co.uk/fab/ is23.html>.

Feline Advisory Bureau, 2008. Vaccinating Your Cat. Available online at: &lt: http://web.ukonline.co.uk/fab/ is23.html>.

Fogle, B., 1990. The Dog's Mind. Macmillan, Basingstoke.

Fogle, B., 1991. The Cat's Mind. Pelham Books, London.

Gwynne-Jones, O., 1983. The Popular Guide to Puppy Rearing. Popular Dogs, London.

Halls, V., 2007. Cat Councellor; How Your Cat Really Relates to You. Bantam Books, London.

Harmar, H., 1974. Dogs and How to Breed Them. John Gifford, London.

Hollings, P., 1996. The Essential Weimaraner. Ringpress Books, Cheltenham.

Karsh, E., 1983. The effects of early handling on the development of social bonds between cats and people. In: Katchere, A., Beck, A. (Eds.), New Perspectives on Our Lives with Companion Animals. University of Pennsylvania Press, Philadelphia, PA, pp. 22–28.

Lyons, L.A., Foe, I.T., Rah, H.C., Grahn, R.A., 2005. Chocolate coated cats: TYRP1 mutations for brown colour in domestic cats. Mamm. Genome 16 (5), 356–366.

Morris, D., 1996. Cat World, a Feline Encyclopaedia. Ebury Press, London.

Muirhead, C., 1996. The Complete English Springer Spaniel. Ringpress Books, Cheltenham.

Rice, D., 1997. The Complete Book of Cat Breeding. Barron's Educational Series, New York.

Roberts, J., 1987. The Irish Setter. Popular Dogs, London.

Robinson, R., 1982. Genetics for Dog Breeders. Pergamon Press, Oxford.

Serpell, J., 1995. The Domestic Dog – Its Evolution, Behaviour and Interactions with People. Cambridge University Press, Cambridge.

Turner, D.C., Bateson, P., 2000. The Domestic Cat – the Biology of Its Behaviour, second ed. Cambridge University Press, Cambridge.

Turner, T. (Ed.), 1990. Veterinary Notes for Dog Owners. Popular Dogs, London.

Vella, C.M., Shelton, L.M., McGonagle, J.J., Stanglein, T.W., 1999. Robinson's Genetics for Cat Breeders and Veterinarians, fourth ed. Butterworth-Heinemann, Oxford.

Recommended reading

Allen, W.E., 1992. Fertility and Obstetrics in the Dog. Blackwell Scientific, Oxford.

Covers all the scientific points associated with reproduction. Easy access bullet points throughout.

Cooper, B., Lane, D.R., 2003. Veterinary Nursing, third ed. Butterworth-Heinemann, Oxford.

Long detailed chapter covering reproduction in dogs and cats.

Evans, J.M., White, K., 2002. The Book of the Bitch. Ringpress Books, Cheltenham.

Covers all aspects of dog breeding.

Feline Advisory Bureau, 2004. Sheet 6 – Feline Vaccines. Available online at: &lt:http://web.ukonline.co.uk/fab/is23.html>.

The Feline Advisory Bureau publish about 50 fact sheets accessible via their web site. They are well written and cover many feline disorders. This particular sheet outlines the nature and regime of vaccinations for cats.

Harmar, H., 1974. Dogs and How to Breed Them. John Gifford, London.

Useful guide to practical dog breeding.

Rice, D., 1997. The Complete Book of Cat Breeding. Barron's Educational Series, New York.

This book on cat breeding is excellent. Although written for the lay person it is worthwhile reading so that the professional is aware of the knowledge base needed by the conscientious breeder to ensure the welfare of the animals. It is very well illustrated.

Turner, D.C., Bateson, P., 2000. The Domestic Cat – the Biology of Its Behaviour, second ed. Cambridge University Press, Cambridge.

This is an excellent book about the biological nature of feline behaviour and how this impinges on their relationships with humans. It is well written and helps towards an understanding of the nature of pets and patients.

CHAPTER 15

The essentials of patient care

Jessica Maughan

Key Points

- While providing nursing care to an animal it is important to consider the whole patient rather then focusing on a particular disease or injury.
- On admission all hospitalized patients should be given a detailed clinical assessment in order to design an effective nursing strategy based on the individual needs of the patient.
- All animals perform certain daily activities that are essential to maintain a comfortable existence and, in some cases to survive. These essential activities, e.g. feeding, drinking and elimination, must be provided for within a hospital environment if the patient is to recover.
- Certain types of hospitalized patient, such as recumbent or geriatric animals, require specific forms of nursing care.

Introduction

The type of nursing care given to a patient depends on the condition being treated and it is important to distinguish between the needs of different types of patient. This chapter aims to describe all the aspects of nursing care required in dealing with hospitalized patients and will provide guidance on assessing the individual needs of patients and implementing effective nursing care.

Models of nursing

Veterinary nursing is beginning a new chapter in its development, much as human nursing did in the 1970s, with nurses becoming registered and more accountable for their actions. A new theroretical approach has been present in human nursing for some time and is an inevitable addition to the veterinary nursing syllabus. This theoretical model not only attempts to set and formalize good standards within veterinary nursing but is also helping to carry the profession forward into being properly recognized. 'If we are to argue that nursing is a profession in its own right, then we need to be able to work out the boundaries of nursing so that we can recognize our field or practice' (Jefferies 2002).

Introduction to nursing models

A nursing model aims to assist nurses and other clinical staff in their role within the hospital or veterinary practice. The idea is that it may act as a guide or template allowing for a comprehensive and high standard of nursing care to all patients:

- The patient must be assessed on an individual basis as a whole and not just part of a disease process
- The model can be used to guide the team's thoughts and actions as they carry out the nursing process
- It is simple and easy to use on paper and in the mind and it aims to be versatile and adaptable.

There are a number of different nursing models present in human nursing, each having a range of philosophical assumptions and approaches. Of the range of human nursing models, the Roper, Tierney and Logan model appears to be the most compatible with veterinary nursing. This was devised by three British nurses in 1976 as part of a research study into human nursing education. It was developed initially as a conceptual framework for individualizing patient care. In 1980 it was published as a theoretical model in a book called *Elements of Nursing* and 3 years later it was applied in clinical situations by human nurses. The authors were keen for it not to be a static model but for it to continue to evolve and develop as knowledge and technology advances.

The conceptual framework

There are five main concepts to the model:

- Activities of living (AOL)
- Lifespan
- Dependence/independence continuum
- Factors influencing AOL
- The nursing process – individualizing care

Activities of living (AOL)

These are a list of 12 activities that living animals have a need and a right to carry out on a daily basis. In context this may be used as a template for the nursing care plan discussed later on in this section. The activities of living are all interrelated and influence one another, so it is important to look at all 12 as a whole. They are as follows:

1. Maintenance of a safe environment
2. Communicating
3. Breathing
4. Eating and drinking
5. Eliminating
6. Personal cleansing
7. Controlling body temperature
8. Mobilizing
9. Working and playing
10. Expressing sexuality
11. Sleeping
12. Dying.

These form the basis of the Roper, Tierney and Logan model. It can be argued that some of these activities hold little relevance to animal patients, e.g. expressing sexuality, while others only apply in a few specialist cases, e.g. most veterinary patients will not be working apart from police and guide dogs but they can actually become quite distressed when they are stopped from working!

Lifespan

This relates to the stages of a patient's time from birth to death – kitten/puppyhood, adolescence, adulthood and senior/geriatric stages. Knowledge, expectation and prediction are the key words in this concept and it is what we need to be good at as nurses! By knowing at which stage each patient is in its lifespan we can predict possible complications associated with each activity of living at that particular life stage and allow appropiate nursing care to be instigated. For example, a newborn kitten and a geriatric dog will share many potential problems even though they are at two different life stages, e.g. maintaining personal clealiness, controlling body temperature and maintaining a safe environment; however, there are big differences in how they are nursed and managed on a day-to-day basis and consequently their care plan should be designed individually.

Dependence/independence continuum

This part of the nursing model brings the previous two concepts together. In the case of a sick animal there will be times when it will not be able to fully perform all the activities of living. The dependence/independence continuum (Fig. 15.1) is used to assess the individual patient's level of competence in carrying out each activity of living. Effective nursing care may then be implemented to help achieve optimum competency for the particular activity. The patient's level of competence should be plotted along the line of each activity to record the degree of dependence or independence for each activity of living. Once this is done, nursing goals can be set, alongside clinical intervention, in order to move the mark further towards independence.

It is important to note that most activities interact and influence one another and so all 12 must be looked at together as well as individually. It is also important to know the patient's normal status and routine at home, so as not to confuse it as an abnormality of the patient's current condition. To minimize disruption and delay in treatment, you

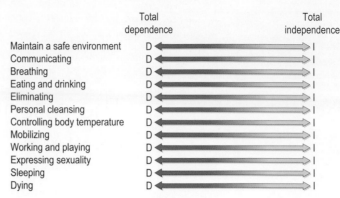

Fig. 15.1 Dependence/independence continuum

must maintain effective communication with the owner to obtain relevant information about the patient's daily routine and any pre-existing conditions. At times this may be difficult to achieve, e.g. when dealing with a canine patient that will only eliminate on grass and the veterinary practice is surrounded by concrete and tarmac.

Factors influencing the activities of living

These factors may influence the nursing care given to the patient. They are:

- Biological
- Psychological
- Sociocultural
- Environmental
- Politico-economic.

Biological – veterinary patients are unique in that there are different breeds within the species which have physiological and anatomical differences and these must be taken into consideration: e.g. a Bulldog may not be able to breathe as well as a Labrador in its 'normal' state; a Siberian Husky may not be able to control its body temperature as effectively in the summer compared to a short-haired Terrier. This allows for the implementation of effective nursing care to maintain health and prevent further disease and deterioration of the patient.

Psychological – illness and injury are both stressful for the patient and owner and can sometimes lead to anxiety and unwelcome behaviour in the patient (and sometimes in the owner!). As well as feeling unwell, the animal has been removed from its familiar environment and it may have also had a previous bad experience at the surgery. Some of the life stages, e.g. a geriatric animal that is blind and deaf, will also have increased anxiety over and above what might normally be expected.

Stress will affect the activities of living and this will present in a variety of manifestations. Cats may become withdrawn, inappetant, unable to relax or sleep or even eliminate. Dogs may become very aggressive and impossible to handle. This will undoubtedly affect the nursing care given and the chances of recovery, and some patients will be impossible to treat within the veterinary practice. A good nurse will anticipate a patient's state of mind, recognize the body language, and adapt the environment and care to suit the patient. A stressed cat will benefit from accommodation away from dogs, in a low-lit, quiet area with a familiar bed in the cage. Any visits from the owners will ultimately be dependent on the individual patient and the nurse is usually the best person to make the decision.

Sociocultural – different cultures have different attitudes to animals as pets and their pain thresholds. People have different ideas as to the perception of their animal in pain. You may recognize the owner who brings in their pet that has had an open wound for a week and it is only when it has stopped eating because the wound is now infected, that they decide to get it treated! You may also recognize the Bichon Frise owner who instantly brings her dog in when it has cut its nail and is spotting blood! Our own perceptions as veterinary nurses influence our approach to the patient and its owner. Their opinions or ideas of their pet in pain may differ from what we recognize or have experienced as professionals in the field.

Our patients cannot tell us if they are in pain so we have to look for outward signs, which can be very subjective. As veterinary professionals we have all dealt with cases of the 'sensitive' owner, who may reflect their own feelings or even experiences onto their pet rather than the animal actually showing outward signs of pain. As veterinary professionals we also consciously or subconsciously relate different breeds to having different pain thresholds and this may also extend to the type of owner that may have these pets as well. This leads on to an idea that a sociologist Talcott Parsons put forward in 1966. He suggested that some human beings may adopt a 'sick role' and can 'act' or give the perception that they are in pain and discomfort in order to obtain a positive response. It may be that animals can adopt a similar role but as yet this has not been proven!

Different cultures and religions may hold ideas and values that extend to their pets: e.g. Jehovah's witnesses do not believe in blood transfusions and may prevent the use of a blood transfusion in their own animal. People also have different ideas about homeopathic medicine, spiritual healing and conventional medicine and may also have different perceptions of the doctors and veterinary surgeons themselves. Some may see them as God-like figures; others may not. All of these will ultimately affect the outcome for the patient.

Environmental – this is particularly significant as this tends to be under the complete control of the veterinary nurse. As nurses we need to be able to adapt the external environment to fit the patient's needs and allow all the activities of living to take place. Environmental factors pertain to light, noise, temperature, humidity, and smell. It also includes cleanliness and the presence of any micro-organisms in the environment, which is particularly significant in cases that require barrier nursing. The environment must be managed to make the patient as comfortable as possible, to increase the chances of it making a full recovery whilst also maintaining the health and safety of the other patients and staff.

Politico-economic – the veterinary industry is based almost entirely on private healthcare so the economic climate at the time has a direct influence on patient treatment and how much clients are able/willing to spend on their animal. In a recession a practice may see a reduction in spending by clients and an increase in debtors. Clients are less likely to invest in preventative health care, e.g. worming, flea

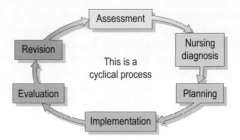

Fig. 15.2 The nursing process (*adapted from Roper, Logan and Tierney model of nursing*)

treatment and vaccination. This in turn affects the level of investment a practice is able to put into staff and equipment. Animal charities will also suffer, with fewer donors and more people seeking financial help. Fewer animals are likely to be insured as monthly premium payments are usually the first thing people drop when tightening the purse strings. All these factors ultimately effect what treatment a patient receives and how effective or successful that treatment is going to be!

The nursing process

Individualizing care

'Care of patients was always planned long before the term "nursing process" was coined, the fundamental difference however, is that the focus of care has changed from tasks to patients' (Jefferies 2002).

There are six main steps involved in the nursing process (Fig. 15.2). This is a cyclical process, allowing nurses to individualize patient care. It can be used in conjunction with the independence/dependence continuum as a template on which to base the resultant nursing care plan.

Assessment

'If we skip on one stage it will be reflected in the quality of the next. This is particularly important for the assessment stage as this forms the basis for the remainder of the nursing stage' (Jefferies 2002).

The assessment stage is used to establish the individuality of the patient and it is only once this has been done that effective care can be given. It is important to gather accurate and relevant information. Wrong or lack of information can result in inadequate action being taken. Veterinary patients, unlike our human counterparts, cannot talk so we have to rely on intuition, experience and recognition of body language and sometimes a bit of detective work is required! The nurse can use both subjective and objective observations in order to determine what state the patient is in. Subjective relates to immeasurable observations that can be made such as demeanour, behaviour, degree of lameness or head tilt. Objective observation relates to measurable factors such as heart rate, body temperature, capillary refill time, blood pressure and blood biochemistry.

Obtaining this information may be done through:

- Effective communication with owner/veterinary surgeon/ other members of staff
- Nurse's own observations
- Hospital sheets/notes and patient files
- Ward rounds.

Some practices have an admittance sheet they go through with the owner, ensuring no important information is left out. Up-to-date hospital sheets/notes are also vitally important if there is a change of shift between members of staff and also for comparison and review of each patient. Ward rounds are also a good exercise in order to allow full collation of information for each patient, but they can be difficult to organize.

Nursing diagnosis

This is not a veterinary diagnosis! It relates to the diagnosis of actual and potential nursing problems that could exist for each individual patient. It requires knowledge, insight and experience in order to identify, predict and diagnose problems.

Planning

This is the problem-solving stage and involves:

- Solving actual identified problems
- Preventing potential problems from becoming actual problems
- Alleviating problems that cannot be solved – effectively managing a patient and owner, allowing them to cope
- Preventing the recurrence of any problems
- Keeping the patient as comfortable as possible even if death is imminent.

Communication is important and should involve all members of staff. It is a good idea to record this as it may be constantly referred to especially in the evaluation stage.

Goal setting is also part of the planning stage and should involve:

- Long- and short-term goals
- Goals set to alleviate each actual and each potential problem
- Goals that may be measured, observed or tested in the evaluation stage
- All goals should be described in enough detail so that they may be used and understoood by other nurses and members of clinical staff.

Implementation

This refers to the active stage of the process and involves taking appropriate action to achieve the goals set in the previous stage. It is what nurses enjoy doing the most as it is what they have been trained to do and allows them to work directly with the patient. Some of the treatments that nurses are able carry out, under the direction of the veterinary surgeon, are:

- Physiotherapy
- Hydrotherapy
- Bathing/grooming
- Nebulization
- Coupage
- Assisted feeding.

Each course of action should have a basis or reason behind it and should be recorded appropriately. This helps to prevent misunderstandings with the owner and other members of staff and to protect oneself against the threat of litigation.

Evaluation

'It is difficult to justify planning and implementing nursing interventions if the outcomes cannot be shown to have benefited the patient or client in some way' (Jefferies 2002)

Evaluation is a crucial stage in the nursing process but not a critical one. It is a re-evaluation of how successful the whole process has been but should not involve criticizing the nursing care given if the goal has not been achieved and the problem not resolved. The whole process is a learning one and can only help to improve nursing skills. This stage can be difficult to do and is dependent on a time frame – either hourly, daily or weekly. It is a comparative exercise and aims to look back at the goals set for each patient and the benefits that have been achieved. It needs to be done honestly by all members of the clinical team involved with the patient.

Some questions to consider at this stage:

- Has the goal been fully achieved?
- Does it require input from another part of the team?
- Should the nursing intervention be changed or stopped?
- Is the problem unchanged or worsening?
- Is the goal to be achieved inappropriate or impossible? (in some cases the situation may have changed due to reduced funding or a change of diagnosis).

Revision

The evaluation stage naturally leads us to revise our nursing plan, the goals we wish to achieve and the ways in which to achieve them. In other words the whole nursing process needs to start again beginning with reassessment of the patient.

Summary

Many nurses may see this approach to nursing as another time-consuming chore, to add to an already long list; however, some nurses may be doing all this in their heads on a daily basis! The aim of this process is to instil a mindset rather than start a paper chase, although some stages do require staff to record information. Using this theoretical approach provides continuity of care as well as individual, finely tuned care and allows a gold standard to be set, to which all clinical staff may work.

The introduction of a theoretical approach to veterinary nursing only serves to compound the idea of veterinary nursing as a separate entity to veterinary medicine and surgery. Whilst still working under and in conjunction with the veterinary surgeon, the two have completely different roles to play in achieving the continued welfare of individual patients.

Patient care

Assessing the patient

The veterinary nurse is usually the person who spends the most time with each patient and so his/her observations are very important in assessing the condition of a patient and the progress of treatment.

When monitoring the condition the SOAP method may be used to ensure completeness. SOAP stands for subjective, objective, assessment and planning:

Table 15.1 Normal clinical parameters in the dog and cat

Parameter	Dog	Cat
Temperature (°C)	38.3–38.7	38.0–38.5
Pulse (beats/min)	60–180	110–180
Respiration (breaths/min)	10–30	20–30
Mucous membrane colour	Salmon pink	Salmon pink
Capillary refill time (s)	< 2.5	< 2.5
Urine production (ml/kg/24 h)	20	20
Fluid intake (ml/kg/24 h)	50–60	50–60
Faeces production (ml/kg/24 h)	10–20	10–20
Acid–base balance (pH)	7.27–7.43	7.25–7.33

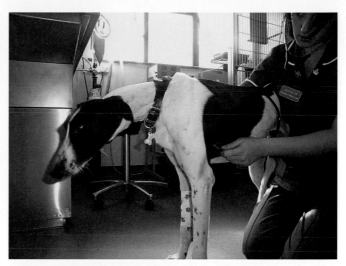

Fig. 15.3 Correct method of auscultation of a dog's heart

- **Subjective** – personal assessment of immeasurable observations, e.g. patient's behaviour, demeanour, posture
- **Objective** – factual assessment of measurable observations, e.g. temperature, pulse and respiration (TPR)
- **Assessment** – a comparative exercise to assess the progress of the patient; may include both subjective and objective observations
- **Planning** – outlines the plan for each patient for that day, whether it is a specific treatment protocol or procedure to be carried out.

Subjective observation relies on the premise that one nurse will be assigned to a specific patient, as interpretation will differ from one person to the next. The assigned person will become familiar with the patient's behaviour and demeanour and any changes are easily identified. Objective assessment relies on the accurate use of equipment, e.g. ability to use a digital thermometer or to auscultate the patient's thorax using a stethoscope. In order to assess accurately and record the progress of a patient it is important to know the normal ranges of the various clinical parameters, e.g. pulse rate, respiratory rate, in healthy patients so that any abnormalities may be identified (Table 15.1). This is also true of behaviour, as in many cases this is the first observation made of a patient's condition or response to treatment.

Vital signs

The vital signs initially assessed in a hospitalized patient are temperature, pulse, capillary refill time and respiration. However, a general assessment should be made of the whole patient, to include eyes, nose, ears, anus, vulva or penis and coat condition. Lymph node enlargement and sensory status, e.g. presence of nystagmus, ataxia and anisocoria, should be assessed and findings should be recorded on to a hospital sheet for each patient.

1. Temperature. Core body temperature is a useful guide to the health status of a patient. A patient may have a high temperature (pyrexia) if infection or sepsis is present or in cases of heat stroke. A subnormal temperature may be recorded in patients who have undergone extensive surgery under general anaesthesia or in cases of hypothermia.

A digital or mercury thermometer is used to take a patient's temperature. Digital thermometers tend to be tolerated slightly better by the patient as the inserted end is slightly narrower than that of a mercury thermometer. If using a mercury thermometer it is important to ensure that the mercury is shaken down to the base before use. The thermometer is then inserted into the anus, using a lubricating gel such as KY jelly, and left in situ for 1 min. The thermometer should be gently twisted as it is inserted and held at a slight angle so as not to record the temperature of any faeces within the rectum.

If a mercury thermometer is broken then the Health and Safety supervisor should be consulted straight away, as mercury is a hazardous substance. It is also important to verify the unit of measurement when recording a temperature. Mercury thermometers record temperatures in both degrees Fahrenheit and degrees Celsius whereas digital thermometers tend to use one or the other.

2. Pulse. This is a basic measurement of heart rate using a stethoscope to auscultate the thorax. This may be done by placing the stethoscope over the lateral aspect of the thorax, just behind and level with the bottom of the scapula (Fig. 15.3). Any irregularities in the heartbeat such as sinus arrhythmias or heart murmurs may also be picked up at this point. Palpation of peripheral pulses gives some indication as to the state of a patient's peripheral circulation.

The pulse may be palpated in several areas of an animal's body. In an anaesthetized animal the lingual pulse may be used. In conscious animals the most commonly used sites are the femoral pulse (medial femur; Fig. 15.4A), digital pulse (palmar aspect of carpus; Fig. 15.4B) and the tarsal pulse (medial aspect, mid tarsus; Fig. 15.4C).

A pulse oximeter may be used to assess pulse rate and the oxygen saturation of the blood. This small machine contains a pair of sensors that may be attached to a membrane or piece of skin such as the interdigital folds, pinna of ear. The tongue may be used in anaesthetized or comatose patients. The measurement relies on a degree of peripheral circulation in order for the sensors to obtain a reading and is of no use in patients with severe circulatory failure.

3. Capillary refill time and mucous membrane colour. These may be used as a measurement of blood volume and circulatory

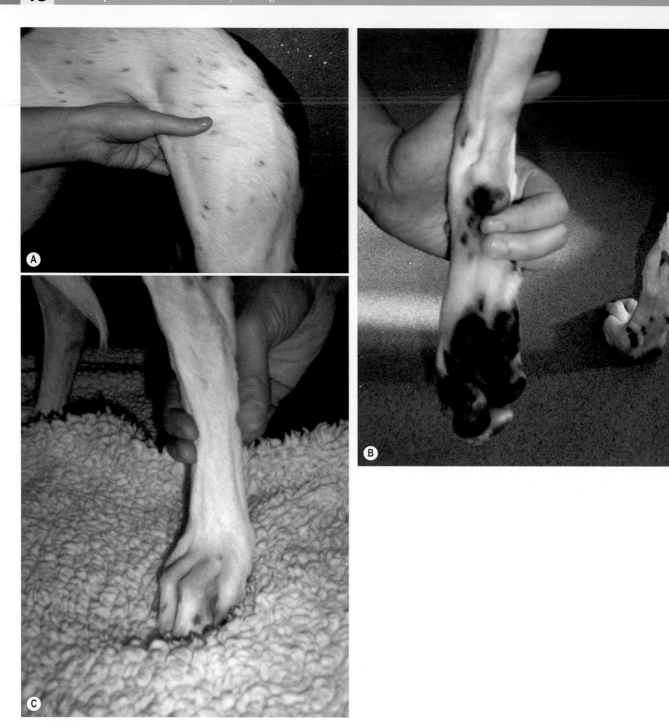

Fig. 15.4 Commonly used sites for palpation of peripheral pulses. (**A**) Femoral pulse. (**B**) Digital pulse. (**C**) Tarsal pulse

status. Capillary refill time is taken by blanching the patient's gum with the tip of a finger and timing how long the gum takes to return to normal colour again. Mucous membrane colour is an observational measurement in which the gums or sclera may be used (Fig. 15.5). Pale mucous membranes may be observed in patients suffering from shock because of the redirection of blood to the body's vital organs. The capillary refill time would also be increased due to the reduction of blood volume in peripheral vessels.

4. *Respiration.* Respiratory rate and pattern may be assessed by observation and auscultation of the thorax. Auscultation

of the thorax is used to listen to a patient's lung to detect chest sounds: e.g. in the case of a chylothorax, the presence of fluid in the chest cavity may be heard. Respiratory rate is calculated by observing and timing the number of times a patient takes a breath over 1 min.

It is important to note the pattern of respiration when observing patients. Dyspnoea is the term given to difficult and laboured breathing. Stridor is used to describe breathing associated with a shrill, harsh sound heard during inspiration. This is usually associated with upper airway complications such as laryngeal obstruction. Cheyne–Stokes respiration is a term given to a particular pattern of breathing

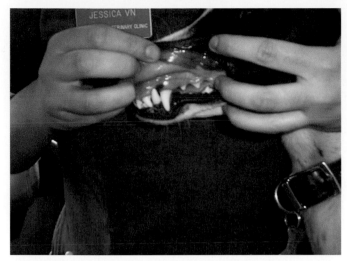

Fig. 15.5 Healthy pink mucous membranes in a canine patient

that usually heralds the onset of death. There is usually a short period of very deep, convulsive breathing which suddenly changes to small shallow breaths or complete termination of breathing, the pattern of which occurs periodically.

Kennelling hospitalized patients

Depending on the layout and design of a kennel area cats and small patients such as rabbits, guinea pigs, rats and birds should be housed separately from dogs. Serious thought should be given to the patient's condition and the effect of the external environment around them: e.g. a dyspnoeic feline patient should not be placed in the kennel above a barking dog. A recumbent patient should not be hidden away in a kennel on its own but accommodated next to an area of activity so that it does not feel forgotten and can be closely monitored.

The size of kennel should be relative to the size of the patient and it should be able to fully stretch out. This is particularly relevant with recumbent and geriatric patients. Placement of equipment within the kennel is also important. A feline patient may be hesitant to eat if its food bowl is directly next to the litter tray. A geriatric patient with spondylosis or a patient with megaoesophagus may benefit from their food and water bowls being raised off the ground.

Essential activities

The needs of a patient encompass all the daily essential activities which a patient performs in order to maintain a comfortable existence and in many cases survive. These relate to the activities of living used in the nursing model discussed earlier and include:

- Elimination, i.e. urination, defecation, vomiting, coughing
- Food intake – maintaining nutritional status
- Fluid intake – maintaining hydration status
- Controlling body temperature
- Mobilization or moving around
- Grooming
- Communication.

In providing nursing care it is important to consider the whole patient rather than focus primarily on a particular disease or injury. By recognizing the ability each patient has to carry out these essential activities an effective nursing strategy may then be planned. Knowledge also plays an important role in the understanding of an injury or disease and the setting of realistic goals when reviewing patient recovery.

Elimination

Urination

Conditions that may cause abnormal urine production include:

- Feline lower urinary tract disease (FLUTD)
- Diabetes mellitus
- Renal disease/failure
- Dehydration
- Bladder rupture.

Useful terminology:

- **Oliguria** – Reduction in daily production of urine
- **Anuria** – Complete cessation of urine production
- **Stranguria** – Passing of urine is painful and uncomfortable
- **Dysuria** – Passing of urine is difficult and uncomfortable
- **Poikuria** – Irregular passage of urine
- **Polyuria** – Passing larger volumes of urine than normal.

Assessing urine production

This may be significant in conditions such as acute renal failure or a ruptured bladder. Note should be made on the hospitalization sheet of when a patient has passed urine, together with volume and appearance of the urine and with a description of its passage, e.g. whether it was difficult or painful.

In cats, a litter tray may be placed in their cage, which also aids the collection of urine, particularly if it is empty of litter. However, stressed cats can deliberately not urinate and cease to pass urine for long periods of time, so manual palpation to check bladder size is sometimes necessary. Dogs should be taken outside to urinate regularly throughout the day as many will be reluctant to urinate in their kennel. Grass is an ideal substrate to encourage urination and a wall or fence is very helpful when encouraging male dogs.

Methods of urine collection

Cystocentesis (cysto- = bladder; -centesis = puncture and aspiration)

Equipment required for this procedure includes:

- Sterile universal plain container (white lid)
- 23 g needle – use as small a gauge needle as possible and a 10 ml sterile syringe
- Sterile gloves
- Chlorhexidine scrub.

The procedure is carried out by a veterinary surgeon and is only usually carried out if the bladder is full, allowing the veterinary surgeon to identify its position. A sterile needle is inserted into the bladder via the patient's flank and correct restraint of the patient is required by one or more assistants. Sterility should be maintained throughout to avoid introducing bacteria into the bladder and to obtain as sterile a sample as possible.

The skin over the area of insertion should be aseptically prepared: the fur clipped and the skin scrubbed with chlorhexidine solution. Sterile gloves should be worn and all equipment used must be sterile. The needle is inserted at a 45° angle to the patient's flank. The urine is then aspirated via the syringe and placed straight into a sterile plain universal pot, identified with the patient's name. As the needle is withdrawn pressure is placed over the site for 10 seconds to seal the point of insertion.

The advantages of using this method are that the urine sample collected is relatively non-contaminated, useful for bacteriology and sensitivity studies, and can be used as a method of urine collection on patients that are unwilling or unable to pass urine normally, e.g. anaesthetized patient. The procedure is also relatively quick and simple and is usually well tolerated. Disadvantages include patient non-compliance, although sedation may be an option. There is also a risk of peritonitis, through poor technique, resulting in fluid leakage from the bladder into the abdomen.

Natural urination – litter tray/midstream sample

With regard to feline patients there are many commercial brands of litter substrate, e.g. Katkor, that may be placed in the tray to encourage urination but will not absorb the urine, allowing it to be collected from the tray via a syringe. The litter may then be disposed of or resterilized. Ideally the litter tray itself should be sterilized, using ethylene oxide sterilization to minimize contamination of the sample.

The advantage of this method is that collection is quick, stress-free and non-intrusive. Disadvantages include poor patient compliance and an increased risk of contamination from passage through the prepuce/vulva and from the patient's coat, paws and collection tray affecting the accuracy of the results obtained. The litter substrate itself can be quite expensive and only a minimal amount of urine may be passed at any one time.

Collection of a canine urine sample requires a collection vessel such as a kidney dish or a sterile plain container. The sample should be collected midstream, which is easier with male dogs. The advantages and disadvantages are similar to those of feline patients. Patient cooperation is essential and gloves should be worn by the collector. Only a minimal amount of urine may be passed at any one time, which may be insufficient to carry out a full urinalysis.

Manual palpation

Gentle pressure is applied on either side of the abdomen in the region of the bladder. This method may be used on anaesthetized patients or those that are unwilling to urinate for no known medical reason. It must not be used if bladder/urethra patency is not known or a blockage is suspected, as excessive force may easily rupture the bladder. A full bladder is required to carry out the procedure and patient compliance is necessary, although it is generally well tolerated.

Urinary catheterization

Not a commonly used method of urine collection as sedation or a full general anaesthetic is usually required for placement of the catheter to avoid damaging the urethra. It can be used in conjunction with contrast studies and indwelling catheterization of hospitalized patients and its many uses include:

- Obtaining a non-contaminated urine sample for bacteriology culture and sensitivity
- Removing urethral blockages by hydropropulsion
- Allowing repeated bladder emptying via an indwelling catheter
- Instilling contrast media and drugs into the urinary tract
- Preventing urine scalding in recumbent animals
- Emptying the bladder in anaesthetized animals prior to surgery.

Insertion of a urinary catheter should be as aseptic as possible to prevent introduction of contaminants into the bladder. A sterile catheter should be used and sterile gloves worn. This procedure may be carried out by a veterinary nurse.

The anaesthetized patient should be placed in an appropriate position. In male cats this is usually in dorsal or lateral recumbency, female cats and bitches in sternal recumbency with legs hanging over the end of a table and in male dogs, lateral recumbency. A catheter may be placed in conscious dogs and bitches, in which case they may be standing.

In females a speculum may be used to expand the vaginal opening, giving a better view of the urethral orifice. Lubrication of the catheter tip aids easy passage into the urethra and reduces the risk of epithelial damage to the urethral tract during passage of the catheter. Depending on the type of catheter and its function, it may be sutured to the patient or the balloon inflated (Foley catheter) to keep it in place. A collection bag may be attached to an indwelling catheter to maintain kennel hygiene, measure the amount of urine production and reduce the risk of introducing infection via the catheter (Fig. 15.6).

Maintenance of indwelling catheters

- Keep the area around the catheter clean from faeces and urine unless a collection bag is used.
- For prolonged use it may be necessary to change the catheter. Commonly used materials are silicone or Teflon, which cause minimal mucosal irritation, making them useful for long-term use.
- In some cases prophylactic antibiotics may be administered to reduce the risk of ascending infection. This is especially important in post-surgical and hospitalized patients where indwelling catheterization is expected. Frequent monitoring is required to check that the catheter is not blocked and in some cases daily flushing with sterile water may be necessary.
- The use of a collection bag is advantageous as it creates a closed system, reducing the risk of ascending infection through an open catheter. The amount of urine produced may also be monitored. Used intravenous fluid bags complete with giving set make ideal collection bags. Care must be taken that the bag is not increasing resistance to flow, especially in smaller patients, and that the urine is flowing freely. The urine may also be inspected to monitor for signs of trauma from placement of the catheter. Figure 15.7 shows a home-made urine collection system using a giving set

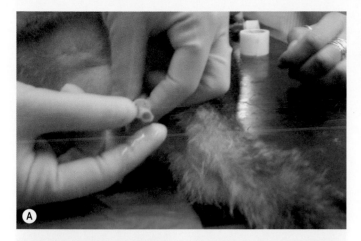

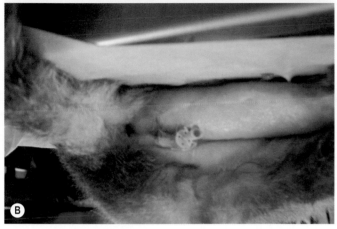

Fig. 15.6 Placement of a Jackson cat catheter into a male feline patient. (**A**) Inserting the catheter. (**B**) Catheter sutured in to be maintained as an indwelling catheter

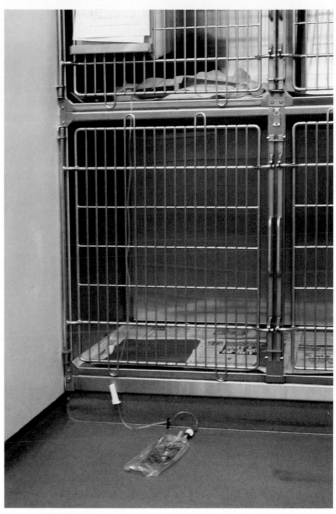

Fig. 15.7 A home-made closed urine collection system

and used intravenous fluid bag into which urine flows with the aid of gravity.

Assessment of urine

Note the volume of urine voided and its appearance. Normal urine should be clear and have a slightly yellow colour. Cloudy or very turbid urine indicates presence of sediment such as white or red blood cells, calculi and casts. Dark red/brown colour urine indicates a large amount of haemoglobin or myoglobin present. A strong brown/yellow colour indicates the presence of bile pigments (Bloxham 1999).

Simple urinalysis tests carried out on urine include measurement of specific gravity using a refractometer. Clinistix (Bayer) may also be used to check pH, presence of blood, ketones, protein and bilirubin within the urine sample. Centrifuging the urine can also determine the presence of sediment and microscopy using Leishman's staining technique can be used to identify the presence of specific crystals, casts or bacteria.

Defecation

Useful terminology

*   **Diarrhoea** – The rapid expulsion of soft, non-formed material from the rectum

*   **Constipation** – Impaction of hard, dry faeces within the large intestine or rectum, which is difficult or may become impossible for the animal to pass
*   **Tenesmus** – Painful, ineffectual straining to pass faeces, seen in cases of constipation
*   **Dyschezia** – Difficult and painful passage of faeces
*   **Melaena** – Production of dark, tarry faeces with or without mucus: evidence of blood loss in the upper gastrointestinal tract
*   **Haematochezia** – Production of fresh, bright red blood in the faeces: evidence of blood loss in the lower gastrointestinal tract
*   **Coprophagia** – When an animal eats its own faeces – usually a vice in a dog.
*   **Steatorrhoea** – Passage of large volumes of pale, fatty faeces, usually associated with exocrine pancreatic insufficiency (EPI).

Diarrhoea

May occur in EPI, dietary intolerance/allergy, bacterial infection due to *Salmonella*, *Campylobacter*, etc., parasitic infection, viral disease due to Parvovirus, etc., malabsorption, colitis.

Diarrhoea can be acute or chronic and can originate in either the small or large intestine. Some cases may be associated with vomiting, anorexia and water and electrolyte losses, particularly potassium, which, if not replaced rapidly can be life-threatening. Other associated signs can include depression and lethargy, abdominal pain, polyphagia (especially in EPI), anorexia and dyschezia. The presence of any of these clinical signs must be noted on the hospitalization sheet when monitoring the patient, as well as colour, consistency, odour, amount and frequency of any diarrhoea passed. If you are unsure, a sample should be kept for the veterinary surgeon to examine. History and hospitalization sheets are important in determining the origin and cause of the diarrhoea.

Nursing considerations

Plenty of opportunity should be given for canine patients to go outside to defecate as many will be unwilling to do so in their kennels. This is especially beneficial in paralysed recumbent patients, as appropriate support, movement and exercise will encourage normal bowel movement and faecal passage.

Maintenance of basic kennel hygiene is important when dealing with these patients. The bedding used should be washable, or disposable in cases of infectious disease, and incontinence sheets are very useful in these cases. Newspaper and towels are also useful bedding materials. Thick blankets and synthetic fleece (Vetbed) should be avoided as they increase the wash load and can harbour bacteria and viruses within the thick fibres. Long-haired patients benefit from having their perianal area clipped to prevent the accumulation of faeces in the surrounding hair, keeping the area clean and hygienic.

Barrier nursing may be indicated if an infectious disease such as Parvovirus is present and all materials in contact with the animal's bodily fluids must be adequately sterilized or disposed of.

Intravenous fluid therapy is commonly administered in patients with diarrhoea because of associated losses of water and electrolytes, especially potassium and bicarbonate. Hartmann's solution (lactated Ringer's) is usually indicated to replace any losses. Further potassium supplementation may be required in severe cases.

The nurse will also play a role in the dietary requirements of these patients. Some cases may require nil per os. Others may benefit from a short-term diet of bland, easily digestible food, low in fat and high in good-quality proteins such as chicken and highly digestible carbohydrates such as rice (McCune 1999). For patients with a dietary intolerance or allergy, the veterinary surgeon will usually recommend a low-sensitivity diet that the patient may have to eat for the rest of its life.

Constipation

May occur in cases of dehydration, neurological disease/trauma, enlarged prostate, inactivity and obesity, and megacolon. Constipation can result in the patient becoming very restless and depressed. Opportunities should be given to canine patients to walk outside as movement and exercise aid the passage of faeces and the patient may be more willing to defecate away from the kennel.

Physical trauma, such as a fractured pelvis, will prevent defecation from occurring, resulting in the faeces within the rectum consolidating and becoming hard and impacted. Oral medication may be administered in the form of lactu-

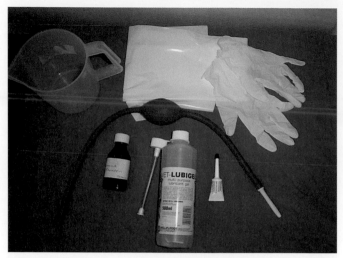

Fig. 15.8 Equipment required for administration of an enema

lose, a natural laxative, to help loosen the faeces, resulting in a relatively pain-free passage. It may also be given to some patients in cases where there is pain around the perianal region, such as after anal gland removal.

Enemas

In some cases where the impaction of faeces is particularly severe an enema may be given. This involves the introduction of a solution into the rectum to help break up the faeces and facilitate the passage of faeces from the rectum. Enemas may also be given preoperatively if surgery is concentrated around the perianal area or involves entering the lower gastrointestinal tract. Patients undergoing abdominal radiography may also be given an enema to allow clear visualization of the caudal abdomen or to introduce contrast agents for lower gastrointestinal contrast studies.

Materials used for enemas include liquid paraffin or warm saline solution. Phosphate enemas or glycerine used in human enemas should not be used in cats as they are toxic; soapy enemas should also be avoided as they are an irritant (Fig. 15.8).

Administration of an enema – most patients will need to be sedated or under general anaesthesia in order to carry out the procedure as it is quite uncomfortable and a relaxed anal sphincter tone is preferable. The veterinary surgeon will usually ensure that there is no physical blockage, such as a foreign body or enlarged prostate, preventing the normal passage of faeces before carrying out an enema.

The warm solution is introduced into the rectum using a Higginson syringe, with one end placed in the solution and the other end inside the rectum (Fig. 15.8). Water is then pumped by squeezing the bulb in the middle of the syringe, which allows the solution to travel one way only into the rectum. The impacted faeces is hydrated and broken down by the pressure from the continual introduction of water into the rectum.

Vomiting

Conditions that can cause a patient to vomit include: gastritis/gastroenteritis; megaoesophagus; viral infection, e.g. parvovirus or feline infectious enteritis; gastric dilation and volvulus (GDV); poisons/toxins; ketoacidosis as seen in diabetes mellitus; pyometra; bacterial infection, e.g. *Salmonella*; pancreatitis.

Useful terminology

- **Vomiting** – An autonomic reflex in which the contents of the stomach are actively ejected via the mouth
- **Regurgitation** – Passage of undigested food from the oesophagus out of the mouth
- **Haematemesis** – Blood present in vomit; may be similar in appearance to coffee grounds or red and fresh
- **Emetic** – An agent that induces vomiting, e.g. apomorphine, soda crystals.

Nursing considerations

Intravenous fluid therapy is usually indicated because of the loss of water and electrolytes, e.g. hydrogen and potassium ions. Fluids containing sodium chloride (saline) or Ringer's solution are indicated as the replacement fluid of choice. Anti-emetics such as metoclopramide, which inhibits the vomiting reflex and increases gastric contractions, may be prescribed by the veterinary surgeon and administered to nauseous and vomiting patients.

Frequency, quantity and appearance of vomitus should be noted and recorded. Fresh or haemolysed blood with the appearance of dark coffee granules or bile, a yellow colour, may be present. Bedding should be easily washable or disposable, as with diarrhoeic patients. Barrier nursing should be applied in cases where an infectious disease has been identified or is suspected.

Nauseous patients are usually depressed and may intermittently lick their lips. If indicated, they should be offered food but avoid leaving it in the kennel for a long period as this may make the patient more uncomfortable and increase food aversion. Many patients will be prescribed 'nil per os' and all medication will be given parentally. Oral fluids should be maintained unless directed by the veterinary surgeon. White and light foods, e.g. chicken and rice, should be introduced gradually, little and often for the first 3–4 days. Normal food can then be gradually introduced over a period of weeks.

Coughing

Coughing is an expulsive mechanism transmitted by the vagus nerve to the thoracic muscles to expel mucus or foreign bodies. Conditions that can induce a coughing reflex include bronchitis/tracheitis/laryngitis, kennel cough or infectious rhinotracheitis, left-sided congestive heart failure, pneumonia, foreign body, laryngeal spasm (in cats following endotracheal tube extubation), malformation, e.g. an overlong soft palate.

Nursing considerations

Instigate barrier nursing to isolate infectious patients such as those with kennel cough. In most cases these are nursed at home but a patient may be admitted from a boarding kennels. Offer warm, palatable food as in some cases the patient may be anorexic.

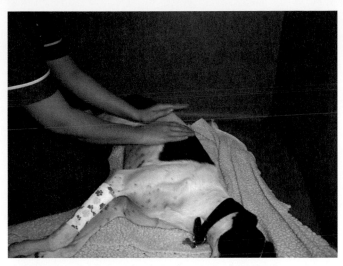

Fig. 15.9 Coupage being administered to a recumbent patient

Ensure appropriate medication is administered. In most cases antitussives or cough suppressants (e.g. butorphanol), antimuscarinic or secretory inhibitors (e.g. atropine) and antibiotics or bronchodilator drugs (e.g. theophylline) may be prescribed. Coupage and nebulization may be used to help loosen up secretions and encourage a more productive cough (Fig. 15.9). Cupped hands should be used to tap firmly on the chest wall, starting caudally and working forward.

Maintaining nutritional status

Conditions that may affect the nutritional status of the patient may be due to:

- Anorexia – e.g. cat flu due to calici/herpesvirus; patients with cervical spine damage or fractured jaw; hospitalized or postsurgical patients in pain; highly stressed patients, usually cats; geriatric patients often have impaired taste bud renewal; olfactory impairment; oncology patients following radiation treatment
- Gastrointestinal compromise – e.g. malabsorption/maldigestion syndromes (e.g. EPI, following gastrointestinal surgery, megaoesophagus).

Useful terminology

- **Inappetence** – Partial reduction in appetite
- **Anorexia** – Loss of desire for food before calorific requirements have been met
- **Starvation** – Long-term deprival of food, resulting in the appearance of associated physical effects such as reduction in fat/muscle mass, loss of skin turgor, lethargy and weakness and hypothermia
- **Pica** – Cravings for unusual items of food, licking and eating at foreign objects; usually seen in animals with nutritional deficiencies
- **Coprophagia** – Ingestion of an animal's own faeces; usually a vice in dogs or cats.

A compromised nutritional intake for whatever reason can seriously affect all body systems which is exacerbated in situations where the animal is also immunocompromised.

A reduction in all nutrients, particularly protein, can result in reduced heart muscle mass and function, compromised pulmonary and immune function and increased catabolism of the body's energy reserves. When applied to hospitalized patients this also results in reduced tissue repair and synthesis, reducing the chance of effective wound healing and recovery. There is also an increased risk of sepsis and altered drug metabolism, resulting in an increase in the risk of drug toxicity. The altered metabolism will also result in an increase in adipose tissue and muscle loss as increased demand for proteins and fat are not being met. Dogs are better at coping with starvation in comparison to cats, who may take up to 6 weeks to recover completely (Agar 2001).

It is vital to ensure that patients are provided with the key nutrients needed for tissue repair and to maintain adequate immune function. Depending on the needs of the individual patient, different forms of assisted feeding will be instigated by the veterinary surgeon to ensure that these nutrients are received. There are two main routes used for feeding:

- Enteral – administration of food or medicines using the gastrointestinal tract
- Parenteral – administration of food and medicines by a route other than that of the gastrointestinal tract, e.g. by intravenous injection (the term literally means the space between the outer surface or skin and the gastrointestinal tract)
- Enteral feeding.

Choice of food

Fats and proteins are absorbed much more easily than carbohydrates. The epithelial cells lining the gut of anorexic or starved patients can be very fragile so provision of an easily absorbable diet will reduce the risk of diarrhoea. Fat also yields twice the calories of carbohydrates and protein so a high-fat diet containing proteins of high biological value is ideal for most hospitalized patients. Proteins and fats further complement one another as non-protein calories are required to oxidize the amino acids during protein catabolism. Contraindications would include patients with EPI or other gastrointestinal problems, which would require a specialized diet low in fat, or renally-compromised patients, which certainly would not benefit from a high-protein diet. A diet rich in arginine (an essential amino acid of the dog and cat) and omega-3 fatty acids is also beneficial, as it is thought to have immunopreservative effects, particularly useful with cancer patients (Agar 2001; see also Chapter 8).

Methods of feeding

Hand-feeding

When faced with the challenge of encouraging an inappetant patient to eat the key is to select highly palatable foods. In feline patients this may be tuna or pilchards in tomato sauce, which can be warmed to increase palatability and is often popular with patients with a reduced sense of smell, such as cats with 'cat flu'. Feeding the same diet that they are given at home may also help. Cats in particular tend to be very texture-sensitive and will prefer what they have been fed before.

Hand-feeding can work very well and should be attempted with all inappetant patients if they are amenable. Spending time with cats and effectively 'playing' with their food usually encourages eating. Care should be taken to avoid force,

however, as this may lead to food aspiration and may even increase food aversion.

Syringe feeding

This is more readily accepted by canine patients and large boluses may be given to amenable patients. Ensure that the patient is sitting upright and that the syringe is positioned at a 90° angle to the jaw. The patient can then take the liquid over the top of the tongue as it is slowly trickled into the mouth, reducing the risk of aspiration. Only liquid foods may be given by this method and they should not be given to recumbent patients as there is an increased risk of aspiration. This method of feeding is not as successful in feline patients and can be a stressful experience for both nurse and patient.

Appetite stimulants

Drugs may be administered under the direction of the veterinary surgeon to stimulate appetite, e.g. diazepam given intravenously in cats has a rapid onset with a short duration of action and may be used for short term only. Cyproheptadine (Periactin), an antihistamine drug, may also be used in cats to stimulate appetite and may be used for up to 1 week (R Giles, unpublished work, 2002).

Tube feeding

There are various types of feeding tube available and the choice depends on which area of the gastrointestinal tract is compromised (Table 15.2). In patients undergoing gastrointestinal surgery the veterinary surgeon will decide which method of feeding will be necessary post surgery and implantation of the feeding tube will usually be done while the animal is still under general anaesthesia.

Maintenance of the feeding tube

When using nasogastric and pharyngostomy tubes it is necessary to check that the tube is still in the oesophagus before each feed as tubes can be dislodged through coughing. This may be done by placing 2 ml of sterile water down the tube beforehand and watching for any signs of coughing, which may suggest that the tube is lying in the trachea. A less common method is to check for a vacuum by attaching a 5 ml syringe to the end of the feeding tube, drawing back the plunger and releasing so that a vacuum is felt. This confirms that the tube is lying in the oesophagus. The feeding tubes must be flushed before and after each feed to prevent blockages. Fizzy drinks have been used, but can cause nausea and vomiting in patients. Cranberry juice works just as well, with few unwanted side effects.

In most cases feeding tubes are used in conjunction with accessories such as stockinettes, abdominal bandages and buster collars to help keep them in place (Fig. 15.10). They may require regular changing or altering and should be closely monitored for any signs of discomfort caused to the patient. The site of entry of a feeding tube should be treated as a surgical wound and will require daily cleaning and dressing to prevent any infection.

Administration of food through the tube

Complete liquid foods, e.g. ready-prepared liquids such as Reanimyl, Fortol and Liquivite, are ideal to administer through the feeding tubes. They are slightly more expensive

Table 15.2 Types of feeding tube

Type of tube	Location of placement	Contraindications	Advantages	Disadvantages
Nasogastric tube	Tube inserted into nostril and passed through pharynx to lie in oesophagus. Tube ends in caudal oesophagus rather than directly into stomach to prevent gastric reflux	Nasal, oral or pharyngeal disease Vomiting or regurgitation Lateral recumbency Oesophageal disease Stomach disease After surgery on the upper gastrointestinal tract	Usually well tolerated Does not require general anaesthetic to place tube Long-term use 3–7 days Allows most of gastrointestinal tract to be used Need to check before each feed that tube is still in the oesophagus	Can be irritating to eyes and nose Patient usually requires an Elizabethan collar to keep the tube in place
Pharyngostomy	Surgical hole made over area of pharynx and tube passed through hole, via the pharynx into the oesophagus. Alternatively a surgical wound may be made directly into the oesophagus	Pharyngeal/oesophageal disease/dysfunction Vomiting patients	Usually well tolerated Allows most of gastrointestinal tract to be used Useful when there is trauma to oral or nasal cavity	Associated complications: • Dysautonomia syndrome (neurological disease) – pharynx/larynx very sensitive • High chance of infection due to associated surgical wound Requires general anaesthetic for placement Wound care maintenance and materials required
Gastrostomy	Placement of feeding tube usually carried out surgically via endoscopy using a percutaneous endoscopic gastrostomy (PEG) mushroom-tipped tube	Gastric/lower gastrointestinal tract disease/dysfunction Vomiting patients Lateral recumbency	Can be used long term and kept in place indefinitely Relatively easy to use and maintain and in some cases patients can be sent home Used in patients with oesophageal, oral, aural or swallowing disease/dysfunction	Requires general anaesthetic for placement Minimum placement time 7 days to allow scar tissue to form around the tube Ischemia may occur within the tissue at the exit point if the mushroom tip of the feeding tube is in contact with the abdominal wall Surgical wound – risk of infection Wound care maintenance Cannot be used for first 24 h to enable a primary seal to form
Jejunostomy tube	Tube placed directly into the small intestine via a surgical hole, to bypass the upper gastrointestinal tract	Patients with lower gastrointestinal tract disease/ dysfunction	Useful in patients with upper gastrointestinal disease/dysfunction, e.g. following gastric surgery	Risk of dislodgement by reverse peristalsis into stomach Can only feed small volumes of food because of small capacity of jejunum Requires general anaesthetic for placement Surgical wound into contaminated area – risk of infection Wound care maintenance

but are more suitable for use in smaller-bore feeding tubes (Fig. 15.11). Non-prepared products, e.g. A/D Diet (Hills) and Convalescence Support (Royal Canin), require mixing with water beforehand but are too viscous, even when mixed with water, to use with small-bore tubes. Ready-prepared products have a short shelf-life once they are opened. Any liquid food should be warmed to body temperature before administering to prevent vomiting. Avoid the use of a microwave, as this can cause uneven heating.

When calculating the volume of food to be given it is necessary to work out how many kilocalories there are per millilitre of food. This information may be found on the label or in a product catalogue and depends on the species and weight of the patient and the length of time the feeding tube has been placed. The food should have a high calorific density as the volume of food administered will be restricted.

The stomach capacity of a cat is 45 ml/kg and of a dog 90 ml/kg.

Feeding requirements will need to be calculated for each individual patient. There are two calculations that can be used when working out the amount of food to administer. The maintenance energy requirement (MER) is the amount of energy required by a moderately active animal. This does not include the extra energy required by the animal for pregnancy, lactation, work or convalescence.

The basic energy requirement (BER) relates to energy required by an animal, in an inactive state, within a thermoneutral environment. This relates closely to the situation of a veterinary patient, and so we tend to use the BER when calculating their energy requirements. Some patients may have undergone trauma, had surgery or be suffering from neoplasia, and will therefore have an increased energy

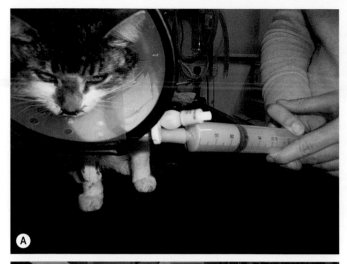

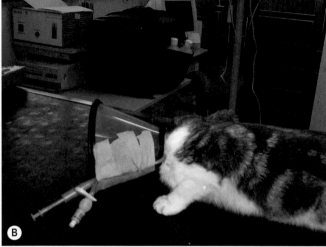

Fig. 15.10 Cat with fractured jaw. (**A**) Feeding via a pharyngostomy tube. (**B**) Placement of an Elizabethan collar securing the pharyngostomy tube

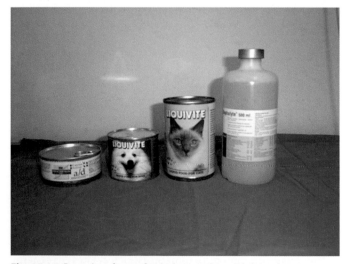

Fig. 15.11 Examples of some foods that may be used through feeding tubes

Box 15.1 Calculation of basic energy requirement for a range of situations

A. **Basic energy requirement (BER) = metabolizable kilocalories (kcal) over a 24-h period**

< 5 kg bodyweight BER = 60 × (bodyweight kg)
> 5 kg bodyweight BER = (30 × bodyweight kg) + 70

Disease factor may be added to the BER:
Hospitalization	BER × 1.3
Major trauma	BER × 1.6
Neoplasia	BER × 1.6
Severe infection	BER × 1.8
Major burns	BER × 2.0

BER × disease factor = amount (kcal) in 24 h

Volume of food in millilitres (ml) or grams (g) may be calculated by dividing the number of kcal/ml or kcal/g of food by the number of kcal to be fed in 24 h

B. **Maintenance energy requirement (MER)**

MER = 2 × BER in dogs
MER = 1.4 × BER in cats

requirement. In these cases a disease factor is added to the BER, increasing the daily energy requirement needed, to aid in convalescence and recovery. Box 15.1 shows how to calculate MER and BER and also lists the various disease factors.

It is not a good idea to feed the full quota of food straight away as this will shock the gastrointestinal system and diarrhoea may result, especially if the patient has been anorexic. By gradually increasing the amount of food over a period of days, the gastrointestinal system will adapt to the new form of feeding. Table 15.3 shows examples of feeding regimes.

Parenteral feeding

Nutrients are administered into the patient's blood stream via a central venous catheter placed in the jugular vein. The technique is particularly useful in patients who are unable to take in nutrients through their gastrointestinal system. It is a technique rarely used in practice because of the high cost of the specialized intravenous infusion fluid and equipment and the nursing care involved.

The intravenous infusion comprises a mixture of amino acids, dextrose, lipid emulsion, water-soluble vitamins, electrolytes and trace minerals and a fresh mixture is prepared aseptically on a daily basis (Fig. 15.11). This is attached to the giving set and an infusion pump and should be administered at a very slow rate. Constant monitoring is required to check for any evidence of precipitate formation in the intravenous infusion and for signs of phlebitis in the jugular vein. Strict catheter management should be adhered to, as there is an increased risk of sepsis (Hurley and Michel 1999).

Fluid intake

Conditions that may cause abnormal hydration status and fluid redistribution include starvation, acute renal failure, diabetes insipidus, diabetes mellitus, toxic shock, pleural effusion, haemorrhage and septicaemia.

Table 15.3 Daily feeding regimes – Where has it gone?

Day 1	1/3 basic energy requirement mixed ratio
	1:2 with water to make up volume given (ml)
Frequency of feeding	3-4 times daily
Day 2	2/3 basic energy requirement mixed ration
	2:1 with water to make up volume given (ml)
Frequency of feeding	4-5 times daily
Day 3	Feed basic energy requirement (ml) with
	Additional water* as necessary
Frequency of feeding	6-8 times daily

*Additional daily water requirement, if not on intravenous fluid therapy, is 50 ml/kg – water provided by food = water intake (ml)

Table 15.4 Clinical signs associated with dehydration

Water deficit (%)	Associated clinical signs
0–5	Concentrated urine, polydipsia, no clear clinical signs
5–7	Reduction in dermal elasticity (tenting), slightly sunken eyes, dry mucous membranes, increased capillary refill time, rapid weak pulse
7–10	Tented skin remains in place, sunken eyes, anuria, extremities, depression, weak pulse
10–12	Progression into shock phase, comatose, death usually inevitable

Assessing hydration status

There are various measurements and observations used to determine a patient's hydration status (Table 15.4), which include:

- Capillary refill time (CRT) – the gum is blanched by finger pressure and time taken for the gum to return to normal colour is recorded; in a dehydrated patient this may take a longer time than a healthy CRT.
- Dry mucous membranes are indicative of a dehydrated patient and can also be assessed while carrying out the above measurement.
- Observing eye position within the socket – retraction of the eye back into its socket indicates that the patient is dehydrated.
- Dermal elasticity – this may be carried out by gently pinching or tenting the patient's skin. In a healthy patient the skin should resume its normal form almost immediately but in cases of dehydration there will be less elasticity within the skin and it will take longer to resume a normal position. This assessment is objective and depends on the age, condition and amount of subcutaneous fat in the patient.
- A packed cell volume (PCV) may be carried out if a blood sample is available. This test is normally used to measure the amount of red blood cells in a given volume of blood but the figure obtained can also be indicative of hydration status. The normal PCV for a cat or dog is 32–45%. A higher PCV (> 45%) would indicate dehydration, as the top layer of the plasma sample, the fluid component of the blood, is reduced so that the relative proportion of red blood cells is greater. When assessing dehydration the rule is that a 1% increase in PCV is equivalent to a water loss of 10 ml/kg.

Maintaining fluid intake

Subcutaneous and intraperitoneal fluid administration

Administering warmed sterile isotonic fluids subcutaneously can be particularly useful in patients where intravenous access would be difficult, e.g. in neonates or in patients where oral administration would be difficult. Absorption of fluids using this method is very slow and should be avoided in severely dehydrated animals. Small boluses should only be administered at any one time and different areas of skin should be used each time.

Warmed sterile hypotonic or isotonic fluids may also be administered directly into the peritoneal cavity. Because of the high absorptive capacity of the peritoneum it is a more efficient way of administering fluids than the subcutaneous route. This method must be carried out in a strictly aseptic manner to avoid introducing infection into the peritoneal cavity.

Intraosseous fluid administration

This method allows administration of fluids into the medullary cavity of a long bone, e.g. the proximal femur or tibia in cats or dogs. It is especially useful in small exotic species, neonates and trauma patients where venous access is fragile or compromised. Absorption of fluids from this route is as rapid as the intravenous route. Placement requires skill and can be painful. Local anaesthetic should always be used in conscious animals. Maintenance of an intraosseous catheter should follow the same strict aseptic technique as intravenous catheter management.

Intravenous fluid administration

Access is gained using an intravenous catheter. Sterile warmed fluids are administered into the vein, commonly the cephalic or saphenous vein. This method is the most rapid and effective way of introducing fluids into a severely dehydrated patient and can be used for continual fluid administration.

Intravenous catheters

There are various types of intravenous catheter available constructed from different materials such as Teflon, polyurethane and silicone (Fig. 15.12). The time a catheter may be left in the vein depends on the patient, the catheter material and the standard of catheter care. Silicone catheters are less likely to cause a reaction within the vein than polyurethane catheters, whereas Teflon catheters have a more rigid structure and are more likely to cause thrombophlebitis (E. Opperman, unpublished work, 2002). Indwelling catheters should not be kept in place for more than 48 hours.

Maintenance of intravenous catheters

- The catheter should be enclosed within a semiocclusive dressing to protect the site of insertion from physical damage and prevent introduction of sepsis into the blood vessel via the catheter.
- The catheter site and surrounding area should be kept as clean and dry as possible to reduce the risk of sepsis.
- Hands should be washed prior to checking all catheters and giving sets. All catheter checks should be done prior to carrying out further checks such as TPR.
- Any sign of patient interference should be dealt with immediately; Elizabethan collars may be used to prevent this, along with close monitoring.
- Ideally catheters should be flushed with sterile heparin saline at every check, to assess patency and prevent thrombus formation; checks should, ideally, be carried out three times a day to ensure there are no complications.
- It is good practice to note, either on the catheter bandage or in the hospital notes, the date each catheter

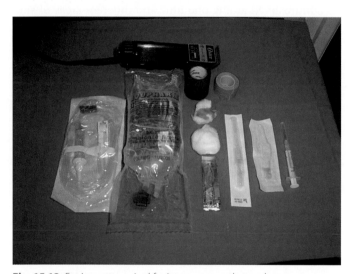

Fig. 15.12 Equipment required for intravenous catheter placement

was placed. This is especially important if there is a change of nursing shift.
- If any medication is introduced directly into the catheter or into the fluid bag, this should be done in a sterile manner. A fresh sterile needle should be placed on the syringe in between collecting the medication from the bottle and placing intravenously (Table 15.5).

Controlling body temperature

Problems in controlling body temperature may be seen in the following conditions: hypothermia, hyperthermia, heat stroke, severe dehydration and/or starvation, systemic infection – pyrexia, underdeveloped thermoregulatory system in neonates, compromised thermoregulatory system in geriatrics, postanaesthesia – recovery phase, recumbent patients, laryngeal paralysis patients.

Nursing considerations

As part of the nursing care there may be cases, such as those outlined in which the patient is unable to fully thermoregulate its body temperature. It is therefore necessary to alter or adapt external temperature or conditions to maintain as normal a temperature as possible.

It is important to note, in patients with a subnormal body temperature, that conserving what heat they already have is insufficient and a direct source of heat is required:

- Heat lamps – care must be taken not to hang the lamp too near to the patient. This form of heating is best suited to small patients such as neonates, as the warmth from the lamp is focused in quite a small area. Larger lamps may be used for larger, walk-in kennels.
- Underfloor heating – some practice kennels have underfloor heating, which provides controlled, continuous warmth directly underneath the patient.
- Heat pads – various commercial heat pads may be warmed in the microwave for a specified length of time and placed under the patient's bedding. They lose their heat eventually and will need rewarming. Latex gloves

Table 15.5 Possible complications resulting from intravenous catheter placement

	Causal agent	Clinical signs	Treatment required
Thrombophlebitis	Inflammation of a vein usually associated with thrombus formation	Swelling of surrounding area, redness, heat and pain	Remove catheter immediately and seek alternative access. Vein should not be used again
Air embolism	Sudden obstruction of a blood vessel due to the introduction of air into the lumen of a blood vessel. An embolism may also be caused by a blood clot or piece of tissue	Temporary paralysis, dyspnoea. Can be fatal if it occurs in the heart or lungs	Catheter should be removed immediately, the catheter insertion site sealed and symptomatic treatment carried out as necessary
Thrombus formation	Formation of a blood clot due to flow of blood being impeded, e.g. by the presence of a catheter within the lumen of the vein, which may lead to an embolism	Engorgement of vein and swelling of associated area (limb), may lead to temporary paralysis, dyspnoe or death from formation of embolism	Administer heparinized saline into the vein to break down clot. Catheter site should be sealed and symptomatic treatment carried out as necessary
Septicaemia/ bacteraemia	Introduction of microorganisms into the vein through poor catheter placement and management	Swelling, redness, pain and discharge from catheter site and surrounding area leading to systemic infection	Remove catheter immediately, flush catheter site with chlorhexidine solution and systemic antibiotics and symptomatic treatment administered as necessary

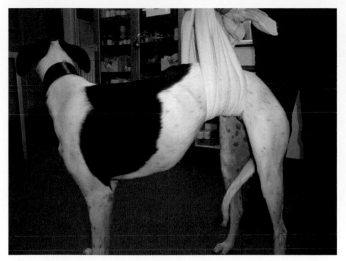

Fig. 15.13 Method of supporting a patient using a towel sling

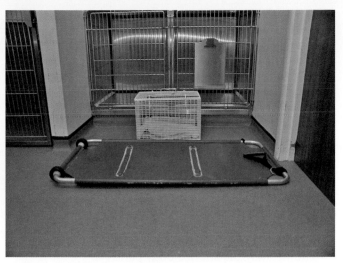

Fig. 15.14 Two methods of patient transport: a stretcher for larger canine patients and a basket for feline patients

may also be used by filling them with hot water, knotting them closed and placing them within the patient's bedding. Care must be taken not to place heat pads or gloves directly in contact with the patient.
- Space blankets may be used to conserve heat, and bubble wrap is often used, especially in neonates, to wrap up limbs and torso.

Mobilization

Conditions that can compromise mobility include: neurological disease, spinal trauma, skeletal limb trauma, ligament and tendon trauma in limbs, e.g. cruciate ligament damage and vestibular disease.

Nursing considerations

Depending on the degree of immobility, various methods of support may be implemented to allow the patient to carry out normal activities as much as possible:

- In cases of hind limb paralysis or paresis, a long towel may be placed under the patient's caudal abdomen and held like a sling to give support to the hind limbs, enabling the patient to walk and toilet (Fig. 15.13). In male dogs it is important not to occlude the penis with the towel. Specialist sling harnesses are available, which do the same job as the towel but are easier to handle.
- Crossed towels may be placed under the chest to support tetra/quadriplegics.
- Small patients such as cats and small dogs may be carried but it may be beneficial for them to use their limbs as much as possible to improve limb circulation and prevent muscle atrophy.
- Care must be taken when supporting large patients and more than one member of the nursing staff may be required! It is important to use the correct physical posture when moving patients, keeping the back straight and taking the weight on bent knees. Do not be afraid to ask for help when lifting a patient, no matter how busy everyone else is!

- Cats may be transported in baskets. This is especially important when moving them within the practice, to prevent escape (Fig. 15.14).

Grooming

Conditions that can compromise a patient's ability to groom include: recumbency, cervical injury, cat flu (calici/herpes virus due to ulcerated tongue), feeding tube placement (usually requires the use of Elizabethan collar), geriatrics with conditions such as spondylosis or arthritis, orphaned neonates.

Principles of grooming hospitalized patients

Grooming is one of the basic activities of general nursing care that can be beneficial to the patient in many ways. Depending on the temperament and condition of patients it allows the nurse to spend time with them, allowing a bond to be formed. It will also reassure the particularly stressed patient that the kennel door opening is not always associated with something unpleasant happening. It can help to relax patients, providing mental stimulation, and improve their general feeling of well-being, especially if they are unable to do it for themselves.

From a health point of view it allows the nurse to assess the patient's body and coat condition, allowing early recognition of problems such as lump formation or reduction in body condition associated with weight loss. The presence of ectoparasitic infection may also be established. Removing dead hair and debris from the coat reduces mat formation and skin irritation while promoting new hair growth. Discharge should also be removed from the eyes and nose to prevent infection arising.

Grooming hospitalized patients also gives a good impression to the owner when a patient is discharged as its appearance portrays the care it has received.

Communication

Effective communication with animal patients can be a rather difficult and misunderstood area and this may be a particular problem when the animal is in pain. Commonly recognized signs of pain in animals can be displayed in obvious behaviour patterns such as vocalization and aggression and in some cases there are specific signs associated with certain diseases; for example, patients with anterior abdominal pain, as seen in cases of pancreatitis and portosystemic shunt, often adopt a noticeable 'prayer' position.

Behavioural signs of pain and discomfort include:

- Restlessness and pacing
- Frequent posture changes
- Paying attention to the site of pain
- Panting and tachypnoea
- Depression
- Appearing lethargic/comatose
- Inappetence
- Attempting to hide away/curl up tightly
- Hiding away the affected body part
- Attention-seeking.

There are also many clinical signs that will indicate a level of pain. These include:

- Tachycardia/bradycardia
- Abnormal body temperature
- Dehydration due to anorexia and lack of drinking
- Abnormal faeces – due to anorexia or gut stasis
- Loss of weight
- Twitching or convulsions
- Abnormal urine/faecal voiding and appearance.

In most cases it is necessary to assess both the behaviour patterns and the clinical signs a patient may be exhibiting, together with its clinical history, to obtain a full picture and a more accurate interpretation.

Nursing specific types of patient

Recumbent patients

Recumbent patients require a demanding amount of intensive care, often for a long period of time. Recumbency is associated with a number of complications, so an effective nursing strategy must be designed to deal with these problems before they arise, reducing the chances of secondary complications and improving the chances of a successful recovery.

Conditions that may cause a patient to become recumbent include neurological disease, spinal trauma, spinal disease (wobbler syndrome), fractures, spinal tumours, poisoning inducing a semi-conscious or comatose state.

Nursing considerations

In many cases the patient may be semi- or fully dependent on the nurse to fulfil a number of essential activities, so you should consider the following:

- Mobility will be severely compromised. Depending on the condition and size of the animal it may be possible to aid mobility by using a towel or specialist support harness. Walking around will help improve circulation to the joints and prevent muscle atrophy, as well as improve the mental well-being of the patient.

- Feeding and fluid intake – intravenous fluid therapy will be instigated in most patients to provide maintenance fluid support. Water should be offered at least every 3 hours and may also be syringed into the mouth to moisten the lips and mucous membranes. Some cases will require assisted feeding through PEG, pharyngostomy or nasogastric tubes while others may be able to feed normally from a bowl. The type of food given should be a low-bulk (reduced fibre), highly digestible diet to reduce faecal matter and allow easy digestion. Energy expenditure is reduced so fewer calories are required.

- Constipation may be a complication and an enema or laxative may be beneficial if faeces have not been passed for more than 3 days. Enabling the patient to go outside will help to encourage natural defecation, as many patients will be unwilling to do so in recumbency.

- The patient's bladder function should be regularly monitored to assess whether voluntary control is present. Many patients will also be unwilling to urinate in recumbency, so supportive mobility to encourage natural urination should be carried out if possible. Gentle pressure on either side of the bladder may also be used to encourage urination but only if a blockage is not suspected.

- Cystitis is another common problem because of reduced water intake, reduced mobility and urine retention. An indwelling urinary catheter may be placed in patients that are difficult to mobilize or are incontinent. A used drip bag may be placed on the end of the catheter to provide a closed urine collection system, preventing urine scalding and reducing the risk of ascending infection. The amount of urine produced may also be measured on a daily basis.

- Self-grooming may be difficult in many of these patients. Grooming the patient will allow the nurse to spend some time with it as well as improving its physical and mental well-being. Some patients with longer coats may require clipping around the perineum or prepuce area to maintain cleanliness.

Potential complications

The successful recovery of these patients depends not only on specialized equipment and resources but also on being able to predict potential complications and implement the correct nursing care to reduce the risk of them occurring.

Skin problems

In recumbent patients common primary skin problems include decubital ulcers (pressure sores) and urine scalding.

Decubital ulcers are primarily caused by a combination of pressure from the weight of the animal, moisture from sweat, and friction caused by movement between the animal and the bedding. These can be difficult to treat once established and common sites tend to be over bony prominences such as the elbows, tarsus/carpus, shoulders and hips. Thin-skinned animals such as greyhounds and lurchers are particularly susceptible.

The occurrence of decubital ulcers may be reduced by providing padded, clean, dry bedding and turning the patient regularly so the potential area is not always under pressure

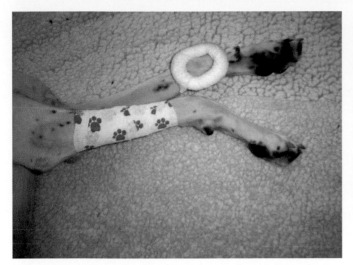

Fig. 15.15 Use of a doughnut bandage to pad bony prominences in a recumbent patient

or in contact with the bedding. Waterproof mattresses are ideal as bedding and duvets may also be used. Towels and blankets are certainly not ideal. Synthetic fleece or Vetbed is useful for a contact layer, as it is soft and highly absorbent. Padded bandages may also be applied to risk areas but care should be taken that this does not put pressure on to other areas. Figure 15.15 shows how a doughnut bandage may be used to pad bony prominences in recumbent patients. The area is elevated without being directly in contact with anything, thus minimizing further abrasion while allowing the air to circulate. This bandage will require to be secured to the area using adhesive tape.

Management of decubital ulcers include clipping the area, bathing in dilute chlorhexidine solution and applying a soothing barrier cream such as Dermisol. Antibiotics may also be prescribed by the veterinary surgeon to prevent secondary skin infections.

Urine scalding is caused by repetitive soiling of the skin by urine. Fur or hair provides little protection and all areas should be protected. By initially applying and frequently reapplying a water-repellent barrier cream such as Vaseline, the urine is prevented from coming into contact with the hair and skin. Placing a well-fitting indwelling urinary catheter can also prevent urine scalding, as the urine is unable to come into contact with the skin.

Hypostatic pneumonia

This can be a complication in laterally recumbent patients, especially those that are geriatric or seriously ill. Pooling of blood and fluids can occur in the lower lung, i.e. the lung closest to the floor, and provides an ideal medium for the growth of bacterial microorganisms. This then reduces the viability of the lung, resulting in the development of pneumonia. Clinical signs include coughing, tachypnoea and a rapid shallow breathing pattern.

Preventative treatment includes turning the patient every 4 hours (Fig. 15.16), if not contraindicated, preventing the lower lung from becoming non-viable. The patient can also be repositioned into sternal recumbency, allowing both lungs to inflate fully. Coupage may also be carried out to aid expulsion of secretions.

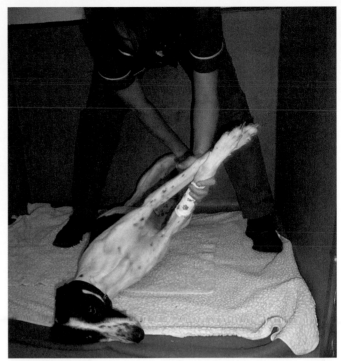

Fig. 15.16 Turning a recumbent patient

Muscle atrophy and joint adhesion formation

Muscle atrophy may be a potential complication through reduced limb use and can lead to joint adhesions and muscle spasms, which can be painful and cause permanent damage. Physical therapy under instruction from the veterinary surgeon, in the form of controlled passive limb movement and voluntary exercise, can help to reduce the risks of these complications occurring (see Ch. 16). Passive limb movement involves the nurse gently extending and flexing the joints in the limbs. Care should be taken not to overstretch the muscles and checks must be made to ensure that all limbs are fully functional and amenable to such activity (Fig. 15.17). Hydrotherapy may be of benefit, as the water provides much of the support for the patient.

Massage has also been shown to increase circulation in immobile limbs, as well as increasing fluid exchange, flushing toxins out of the tissues via the pulmonary and lymphatic drainage system and reducing the presence of oedematous fluid formation. Massage can prevent fibrous adhesions occurring between connective tissue in the limbs and provide mental relaxation for the patient. In spinal cases, massage has been beneficial in alleviating painful spasms associated with spinal disease and trauma (A. Sutton, unpublished work, 2002).

Psychological needs

In most cases the patient will be physically unwell, in pain or discomfort, and may become depressed. Bonding with the patient is important so that changes in behaviour or improvements or decline in its condition may be recognized quickly. Ideally, these patients should be kennelled in busy areas where they can observe people and other animals. Visits from owners can be beneficial and if a favourite toy or piece of clothing can be left in the kennel with the patient it will provide additional reassurance.

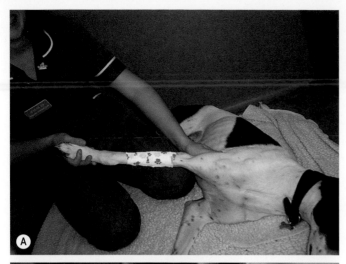

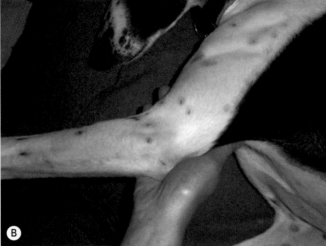

Fig. 15.17 A shoulder joint extended (**A**) and the shoulder joint flexed (**B**) in a recumbent patient as part of a passive physiotherapy routine

Neonatal and juvenile patients

Neonates requiring hand-rearing by the veterinary nurse may have been abandoned or orphaned at birth. Their care can be very time-consuming but also extremely rewarding. The type and intensity of care varies greatly over a relatively small age range. A patient of 6 weeks and under will require a greater amount of care compared to that required by a 10- or 11-week-old patient, which will be more independent and able to carry out most essential activities by itself. Consider the following factors:

Feeding and fluid intake

From birth to 7 days healthy neonates will require feeding approximately every 2 hours. This will then increase to every 3–4 hours up to 5 weeks old. At this stage weaning should be actively encouraged by offering semi-solid, highly palatable, high-caloric-density food and allowing the patient to lap. Bottle-fed neonates can find this transition difficult and a syringe may be used initially.

Neonates born by caesarean section should be reunited with their mother as soon as possible to enable them to suckle. This is important as they require the colostrum, rich in maternally-derived antibodies, which may only be absorbed effectively by their gastrointestinal system within the first 24 hours of life.

Once fully weaned the young animal will benefit from frequent small meals especially prepared for their life stage. Close checks on weight gain should be made on a daily basis. If necessary, fluids may be administered subcutaneously in small quantities to very young patients. The intraosseous route may also be used for more rapid fluid administration. Intravenous access can be difficult in these patients as the veins are fragile and small.

Elimination

Up to about the age of 4 weeks stimulation is required to induce the neonate to defecate or urinate. A damp piece of cotton wool may be used to rub the prepuce or vulva and perianal area after each feeding. Juvenile patients may be partially, fully or not toilet-trained at all, so an initial assessment will need to be made as to what stage the patient is at so that it can be nursed accordingly.

Temperature regulation

A combination of an underdeveloped thermoregulatory system, minimal subcutaneous fat deposits and a high body surface area to volume ratio increases the potential risk of significant heat loss in neonatal patient, so maintaining a warm environmental temperature is essential. The temperature for the first 7 days should be 29°C, decreasing to 26°C for the following 7 days and then 20°C until the animal is about 6 weeks of age. Hot water bottles and microwave heat pads can be used within the bedding to provide warmth. Heat lamps can be used carefully at the recommended distance.

Communication and behaviour

Neonatal and juvenile patients require a stimulating environment but they should also have a quiet area for sleep. They should be housed in an area of activity unless incubating a contagious disease, in which case they should be isolated. The kennel should be secure and free from draughts.

Toys and bedding from home should be provided to allow play and make them feel a little more secure and happy in a strange environment. An alarm clock placed under the bedding of orphaned neonates to simulate the heartbeat of the mother provides comfort and contentment.

Unfortunately, long periods of hospitalization during the prime socialization period between 8 and 14 weeks of age can have an effect on behavioural development, with resultant undesirable behaviour patterns emerging in these patients. This can be seen in puppies with canine Parvovirus that have to be isolated for long periods of time, which restricts normal developmental interaction with other dogs and people (Hobbs, unpublished work 2004). Hand-reared kittens can also become difficult to handle when they become adults because of their lack of discipline and teaching from the mother cat during kittenhood (Hewitt, unpublished work 2004).

Nursing considerations

Neonatal and juvenile patients have an undeveloped immune system so, as with any other hospitalized patient, a high level of cleanliness and hygiene must be maintained. This is even more significant in sick neonates and juveniles, especially if the primary vaccination has not yet been given and levels of maternally derived antibody levels are waning, which usually occurs around 8–12 weeks of age. All feeding bowls and litter trays should be disinfected and sterilized. Barrier nursing should be implemented in the case of a contagious disease.

There are very few veterinary drugs licensed for use in neonates and juveniles because of their potential toxicity and low therapeutic index. It is therefore very important to obtain an accurate weight on which to base correct drug dosages.

Always check for potential congenital defects in neonates and juveniles, e.g. cleft palate, umbilical and inguinal hernias, heart problems such as patent ductus arteriosus, and over- or undershot jaw. Most may be obvious and diagnosed in the early stages, but other complications, such as heart defects, may not become apparent until the patient is older.

Geriatric patients

Geriatric patients usually require intensive nursing because their ability to recover from disease or surgery will be significantly reduced compared to that of younger patients. There may also be some sensory deprivation in the form of blindness or deafness, which may make the elderly patient disorientated and anxious.

Common conditions in these patients include cancer, cardiac disease, cataracts, hepatic and renal disease, pulmonary disease, osteoarthritis, spondylosis, degenerative joint disease and dental disease. Consider the following factors:

Feeding and fluid intake

A significant proportion of hospitalized geriatric patients will be suffering with one or more conditions, so the history is a significant factor when formulating a nursing plan. Part of the treatment will be achieved through effective dietary management. Common examples include elderly dogs with heart disease or old cats with renal or hepatic disease (see Ch. 8).

Obesity may also be a problem, particularly in geriatric dogs, who usually take less exercise but their owners continue feeding the same amount and type of food the patient was fed when it was 2 years old. The energy requirements of a senior dog are approximately 20% less than its younger counterpart (McCune 2003). In some cases, owners in fact increase the food as a loving gesture! The resultant problems include the onset of joint disease such as arthritis, which, although a common condition in geriatrics, may be exacerbated by extra weight and strain on the joints. In general, a reduced-calorie, highly digestible and palatable diet with individual adaptations for particular conditions is recommended for these patients. Palatability is an important factor in feeding geriatric patients because of the reduction in olfactory senses and impaired renewal of the taste buds. There is also a commercial diet specifically designed to reduce the amount of free radicals in the brain, claiming to reduce the behaviour patterns associated with geriatric senility.

Elimination

Reduced bladder or anal sphincter tone is a common condition associated with ageing and patients should be offered more frequent opportunities to defecate and urinate outside, as many will be reluctant to do so in their kennels. Defecating indoors in the kennel or on the bedding can be as a result of mental ageing and the onset of senility. These patients may benefit from disposable padded incontinence sheets over their bedding.

Nursing considerations

When preparing a kennel for a geriatric patient, well-padded bedding is essential, especially if the animal is suffering from joint disease. This will provide support and comfort and prevent further joint stiffness and the development of decubital ulcers.

Water should be available at all times, unless it is contraindicated and intravenous fluid therapy has been put in place. These patients are less able to deal with water deprivation, compared to younger patients, and it may result in severe renal compromise.

Drug toxicity can occur because a reduction in renal and hepatic function makes metabolism of the drugs less efficient and overdosing can become a significant risk. Accurate body weights should be taken to enable accurate dosage calculations to be made.

Sensory compromise may make these patients anxious and disorientated. They should be approached gently and attempts should be made to attract their attention before entering the kennel and touching them, as they may bite if startled. An item of the owner's clothing, a familiar toy from home or visits from the owner may make them feel happier. However, some patients may find the departure of the owner too upsetting and stressful and this should be taken into consideration when planning the individual nursing care of these patients.

Bibliography

Agar, S., 2001. Small Animal Nutrition. Butterworth-Heinemann, Oxford.

Blood, D.C., Studdert, V.P., 1999. Comprehensive Veterinary Dictionary. W B Saunders, London.

Bloxham, P.A., 1999. Laboratory diagnostic aids. In: Lane, D., Cooper, B. (Eds.), Veterinary Nursing, second ed. Butterworth-Heinemann, Oxford.

Hurley, K., Michel, K., 1999. Manual of Feline And Canine Emergency Critical Care. British Small Animal Veterinary Association, Cheltenham.

Jefferies, A., 2002. Lecture notes, University Of Bristol (personal communication).

McCune, S.. Nutrition. In: Lane, D., Cooper, B. (Eds.), 2003. Veterinary Nursing, third ed. Butterworth-Heinemann, Oxford.

Simpson, G., 1994. Practical Veterinary Nursing. British Small Animal Veterinary Association, Cheltenham.

Williams, L., 1992. Care of the paraplegic patient. Veterinary Practice Nurse 4, 17–20.

Recommended reading

Agar, S., 2001. Small Animal Nutrition. Butterworth-Heinemann, Oxford.

An easy-to-read and informative book covering all aspects of small animal nutrition. Good as a quick reference guide.

Aspinall, V., 2008. Clinical Procedures in Veterinary Nursing. Butterworth-Heinemann, Oxford.

Good step-by-step guide to all procedures involved in nursing patients.

Chandler, S., 1999. General nursing. In: Lane, D., Cooper, B. (Eds.), Veterinary Nursing, second ed. Butterworth-Heinemann, Oxford, Ch. 16.

Useful text and photographs on urinary catheterization, types of catheters used and their management.

Park, F.S., 1999. Reproduction and care of the neonate. In: Moore, M. (Ed.), Manual of Veterinary Nursing. British Small Animal Veterinary Association, Cheltenham.

Informative section on nursing geriatric, neonatal and recumbent patients. Also a very good practical section on basic physiotherapy and massage.

Simpson, G. (Ed.), 1996. Practical Veterinary Nursing. British Small Animal Veterinary Association, Cheltenham.

Useful diagrams demonstrating urinary catheterization in dog, bitch, tomcat and queen.

Van der Heiden, C.A., 2003. Management of kennels and catteries. In: Lane, D., Cooper, B. (Eds.), Veterinary Nursing, third ed. Butterworth-Heinemann, Oxford, Ch. 5.

Useful section on grooming, including coat management and broad range of useful equipment displayed.

CHAPTER 16

Physiotherapy techniques

Kirsty Gwynne

Key Points

- Physical therapy or physiotherapy in animals is a relatively new branch of veterinary medicine which involves the use of natural forces such as movement, water, light and heat.
- There are many different types of physiotherapy but they all aim to improve the range of movement of joints and limbs and help with pain management so that, ultimately, the patient returns to normal locomotory function.
- Any physiotherapy regime must be preceded by detailed assessment of the patient based on a full history and a thorough physical examination.
- While the patient is undergoing physiotherapy, the type and duration of the sessions must be constantly monitored and evaluated and, if necessary, the regime must be altered to suit the condition of the patient.

Introduction

The size of the patient population has changed dramatically over the last 10 years and veterinary medicine has made real progress in the diagnosis and treatment of surgical and medical locomotor disorders. Physiotherapy, or physical therapy as it was originally known, is becoming an increasingly important component of veterinary care.

Physiotherapy can be described as medical treatment in which exclusive use is made of natural forces such as light in the form of lasers, water, electric current, thermal agents, movement, therapeutic ultrasound and magnetic fields. The use of most types of physiotherapy should ideally be restricted to qualified professionals, and the Royal College of Veterinary Surgeons (RCVS) Code of Professional Conduct advises that the veterinary surgeon, with the care of the animal, must be satisfied that the person carrying out the procedure is suitably trained and experienced. The use of hydrotherapy can theoretically be done by any untrained lay person, but it is to be hoped that any responsible veterinary practice will recommend the use of trained and reliable hydrotherapists in order to ensure the safety and welfare of their patients. For physiotherapy to be successful, it is essential that all persons involved, principally the owner, nurse and veterinary surgeon, are fully aware that treatment may be a long-term commitment and is not a 'quick fix'.

The aim of physiotherapy

Physiotherapy for companion animals presents multiple therapeutic benefits, improves the quality of life and speeds up functional recovery. It can be helpful in:

- Pain management
- Combating acute and chronic inflammatory processes
- Improving the range of motion of affected joints
- Improving blood perfusion and consequently tissue growth
- Reducing muscle contraction and tension
- Maintaining and strengthening muscles
- Stimulating the nervous system
- Encouraging proprioceptive rehabilitation and re-learning of motor patterns
- Improving cardiorespiratory capacity
- Reducing oedema
- Weight management in overweight patients.

Successful veterinary physiotherapy is directly related to the assessment of the patient and requires knowledge of functional anatomy and physiology, excellent communication skills and the ability to observe and assess movement patterns.

Patient assessment

When performing any clinical examination, it is essential that it is approached in a systematic manner that prevents essential signs being missed and prevents symptoms being confused with potential behavioural issues. When dealing with a patient, the physiotherapist, nurse and veterinary surgeon must take into account the animal's normal behaviour, e.g. normal gait and positioning of the limbs. This information can only be elicited by asking the client/owner the correct questions and by unobtrusive observation of the animal. The physiotherapist must consider the individual animal's nature, any underlying genetic influence, e.g. hereditary breed conditions, previous injuries or experiences, and current mental state: e.g. is the animal very fearful, all of which may affect its response.

The following points are worth noting:

1. The initial part of the patient assessment should include taking a full history from the owner, noting any subjective information.
2. The animal must be handled sensitively at all times to prevent the development of an aversion to handling and treatment.
3. While performing any examination or subsequent physiotherapy, it is essential that the patient is continuously monitored in terms of its pain response, behaviour, efficacy of the treatment and any potential changes in the treatment protocol. A lack of response from a patient to a technique or aggravation of a condition may indicate that the treatment protocol needs revising. Any improvement in range of motion, function and pain response should be noted, and these changes should be recorded.
4. The vet should observe the animal's conformation and gait, any soft tissue pain, assessed by palpation, and the response of both the peripheral and central nervous systems. This is done by active and passive movement tests and by neurological examination.
5. Note whether the animal distributes its weight evenly and whether the limbs are in correct alignment and correctly angulated. Check that the trunk is held symmetrically with evenly arranged musculature.
6. The head should be observed for any degree of tilt and that mentation appears to be normal.

Pain

When considering a physical therapy regime for a patient, it is vital that a pain assessment or scoring is conducted, and this is essential when deciding the type of treatment and formulating a treatment plan. In humans, it is relatively easy to score pain because they can self-assess and tell the doctor; however, in animals, it can only be measured indirectly. Pain in animals can lead to detrimental actions, such as biting or aggression, reluctance to move or use an affected limb, or even becoming anorexic. The nurse is vital in identifying a patient who may be experiencing pain by careful observation. It is prudent to remember that pain will be experienced differently in animals who are suffering from different types of injury. The role of the owner may also be important in helping the nurse, veterinary surgeon or physiotherapist assess the level of pain because they are familiar with the animal's normal behaviour patterns and temperament.

Animals may be able to experience anticipatory pain and may have symptoms of anxiety when faced with a painful stimulus, so when approaching a patient, a person should take into consideration that this may appear to be a threat to the animal.

A pain sensation is when sensory information is transmitted to the central nervous system (CNS) from afferent neurons. The process is called nociception. The pain sensation is detected by sensory receptors and transmitted through the dorsal horn of the spinal cord into the grey matter and results in a reflex action or arc in which the limb is withdrawn from the stimulus (see Ch. 4). The pain sensation also travels up the spinal cord in the white matter to the brain where it is interpreted as conscious pain. This may teach the animal to avoid that painful stimulus in future. Pain reflexes work closely with the fear response, which is important in recognizing potentially dangerous stimuli. As a result, the animal develops avoidance methods such as reluctance to use a limb. Pain is a complex mechanism that merits further reading (see 'Recommended Reading').

Behaviour indicators such as inappetance, recognition of pain and distress (e.g. vocalization, paying attention to the injured area or withdrawal from the group), and mentation levels are commonly used to monitor or score the level of pain. Clinical signs such as cardiovascular function, pupil dilation, temperature, respiratory rate and pattern, neurological and musculoskeletal signs, and digestive system function are also essential indicators of pain. Many of these indicators are subjective and opinions may differ between personnel – the owner who is most familiar with the animal remains the most useful assessor. There are a number of different pain scoring charts that have been designed for use with animals and provide a more objective scale by giving numerical value to the behavioural and clinical signs. The Glasgow Composite Pain Scale, which has been designed by the University of Glasgow, is a useful and comprehensive tool in identifying pain levels in animals.

If a patient has been identified as experiencing pain, there is an ethical obligation to reduce or eliminate the pain that is being experienced (see Ch. 1). Physiotherapy can help reduce the pain that an animal may be experiencing, and this may be assisted by the concurrent use of pharmaceutical agents, e.g. non-steroidal anti-inflammatory drugs (NSAIDs), opioids.

Techniques used in physiotherapy

Massage

There are many forms of massage that can be used to assist the patient to relax, reduce tension and pain in the muscles, improve lymphatic and venous circulation, stimulate the nervous system, and encourage the elimination of metabolic waste.

Contraindications include pyrexia, tumours, in case the actions result in metastatic spread, inflammation and open wounds. Massage helps prepare the muscles before other forms of physiotherapy are used.

The following techniques are all classified as massage:

a. **Effleurage** – this is a gentle form of massage that should be used prior to other forms of physiotherapy and familiarizes the animal to being touched. The technique can be performed all over the body. The therapist makes gentle contact with the patient's skin using the palm of the hand and strokes towards the heart, which encourages lymphatic and venous return. When massaging the limbs, effleurage should be performed from the distal to proximal limb. A session of effleurage should last for approximately 10 minutes.
b. **Petrissage** – when performing petrissage, the therapist rolls, squeezes, compresses and kneads the skin and muscles to increase the circulation. This increases the supply of oxygen and nutrients to the tissues, while

Table 16.1 Indications for the use of coupage or respiratory physiotherapy

Indications for respiratory physiotherapy	Example
Pulmonary oedema	Cardiac disease
Upper respiratory tract obstruction	During and post anaesthesia recovery in brachycephalic dogs
Pneumonia	Bacterial infections
	Viral infections
	Fungal infections
Aspiration pneumonia	Poisoning
	Laryngeal paralysis
	Megaoesophagus
	Myasthenia gravis
	Forced feeding

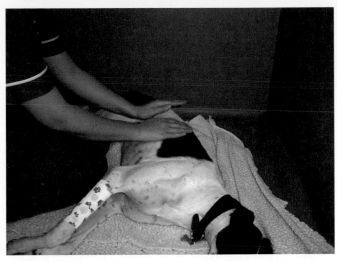

Fig. 16.1 Coupage being administered to a recumbent patient

encouraging muscle relaxation. Petrissage is used to encourage the breakdown and mobilization of adhesions in damaged tissues, soften fascia and prevent injury. It is very important for the therapist to observe the patient closely while doing this to assess pain levels and tolerance.

Procedure:

- The therapist should start petrissage at the distal limb and move in a proximal direction or from the tail, working cranially.
- Fingertips or the palm of the hand are applied to the muscles and skin with differing amounts of pressure according to the condition of the tissues and the purpose of the massage.
- In the hospitalized patient, petrissage should be performed for 10–20 minutes, three to four times a day.

c. **Percussion** – this involves gently tapping the skin with the palm or the side of the hand – large areas of muscle can be treated in this way. Percussion increases blood supply to the surrounding tissues and also aids relaxation of the muscles.

d. **Vibration** – this is a useful technique in which a group of muscles are slowly moved in a to-and-fro movement or by holding the paw to stimulate the whole limb. Vibration is useful at the end of a massage session because it relaxes the muscles. Effleurage may also be used at the end of the massage session.

Coupage

Coupage, which is also known as respiratory physiotherapy, is important in recumbent animals and those suffering from pulmonary disease because this type of patient is likely to suffer from reduced lung volume and pooling of pulmonary secretions. Coupage is used to maintain optimal respiratory function by loosening secretions and assisting airway clearance by encouraging coughing (Table 16.1).

Coupage is performed by rhythmically patting or clapping with cupped hands over the walls of the thorax for approxi-

mately 5 minutes, working from the caudal to the cranial lung fields (Fig. 16.1). This rhythmic patting loosens pulmonary secretions. The technique is contraindicated in cases where there are fractured ribs or other thoracic trauma. Patients suffering from pulmonary disease are liable to have a reduced lung capacity and function, and it is therefore important not to stress the patient prior, during or after the treatment.

Procedure:

- The patient should be positioned in sternal recumbency, which ensures that the patient has the maximum available lung capacity and a more effective cough reflex. It may be useful for the nurse to use foam wedges or blankets to support the patient in this position.
- Coupage may be performed for 2–10 minutes, three to five times a day depending on the condition and tolerance of the animal.
- After the procedure is over, the animal should remain in sternal recumbency for at least 10 minutes or until any secretions have been coughed up and expelled.

More than 90% of the respiratory secretions are water. They may be quite mucoid or viscous, and they have to be expelled via the relatively narrow bronchi and trachea. It is essential that the patient is not dehydrated as this will increase the viscosity of the secretions, making elimination harder for the patient. Unless respiratory distress is observed, avoid the administration of diuretics as this will only cause an increase in viscosity. It is important to note that animals that require coupage may be hypoxic and tachypnoeic and should be treated with the relevant medications and oxygen therapy at the direction of the veterinary surgeon. In some patients, mucolytics or nebulization may be required. The patient should be monitored closely and the nature and colour of the secretion observed.

Postural drainage – this refers to the position in which the patient is placed to drain the fluid from the lungs by coupage. This depends on the location of the fluid (Table 16.2). To be successful, the patient should be cooperative, and this is more likely to be achieved in the more compromised animal.

Table 16.2 Postural drainage positions (from McGowan et al. 2007)

Areas of lung to be drained	Postural drainage position
Lateral segment of the left caudal lung lobe	The patient is placed in left lateral recumbency, with the hind end elevated to 40°
Left and right caudal dorsal lung fields	The patient is in sternal recumbency, with the hind end elevated 40°
Left and right caudal ventral lung fields	The patient is in dorsal recumbency, with the hind end elevated 40°
Left and right cranial ventral lung fields	The patient is in dorsal recumbency, with the front end elevated 40°
Left and right cranial dorsal lung fields	The patient is in sternal recumbency, with the front end elevated 40°
Right middle lung lobe	The patient is in dorsal recumbency and a pillow is placed under the right-hand side of the thorax (so that the right side is higher than the left). The hind end is elevated 40°, and the front end in rotated a quarter turn to the right
Lateral segment of the right caudal lung lobe	The patient is in left lateral recumbency, with the hind end elevated 40°

When deciding on the position, consider any underlying conditions that may cause discomfort. It is essential that all patients should be closely monitored during treatment, paying particular attention to the respiratory and heart rates and the levels of oxygen saturation.

The use of positioning aids such as sandbags, rolled-up blankets or foam wedges will help to keep the animal in position. The body must be fully supported and comfortable to prevent ischaemia of the tissues, which potentially may result in decubital ulcers on prominent projections such as the hock and point of the hip. Once the patient is comfortable and in a secure position on the table, coupage can be performed on the appropriate area of the chest.

Passive joint mobilization and stretching

Mobilization and stretching preserves or increases the flexibility of joints and stimulates the muscles and nerves, improves coordination and range of motion and is suitable for the recumbent patient. The procedure should never cause any pain to the patient; the joints should not be over-extended and the animal should be carefully restrained to prevent any injuries.

Procedure:

- The animal should be positioned in lateral recumbency.
- Heat may be applied to the appropriate joints and muscles to achieve better relaxation.
- All joints in the affected limb should be supported and gently flexed and extended through the full range of motion.
- The limb being worked on should be held parallel to the ground to prevent torque of the joints.
- Flex the most proximal joint first and work distally (Fig. 16.2).

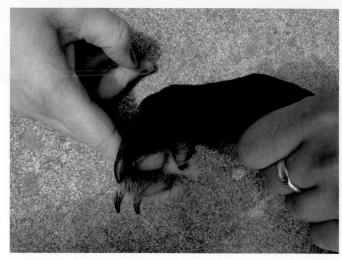

Fig. 16.2 Flexion of the phalanges

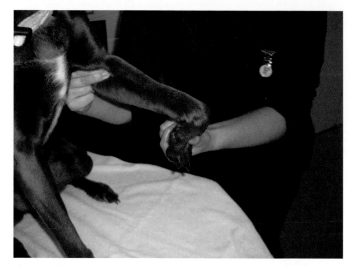

Fig. 16.3 Flexion of the carpus

- Guide the limb, do not pull it.
- Do not hyperextend the carpus or tarsus; these joints should be flexed and relaxed, unless there is a tendon contracture problem (Fig. 16.3).
- The hip and shoulder joint have rotation as well as flexion and extension. Start with small circles and gradually increase the motion.
- The affected limb/joint should be manipulated 10–20 times, three to four times daily.
- The final extension or flexion position is maintained for approximately 10 seconds before relaxing.
- The exercise can be completed by mobilizing the entire limb in a 'bicycle' movement, which stimulates the entire nerve pathway to the area.

Active therapeutic exercise

Animals, unlike humans, are usually keen to attempt to return to normal limb function as soon as they can after injury or disease, so, as soon as it is safe for a limb to be used, active therapeutic exercises can be gradually intro-

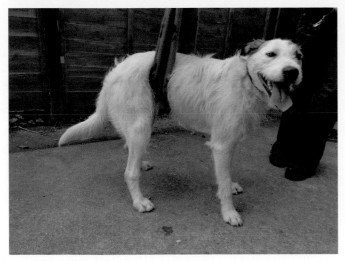

Fig. 16.4 Support being provided to a dog using a towel

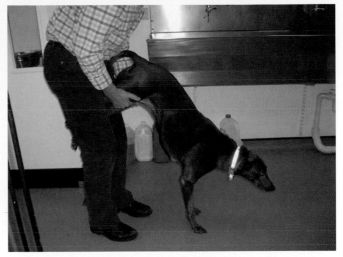

Fig. 16.5 The use of 'wheelbarrow walking' in a dog

duced to increase the strength, range of movement and proprioceptive function. These exercises are often better tolerated by the patient than passive exercise.

Active therapeutic exercise encourages the patient to make limb movements and for the limbs to become weight bearing. They help reduce pain and also stimulate the complete locomotor system, improve cardiorespiratory capacity and increase activity. The exercises should be started as soon as possible but the intensity, duration, frequency and type of exercise must be determined by the animal's clinical signs. Contraindications include disorders of the cardiovascular and respiratory systems, weakening of the bone structure, e.g. osteoporosis, and injuries resulting from trauma.

Procedure:

- Ensure that the animal is standing on an appropriate floor surface – rubber matting is a good non-slip surface.
- Support the animal's weight using slings or hoists. The use of towels is often the easiest method (Fig. 16.4).
- The weight of large dogs must always be supported by two nurses.
- Support the animal in a standing position so that all four feet are touching the floor.
- The animal should be gently raised off the floor and lowered back down – this encourages the animal to take its weight and increases proprioception.
- Once weight bearing improves and muscle strength increases, the animal can be encouraged to stand and walk on its own.
- The duration of the exercise will depend on the animal's condition. Recommended session length is 2–10 minutes, repeated three to four times a day.
- Observe the patient closely to monitor and record progress and to ensure that the treatment session has not gone on for too long.

Walking is the simplest and most essential form of exercise for an animal. Slow lead walking encourages natural posture and weight distribution and involves little or no financial cost for the client. The nurse or physiotherapist can teach the client the different types of walking, e.g. incline walking, stair walking and the speed, and duration that are required.

A treadmill is a useful piece of equipment because as the floor moves under the animal's feet, it encourages weight bearing, which the patient may refuse to do. The speed and height of the treadmill can be adjusted according to the patient's tolerance and condition. Galloping on a treadmill is not recommended as it increases shock to the joints and may cause uncontrolled movements. Any resistance to the exercise may be helped by the nurse walking beside the patient or encouraging it from the front of the treadmill. The use of a harness will help prevent the animal from walking off the side of the treadmill.

Other forms of active exercise include:

- 'Wheelbarrow walking', which forces the use of the forelimbs and increases the extension of the shoulders and hip joints (Fig. 16.5).
- Stair walking to induce hip and knee flexion and extension. The height and depth of the steps should be assessed to ensure that the patient is exercised appropriately. Stair walking should be slow and controlled to encourage the use of all limbs rather than allowing the animal to hop or jump up the stairs.
- Obstacles such as stones/rocks or boxes for the patient to step over to encourage flexion of the joints.
- Sitting/standing exercises to strengthen the hind limbs. Encouraging a sitting patient to stand up uses the hind limb and lumbar muscles and improves muscle tone and proprioception. This can be extended to lying/ standing exercises.
- Walking in a circle or a figure of eight to stimulate proprioceptive function.
- Voluntary flexion and extension of the neck by tempting the animal with a ball or a bowl of food and moving it up or down, or left and right.
- Weight shifting, which involves a nurse supporting the animal's pelvis and gently pushing the hindquarters to the left or the right. This causes the animal to lose its balance so it must move its feet to keep upright. This helps improve proprioception and muscle tone.
- Pole walking requires the placing of four to five poles horizontally on the ground, a set distance apart that corresponds to the length of the patient's stride – a

horizontal ladder may also be used The animal is then led on a lead over them. This encourages proprioception to maintain balance and extension and flexion of the fore and hind limbs. Pole walking uses muscle activities different from that used in simple walking and is also good for patients recovering from neurological dysfunction.

- Exercises using exercise/gym balls or peanut balls (inflatable balls shaped like a peanut) can be used in patients with spinal or locomotor injuries or patients recovering from surgery to the spine. This type of physiotherapy should be performed at the direction of the veterinary surgeon or the physiotherapist. The exercise ball can be used to support a patient who can stand actively or passively for a short period of time. The patient is laid on its abdomen on the ball with its feet on either side and is closely supported by the nurse. The ball is then gently rolled forwards, backwards and sideways and the aim is for the patient to keep its balance. This gentle motion helps the animal maintain neurological proprioception and muscle tone of its limbs and abdomen while the spine is fully supported, preventing hyperflexion or extension.

Active and passive joint movement and other forms of exercise should not be used in patients with acute arthritis. These patients should be rested and confined; however, they would be suitable for simple forms of massage.

Thermotherapy

Thermotherapy is the application of heat and cold for the treatment of pain and injury.

a. **Heat** – the application of heat causes dilation of the blood vessels, increasing the blood flow to the muscles and bringing about relaxation of the muscle fibres. This allows for increased extension of fibrous tissues and accelerates nerve conduction.
   Heat application is a very useful therapy prior to walking, exercise and physical therapies. It may be applied to the distal limbs and provided in the form of heat pads, hot water bottles and infrared lamps that will warm the superficial surrounding tissues to approximately 1 cm in depth. It should be noted that all heat sources should be wrapped in towels and heat lamps should be monitored carefully to avoid any burns to the skin. For deeper heat, e.g. around the hip, shoulder and vertebral column, it is recommended to use therapeutic ultrasound, which should only be used by the nurse at the direction of the veterinary surgeon or physiotherapist.
b. **Cold** – known as cryotherapy – this may be applied to an area in the initial post-injury phase to reduce haemorrhage and swelling of affected muscles and joints. Cold can be provided in the form of icepacks or ice cubes in a plastic bag, and in an emergency, bags of frozen peas provide a perfectly acceptable alternative. It is essential that the icepack is covered in a towel to prevent cold burns to the patient's skin.

Superficial heat and cold can be applied for 15–20 minutes, one to three times a day or several times per week depending on the condition. When using direct sources of heat or cold, it is essential that the temperature is monitored closely to prevent heat or cold burns.

Hydrotherapy

Hydrotherapy provides exercise in water in the form of swimming or just walking. It has become popular in the last few years as form of physiotherapy for dogs but is not generally popular with cats. It is mainly used in the form of a bath or pool and the therapeutic value is related to the physical properties of water, i.e. the hydrostatic pressure it exerts on tissues and the resistance that it provides to movement within the water, thus slowing down the animal's movements. The body is supported by the water and the combination of reduced velocity and buoyancy results in low-impact activity, which is much less damaging to limbs than comparable activity on land.

Hydrotherapy is useful for rehabilitation following orthopaedic surgery, promoting joint work and function, rehabilitation after neurological injury, for muscle strengthening and development and cardiorespiratory function. Hydrostatic pressure, i.e. the pressure exerted by the water, will also reduce swelling and oedema within tissues; however, water also produces pressure on the thorax, which may increase the physical exertion of breathing, so the cardiovascular and respiratory health of a patient must be assessed before prescribing the use of hydrotherapy.

Hydrotherapy is not suitable for those animals with skin disease, open wounds and surgical incisions, pyrexia, cardiovascular or respiratory system disease, uncontrolled epilepsy, or viral infections.

It has been suggested that hydrotherapy may have the following benefits:

- Increasing muscle mass and strength
- Allows gradual progression and full return to normal function for joints and muscles
- Reduction of pain in patients with degenerative joint disease
- Reduction of oedema
- Prevention of muscle atrophy
- Allows the continuation of exercise when land-based exercise is difficult or contraindicated
- Increased circulation, which assists healing
- By building up the animal's fitness, it reduces the likelihood of injury to muscles, tendons and ligaments.

Types of hydrotherapy pool

There are two main types of pool, which have various advantages and disadvantages, but experience will eventually influence the final choice.

1. **Underwater treadmills** (Fig. 16.6) – these are better for developing an animal's fitness rather than providing a 'fun' experience. They consist of a tank that is filled and emptied according to use, through which runs the treadmill. They occupy less space than a pool and require a filler tank and a filter system. The water level can be easily altered to suit the patient either by pumping water in or out or by adjusting the height of the treadmill. The speed of the treadmill can also be varied. One of the main advantages is that the window

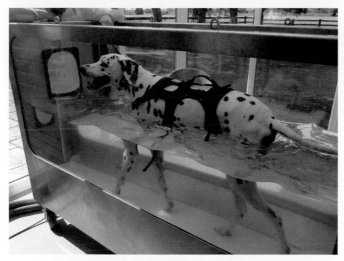

Fig. 16.6 Dalmatian using an underwater treadmill

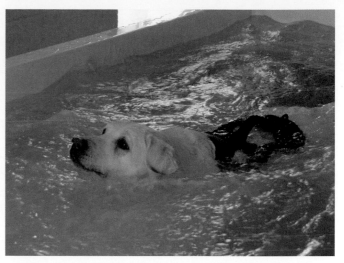

Fig. 16.8 Labrador swimming against the force of a current created by jets within the walls of the pool

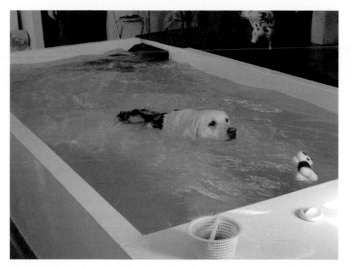

Fig. 16.7 Labrador swimming in pool and encouraged to move by the presence of his toys

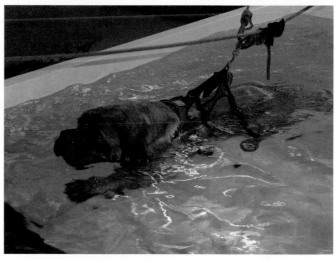

Fig. 16.9 Large mastiff assisted by a hoist

in the side allows limb movements to be easily observed.

2. **Pools** (Fig. 16.7) – these consist of a large pool with ramps to allow the dog to walk up to the level of the surrounding wall and to get down into the water. The incline of the ramps can be altered to suit the patient. There is often a submerged platform within the pool to allow resting. Some pools also have jets set within the walls, which are used to increase the workload of the dog (Fig. 16.8).

Pools are generally more versatile as they allow access to the animal from every angle and the hydrotherapist may remain outside the pool to monitor progress or get into the pool with the dog. This is useful to persuade the dog to use proper limb movements – some dogs may only use their front feet to paddle – help support the hind limbs by placing a hand under the abdomen and encourage the dog to move using various toys. Hoists are often used to help large dogs (Fig. 16.9) up the inclined ramps into and out of the pool, but some dogs panic and care must be taken with patients with spinal injuries.

The temperature of the water in the pool must be controlled and is usually set between 26 and 28 °C – this provides sufficient warmth without causing heat-related problems. Temperature can be varied and is an important aspect of thermotherapy. Cold has an analgesic effect and causes vasoconstriction, whereas heat causes vasodilation, muscle relaxation and stimulates tissue metabolism. The temperature of the water also depends on the amount of the animal's body fat. The age of the dog and the type and duration of the activity in the pool must be taken into consideration and the rectal temperature must be monitored periodically to prevent hypothermia.

To perform hydrotherapy successfully, there are several pieces of additional equipment that may be used to increase the effectiveness of the therapy (Table 16.3).

Walking in water and swimming are extremely useful active exercises for overweight or arthritic animals, but hydrotherapy should not be used if an animal is suffering from acute arthritis. Swimming induces a state of relative weightlessness or buoyancy, which forces the animal to move its entire locomotor system to maintain its position

Table 16.3 Equipment used in hydrotherapy and its indications

Equipment	Indications
Buoyancy vest or jacket	For initial swimmers and anxious dogs
	To assist in the reduction work load on the heart and lungs
	Enables the patient to exercise for a longer period
Harness	Provides support and assistance to some body areas (e.g. holding hind end or fore end higher, allowing the dog to use trunk muscles to control body rotation)
	Provide resistance from the front or rear of the dog
Hoists	Assisting large dogs in and out of the pool
Aquatoys	Motivation to encourage swimming
Steps	Provide an alternative terrain for the animal to negotiate when walking through the water
Dynamic band	Provides assistance or resistance to movement; the band can be looped behind the hind limbs to increase the workload while walking through water

and balance. The support of the water is less stressful to muscles, while the increased resistance of the water makes the muscles work harder. The resistance can be increased by using water jets for the animal to swim against (Fig. 16.8).

It should be noted that the density of the water and the animal itself has a direct effect on whether the animal floats or sinks. Before putting the animal in the water, its body type must be assessed:

- An animal that is lean or heavily muscled has a high specific gravity and will be liable to sink, so a buoyancy vest or jacket may need to be used to reduce the effort expended in keeping the head above water.
- An animal with increased body fat or osteoporosis (thinning and lightening of the bony skeleton) will have an overall lower specific gravity and will tend to float more easily, resulting in the possible need for weights to be used to get the animal to lie lower in the water, so increasing the effort required to keep the head above water.

When considering whether hydrotherapy is suitable for a patient, it is essential to consider centres of gravity and buoyancy because it will have a direct implication on some patients. For example, if a patient has had a limb amputated, then the body will rotate to the opposite side and a patient with a spinal injury and asymmetrical musculature may not be able to control any rotation in the trunk. To counterbalance the effects of rotation, it may be necessary to use a buoyancy vest and later progress to exercising against movement, e.g. modular jets.

Hydrotherapy sessions can be performed two to three times a week and last for 5–20 minutes depending on the condition and compliance of the patient. Sessions usually continue for 4–6 weeks. For orthopaedic cases, they are then reduced to one to two sessions per week for a further 6 weeks. For patients suffering from neurological conditions, daily hydrotherapy is recommended for the first 2–3 weeks. It should be emphasized that the exact details of the therapy depend on the patient, its rate of progress, and the recommendations of the veterinary surgeon and the hydrotherapist.

Therapeutic ultrasound

Therapeutic ultrasound is a form of electrotherapy and is used to treat diseased and dysfunctional joints and certain muscular disorders. The ultrasound waves are at a frequency of 1 MHz, and the technique is mainly used in collagen-rich tissues such as tendons, ligaments, cartilage and muscles because they have a high absorption of this form of energy. Diagnostic ultrasound uses frequencies between 5 and 10 MHz. Within the tissues, the energy is converted to heat, resulting in the heating of deeper tissues, which cannot be warmed by superficial methods, e.g. heat pads. Treatment by this method improves the elasticity of fibrous structures, increases blood flow, improves tissue nutrition, increases the range of movement, and reduces pain and muscle tension.

Therapeutic ultrasound is used in patients suffering from tendon and ligament injuries such as bursitis, tendonitis and joint contracture. It promotes healing by increasing blood flow and reducing pain. It also reduces any scar tissue by heating and stretching the affected tissue, and in wound healing, it encourages the inflammatory processes. Therapeutic ultrasound can be used at any time during the healing process, although during the acute stages following injury, it should be used only at low intensities as there is the potential to exacerbate oedema. The areas of the body that are either unsuitable for its use or in which it should be used only with great care are shown in Table 16.4.

Therapeutic ultrasound can also be used to enhance the application of topically applied medications such as dexamethasone, hydrocortisone and lidocaine. This technique is called phonophoresis. Ultrasound changes tissue permeability by warming the surrounding tissue, which helps dilate the point of entry, hair follicles and sweat glands and increases cell diffusion. The administration of these drugs is achieved by applying a specially prepared water-soluble coupling agent to the skin.

When using this technique, care must be taken to avoid burning the deep tissues. Make sure that the settings for the power rating and frequency of the ultrasound unit are appropriate and correct. Treat for no more than 4 minutes in any one position, and in one treatment session, use no more than four adjacent positions. Keep the transducer moving at a rate of 4 cm/s to avoid localized overheating of the area. Any behaviour by the patient, e.g. vocalization or trying to move away, should be taken as an indication of discomfort and the treatment should be stopped or reduced.

Transcutaneous electrical nerve stimulation (TENS)

TENS is another form of electrotherapy. An electrical stimulus is delivered by a TENS unit via flexible surface electrodes and is used to stimulate muscles, promote tissue repair and reduce acute, chronic muscular and skeletal pain. TENS works by blocking (depolarizing) sensory nerves, which carry pain information to the thalamus and cortex of the CNS, causing a release in endorphins or natural analgesics,

Table 16.4 Areas of the body in which use of therapeutic ultrasound is limited

Do NOT use therapeutic ultrasound in the following areas:	Take CARE with the use of therapeutic ultrasound in the following areas:
• Cardiac pacemakers • The eyes • A gravid uterus • Neoplasia • Contaminated wounds or infection • The testes • Areas where thrombophlebitis has occurred	• Over fracture sites and bony prominences • Areas of decreased circulation • Decreased pain or temperature sensation • Epiphyses in immature animals • Where plastic or metal implants have been inserted

and by depolarizing motor nerves to the muscles, resulting in muscle contraction.

TENS can be used in two modalities:

a. **High frequency (80–100 Hz)** – the intensity of the current should remain constant and beneath the threshold of motor neuron stimulation, i.e. without triggering muscular contraction. This type generates rapid, but short-term, analgesia (one to several hours). High-frequency TENS is indicated mainly for acute and super acute pain.

b. **Low frequency (2–8 Hz)** – the intensity of the current is just above the muscular contraction threshold and provides gradual and longer-lasting pain relief (up to 8 hours). Low-frequency TENS is indicated for subacute and chronic pain. The electrode should be applied over the affected muscle and the intensity increased until a muscle contraction is obtained.

The TENS current can be applied for initial treatments of 10–15 minutes to reduce anxiety and to allow the animal to become familiar with the sensations. Subsequent treatment sessions may last for up to 1 hour at a time. The most common application sites for the electrodes are directly over the site of pain, directly over the nerve that supplies the affected area, or on either side of the affected joint or nerve root. The electrodes can also be placed over acupuncture sites as a practical and effective alternative to acupuncture, which may present difficulties in some animals. Conduction of the electrical stimulus through the skin is facilitated by the use of a conducting gel.

Contraindications for the use of TENS include:

• Patients with a pacemaker or over the heart area
• Patients with seizure disorders
• Over areas with decreased pain or temperature sensation
• When active motion is contraindicated
• Sites of infection
• Neoplasia
• Over areas of thrombophlebitis.

Laser therapy

Laser therapy uses electromagnetic radiation that is in the visible or near-visible part of the electromagnetic spectrum and should only be used under the direction of a physio-therapy practitioner or veterinary surgeon. The energy produced by low-intensity lasers causes tissue reactions that can stimulate tissue repair and cause changes in blood flow circulation. Laser treatment may also help reduce pain by releasing endogenous opiates.

Lasers can be specifically used in the treatment of:

• Decubital ulcers and wounds
• Arthritis and acute and chronic inflammation
• Musculoskeletal conditions and injuries that are acute and chronic (e.g. tendon and muscle tears, soft tissue injuries).

Laser therapy is contraindicated in cases with haemorrhage, used over a gravid uterus, or in patients with diagnosed or suspected carcinomas.

Physiotherapy in practice

For physiotherapy to be a success, it is essential that a care plan is carefully designed for the individual patient and implemented by all members of staff. It is essential that detailed physical examinations are undertaken on a regular basis to ensure that the treatment is progressing satisfactorily and that any changes that may be required are identified and put into practice.

The role of the owner

Before the physiotherapy programme begins, owners must understand exactly what will be done to their animal and how they will be involved. For example, are they expected to attend the session and watch or help, or will the animal be admitted to the practice and the treatment carried out in the kennels or operating theatre; is there anything that they can do at home with the animal; are any additional drugs to be given; how often must the exercises be done and for how long; how long will the programme go on for. Client understanding, support and compliance are vital if the programme is to be successful, and it may be the job of the nurse to explain all the procedures.

After the first physiotherapy session, and then before every subsequent session, the following information must be obtained and recorded:

• How is the animal today and what exercise has been done before coming in for the appointment?
• Has the animal been given any form of pain relief?
• Has the animal had any treatment at home such as massage or heat or ice therapy?
• Has the owner made any changes to the animal's exercise regime at home, which may be a contributory factor in any improvement or deterioration?
• If the animal has been more lame, then how severe was it and how long did this last?

Asking these questions will allow the physiotherapist or the veterinary surgeon to decide how to progress with the patient's exercise programme and what advice to give to the client about any continuing care in the home.

Some treatments may be able to be performed by owners in their own home as long as direct instruction and demonstration of the techniques has been undertaken and the clients are confident and competent. If treatments are to be performed by the client, then it is imperative that the client keeps a detailed record of the treatment session and any improvement or deterioration of the condition.

After any physiotherapy session in which the patient is returning home, it is essential that the owner monitors the animal very closely for at least 24 hours, taking particular note of any changes and anything that may indicate that the treatment was too intense e.g. stiffness, muscle soreness and an increase in lameness.

Acknowledgement

I would like to thank Hereford Canine Hydrocare for the use of their facilities and their support.

Bibliography

Brockstahler, B., 2006. The orthopaedic patient: conservative treatment, physiotherapy and rehabilitation. Clinical Nutrition Symposium.

Grubb, T., 2006. Non-pharmacologic pain relief in sporting dogs. International Veterinary Information Service. NAVC Proceeding.

McGowan, C., Goff, L., Stubbs, N., 2007. Animal Physiotherapy: Assessment, Treatment and Rehabilitation of Animals. Blackwell Publishing, Oxford.

Owen, M.R., 2006. Rehabilitation therapies for musculoskeletal and spinal disease in small animal practice. Eur. J. Companion Anim. Pract. 16 (2), 137–147.

Piras, A., 2006. Muscle and tendon injuries and diagnosis, treatment and prognosis. European Society of Veterinary Orthopaedics and Traumatology Congress. pp. 121–127.

Piras, A., 2007. Muscle and tendon injuries: diagnosis, treatment and prognosis. North American Veterinary Conference.

Prankel, S., 2008. Hydrotherapy in practice. In Pract. 30, 272–277.

Rivier, S., 2007. Physiotherapy for cats and dogs applied to locomotor disorders of arthritic origin. Vet. Focus 17 (3), 32–36.

Vannini, R., 2006. Muscle and tendon injury in cats. European Society of Veterinary Orthopaedics and Traumatology Congress. pp. 151–152.

Recommended reading

McGowan, C., Goff, L., Stubbs, N., 2007. Animal Physiotherapy: Assessment, Treatment and Rehabilitation of Animals. Blackwell Publishing, Oxford.
This is an excellent book. It details many of the physiotherapy techniques that are available to the veterinary nurse while providing an insight into the different treatment protocols for dogs and horses.

I also strongly suggest that the reader obtains bibliography from scientific veterinary journals (e.g. In Practice *and the* European Journal of Companion Animal Practice*) because they provide information on recent and current research/writing.*

Owen, M.R., 2006. Rehabilitation therapies for musculoskeletal and spinal disease in small animal practice. Eur. J. Companion Anim. Pract. 16 (2), 137–147.

CHAPTER 17

Fundamental pharmacology

Sally Bowden

Key Points

- When a drug is administered to the body it moves through the tissues to its designated site of action – this is the study of pharmacokinetics.
- The speed at which a drug reaches its site of action is determined by the route of administration.
- The body metabolizes drugs, mainly in the liver, during which process the drug is converted into a form that can be excreted.
- Different types of drug have differing effects, which are determined by their formulation and determine their therapeutic use.
- Drugs and other chemicals in the body may interact with each other, resulting in unpredictable and sometimes adverse reactions.
- The production of drugs by pharmaceutical companies, the dispensing of drugs by veterinary surgeons to their clients and the subsequent disposal of the surplus drug are subject to many pieces of legislation. These are all designed to protect the patient, the owner giving the drug, the general public and the environment.

Introduction

This chapter aims to provide veterinary nurses with a broad, basic understanding of various aspects of pharmacology. It encompasses a range of subjects, from general pharmacokinetics and pharmacodynamics, through the classification of commonly used drugs, to practical aspects of handling and dispensing medication.

What is pharmacology?

Pharmacology is the study of the properties of drugs and their effects on living organisms. It is derived from the Greek word *pharmakon,* meaning 'drug', and the suffix -logy, meaning 'study of'. Clinical pharmacology, or pharmacotherapeutics, is concerned with the effects of drugs in treating disease. The term 'drug' may be defined in various ways but, put simply, describes any substance that, when administered, has a specific effect on the body.

The origins of drugs

Drugs have been used for religious, recreational and medicinal purposes throughout the course of history. Alcohol and opium are among the earliest examples of drugs. Other plant-derived drugs such as tobacco, strychnine, digitalis and atropine, to name but a few, have also been used for several hundred years. More recently, around the beginning of the 19th century, scientists discovered methods of modifying natural substances, or synthesizing drugs, to provide safer and more effective treatments. Drugs from animal and mineral sources began to be used. In the modern age, genetically engineered drugs are the latest pharmacological development in a burgeoning pharmaceutical industry.

Pharmacokinetics

The word pharmacokinetics literally means 'drug movement'. It pertains to what happens to a drug when it enters the body, i.e. what the body does to the drug. This section traces drug movement through the body and examines how it gets in, where it goes, what happens to it along the way and how it leaves. Pharmacokinetic processes are often categorized into four main areas – absorption, distribution, metabolism and elimination.

Drug absorption

The route of administration, the disease status of the patient and the formulation of the drug affect drug absorption into the body.

Route of administration and its effect on absorption

There are many routes of drug administration, but the most commonly used ones in veterinary medicine are the oral, subcutaneous, intramuscular and intravenous routes. Generally, in order for a drug to reach its site of action and have an effect, it must enter the systemic blood circulation. The exceptions to this are drugs that act locally, i.e. in the area they are applied. An example of a locally acting drug that

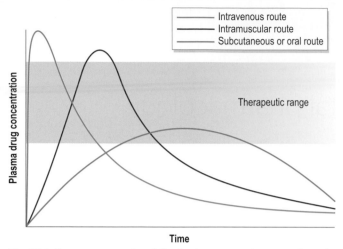

Fig. 17.1 Plasma concentrations following intravenous, intramuscular and subcutaneous injections *(Redrawn from Bill 1997)*

does not need to enter the circulation in order to reach its site of action is lidocaine hydrochloride.

The amount of drug that reaches the circulation intact (i.e. unaltered) determines the drug's **bioavailability.** For example, if the entire administered dose reaches the circulation intact, that drug has 100% bioavailability. This is also known as a bioavailability of 1. Consider the intravenous route of drug administration – drugs given by this route have a bioavailability of 1 as the drug enters the bloodstream directly and there is no absorption phase. Drugs given by all other routes of administration are said to have a bioavailability of less than 1, as less than 100% of the dose will reach the circulation intact.

Bioavailability is affected by the rate at which the drug is absorbed and also the ease of absorption. Generally, the better the blood supply to an area, the quicker the rate of absorption (Fig. 17.1). Drugs administered intramuscularly are usually absorbed quickly. Of the commonly used parenteral routes of administration, subcutaneously administered drugs have the lowest bioavailability because the skin is a less vascular part of the body.

Orally administered drugs travel through the gastrointestinal tract and most are absorbed in the small intestine. Solid oral preparations, including tablets, capsules and granules, undergo a process of dissolving known as dissolution prior to being absorbed. Liquid preparations do not need to undergo dissolution and so are usually absorbed more quickly than the solid oral preparations. Some drugs are formulated as a 'sustained release' preparation, where dissolution and subsequent absorption is slowed down. Note that this is not the same as an 'enteric-coated' tablet, which has a protective coating to prevent the destruction of the drug in the highly acidic environment of the stomach.

Once absorbed across the intestinal wall, orally administered drugs enter the hepatic portal circulation and are routed directly to the liver. One of the roles of the liver is to remove potentially toxic substances before they reach the systemic blood circulation and drugs may be partially or completely broken down because of this mechanism. This is known as the first-pass effect. The first-pass effect is one reason that some drugs cannot be administered orally, or

that the dose rate of an oral preparation when compared with a parenteral preparation of the same drug is much higher. Because of the need for dissolution, time taken to reach the site of absorption and the first-pass effect, orally administered drugs tend to have a comparatively low bioavailability. Other factors also affect the rate of absorption:

Tissue perfusion

Tissue perfusion directly affects the rate of absorption; for example, a drug injected into an active, well-perfused muscle will be absorbed more quickly than one injected into an inactive muscle, which will have a poorer blood supply. Vasoconstriction or vasodilation will cause reduced or enhanced blood flow to an area so, when injecting subcutaneously, exposing the patient to cold or hot environmental temperatures will affect the absorption rate. Disease conditions affecting perfusion have the same effect.

Drug formulation

The drug formulation can also have an effect on absorption. Drugs that dissolve more easily in water are termed hydrophilic, which literally means 'water-loving'. Drugs that dissolve more easily in fat are termed lipophilic or 'fat-loving'. Drugs administered intravenously or intramuscularly enter the extracellular fluid and, in the case of the intramuscular route, must diffuse through it to reach the circulation. Therefore, hydrophilic drugs are more readily absorbed via these routes. Drugs administered via other routes, e.g. orally or subcutaneously, must diffuse through cell membranes in order to reach the circulation. As cell membranes are mostly made up of phospholipids, lipophilic drugs are able to diffuse through them more readily.

While most drugs are formulated to facilitate absorption, there are some drugs deliberately designed to provide a 'slow-release' or 'depot' formulation. An example of this is nandrolone laurate, which is lipophilic and so not easily diffused into the interstitial fluid surrounding muscle fibres. Some drugs are formulated for slow absorption because they exert their effect where the drug is introduced. A prime example of this is piperazine, which is hydrophilic and therefore is not easily absorbed from the gut, as it must cross the cell membranes of the intestinal wall. This means that sufficient concentration remains in the gastrointestinal tract for the drug to be effective at this site. The pH of the drug and of the environment can affect absorption because it can affect the drug's hydrophilic or lipophilic tendency.

Drug distribution

The movement of drug from the systemic circulation into the body tissues is known as **distribution.** Most drugs must reach a specific area or target tissue in order to have their desired effect, known as the **therapeutic effect.**

When a drug enters the systemic circulation, drug molecules attach themselves to a certain site on plasma proteins (notably to albumin). This is called **protein binding.** Once attached, the drug molecule is inactive, i.e. unable to move into the body tissues. In order for a drug to be active, it must become unbound or 'free' – in other words, detach itself from the plasma protein. The amount of bound drug in the circulation is always the same as the amount of unbound drug in the circulation, so, as free drug molecules move into the body tissues, more bound drug molecules are released to maintain this balance. Likewise, the amount of unbound drug in the circulation and the amount of drug in the tissues will always equalize along a concentration gradient.

Factors affecting drug distribution

Some drugs bind more strongly to plasma proteins than others – these are termed highly protein-bound. The more highly protein-bound a drug is the less free drug is available to distribute into the body tissues. This means that it is often necessary to give high doses of drugs that are highly protein-bound in order for them to have a therapeutic effect. Disease conditions that cause a decrease in blood plasma protein levels, e.g. hypoalbuminaemia due to liver failure, can mean that a higher than normal amount of free drug is available for distribution and this can result in toxicity. Some drugs bind to the same site on plasma proteins. If administered together, this can result in the less highly bound drug lacking binding sites and, again, a higher than normal amount being available as free drug for distribution, so toxicity can occur. For this reason, some drugs, e.g. methotrexate and phenylbutazone, must not be administered together.

Natural barriers to the circulation exist in the body. These are the blood–brain, placental and testicular barriers. They are present to protect these areas of the body from dangerous toxins in the blood circulation. The capillary walls in the brain have a different structure from others, which means that only highly lipophilic drugs are able to cross into the brain tissue. Drugs that must reach the brain to have an effect, e.g. general anaesthetics, must be sufficiently lipophilic to be able to cross the blood–brain barrier. The placental barrier is not as efficient at preventing drugs passing into the fetal circulation and so caution should be exercised when treating pregnant animals.

Tissue perfusion in the target organ or organs will also affect distribution. Well perfused organs will receive the drug quickly. After a time, the drug will also distribute into the poorly perfused areas and drug concentration levels will drop in the blood plasma. Because distribution of drug occurs along a concentration gradient, this can cause the drug to leave the well-perfused organs and re-enter the circulation, then move into a less-well-perfused area until equilibrium is reached. This is called **redistribution**. An example of this is the anaesthetic thiopental, which is lipophilic and redistributes to the adipose tissues, causing the animal to regain consciousness (Fig. 17.2). Reduced blood flow to an organ or ischaemia caused by disease must be taken into consideration when monitoring the effects of drug therapy.

Drug metabolism

The body will metabolize or biotransform drugs as it would attempt to do with any foreign substance in the circulation. The resultant product of metabolism is known as a metabolite. This mainly occurs in the liver, although sometimes other organs, including the lung and the kidney, are involved.

Biotransformation does not simply mean that the body turns potentially harmful substances into less harmful ones

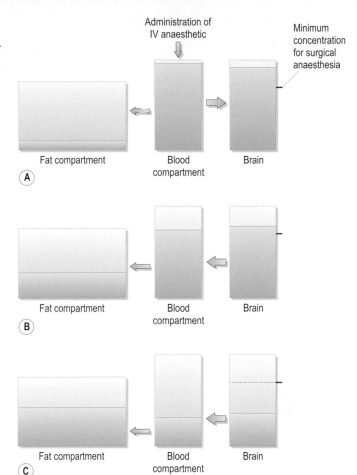

Fig. 17.2 Redistribution of an anaesthetic drug from the brain to other tissues. (**A**) The drug moves quickly from the blood to the brain, causing anaesthesia. (**B**) The brain concentration of anaesthetic then drops until it is too low to maintain anaesthesia. (**C**) When the animal begins to awaken *(Redrawn from Bill 1997)*

– it is the process by which drugs are changed into a form that is more readily excreted by the body. In some cases, the metabolite can be more active in the body than the original drug molecule. This can be an advantage if it is not possible to give the active form of the drug in the first place, and is known as giving a prodrug; for example, the corticosteroid prednisone is metabolized into prednisolone. Alternatively, the metabolite can be as active as the original drug, or even more toxic than the original drug.

The metabolic process

As elimination of drugs from the body occurs via body fluids, this means that drug metabolites must be hydrophilic to be excreted. There are two phases of drug metabolism:

- **Phase I metabolism** – enzymes act on the drug to transform it; the processes that occur are hydrolysis, reduction and/or oxidation
- **Phase II metabolism** – the metabolite is joined with another molecule to make it more hydrophilic. This is known as conjugation.

Most drugs undergo both metabolic phases but some only undergo phase II.

Factors affecting drug metabolism

Metabolic systems

A key metabolic system found in the liver is known as the mixed function oxidase system. The enzyme involved, cytochrome P450, is induced by the presence of one or more of the drugs it metabolizes. This means that consistent exposure to drugs metabolized by P450 will increase the rate of metabolism and result in ever-increasing doses being required to have a therapeutic effect. An example of this is the drug phenobarbital, used for controlling epileptic seizures. Other drugs affected by P450 would also be metabolized more quickly, so the dose rate of these would also have to be increased.

Drug interaction

Other enzyme systems are not induced by the presence of the drugs they metabolize, resulting in a fixed amount of enzyme available at any one time. If two or more drugs are administered that use the same enzyme system, this can cause a delay in drug metabolism, resulting in drug toxicity if the dose of the drugs involved is not reduced.

Some drugs cause the inhibition of certain enzymes, which could result in the metabolism of that drug, or another drug, being slowed. Inadequate liver function can also have an effect of drug metabolism, as production of the necessary enzymes may be impaired. This could be due to disease but it should be borne in mind that neonatal and geriatric animals may also have reduced liver function.

Species variation

Species variation must also be taken into account when considering drug metabolism. Most notably, cats do not possess the ability to conjugate certain drugs and so elimination from the body is slowed. This increases the likelihood of toxicity in this species from drugs that are well tolerated in other species.

Drug elimination

Drugs are eliminated from the body via a number of routes. The two main routes of elimination are in the urine via the kidney and in the faeces via the liver (in bile). Other routes of elimination include the breath, saliva, sebum and milk. The rate at which a volume of fluid can be completely cleared of drug is called the **drug clearance rate** and is measured in litres/hour. The rate at which a drug is eliminated from the body is called the **elimination rate** and is measured in mg/hour. Rapid clearance occurs when the elimination rate is high.

Elimination half-life and the therapeutic range

The elimination half-life of a drug is the amount of time required for the concentration of a drug in the blood to decrease by 50% by metabolism and elimination. It is not as easy as saying that the same length of time again will equal total clearance, as the elimination rate does not continue at the same pace, although it is usually constant. For example, if a drug had a blood concentration of 40 µg/l and after 2 hours blood concentration was 20 µg/l, that drug's half-life is 2 hours. In a further 2 hours, the blood

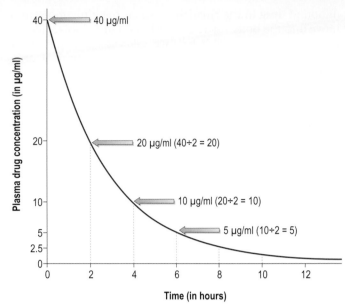

Fig. 17.3 Decrease in plasma concentrations of a drug with a half-life of 2 h *(Redrawn from Bill 1997)*

concentration would be 10 µg/l; in another 2 hours it would be 5 µg/l and so on. The symbol for elimination half-life is $T_{1/2}\,\beta$ (Fig. 17.3).

Elimination half-life is important because it can be used to determine when repeat doses of a drug are required in order to maintain the drug concentration in the blood at a sufficiently high level to ensure that enough is available for distribution to the tissues for there to be a therapeutic effect. Giving repeat doses too frequently will result in drug levels climbing too high, causing toxicity. Leaving too long a time interval between repeat doses means that the blood concentration levels will drop too low to have a therapeutic effect in the tissues. Maintaining optimal amounts of drug concentration in the blood so that neither toxicity nor ineffectiveness is created is known as keeping the levels within the therapeutic range or margin. Some drugs have a wide therapeutic range – this means that a large overdose would have to be administered before toxicity occurred. An example of a drug with a wide therapeutic range is ampicillin. Drugs with a narrow therapeutic range are those that cause toxicity with even the smallest overdose, such as digoxin. Therapeutic range can be measured by using the calculation below and this is termed the **therapeutic index**. The greater this figure, the safer the drug:

$$\text{Therapeutic index} = \text{Toxic dose}/\text{Effective dose}$$

When drug therapy is initially instigated, peak and trough blood concentrations are low. After approximately five half-lives the rate of administration is equal to the rate of elimination and so the peak and trough levels increase and remain more constant. This is known as the steady state (Fig. 17.4). When monitoring drug concentrations in the blood, it is important that the steady state has been reached to ensure that peak and trough blood plasma concentrations are within the therapeutic range. Thus, knowing the elimination half-life of a drug is important. A common example is monitoring blood concentrations of phenobarbital. As this drug

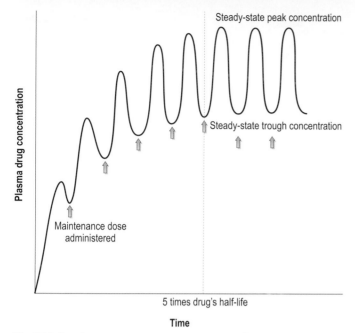

Fig. 17.4 Steady-state concentration *(Redrawn from Bill 1997)*

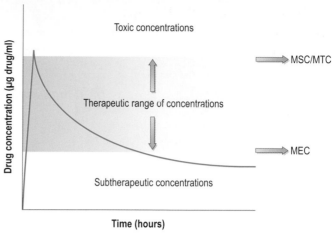

Fig. 17.5 Therapeutic range of plasma drug concentrations *(Redrawn from Bill 1997)*

has an elimination half-life of 2 days, the steady state is not reached until day 10. Measuring blood plasma concentration prior to day 10 of treatment would give an inaccurately low measurement.

Some drugs with very long half-lives will not reach the steady state, and therefore are not fully effective, for many days. To combat this problem a higher than normal amount of drug is given initially, which is known as a **loading dose**.

Drugs licensed for use in food animals have a **withdrawal period**, which is the clearance time calculated using the elimination half-life of the drug. Withdrawal periods are usually present on drug labels and state the period of time after the last dose of each drug that the animal or its produce e.g. milk cannot be used for human consumption. Withdrawal periods prevent drug residues entering the human food chain.

Factors affecting drug elimination

Renal elimination

Renal elimination, in which a drug is carried to the kidney by the blood and excreted via the urine, is dictated by the glomerular filtration rate (GFR), among other factors. Conditions causing reduced blood flow to the kidney, e.g. hypotension and hypovolaemia, will decrease elimination rate, which could result in toxicity. Geriatric animals often have a degree of renal compromise and the dose rates of renally excreted drugs may need to be reduced to allow for this.

Hepatic elimination

In hepatic elimination a drug is secreted into the bile in the liver. It is then emptied into the gastrointestinal tract and excreted in the faecal matter. Disease conditions affecting liver function can decrease the elimination rate via this route in addition to affecting metabolism. Some drugs are lipophilic after emptying into the gastrointestinal tract – this means that they may be reabsorbed through the gut wall and

into the hepatic circulation, then return to the systemic circulation, where they can exert an additional therapeutic effect. This is known as enterohepatic circulation.

Pharmacodynamics

The word pharmacodynamic literally means 'drug action'. It pertains to what effect a drug has on the body, i.e. what the drug does to the body. This section traces drug movement through the body and examines how drugs exert their effects.

The basic principle of drug therapy is to maintain concentrations within the therapeutic range. The higher the dose, the greater the pharmacological effect – too small a dose and the concentrations will be subtherapeutic; too great a dose and the concentrations may cause toxicity. The lowest level at which concentrations are therapeutic is termed the minimum effective concentration (MEC). The highest therapeutic level is usually the same concentration at which toxicity could occur. This is sometimes termed the maximum safe concentration (MSC) or minimum toxic concentration (MTC) (Fig. 17.5).

Receptor-mediated pharmacodynamics

The main mechanism of drug action is via receptor sites, which are specific protein molecules on a cell membrane. There are several different receptors, differentiated by their molecular structure or shape. Cells do not have all receptor types – different cells have a different range and number.

Agonist and antagonist effects

Receptors normally interact with natural substances called endogenous ligands, e.g. neurotransmitters and hormones that have an effect on the cell. When a drug is present in the body tissue it combines with the receptors into which it 'fits'; in other words, the molecular shape of the drug is similar to certain endogenous ligands and therefore compatible with its receptors (Fig. 17.6). Combining with the receptor causes a change in the activity of the cell – this is how the drug actually exerts an effect. The effect it has may be to stimulate

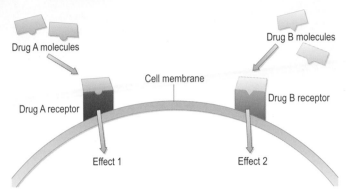

Fig. 17.6 Drug molecules have specific shapes that allow them to combine with specific receptors on the cell membrane surface *(Redrawn from Bill 1997)*

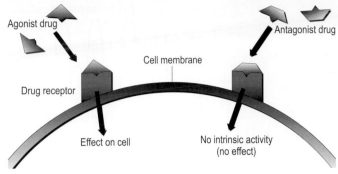

Fig. 17.7 Agonist and antagonist drug reactions *(Redrawn from Bill 1997)*

the cell in a similar way to the endogenous ligand – this is known as an **agonist effect**. Conversely, it may combine with the receptor site and 'block' the endogenous ligand but produce no effect itself – this is known as an **antagonist effect**.

Some drugs 'fit' poorly but still partly combine with a receptor site. The effect of this is to block the endogenous ligand but not necessarily produce a particularly strong effect itself. This is known as **partial agonism**. There are drugs that have an agonist effect at some receptor sites and an antagonist effect at others – these are known as agonist/antagonist drugs.

Affinity and competitiveness

The majority of drugs combine only temporarily with receptor sites and when present in sufficient quantity they 'win' the competition with the endogenous ligand for the receptor site. As soon as the concentration diminishes the endogenous ligand 'wins' the competition and the drug comes off the receptor site. In other words, competitive drugs have **reversible** effects. There are some drugs that do not come off the receptor site once they have combined with it – these are termed **non-competitive or irreversible.** Their effects do not diminish until the drug actually breaks down. An example of a non-competitive, irreversible drug is suxamethonium.

For a drug to combine with a receptor site, it must be attracted to that receptor. This attraction is known as **affinity**. Drugs with a strong affinity for the receptor site are usually highly effective and produce a good therapeutic response. However, they may remain on that site for a long time and therefore the potential for toxicity is higher. Drugs with a weak affinity for a receptor site tend to have a weaker therapeutic response as they leave the receptor site more quickly. However, these drugs are less likely to cause toxicity.

When more than one drug is administered that 'fits' the same receptor site, they may compete (Fig. 17.7). The drug with greater affinity for the site, or that is present in greater amounts, will 'win'. This could mean that the drug with weaker affinity or that is present in smaller amounts does not exert a therapeutic effect and is the reason why some combinations of drugs, e.g. morphine and buprenorphine, cannot be administered. This mechanism is sometimes used to control the effects of drugs; for example, atipamezole is used to antagonize the effects of medetomidine.

Downregulation and upregulation

Continual and prolonged exposure to agonist drugs can cause the number of receptor sites to decrease – this is known as downregulation. The result of this is that there is a decrease in therapeutic response. This is one reason why drug therapy should not be continued unnecessarily. Continual and prolonged exposure to antagonist drugs can cause the number of receptor sites to increase – this is known as upregulation. The result is that, if the drug is suddenly withdrawn, the endogenous ligand that was being blocked by the antagonist suddenly has an excessive number of binding sites and its effect is enhanced. This is the reason why some drugs, e.g. beta-blockers, must be withdrawn slowly after a course of treatment.

Specificity, potency and efficacy

Drug specificity or selectivity relates to the ability of a drug to act on a small number of receptors. Generally, it is desirable to have a highly selective drug as it is possible to target and treat the affected tissue or organ without affecting receptor sites in other parts of the body, which could cause side effects.

Potency refers to the amount of drug that has to be present to produce a therapeutic effect. Efficacy refers to the ability of the drug to produce the therapeutic effect. It is easy to confuse these two terms, but they do have different applications. Potency would be used to compare two drugs of the same type: for example, the one required in a smaller amount is more potent. Efficacy is used to compare two drugs of different types that produce a similar response: i.e. the drug that produces the more satisfactory response is more efficacious.

Non-receptor-mediated pharmacodynamics

Not all drugs exert their effects via receptors. There are several other pharmacodynamic mechanisms. Antimicrobial drugs exert their action on the pathogenic microorganisms in the body and, unfortunately, sometimes on the commensal microorganisms too. Chelating agents act by combining with metals to create less-harmful substances. An example is EDTA, given for lead poisoning. Some drugs work by chemical action, e.g. antacids such as aluminium hydroxide. Some drugs work by physical action, e.g. charcoal, used in poisoning cases to adsorb toxins, or mannitol, used as an osmotic diuretic.

Drug interactions and adverse reactions

Drugs or other chemicals can combine so that one has an effect on the other or so that they each affect one another. These occurrences are known as **interactions**. Drug interactions can occur outside the body, after administration or at any stage in the pharmacokinetic process.

Most drugs, if administered correctly, will have a predictable effect on most patients. However, on occasion, drugs will not have the usual effect. This may be because of the drug, its administration or because of the patient. When a drug has a harmful effect on the body it is known as an **adverse reaction.** This is not the same as a side effect, which is a predictable but unwanted effect of normal drug administration, usually related to its actions in parts of the body other than the area being treated.

Drug interactions

Using a combination of many drugs to treat a patient is known as **polypharmacy**. As the possibility that a drug interaction will occur increases with the number of drugs administered to a patient at any one time, polypharmacy should be undertaken with extreme care.

The use of interactions to treat patients

Sometimes, a known drug interaction is deliberately employed as it has therapeutic value. A well-known example of this is giving oral drugs with certain types of food to enhance absorption, e.g. giving griseofulvin tablets with corn oil or cheese. Two drugs with a different action can be given together to increase the therapeutic response – this is known as **synergism** (Table 17.1). If the response is the same as the sum of the two individual drugs, the effect is known as **summation**. However, in some cases, the response is greater than the sum of the two individual drugs. This effect is known as **potentiation**. Another therapeutic interaction is when the rate of metabolism or excretion from the body is altered to prolong the therapeutic effect, or conversely to increase clearance rate.

Unwanted drug interactions

Drug interactions often have an unwanted effect. This may be to inhibit the effect of the drug (antagonism) or to cause toxicity due to potentiation or alteration in the rate of metabolism or excretion.

Interactions can occur before the drug has entered the body. Sometimes, a drug can react with the carrier substance it is combined with in order to create the formulation, known as the excipient, or even the packaging. Drug manufacturers must be very careful to ensure that any changes to the excipient or packaging do not cause an interaction. On the pharmacy shelf, drugs exposed to inappropriate light levels, moisture levels or temperature extremes can alter in their effect.

Some drugs interact with certain foods to cause an unwanted effect. For example, oxytetracycline should never be given with milk or cheese as it binds to calcium and will not be absorbed from the gastrointestinal tract. Drugs can also interact with other drugs even if they are of different types and have been administered via different routes.

Adverse reactions

Adverse reactions may be the result of a number of factors. The dose given to the patient may be inappropriate, either because it has been miscalculated or because the patient's MTC level is reduced because of concurrent drug treatment or disease. Other drug reactions are not dose-dependent – these are known as idiosyncratic reactions. Idiosyncratic reactions are far less common but are more dangerous as they are unpredictable and do not tend to be proportional to the dose. Adverse reactions are often classified according to their suspected cause (Table 17.2).

Table 17.1 Definitions of drug interaction terminology

Definition	Numerical explanation
Summation – response is equal to the combined responses of the individual drugs	1 + 1 = 2
Synergism – response is greater than the combined responses of the individual drugs	1 + 1 = 3
Potentiation – one ineffective drug enhances the effect of another drug	0 + 1 = 2
Antagonism – one drug inhibits the effects of another drug	1 + 1 = 0

Table 17.2 Classification of adverse reactions

Reaction type	Description	Details
A	Augmented – enhanced drug effect	Predictable, dose-dependent, common, low mortality
B	Bizarre – allergic reactions	Unpredictable, not dose-related, high mortality
C	Chronic – due to continuous therapy	e.g. iatrogenic Cushing's disease from long-term prednisolone therapy
D	Delayed – occurring a long time after treatment	e.g. teratogenicity of griseofulvin, carcinomas
E	End of treatment – occurring on withdrawal of therapy	e.g. seizure after phenytoin withdrawal; adrenocortical insufficiency after prednisolone therapy

Nurses should …

- Be familiar with common interactions and reactions to the drugs frequently used in the practice
- Instigate appropriate patient observation and monitoring systems to ensure early detection of a reaction
- Report suspected drug reactions to the veterinary surgeon immediately
- Store drugs according to the manufacturer's instructions
- Ensure that stock is rotated correctly
- Monitor the environmental temperature in the pharmacy
- Vary parenteral administration sites for different drugs
- Consider staggering oral dosing intervals for different drugs
- Ensure that suspected drug reactions are reported to the Veterinary Medicines Directorate
- Prepare drugs for administration immediately prior to use and not in advance, e.g. the night before
- Use separate equipment for each drug – do not mix drugs in the same syringe
- Ensure the case notes clearly indicate any history of a drug reaction
- Advise owners to keep a note of any prior drug reaction or have a collar disc engraved with the necessary information in case of straying or illness on holiday

Patients prone to adverse reactions

In common with drug interactions, the possibility that an adverse drug reaction will occur increases with the number of drugs administered to a patient at any one time, so polypharmacy should be undertaken with extreme care (Box 17.1). Patients who are underweight, and therefore have less adipose tissue for drug distribution, are more prone to type A reactions, as are hypoproteinaemic animals, which have less plasma protein for the drug to bind to in the circulation. Dose rates for such patients should be reduced accordingly.

Toxicology

Toxicology is the study of the harmful effects of chemicals. Any substance that has a harmful effect on the body is known as a poison or toxin. We often think of poisons as substances that have been accidentally ingested or absorbed by an animal, e.g. metaldehyde or slug bait. However, toxicity can also be caused by therapeutic substances, i.e. a drug used to treat one or more conditions in animals, if the dose rate is too high, the animal's response to the drug is not usual or a drug interaction has occurred.

Toxicity can be acute, i.e. when symptoms develop quickly after exposure and are severe. Chronic toxicity can result from repeated exposure of small amounts of a toxin over a long period of time. A common example of chronic toxicity occurs with prolonged prednisolone therapy.

The effect of toxins on the body

Most chemicals introduced to the body have some sort of physiological effect – this is the basis on which therapeutic

Table 17.3 Factors affecting the toxicity of a substance

Substance-related factors	Animal-related factors
Time between exposure to toxin and treatment of toxicity	Species
Formulation of drug or substance	Age
Action of drug or substance	Genetic individuality
Dose or amount animal has been exposed to	Disease status
Route of administration, metabolism and excretion	
Quality and age of drug (if applicable)	
Concurrent treatment	

drugs work. However, toxins tend to have an extreme effect on the body, resulting in an unwanted alteration in function that can be life-threatening.

All organs in the body are susceptible to toxins. However, because of their role in drug metabolism and excretion, the liver and kidney are most at risk from damage. The mechanisms of action vary but include interfering with cellular function, alteration or destruction of vital enzymes, or competing for receptor sites, preventing the endogenous ligand from binding. Drug interactions can cause toxicity in this way, increasing the plasma concentration levels of the drug with less affinity for the binding site.

As there are many factors to take into consideration, the effect of an individual toxin on the body is only predictable to a certain extent. These factors are outlined in Table 17.3.

Treatment protocols

(For further details see Ch. 18)

Similar methods of treatment can be grouped together to give an overview of the management of poisoning cases:

- Prevention of absorption – washing, clipping, emesis, adsorbents
- Prevent action by using chelator/antidotes
- Increase clearance by inducing diuresis, dialysis
- Palliative and symptomatic treatment, ABC – life support.

Drug formulations, names and commonly used drugs for specific conditions

Once a condition has been diagnosed, the veterinary surgeon must decide the type of treatment necessary. This involves three stages:

1. The type of drug must be prescribed
2. The formulation to be administered must be selected
3. The dose rate must be decided.

It is essential for veterinary nurses to have a sound understanding of the various categories of drugs available, their mode of action and common side effects, in order to manage patients and support owners effectively. It is also vitally important that nurses can calculate drug dosages accurately in order to safely interpret the veterinary surgeon's instructions (see Appendix 1).

There are so many drugs on the market that a comprehensive knowledge of all of them is not realistic. With experience, nurses tend to develop a good understanding of the commonly used medications, but must always refer to the veterinary surgeon, senior nursing staff or the drug data sheet if they are unsure of anything relating to a patient's medication.

Drug formulations

There are several factors to take into account when considering in which formulation a drug is to be used. Drug manufacturers must calculate what a drug can actually achieve – for example, some drugs would be ineffective if given orally because of the first-pass effect; others may be inactivated by the additives needed for certain forms of medication. The target species must also be considered, as it may be easier to administer certain formulations to some species than others, e.g. oral tablets for hamsters! In recent years drug manufacturers have become more aware of the need to increase the ease of administration, especially for owners, in order to improve compliance. Many medicines indicated for long-term use are now offered in palatable or easy-to-give formulations (Table 17.4).

Table 17.4 Drug formulations and nursing considerations

Formulation	Variations and routes of administration	Description	Nursing considerations
Tablets	Non-palatable oral tablets	Powdered, compressed discs. May be coated. Many different shape, size and colour combinations	Never crush or split an enteric-coated tablet, as this will expose the drug prematurely. If tablets are split, round off any sharp edges prior to administration to prevent scratching the patient's mouth or throat and wear protective equipment to prevent absorption, inhalation or ingestion of the drug when handling
	Palatable oral tablets	Flavoured, shaped tablets	Ensure these are stored carefully to prevent patients helping themselves!
Capsules	Hard capsules for oral administration	Made up of two halves containing the drug in a powder or granule form. Many different colours and sizes	In some cases, it is possible to open or puncture the capsule and give the contents on food, or mixed with water as a paste. Check the drug data sheet to ensure that this is not contraindicated and wear protective equipment to prevent absorption, inhalation or ingestion of the drug when opening the capsule
	Soft capsules for oral administration	Sealed pouches containing liquid	
	Sustained-release capsules for oral administration (see section on Pharmacokinetics for further detail)	Hard gelatin capsules containing individual granules of drug	Never open or puncture a sustained-release capsule as this will affect the absorption of the drug. Sustained-release preparations licensed for humans only do not always have the same effect because of differences in transit time. There is more likelihood of the drug not reaching therapeutic levels in the bloodstream and in some cases more likelihood of toxicity
Solutions	For parenteral injection	Available in single- or multi-dose vials	Many drugs are unstable in solution so they need to be reconstituted from a powder immediately prior to use. Care must be taken when undertaking this task to use the correct volume of liquid and to adopt an aseptic technique. Never keep reconstituted solutions longer than the recommended time
	Linctus (syrup) for oral administration	Drug dissolved in a sugar solution	There are few veterinary-licensed products of this nature in the UK
	Elixir for oral administration	Drug dissolved in an alcohol solution	Never dilute elixirs with water as the alcohol and water will not mix together
Suspensions	For parenteral injection	Available in single- or multi-dose vials or bottles	Must be shaken thoroughly before use to ensure that the particles are fully and evenly distributed throughout the liquid
	For oral administration		Suspensions must never be given intravenously as they contain solid particles

Table 17.4 Continued

Formulation	Variations and routes of administration	Description	Nursing considerations
Long-acting solutions or suspensions (see Pharmacokinetics for further detail)	For parenteral injection	Either the drug or the carrier contents are not readily absorbed from the injection site	Sometimes referred to as LA, depot or repository injections. Suspensions must never be given intravenously as they contain solid particles
Creams	For topical administration	Water and oil emulsion base	Designed to liquefy at body temperature
Ointments	For topical administration	Oil base	Ensure gloves are worn when handling as absorption through the skin is possible with many drugs
Gels	For topical administration	Alcohol base	Some patients may need Elizabethan collar or similar to prevent them licking the medication
Pastes	For oral administration	Usually available in a pre-filled dosing syringe	If dosing several animals with the same syringe, disinfect the outside of the syringe to avoid cross-infection. Clients may need careful instruction on how to set the dial to the correct dose
Powders and granules	For topical administration	Often available in single-dose sachets	Now infrequently seen – many lost their product licences because of operator health and safety concerns, as inhalation and absorption of the products during administration is difficult to avoid
	For oral administration		Ensure that the correct dose is administered and ingested within a short time period or therapeutic levels may not be reached
Aerosol sprays	For topical administration	Pressurized or non-pressurized multi-dose bottles	Ensure that correct protective equipment is used to prevent inhalation or absorption of airborne drug particles. Use in a well-ventilated area
	For administration via inhalation	Liquids administered via a nebulizer	Ensure a quiet and calm environment to reduce stress levels when administering medication via nebulization
Shampoos	For topical administration	Usually presented in plastic bottles	Clients may need careful instruction on the safe use of these products and must also be made aware of the difference between medicated shampoos and cleansing or cosmetic shampoos
Drops	For oral administration	Usually solutions or suspensions presented with a precalibrated dosing syringe or dropper bottle	Some oral drops need to be reconstituted prior to use (see notes under solutions). Some drops require refrigeration once opened and/or reconstituted
	For administration to the mucous membranes	Unusual method of administration with limited applications	May be used to administer desmopressin. The most common site is the conjunctival sac. Ketamine is also absorbed easily across the mucous membranes (see section below and Ch. 25)
	For topical administration	Usually single-dose vials contained in a multipack for sale to clients	An increasingly common method of administering antiparasitic agents. Most commonly used to treat ectoparasites, but some products also treat endoparasites
	For administration to the eyes or ears	Dropper bottles containing aqueous solution	Often have a short use-by date once opened – some need refrigeration. Bottles should not be shared between patients because of the risk of cross-contamination
Patches	For transdermal administration	Unusual method of administration with limited applications. Gel impregnated with the drug is placed on skin. Protective cover may be placed on top	May be used to administer fentanyl or glyceryl trinitrate
Enemas	For rectal administration	Unusual method of administration with limited applications	May be used to administer diazepam to control seizures

What else is in a medicine apart from the drug?

All formulations are made up using the correct amount of drug, plus certain additives used for various reasons. As most drugs are divided into very small quantities, another substance is added to render the drug visible and easier to handle; this is called the **excipient**. Tablets also contain a **binder,** which is a substance that holds them together until they are administered. However, once ingested, they must be able to dissolve in the gastrointestinal tract, so tablets often contain a substance such as starch, which aids disintegration. Think about the colourful array of drugs on the pharmacy shelf – most drugs also contain colouring and some sort of **preservative.** Drug manufacturers must be very careful to ensure that all of these substances are inert, i.e. have no pharmacological action. However, sometimes a substance is combined with a drug to enhance its effect – this is known as an **adjuvant**.

Oral tablets may have an outer coating, which is often added to protect the tablet prior to use, or disguise a bitter taste to ease administration. Coatings are also used on some tablets to delay disintegration until they have passed through the stomach. This may be because the contents will irritate the gastric mucosa, or because gastric acid would destroy the drug. These medicines are called enteric-coated. Drugs are sometimes given in capsule form; the capsule is usually made of gelatin.

Drug names

Most drugs have several names. On discovery, a drug is given a **chemical name**, which describes its atomic or molecular structure. The chemical name is usually too long and complicated for general use, so an abbreviated code name or number is often used by researchers. When a drug is issued with a Marketing Authorization (MA), it is given a **generic** (official) name and a **trade** (proprietary or brand) name. The trade name is chosen by the company holding the MA for the drug and identifies it as the exclusive property of that company. Protection from competition is afforded to the company for a time, providing the opportunity for scientific innovation to be rewarded by a financial return on their investment. Once this period has expired, legislation permits competition from other manufacturers – providing they can demonstrate their product is equivalent to the pioneer product. Other companies filing for approval to market the drug must use the same generic name but can create their own trade name. As a result, the same generic drug may be sold under either the generic name or one of many trade names. Table 17.5 gives an example. It is standard practice to use the generic name when referring to drugs in text.

Drug types

There are hundreds of drugs available to treat animals in the UK. The list below is not exhaustive but describes drug groups that are commonly used in modern veterinary practice. The drugs have been categorized into groups depending on their action.

Anaesthetics

Anaesthetics are drugs that induce loss of sensation in all or part of the body.

- **General anaesthetics** involve the central nervous system (CNS) and cause unconsciousness. Injectable barbiturates, such as thiopental, are beginning to be superceded in general practice by non-barbiturate drugs, such as propofol and alfaxalone. Commonly used inhalational general anaesthetics include halothane and isoflurane, although sevoflurane and methoxyflurane are increasing in popularity (see Ch. 25).
- **Dissociative anaesthetics** derive their name from human patients describing a feeling of being separated from their body. These also affect the CNS but do not cause muscle relaxation and loss of reflexes to the same extent as general anaesthetics. Ketamine is a dissociative anaesthetic.
- **Local anaesthetics** cause loss of sensation around the site of administration. The most commonly used local anaesthetic is lidocaine.

Analgesics

Analgesics are drugs that prevent or relieve pain without loss of sensation. There are two main types of analgesic:

- **Narcotic analgesics** – are so-called because they tend to cause narcosis (sleepiness). They are opium-related agents and are sometimes called opioid analgesics. Narcotic analgesics, e.g. morphine and pethidine, exert their analgesic effect primarily by occupying the endogenous opioid receptor sites in the brain. They also occupy receptor sites elsewhere in the body, which can cause side effects. Buprenorphine is also a narcotic analgesic, although it is a partial agonist rather than a pure agonist like most others. Narcotic analgesics can be combined with a sedative to produce a state of semiconsciousness and drowsiness known as neuroleptanalgesia. Buprenorphine combined with acepromazine is a commonly given neuroleptanalgesic combination.
- **Non-steroidal anti-inflammatory drugs (NSAIDs)** – work in a different way from narcotic analgesics.

Table 17.5 Example of the names given to a drug during its development

Chemical name	Generic name	Trade names	MA holder
(2S,5R,6R)-6-{[(2R)-2-amino-2-(4-hydroxyphenyl)-acetyl]amino}-3,3-dimethyl-7-oxo-4-thia-1-azabicyclo[3.2.0]heptane-2-carboxylic acid	Amoxycillin trihydrate	Clamoxyl™ Amoxycare™ Duphamox™	Pfizer Limited Animalcare Ltd Fort Dodge Ltd

Instead of affecting the central nervous system (CNS), they have a pharmacological action at the site of the pain. Most work by inhibiting the production of cyclooxygenase (COX). Two types of COX have been discovered to date, known as COX1 and COX2. COX1 mainly plays a role in the normal functioning of a wide variety of body tissues, including the kidneys, stomach and intestine. COX2 mainly plays a role in the inflammatory process. NSAIDs that are not selective for COX2 (e.g. aspirin, phenylbutazone) can induce certain side effects, including gastric ulceration and diarrhoea.

COX2-selective NSAIDs (e.g. carprofen, meloxicam, firocoxib) are thought to be safer and have less effect on other body tissues.

Antacids

These are agents used to reduce acidity in the stomach, in order to prevent, manage or reverse damage to the intestinal tract. There are two types of antacids:

- **Non-systemic antacids** – work locally in the stomach to raise the pH of gastric juices. The most commonly used products contain aluminium hydroxide and magnesium carbonate. Because of the alteration of pH in the stomach these products can affect the dissolution and absorption of other drugs such as corticosteroids, tetracyclines, acepromazine and digoxin. Allow a 2–3 hour interval between doses. Increasingly, the drug sucralfate is being used when ulcers are present, as this drug forms a protective barrier over their surface. Sucralfate should not be given in combination with other antacids or meals, as it needs the acid environment of the stomach to exert its effect.
- **Systemic antacids** – there are several types and they act in a number of different ways. All aim to reduce gastric acid secretion. The most common example is cimetidine, which is an H2-receptor antagonist. These drugs block the effect of histamine in the stomach, which is to increase gastric acid production. (Do not confuse with antihistamines, H1-receptor antagonists, which are used to treat allergies.) Other systemic antacids affect more than gastric acid production – the prostaglandin misoprostol also increases mucus production and increases blood flow to the gastric area, thus promoting healing.

Antiarrhythmics

These are agents used to treat arrhythmia, an abnormality in the rhythm of the heart. There are many types and causes of arrhythmia and the choice of drug depends on the diagnosis:

- **Beta-blockers** – work by blocking stimulation of the β1 receptors in the heart, which decreases the heart rate and strength of contraction (drugs that cause the latter are also known as negative inotropes). A commonly used example is propranolol. Because of upregulation, animals treated with beta-blockers may need increasing doses to maintain the therapeutic effect. For the same reason, treatment should not suddenly cease: the sudden availability of β1 receptors to endogenous β1

stimulators such as adrenaline (epinephrine) could have a serious effect on the patient.
- **Calcium channel blockers** – reduce the rate of impulse generation and conduction across the heart. Examples are amlodipine, verapamil and diltiazem. The latter is also used to treat hypertrophic cardiomyopathy in cats.
- **Sodium channel blockers** – these are drugs with local anaesthetic action, which act to reduce contractions from occurring outside of the normal heartbeat. An example is lidocaine, which must be administered by slow intravenous injection. The presentation containing adrenaline (epinephrine) that is available for use as a local anaesthetic is not suitable to treat arrhythmias and using it for this purpose could be life-threatening for the patient.

Anticonvulsants

These are drugs used to prevent or control convulsions. The most commonly used drug for this purpose is the barbiturate phenobarbital, which stabilizes the brain cells, making them less likely to begin abnormal activity, and also tends to lessen the severity of convulsions if they do occur. It is sometimes used in conjunction with potassium bromide to reduce the dosage required.

Phenobarbital is metabolized by the mixed function oxidase system, so animals on long-term treatment develop tolerance and may need increasing doses in order to achieve the same therapeutic effect. Periodic testing of blood plasma levels will provide the necessary information to increase the dose safely. Phenobarbital acts too slowly to be used in emergency situations, when diazepam may be used intravenously. Diazepam can also be administered rectally, which is a useful route for owners to use if the animal convulses at home.

Antidepressants

Relatively new to veterinary pharmacology, three main types of antidepressant are used – tricyclic antidepressants, selective serotonin reuptake inhibitors (SSRIs) and monoamine oxidase inhibitors (MAOIs). All work by increasing the amount of neurotransmitter chemicals, e.g. serotonin, at the synapses. Clomipramine, nicergoline and l-deprenyl are examples of each type, respectively.

Separation-related problems, anxiety, stereotypies and geriatric cognitive dysfunction are sometimes treated with antidepressants. With these problems and other behaviour-related conditions, accurate diagnosis and an holistic approach, e.g. educating clients, altering routines and modifying animal and human behaviour, are usually needed for satisfactory results.

Antidiarrhoeals

These are drugs that combat diarrhoea. Diarrhoea is a symptom caused by an underlying condition or toxic substance and the drug of choice will depend on the cause of the diarrhoea. There are four main types of antidiarrhoeal drug:

- **Adsorbent/protectants** – these adsorb bacterial enterotoxins that cause hypersecretion of intestinal fluid and prevent them from contacting the intestinal lining. Examples include charcoal and bismuth. Some formulations, e.g. kaolin and pectin, also coat the gut wall, although this formulation has questionable efficacy.

- **Intestinal motility modifiers** – opioid drugs increase segmentation (mixing) movements and decrease peristaltic movements of the gut. Low doses of oral codeine, morphine combined with kaolin and diphenoxylate are all used to slow the passage of intestinal contents.
- **Anti-inflammatory drugs** – these are most commonly used for treating the chronic diarrhoea caused by inflammatory bowel disease. The antimicrobial drug sulfasalazine is used as it is not well absorbed through the gut wall and has an anti-inflammatory effect on the colon. Sometimes, corticosteroid therapy is instigated. It should be remembered that a diarrhoeic patient may not absorb any orally administered drugs to the same extent as a healthy patient, so parenteral routes of administering drugs may be preferential. Some antidiarrhoeal agents, particularly the adsorbents and protectants, may also affect the constitution and absorption rate of other drugs, so should be given at 2–3 hour intervals.

Antiemetics

These are agents used to prevent or decrease vomiting. Vomiting is a symptom caused by an underlying condition or toxic substance. Three examples of antiemetic drugs are metoclopramide, acepromazine and cisapride. Metoclopramide works by affecting the vomiting centre in the brain. It causes an increase in oesophageal and gastric muscle tone, relaxes the pyloric sphincter and increases intestinal motility. Acepromazine, part of the phenothiazine family, is sometimes used to control motion sickness as it reduces the amount of histamine, a powerful emetic, produced by vestibular stimulation. Cisapride is sometimes used to treat vomiting caused by megaoesophagus and gut stasis as it increases oesophageal tone and peristalsis.

Antihistamines

Histamine is a substance present in large quantities in the gastrointestinal, lung and skin tissue and plays a role in the immune response. In humans, this response is triggered by certain antigens, e.g. pollen, to cause allergic symptoms and in extreme cases, anaphylaxis. In contrast, histamine does not appear to play a major role in many of the allergies seen in animals, with the exception of certain feline and equine respiratory conditions. In these cases antihistamine drugs may be used to combat the bronchoconstriction caused by histamine in the lungs. These drugs work by antagonizing the H1 receptors in the smooth muscle of the bronchioles. So-called 'first-generation' antihistamines such as chlorpheniramine and cyproheptadine are sometimes used effectively, although they may cause sedation as a side effect. The so-called 'second-generation' antihistamines, such as astemizole and terfenadine, are more expensive and some have been linked to heart problems but they do not have a sedative side effect.

Antimicrobials

These are drugs that destroy, or facilitate the destruction of, microorganisms. The term antibiotic is sometimes used instead, although this is not strictly correct terminology as an antibiotic refers to a substance produced by one microorganism that affects another and most modern antimicrobials are synthetically produced.

Antimicrobials are broadly divided into two categories – those that destroy the target pathogen, defined by the suffix -cidal, and those that inhibit the growth of the target pathogen, defined by the suffix -static. They are further defined by the type of microorganism they affect – this may be bacteria, viruses, fungi or protozoa. So, for example, a substance that inhibits the growth of bacteria is called bacteriostatic. A substance that destroys fungi is called fungicidal, etc. Some drugs have a -static effect at a certain dosage, which becomes -cidal at a higher dosage. Table 17.6 describes the way in which antimicrobial drugs work.

Acquired resistance to antimicrobial drugs is an increasing problem, brought about by changes or mutations to the DNA of the microorganism in question. This allows the microorganism to survive in the presence of a drug designed to destroy it. Inappropriate use of antimicrobial agents may exacerbate this problem. Table 17.7 identifies key points to consider when using such products to reduce the problem of acquired resistance to a minimum.

Antineoplastics

These are drugs used to treat neoplastic or cancerous tissue. Most of them are cytotoxic, meaning that they kill cells. The term 'chemotherapy' is often reserved for this type of treatment, although this term literally means 'drug therapy' so could be used to describe any type of drug therapy. The aim of an antineoplastic agent is for it to be selectively toxic towards the neoplastic cells while sparing the normal healthy cells. It is the property of accelerated reproduction of neoplastic cells that allows this to happen. Unfortunately, other healthy cells in the body that tend to divide fairly rapidly, e.g. hairs, can also be affected by the agent which is why these types of drugs have so many side effects, e.g. suppression of bone marrow cells.

Veterinary nurses must be aware that accidental ingestion, absorption or inhalation of cytotoxic drugs can seriously affect their health. Local health and safety rules for dispensing and administering this type of medication must be observed at all times and clients must be made fully aware of the dangers of these drugs (Table 17.8). Vincristine, cyclophosphamide and doxorubicin are all examples of antineoplastic agents.

Antiparasitics

These are drugs used to treat infection by parasites. There are several categories, which are divided according to their action:

- **Endoparasiticides** – agents that treat internal parasites. Divided into anthelmintics – agents that treat helminths (roundworms, tapeworms and flukes) and antiprotozoals – agents that act against protozoa. Anthelmintics can be further divided into antinematocides (act against roundworms),

Table 17.6 Mode of action of antimicrobials

Mode of action	Description	Example
Inhibition of cell-wall synthesis	Prevent bacterial cell wall forming correctly	Penicillins, e.g. ampicillin, amoxicillin
		Cephalosporins, e.g. cefalexin
		Terbinafine
Disruption of microbial cell membrane	Change membrane permeability and so affect transport in and out of microorganism	Polymyxin-B
Inhibition of protein synthesis	Affect either protein synthesis in the ribosomes or in the nucleus, preventing effective replication of the microorganism	Tetracyclines, e.g. oxytetracycline, doxycycline
		Aminoglycosides, e.g. gentamicin, neomycin, streptomycin
		Metronidazole
		Erythromycin
		Quinolones, e.g. enrofloxacin
Interference with metabolic processes	Many microorganisms must manufacture folic acid in order to replicate – they cannot obtain it from food sources as animals can. These agents either interfere with or inhibit folic acid production	Trimethoprim, sulphonamides, e.g. sulfadiazine

Table 17.7 Actions to be taken to reduce the risk of antimicrobial resistance

Key area	Nursing implications
Always try to identify the pathogen in order to select the most appropriate drug to treat	Nurses may be involved in undertaking sample cultures and/or sensitivity testing. Ensure this is accurately carried out and interpreted
Avoid broad-spectrum drugs where possible	Monitor the volume of broad-spectrum antimicrobial drug used – report excessive use to relevant person or authority
Select the lowest optimal dose	Ensure adequate availability of suitable literature to access recommended doses – keep drug data sheets within easy reach. Calculate drug dosages carefully
Select route carefully, ensuring that an adequate dose can reach the affected site	Ensure adequate availability of suitable literature to access recommended routes
Do not use antimicrobial drugs unnecessarily	Discourage clients from retaining unused medication to use on another occasion or for another animal – consider an 'easy disposal' system in the practice to encourage them to return unused medicine
Limit the use of new products	Consider the stock of drugs in the pharmacy carefully and select new products on the basis of need
Always complete the prescribed course of treatment	Ensure clients are fully aware that they should always treat the patient at the prescribed dose, route and time and should always complete a course of treatment even if the symptoms have gone
Religiously observe drug withdrawal times in food-producing animals	Ensure adequate literature is available in order to advise clients accurately

anticestocides (act against tapeworms) and antitrematocides (act against flukes). Not all drugs will kill every parasite in a group but, conversely, some drugs have action against more than one group of helminths and are termed broad-spectrum anthelmintics. Anthelmintics may act as either a vermicide, which kills the parasites, or a vermifuge, which paralyses the parasite, which may then be passed out of the host's body alive. Some drugs are both vermicidal and vermifugal. Piperazine citrate, fenbendazole, febantel, praziquantel and levamisole are all commonly used anthelmintics.

It is important to understand the lifecycle of the parasites (see Ch. 27) being treated, as most anthelmintics act mainly in the gut lumen and may not treat migrating larvae or eggs elsewhere in the body.

Antiprotozoals are often antimicrobials, e.g. sulfadimidine, although fenbendazole, an anthelmintic, has also been proved to be effective against the protozoan *Giardia* spp.

- **Ectoparasiticides** – agents that treat external parasites. May be acaricidal, i.e. act against acarids such as mites and ticks, or insecticidal, i.e. act against insects such as fleas, or have both properties. In the past, organophosphorus products such as dichlorvos and pyrethroid products such as permethrin were commonly used as insecticides but, more recently, products such as fipronil and imidacloprid have

Table 17.8 Methods of reducing the risk of contamination when using cytotoxic drugs

Action	Method of reducing the risk
Preparing, dispensing and administering	Always wear gloves, apron and mask when preparing these products for use, administering or dispensing. It may also be necessary to wear eye shields if handling liquids or powdery tablets
	Never cut or break tablets, unless the dose rate makes it necessary. Do not expect the client to do this at home. Clear away spillages carefully
	Keep a separate 'cytotoxic kit' in the pharmacy, for use with these products, so all personal protective equipment is readily available – replenish after each use, as gloves, masks and apron should be single-use only
	Provide clients with a verbal and written explanation of the dangers of their pet's medication and how to reduce the risks to them
Nursing a patient	Remember that body fluids, vomit and faeces will sometimes be contaminated with the cytotoxic drug. The patient should urinate and defecate in an area that is easily cleanable. Avoid urine splashes onto clothing. Ensure that the client understands the dangers of this route of contamination
Disposal	Clear away all empty packaging and excess drug carefully and dispose of it according to health and safety guidelines. Encourage clients to return any empty packaging or unused drug to the surgery for correct disposal

become the treatments of choice because of their relative safety compared with the former and efficacy compared with the latter. Products that interfere with insect growth and development have become popular as a useful adjunct to insecticides to treat fleas in dogs and cats. Examples include S-methoprene and lufenuron.

Antitussives, mucolytics, expectorants, decongestants

Antitussives are used to suppress coughing. In veterinary medicine, these are centrally acting, i.e. act on the 'cough centre' in the brain. Examples include butorphanol and codeine. Locally acting antitussives work by soothing the mucous membrane in the respiratory tract – they are not appropriate for use in veterinary medicine, as animals will not suck lozenges or gargle liquids as human patients will. Mucolytics and expectorants, e.g. bromhexine and eucalyptus oil, break down and thin out respiratory mucus. Decongestants, such as phenylephrine, act by causing vasoconstriction and a subsequent reduction in oedema and mucus production of the nasal mucous membranes. Care should be taken as this drug can have cardiovascular effects, which may prove deleterious to animals with pre-existing cardiovascular or respiratory disease.

Astringents and keratolytics

These agents are usually available as medicated shampoos, lotions or drops. Astringent products, such as zinc oxide, harden and protect the skin by causing proteins to precipitate on its surface. Keratolytics such as benzoyl peroxide enhance desquamation and are therefore used to reduce scaling on the skin surface.

Bronchodilators

These are agents that cause the smooth muscle of the terminal bronchioles to relax, thus counteracting bronchoconstriction and narrowing of the airway diameter. Two main types of bronchodilator are used in veterinary medicine:

- **Beta-agonists** – stimulate β receptors. There are two types of β receptor – β1 and β2. The former are found elsewhere in the body, including in the heart, so non-selective beta-agonists may have unwanted side effects, such as arrhythmias and tachycardia. β2 receptors are found in the smooth muscle of the bronchioles. Their stimulation causes bronchodilation. The more β2-selective agonists such as terbutaline minimize cardiac side effects and are usually preferred over the non-selective drugs such as adrenaline (epinephrine).
- **Methylxanthines** – work on the smooth muscle cells by interfering with their chemical composition, discouraging bronchoconstriction. They are not selective, so can cause a range of stimulatory side effects as they affect many other cells in the body. Examples include theophylline. As methylxanthines are metabolized by the mixed function oxidase system, the dose may need to be increased in patients concurrently being treated with other drugs metabolized by the same system.

Central nervous system stimulants

These agents are commonly used to reverse the action of a sedative or anaesthetic, or to stimulate respiration in a patient. Two of the most commonly used CNS stimulants are atipamezole, an α2-agonist, and doxapram, a drug that works primarily in the medulla oblongata to stimulate respiration. The methylxanthine drugs are also CNS stimulants.

Corticosteroids

Corticosteroids are hormones that are naturally produced by the adrenal cortex. They are divided into two main groups depending on the main action they exert: **mineralocorticoids** mainly affect the mineral balance of the body and **glucocorticoids** mainly exert an anti-inflammatory effect on the body as well as affecting glucose metabolism. The mineralocorticoid fludrocortisone is used in animals to treat Addison's disease, which is atrophy of the adrenal cortex, resulting in hypoadrenocorticism.

Glucocorticoids are far more widely used. They can be divided into three groups depending on their duration of action:

Table 17.9 Side effects of glucocorticoids

Side effect	Nursing considerations
Inhibition of fibroblasts can cause delayed healing	Ensure that records of animals on corticosteroid therapy are clearly marked to prevent this fact being missed. Clients may need advice on temporary cessation of corticosteroid therapy prior to surgery
Immunosuppression due to inhibition of T cells and immune responses	Advise clients of patient's increased risk of infection. Take extra care not to expose hospitalized patients to infection
Increase of gastric acid and decrease of gastric mucus production	Advise clients never to give concurrent NSAID therapy. Do not give premedication on admission to hospital if it contains an NSAID
Catabolic effects – protein breakdown	Ensure adequate bedding for patients with thin skin and haircoat. Those with muscle atrophy may need physical support if standing for long periods. Do not use corticosteroid preparations on ulcerated tissue, e.g. corneal ulcers
Prolonged continuous use may cause hyperadrenocorticism – iatrogenic Cushing's syndrome or diabetes mellitus	Observe patients closely for symptoms of these iatrogenic diseases. Ensure that clients understand that a higher dose of corticosteroid every other day is safer than a lower dose of daily therapy, so they do not revert to the latter without consultation with the veterinary surgeon
Exogenous sources of corticosteroid suppress the endogenous release from the adrenal cortex	Ensure that clients taper doses at the end of treatment to prevent hypoadrenocorticism
Polyphagia, polydipsia and polyuria	Advise clients of these potential side effects and how to manage them to prevent obesity and inappropriate elimination

- Short-acting, e.g. hydrocortisone, which is commonly found in topical formulations; these have a 12 hour duration of action
- Intermediate-acting, e.g. prednisolone – commonly given as an oral medication; these have a 12–36 hour duration of action
- Long-acting, e.g. dexamethasone – duration of action more than 48 hours.

Glucocorticoids are mainly used for their anti-inflammatory actions. They affect many of the body's cells and so, although they are useful for a variety of inflammatory diseases, they also produce a wide variety of side effects. Table 17.9 describes some of these side effects and the nursing considerations that arise from them.

Diuretics

These are agents that promote water loss by increasing urine production. They are usually used to reduce fluid retention caused by congestive heart failure, but are also indicated for certain respiratory diseases and acute renal failure. There are several types of diuretic, which are classified according to their action:

- **Loop diuretics**, e.g. furosemide – act on the loop of Henle to prevent the reabsorption of sodium, so that water remains in the urine by osmosis. Sodium is later exchanged for potassium; thus long-term use of loop diuretics can result in hypokalaemia.
- **Potassium-sparing diuretics**, e.g. spironolactone – work by antagonizing the action of aldosterone. As the name suggests, they do not cause potassium loss.
- **Osmotic diuretics**, e.g. mannitol – a sugar-based substance that works by increasing the osmotic pressure within the renal tubule, thus drawing water into the urine from the plasma and increasing its volume. It is used to reduce cerebral pressure after head trauma and to increase elimination of a toxin from the body.

- **Carbonic anhydrase inhibitors**, e.g. acetazolamide – are used to treat glaucoma.
- **Thiazide diuretics**, e.g. chlorothiazide, are infrequently used as they are less potent than the loop diuretics yet can still cause hypokalaemia. They can be used to treat nephrogenic diabetes insipidus.

Hormones

Endogenous hormones are substances produced by endocrine glands that reach their site of action via the bloodstream. Exogenous hormones (natural or synthetic in origin) are sometimes used to test for or treat disease of the endocrine gland that has caused an imbalance of one or more of the endogenous hormones. In addition to the use of corticosteroids, several other hormones are used for therapeutic reasons:

- **Adrenocorticotrophic hormone (ACTH) and thyroid-stimulating hormone (TSH)** are both anterior pituitary hormones. They are used diagnostically to measure the response of the adrenal cortex and thyroid gland, respectively.
- **Desmopressin** – this is a synthetic version of the posterior pituitary hormone antidiuretic hormone (ADH) and is used to treat central diabetes insipidus.
- **Insulin** – there are various types of insulin derived from various sources and available to treat diabetes mellitus. Each type has a different duration of action, allowing regimes to be tailored to individual patients depending on their blood glucose responses.
- **Oestrogens** – used in some species to induce oestrus, this group of hormones also includes diethylstilboestrol, which is sometimes used to treat misalliance and urinary incontinence.
- **Progestagens** – this group of drugs are progesterone-like in their activity. They can be used to suppress oestrus but should be used with caution as they predispose entire females to uterine disease.

- **Levothyroxine (thyroxine)** – also known as T4, this synthetic product replaces the naturally occurring thyroxine normally produced by the thyroid gland but lacking in cases of hypothyroidism. The drug methimazole, used to treat hyperthyroidism, works by blocking the ability of the thyroid gland to produce natural thyroxine.
- **Anabolic steroids** – this term relates to a group of drugs that promote increased mass of body tissues. They are most frequently used in convalescing, geriatric or chronically ill patients. In food-producing animals they have been used to increase the animal's weight and muscle condition. A commonly used example is the testosterone derivative nandrolone, but some progestagens and oestrogens also fall into this category.

Laxatives

These are agents used to facilitate defecation. There are three main types of laxative:

- **Bulk laxatives** – these increase the bulk of faeces by retaining or drawing water into the gut lumen. Indigestible fibre such as bran or isphagula husk and hypertonic substances such as phosphate salts are commonly used.
- **Lubricant laxatives** – these products, e.g. liquid paraffin and glycerine, may be useful to facilitate the passage of faeces following pelvic trauma.
- **Stimulant laxatives** – these products tend to have a stronger effect than other laxatives and can be irritant, so should be used with care. They work by increasing local gut motility, e.g. dantron.

'Natural' supplements

Increasingly, clients are showing a preference for products that they perceive to be 'natural', such as fish oils, garlic and chondroitin. Some of these products are proving extremely useful as a treatment or adjunct to certain conditions. However, clients should be advised to exercise caution as the fact that they do not fall within the definition of veterinary medicines and may be freely available does not necessarily mean that they cannot cause harm if incorrectly administered. It is not unusual for a client to use the same product (and dose!) that they take themselves – remember that not all products safe for use in humans are equally safe for animals. In addition, instruct the client of the correct methods of handling these products as they may be easily absorbed, ingested or inhaled. This is particularly true of essential oils, which can have serious effects if incorrectly handled and administered.

Recently, there has been a lot of interest in the use of nutrients with therapeutic properties, which may be given as powder, tablets, capsules, etc., and may be included in a commercial diet or presented as a food product. These products are known as nutraceuticals. Examples of nutraceuticals include glucosamine, essential fatty acids and probiotics.

Herbal and homeopathic remedies are generally considered to be entirely discrete treatment systems. Many herbal and homeopathic remedies are defined as veterinary medicines and as such are subject to regulation and licensing legislation. Homeopathic remedies are listed in the *British Homeopathic Pharmacopeia*.

Parasympathomimetics and parasympatholytics

These are agents that mimic the effects and inhibit the effects of the parasympathetic nervous system, respectively. An example of a parasympathomimetic is the miotic (pupil constricting) drug, pilocarpine. An example of a parasympatholytic drug is atropine.

Sympathomimetics and sympatholytics

These are agents that mimic the effects and block the effects of the sympathetic nervous system, respectively. They are also known as adrenergic agonists and antagonists. They are used for conditions where sympathetic stimulation is excessive or inadequate and causes problems. Examples of sympathomimetic drugs are those used to stimulate the β1 receptors in the heart, to increase its rate and contraction (known as positive inotropes). This group includes isoprenaline and pimobendan. An example of sympatholytic drugs is the β-blocker.

Tranquillizers and sedatives

This encompasses a range of drugs that have some effect on the animal's awareness or perception of its surroundings. There are several terms used in relation to this group of drugs that may appear confusing as some are interchangeable. Many drugs of this type can produce a variety of effects depending on the dose given.

Tranquillizers or ataractics tend to reduce anxiety (have an anxiolytic effect) and produce a mentally relaxed state.

Drugs that produce a more profound drowsiness are termed sedatives. Potent sedatives that induce sleep or reduced consciousness are termed hypnotics or narcotics.

Neuroleptic drugs produce a state of mental detachment. Commonly used tranquillizers and sedatives are the phenothiazine, acepromazine, benzodiazepines such as diazepam and midazolam and α2-agonists such as medetomidine and xylazine.

Urinary pH modifiers and antiseptics

The pH of urine can cause or precipitate certain conditions, most notably urolithiasis. The use of agents that modify urinary pH is often indicated in the treatment of such conditions and to prevent recurrence. Modern veterinary practice makes full use of diets that have been formulated to maintain a certain pH but it is also possible to achieve this using drugs. Urine acidification can be achieved using ascorbic acid (vitamin C) and alkalinization can be achieved using sodium bicarbonate. Excessive use of these products can cause metabolic disturbances. The use of a urinary antiseptic, such as methenamine hippurate, may be indicated for use in patients with recurrent urinary tract infections.

Vaccines, toxoids, antitoxins and antisera

A vaccine is a substance given to stimulate active immunity against a known disease or diseases (see also Ch. 19). They may be live, containing microorganisms that are similar to the pathogen, or the pathogen may have been manipulated to render it safe for use (attenuated) so that it stimulates a suitable immune response but does not cause the disease.

Killed or dead vaccines contain inactivated pathogen – these tend to be less effective than live vaccines and may contain an adjuvant to enhance their effect. Some inactivated vaccines contain purified versions of toxins produced by the pathogen in question, in order to stimulate immunity to that toxin. These products are called toxoids.

In certain circumstances, it may be necessary to give immediate protection against a disease rather than waiting for the animal's own immune system to respond to a vaccine. This type of passive immunity is achieved by administering antibodies to an animal that have been produced by another animal (usually of the same species). These antibodies are known as antitoxins and they are administered in fluid known as antiserum. Although passive immunity is immediate, it does not last long.

Vasodilators

Certain conditions, e.g. congestive heart failure, cause vasoconstriction or a decrease in the diameter of blood vessels. This increases the resistance of blood flowing through the vessels and increases strain on the heart. Vasodilators increase the diameter of blood vessels, thus decreasing resistance and making it easier for the heart to pump blood around. These drugs exert their action by relaxing vascular smooth muscle – some on arterial vessels, e.g. hydralazine; some on venous vessels, e.g. glyceryl trinitrate, and some on both, e.g. the angiotensin-converting enzyme (ACE) inhibitor enalapril. This group of drugs is commonly used in animals with cardiac disease as it blocks the formation of angiotensin II, a potent vasoconstrictor. Other commonly used ACE inhibitors include benazepril and ramipril. Vasodilators can cause hypotension or low blood pressure, so ataxia and syncope may be seen, especially when treatment begins.

Vitamins and minerals

Nutritional science is so well advanced today that dietary supplementation is rarely necessary for healthy animals. Careless addition of vitamin and/or mineral supplements to the diet could cause dangerous imbalances or excesses. However, there remains a role for certain vitamins and minerals in the veterinary pharmacy:

- Exotic animals, e.g. reptiles in particular, may require certain supplements in order to maintain their health. It is possible to buy proprietary powders and liquids in suitable combinations.
- Calcium gluconate should always be available as it is necessary to administer this mineral quickly in cases of hypocalcaemia, e.g. in eclampsia or damaged parathyroid glands.
- Potassium chloride supplementation may be necessary for patients receiving treatment for dehydration and anorexia and those on loop diuretics.
- Vitamin K (phytomenadione) is used as an antidote for warfarin poisoning.

Dosage calculations

Veterinary professionals must be able to calculate drug dosages correctly. Inaccurate calculations could lead to under- or overdosage of medication, with disastrous consequences. Most drug calculations are based on one or more commonly used formulae. Once the concept of these formulae has been mastered, drug calculations are relatively straightforward. It is, however, important to recognize your own limitations, and if in doubt, calculations should be checked by an experienced person (see Appendix 1).

Licensing, prescribing and dispensing medication

Introduction to veterinary pharmaceutical legislation

There are two main pieces of legislation governing the use of drugs in veterinary practice. These are The Veterinary Medicines Regulations (VMR) 2009 and The Misuse of Drugs Act 1971 (with associated Regulations). The Supply of Relevant Medicinal Products Order 2005 also specifies some legal aspects of prescribing and supplying veterinary medicines. Table 17.10 describes these pieces of legislation and which area is covered by veterinary pharmaceutical practice. Other significant legislation includes:

- The Health and Safety at Work Act 1974, The Management of Health and Safety at Work Regulations (amended 1999) and The Control of Substances Hazardous to Health Regulations 1999 (COSHH), which relate to safe storage, transporting and handling of medicines.
- The Control of Pollution Act (1974), The Controlled Waste Regulations (1992) and The Environmental Protection Act (1990), which relate to safe disposal of medicines.

The Royal College of Veterinary Surgeons (RCVS) Guides to Professional Conduct also specify some requirements with which veterinary surgeons and registered veterinary nurses must comply. Failure to do so could result in disciplinary action being taken.

Changes in veterinary pharmaceutical legislation

For some years, there has been a drive towards producing a uniform approach to drug legislation for all European Union (EU) member states. In addition to this, there have been two reports published which have investigated the supply of veterinary medicines and have had an impact on recent legislative changes.

The 'Independent Review of Dispensing by Veterinary Surgeons of Prescription Only Medicines' (The Marsh Report) was published in May 2001. Amongst its recommendations were the reclassification of drugs into different prescribing categories and the suggestion that more outlets should be allowed to supply prescription-only medicines (POMs). The latter recommendation was also made by the 'Report on the Supply Within the United Kingdom of Prescription-only Medicines', published by The Competition Commission in April 2003, which also recommended that veterinary practices should provide clearer drug pricing information and offer all clients the choice of a prescription should they wish to purchase their medication elsewhere. These recommendations were incorporated into The VMR 2005. The Supply of

Table 17.10 Legislation covering the use of veterinary medicines

Legislation	Function	Areas covered
The Veterinary Medicines Regulations 2009	• Governs the licensing, prescribing, supply and labelling of veterinary medicinal products in the UK • Brings UK legislation in line with other European Union member states	Issue and review of marketing authorizations (MAs) to manufacturers
		Exemptions for the requirement for medicines used to hold a MA (e.g. small animal exemption scheme)
		Use of unauthorized ('unlicensed') products (the prescribing cascade)
		Provisions for wholesale supply of veterinary medicinal products
		Provisions for retail supply of veterinary medicinal products, including prescribing classes and issue of prescriptions
		Advertising of veterinary medicinal products.
		Restricts the advertising of POM-V, POM-VPS and NFA-VPS products
The Misuse of Drugs Act 1971 (Including The Misuse of Drugs Regulations 2001 and The Misuse of Drugs (Safe Custody) Regulations 1973)	• Controls the production, supply, possession and storage of dangerous drugs • Deals with controlled drugs (CDs), a special category of POM-V medicines • Refers to 'classes' of drug, i.e. class A, class B, class C. These classes are not referred to in veterinary medicine • Also promotes education and research into drug dependency and addiction	Place CDs into one of five schedules (which are different from the drug prescribing classes)
		Relate to the storage of CDs. States that a locked car is not considered an acceptable place to store CDs
The Supply of Relevant Medicinal Products Order 2005	• Implements recommendations from discrimination of charges between clients who request prescriptions and those who do not, for other veterinary services (see section entitled, 'writing prescriptions'). The Competition Commission	Prohibit discrimination of charges between clients who request prescriptions and those who do not for other veterinary services (see section on 'writing prescriptions')
The RCVS Guide to Professional Conduct	• Implements recommendations from the Competition Commission	Stipulates that a transparent pricing structure is necessary, including itemized invoices, information about charges for further examination of the animal and waiting room displays showing the availability of prescriptions, costs involved and prices of the 10 most frequently prescribed drugs

Relevant Medicinal Products Order 2005 and The RCVS Guide to Professional Conduct for Veterinary Surgeons. Since 2005, The VMR have been updated annually, although there will be no VMR 2010 due to time constraints. Currently, the VMR 2009 are in effect, although drafts of the VMR 2011 are underway. The RCVS Guide to Professional Conduct for Veterinary Nurses now also incorporates the recommendations.

Licensing of veterinary drugs in the UK

Veterinary medicines must only be administered to an animal if they have a product 'licence', called a marketing authorisation or MA, for the treatment of that particular species and condition. These regulations apply to both food-producing and non-food-producing animals. There are exceptions which are discussed in the next section.

Obtaining an MA requires the undertaking of a series of pharmacological and toxicological tests and clinical trials. The drug manufacturer must be able to prove by scientific means the product's safety, quality and efficacy. MAs are issued for a period of 5 years, after which time the granting of the MA is reviewed. In certain situations, provisional, or

'exceptional', MAs are issued. This would be in circumstances where a new disease was discovered or the existing treatment was no longer effective or available. These are issued annually.

Manufacturers wishing to obtain an MA can apply through one of three routes:

- Centralized – via the European Medicines Agency. MA would be valid in all EU member states
- National – via the Veterinary Medicines Directorate. MA would be valid in the UK only
- Decentralized – known as 'mutual recognition', the holder of a MA in another EU member state can apply for identical MAs in one or more other member states.

Prescribing veterinary drugs

When an MA is obtained the drug will be placed into one of four main categories, which have varying restrictions placed on the product with regard to who may supply it. Which category they fall into will be determined by the potential of the drug to cause harm, the type of animal (food-producing vs non-food-producing) and the

Table 17.11 Drug categories under the Veterinary Medicines Regulations 2009

Abbreviation	Category name	Prescribing and supply restrictions	Notes
POM-V	Prescription-only medicine – veterinarian	To be prescribed only by a veterinary surgeon following diagnosis for an animal under his/her care*	Another veterinary surgeon or pharmacist may dispense the medicine against a prescription but only from registered premises.* Advertising is restricted to veterinary surgeons, veterinary nurses, pharmacists and professional keepers of animals (e.g. farmers)
POM-VPS	Prescription-only medicine – veterinarian, pharmacist, suitably qualified person** (SQP)	To be prescribed only by a veterinary surgeon, pharmacist or SQP. The animal need not be under his/her care*	Relates to livestock. Mainly antiparasiticides. Advertising is restricted to veterinary surgeons, pharmacists, professional keepers of animals and other veterinary professionals, including VNs.*** Another veterinary surgeon, pharmacist or SQP may dispense the product against a prescription* but only from registered premises
NFA-VPS	Non-food animal – veterinarian, pharmacist, SQP	To be supplied only by a veterinary surgeon, pharmacist or SQP*	Relates to companion animals, including horses, who are registered in their passport as not intended for human consumption. Mainly antiparasitic products. Can only be supplied from registered premises
AVM-GSL	Authorized veterinary medicine – general sales list	May be supplied by any retailer	Veterinary medicines deemed to be extremely safe. Includes some shampoos and other products with very small amounts of active ingredient

*Those prescribing or supplying veterinary medicines must provide advice on safe administration and warnings or contraindications. They must also be satisfied that the person supplied is competent to use the product safely and intends to use it for its authorized purpose.
**A suitably qualified person (SQP) is one deemed to have successfully undergone a course of training approved by the Animal Medicines Training Regulatory Authority (AMTRA). Currently, this does not include the RCVS veterinary nursing syllabus, although qualified veterinary nurses (VNs) are eligible for a partial cross-credit.
***VN, veterinary nurse.

importance of receiving regular veterinary attention to prevent harm and/or suffering to the animal concerned. The prescribing categories are detailed in the Table 17.11.

Veterinarians and suitably qualified persons (SQPs) supplying veterinary medicines may only do so from registered premises. The register of veterinary practice premises is held by the RCVS. Registered premises are subject to inspection to monitor compliance.

Controlled drugs

Drugs that have the potential for abuse are placed in a sub-category of POM-Vs, known as controlled drugs (CDs). There are five schedules of CDs, which have controls that decrease in their stringency. Table 17.12 shows the five schedules and their requirements and gives some examples of CDs that may be used in veterinary practice.

In 2006, ketamine became a Schedule 4 CD. Although there are no special storage requirements set out in the legislation, the RCVS recommends that ketamine should be stored in a secure receptacle and have its usage recorded in an informal register.

The prescribing 'cascade' (Fig. 17.8)

There are occasions when the veterinary surgeon is faced with a diseased patient for whom no product exists that is authorized in the United Kingdom (UK) to treat that species and condition; this probably happens most frequently in the treatment of exotic animals. The VMR 2009 allow for such circumstances by setting out the rules of the prescribing

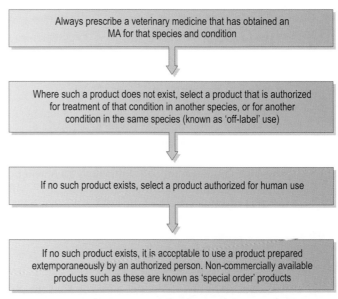

Fig. 17.8 The prescribing cascade (MA – marketing Authorisation)

'cascade' (Fig. 17.8). Use of unauthorized medicines for food-producing animals have additional restrictions; only products approved for use in food animals can be used and minimum withdrawal periods apply.

It is a criminal offence for a veterinary surgeon to prescribe an unauthorized product where one that is authorized in the UK for that species and condition exists without valid clinical reason (subject to exemptions, e.g. small animal

Table 17.12 Classification, restrictions and examples of controlled drugs

Schedule	Requisition restrictions	Storage restrictions	Dispensing restrictions	Nature of drugs included	Examples
S1	Veterinary surgeons are not generally authorized to possess S1 drugs – the only exception is for research purposes, when a special licence must be obtained	—	—	Highly addictive substances with no therapeutic indication in veterinary practice	Cannabis LSD Raw opium
S2	Can only be obtained with a written requisition signed by the veterinary surgeon. All requisitions must be entered into a bound register (commercially available). Entries must be written in indelible ink and made in chronological order, with a separate section for each drug. Mistakes should not be written over – a marginal note should be made, dated and signed	Most must be stored in a locked receptacle that can only be opened by a veterinary surgeon or person authorized by them to do so	Each time a drug is administered and dispensed, a record must be made in a bound drug register. S2 recording requirements are as stated in 'supply restrictions'. The register must be kept for a minimum of 2 years. S2 drugs used in the practice cannot be destroyed, except in the presence of a person authorized by the Secretary of State. S2 drugs returned to the practice by clients for disposal are also subject to specific requirements	Substances with significant potential for abuse, but have a therapeutic indication in veterinary practice, e.g. some opiate analgesics	Morphine Methadone Fentanyl Pethidine
S3	Can only be obtained with a written requisition signed by the veterinary surgeon. All requisitions must be entered into a bound register (commercially available). Entries must be written in indelible ink and made in chronological order. Mistakes should not be written over – a marginal note should be made, dated and signed	Most S3 drugs commonly used in veterinary practice are not subject to special storage requirements, although buprenorphine must be kept in a locked receptacle	Administration and dispensing does not have to be recorded in a drug register	Barbiturates and opioid analgesics with less potential for abuse	Buprenorphine Phenobarbital Pentobarbital Pentazocine
S4	No special requisition requirements	No special storage requirements	No dispensing restrictions	Anabolic substances and benzodiazepines	Diazepam Nandrolone. Also includes ketamine.
S5	No special requisition requirements, although invoices of purchase should be kept for 2 years	No special storage requirements	No dispensing restrictions	Preparations containing less than a stated volume of substance, e.g. less than 0.2% morphine	Kaolin and morphine Codeine cough linctus

exemption scheme). The Veterinary Medicines Directorate Guidance (2008) suggests that, whilst the consequences of use of unlicensed medicines is a matter for the courts, issue of an unauthorized veterinary medicine where cost is the only factor is unlikely to be defensible. Veterinary Medicines Directorate Inspectors have the power to seize unlicensed products without compensation.

A veterinary surgeon can only prescribe unauthorized products to animals under his/her direct personal responsibility and to avoid causing unacceptable suffering to that animal. If such products are to be used, the veterinary surgeon should inform the owner and obtain written consent. Records must be kept for a minimum of 5 years, which must include:

- Date of examination of the animal
- Name and address of the owner
- Identification and number of animals treated
- Diagnosis
- Trade name of the product if there is one
- Batch number if there is one
- Name and quantity of active substance
- Dose administered or supplied
- Duration of treatment
- Withdrawal period if applicable.

There are also specific labelling requirements if the medicine is to be dispensed for a client to administer at home.

Writing prescriptions

A prescription may be needed to obtain a supply of drugs, or may be made out in order that owners can obtain medication elsewhere. A prescription may be oral or written, but it must be written if the medication is to be obtained elsewhere. In many cases, recognized abbreviations are used which are often based on Latin (Table 17.13). The VMR 2009 allow another veterinary surgeon, pharmacist or SQP to dispense against a veterinary prescription, but only from registered premises. According to The Supply of Relevant Medicinal Products Order 2005, it was illegal to charge a fee to issue a veterinary prescription for a 3-year period from October 2005 to October 2008, but the ban on prescription charging has now been lifted. However, it is important to remember that prescription fees should be reasonable and transparent. Clients not receiving a prescription must not be charged for one and also, there should be no discrepancy between those issued with a prescription and those not issued with prescription with regard to costs of other services (in other words, one cannot simply increase the consultation fee for one or both groups of people to recover the cost of prescription writing).

Table 17.13 demonstrates some commonly used prescription abbreviations. Prescriptions for POM-V and POM-VPS products have specific legal requirements. Prescriptions for CDs have additional requirements over and above those for other POMs. In addition, there are some recommendations regarding prescription writing, which it would be good practice to take into account. Table 17.14 demonstrates legal and recommended guidelines for prescription writing. Prescriptions for POM products should not be dispensed any more than 6 months from the date of issue. Prescriptions for CD products should not be dispensed any more than 28 days from the date of issue. Under the VMR 2009, it is a criminal offence to alter a written prescription unless authorised to do so by the person who signed it.

Table 17.13 Abbreviations commonly used in dispensing and prescription writing

Abbreviation	Meaning
ad lib.	Take freely
b.i.d.	Bis in diem – take twice a day
o.m.	Omni mane – every morning
o.n.	Omne nocte – every night
p.c.	Post cibum – after food
p.o.	Per os – by mouth
p.r.n.	As required
q.i.d.	Quattuor in diem – take four times a day
q.4h	Every 4 hours
t.i.d.	Tres in diem – take three times a day
cc	Cubic centimetre
mg	Milligram
ml	Millilitre
a.c.	Ante cibum – before food
t.d.s.	Ter die sumendum – three times a day
q.d.s.	Quater die sumendum – four times a day
o.d.	Omni die – once daily
u.d.	Ut dictum – as directed
s.i.d.	Semel in die – once daily
q.q.h	Quater quaque hora – every four hours
s.o.s	Si opus sit – if necessary

Dispensing veterinary drugs

Dispensing procedure

In many veterinary practices, the veterinary nurse plays a key role in dispensing medicines to clients. It is important that this procedure is carried out accurately and carefully, in order to avoid mistakes by both the nurse and the client. According to The VMR and COSHH regulations, the prescribing veterinary surgeon, pharmacist or SQP must be satisfied that the owner is competent to administer the medicine and has a duty of care to ensure that the owner using the product knows how to do so safely. If they are not personally dipsensing the medication, they must be satisfied the person handing over the medication is competent to do so.

Each practice should have a standard operating procedure, designed to minimize the number of errors, maximize client and animal safety, and comply with legislative requirements. This should incorporate a mechanism whereby dispensed medication can be double-checked, either by a second person or by a computer. Clients not only need to fully understand how to dose the patient but also they need to be given sufficient information regarding contraindications, adverse reactions, storage, handling and safe disposal of medicines. They should receive written instructions regarding these issues to reinforce the advice given at the time of

Table 17.14 Legal and recommended guidelines for prescription writing

Legal	Rec'd	POM	POM CD
In ink or other indelible format	X	X	X
Name and address of prescriber (may be letterheaded paper)	X	X	X
Name and address of client or keeper	X	X	X
Premises where animal(s) is/are kept if different from owners address	X	X	X
Species, identification and number of animal or group of animals (if applicable)	X	X	X
Date	X	X	X
Name(s) and amount(s) of drug	X	X	X
Dosage and administration instructions	X	X	X
Any necessary warnings	X	X	X
Withdrawal period if relevant	X	X	X
Prescriber's signature and professional qualifications	X	X	X
Number of times the prescription is to be repeated if more than once	X	X	X
Written in veterinary surgeon's own handwriting	X		X (except phenobarbital)
Form of drug to be dispensed	X		X
Amount to be prescribed written in words and figures	X		X
The wording, 'For animal treatment only'	X	X	X
Decimal points to have a figure in front of them, e.g. 0.5 instead of .5	X	X	X
Names of drugs should be written in English without abbreviation	X	X	X
Directions should be written in English without abbreviation (except the standard Latin abbreviations)	X	X	X
Quantities of less than 1 g to be written in milligrams	X	X	X
Millilitres to be used instead of cubic centimetres	X	X	X

dispensing. Table 17.15 identifies the routes by which those dispensing and administering medication may become contaminated (see also sections on handling and use of cytotoxic drugs and on pharmacy management).

When dispensing, ensure that the client is confident to administer the medication and has fully understood the instructions. In some cases, a practical demonstration may be advisable, asking them to repeat the procedure after the demonstration. Clients must be made fully aware of any restrictions regarding the medication, e.g. only give with food, do not crush, give at a separate time to other medications, etc.

Occasionally, it may be necessary to send medication by post. This is permitted by Royal Mail, provided that the medication has been sent by, or at the request of a veterinary surgeon, is not hazardous to the public, e.g. corrosive to the touch, has been packaged using a strong inner container and wrapped in sufficient outer layers to absorb any leakage. The total volume of any aerosol must not exceed 50 ml and Medication must be sent via a traceable route, e.g. Royal Mail Special Delivery Service. It is not permitted to send CDs, narcotics or psychotropic substance by post.

Packaging and posting a drug should not contravene any storage requirements as stipulated on the product data sheet, e.g. it would not be acceptable to post a drug that requires refrigeration unless you could guarantee that the product would kept at the required temperature during transportation.

Dispensing containers

According to The VMR 2009, any specific packaging instructions supplied by the MA holder on the data sheet must be adhered to by the dispensing premises. If there are no specific instructions, The Royal Pharmaceutical Society of Great Britain (RSPGB) issues guidelines for suitable containers. Table 17.16 outlines their recommendations.

Labelling medication

According to The VMR 2009, labels may be amended in accordance with a prescription, provided the product is still being used legally within the confines of UK legislation and the instructions are clear. There must be sufficient information on the label to enable the product to be used safely. There is currently no other restriction regarding labelling a product in a veterinary practice, i.e. when it is dispensed to a client, with the exception of medicines prescribed under the 'cascade' (see relevant section above); however, it is good practice to ensure that all medication is labelled clearly and BVA guidance regarding this subject is a good source of information. Table 17.17 below incorporates this guidance.

Table 17.15 Health and Safety recommendations for safe handling of medication

Route of contamination	Method of prevention	Note
Via skin	Always wear gloves when handling drugs	Some people have idiosyncratic hypersensitivity or allergy to a specific drug, e.g. penicillin allergy. However, even if this is not the case, it should be remembered that some drugs are very effective at entering the body via the transdermal route. Some may have an accumulative effect, so constant contact with the drug over a long period of time may cause problems
Via mucous membrane or by inhalation	Wear goggles and a mask. Dispense in a draft-free room, but ventilate the area thoroughly after use. Wear gloves and wash hands thoroughly after use. Do not rub face or eyes	This particularly applies to powders, but could also occur with very dry tablets that tend to accumulate loose powder in the bottom of the container
Open wounds	Cover open wounds with an appropriate waterproof dressing	More likely to occur when dispensing liquids or semi-solid medication such as cream
Ingestion	Do not eat or drink in the dispensary. Do not wipe face with hands. Keep work surfaces tidy and do not dispense medication on top of books, records or other equipment	Drug residue could be left on another object, then transferred to another part of the building, e.g. the rest room, where it could come into contact with food
Accidental injection	Observe strict rules relating to use of needle guards and swift disposal of sharps	It is unlikely that large quantities of drug could be accidentally injected, but residues in the needle, or trauma from the sharp point, could cause a nasty reaction or injury

Table 17.16 Royal Pharmaceutical Society of Great Britain (RPSGB) guidelines for suitable medicine containers

Medicine	Suitable container	Exceptions/additional rules	Note
Loose-supplied medications, e.g. tablets, liquids	Supply in child-proof container. Oral liquids should be dispensed in a non-fluted container	Discretion may be exercised in the use of child-proof containers – aged and infirm clients may need an easy-to-open container. Also, there may not be a suitable child-proof container available for certain preparations, e.g. liquids	The RPSGB recommends that a notice is displayed in the waiting room, indicating that medication will be dispensed in child-proof containers, but plain containers are available on request
Blister-packed preparations and sachets	Paper board cartons, wallets, or paper envelopes	Paper envelopes should not be used as the sole container	Removing medication from its blister-pack is not advisable as it may damage the medication, or expose it to environmental conditions that affect the medication
Medicines for external application	Fluted bottles	According to the RPSGB, this should be carried out so that medication is not inadvertently ingested by a visually impaired person	It may not always be possible to dispense large volumes and pre-packaged eye and ear preparations (already in plastic bottles) in fluted containers
Creams, ointments, powders and granules	In the original container if suitable, or in wide-mouth containers made from glass or plastic	Most creams and ointments are packaged for individual use. There are few powders on the market – again, most do not need repackaging	If repackaging, care must be taken not to contaminate the medication, expose it unnecessarily to air or moisture or absorb/inhale the medication

Safe disposal of medicines

Clients should be discouraged from keeping medication indefinitely and made aware that any surplus or unused medication should be disposed of carefully to avoid risk to themselves, other people, animals or the environment. The ideal system is to request that they return unused medication to the veterinary practice and some product data sheets will stipulate this. Returned medication should not be redispensed as appropriate storage conditions in the client's home cannot be guaranteed. Clients who will generate sharps and other hazardous waste, e.g. owners of diabetic animals, should be supplied with an appropriate bin or clinical waste bag which can be returned at suitable intervals.

Returned Schedule 2 CDs are subject to very specific disposal requirements. They must be destroyed in the presence of an Animal Medicines Inspectorate (AMI) or RCVS Practice Standards Scheme Inspector, a witnessing veterinary surgeon who is independent of the practice concerned (this excludes locums who have or are acting in the practice, family members or any relationship that may pose a risk of collusion), or another person authorised to witness the

Table 17.17 Recommendations for labelling medication

Item	Recommended method/information
Type of printing or writing to use	Must be indelibly and legibly printed or written. Mechanically printed lettering is ideal. Pencil and non-water-resistant ink are not acceptable
Expiry date	The label should not obscure the expiry date
Instructions on the product packaging	Every effort should be made not to obscure product information. There must be sufficient information visible so that the product can be used safely.
Manufacturer supplied product information sheets, inserts and leaflets	These should be passed on to the client. (The VMR 2009 state that the user must be informed of administration method/s, risks, warnings and contraindications so omitting the leaflet could be illegal if no other information is given)
Recommended information	• Name and address of owner/keeper • Name and address of veterinary surgeon • Date of dispensing • The wording 'For animal treatment only' and 'Keep out of the reach of children' or similar • The wording 'For external use only' where relevant • The withdrawal period, where relevant (even if it is nil) for food-producing animals • Animal name • Drug name • Drug strength and quantity • Dose • Special precautions • Initials of person dispensing

destruction of controlled drugs under the Misuse of Drugs Regulations 2001 or the Misuse of Drugs Regulations (Northern Ireland) 2002 such as a Police contact. A record must be made of the date of destruction and the quantity destroyed, which the witness must sign. It is good practice to also record the name of the controlled drug, form, strength and quantity, date it was destroyed and the signature of the witness and the person destroying it.

Pharmacy management

As in many areas of a veterinary practice there are a multitude of health and safety risks inherent in the veterinary pharmacy. Thorough assessment, evaluation and reduction of these risks is important. Apart from the health and safety considerations, there are other aspects of pharmacy management to consider: minimizing drug error, wastage of stock (and therefore money) and providing an efficient service to the client. With the introduction of tighter regulation on the storage and supply of medicines, including the registration and inspection of veterinary practice premises, those involved with pharmacy management must ensure they are up to date with the latest requirements in order to keep within the boundaries of the law.

Key considerations for effective pharmacy management

It is unlikely that veterinary nurses will be able to design a pharmacy from scratch and, quite frequently, they must 'make do' with the basic environment and position of the pharmacy. It is, however, still possible to undertake a full review of the pharmacy and make changes in order to improve this area of the practice. Table 17.18 illustrates some of the key considerations when reviewing pharmacy facilities and practice.

Client compliance

What is client compliance?

Client compliance is the extent to which the actions of the owner coincide with the instructions of the veterinary team with regard to the care of an animal. It can be used to describe any aspect of treatment but is most commonly referred to when discussing drug therapy and the likelihood that the owner will give prescribed medication correctly. Some human-centred nursing texts dislike the use of the word 'compliance', as it implies that people are being ordered to do as they are told, rather than following a course of treatment that has been negotiated and agreed. The terms 'adherence' and 'concordance' are preferred.

The importance of client compliance

Studies in human medicine show that patient non-compliance is a major cause of ineffective treatment. Recently, some studies have been undertaken in the veterinary field and it appears that the situation there may be similar. Ensuring client compliance will improve the health and welfare of the patient and the veterinary professional should facilitate this. Table 17.19 provides the details of factors that affect compliance.

The nurse's role in improving compliance

The veterinary nurse is ideally placed within the team to play a major role in increasing compliance and, in doing so, improving the well-being of patients. The following lists some suggestions as to how a dedicated veterinary nurse can achieve this:

• Ensure the client clearly understands the recommendations that have been made for their pet.

Table 17.18 Considerations in designing and running a pharmacy

Area/issue	Suggested action
Environmental conditions	Purchase a thermometer and hygrometer to monitor the environmental temperature and humidity. Additional heating or a dehumidifier may be necessary. Windows are a security risk and not desirable in a pharmacy, but if present they should be shuttered if possible. Heavy blinds could be used as an alternative, to reduce excessive heat, draughts and light entering the pharmacy. Ensure that light-sensitive drugs are kept in dark containers and stored in a light-proof receptacle. Review the ventilation system to ensure that minimal dust and particles enter
Shelving	Check that there is adequate shelving to hold all stock. Cluttered shelves are difficult to keep clean and may interfere with stock rotation, as well as making it hard to locate drugs ind increasing the risk of a dispensig error. Install additional shelving if needed or reduce the volume of stock kept
Position of stock	Drugs should be kept in alphabetical order on the pharmacy shelf. Ensure that all personnel involved with the pharmacy are familiar with the system so they can locate drugs easily. Heavy items should not be stored on very high or low shelves. Controlled drugs must be stored according to legislative requirements
Stock rotation	Ensure that stock is appropriately rotated. Only have one bottle or packet open at a time and mark each product 'OPEN', with the date of broachment when in use. Ensure that there is an effective system for recording batch numbers of stock once opened. Despite effective rotation, packaging often gets dusty and it is important to vacuum and clean regularly to avoid spoilage of stock. Monitor stock usage – drugs tend to fall in and out of 'favour', so the types and amounts of each type will change as time goes by. Avoid stocking duplicate products, i.e. the same drug made by two different manufacturers. Unused drugs from an open pack or bottle should be discarded within 28 days of opening, unless the product information stipulates a shorter time frame
Dispensing	Ensure that an adequate supply of Personal Protective Equipment (PPE) is within easy reach of those dispensing drugs. It is advisable to assemble a 'cytotoxic kit' especially for dispensing these drugs. Ensure that suitable waste bins are within easy reach. Ensure that clients are supplied with PPE as per practice policy. It may be necessary to supply written instructions to accompany these
Prevention of contamination	Never allow food or drink into the pharmacy. Remove unnecessary equipment and literature. Ensure that hand-washing facilities, first aid kit and eye-washing facilities are easily accessible. Ensure that staff clean the outside of drug containers (including swabbing the tops of multi-dose vials) as necessary
Prevention of theft	Stock should not be kept where the general public can gain access to it. Ensure that pharmacy desks or serving hatches are staffed at all times when the surgery is open. CD receptacles should be out of sight of the public and kept locked at all times. Ensure that clients pay for their treatment prior to collecting it from the pharmacy
Record keeping	Annual audit is a legal requirement. This must include a reconciliation of all incoming and outgoing stock., including disposal of out-of-date and damaged items. An efficient system of recording batch numbers is also required to conform with legislation. The exact requirement varies, depending oin the type of animals being treated, i.e. food-producing or non-food-producing. Keep documentation relating to the RCVS registration of the practice premises updated and ensure fees are paid on time. Ensure all records of stock, material safety data sheets, risk assessments and suspected adverse reaction report forms are kept up to date and in an orderly fashion
Minimizing dispensing errors	Ensure that adequate literature is available to enable staff to check dosages, etc., e.g. *Veterinary Data Sheet Compendium* from the National Office of Animal Health, *Small Animal Formulary* from the British Small Animal Veterinary Association. Clearly differentiate between drugs of similar names and strengths, e.g. by placing them in different-coloured outer receptacles, especially if the manufacturer's packaging is similar. Ensure that staff dispensing medication are adequately trained and, if necessary, supervised. Introduce a system of 'double-checking' dispensed medication. Request that staff initial the labels of dispensed drugs, so that errors may be traced. This is not to apportion blame but to enable any problems to be identified and rectified. Encourage staff to be open and honest about mistakes – remember that this may prevent the death of a patient
Minimizing administration errors	Produce client handouts about drug administration – these may be generic or specific to certain drugs, e.g. cytotoxic drugs or those with complex administration regimes. Ensure an adequate supply of effective administration aids, e.g. pill crushers
Adverse reactions	Ensure all veterinary surgeons, SQPs and other relevant staff are fully aware of the action to take in the event of a suspected adverse reaction to a veterinary medicine

Nurse consultations for patients diagnosed with long-term conditions

- Demonstrate how to give medication and encourage the owner to repeat the dosing technique while in the practice
- Offer medication aids such as reminders and pill givers
- Use written instructions and take advantage of commercially produced literature and videos
- Assure clients that they can return to check progress or discuss treatment at any time
- Consider a system of allocating a named nurse to each chronically ill patient to encourage confidence
- Check that repeat prescriptions are being ordered at the correct time intervals
- Ask clients if they are able to manage the treatment programme easily when they call for a repeat prescription.

Table 17.19 Factors affecting client compliance

Factors	Description
Patient characteristics	The patient's temperament and lifestyle – animals who are aggressive or spend time away from the house may be less likely to receive regular treatment
Treatment regime	The complexity of the treatment regime – frequent dosing intervals and polypharmacy may reduce compliance
Disease nature	There is evidence from human studies that prophylactic treatment regimes and treatment regimes for chronic or terminal patients may be less likely to be administered as instructed
Client characteristics	Aged clients or those who have disabilities or illnesses may be less likely to comply with treatment regimes
Relationship with the veterinary team	A clear recommendation for the client about the patient's treatment from the veterinary team is crucial. A good relationship with the veterinary team will enhance the possibility that clients will return for assistance if they encounter difficulty in adhering to a treatment regime

Bibliography

Bill, R., 1997. Pharmacology for Veterinary Technicians, second ed. C V Mosby, St Louis, MO.

Bishop, Y., 2000. BVA Code of Practice on Medicines. BVA Publications, London.

British Homeopathic Pharmacopeia, 1876. British Homeopathic Society, 2008.

Compendium of Data Sheets for Veterinary Products 2003–2004. National Office of Animal Health, Enfield.

Competition Commission 2003 Report on the supply within the United Kingdom of prescription-only medicines. Available from: <http://www.competition-commission.org.uk/inquiries/completed/2003/veterinary/>.

Galbraith, A., Bullock, S., Manias, E., Hunt, B., Richards, A., 2007. Fundamentals of Pharmacology, second ed. Pearson Education Limited, Harlow.

Marsh, J. (chairman), 2001. Report of the independent review of dispensing by veterinary surgeons of prescription only medicines. Available from: <http://www.vmd.gov.uk/ird/irdfinal.pdf>.

RCVS Guides to Professional Conduct for Veterinary Surgeons and Veterinary Nurses.

Tennant, B., 2002. BSAVA Small Animal Formulary, fourth ed. British Small Animal Veterinary Association, Cheltenham.

Veterinary Medicines Directorate 2008 Guidance notes on the prescribing cascade (guidance note 15). Available from: <http://www.vmd.gov.uk>.

Wanamaker, B., 2004. Applied Pharmacology for the Veterinary Technician, third ed. W B Saunders, Philadelphia, PA.

Recommended reading

Animal Medicines Training Regulatory Authority website. Available from: <http://www.amtra.org.uk>.

Bill, R., 2006. Clinical Pharmacology and Therapeutics for the Veterinary Technician, third ed. C V Mosby, St Louis, MO.
An excellent general pharmacology book. Particularly good for pharmacokinetics and drug types; however, as it is a US publication, some drugs are different and the legislation is not applicable.

Compendium of Data Sheets for Veterinary Products. National Office of Animal Health, Enfield.
Contains the data sheets for all licensed medicinal products used in the OK.

Galbraith, A., Bullock, S., Manias, E., Hunt, B., Rickards, A., 2007. Fundamentals of Pharmacology, second ed. Pearson Education Limited, Harlow.
A human pharmacology book which gives some useful information regarding legislation and may be useful to obtain a nursing perspective on the management of patients on certain medications.

Rock, A., 2007. Veterinary Pharmacology: A Practical Guide for the Veterinary Nurse. Butterworth-Heinemann, Oxford.

Royal College of Veterinary Surgeons Guide to Professional Conduct for Veterinary Nurses.

Tennant, B., 2008. BSAVA Small Animal Formulary, sixth edn. British Small Animal Veterinary Association, Cheltenham.
Excellent guide to the drugs in common use in the UK small animal practice including side effects, contraindications and dose rates.

Veterinary Medicines Directorate website. Available from: <http://www.vmd.gov.uk>.

Wanamaker, B., Massey, K., 2008. Applied Pharmacology for Veterinary Technicians, fourth ed. W B Saunders, Philadelphia, PA.
A good book for general information about all aspects of pharmacology.

CHAPTER 18

First aid

Wendy Miller Smith

Key Points

- Anyone may carry out first aid provided that it is aimed at preserving life, preventing suffering and preventing the deterioration of the animal's condition.
- The patient must be assessed in the order of ABC – airway, bleeding and circulation.
- Common first-aid situations include dealing with wounds, burns and scalds, insect stings and poisoning.
- Shock, in which the tissues suffer from inadequate perfusion, is a common sequel to many first-aid emergencies and is often the cause of death. Shock should never be underestimated.
- There are several types of fracture and the first action should be to provide support by means of the appropriate splint or support bandage (e.g. Robert Jones bandage).
- The sensory organs may be damaged in a variety of ways and as they are vital to the wellbeing of the animal it is important that their function is restored as soon as possible.
- Damage to the major organs may result in death but if the rules of first aid are applied the life of the patient may be saved.

Introduction

First aid is the critical first action carried out when a patient suffers an incident. What occurs at this stage will have an effect on the animal's treatment and subsequent recovery and it is vital that any actions are carried out with care and precision. It is essential that any first aid is carried out not only rapidly but also with some consideration as to what the outcome is likely to be. The first important action is 'Don't Panic!'

Under the Veterinary Surgeons Act 1966 (see Ch. 3) anyone may perform first aid to an animal provided that it is:

- To preserve life
- To prevent suffering
- To prevent the deterioration of the patient's condition.

There are five rules one must remember when dealing with first aid – remember ABC:

- Keep calm – ensure it is safe to approach the patient – you will be no good to the animal if you are also hurt by the surroundings or situation
- Airway – ensure that the patient has a clear airway so that oxygen can pass into the respiratory system
- Bleeding – control any haemorrhage
- Circulation – check to see that the blood is circulating around the body
- Contact the veterinary surgeon as soon as you can.

Handling the emergency telephone call

As a veterinary nurse it will be your role to carry out first aid in the surgery until the veterinary surgeon arrives and also, very importantly, if the first contact is made by telephone to explain clearly to the owner what they should do to help the animal before they arrive at the surgery. This must be done calmly and as quickly as possible while at the same time determining the level of the emergency.

In order to do this you must:

- Listen carefully – pay full attention to the caller
- Be patient – the caller may be distressed and panicking.
- Ask the caller's name, address and telephone number as soon as possible in case they are cut off. Check whether they are the owner or ringing on behalf of the owner
- Ask the species and name of the animal in question. If you do not know the animal ask for other details such as sex, breed and age
- Get a brief history of the current situation by asking clear and concise questions.

Write everything down, as you may forget it 'in the heat of the moment' and you will later have to tell the veterinary surgeon. Once you have this information you can decide on the degree of severity of the problem and advise the owner accordingly. This must be done calmly and patiently, ensuring that they understand your advice and why it is necessary.

Table 18.1 Examples of some types of emergency

Life threatening	Immediate attention
Serious haemorrhage	Conscious collapse
Severe burns	Dyspnoea
Poisoning	Fracture and dislocations
Unconsciousness	Gaping wounds
Prolapsed eye	Dystocia (birthing problems)
Road traffic accident	Convulsions
Gastric dilation and torsion	Less severe haemorrhage

First-aid situations can be broken down into two categories (Table 18.1)

- Life threatening – these need immediate action by the caller and the animal must be brought to the surgery straight away for treatment
- Minor emergencies – in which the animal needs immediate treatment at the surgery but its life is not in danger.

If you are aware of the imminent arrival of a first-aid case, get ready to receive it by:

1. Preparing a kennel in a suitable location
2. Making sure that any equipment needed to maintain the airway, including a readily accessible oxygen supply, is ready and working
3. Prepare bandaging material to control any haemorrhage.

Handling and restraint

Always remember that an animal in pain may be aggressive!

Care must be taken to ensure that no further damage and distress is caused to the patient and that the handler is not injured while attending to it.

It is important to talk to the animal, approach it calmly and then restrain it in a suitable manner; for example, for cats and small dogs use cages or baskets, for larger dogs attach a lead and loop it around the neck so that it cannot escape and further injure itself. All cages and baskets must be escape-proof and provide ventilation for the patient. A muzzle may be necessary for some dogs and a soft muzzle made from a bandage is often the best in these situations (see also Ch. 10).

Large dogs may be difficult to move and ideally this should be achieved by using a rigid stretcher such as a board, which will support the animal and help to support any spinal injuries. If there is no such object at hand, a makeshift stretcher can be created using a blanket or large towel placed under the dog and lifted by the corners by two or more people. This does not provide the best support for the animal but it is more likely to be readily available.

Assessing the patient

Respiratory competence

Once the animal is in your care you must first assess its ability to breathe. Initially this is be done by observation, which can be achieved very quickly.

Questions to ask yourself:

- Is the patient breathing? Watch for chest movements or nose/mouth movements. Put your ear to the nose and mouth and listen. Place your hand lightly on the chest and feel the movements
- Is the breathing laboured? This could indicate a blockage to the airway and it is vital that you act quickly to remove or alleviate the blockage. Care must be taken at all times in removing a visible blockage in a conscious animal, as removing it may cause further injury or injury to the first aider. If the animal is recumbent it may be possible to alleviate the blockage by extending the neck
- Is the breathing shallow? This might indicate that the animal is in shock or pain
- Is the animal conscious? If the animal is aware of its surroundings, it is less likely to be a life-threatening situation and you may have time to tend to other injuries. However, always monitor respiration in case of any change.

Haemorrhage

Any blood loss can result in a serious outcome and should be treated as an emergency (Table 18.2). In first aid the methods used to stop haemorrhage include:

- **Direct pressure** – pressure is applied directly to the haemorrhage site to aid the natural clotting process. This is done either by pressing with clean fingers, known as direct digital pressure, or by using a bandage or dressing. The latter has the advantage of releasing the first aider's hands to further attend to the patient; also if the wound is very large or there are several wounds, digital pressure will not be suitable. You should ensure that the material you use as a bandage or dressing is not fluffy, as this will adhere to the wound. The material should also be clean so that the wound is not contaminated. If the bleeding persists and goes through the original dressing, the dressing should not be removed but another should be placed on top. In this way the clots that have started to form are not disturbed or destroyed.
- **Indirect pressure** – the use of pressure points around the body. These occur in places where it is possible to press an artery against a bone and reduce the blood flow to a wound. It is often easier to use pressure points in small animals than in larger ones. Three arteries are generally used:
  1. **Brachial artery** – lies on the medial side of the humerus and the pulse can be felt at the distal end of the humerus. By applying pressure, blood flow to the lower forelimb is significantly reduced

Table 18.2 Comparison between the methods of controlling haemorrhage

Method	Risks	Advantages	Disadvantages
Direct digital pressure	What is under the wound? For example, foreign body or fracture?	Quick, effective, no other equipment required Can be applied around the foreign body	It is only a temporary treatment and haemorrhage may start again once the pressure is released
Pressure bandage	Is there a protruding object or anything that you may push further into the wound by applying the dressing?	Easy to apply Can be left in place	Some areas of the body are difficult to bandage
Indirect pressure	Locating the pressure point may be difficult	Equipment always available, e.g. fingers. Can reduce the pain for the animal	Response is not immediate Temporary treatment
Tourniquet	Cuts off the circulation to the limb and tissues will start to die if left too long It should never be in place for more than 15 min	Quick and easy; no special equipment required	Blood supply is cut off and tissues are damaged

2. **Femoral artery** – found on the medial aspect of the femur. Pressure applied here will affect the blood flow to the lower hind limb
3. **Coccygeal artery** – found on the ventral aspect of the tail (Fig. 18.1).

- **Tourniquet** – the aim is to fix the tourniquet or tie a strip of soft material above the wound on the limb and gradually tighten it until the haemorrhage is controlled (Fig. 18.2). Tourniquets are commercially available in many forms, although they can be constructed from bandages or thick elastic. They should only be used for short periods of time as their use not only reduces the haemorrhage but also affects the circulation to all the tissues below it. For this reason the tourniquet must be in place for no more than 15 min and once removed should not be replaced for at least 1 min; this time allows the blood to recirculate within the affected area. On no account should a tourniquet be covered with a dressing and at all times it should be constantly under observation and the time it is on monitored.

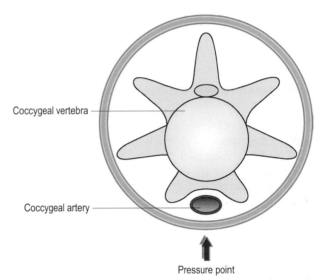

Fig. 18.1 Cross-section through a tail – site of the pressure point on the ventral aspect

Wounds

Wounds can be divided into two groups – open and closed.

Open wounds

An open wound is one where the skin surface is broken. Open wounds include the following types:

- **Incised wounds** – have clean edges and are caused by sharp implements such as glass or a knife. They generally heal quickly and result in very little scar formation
- **Lacerated wounds** – have irregular edges and are often caused by fights or road traffic accidents. Healing is generally slow and scars are often formed
- **Punctured wounds** – have small visible sites of entry but can travel deep into the underlying tissues and are often caused by objects such as nails, stakes, gunshot or cat bites. The depth of puncture wounds may track bacteria and debris deep into the body. For healing to occur successfully the wound must heal from the bottom upwards and this can take a long time

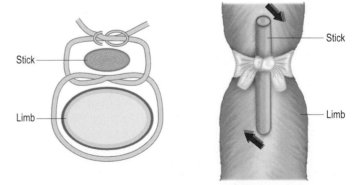

Fig. 18.2 Method of placing and tightening a tourniquet

- **Abrasion** – often described as a graze or a scrub. In these cases the skin surface is not broken and, although they are not deep wounds, abrasions are generally very painful because of the exposure of nerve endings. They often occur in road traffic accidents, when the body may have been dragged.

Treatment of open wounds

First, stop the haemorrhage using one of the methods already described. If you are in the surgery the following steps must now be followed:

1. Remove any dressings. Although the wound may start bleeding again it is vital that this is done in order to examine the wound and assess the degree of damage
2. Remove any obvious foreign bodies, providing their removal will not cause additional damage. Any protruding foreign bodies should be shortened so that a dressing can be applied around them, preventing further damage if the patient knocks the area
3. Clip the hair around the wound. Avoid contamination of the wound site by using saline on the hair. This helps clipping and reduces the chance of it getting in the wound
4. Clean the wound, working from the wound outwards
5. Apply a non-adhesive dressing
6. Apply a bandage.

Closed wounds

Here there is no break in the skin surface but the underlying tissues are damaged. They include the following types:

- **Haematoma** (pl. haematomata) – a pocket of connective tissue under the skin that fills with blood. Common sites are in the ear pinna, due to excessive shaking of the head, and at injection sites. Gradually the clots contract and the wound becomes hard. The first-aid action in these cases is to dress the area firmly as soon as possible to reduce further haemorrhage into the pocket
- **Contusion, or bruise** – Contusions are caused by a blow to the skin surface that damages the underlying capillaries, causing them to rupture and allow blood to leak from the vessels. The skin becomes warm to the touch and discoloration gradually follows because of the breakdown of the haemoglobin pigment, which gives rise to the classic purple, yellow and green colours
- **Injuries to internal organs** – these must be treated in specific ways, depending on the organ injured, and will be discussed later.

Treatment of closed wounds

Apply cold compresses to reduce the blood flow to the damaged capillaries, causing them to constrict. Dressing and bandaging the area will provide support for the wound and protect the nerve endings, which should make the patient more comfortable.

Bandaging techniques

Completing a well-placed bandage that will neither come off nor cause the circulation to be cut off is an art that can only be achieved by practice. The importance of bandages is listed in Box 18.1. A loose bandage will not be of any therapeutic advantage and will quickly fall off, while if it is too tight either the underlying tissues will become damaged or the animal will try to remove it and cause further complications.

Bandaging techniques are illustrated on the website.

Box 18.1 Why are bandages important?

Bandages have a number of roles, which include:

Support	For fractures, dislocations, sprains, strains, healing wounds. This support will help to:
	• Reduce pain levels and swelling
	• Assist in movement
	• Give additional support to internal fixation of fractures
Protection	From infection or other contaminates
	From self-mutilation
	Holds dressings in place
Pressure	To arrest haemorrhage
	To reduce swelling
Immobilization	To restrict the movement of joints or soft-tissue injuries
	To reduce pain levels
	To provide comfort
	To reduce a dislocation
Security	To protect intravenous cannulae

Bandaging rules

1. Before you start, wash your hands and make sure that you have all the equipment ready close at hand
2. Remove all soiled bandages and dispose of them in the clinical waste bin
3. If bandaging a lower limb, always include the foot
4. If including the foot, place cotton wool padding between the toes for comfort and to absorb sweat (Fig. 18.3)
5. Keep the bandage rolled up while using it as this helps to maintain tension
6. Only unroll a small amount at a time – to achieve an even tension and to allow you to control the bandage
7. Always overlap the bandage
8. When bandaging limbs or tails work from the distal end upwards to prevent blood from 'pocketing' at the end
9. Secure the ends with tape – do not use safety pins, which may be swallowed by the patient
10. Always include the joint below and above when immobilizing a fracture
11. On completion all bandages must be checked to ensure they are not too tight or loose
12. The finished result should be neat and serve the purpose for which it is designed.

Burns and scalds

A **burn** is an injury caused by any of the following:

- Dry heat such as fire or contact with a hot surface
- Electricity
- Excessive cold, including cryosurgery
- Corrosive chemicals.

A **scald** is an injury that has been caused by moist heat such as:

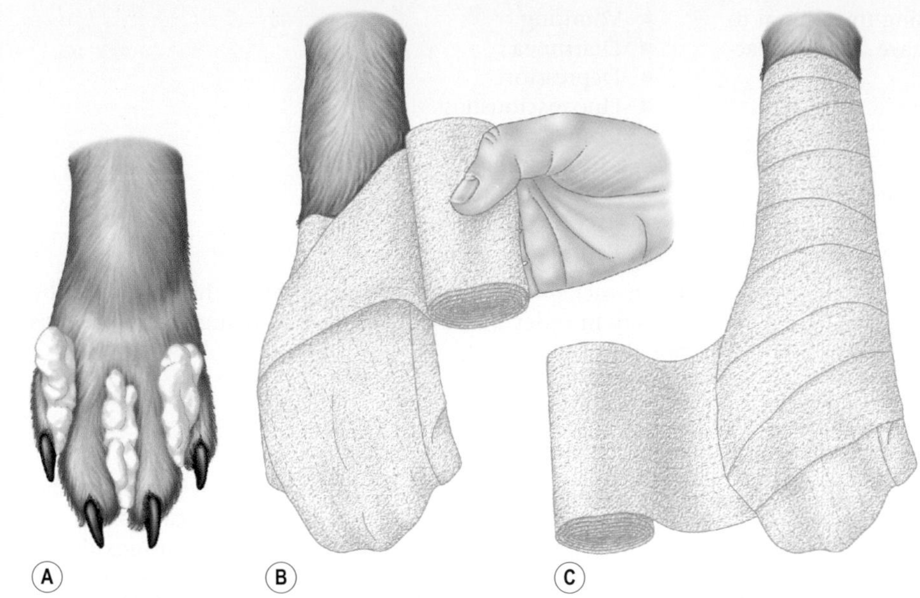

Fig. 18.3 (A–C) Basic bandaging technique

- Boiling water
- Hot tar
- Hot oil.

Classification

These wounds are classified according to:

- Depth of injury
  Superficial burns are those that infiltrate no deeper than the skin surface
  Deep burns are those that penetrate though the skin into the tissues below.
- Size of area affected – this is an estimation of the amount of the patient's body that has been affected by the burn or scald, e.g. if one side of a patient's body is affected, this is estimated as a 40% burn.

Treatment of burns and scalds

1. Cool the area – this should be done with running water or saline, which reduces the heat in the tissues and reduces the pain and damage to the cells
2. Warm the patient – it is important to maintain the animal's body temperature so that it does not become hypothermic
3. Dress the wound – these dressings prevent further fluid loss from the site. They should be sterile and non-adherent. They should also be covered with warm saline swabs to keep the site moist and cool
4. Replace fluid loss by intravenous infusions – dehydration may result from fluid loss from the site of the injury.
5. Provide analgesia
6. Treat for shock.

Electrical burns

These should be treated in the same way as other burns and scalds. It is vital that you do not touch the animal until the electricity supply has been disconnected. Use a wooden implement such as a broom handle to move the patient away from the source.

Chemical burns

If the identity of the chemical is unknown, wash the site thoroughly with water or saline to remove the chemical. This should be done wearing suitable protective clothing. If the chemical is known to be alkaline, then prepare an acidic solution to neutralize the chemical, e.g. mix vinegar with water and use it to remove the chemical from the coat; if it is acidic, prepare an alkaline solution of bicarbonate of soda and water.

Complications of burns and scalds

- **Shock** – this may severe and in some cases may lead to death. It is caused by:
  - Tissue damage
  - Fluid loss
  - Pain
  - Infection after the injury
- **Dyspnoea** – patients that have been exposed to house fires become dyspnoeic because of smoke inhalation into the respiratory tract. The outcome is often seen as pneumonia or bronchitis, which occurs 2–3 days after the event
- **Infection** – occurs because the moist conditions attract bacteria. Delays in wound healing will result
- **Poisoning** – may occur in chemical burns due to the fact that the patient has licked the chemical from its coat.

Insect stings

In the UK wasp and bee stings are the most common, although hornet stings may also be seen. Stings are generally not severe unless they occur in areas where swelling causes problems, e.g. in the pharyngeal area causing the animal to become dyspnoeic. Some patients may have allergic reactions to stings, causing collapse.

Treatment of insect stings

- **Bee stings** – are acid, so bathe the area in dilute bicarbonate of soda
- **Wasp stings** – are alkaline, so bathe the area in dilute vinegar.

Poisons

Poisoning is said to have occurred when a poison or toxin enters the patient's body either by the enteral or oral route or via the skin and is in sufficient quantity to cause a harmful effect. Potential poisons include: many chemicals, e.g. ethylene glycol or antifreeze, which may cause irreversible kidney damage even if the animal has only consumed a small amount; drugs, e.g. meloxicam, which causes gastro-interstinal irritation if taken in excess; and plants found within the house and garden, e.g. yew (*Taxus baccata*) or foxglove (*Digitalis lanata*).

Other poisons include:

- Pesticides, e.g. slug bait (metaldehyde), rat bait (warfarin and its derivatives)
- Fungicides
- Household chemicals, e.g. bleach, white spirit
- Plants, e.g. daffodil bulbs, poinsettia, rhododendron.
- Medicines, e.g. aspirin – poisonous to cats, although it can be given to other animals in small doses – phenobarbital, diazepam.

In poisoning cases it is vital that an accurate history is taken to ascertain the following facts:

- **When did the animal take the poison?** Different poisons will act within a variety of timescales – some will act instantly; others may take several hours to have an effect. The time will also influence the treatment – if the poison was ingested more than 4 hours previously it will already have been absorbed into the bloodstream and inducing the animal to vomit will not reduce the effect.
- **What poison was eaten?** Encourage the owner to bring the packet, label or data sheet with them when they visit the surgery. Knowing the name of the poison will affect the type of treatment.
- **How much of the poison was eaten?** A small quantity of chocolate may have no effect on a dog but a large bar may be very toxic; however, only a small amount of slug bait could be fatal.
- **Did it definitely eat the poison?** A panicking owner may assume that a broken packet means that the material has been eaten.
- **What are the species, breed and age of the animal?** Different poisons affect different species in different ways: e.g. phenolic compounds and aspirin are toxic to cats; young animals may be more affected than older animals.
- **What symptoms (if any) is the animal exhibiting?** These vary according to the poison but may include:

- Vomiting
- Diarrhoea
- Depression
- Unconsciousness
- Convulsions
- Muscle tremors
- Abdominal pain
- Excessive salivation
- Panting.

The owner should be encouraged to bring the animal to the surgery in order that treatment can be instigated as soon as possible.

Treatment of poisoning

1. Prevent further exposure to the poison by removing the source or by removing the patient. In the case of inhaled poisons such as smoke or carbon monoxide take the patient into the fresh air or administer oxygen. If the coat is contaminated it should be washed to prevent the patient grooming or licking itself. An Elizabethan collar may be also used to limit access to the chemical. Make sure that in future the poison is kept locked away in a cupboard.

2. Identify the poison and administer the antidote if one exists: e.g. the effect of warfarin poisoning may be limited by administering vitamin K. In the majority of cases there is no antidote.

3. Contact the Veterinary Poisons Information Service – this service provides 24 hour information on the treatment of poisons and possible antidotes. You may also use other sources such as the internet.

4. Prevent absorption of the poison by the stomach and small intestine by:

   a. **Induce vomiting** by the use of emetics, e.g. two teaspoons of mustard in a cup of warm water or one or two pea-sized crystals of washing soda placed on the back of the tongue – both can be administered by the owner. A veterinary surgeon may use apomorphine (0.1 mg/kg s/c) or xylazine (3.0 mg/kg im). Never use salt solution, as salt in excess may also cause poisoning.

   Do **not** induce vomiting if:

   - The poison is known to be corrosive, e.g. creosote, petrol – the tissues of the mouth and oesophagus will be burned both on the way down and when the poison is regurgitated
   - The patient is unconscious or having a fit
   - The poison was ingested more than 4 hours ago – absorption may already have taken place.

   If the owner is unable to induce vomiting they must bring the animal into the surgery as soon as possible.

   b. **Use gastric lavage** to wash the ingesta from the stomach. This must be done under the direct supervision of the veterinary surgeon. The patient should be anaesthetized or unconscious and warm water or saline is introduced into the stomach via a stomach tube. The stomach is washed out several times until the draining solution is clean. Replace with absorbent charcoal granules to remove any remaining ingesta.

c. **Use a saline purge** – if the poison is corrosive the passage of the ingesta can be hurried through the tract by the use of a saline purge – this is not recommended if the patient is shocked or the digestive tract is inflamed.

d. **Use a demulcent** – if the poison is irritant then the digestive tract may be soothed by the use of a demulcent which coats the lining of the stomach, e.g. raw egg beaten with a little milk and sugar.

5. If the coat or skin is contaminated then it should be washed as soon as possible. This is a problem in cats, as they hate being bathed and many poisons are toxic to cats. If necessary they should be anaesthetized for the procedure. Keep under observation during recovery and take care that the heat source used to dry the coat does not burn them:

- **Liquid oily compound**, e.g. creosote or sump oil – wash the coat in Swarfega, cooking oil or liquid paraffin. Rinse thoroughly until all smell has gone.
- **Non-oily compounds**, e.g. disinfectants – wash in warm water. The use of detergents will increase the absorption of the disinfectant by the skin.
- **Solid oily compounds**, e.g. tar. Clip affected areas of hair. Massage vegetable oil, butter or liquid paraffin into the area to soften the tar and wash thoroughly. Bandaging the area for 15 min after applying the butter will encourage the heat of the body to soften the tar.

Many poisons are corrosive or carcinogenic and precautions must be taken for the health and safety of the handler – always wear gloves and protective clothing.

Collection of samples

Samples discharged from the body such as vomit, faeces and urine are often the only real indicators of what poison has been ingested. The colour may be abnormal, as many domestic poisons contain bright colourants. If the veterinary surgeon is unsure as to which poison is involved, samples can be sent away for analysis and should be labelled clearly with the following details:

1. Name and address of the owner
2. Animal's details, including species, name, sex and age
3. Time and date of collection
4. What the sample contains.

Shock

Shock may be explained as the state that results from inadequate perfusion of the tissues, which affects the supply of oxygen and nutrients to the tissues and the removal of waste products formed by the tissues. If the state of shock continues, the tissues are damaged and the patient may die. Patients that require first aid are likely to be suffering from some degree of shock. This is a potentially life-threatening condition, which can progress unless action is taken. There are several types of shock:

1. **Hypovolaemic shock** – this is the most common type and is the result of reduced circulating blood volume in the body. It may be due to:
   - Haemorrhage
   - Loss of tissue fluid and electrolytes, e.g severe vomiting and diarrhoea.

   The body responds to hypovolaemic shock by vasoconstriction, so that blood pressure rises and blood is redistributed to the vital organs, such as the brain. This is a short-term solution which will only result in full recovery by the application of fluid therapy before irreversible cell damage has occurred.

2. **Traumatic shock** – results from the release of inflammatory mediators released as a result of trauma and tissue damage. It may be complicated by haemorrhage and sepsis and hypovolaemia may follow. Initially cardiac output and heart rate increase; vasodilation occurs followed by intense vasoconstriction.

3. **Cardiogenic shock** – results from failure of the pumping mechanism of the heart. Blood volume remains normal but cardiac output is reduced. Pressure rises in the atria of the heart, leading to oedema and congestion of the dependent tissues, e.g liver and lungs. Blood pools in the tissues and blood pressure falls. Cardiogenic shock results from myocardial disease, pericardial problems and valvular dysfunction.

4. **Distributive shock** – results from the release of inflammatory mediators which interfere with the normal mechanisms that regulate blood pressure. There is no fluid loss, just redistribution of the body fluids, which results in hypotension and vasodilation. Clinical signs are **different** from those of other types of shock and include warm extremities, a bounding pulse, rapid capillary refill time and hyperaemic (brick red) mucous membranes. There are two types:
   - **Anaphylactic shock** – occurs when the body has an allergic reaction to an antigen to which the patient has become sensitized. Signs of shock may be accompanied by urticaria, laryngeal oedema and bronchospasm.
   - **Septic shock** also called endotoxic shock – occurs when bacteria or their toxins are present in the circulation. Also seen in fungal, viral and protozoal infections. Clinical signs begin as pyrexia followed by signs of shock.

Clinical signs of shock

These include:

- Pale/dry mucous membranes
- Slow capillary refill time
- Weak, rapid pulse
- Cold extremities
- Increased heart rate
- Rapid, shallow respiration
- Subnormal temperature
- Poor skin turgor
- Decreased urine output
- Reduced level of consciousness
- Collapse
- Convulsions.

Treatment

1. It is vital that any haemorrhage is controlled as soon as possible.
2. Warm the animal using towels and blankets. Direct heat must not be applied as this will dilate the peripheral blood vessels, taking the blood away from the organs, where it is needed most.
3. Make the animal comfortable in a safe and secure environment – reduce the lighting and keep noise to a minimum.
4. Prepare the equipment for intravenous fluids to be administered. The choice of fluid depends on the type of shock (see Ch. 21).
5. Check any dressings that are already in place for signs of continuing haemorrhage and for any self-inflicted damage.
6. Observe the patient constantly, as the condition of a patient in shock can deteriorate quickly.
   Monitor the following parameters at 5–10 min intervals:
   - Pulse
   - Respiration
   - Capillary refill time
   - Mucosal colour
   - Papillary reflex
   - Palpebral reflexes
   - State of consciousness.
   Notes of these observations should be placed on the hospital chart for reference.
7. Provide 'TLC' to the patient by stroking and talking to it. This will make it feel more comfortable and confident. Remember that the animal has been through a traumatic experience and is now in unfamiliar surroundings.

Unconsciousness and collapse

Unconsciousness is often misinterpreted as death. When an animal is unconscious the brain is affected in such a way that the animal is unaware of its surroundings or external stimuli such as sound or touch (Table 18.3). A good stimulus to use to assess the state of unconsciousness is to call the patient's name.

Unconsciousness is measured in depths:

- Stupor – the patient will attempt to be aware of its surroundings, but with some difficulty
- Coma – all body functions are present but the patient cannot be roused.

Treatment

1. If possible, establish the cause of the unconsciousness and ensure that you will not be endangered by approaching the patient.
2. Check that the airway is patent. Loosen a tight collar and examine the oral cavity to establish if there is any obstruction. Pull the tongue forward and extend the neck.
3. Observe the patient for evidence of a heart beat and respiratory movements. If these are not obvious, place your hand at the base of the patient's chest and feel the chest movements; if the patient is small it may be better to use two fingers.

Table 18.3 Comparison between the signs of unconsciousness and death

Signs of unconsciousness	Signs of death
Heart beat is present but may be slow	No heart beat
Respiration present	No respiration
Muscles are flaccid	Muscles are rigid
Body temperature is stable	Body temperature gradually falls
Cornea is moist	Cornea is dry and the pupil is fixed and dilated
Pupillary light response is present but may be sluggish	Mucous membranes become cyanotic
Fits may occur	Bladder and anal control may be lost at the moment of death
Bladder control may be lost	Rigor mortis sets in after a few hours

4. Check the colour of the mucous membranes.
5. If you are in the surgery, provide oxygen if necessary.
6. Keep the patient warm but do not use direct heat (see Shock).
7. Make the animal comfortable.
8. Monitor and record temperature, pulse and respiration every 5–10 min.

Resuscitation of a patient

Artificial respiration

If respiratory movements appear to be absent, the patient must be supplied with oxygen artificially. Ideally, the patient should be intubated and the cuff of the tube should be inflated, which will ensure that the airway remains patent, that fluids cannot be inhaled and that the oxygen supplied is going straight into the lungs.

Once intubated, the patient should be given oxygen via a closed anaesthetic circuit (see Ch. 25). Gentle pressure should be applied to the rebreathing bag. If there is no anaesthetic machine available, the lungs can be inflated by gently blowing down the tube. Alternatively, if you are not in the surgery, mouth-to-nose resuscitation can be achieved in the following manner:

1. Place the patient on its side and extend the neck
2. Pull the tongue forward
3. Take hold of the nose firmly and hold one hand under the jaw to seal the mouth
4. Blow into the nose, making sure you remove your mouth when you inhale, thus avoiding taking in any saliva or mucus from the patient
5. The blowing action must be done gently so as not to overinflate the lungs, as animal patients have a smaller lung capacity than a human.

Cardiac massage

If it is not possible to detect a heartbeat it may be possible to stimulate the heart by manually compressing the ribcage.

If this is necessary the patient should also be supplied with oxygen by either of the methods above. When both the heart and the respiration have stopped, this is referred to as cardio-pulmonary arrest.

The procedure for cardiac massage is as follows:

1. Place the patient in lateral recumbency, extending the neck and forelimbs forwards.
2. For small individuals, place your hand ventrally around the chest with the finger tips on one side and thumb on the other side of the chest wall just behind the elbows and apply even pressure squeezing the thumb and fingers together. This should be repeated about 120 times per minute.
3. For larger patients this method may be more difficult, so use the heel of the hand and, with your other hand underneath the chest, apply pressure over the region of the heart.
4. Stop massaging the heart at regular intervals (every 20–30 seconds) and observe whether or not the heart has started to beat on its own again.

Epilepsy

Epilepsy is said to occur when the patient has an epileptic fit. This is caused by waves of disorganized electrical activity within the brain. The sight of their animal having a fit can be very distressing for owners. There are many causes of fits but very often they are idiopathic, i.e. there is no known cause.

Specific causes include:

- Brain damage caused by disease or trauma
- Poisoning
- Viral or bacterial infections
- Metabolic disease, such as chronic liver or kidney failure
- Cerebral anoxia, e.g. due to anaesthetic accidents.

Clinical signs

Clinical signs of fitting can be divided into three phases:

1. **Pre-ictal phase** – the patient may become hyperexcited or overanxious and may have an 'aura' or an apparent awareness that something is about to happen.
2. **Ictal phase** – the patient becomes recumbent – usually laterally. The body is tense, with the limbs extended and sometimes the patient will 'paddle'. Eyes are fixed and staring. Drooling and frothing at the mouth can be seen. Bladder and rectal control may be lost. The patient is unaware of its surroundings
3. **Post-ictal phase** – the patient is usually dazed, unsteady and appears to be exhausted. It may sleep for long periods after the event.

The timescale varies with the individual but the average time for a single fit is about 5 min. In some cases, the animal may have one fit after another – a condition known as **status epilepticus**.

Telephone advice

The most common situation will be that the owner of the animal will telephone the surgery for advice. The owner will be distressed and panicking and you must remain calm and patient. Very little can be done to the animal while it is having a fit. However, the following should be recommended:

- Ensure that only one person is left with the patient.
- Do not touch the patient.
- Remove any objects that could fall on to the animal and cause further harm.
- Reduce the light and noise levels.
- Once the fit has subsided, allow the patient to rest.
- Make a note of how long the fit lasted, what the symptoms were and any occurrences that might have stimulated the fit. When the fit has subsided the owner should arrange for the veterinary surgeon to check the animal. If the fit persists, the veterinary surgeon will ask the owner to bring the animal into the surgery so that treatment can be started as soon as possible.

Fractures

Fractures are breaks in the bone and are named according to the type of damage that has occurred (Fig. 18.4). A fracture may be:

- **Simple** – the bone is broken cleanly into two pieces
- **Compound** – a skin wound leads to the fracture site and the risk of infection is high
- **Complicated** – organs and vital structures such as major blood vessels and nerves are damaged around the fracture site
- **Multiple** – there is more than one fracture site with a distance between them
- **Comminuted** – the bone is shattered and there are splintered fragments
- **Greenstick** – an incomplete break usually seen in the bones of young animals
- **Spiral** – the fracture line spirals around the shaft – commonly associated with the humerus.

Clinical signs

- Pain at the site – this may not occur until the animal moves the affected part of the body.
- Swelling – due to the bruising of the surrounding soft tissues.
- Deformity – the limb is often held at an abnormal angle. This may be less obvious in fractured bones that are deep within muscles, such as the pelvis or spinal vertebrae.
- Loss of function – may be complete or partial.
- Crepitus – the grating sound of broken bone moving against other bones.
- Unnatural mobility.

Treatment

1. Do not handle the fracture site, as this will cause pain and discomfort, with the added risk of more damage to the bones or organs in the region of the fracture.
2. Provide support to the area using a dressing and bandage to prevent further damage. This support must include the joints above and below the fracture.

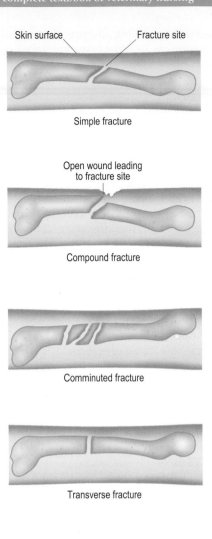

Skin surface   Fracture site

Simple fracture

Open wound leading
to fracture site

Compound fracture

Comminuted fracture

Transverse fracture

Greenstick fracture

Spiral fracture

Fig. 18.4 Types of fracture

3. Control the haemorrhage, ensuring that pressure is not placed directly on the fracture site.

Supporting the fractured limb

Support methods include splints and the use of padded support bandages such as the Robert Jones bandage. Both these methods require a degree of skill and there is a risk that they may be more of a hindrance to healing than a help.

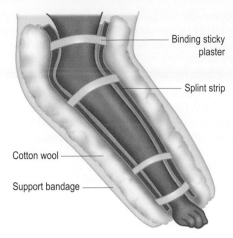

Binding sticky
plaster

Splint strip

Cotton wool

Support bandage

Fig. 18.5 Supporting a fracture – placing a splint

Splints

Many splints may be adapted from household objects such as broom handles, lolly sticks, or rolled-up newspapers or magazines. Others are manufactured specifically for the job and are made of wood, metal, plastic or resin/plaster and air bags.

Application of a splint:

1. Ensure that any wounds are covered with a suitable dressing
2. Apply a layer of protective padding, e.g. soft bandage or cotton wool. This should be thick enough to prevent the splint pressing on the skin and causing damage
3. Select the most suitable splint for the limb and fracture site
4. Place the splint on the limb so that the joints above and below the site of the fracture are included. This may mean that the splint has to be bent to conform to the angle of the joints
5. Bandage the splint in place – working initally from the distal end of the limb towards the proximal direction
6. Apply further padding to the limb
7. Finally, apply an outer support bandage to hold the padding in place, prevent self-inflicted damage to the area and provide a degree of waterproofing (Fig. 18.5).

Robert Jones bandage

This dressing is commonly used in first aid but does require a degree of expertise in order to work effectively (Fig. 18.6). The bandage creates a rigid dressing that provides support to the limb, and involves the use of large quantities of padding.

1. Ensure that any wounds are covered with a suitable dressing
2. Place cotton wool padding between the toes, making sure that these pieces are not too large or they will cause discomfort. This prevents the toes rubbing and helps to absorb any sweat
3. Take two strips of zinc oxide tape and place them on opposite sides of the limb, avoiding the wound site. They should extend several centimetres further than the toes

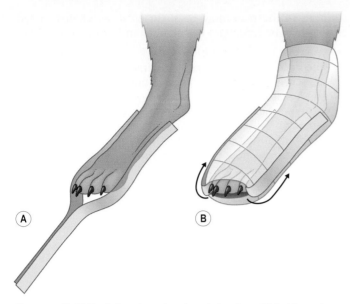

Fig. 18.6 (A, B) The Robert Jones bandage *(taken from Clinical Procedures in Veterinary Nursing 2e)*

4. Wrap the roll of cotton wool or padding evenly around the limb and including the joints above and below the fracture. Apply a number of layers until the limb is fully supported

5. Apply the conforming bandage over the padding working from the toes upwards – the toes should still be able to be seen. While doing this, tension should be applied to compress the padding layer

6. Take the zinc oxide strips that are protruding from under the padding and twist them so they can be stuck upwards on the dressing. These 'stirrups' will prevent the dressing from slipping down the limb

7. Apply a protective outer layer of adhesive bandage, working upwards from the toe

8. Test the tension of the dressing by flicking it with your fingers – a hollow sound like that of a ripe melon should be heard

9. Check the toes, making sure you can see them in case the dressing is too tight. In this case they will become cold because of the lack of blood flow

10. If the patient is exercised outdoors, this limb must be covered with a plastic bag or old drip bag to protect the bandage. A commercial sock or boot may be used.

First aid for injuries to the sensory organs

The eye

The eye may be injured either on the eyeball itself or on the eyelid but the clinical signs are generally similar and include:

- **Conjunctivitis** – reddening and inflammation of the sclera and conjunctiva. The patient will rub the eye with a paw or on the floor/furniture and thus cause further damage.
- **Epiphora** – increased tear production.
- **Photophobia** – avoiding bright light by closing the eye or burying the head.

- **Blepharospasm** – scrunching up the eye to avoid the light.

Eyeball injuries

1. Corneal injury – care must be taken to avoid touching the cornea, as this may cause ulceration:
   The cornea may be injured by:
   - Penetrating wounds – during fights or road traffic accidents. These cause a loss of aqueous humour and subsequent intraocular pressure, and the cornea may take on a shrunken, wrinkled appearance. It is vital that the eye is disturbed as little as possible.
   - Non-penetrating wounds, e.g. ulcers, which may have been caused by foreign bodies, such as thorns or claw scratches.
2. Direct trauma to the eyeball, causing haemorrhage within the eye – known as hyphaema.
3. Fractures to the skull – can cause the eye to be bruised, which is often seen as a red blister on the sclera, or the eye may protrude slightly from the socket as a result of haemorrhage in the soft tissues behind the eyeball – retrobulbar haemorrhage.
   General treatment of eyeball injuries – this includes the following:
   - Flush with saline to clean the area
   - Place a sterile gauze swab over the eye and attach loosely in position with adhesive tape
   - Reduce any possibility of self-trauma by applying an Elizabethan collar
   - Place the patient in a darkened area to help with photophobia
   - Keep warm
   - Monitor for any changes or signs of shock.
4. Prolapse of the eyeball – the eye becomes dislodged from the socket and is exposed. This may result from fighting and is more likely in breeds with more protruding eyeballs, e.g. Pekinese. In this state the eyeball is unprotected and may dry out, causing the cornea to ulcerate, and damage to the optic nerve may also result.
   Treatment
   - Although it is vital that the eye is replaced as soon as possible, this must not be attempted by anyone other than a veterinary surgeon.
   - Lubricate the eye using false tears or contact lens fluid. If neither of these is available, boiled and cooled water can be used.
   - Prevent self-trauma, e.g use of an Elizabethan collar or cover the feet in socks or bandages.

Eyelid injuries

The eyelid may be injured by:

1. Foreign bodies – the most common are grass seeds, which become lodged either under the eyelids or beneath the third eyelid. They cause excruciating pain and the patient will keep the eye tightly shut, making an examination very difficult. They may also cause trauma to the eyeball by scratching it.
   Foreign bodies may be treated in a number of ways depending on their size. If they are large enough to be

removed, then do so taking care not to cause any further damage. However, removal should not be undertaken if the cornea is penetrated. If the foreign body is small it can be flushed out with warmed saline.

2. Wounds – due to trauma such as fights and road traffic accidents or as a result of self-trauma. Wounds should be cleaned to remove any contaminants by flushing with warmed saline.

3. Inflammatory or allergic reactions – cause oedema to the conjunctiva which can be seen as the conjunctiva bulging from under the eyelid – chemosis. The pain caused by all eyelid injuries can be reduced by applying ice packs to the eye, but take care to ensure that the ice is covered in a soft, non-abrasive material to reduce the possibility of damage to the cornea.

The ear

External injuries

The most common injuries are those to the ear pinna. They may be caused by scratches, bites and stings or self-trauma resulting in aural haematomata or blood blisters.

Clinical signs

- Haemorrhage – the pinna can bleed profusely, which can be very alarming to the owner
- Shaking of the head – leads to wide distribution of blood droplets
- Self-trauma – rubbing and scratching at the ear
- Swelling – formation of a haematoma within the tissue of the pinna.

Treatment

1. Stop the haemorrhage – apply a pressure pad to the wound. The owner can use a folded handkerchief or similar bandage. In the surgery the pinna can be held back over the head with a bandage – care must be taken not to wrap the bandage too tightly under the head as this will cause asphyxia.
2. Pain may be reduced by the use of ice packs held against the ear pinna.
3. Treat insect stings according to their cause.
4. Aural haematoma – this must be treated surgically by the veterinary surgeon.

Internal injuries

Foreign bodies such as grass seeds are the most common cause of inner ear problems. Grass seeds are most often seen in the summer and are able to travel down the ear canal and become lodged deep in the ear, causing severe irritation and pain. A general anaesthetic is required to locate the foreign body and remove it without causing further damage; owners should not try to remove the object themselves.

The nose

As the nose is part of the respiratory tract any injury may restrict the oxygen supply to the body and could be fatal. Any difficulty in breathing should always be investigated.

Injuries to the nose may result in epistaxis or nose-bleed, which may be unilateral or bilateral and can be caused by:

- Trauma, e.g. a direct blow. Check for crepitus around the nose, indicating a possible fracture
- Presence of a foreign body, e.g. grass seed or blades of grass – also cause persistent sneezing and rubbing the nose on the ground or with the paw
- Infection – due to bacterial, viral or fungal infections
- Tumours in the nasal cavity – if these are very large the patient may show mouth breathing or snoring respiration.

Treatment

1. If the nose is injured, avoid muzzling the animal as this may cause further complications.
2. Cold compresses can be applied to the nose to alleviate haemorrhage. Pressure placed on the nose should be gentle, as it may make the situation worse and compromise the respiratory tract.
3. Place the patient in a quiet, darkened kennel – this will reduce the stress to the animal, allowing the heart rate and blood pressure to return to normal, which may assist with the haemorrhage.
4. Observe the patient. Watch out for signs of dyspnoea and vomiting, which may be caused by swallowing blood. Concussion may also be seen in cases where a serious blow or other trauma has occurred.

The mouth

The mouth is often injured, as animals use it for investigating and in searching for food. Injuries include:

- Foreign bodies – these are a common problem, e.g. sticks caught in the back of the throat, fish hooks, various 'chews' and bones wedged across the hard palate
- Fractures – following direct blows, as seen in road traffic accidents
- Insect stings – most often on the lips but sometimes inside the mouth.

Clinical signs

- Pain and swelling of the affected area
- Pawing or rubbing at the face
- Salivation and drooling
- Dysphagia – difficulty in eating – the animal may go to the food and sniff it but walk away leaving it uneaten or the food may drop out of the mouth.

Treatment

1. Foreign bodies must be removed quickly in order to reduce the distress caused to the animal. However, retrieval in a conscious animal is not always a safe option! These cases should be brought to the surgery as soon as possible and anaesthetized by the veterinary surgeon so that the foreign body can be removed.
2. Fractures are difficult to treat using first aid and should be treated under a general anaesthetic. Bandaging the

jaws together to provide support could compromise the respiratory tract.

3. Insect stings are treated as appropriate.

First aid for injuries to the major internal organs

Some of the organs of the body are so essential to life that if they are seriously injured the death of the animal is almost inevitable. However, if first-aid procedures are followed correctly the animal's chances of survival are significantly increased.

Gastric dilation and volvulus (GDV)

This is a very serious, life-threatening condition that often affects deep-chested breeds, e.g. Great Danes and Greyhounds. The cause is not always known but the condition can sometimes be triggered by large intakes of dry food eaten quickly, often followed by exercise. The stomach fills with methane gas formed by fermentation of the food, becomes unstable within the abdomen, and then twists, usually at the cardiac sphincter. This prevents the escape of the gas. Fermentation continues to occur and the problem becomes worse. Eventually the animal will go into shock and the condition may be fatal within a few hours.

Clinical signs

- Distension of the stomach, which feels hard to the touch and sounds hollow when tapped
- Signs of discomfort and restlessness – the dog may belch to relieve gas build-up
- Dyspnoea – the diaphragm is pressed upon by the distended stomach and the size of the thoracic cavity is reduced
- Collapse due to the respiratory distress
- Shock – the stomach pushes on the caudal vena cava and portal veins, slowing the blood flow to the heart and reducing circulating blood volume.

Treatment

This is a genuine emergency and the animal must be seen by the veterinary surgeon as soon as possible:

- The operating theatre, suitable anaesthetic and surgical equipment should be prepared.
- The gas pressure in the stomach must be relieved by attempting to pass a stomach tube. This may not be possible if the oesophagus is occluded, but avoid forcing the tube down as you may rupture the oesophagus.
- Gas pressure may be also relieved by introducing a suitably sized trocar and cannula into the stomach via the left dorsal abdominal wall. This should not be carried out by anyone other than a veterinary surgeon, who will take steps to avoid puncturing the spleen. If the stomach has twisted, the spleen may be lying in an abnormal position.
- The patient should be treated for shock.
- When the patient is stable the veterinary surgeon may perform a laparotomy to correct the twist and then suture the stomach wall to the abdominal wall – a technique known as a gastropexy – to prevent recurrence of the GDV.

Ruptured diaphragm

This condition is seen more often in cats than in dogs and is generally caused by a road traffic accident. The animal may be hit violently and the diaphragm is torn by a crushed rib or ruptured by the pressure within the thoracic cavity at the time of the accident. The abdominal organs are then able to move into the thoracic cavity, causing dyspnoea or, in extreme cases, total lung collapse.

Clinical signs

- If the tear is small, problems may not be seen at all and the animal may adapt to live a normal life
- If the abdominal organs move into the thorax, the animal will show varying degrees of dyspnoea. In some cases this may only become apparent when the animal is excited or during exercise
- Some affected animals will prefer to sit upright so that the abdominal organs fall downwards away from the area of the diaphragm, making breathing easier
- Severely affected cases may breathe showing orthopnoea – breathing with the mouth open.

Treatment

This condition must be seen by a veterinary surgeon and surgery is required to repair the diaphragm. However, it is important to stabilize the patient before surgery is performed and this may take several days:

- Place the animal in a warm, quiet kennel. It should be moved and stressed as little as possible
- If necessary, be prepared to administer oxygen – it may be useful in severely affected cases to place the animal in an oxygen tent
- Allow the animal to adopt a position in which it is comfortable
- Observe the animal, monitoring respiration and pulse closely
- Withhold food in preparation for surgery.

Splenic injuries

The spleen is a blood-filled organ that is capable of profuse haemorrhage and in many cases this leads to a rapid death. Damage to the spleen may be caused by:

- Trauma, e.g. due to road traffic accidents
- Tumours, e.g. haemangiosarcoma – often undetected until the late stages, when the patient may suddenly collapse as a result of internal haemorrhage
- Torsion of the spleen – often a complication of GDV when it becomes twisted, causing congestion and swelling.

Clinical signs

- Sudden collapse
- Rapid respiratory rate

- Pale mucous membranes and weak pulse
- If there is torsion the abdomen will be swollen, hard and extremely painful.

Treatment

In cases where the spleen has ruptured very little can be done and the animal is likely to die of internal bleeding. If the animal is able to be treated, then treat as for shock. Give intravenous blood transfusion or colloids to replace the loss of blood.

Kidney injury

The kidney has a large blood supply and if damaged by a road traffic accident or a violent blow such as a kick it may be ruptured, which results in extensive loss of blood into the abdomen and subsequent death. If the trauma is less severe, the kidney may be bruised and the animal may recover because the second kidney should be able to maintain sufficent kidney function.

Clinical signs

- The animal will show signs of pain and will stand in a 'hang dog' position, with its head down and back arched
- A urine sample may show haematuria
- Oliguria – reduced volume of urine.

Treatment

Place the patient in a warm, dark kennel and treat for shock before the veterinary surgeon diagnoses the extent of the damage.

Bladder injuries

The bladder may be ruptured, bruised or displaced by severe trauma such as a road traffic accident. The animal may also suffer from cystic calculi or bladder stones, which may either irritate the mucosal lining of the bladder or cause a blockage of the urethra. If a blockage is not detected there is a risk that backflow of urine up the urethra will cause kidney damage or that the bladder will rupture. In any case of bladder injury, a urine sample should be collected for analysis.

Clinical signs

- **Anuria** – lack of urine being passed may indicate a ruptured bladder or a blockage
- **Haematuria** – blood in the urine may indicate infection or irritation of the bladder wall
- **Dysuria** – difficulty or straining to pass urine may indicate a partial blockage
- **Oliguria** – small amounts of urine passed at intervals.

Treatment

- Closely monitor the production of urine
- Collect a sample of urine for analysis
- Prepare equipment for catheterization – may need to be used in cases of a blocked urethra
- Prepare radiography equipment for visualization of the bladder and kidneys. May also need to use contrast media.

Bibliography

Aspinall, V., 2003. Clinical Procedures in Veterinary Nursing. Butterworth-Heinemann, Oxford.

Bowden, C., Masters, J., 2003. Textbook of Veterinary Medical Nursing. Butterworth-Heinemann, Oxford.

Dallas, S., 2000. Animal Biology and Care. Blackwell, Oxford.

Lane, D.R., Cooper, B., 2003. Veterinary Nursing, third ed. Butterworth-Heinemann, Oxford.

Recommended reading

Aspinall, V., 2007. Clinical Procedures in Veterinary Nursing, second ed. Butterworth-Heinemann, Oxford.

Contains a chapter on first-aid procedures in a step-by-step format.

Bowden, C., Masters, J., 2003. Pre-Veterinary Nursing Textbook. Butterworth-Heinemann, Oxford.

Clear, no-fuss text which is ideal to remind you of those key areas for revision.

BVNA, 2004. First Aid Revision Booklet. British Veterinary Nursing Association, Harlow.

Ideal key facts needed for examination revision.

Dallas, S., 2000. Animal Biology and Care. Blackwell, Oxford.

Clear and concise with excellent pictures to demonstrate facts.

Lane, D.R., Cooper, B., 2003. Veterinary Nursing, third ed. Butterworth-Heinemann, Oxford.

Contains the basic knowledge for any veterinary nurse.

CHAPTER 19

Prevention of the spread of infectious diseases

Helen Harris and Amanda Rock

Key Points

- Infectious diseases are caused by pathogenic microorganisms, including bacteria, viruses, fungi and protozoa.
- Pathogens are able to leave the body via any of the normal orifices and within any of the body secretions.
- To cause infection, a pathogen must be transmitted by a method that ensures that it reaches the susceptible animal as quickly as possible or ensures its survival in the environment before it enters the animal.
- Methods used to control the spread of disease are mainly aimed at preventing transmission of the pathogen.
- Once a pathogen enters the body, the immune system initiates a series of responses aimed at overcoming the pathogen and preventing the development of clinical signs.
- Immunity can be divided into innate factors, which produce the same response to every type of 'attack', and acquired factors, which produce a specific response to the individual pathogen.
- Vaccination is based on the acquired immune response and results in lifelong immunity to a disease without suffering the symptoms of the disease.

Introduction

An infectious disease is one that is caused by the invasion of harmful microorganisms or pathogens, which will establish and grow in the body tissues. The pathogens are then transmitted between individuals and the disease spreads. When dealing with infection, it is important to understand how the pathogen leaves the infected animal, how it transfers and how it enters the susceptible animal or new host. Each pathogen has its own pattern, evolved to achieve optimum pathogen survival and virulence. Through training and experience, the nurse will play an important role in the survival of the animal and elimination of the disease. A list of useful definitions relating to infectious diseases are included in Box 19.1.

Spread of infectious diseases

Causal agents

Microorganisms are living creatures seen only with the aid of a microscope or macroscopically when grown in colonies. They come in many forms and have varying forms of transmission and effects on the body. Not all microorganisms are pathogenic, i.e. capable of causing disease; some are normal inhabitants of the living body and live in harmony with the host without causing disease (see Ch. 28 for further details). Pathogenic microorganisms are categorized as follows:

Bacteria

Bacteria are single-celled organisms that range in size from $0.5 \, \mu m$ to $5 \, \mu m$ in length. They can replicate outside the living cell, ensuring their survival and making them difficult to eliminate. There are three basic shapes that are recognized:

- Bacilli (cylindrical or rod-shaped), e.g. *Salmonella* spp.
- Cocci (spherical), e.g. *Streptococcus* spp.
- Spirochaetes (spiral), e.g. *Leptospira* spp.

They are further divided into groups depending on whether or not they stain with Gram stain (see Ch. 29). For example:

- Gram-negative *Salmonella* spp. live within the intestines
- Gram-positive streptococci cause respiratory disease
- Gram-variable *Leptospira canicola* causes leptospirosis.

Most bacteria reproduce most effectively at body temperature but are not always pathogenic. They may be:

- Commensals – live on or in the animal and do not normally cause disease
- Facultative pathogen – become pathogenic within immunosuppressed animals
- Obligate pathogens – will always cause disease.

In addition:

- Saprophytic bacteria will only replicate on dead tissue and are responsible for the decay of dead animals and plants

- Symbionts or mutualistic bacteria are organisms that both provide a benefit to the host and derive a benefit for themselves – this process is known as symbiosis or mutualism.

Viruses

Viruses are extremely small, simple structures incapable of replicating outside the body cell. They are obligate intracellular parasites and are sometimes classified as non-living. Viruses vary in their stability and, with the exception of poxvirus, parvovirus and rotavirus, they do not survive well outside the host. They are difficult to treat once established, as they are protected within the host cells and the chosen methods of treatment are prophylactics, vaccination and good nursing. Examples of viruses include canine adenovirus (CAV-1), which causes canine infectious hepatitis, and feline parvovirus, which causes feline infectious enteritis.

Chlamydias and rickettsias

This group have characteristics of both bacteria and viruses and cause such diseases as psittacosis in birds, chlamydiosis in cats and Q fever in a range of mammals, including humans.

Parasites

Parasites are defined as eukaryotic organisms that live off another organism to the advantage of the parasite (see Ch. 27). They may be:

- **Ectoparasites** – living on the outside of the body. They may cause discomfort and sometimes they act as vectors of disease, e.g. *Ctenocephalides* spp. and *Trichodectes canis* transmit the tapeworm *Dipylidium caninum*; *Ctenocephalides felis* transmits *Haemobartonella*, the causal agent of feline infectious anaemia; ticks carry *Borrelia burgdorferi*, the bacteria which causes Lyme disease
- **Endoparasites** – living inside the body. Any detrimental effects on the animal's health will depend on the species. Some may also be zoonotic, i.e. they can be transmitted from the animal to humans; for example, *Toxocara canis*, the roundworm of the dog, may cause visceral larva migrans and *Echinococcus granulosis*, a dog tapeworm, causes hydatidosis in humans.

Protozoa

Protozoa are single-celled organisms causing varying levels of disease within animals depending on the species. Some may also be zoonotic, e.g. *Toxoplasma gondii*, found in cats, may cause cysts within body tissues and abortion and birth defects in humans. Certain species of *Coccidia* live within the intestines of rabbits and poultry but can become pathogenic in intensively managed animals, causing coccidiosis, which may be fatal.

Fungi

Most fungi are non-pathogenic but some are able to invade healthy tissues and cause disease. They can be divided into yeasts, e.g. *Malassezia pachydermatis*, a common cause of skin

---

> **Box 19.1** Useful definitions
>
> - **Infectious disease** – a disease caused by microorganisms that can be spread between individuals.
> - **Non-infectious disease** – a disease that is not caused by microorganisms but is usually due to a disturbance in the normal metabolism of the animal, e.g. diabetes mellitus, neoplasia, poisoning.
> - **Contagious disease** – a disease that is able to spread from one animal to another via direct or indirect contact.
> - **Direct contact** – physical contact between animals. Skin surfaces of animals will come together during licking, grooming, sleeping, fighting and, in rare circumstances, coitus. Microorganisms transmitted via this route need to live in or on an animal to survive. Pathogens spread in this way are frequently fragile and easily destroyed.
> - **Indirect contact** – no physical contact between animals. Transmission occurs when the animal contaminates the environment with body fluids, e.g. urine or faeces. The microorganism is transported on fomites or by vectors and can survive in the environment for varying periods depending on the species.
> - **Fomite** – a contaminated, inanimate (non-living) object, e.g. feeding bowls or litter trays.
> - **Vector** – an animate object that carries the microorganisms. These can be further grouped into:
>   - **Biological vector** – acts as intermediate host in the lifecycle of some microorganisms or parasites. Some of the organism's development occurs within the intermediate host before it is eaten by the final/definitive host. For example, the cat flea is the vector for the larval form of the dog and cat tapeworm *Dipylidium caninum*.
>   - **Non-biological vector/mechanical vector** – these play no role in development of the microorganism or parasite and simply transfer the disease from one animal to another. There are two types:
>   - **Transport host** – will carry the infection to another animal without becoming affected by it at all. They maintain the viability of the microorganism; for example, the cat flea transports the virus that causes feline panleukopenia and the rickettsia *Haemobartonella felis*, which causes feline infectious anaemia.
>   - **Paratenic host** – must be eaten by the final host to continue the lifecycle and spread the infection. The microorganism lives within the paratenic host's tissue but there is no further development; for example, cats eating raw lamb from individuals infected with the protozoon *Toxoplasma gondii* will then become infected.

---

disease in dogs, and dermatophytes, e.g. *Microsporum canis*, which is a cause of ringworm in many species.

Routes of transmission

In order to cause disease a pathogen must leave the host animal, be transmitted between the host and the susceptible animal and then enter the susceptible animal.

Pathogens are able to leave the host through any of the body orifices (Fig. 19.1) and within any of the body secretions – the choice depends on the species of pathogen (Table 19.1).

When the pathogen has left the body it must be transmitted to a susceptible animal. This may be almost instant, e.g.

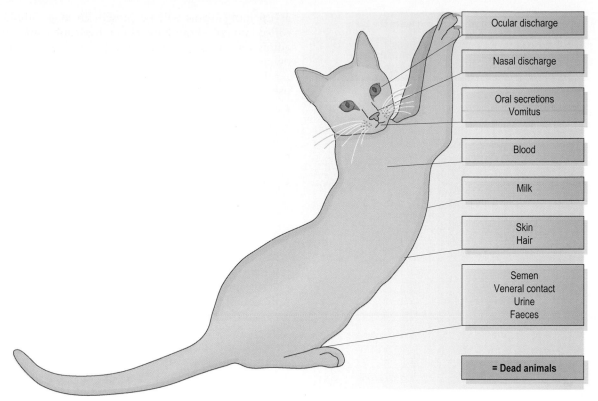

Ocular discharge

Nasal discharge

Oral secretions
Vomitus

Blood

Milk

Skin
Hair

Semen
Veneral contact
Urine
Faeces

= Dead animals

Fig. 19.1 Methods by which pathogens leave the infected animal

droplets transmitted by sneezing or coughing, or may take many weeks or even years, e.g. eggs of *Toxocara canis* may survive in grass for up to 2 years ready to be ingested by a susceptible dog. The following list shows the methods of transmission used by different groups of pathogens.

- **Direct contact** – the host animal touches the susceptible animal, e.g. during grooming, licking, etc., and the pathogen is transferred from one to the other. Commonly occurs in the transmission of ectoparasites
- **Indirect contact** – the host and the susceptible animal may be some distance apart and the pathogen requires a means of transport and a means of survival – often protection from drying out. The following are examples of indirect contact:

1. **Aerosol droplets** – pathogens that cause respiratory diseases survive within the water droplets coughed or sneezed into the environment. The contaminated atmospheric air is inhaled and the pathogen will reach the nasal chambers and the pharynx
2. **Topical (inoculation)** – via bites or scratches. The skin is penetrated, allowing the pathogen to enter the body systems, e.g. *Staphylococcus* spp.; the hookworm *Uncinaria stenocephala* is able to burrow through the footpads of the dog; feline leukaemia virus is spread by bites and scratches during cat fights
3. **Faeces** – contains many pathogenic organisms, e.g. worm eggs and viruses such as parvovirus
4. **Vomit** – may carry parvovirus, salmonella or distemper virus
5. **Saliva** – may carry rhabdovirus, causing rabies, or feline leukaemia virus

6. **Blood** – may transmit feline immunodeficiency virus or *Haemobartonella felis*
7. **Oral** – a common route for the ingestion of pathogens that affect the digestive tract, e.g. roundworms, *Toxoplasma gondii*, *Salmonella* spp., *Cryptosporidium* spp.
8. **Venereal** – occurs during coitus, e.g. *Brucella canis* and transmissible venereal tumours.

Carriers

Some diseases may be transmitted by carriers. These are animals that secrete the pathogen at intervals and are a risk to contact animals. They may be classed as:

- **Convalescent carriers**, i.e. animals that have recovered from the disease, e.g. cat flu, canine infectious hepatitis, but secrete the pathogen, particularly when they are stressed
- **Healthy carriers**, i.e. animals that have apparently never had the disease and may be immune to it. Healthy carriers, e.g. of ringworm, are a particular risk, as there is no history of having had the disease.

Once the pathogen has entered the susceptible animal it must establish itself and replicate within the tissues. The most common site is in the lymph nodes local to the point of entry. When sufficient numbers of pathogens have been produced they are carried around the body by the blood or the lymph to their favoured site of action and symptoms will develop. The time lag between the entry of the pathogen into the body and the development of symptoms is known as the **incubation period**. The length of the incubation period varies according to the type of infection.

Table 19.1 Methods by which pathogens can leave the body

Part of the body	Secretion	Examples of disease
Eyes	Ocular discharge	Cat flu
		Chlamydia
		Myxomatosis
Nose	Serous nasal discharge	Cat flu
		Kennel cough
		Distemper
Mouth	Oral discharge: saliva Vomit	Rabies
		Feline leukaemia virus
		Feline immunodeficiency virus
		Salmonella
Ear	Wax	*Otodectes cynotis*
Skin	Ectoparasites	*Ctenocephalides felis*
		Linognathus setosus
		Trichodectes canis
Mammary glands	Milk	*Toxocara canis*
		Feline leukaemia virus
Circulatory system	Blood	*Haemobartonella felis*
Gastrointestinal tract	Faeces	*Toxocara* spp.
		Toxoplasma gondii
		Salmonella spp
		Campylobacter spp.
Urinary	Urine	*Leptospira canicola*
		Canine infectious hepatitis
Reproductive	Vaginal discharge	*Brucella canis*

Disease control

The transmission of microorganisms can be minimized with the use of prophylactics, good nursing care and client education. The following are examples used within veterinary practice:

Treatment

Rapid diagnosis followed by rapid effective treatment will prevent the spread of infectious disease to susceptible animals. In some cases euthanasia may be used as a means of prevention of spread.

Hygiene

Hygiene, involving cleaning, disinfection, sterilization and personnel hygiene, is vital if the spread of disease is to be prevented within a veterinary practice. All urine, faeces, blood and discharges should be removed and incinerated, as microorganisms will be present in large numbers. The soiled animal should be clipped, cleaned and dried on admission, prior to surgery and before it is returned to its owner.

All surgical equipment must be sterilized between each use:

- Cleaning – reduces the number of pathogens and physically removes them by the use of water and detergents
- Disinfection – kills all pathogens with the exception of bacterial spores by the use of disinfectants
- Sterilization – kills all pathogens and bacterial spores by the use of heat, ethylene oxide gas or radiation.

Disinfectants

When controlling microorganisms within the hospital environment it is essential to clean and disinfect correctly to prevent the transmission of pathogens between animals. **Antiseptics** are disinfectants designed for use on skin and are used for scrubbing up prior to surgery and for preparation of the surgical site. Removal of organic matter, e.g. faeces, blood, dust and hair, will ensure that disinfectant agents are not inactivated before they reach the microorganisms. Most disinfectants are used at a lower strength for routine use and higher concentrations for specific disease-causing conditions, but it is important to read the manufacturer's instructions.

Each disinfectant will have different properties and may be classified as either bactericidal, i.e. it will destroy the microorganisms, or as bacteriostatic, i.e. it will inhibit their replication for a period of time.

As a guide:

- Most disinfectants are effective against Gram-positive bacteria, as they are easily destroyed
- Gram-negative bacteria are more resistant, as are bacterial spores. The aldehyde and halogen groups are most effective against them
- Halogens (hypochlorites) are used for viral infections
- Fungi should be eradicated with a designated fungicide to ensure elimination of fungal spores
- Pine oil disinfectants have no activity against the major microorganisms and should never be used, especially if fungi are present.

Isolation and quarantine

Animals suspected of having an infectious disease should be isolated to prevent kennel mates acquiring the disease as a nosocomial infection, i.e. an infection acquired during hospitalization.

Two techniques are used to nurse the infectious patient:

- **Isolation** – segregation of infected patients to reduce transmission of disease to susceptible animals
- **Quarantine** – isolation of animals that may be incubating an infectious disease. This is sometimes compulsory, as in quarantine for rabies. Animals recently acquired or new to an establishment should also be quarantined, and the period of time will be dependent on species and the incubation period of the suspected disease.

An isolation area should be set up within the practice. If possible, this should have a separate entry door from the outside and services such as water, waste disposal and ventilation should be separate from those of the main practice. In reality, the isolation area is often a cage within an area not used by other animals. Basic nursing protocols should be applied to all patients housed in the isolation area and strict clothing changes and hygiene regimes should be rigorously followed (see Ch. 15).

Barrier nursing

This is a set of special nursing requirements that mean that an effective 'barrier' is created preventing the transmission of a pathogen by a fomite, e.g. clothing or cleaning equipment:

- Keep the animal in strict isolation
- Use the same kennel, if possible, for the duration of the stay
- Clean and treat the patient after all others
- Keep separate equipment, e.g. cleaning and feeding equipment, for each patient
- Disinfect all animal areas after use
- Use disposable gloves, apron and foot baths if necessary.

Parasiticides

Routine eradication of parasites will prevent their transmission to other animals, reduce the effects, such as anaemia, emaciation and failure to thrive, and improve the animal's immune system. It will also minimize the chances of the owner developing a parasitic zoonotic infection, e.g. visceral larva migrans.

Vaccination

Vaccines are given to stimulate antibody production, so preventing a specific disease. Hyperimmune serum contains ready-made antibodies and can be given to the animal where there is a high and immediate risk of contracting a disease. The level of immunity must be kept up by the use of regular booster vaccinations.

Balanced diet

An animal receiving the correct nutrients will develop a healthy immune response, which will enable the body to fight any disease with which it comes into contact.

Client education

Clients must be educated as to what is required when looking after an animal. This should include vaccination, parasite control and basic hygiene, all of which will help in the control of disease.

Zoonoses

A zoonosis is the term used to describe any disease transferable from animal to human, its opposite being an anthroponosis, which is a disease transferable from human to animal, e.g. gorillas may be infected by human measles. An increasing number of households now own a pet, so animal owners and veterinary personnel are at increased risk of contracting a zoonotic disease. Unsuspecting owners may show moderate to severe illness, which may, on occasion, be fatal. Some examples of zoonotic diseases are shown in Table 19.2. They include:

- Leptospirosis – Weil's disease
- *Cheyletiella* spp. – mange
- *Sarcoptes scabiei* – scabies/mange
- Ringworm
- *Toxocara canis* – roundworm
- Toxoplasmosis
- Salmonellosis
- *Chlamydia psittaci* – psittacosis.

The main defence against zoonoses are education and basic but rigorous hygiene routines. The veterinary practice must devise its own rules and ensure that all staff are aware of them. Care must be taken when handling infected animals and their secretions. General guidelines to protect against contracting a zoonotic disease include:

- Owner education – make sure that they are aware that such diseases exist
- Wear protective aprons, gloves and, in some cases, eye protection when dealing with infected patients
- All faecal and urinary samples for testing should be treated with care and disposed of correctly without contaminating personnel
- Always wash hands with chlorhexidine or povidone-iodine after handling animals or their products
- Change infected clothing immediately after dealing with the animals
- Keep kennel runs, gardens and children's sandpits free from faeces.

Infectious diseases

The dog

Canine parvovirus

Aetiology: Canine parvovirus 2 (CAV-2).
Very infectious disease. Virus mutated from feline parvovirus or panleukopenia in the 1970s. The virus is shed in the faeces during the incubation period and is very stable, surviving within the environment for over 6 months. Barrier nursing and correct use of virucidal disinfectants are essential in controlling nosocomial infections within the hospital. The most critical stage of the disease for the animal is the first 3–4 days.
Transmission: via direct or indirect contact with faeces.
Incubation period: 4–7 days
Pathogenesis: Virus can only replicate in rapidly dividing cells such as lymph nodes, bone marrow, epithelial linings of lung, liver and intestines, which makes this disease very common in young, developing puppies. Rottweilers, German shepherd dogs and dobermans have a greater susceptibility to this disease.
Clinical signs: Depression, vomiting, anorexia. Vomiting follows 48 hours after the onset of profuse, watery, haemorrhagic diarrhoea. Loss of body fluids leads to

Table 19.2 Zoonotic diseases

Zoonosis	Causal agent	Body system affected	Clinical symptoms	Incidence/ prevalence	Transmitted within	Symptoms found in humans
Campylobacter	*Campylobacter jejuni*	Gastrointestinal (GI) tract	Tenesmus diarrhoea: • Mucoid • Watery • Bloody • Bile streaks Occasional fever Anorexia Intermittent vomiting	Dogs Higher in puppies Less commonly affects adult cats but kittens up to 6 months of age	Faeces Poorly sanitized kennels Asymptomatic carriers	Fever Abdominal pain Diarrhoea
Cat scratch fever	*Pasteurella*	n/a	(none, as *Pasteurella* is a commensal bacterium – unless immunosuppressed)	Cats	Bites Scratches	Inflammation at scratch/bite wound Cellulitis Occasional fever Regional lymphadenopathy
Cheyletiellosis	*Cheyletiella* spp.	Skin/exocrine	Pruritus Scaling	Animals within shelters Boarding and grooming establishments	Hair and dander	Pruritus Urticarial weals on trunk and arms
Chlamydiosis	*Chlamydia psittaci*	Ophthalmic Respiratory GI tract Reproductive tract	Unilateral conjunctivitis leading to bilateral Nasal discharge	Adult cats Kittens between 2 and 6 months of age Birds	Ocular discharge	Mild conjunctivitis
Cryptosporidiosis	*Cryptosporidium* spp.	GI tract	Diarrhoea	Dogs (esp. > 6 months of age) Cats	Faeces	Vomiting Diarrhoea Headache Abdominal pain
Hydatidosis	*Echinococcus* spp.	GI tract	Malnutrition	Dogs fed on raw meat	Faeces	Abdominal pain Jaundice Chest pain Cough
Leptospirosis	*Leptospira canicola* *Leptospira hardjo*	Primarily: • Renal • Hepatobiliary Can also affect: • Nervous • Respiratory • Cardiovascular • Reproductive • Ophthalmic	Pyrexia Jaundice Vomiting Diarrhoea	Unvaccinated dogs Rarely found in cats	Urine Contaminated bedding	Fever Vomiting Headache Muscle ache Jaundice Nephritis
Rabies	Rhabdovirus	Nervous system Salivary glands	Change in attitude and behaviour depending on dumb or furious Mandibular and laryngeal paralysis Dropped jaw Hypersalivation	Dogs Bats Foxes	Saliva	Fever Anxiety Headaches Dysphagia Hydrophobia Convulsions Death
Ringworm	*Microsporum canis*	Skin/exocrine	Alopecia Crusty lesions Erythema Hyperpigmentation Pruritus	Dogs Cats – especially long-haired breeds	Skin and dander	Dermatitis Alopecia Erythema Ring-shaped crusty lesions

Table 19.2 Continued

Zoonosis	Causal agent	Body system affected	Clinical symptoms	Incidence/ prevalence	Transmitted within	Symptoms found in humans
Roundworm	*Toxocara canis*	GI tract	Abdominal distension Cachexia Coughing Diarrhoea	Dogs, especially puppies	Faeces containing L2 larvae	Can cause blindness (temporary or permanent) in young children
Salmonellosis	Gram-negative bacteria	GI tract	Vomiting and diarrhoea Systemic disruption Organ infarction Anorexia Malaise	Dogs – young, pregnant Cats normally have a high resistance but stressed, hospitalized cats	Faeces Densely populated areas Pig ear treats Exposure to carrier animals Exposure to raw meat	Watery diarrhoea Dehydration Abdominal pain Fever
Sarcoptic mange	*Sarcoptes scabiei*	Skin/exocrine	Pruritus Scaly lesions Alopecia	Dogs	Skin lesions	Intense pruritus Red lesions at site of contamination or between fingers, under breasts or in groin region
Toxoplasmosis	*Toxoplasma gondii*	Reproductive	Normally asymptomatic	Cats	Faeces Infected hair	Fever Headache Lymph-adenopathy Cough, although symptoms often ignored **Pregnant women:** Fetal changes, abortion

dehydration, which is the most common cause of death in these patients.

Diagnosis: History, clinical signs leading to enzyme-linked immunosorbent assay (ELISA) testing for CAV-2 antigen during early stages of infection, as this is when the virus will be shed.

Treatment: Isolation and barrier nursing. Rehydration and maintenance fluids to replace the fluid deficit. Antibiotics to treat secondary infections.

Prevention: Vaccination of dam before mating and puppy from 8 weeks of age using a live vaccine. In high-risk areas the dam can be given a killed vaccine during gestation and puppies can receive antiserum or start early vaccination at 6 weeks of age, followed by the usual primary vaccine course. Puppies who survive the disease will develop very good immunity, which may last a number of years.

Canine distemper

Aetiology: Canine distemper virus – a morbillivirus related to rinderpest and measles.

A multisystemic viral disease that can become chronic, affecting the dog several years after infection. The virus is labile and is easily destroyed by sunlight, heating and drying. Poor hygiene is normally to blame for disease outbreak.

Transmission: Via aerosol droplets and ingestion.

Incubation period: 7–21 days.

Pathogenesis: The virus replicates in the tonsils and lymph nodes, causing a viraemia. The next stage depends on the animal's immune response. In animals with poor immunity, further replication occurs within the epithelial cells of the respiratory and gastrointestinal cells. The skin can also become affected, leading to the 'hard pad' syndrome. In animals with more established immunity, mild signs may be observed but in each the virus will affect the nervous system.

Clinical signs: Pyrexia, nasal discharge, coughing, vomiting, diarrhoea, chorea (twitching) and hyperkeratosis of the pads. Fifty per cent of patients will be subclinical cases. Chronic signs include encephalitis and rheumatoid arthritis.

Diagnosis: Blood samples show red and white blood cell inclusions and lymphopaenia. Lymph nodes will harbour the virus and are normally viewed during post-mortem examination.

Treatment: Good nursing care and symptomatic treatment – fluid therapy, antibiotics, antiemetics, anticonvulsants, antitussives. Euthanasia may be considered in some cases.
Prevention: Vaccination.

Canine leptospirosis

Aetiology: Bacteria – *Leptospira canicola* (affects the kidney) and *Leptospira icterohaemorrhagiae* (affects the liver).
A zoonotic bacterial disease contracted from contaminated water, especially stagnant woodland pools where rats drink and bathe.
Transmission: Direct or indirect contact with contaminated water or urine. Can also be spread via transplacental and venereal infection.
Incubation period: Up to 7 days.
Pathogenesis: Bacteria penetrate broken skin and mucous membranes and replicate in the liver and kidney, causing hepatitis, acute renal failure and intravascular coagulation. *Leptospira* can be excreted in the animal's urine for months or years after recovery.
Clinical signs: Pyrexia, vomiting, shock, interstitial nephritis and hepatitis. Signs dependent on animal's age, immunity and environmental factors.
Diagnosis: Blood samples show elevated urea and creatinine and elevated liver enzymes alanine aminotransferase (ALT) and alkaline phosphatase (ALKP).
Treatment: Rehydration fluids, to include plasma or blood to correct the intravascular coagulation. Antibiotics, antiemetics and dietary management to assist with liver and kidney function.
Prevention: Vaccination, especially in high-risk animals – working or outdoor dogs. Good hygiene procedures to prevent spread and development of a zoonosis.

Infectious canine hepatitis

Aetiology: Canine adenovirus (CAV-1).
Also known as Rubarth's disease.
Transmission: Direct or indirect contact with faeces, urine, saliva and fomites.
Incubation period: 5–9 days.
Pathogenesis: Virus enters the mouth and replicates in the tonsils and lymph nodes via the thoracic duct. Viraemia results and further replication occurs within the vascular endothelium, causing pericardial effusions, hepatitis and vasculitis.
Clinical signs: Anorexia, pyrexia, vomiting, diarrhoea, hepatomegaly, conjunctivitis, photophobia, petechiae and jaundice. Death can occur within 24 hours.
Diagnosis: Blood samples show increased liver enzymes ALKP and ALT and bile salts.
Treatment: Supportive therapies – fluids, antibiotics for secondary infections, antiemetics, good nursing care.
Prevention: Vaccination. Live CAV-2 vaccine is used to protect against CAV-1 and CAV-2. Live CAV-1 will cause mild symptoms and 'blue eye'.

Kennel cough

Aetiology: Numerous pathogens can be responsible, including *Bordetella bronchiseptica*, parainfluenza (pi) virus 2, CAV-2, reovirus, herpes virus and secondary bacterial infections.

Also known as canine infectious tracheobronchitis or canine contagious respiratory disease (CCRD).
Transmission: Aerosol droplets, via direct or indirect contact. This is a common disease found where several animals share the same air space, e.g. boarding kennels and hunt kennels.
Incubation period: 5–7 days.
Pathogenesis: Organisms replicate within the upper respiratory tract (parainfluenza virus is unable to replicate in macrophages). Secondary infection attacks the damaged tracheal epithelium. Ciliostasis (paralysis of the cilia on the mucous membranes) can occur, due to toxins that are produced in response to a *Bordetella* infection.
Clinical signs: Dry, hacking cough, with or without a terminal retch, which is precipitated by exercise, excitement or palpation of the trachea. Animals are not normally pyrexic unless a secondary infection is evident. A mucopurulent nasal and ocular discharge and bronchopneumonia can result from serious infection.
Diagnosis: Clinical signs and history. Further tests are of limited value.
Treatment: Antibiotics, antitussives, restricted exercise, rest. Most animals recover well and quickly.
Prevention: Vaccination – parenteral and intranasal.

Lyme disease

Aetiology: *Borrelia burgdorferi* – a bacterium.
Transmission: Via deer tick (*Ixodes scapularis*). This is now the most common arthropod-borne illness in man in the USA and is becoming more common in the UK, particularly in areas where ticks are found in large numbers, e.g Exmoor, Dartmoor and parts of Scotland. May affect dogs walking in these areas.
Incubation period: Not known, as the bacteria may lie dormant for several months.
Clinical signs: This is a multisystem inflammatory disease that affects the skin and then spreads to the joints, nervous system and other organs in the later stages. Symptoms include lameness, pyrexia, lethargy, lymphadenopathy, cardiac arrhythmias.
Diagnosis: Blood tests.
Treatment: Removal of any ticks. Antibiotics and supportive therapies.
Prevention: Regular treatment with a recognized ectoparasiticide, especially before visiting wooded areas that the tick may inhabit. Transmission of *B. burgdorferi* does not begin until the tick has been attached for 36–48 hours, so after walking the dog it should be checked for the presence of ticks, which should be removed immediately.

The dog and cat

Rabies

Aetiology: Rhabdovirus belonging to the genus Lyssavirus. This notifiable zoonotic disease affecting all warm-blooded animals has been eradicated in the UK because of our strict quarantine regulations.
Transmission: Saliva within bite wounds.
Incubation period: Variable between 1 and 6 months – depends on the area bitten and its proximity to the central nervous system, the immune status of the animal and the strain of the virus.

Pathogenesis: Replication of virus in the injured muscle tissue before it enters the peripheral nervous system and central nervous system. Antibodies can attack the virus while in the muscle tissue but once the virus has entered the nervous system nothing can be done.

Clinical signs: There are two forms – furious and dumb. Both follow a prodromal period in which general character changes are seen within the animal before specific clinical signs develop. Some cases may be atypical:

- Furious form: Hyperexcitability, interspersed with periods of calm, pica, biting and 'snapping' – often at imaginary objects, ataxia, progressive facial paralysis, drooling, dysphagia, frothing of saliva. Death normally occurs after convulsions. This form is most likely to be seen in carnivores such as the dog and cat.
- Dumb form: Animals are timid, often affectionate, and have a generalized paresis leading to paralysis and ataxia. Death normally results from paralysis of the respiratory muscles. This form is most likely to be seen in herbivores such as the cow.

Diagnosis: Clinical history. Histopathological examination of the brain following death demonstrating the presence of Negri bodies, which are seen in 75% of cases.

Treatment: None. Supportive therapies are not used because of the zoonotic potential and disease prognosis. DEFRA and the police must be contacted by the veterinary surgeon as soon as a case of rabies is suspected. The animal must be kept in the practice until the DVO arrives; then it will be destroyed and taken away for tests.

Prevention: Animals in the UK are not routinely vaccinated against rabies unless they are to travel abroad under the Passports for Pets Scheme (PETS).

Salmonellosis

Aetiology: Salmonella typhimurium – a bacterium.
This zoonotic disease is caused by a facultative bacteria living within the intestines of the animal.

Transmission: Raw, uncooked meat. Immunosuppressed animals may precipitate their own illness.

Incubation period: Impossible to specify, as the bacteria have permanent residency within the gut.

Clinical signs: Depending on the severity – acute or chronic gastroenteritis, drooling saliva, pyrexia, abdominal pain, slight icterus, breeding problems.

Diagnosis: Faecal or saliva sampling to isolate high numbers of the microorganism.

Treatment: Isolate and barrier-nurse. Rehydration and maintenance fluids. Rest and allow the animal to recover to encourage its own immunity to develop. Antibiotics are not normally used as they can destroy healthy bacteria living within the gut.

Prevention: Reduce the use of unnecessary antibiotics as this may lead to the development of antibiotic resistance. Ensure that all food offered to animals is fresh and cooked.

The cat

Feline upper respiratory tract disease (FURTD)

Aetiology: Feline calicivirus (FCV) and feline herpes virus (FHV).

Also referred to as cat flu or feline influenza. Once recovered, cats can become carriers and reinfect themselves and other cats, especially at times of stress.

Transmission: Aerosol droplets via the oral, nasal and conjunctival route. Can be direct or indirect contact.

Incubation period: 2–12 days.

Pathogenesis: The virus will replicate in the tissues of entry into the body, e.g. mouth and nares (Fig. 19.1).

Clinical signs: These are slightly different depending on the causal virus:

- FCV – sneezing, oral ulceration, chronic stomatitis, pyrexia and occasional intermittent lameness
- FHV – symptoms are more severe – sneezing, pyrexia, conjunctivitis, keratitis, corneal ulceration, anorexia, depression.

Secondary infections can cause damage to intranasal structures and chronic illness.

Treatment: Antibiotics, fluid therapy and good nursing to include ensuring that the animal's airways are patent. Encourage the animal to eat, using smelly foods such as sardines or by placement of a naso-oesophageal tube if anorexic. It is important to remember that cats will not eat if they cannot smell the food.

NB. Recovered cases can become carriers and therefore a source of infection. Overt signs of sneezing may begin to show as a result of stress such as being put into boarding kennels or being taken into the veterinary surgery for procedures such as castration or spaying.

Prevention: Annual vaccination. Owners should ensure that the boarding cattery they use has strict procedures for vaccination and isolation. Sneezing cats should be isolated immediately or discharged if there is no secondary infection evident.

Chlamydiosis

Aetiology: Chlamydia psittaci.
Also called feline pneumonitis. This disease is potentially zoonotic and the persistent conjunctivitis often gets overlooked. It often occurs as part of FURTD.

Transmission: Direct contact with ocular discharges.

Incubation period: 3–10 days.

Pathogenesis: The virus replicates within the point of entry, the eyes and mouth (Fig. 19.1).

Clinical signs: Unilateral conjunctivitis, which can become bilateral. Mild rhinitis.

Diagnosis: Conjunctival scrapes/swabs.

Treatment: Topical and systemic antibiotics – to be given over a period of weeks. All in-contact cats should be treated to control further outbreaks. *Chlamydia* is sensitive to disinfectants, so kennels must be thoroughly cleaned.

Prevention: Vaccination of animals in contact with *Chlamydia* carriers.

Feline infectious peritonitis (FIP)

Aetiology: Feline coronavirus (FeCoV).
This disease predominantly affects young cats, causing the body cavities to fill up with effusions.

Transmission: Intrauterine.

Incubation period: Variable.
Pathogenesis: Virus replicates within the lymph nodes of the gut, then transfers to endothelial layers of the body, to include pleura, peritoneum, meninges and the kidneys, eyes and blood vessels.
Clinical signs: There are two forms:
- Effusive (wet) – this is the acute form of the disease: signs include ascites, pleural effusions, dyspnoea, pyrexia, weight loss, jaundice
- Non-effusive (dry) – the more chronic form of the disease: weight loss, neurological signs, ocular lesions, hepatomegaly.

Diagnosis: Serology, haematology and biochemistry, analysis of ascitic/pleural fluid.
Treatment: None, although steroids may be used in the short term. Symptomatic nursing by the owner is beneficial.
Prevention: Isolate breeding queens before kittening.

Feline infectious anaemia (FIA)

Aetiology: *Haemobartonella felis*, now known as *Mycoplasma haemofelis* – a chlamydia.
Transmission: *Ctenocephalides felis*, the cat flea, ingests blood as it bites. It then passes on the organism at its next bite.
Incubation period: Unknown.
Pathogenesis: Severe anaemia can occur in immunosuppressed or debilitated animals. Parasitized red blood cells are phagocytosed by macrophages within the spleen.
Clinical signs: Sudden onset of weakness, lethargy and anorexia. Pale mucous membranes with associated tachycardia, tachypnoea and splenomegaly.
Diagnosis: Examination of a blood smear – blood to be collected within an EDTA coagulant as this will free the parasite from the red blood cells.
Treatment: Antibiotics and steroids.
Prevention: Unknown.

Feline leukaemia virus (FeLV)

Aetiology: A retrovirus.
Most common in younger cats in multicat households, where direct contact occurs during social grooming.
Transmission: Vertically – via the placenta to the kittens; horizontally – in milk or saliva via bites and scratches.
Incubation period: Unknown.
Pathogenesis: Virus replicates in the oropharynx and related lymph tissues, leading to viraemia. Some animals may recover but in others the virus will further replicate in the lymph nodes and bone marrow. Some cats have a latent infection; others will be persistently viraemic and continue to shed the virus in their saliva.
Clinical signs: Many remain asymptomatic for years before showing immunosuppressive signs and related disease conditions. Reproductive problems such as resorption, abortion or stillbirth can be apparent before diagnosis.
Diagnosis: ELISA tests detect the p27 protein.
Treatment: There is no known cure. As infected cats shed the virus they are a continual threat to others and euthanasia may be the best option.
Prevention: Vaccination is available.

Feline immunodeficiency virus (FIV)

Aetiology: A retrovirus.
This disease is common in free-roaming, older male cats, with the highest incidence at the age of 5–9 years.
Transmission: Via bite wounds.
Incubation period: A few weeks to a few months.
Pathogenesis: The virus replicates at the site of the bite wound, causing viraemia which cannot be eliminated from the body. A permanent infection remains, leading to a further depletion of T lymphocytes and resultant immunodeficiency.
Clinical signs:
- Primary infection – pyrexia, neurological signs, weight loss, lymphadenopathy, lymphopenia, increased risk of neoplasia
- Secondary infection – chronic stomatitis, upper respiratory tract infections, skin changes, diarrhoea.

Diagnosis: ELISA tests can detect the viral antibodies, although early infections may not be very reliable.
Treatment: Nothing is effective, although low-dose steroids may be beneficial for a short time.
Prevention: Control breeding of infective cats by neutering. Keeping cats housed indoors will significantly reduce the risk. There is no vaccine available.

Toxoplasmosis

Aetiology: *Toxoplasma gondii* – a protozoon.
Transmission: After 3 days infected cat faeces containing sporulated oocysts, which are ingested by a variety of intermediate hosts, e.g. cattle, horses, sheep, mice and humans. Within the intermediate host the parasite settles mainly in the musculature and causes few if any symptoms. If cats are fed raw meat from an infected animal, the disease is transmitted (see Ch. 27).
Incubation period: 2–5 weeks.
Pathogenesis: The end host for *T. gondii* is the cat, where it is found within the small intestine.
Clinical signs: Normally asymptomatic, although mild cases of diarrhoea, lethargy, jaundice may show if cysts are present.
Diagnosis: Blood test to detect antibodies.
Treatment: Antibiotics.
Prevention: Cook meat before feeding, clean litter trays regularly before the faeces reach the infective stage. There is no vaccine available in the UK. This disease is zoonotic and pregnant women are at risk – infection may result in fetal deformities, although this is rare.

The rabbit

Respiratory disease

Aetiology: The most common bacterial cause is *Pasteurella multocida*; however, other organisms such as *Staphylococcus aureus*, *Enterobacter* spp. and *Pseudomonas aeruginosa* are not uncommon pathogens cultured from the respiratory tract. *Bordetella bronchiseptica* has also been isolated from some severe cases.
Often the only sign of respiratory disease is a small amount of discharge matted on the medial aspect of the forepaws where the rabbit has rubbed it nose with its

paws. Infection may progress rapidly and cause abscesses in the rabbit's chest, significantly compromising the lung capacity.

Transmission: Both direct and indirect contact. Rabbits develop little effective immunity following infection and many are asymptomatic carriers, which perpetuates the infection in the community.

Pathogenesis: After initial replication in the upper respiratory tract, the organisms may spread to associated structures such as the nasolacrimal ducts or the middle ear. The condition may end in septicaemia, bronchial congestion, tracheitis, splenomegaly and subcutaneous haemorrhages. Pneumonia is a secondary and complicating factor, which causes pleuritis, pyometra and pericardial petechiae.

Clinical signs: Upper respiratory tract infection is usually characterized by a serous exudate from the eyes and nose, which later becomes a mucopurulent discharge. Infection may manifest as any of the following: rhinitis (snuffles), pneumonia, otitis media, conjunctivitis, abscesses, genital infections or septicaemia.

Diagnosis: Culture a sample of discharge taken from at least 2 cm into the nasal cavity. The retracted swab can be used in an indirect fluorescent antibody test or plated into a culture medium. There is an ELISA test for detecting antibodies against *Pasteurella multocida*. When culturing abscesses, the capsule wall should be sampled rather than the contents, which are often sterile.

Treatment: Therapeutic agents must be carefully considered, as severe dysbiosis (loss of intestinal flora responsible for digestive function) and life-threatening enteritis can occur if the wrong antibiotic is chosen. Safe antibiotics include the fluoroquinolones, enrofloxacin, chloramphenicol or trimethoprim/sulfadiazine (Tribrissen) given orally once daily for 10–14 days. Penicillin G is an effective treatment given every 3–4 days to reduce the gastrointestinal effects. Pasteurellosis is considered an essentially incurable infection, so the aim is to alleviate clinical signs. In cases where there is improvement, therapy may be indicated for several months. A useful adjunct to systemic therapy is the use of nebulization. Antibiotics, a mucolytic agent, a bronchodilator and saline to moisten the turbinates can all be combined for this therapy. The nebulization is usually well tolerated through a mask over the rabbit's nose.

Prevention: Isolation of new rabbits until testing has been performed. Detection and culling of carriers. Rabbits with exudative rhinitis should be isolated from others.

Myxomatosis

Aetiology: A pox virus.

Myxomatosis is a fatal disease of all breeds of domestic rabbits and the European wild rabbit.

Transmission: Biting by mosquitoes, biting flies and fleas, and by direct contact.

Pathogenesis: The virus replicates and does its damage in the dermis, and lesions are seen in the mucous membranes as well as fibrotic nodule formation over the nose, ears and forefeet. There are few other characteristic lesions found at necropsy, although the spleen is occasionally enlarged and is almost always devoid of lymphocytes when examined histologically.

Clinical signs: Conjunctivitis develops, rapidly becomes more marked and is accompanied by a milky ocular discharge. The animal is listless and anorexic and the temperature reaches over 42 °C. In acute outbreaks some animals die within 48 hours while those that survive become progressively depressed and develop a rough coat. The eyelids, lips, ears and coat become oedematous and the vulva and scrotum swell. A purulent nasal discharge appears and breathing becomes laboured. Death occurs within 1–2 weeks of the appearance of clinical signs.

Diagnosis: The clinical appearance and the high mortality are of diagnostic significance. Large, eosinophilic, cytoplasmic inclusion bodies in the conjunctival epithelial cells are also helpful.

Treatment: Supportive therapy is often tried but, as the disease is invariably fatal, euthanasia is recommended.

Prevention: An attenuated vaccine is available. This should be given every 6 months using a 25 gauge needle. 10% of the vaccine should be deposited intradermally and the rest administered subcutaneously.

Viral haemorrhagic disease (VHD)

Aetiology: A parvovirus thought to be related to porcine parvovirus.

VHD is an acute, highly contagious infection first described in 1984.

Transmission: Aerosol transmission seems to be important, although all secretions and excretions are sources of infection. Mechanical transmission by fomites, rodents and other vermin, rabbit by-products and humans are all implicated in spread of the disease. Insects do not seem to be important vectors.

Pathogenesis: Replication is rapid, the incubation period being only 24–72 hours, and animals are found dead but in good condition. Gross lesions are subtle and generally restricted to congestion of the respiratory tract and liver. There is intense congestion of the lungs and trachea, which may be filled with froth. Haemorrhage in the thymus is common and there is congestion of the liver, spleen and kidneys. Histologically there is a massive, focal, coagulative hepatic necrosis.

Clinical signs: In protracted cases, dyspnoea, congestion of the eyelids, orthopnoea, abdominal respiration and tachycardia are seen. Before death there is violent cage activity, with rapid turns and flips that resemble convulsions or mania. Some cases show a blood-tinged nasal discharge.

Diagnosis: The peracute course of the disease is the most important feature. Symptoms of respiratory distress, high mortality and rapid spread are all significant. Fluorescent antibody techniques and immunostaining techniques can be used to identify the viral antigen. Liver, spleen and lung are the specimens of choice as they contain a high number of virus particles.

Treatment: The disease is always fatal and death often occurs before a diagnosis is made.

Prevention: There is a vaccine for use in countries where the disease is already widespread and eradication efforts are difficult to employ. Quarantine measures must be applied to rabbits entering from countries where VHD is present. There is documented evidence to suggest increased resistance among young rabbits, which may be due to passive immunity acquired from ingesting colostral antibodies against the apathogenic strain of lapine parvovirus.

Encephalitozoon cuniculi

Aetiology: A protozoan that affects many mammals including man.
Transmission: Organisms are shed in the urine and spread by ingestion, inhalation or to the developing fetuses by the transplacental route.
Pathogenesis: Levels of serum antibodies rise 21 days post infection and peak at 63 days. Protozoal spores are shed in urine for 9 weeks. The target organs are the liver, kidney, lung, heart and brain.
Clinical signs: The infection may be latent and cause no clinical signs; however, a range of signs may be seen including those of renal disease, ataxia, weight loss, polyuria and polydipsia, torticollis, convulsions and death. Cataract formation may also occur.
Diagnosis: Serological tests are reported back as titre levels.
Treatment: Rarely successful in neurological cases. Fenbendazole given at 20 mg/kg for 4 weeks is recommended.
Prevention: The use of fenbendazole for 9 days, 2–4 times a year is recommended as this disease is widespread and potentially zoonotic.

The horse

Equine herpesvirus

Aetiology: There are four equine herpes viruses (EHV). EHV-1 is associated with respiratory disease and is the most commonly diagnosed infectious cause of abortion. EHV-2 does not seem to cause disease. EHV-3 causes genital problems and EHV-4 is primarily a respiratory pathogen. These viruses are endemic worldwide. They result in abortion and respiratory disease, resulting in a significant financial loss to breeders, and are a major cause of loss of performance in racehorses.
Transmission: The virus is easily spread through respiratory tract secretions and morbidity may be 100%. Fetuses aborted are heavily contaminated with virus and serve as a source of infection to other in-contact horses.
Pathogenesis: After respiratory infection with virus, it travels transplacentally in pregnant mares by migrating leukocytes within which it can establish latent infection.
Clinical signs: Respiratory disease is characterized by a transient elevation of temperature to 40°C, inappetence, nasal discharge, pharyngitis, depression and sometimes limb oedema.
Diagnosis: Serological diagnosis can be made on the basis of a rising antibody titre (i.e. a fourfold rise in antibody levels over a 2-week period). Diagnosis of abortion is usually made on post-mortem examination of the fetus and on virus isolation.
Treatment: Symptomatic treatment, including antibiotics to prevent secondary bacterial infection. Minimizing stress is also important.

Prevention: Both killed and live attenuated EHV-1 vaccines are available. There is also a vaccine containing inactivated EHV-4.

Equine influenza

Aetiology: Viruses of the orthomyxovirus group. They are subject to constant change, known as antigenic drift.
Transmission: Droplet infection and inhalation. The short incubation period of 1–5 days and the persistent coughing that releases large amounts of virus into the air contributes to the rapid spread of the disease.
Pathogenesis: The virus infects the ciliated respiratory epithelial cells, which lose their cilia and become oedematous. The impaired clearance mechanism results in susceptibility to secondary infection.
Clinical signs: Elevation in temperature to 41°C followed by a deep cough. Serous nasal discharge, which soon becomes purulent, inappetence and enlarged mandibular lymph nodes. Occasionally there is oedema of the legs and scrotum.
Diagnosis: Isolation of the virus from nasopharyngeal swabs or serological examination.
Treatment: One week of complete rest for every day of elevated temperature. Non-steroidal anti-inflammatories and antibiotics to prevent secondary infection.
Prevention: Inactivated vaccines. Safe live attenuated vaccines are difficult to manufacture as the virus is capable of rapid mutation.

Equine viral arteritis

Aetiology: A coronavirus-like viral agent that causes international concern because of its abortigenic potential.
Transmission: The virus is spread through respiratory and venereal routes and through indirect contact with fomites. Aborted fetuses are heavily contaminated with virus.
Pathogenesis: There is a predilection for the arterial walls, so the main lesions seen are necrotizing arteritis.
Clinical signs: Variable range and most infections are subclinical. Fever, depression, inappetence, limb oedema, stiffness in gait, inflammation of the conjunctiva (pink eye) and ocular and nasal discharges.
Diagnosis: Virus isolation and/or serology.
Treatment: Supportive therapy and rest. Most horses make a speedy and uneventful recovery.
Prevention: Restriction of movement of horses from infected premises and, where permissible, by vaccination with a modified live vaccine.

Tetanus

Aetiology: *Clostridium tetani* – a bacterium.
This is a disease which can affect many warm-blooded species including man.
Transmission: Abundant in equine faeces and occurs in the gut of other herbivores and in the soil. The organism is anaerobic and is only able to multiply in damaged tissue where necrosis and lowered oxygen tension combine.
Pathogenesis: A toxin is released by the organism within deep wounds, which enters the local motor and sensory nerves. Free toxin may enter the capillaries and lymphatic channels.

Clinical signs: Incubation period varies from 1 to 3 weeks. Inability to retract the nictitating membrane and spasms in the facial muscles. The ears are pricked; there is stiffness, trembling, difficulty in eating and chewing. Muscular responses become exaggerated. Sweating is profuse and the heart rate is elevated. The mortality rate is about 80%; death occurs within 1 week of the start of clinical signs.
Diagnosis: Based on clinical signs. The bacteria can be readily grown in the laboratory.
Treatment: Large doses of antitoxin prevent the toxin from damaging further nervous tissue. Prognosis is poor.
Prevention: Immunoprophylaxis is essential in horses as the risk of tetanus following injury is so great. Vaccination with tetanus toxoid, regular boosters and the use of antitoxin when a horse is wounded are all essential.

African horse sickness (AHS)

Aetiology: An orbivirus which causes a highly fatal disease, last seen in Europe in the late 1980s.
Transmission: Climate change has sparked significant concern in the UK about AHS as it is transmitted by the same insect species as the recently problematic Bluetongue virus in cattle and sheep. The biting insects responsible are midges (*Culicoides* spp.).
Clinical signs: Respiratory and circulatory damage, fever, loss of appetite; 70–90% mortality.
Diagnosis: Based on clinical signs and virus identification.
Treatment: None as infected animals should be culled.
Prevention: Almost no horses have antibodies against foreign diseases, because they have never been exposed to them. This results in a large, highly susceptible population and an ideal scenario for a major outbreak. The AHS outbreak in Spain and Portugal was eradicated by slaughtering infected animals, movement restrictions, vector (insect) control, and horse vaccination. No vaccine for AHS is currently licensed in the EU. Use of a modified live vaccine for AHS carries a risk of vaccine virus reversion to wild type (i.e. the virus used in the vaccine can potentially undergo changes that mean it could actually infect vectors, and subsequently susceptible Equidae). Thus at the present time, the vaccine will not be considered for use in the UK other than in an emergency situation.

Immunity

Also called functional or protective immunity, this describes security against a particular pathogen, which makes the animal non-susceptible to certain specific diseases. It involves the introduction of a foreign body, usually a protein or antigen, into the body and the body responds by enabling the lymphocytes (white blood cells) to produce specific antibodies or immunoglobulins (Fig. 19.2) to fight against that antigen. Antibodies are Y-shaped proteins with specific binding sites on the tips of the 'Y' which are formulated to attach to a specific antigen and by a variety of methods they then inactivate the antigen.

Lymphocytes are the key constituents of the immune system which can produce antibodies against millions of invading foreign agents. All microorganisms carry on their

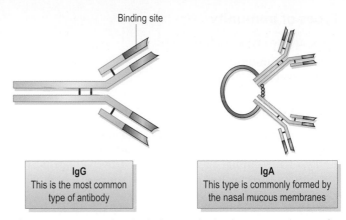

Fig. 19.2 Two types of antibody showing the binding sites on the tips of the Y-shaped proteins

surface or secrete large protein molecules (the antigens), which initiate the immune response. B lymphocytes, cells originating in the bone marrow, have proteins on their surface that bind to the antigens. Binding, in turn, stimulates the B lymphocytes to mature into plasma cells and secrete antibodies at the rate of 2000 per second from each cell, which are then released into the blood circulation in response to the enemy invasion. These mature cells develop a memory of that particular invader and, if the antigen re-enters the body later in the animal's life, it will be recognized by the memory cells, specific antibodies will be produced and the antigen will be attacked and eliminated before clinical symptoms are observed. This is humoral immunity. Immature lymphocytes within the bone marrow are not competent to carry out their immune functions.

In addition, cells of another type, T lymphocytes, may bind to the antigen surface and assist with the immune response. T lymphocytes, which mature within the thymus gland, have proteins on their surface called T-cell receptors, which bind directly to the antigen. They are responsible for cell-mediated immunity. There are three types of T cell involved: the cytotoxic or killer T cells, which bind to and destroy other cells displaying antigens on their surface; the helper T cells, which assist B cells to stimulate antibody production; and suppressor T cells, which reduce B-cell activity, reducing the possibility of an autoimmune response.

Lymphoid organs, e.g. spleen and thymus gland, are responsible for filtering bacteria and other foreign substances into the lymph nodes and for producing lymphocytes to combat infection. The thymus gland, in the neck, contains macrophages and immature and mature T lymphocytes. The spleen, found in the cranial abdomen, acts as a defensive filter for blood and as a site of B- and T-cell function. Other areas of lymphoid tissue, such as the palatine, pharyngeal and lingual tonsils, are permanent sites of lymphocyte aggregation, meeting and fighting microorganisms that enter via the oral or nasal route.

Lymph nodes are found at portal sites throughout the body and act as a defensive filter for lymph and a site of B- and T-cell function. The cortex of each node is densely packed with B lymphocytes, the medulla consists of lymphocytes and plasma cells and the paracortex (junction of cortex and medulla) contains T cells.

Types of immunity

There are two types of immunity:

- Innate immunity
- Acquired immunity.

Innate immunity

Innate immunity is hereditary and congenital, i.e. present at birth. There are many non-specific factors that affect the ability of the animal to resist invasion by pathogens. The response of these factors is always the same no matter what the injury or type of pathogen. They include the following:

- Genetic factors – may be due to the animal's species, breed or strain
- Physical barriers – external or mechanical defence of the body
- The inflammatory response – a non-specific response to tissue damage

Genetic factors

Animals are automatically immune to certain diseases that affect some species but not others. For example, myxomatosis affects rabbits but not dogs or cats, while foot and mouth disease only affects cloven-hoofed animals. This may even be extended to certain strains or families of animals which may carry a predisposition to a particular disease while other strains are not. The colour of an animal may also be a genetic factor in its protection. White animals, e.g. horses, and the white ears of cats may be more susceptible to damage by the ultraviolet rays of the sun which may result in some types of tumour.

The physical barrier

Often referred to as the external or primary defence mechanism. Providing they are not damaged and the animal is healthy, the following will create an external and internal barrier to prevent 'invasion' of the body:

- Skin – the largest organ in the body provides protection as the external covering of the body. The sebaceous glands produce sebum, which creates an acid surface pH that prevents replication of pathogenic bacteria while creating an environment for the survival of normal commensal bacteria. Sweat glands release sweat, which contains lysozymes with antibacterial properties.
- Mucous membranes – produce secretions, which wash away any foreign material. The conjunctiva keeps itself clear by producing tears, the respiratory tract produces mucus and saliva contains more lysozymes.
- Hairs – microscopic hairs or cilia are found as part of epithelial tissues in selected areas of the body, in particular within the respiratory system. They are found in association with mucus-producing glands and are collectively termed 'ciliated mucous epithelia' (see Ch. 4). Their function is to trap bacteria or foreign particles within the mucus and the hairs then sweep them away from susceptible organs.
- Secretions – in addition to the above, semen contains antibacterial proteins and zinc; the vagina maintains an acidic environment that inhibits bacterial growth;

and stomach acids provide an inhospitable environment for any pathogen that is swallowed.

The inflammatory response

When the body is damaged, e.g. by wounds or by infection, it responds by releasing histamine from mast cells within connective tissue. Histamine causes vasodilation of blood capillaries, increasing the blood supply to the area, and the area becomes reddened. It also changes the permeability of blood capillaries so that plasma proteins and tissue fluid leak out into the surrounding tissues, which then become swollen. Chemical mediators are transported by the tissue fluid to the site and attract white blood cells, in particular the polymorphonuclear leucocytes (PMNs), which are able to phagocytose dead and damaged tissue and bacteria to fight the infection. The inflammatory response is essential in the elimination of the initiating factor but it can lead to chronic problems if not controlled.

Acquired immunity

This form of immunity is acquired by the animal continuously throughout its life. It is also referred to as specific immunity, as it has a definite role to play in combating specific infectious diseases. Acquired immunity involves the development of specific antibodies in response to attack by specific antigens. For example, canine parvovirus antibodies will be produced by the lymphocytes in response to infection with canine parvovirus. It can be further classified as follows:

a. **Natural active immunity** – antibodies are produced in the body by lymphocytes in response to the animal actually having had, and survived, the disease. This type of immunity is more pertinent to viral disease conditions than to bacterial or protozoal infections and the antibodies produced following eradication of a pathogen give lifelong protection.

b. **Artificial active immunity** – this involves the introduction of an inactivated form of the disease into the animal's body to encourage the lymphocytes to produce specific immunoglobulins but without actually causing clinical symptoms. This is the basis of vaccination: a vaccine is an inactive form of a disease.

c. **Artificial passive immunity** – the animal acts as the recipient for antibodies via antiserum or hyperimmune serum, which have been already been produced within a donor animal. The transfer of this protection is vital for animals with a poor or undeveloped immune system. It gives them instant protection against diseases that they may be susceptible to because they are too young to form their own antibodies or because they have had no previous exposure in the form of the disease or through vaccination. This form of immunity lasts for only a few days because the antibodies themselves are foreign protein and are broken down by the body's defence system.

d. **Natural passive immunity** – neonatal animals have an inherent ability to respond immunologically to some antigens but the response is much slower and weaker than in an older animal that has been exposed to many pathogens during its life. This means that a neonate is at risk of contracting a disease until it develops the ability to produce its own antibodies. Maternally derived antibodies, supplied to the neonate in the colostrum or first milk, provide protection for the first 8–12 weeks of life (Fig. 19.3).

Neonates must consume the colostrum within hours of birth, as at this stage there is an absence of digestive enzymes and the large antibody protein molecules will be able to pass undigested through the intestinal wall into the blood stream. A small percentage of maternal antibodies also reach the fetus via the placenta. The dam can only supply the level of protection that she has accumulated over her life via regular vaccination and disease exposure. Her reaction to antigen identification and antibody formation rely on a healthy immune system and vaccination prior to coitus or during early gestation. Any neonate deficient in colostrum will be susceptible to illness until its own immune system has developed.

The timing of the administration of the first vaccine to the young animal is related to the levels of maternal antibodies remaining in the body. If the levels are too high they will destroy the antigen which is injected to stimulate the immunity of the animal; if the animal is not given its first vaccination until the levels of the maternal antibodies have becomes very low, then the animal is at risk of disease. The recommended time for the first vaccination is at about 8 weeks (Fig. 19.3).

Immune response time

The first time that an animal encounters a specific pathogen, antibodies will be produced within 7–10 days – known as the primary response. By this time the animal may already have developed symptoms; however, if the animal meets the antigen later in its life the immune system, having retained the memory of the first response, is able to produce the antibodies within 24 hours, long before symptoms develop. This secondary response is 10–50 times greater than the primary response and is the principle behind the idea of regular booster vaccinations (Fig. 19.4).

Vaccination

Young animals have an insatiable curiosity and, as they investigate the world around them, will come into contact with infectious diseases. The purpose of vaccination is to provide immunity to the susceptible animal by introducing a disrupted and harmless version of the pathogen into the body. This stimulates the defence system to produce an immune response in the absence of clinical disease. Although it has not been proved that vaccination will completely protect the animal, it will protect the animal from expressing all clinical symptoms when naturally exposed to the disease. Vaccines are available against most of the common infectious diseases of companion animals and horses (Table 19.3). A list of useful definitions relating to vaccines is shown in Box 19.2.

Types of vaccine

There are two types of vaccine used within current veterinary practice and they both have advantages and disadvantages (Table 19.4):

- Live attenuated (modified) vaccine– contains live organisms that have been attenuated by culturing the pathogen in controlled conditions, e.g. canine parvovirus, feline infectious enteritis. These stimulate a good immune response but have the risk of causing the disease
- Killed (inactivated) vaccine– contains dead organisms killed by ultraviolet, heat or sublethal chemicals such as formalin, e.g. leptospirosis. As the dead organisms cannot replicate within the body and are gradually removed by phagocytosis, several doses are required to produce sufficient antibody levels. Killed vaccines may be made more potent by the addition of an adjuvant such as oil or aluminium. This slows the release of the vaccine and delays its removal from the body by phagocytosis. Adjuvenated vaccines stimulate better immunity and in some cases remove the need for additional boosters.

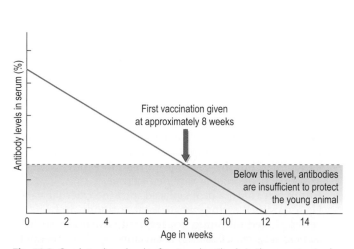

Fig. 19.3 Graph to show levels of maternal antibody in the young animal

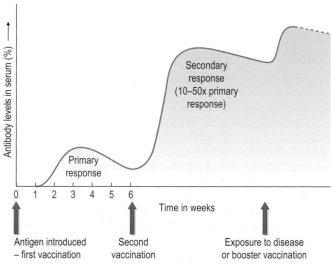

Fig. 19.4 Graph to show antibody response to the introduction of an antigen by natural exposure or vaccination

Table 19.3 Vaccines available for the prevention of infectious diseases in the dog, cat, rabbit and horse

Species	Infectious disease	Form available	Route
Dog	Distemper	L or ML	Subcutaneous
	Hepatitis	L (CAV-2)	Subcutaneous
	Parvovirus	L or ML	Subcutaneous
	Leptospirosis	K	Subcutaneous
	Parainfluenza virus	L or ML	Subcutaneous
	Bordetella bronchiseptica	L	Intranasal
	Rabies	K	Subcutaneous
	Tetanus	K	Subcutaneous
Cat	Feline infectious enteritis	L, ML or K	Subcutaneous
	Feline influenza	ML or K	Subcutaneous
	Feline leukaemia	L (non-replicable) K or subunit	Subcutaneous
	Feline *Chlamydia* virus	K	Subcutaneous
	Rabies	K	Subcutaneous
	Tetanus	K	Subcutaneous
Rabbit	Viral haemorrhagic disease	K	Subcutaneous
	Myxomatosis	L	Subcutaneous
Horse	Influenza	K	Subcutaneous
	Herpes virus	Inactivated EHV-1	Subcutaneous
	Rotavirus	K	Subcutaneous
	Tetanus toxoid	K	Subcutaneous
	Rabies	K	Subcutaneous

Data taken from Mueller P 2004 Henston Companion Animal & Equine Veterinary Vade Mecum, 22nd edn. Henston, Peterborough
K, killed; L, live; ML, modified live.

Box 19.2 Vaccine terminology

- **Vaccine** – a preparation containing a small inactivated quantity of an organism that would normally cause disease.
- **Toxoid** – a chemically or heat-treated toxin that has a reduced pathogenicity but is still able to stimulate the production of antibodies.
- **Hyperimmune serum/antiserum** – serum containing antibodies to a particular disease. The antibodies are extracted from an animal that has produced high quantities as a result of vaccination. Used when an animal is in contact with the disease and requires instant protection, e.g. in a canine parvovirus outbreak.
- **Autogenous vaccine** – a vaccine made from the animal's own cells. A sample is taken and prepared by a laboratory before being injected back into the donor animal. Used in cases of skin infection where traditional therapies have not been successful.
- **Adjuvant** – a substance that is added to an inactivated vaccine to increase its efficacy and prolong its action.
- **Attenuation** – the virulence of an organism can be reduced (attenuated) to a point where it is able to replicate but is no longer pathogenic.
- **Subunit vaccine** – contains only a component of the microorganism, which is enough to produce an immune response but cannot cause the disease, e.g. FeLV vaccine.

Table 19.4 Comparison between live and killed vaccines

Modified live (attenuated)	Killed (inactivated)
One dose required	Two doses required
Allows controlled virus replication	No viral activity
Low antigen numbers required	High antigen numbers
Adjuvant not used	Adjuvant used – a reaction may be noted
Mild clinical signs may be observed	Killed so no risk of clinical signs
Contraindicated in immunocompromised animals	Safe in immunocompromised animals
Contraindications in pregnant animals – may affect the fetus	Safe to use in pregnant animals
Gives rapid and long-lasting protection	Shorter protection

Vaccine management

A course of two or sometimes three vaccinations are given to provide protection to the vulnerable young animal whose immune system is underdeveloped. The first vaccination is given as the maternally derived antibody levels begin to fall (Fig. 19.3), and antibodies will be formed within 7–10 days. A second dose is given 2–3 weeks later, stimulating the production of yet more antibodies with a quicker response time of 12–24 hours (Fig. 19.4). This initial course provides antibodies for several months and should be reinforced 1 year later with a 'booster' vaccine to 'top-up' the acquired immunity. Failure to present the animal for the initial booster may result in a two-dose vaccine programme comparable to the primary course. In addition, the animal can gain natural active immunity when exposed to disease, creating further antibodies and protection.

The vaccines are administered by the following routes:

- **Subcutaneous route** – this is the most common route and is given in the scruff. The site of injection needs to be varied to prevent skin irritation if this route is to be used for a course of injections. Sterile equipment will be required but the use of a spirit swab is not advised, as it may precipitate a vaccine reaction
- **Intranasal route** – drops placed into the external nares via a modified syringe create local antibody and cell-mediated immunity for respiratory diseases such as *Bordetella bronchiseptica,* a causative agent for kennel cough

- **Oral route** – available for some European vaccines, e.g. rabies vaccine used in wild foxes.

Vaccines will only be effective if they are stored in a refrigerator at 2–4°C and remain cold. Warmth will kill the microorganisms within a live vaccine. Stock control should be observed and those with the shortest expiry date should be used first. The veterinary surgeon or nurse should understand how to reconstitute vaccines and know which vaccines can be mixed to reduce the number of injections to be given. The veterinary nurse can prepare the vaccination certificate but the veterinary surgeon is responsible for the document and must check all details and sign to authenticate it.

Failures in vaccination

Vaccines may be ineffective for various reasons and owners must be aware that the veterinary surgeon may refuse to vaccinate their animal if an underlying illness or complications are suspected. Newly acquired puppies should not be brought to the surgery until they have had time to settle, as stress will have a negative effect on the immune system, causing vaccine failure. Older animals presented for vaccination without a current vaccine certificate will, depending on age and health, be given a full booster vaccination to ensure that the animal is truly protected against all infectious diseases (Table 19.3).

Primary vaccine courses should be administered when the passive immunity received from the mother has decreased, as maternally derived antibody (MDA) interferes with the neonate's ability to respond to a vaccine (Fig. 19.3). Delaying vaccination until MDA wanes may result in some puppies or kittens becoming infected and suffering the disease. Animals suffering systemic disease will suffer from immunosuppression and protective antibodies will not be produced in response to the antigen. A risk of clinical disease within patients suffering from FeLV and FIV has resulted in an abandoned vaccine schedule.

Other causes of vaccine failure include:

- Animal has been exposed to the disease shortly after vaccinating – before the body has produced sufficient antibodies
- Animal was actually incubating the disease at the time of vaccination
- Vaccine has passed the expiry date
- Vaccine was not stored correctly
- Incorrect administration route

- Use of antibiotics or corticosteroids at the same time
- Incorrect timing of primary vaccine course
- Failure to boost the vaccine
- Animals may have a poor immune system
- Excessive use of alcohol or disinfectant on the skin.

Adverse reactions

When introducing any foreign substance into the body there is a risk of an allergic reaction. Owners should be made aware of possible effects and asked to report to the veterinary surgeon if any are observed. Symptoms may range from mild lethargy to severe shock and may include:

- Swelling of injection site
- Urticaria
- Vomiting
- Diarrhoea
- Depression
- Ataxia
- Shivering
- Collapse.

Corticosteroids may be given as treatment and, if there are signs of shock, supportive therapy must be administered. The reaction should be recorded on the animal's treatment card and a different type of vaccine should be used for the next dose.

Diagnostic use of antibodies – ELISA tests

Enzyme-linked immunosorbent assay (ELISA) is based on the ability to produce monoclonal or polyclonal antibodies to a specific antigen or isolation and production of a specific antigen. In kits to detect antigens, antibodies specific for the antigen are bound to the wall of the test well, wand or membrane. The blood, serum or plasma sample is then added and any antigen present will bind to the antibody present. Washing of the test kit removes any unbound antibody. A second enzyme-labelled antibody is added, followed by a second washing. To finish, a substrate is added to develop a specific colour if the antigen is present.

At present there are commercial tests kits available to recognize the p27 protein found in FeLV and to test for antibodies in FIV cases. Fewer steps within the kits reduce the likelihood of human error and for further accuracy most tests contain a positive and negative control. These kits are of most use in cats showing suspected clinical symptoms, animals that have been in contact with a suspected case and as a precaution prior to breeding.

Bibliography

American Lyme Disease Foundation. Available from: <www.aldf.com/lyme.shtml>.

Bowden, C., Master, J., 2003. Textbook of Veterinary Medical Nursing. Butterworth-Heinemann, Oxford.

Cooper, B., Lane, D.R., 1999. Veterinary Nursing, second ed. Butterworth-Heinemann, Oxford.

Davol, P.A., 2002. Vaccines, Infectious Diseases and the Canine Immune System. Available from: <http://www.labbies.com/immun.htm>.

Fraser, C.M., 1991, The Merck Veterinary Manual, seventh ed. Merck & Co., Inc., Whitehouse Station, NJ.

Higgins, A.J., Wright, I.M., 1994. The Equine Manual. Baillière Tindall, London.

Kelleher, S., 2003. Respiratory disease in the rabbit. In: British Small Animal Veterinary Association Congress 2003 Scientific Proceedings. British Small Animal Veterinary Association.

Lightfoot, T.L., 2002. Hyaluronidase: therapeutic applications including egg-yolk disease, In: Proceedings of the Association of Avian Veterinarians.

Mackean, D., Jones, B., 1985. Human and Social Biology. John Murray, London.

Mueller, P., 2004. Henston Companion Animal & Equine Veterinary Vade Mecum, twenty-second ed. Henston, Peterborough.

Pratt, P.W., 1998. Principles and Practice of Veterinary Technology. C V Mosby, St Louis, MO.

Tilley, L.P., Smith, F.W.K., 2004. The 5-minute Veterinary Consult: Canine and Feline, version 3. (Available as CD-ROM). Lippincott Williams & Wilkins, Philadelphia, PA.

Recommended reading

Bowden, C., Master, J., 2003. Textbook of Veterinary Medical Nursing. Butterworth-Heinemann, Oxford.
Entire book dedicated to the subject designed for veterinary nurses and those taking more advanced courses.

Ramsey, I., Tennant, B., 2001. Manual of Canine and Feline Infectious Diseases. BSAVA, Quedgeley, Gloucester.
Written for the veterinary surgeon but information is comprehensive and approachable.

Access to all of the equine disease surveillance reports can be obtained from the Animal Health Trust website on www.aht.org.uk or from the DEFRA website www.defra.gov.uk or the BEVA website www.beva.org.uk.

CHAPTER 20

Common medical conditions of the body systems

Paula Hotston Moore

- Medical conditions described in this chapter are defined as those that result from an abnormality or malfunction within one of the body systems and are neither infectious nor generally require surgery to correct them.
- A detailed history of the patient followed by a thorough clinical examination will elicit a list of potential causes of the clinical signs, i.e. a differential diagnosis.
- Diagnosis may be confirmed by using the appropriate tests and diagnostic procedures, which include: laboratory tests, e.g. blood biochemistry, urinalysis; radiography; ultrasonography; endoscopy.
- Confirmation of the diagnosis will lead to the formulation of a treatment plan.
- Many conditions do not have a specific treatment and the patient is treated symptomatically.

Introduction

The common medical conditions covered in this chapter may be described as those which result from an upset within one of the body systems and are neither infectious nor require surgery to correct them. Many of these conditions elicit a differential diagnosis, which is a list of potential causes of the condition. A veterinary surgeon will work through each condition on the list and undertake various diagnostic tests that will eventually confirm the diagnosis.

Respiratory system

Acute respiratory distress

Acute respiratory distress is a true respiratory emergency and has many possible causes which include:

- Airway obstruction (Fig. 20.1), e.g. by a foreign body such as a ball
- Trauma, e.g. road traffic accident
- Laryngeal paralysis

- Poisoning
- Neoplasia
- Overdose of anaesthetic
- Pneumonia.

Treatment

1. A patent airway must be maintained in order that air can pass through the trachea to the lungs
2. The use of suction will remove secretions such as haemorrhage or excess saliva
3. Intubation will maintain an open and clear airway in the unconscious patient
4. Placement of a tracheostomy tube is a semi-permanent solution to maintain a patent airway
5. Oxygen therapy will ensure that air reaching the alveoli is rich in oxygen and thus aid oxygen exchange.

Oxygen may be administered in several ways – select the method that is readily available and is most easily tolerated by the patient (see also Ch. 23):

- A commercial oxygen cage is the ideal way to administer oxygen as this provides an enclosed environment that prevents the oxygen leaking away. Cage fronts can be purchased that can be fitted on to the front of an existing cage when oxygen therapy is required. As it is transparent, the oxygen cage allows observation of the patient and prevents the animal from feeling enclosed. An oxygen tube is fed into the cage via a hole in the cage front. This type of cage is not available in all practices
- A Hall's anaesthetic mask is placed on or near the patient's nose and mouth to allow it to inspire oxygen-rich air (Fig. 20.2)
- An oxygen tent can be made from a large plastic bag, with the patient placed inside and an oxygen tube leading into it. A clear plastic bag allows the patient to see out and helps to prevent the animal from struggling. If only a coloured or black plastic bag is available, then cut a hole in the bag and reseal it with cling film to provide a 'viewing hole' for both observer and patient. Some animals, but not all, will tolerate this technique

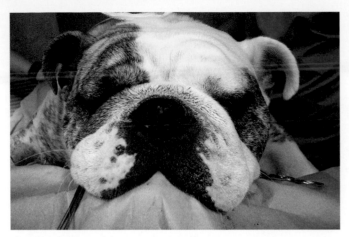

Fig. 20.1 Bulldog exhibiting respiratory obstruction caused by stenotic nares

- Breed of animal (some breeds are predisposed to certain conditions)
- Age of animal
- Presence of exercise intolerance
- Length of time the cough has been present
- Type of cough – dry/hacking or moist and productive
- History of any trauma
- Presence of any other medical conditions
- Exposure to possible infections
- In contact animals showing similar clinical signs
- Time of day when cough occurs or is worse

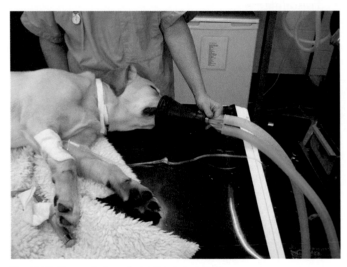

Fig. 20.2 Oxygen being administered via a mask

- An alternative is to place an Elizabethan collar on the patient and cover the front with cling film. An oxygen tube is placed through the neck opening of the collar. This creates an almost enclosed area in which to deliver oxygen therapy
- Nasal prongs deliver oxygen to the patient and cause minimal stress
- Respiratory stimulants such as doxapram hydrochloride may be given to patients that do not have respiratory obstruction
- Bronchodilators may also help in cases of acute respiratory distress.

Coughing

A cough is defined as 'a reflex action causing sudden expulsion of air from the respiratory tract'. Coughing is a common clinical sign that occurs in several medical conditions and it is important to determine whether the cough is dry and hacking or whether the cough is moist and productive because this will determine the differential diagnosis. Animals do not often expectorate but usually swallow the material instead. A comprehensive history from the client together with a thorough clinical examination will ascertain the type of cough. Box 20.1 shows some of the points that must be considered.

Coughing may be caused by:

- **Heart failure** – in left-sided congestive heart failure the patient may present with a moist cough caused by pulmonary oedema. Thoracic radiographs will show the severity of pulmonary congestion and help to decide the treatment regime. Thoracic radiographs should be taken with the patient in right lateral recumbency if possible. Alternatively, a dorsoventral thoracic radiograph will still be diagnostic and will also be more comfortable for the patient if severe coughing or respiratory distress is present. During radiography it is vital to cause a minimum of stress to the respiratory-challenged patient. It may be advisable to sedate the patient rather than administering a general anaesthetic and allowing the animal to adopt a near-natural position will help to prevent further respiratory distress
- **Upper airway obstruction** – may be due to laryngeal paralysis or an inhaled foreign body. Laryngeal paralysis is paralysis of the vocal folds, usually bilateral, and is often a degenerative condition of the older dog. Laryngeal paralysis responds well to a surgical procedure known as a laryngeal tieback
- **Viral or bacterial infection** – for example, kennel cough causes a dry hacking cough
- **Feline asthma**
- **Tracheal collapse** – most commonly a condition of toy and small breeds of dog. The tracheal rings collapse inwards and cause coughing on exercise, often accompanied by dyspnoea. Manual palpation of the trachea in the neck and the use of radiographs and endoscopy will confirm the diagnosis (Fig. 20.3). Most cases are managed medically by treatment of underlying causes, e.g. bronchitis
- **Allergies**
- **Aspiration pneumonia** – may be linked to forced feeding or feeding neonates
- **Bronchitis**
- **Pulmonary oedema**
- **Lungworm infection** – caused by *Aelurostrongylus abstrusus* in the cat. *Angiostrongylus vasorum* is the more common

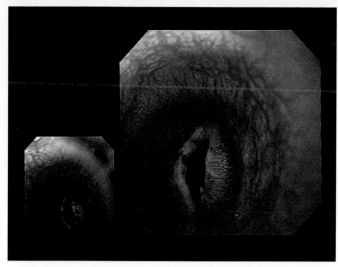

Fig. 20.3 Tracheal collapse shown on endoscopy

parasitic infestation in the dog and slugs and snails act as the intermediate host. Dogs ingest larvae from eating the molluscs or from eating grass contaminated with slug trails, drinking from outside water bowls or playing with outside toys contaminated with larvae from slugs or snails. Larvae are coughed up and swallowed and are then passed out in faeces (see Ch. 27). Clinical signs in the dog include coughing, dyspnoea, tachypnoea, wheezing, blood clotting problems (coagulopathy) anaemia, annorexia and depression. Faecal tests are performed to confirm the diagnosis (see Ch. 29). Treatment includes imidacloprid/moxidectin, fenbendazole, milbemycin or ivermectin.

- **Respiratory neoplasia** – confirmed by radiography
- **Inhalation of a foreign body** – patient will show severe distress
- **Tuberculosis.**

Nursing care

- Allowing the patient to adopt a natural position in which it feels comfortable and does not struggle, often sternal recumbency, will let it breathe calmly and efficiently between episodes of coughing
- Antitussives, e.g. butorphanol, suppress coughing and are useful if coughing is causing distress but must only be used in patients where suppressing the cough will not cause further harm. Alternative drugs are other opiates, such as codeine or theophylline
- Nebulization is an effective way of hydrating the patient's respiratory tract and will increase the effectiveness of coupage (see Ch. 16). A commercially available nebulizer is used to deliver sterile water to the patient via a mask or with the patient restrained in a cage
- The living conditions of the animal must be thoroughly investigated. Environmental factors should be examined and adjusted if necessary. Dusty or fluffy bedding material such as straw or old-type blankets must be exchanged for bedding materials that do not

separate into particles. A dusty or damp atmosphere will worsen a cough
- Owners should be advised that animals are susceptible to passive smoking, so a smoke-free home environment is essential.

Dyspnoea

Dyspnoea is defined as 'laboured or difficult breathing'. This implies that oxygen supply is insufficient to meet the demands of the body. Dyspnoea can be seen on close observation of the animal or by auscultation of the thorax. It may be caused by:

- **Upper airway obstruction**, e.g. by a foreign body, will not allow sufficient air to pass into the trachea, causing the patient to become dyspnoeic
- **Laryngeal paralysis** – this will present as inspiratory dyspnoea as the paralysed vocal folds obstruct the passage of air into the trachea
- **Tracheal collapse**
- **Feline asthma**
- **Pulmonary oedema**
- **Pulmonary neoplasia**
- **Pneumonia**
- **Brachycephalic upper airway syndrome** – commonly affected brachycephalic breeds include the bulldog, pug, Pekinese and Cavalier King Charles spaniel. The condition presents as dyspnoea due to problems such as an extended soft palate, stenotic nares and laryngeal deformities. These conditions interfere with the inflow and outflow of air into the upper respiratory system
- **Heart failure**
- **Smoke inhalation** following a house fire causes dyspnoea because there is little or no oxygen in the inhaled air during the fire. The smoke also irritates the respiratory system, causing inflammation and the release of inflammatory fluid into the alveoli. Fluid in the alveolar spaces prevents air entering the alveoli and interferes with gaseous exchange
- **Poisoning**, e.g. from chemicals such as paraquat or chlorates (weed killers), paracetamol and carbon monoxide (exhaust fumes/poorly ventilated gas fires or boilers). Ingestion of paracetamol and chlorates causes haemoglobin to change into methaemoglobin, which is unable to transport oxygen around the body and leads to dyspnoea. In cases of carbon monoxide poisoning, the haemoglobin combines with the carbon monoxide rather than with the oxygen, resulting in a much lower oxygen content of blood
- **Pain** caused by compression of the thorax, e.g. during gastric dilation and volvulus. The abdominal contents press on the diaphragm and restrict the expansion of the thoracic cavity
- **Thoracic wall injury**, e.g. diaphragmatic hernia or invasive foreign body – leads to dyspnoea, as air enters the pleural cavity and prevents the lungs from fully expanding.

Nursing care

- Keeping the animal free from distress and anxiety will avoid making the dyspnoea worse

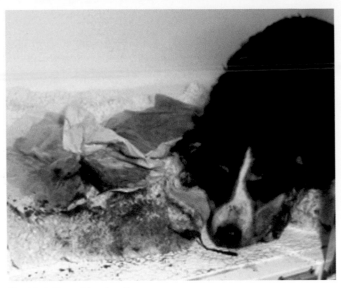

Fig. 20.4 Dog with epistaxis

- Confine the animal to a small space where it can adopt a comfortable position and not become agitated or move excessively
- Avoid handling the patient unless it is absolutely necessary, to avoid a possible struggle
- Oxygen therapy, as described above, may be helpful
- Monitor and record the patient's vital signs, e.g. temperature, pulse and respiration.

Epistaxis

Epistaxis is defined as 'haemorrhage originating from the nose', i.e. a nosebleed (Fig. 20.4). The original source of the blood is not necessarily the nose but may be some other part of the respiratory system. Epistaxis is usually bilateral. Unilateral epistaxis may be caused by a foreign body, neoplasia or trauma.

Causes of epistaxis include:

- **Direct trauma**, e.g. road traffic accident
- **Nasal neoplasia** – often unilateral. Confirm diagnosis by radiography of the affected area
- **Foreign body**, e.g. grass seeds, blades of grass, etc. – will cause trauma to the nasal lining
- **Ulceration of nasal epithelium** – may be due to fungal infection caused by *Aspergillus* spp. or diseases affecting the mucocutaneous function. A long-term condition such as cat flu may also cause ulceration of the nasal epithelium
- **Blood clotting problems** – haemophilia is the most common in small animals
- **Severe skull fractures** – rare but may cause epistaxis.

Nursing care

- Where dyspnoea accompanies epistaxis, treatment must be given for dyspnoea
- If a foreign body is visible then it should be removed. In some more difficult cases it may be better to remove it when the animal is sedated or anaesthetized

- A cold compress applied to the nose will alleviate pain and aid haemorrhage
- Topical vasoconstrictor drugs may be squirted into the nose to prevent haemorrhage.

Discharges

Discharges involving the respiratory system are usually nasal in origin. Serous discharges are clear in colour and often due to a viral infection. Mucopurulent discharges are thicker in consistency and often yellow or green in colour. These are often a result of a secondary bacterial infection following an initial viral infection.

Fungal infections

The most frequent fungal infection of the respiratory system is due to *Aspergillus fumigatus*, which invades the nasal mucosa. It is more common in long-nosed or doliocephalic breeds of dog and very rare in cats. Clinical signs are a mucopurulent nasal discharge, which may become blood-stained, sneezing and pain. Diagnosis is confirmed by radiography, nasal culture, rhinoscopy and nasal biopsies. Surgical treatment is usually successful, using indwelling catheters placed in the frontal sinuses and then flushing the nasal chambers with fungicides, e.g. clotrimazole.

Nursing care

- The administration of a fungicide via indwelling nasal catheters is often performed at a referral centre
- Monitor the vital signs regularly
- Prevent patient interference with the nasal catheters, e.g. use an Elizabethan collar
- Clean the nostrils to maintain patient comfort
- Tempt the patient to eat with warmed food or by hand feeding
- Coupage (see Ch. 16) is used to loosen mucus in the lungs, which is then coughed up by the animal. Percussion of the chest is ideally performed with the animal in sternal recumbency or in a standing position. Cupped hands are placed on either sides of the lateral thorax, starting at the diaphragm. Maintaining cupped hands and loose wrists, the hands move along the length of the thorax, progressing cranially, percussing the chest along its length. Coupage should be performed for 10 minutes, three to four times a day. It is typically well tolerated by the patient. Using nebulization prior to coupage may help loosen dehydrated mucus.

Pleural disorders

These are summarized in Table 20.1.

Pneumothorax frequently occurs as a result of trauma, e.g. a road traffic accident, gunshot wound, bites to the chest wall or impaling injury. A patient with pneumothorax will show signs of dyspnoea and, depending upon the severity of the case, asphyxiation and unconsciousness leading to death (Table 20.2).

Diagnosis may be confirmed by the use of radiography (Fig. 20.6). The removal of the air or fluid from the thoracic

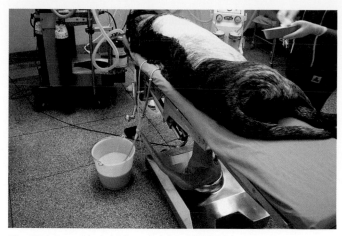

Fig. 20.5 Dog with chylothorax prepared for fluid drainage

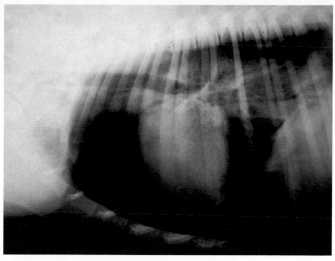

Fig. 20.6 Pneumothorax – lateral radiograph of a dog

Table 20.1 Conditions affecting the pleural cavity

Condition	Definition
Pneumothorax	Presence of air in the pleural cavity
Pyothorax	Accumulation of pus in the pleural cavity
Haemothorax	Accumulation of blood in the pleural cavity
Chylothorax (Fig. 20.5)	Accumulation of chyle in the pleural cavity
Hydrothorax	Accumulation of serous fluid in the pleural cavity

Table 20.2 Types of pneumothorax

Type of pneumothorax	Definition
Open pneumothorax	An opening into the thoracic cavity is present, e.g. from a penetrating wound. Air enters the thoracic cavity, thus destroying the negative pressure within the pleural cavity, leading to lung collapse
Closed pneumothorax	Lung tissue is torn or crushed, e.g. by a fractured rib, allowing air to escape into the pleural space and destroying the normal vacuum. The lungs are then unable to expand in the normal way and the animal becomes dyspnoeic
Tension pneumothorax	A type of closed pneumothorax in which the air pressure in the pleural space increases every time the animal breathes in, resulting in progressive lung collapse

cavity by thoracocentesis is essential in both the diagnosis and treatment of these conditions.

Urinary system

Renal disease

Renal disease is only noticed clinically when 75% of the renal tubules are functionally impaired. Until this happens the kidney is able to compensate and function normally, so by the time clinical signs are evident the condition is already severe. All parts of the kidney work together, so, if any part is diseased, kidney function as a whole will be affected.

Causes of renal disease include:

- **Poisoning**, e.g. mercury, ethylene glycol, sulphonamide
- **Nephritis** – to any inflammatory condition of the kidney
- **Glomerulonephritis** – often immune-mediated, affecting the renal glomerulus and thus renal filtration
- **Pyelonephritis** – infection of the renal pelvis, usually due to an ascending bacterial infection from the lower urinary tract
- **Interstitial nephritis** – affects the tissue between the nephrons but clinical signs are similar to those of any

type of nephritis; associated with blood-borne infections, e.g. leptospirosis, canine adenovirus
- **Urinary calculi** – the formation of calculi or 'stones' within the bladder
- **Urinary obstruction** – if the calculi move along the urinary tract they may cause obstruction
- **Neoplasia**
- **Trauma**.

Acute renal failure

May be due to severe dehydration, circulatory failure, poisoning, urinary tract obstruction or trauma. The patient shows signs of acute abdominal pain, anorexia, pyrexia, vomiting and oliguria, which may become polyuria at a later

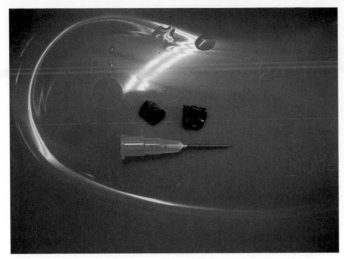

Fig. 20.7 Bladder stones from a cat

stage. Acute renal failure can usually be reversed. Treatment of the underlying cause, e.g. poisoning, obstruction, is essential. Correction of dehydration status by intravenous fluids is required, together with supportive therapies such as antibiotics and nursing care.

Chronic renal failure

May be due to congenital problems, interstitial nephritis, glomerular nephritis, pyelonephritis or long-term urinary obstruction. Usually seen in older animals, where onset is gradual and the condition may not be diagnosed until the kidney fails to compensate. Presents as polydipsia and polyuria, anorexia and weight loss, anaemia, gingivitis, oral ulceration, halitosis and hypertension. Treat symptomatically but, once the condition is established, very little can be done.

Urinary obstruction

Commonly caused by 'stones' (calculi or uroliths; Fig. 20.7). The formation of calculi, or urolithiasis, is complicated but is considered to be due to high concentrations of salts in the body. In dogs and cats 50% of uroliths are struvite, composed of magnesium ammonium phosphate salts known as triple phosphate. Other calculi may be made of oxalate, urate, uric acid or cystine (Table 20.3).

The presence of urinary calculi may or may not cause clinical signs. Where clinical signs do occur, the patient will show varying signs of local pain and discomfort, haematuria, urinary tenesmus, dysuria or possibly anuria or urinary incontinence. Urinary calculi may obstruct the urethra, often at the ischial arch in male dogs, or they may cause irritation of the lining of the bladder.

A diagnosis is reached from interpretation of the clinical signs and the inability to pass a urinary catheter and it is confirmed by the use of radiography, particularly the use of contrast media (see Ch. 30).

Surgical removal of the calculi is often necessary, followed by prophylactic measures to avoid recurrence, e.g. control of urinary infection, increasing water intake, dietary changes and using urinary acidifiers. Encouraging the patient to pass urine frequently discourages re-formation of calculi. Renal

Table 20.3 Common types of urolith

Type of urolith	Found in acidic/ alkaline urine	Notes
Struvite/triple phosphate	Alkaline	Often an incidental finding in dogs and cats. More common in bitches than male dogs. Bacterial infection often present in dogs. Most common in cats
Calcium carbonate	Alkaline	Less common in dogs and cats but common in herbivores, e.g. rabbits
Uric acid	Acidic	Common in dalmatians
Ammonium urate/ Ammonium acid urate	Acidic	Common in dalmatians. In other breeds often accompanies liver failure. Often poorly radiopaque so not always identified on plain radiographs
Calcium oxalate	Acidic	Sometimes an incidental finding in dog and cat urine
Cystine	Acidic	Less common urolith, almost always found in male dogs

function must also be checked in such cases by performing routine biochemistry. Chemical analysis of the removed urinary uroliths will help in the treatment and prevention of recurrence. Urinary acidifiers, such as methionine or ammonium chloride, are either added to the patient's food or administered orally. Some diets used in the treatment of uroliths contain urinary regulators, so care must be taken not to 'double-dose' the patient.

Other urinary problems

Neoplasia

Uncommon. Surgical removal of the tumour is possible but this condition offers a poor prognosis. Diagnosis is confirmed by radiography.

Trauma

Trauma, e.g. a road traffic accident or a kick, may cause haematuria, anuria and the patient may show signs of acute renal failure. Diagnosis is confirmed by radiography and paracentesis – removal of fluid from the abdomen. A ruptured bladder will require surgical repair. Milder trauma will resolve with medical management, e.g. fluid therapy and supportive treatment.

Cystitis

This is caused by a urinary tract infection, which is often ascending. It is more common in females than males because

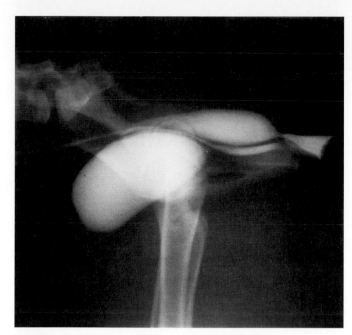

Fig. 20.8 Radiograph showing an ectopic ureter in a dog

of the position of the opening of the tract in relation to the anus – often caused by faecal contamination. An infection is more likely if a urinary obstruction is present or where trauma to the urinary tract has occurred. The animal will pass smaller amounts of urine more frequently, often showing signs of tenesmus and haematuria. Treat with antibiotics following a urinary bacterial culture and sensitivity test.

Urinary incontinence

This is the involuntary passage of urine. Diagnosis is made from an extensive client history, radiography and urinary catheterization. Causes include:

- Congenital anatomical malformation, e.g. ectopic ureter (Fig. 20.8) – can be corrected surgically
- Neoplasia
- Hormonal – in spayed bitches; treat with oestrogens
- Displacement of the bladder, e.g. after a road traffic accident
- Prostate disease
- Neurological disorders, e.g. spinal trauma or disease
- Senility
- Psychological, e.g. excitement or fear.

Urinary catheterization

Urinary catheterization is performed for many reasons (see also Ch. 15).

An aseptic technique must be used to place the urinary catheter to avoid introducing infection into the bladder. The use of antibiotics in a patient with a urinary catheter in place is controversial. There is more likelihood of a urinary tract infection following catheterization if the patient is immunosuppressed, if recurrent catheterization is necessary or if there is already trauma to the urinary tract. To avoid damaging the urethra the catheter should always be introduced

with care and not forced into the urethra. In cases of urolithiasis and sediment in the urethra the catheter will not pass easily and an alternative means of treatment must be sought. If the catheter becomes blocked, flushing with sterile water or sterile saline may clear the blockage.

Urinary catheters are purchased pre-sterilized (Table 20.4). Other than the metal urinary catheter, all urinary catheters are for single use only. Catheters should be stored flat and not allowed to curl, since this will hinder catheter placement. All urinary catheters must be lubricated and checked prior to use, maintaining the sterility of the catheter. The stylet, if present, is checked for ease of movement and the balloon in the Foley catheter is inflated prior to use to check for holes and then deflated for insertion. Where indwelling urinary catheters are in place, patient interference must be avoided. A buster collar is commonly used.

Cystocentesis

In some cases cystocentesis may be used as an alternative method of draining the bladder. An area of hair on the ventral abdomen, over the site of the bladder, is clipped and surgically prepared. Locate the bladder by palpation and hold it firmly. A sterile needle with attached syringe is inserted through the abdominal wall into the bladder and urine is withdrawn. This procedure can be performed in a conscious animal in either lateral recumbency or in a standing position. Cystocentesis is well tolerated in most patients.

Cardiovascular system

Heart disease

Heart disease may be:

- Congenital – present at birth but usually detected at the time of first vaccination. Congenital heart lesions represent about 5% of canine cardiac disease (Detweiler & Patterson 1965). They are commonly diagnosed when the heart is auscultated during the check-up prior to the first vaccination consultation. Table 20.5 describes the range of conditions and their treatment.
- Acquired – may develop as the animal ages. Acquired heart disease represents approximately 95% of canine cardiac diseases (Detweiler & Patterson 1965). Table 20.6 describes the range of conditions and their treatment.

Arrhythmia

The term arrhythmia indicates an abnormality in the normal rhythm of the heart. Table 20.7 describes types of arrhythmia and their treatment.

Heart failure

Heart failure is defined as 'an inability of the heart to provide sufficient output to maintain the blood circulation'. Heart failure is either acute, with a sudden onset, or chronic, having a gradual onset over a period of time. Numerous

Table 20.4 Types of urinary catheter

Types of urinary catheter	Dog/cat	Comments
Jackson cat catheter	Cat Commonly used in male cats but can also be used in female cats	Can be used as an indwelling catheter
		Has a Luer fitting
		Available in two sizes: 3 and 4 FG
		Has a stylet to aid insertion
Plastic plain urethral catheter	Dogs, bitches and female cats	Longer than the Jackson cat catheter
		Has no stylet
		Available in a variety of diameters and lengths
		Has a Luer fitting
		Can be used as an indwelling catheter
Foley catheter	Bitches	Can be used as an indwelling catheter
		Available in a variety of diameters and lengths
		Catheter does not come with a stylet but a separate stylet is often necessary to aid insertion
		Does not have a Luer fitting so a connector is required to attach the catheter to the urinary drainage system
		When used as an indwelling catheter the balloon is inflated with sterile water or sterile saline. The amount of fluid required to inflate the balloon is stated on the end of the catheter
		Care must be taken with lubricants and latex rubber – KY jelly is the lubricant of choice
Tieman's catheter	Bitches	Not used as an indwelling catheter as impossible to suture in place effectively
		Curved tip aids insertion
		Has a Luer fitting
		Has no stylet
Metal catheter	Bitches	Now considered outdated. Difficult to use as made of inflexible material. Other catheters have now superseded this type

diseases or conditions affecting the heart lead to heart failure. The heart is able to compensate for any defects so many heart conditions go unnoticed until the condition severely affects cardiac output.

The heart may compensate in the following ways:

- Peripheral vasoconstriction – increases circulating blood volume
- Tachycardia – increases cardiac output
- Enlargement of the heart chambers
- Myocardial hypertrophy
- Decreased renal perfusion, leading to:
  - Aldosterone release and an increase in plasma volume
  - Followed by angiotensin release, peripheral vasoconstriction and thus hypertension.

Many factors can affect the ability of the heart to compensate, including:

- Myocardial disease
- Heart valve disease
- Obesity

- Sudden excessive exercise or activity
- Excessive environmental temperature, leading to hyperthermia
- Pregnancy
- Respiratory disease
- Shock
- Haemorrhage
- Anaemia.

Heart failure may affect one particular side of the heart and is then referred to as right-sided heart failure or left-sided heart failure:

a. Left-sided heart failure – may be caused by:
  - Aortic stenosis
  - Mitral valve dysplasia
  - Endocardiosis
  - Cardiomyopathy
  - Obstruction of aorta
  - Dysrhythmias.
The clinical signs include pulmonary oedema and congestion, tachypnoea, dyspnoea, coughing, lethargy,

Table 20.5 Congenital heart conditions

Congenital condition	Clinical signs	Diagnosis	Comments	Treatment
Pulmonic stenosis	Exercise intolerance Syncope	Radiography	This is a narrowing of the pulmonary semilunar valve Will lead to right-sided congestive heart failure	Surgical correction
Aortic stenosis	Syncope Exercise intolerance	Radiography	This is a narrowing of the aortic semilunar valve	Surgical correction
Patent ductus arteriosus (PDA)	Stunted growth Sudden death Exercise intolerance Coughing Dyspnoea Heart murmur	Radiography	Persistence of a small vessel which links the aorta to the pulmonary artery – normally closes over at birth. Seen in young animals, commonly detected at vaccination consultation Breed predisposition – German shepherd dogs, Irish setters and crossbreeds	Surgical ligation
Ventricular septal defect (VSD)	Exercise intolerance Signs of congestive heart failure	Radiography	Commonly known as 'hole in the heart' – this is a hole in the interventricular septum	Requires heart bypass – not generally available in the UK
Mitral or tricuspid valve dysplasia	Heart murmur	Clinical examination	A common congenital condition	Requires heart bypass – not generally available in the UK
Tetralogy of Fallot	Heart murmur Exercise intolerance Weight loss Cyanosis	Clinical examination	A combination of ventricular septal defect, pulmonary stenosis, a displaced aorta and hypertrophy of the right ventricular wall	Surgery possible but not often performed Very guarded prognosis
Persistent right aortic arch/vascular ring anomaly	Usually no cardiac signs are present Regurgitation Oesophageal diverticulum cranial to the stricture Possibly aspiration pneumonia	Radiography	Causes oesophageal constriction	Surgical ligation

tachycardia and pulmonary râles. All signs will become worse with exercise and in severe cases exercise must be limited to avoid precipitating cardiac arrest and death.

b. Right-sided heart failure – may be caused by:
- Pulmonic stenosis
- Tricuspid dysplasia
- Endocardiosis
- Congestive cardiomyopathy
- Pericardial effusions
- Neoplasia
- Myocarditis
- Following long-term left-sided heart failure.

The clinical signs include pooling of blood in the veins leading to oedema, hepatomegaly, splenomegaly, ascites, muffled heart sounds and dysrhythmias.

Congestive heart failure occurs when both the left and the right sides of the heart fail simultaneously. This can often happen following a one-sided heart failure.

Treatment

The main treatment of heart failure is by using drugs and Table 20.8 shows the main groups of drug that are commonly used. In addition to drugs, the following may also be used:

- **Diuresis** – in heart failure, fluid is retained and accumulates in the body tissues because the heart is unable to pump effectively. This results in pooling of fluid in the tissue spaces, leading to oedema, ascites and pulmonary congestion (Fig. 20.9). Diuretic drugs are used to overcome fluid retention (Table 20.8)
- **Dietary management** – this plays an important role in the longer-term management. Sodium is the main cation of extracellular fluid and leads to the retention of fluid, which increases blood volume and increases the workload of the already failing heart. A low-sodium diet will reduce fluid retention and assist in treating heart failure. Many proprietary diets have a high sodium content, so a specific cardiac

Table 20.6 Acquired heart disease

Acquired condition	Clinical signs	Diagnosis	Comments	Treatment
Endocardiosis	Left-sided heart failure leading to congestive heart failure Heart murmur	Clinical examination Client history	Valvular disease Valves leak when closed Common in small breeds of dog Mitral valve commonly affected and occasionally the tricuspid valve	No specific treatment Management of heart failure
Endocarditis	Weight loss Anorexia Lethargy Inflammation of other body parts, e.g. lameness, joint pain Pyrexia Bounding pulse	Electrocardiography (ECG) Clinical examination Haematology	An uncommon disease Associated with a bacterial infection present elsewhere in the body and having spread to the heart valves	Antibiotics Supportive therapy, e.g. rest, warmth, TLC Guarded prognosis
Myocarditis	Pyrexia	Clinical examination	Very rare Infection of heart muscle	No specific treatment but treat underlying cause – antibiotics and corticosteroids
Pericardial disease	Ascites Muffled heart sounds	Auscultation Clinical examination Radiography	Leads to right-sided heart failure Usually accompanied by pericardial effusion	Aspiration of fluid
Bradycardia	Incidental finding on clinical examination while investigating ECG underlying medical disease, e.g. Addison's disease	Auscultation	Usually defined as a heart rate < 60 beats per minute	Treat the underlying disease
Tachycardia	Incidental finding on clinical examination while investigating underlying medical disease, e.g. feline hyperthyroidism or adrenal neoplasia	Auscultation	Usually defined as a heart rate of > 150–200 beats per minute Commonly found in congestive heart failure Remember that environmental and physical factors, e.g. fear, pain, excitement, can cause tachycardia	Treat the underlying disease
Arrhythmias	Vary from none through syncope to sudden death	ECG	A deviation from the normal heart rhythm	Medical therapy, e.g. lidocaine

Table 20.7 Types of arrhythmia

Type of arrhythmia	Diagnosis	Comments	Treatments
Sinus arrhythmia	Auscultation	Commonly found in normal dogs. Related to breathing: heart quickens on inspiration and slows on expiration	A normal finding in dogs
Premature beats/missed or dropped beats	Auscultation Electrocardiography (ECG)	Caused by ventricles beating prematurely	Medical drug therapy, e.g. propranolol
Atrial fibrillation or 'flutter' (tumultuous heart)	Auscultation ECG	A random variation in heart rhythm More common in large and giant breeds In dogs, may develop as part of congestive heart failure Often accompanies cardiomyopathy	Medical drug therapy, e.g. propranolol
Heart block	Auscultation ECG	Conducting system of heart fails, producing slower and less forceful contractions Varies in severity, most important is third-degree block, resulting in severe bradycardia	Surgical implantation of a pacemaker

Table 20.8 Drugs used in the treatment of heart failure

Drugs used in the treatment of heart failure	Effect of drug	Example of drug
Glycosides	Affect heart muscles, cause stronger contractions	Digitalis
Vasodilators/ACE inhibitors	Increases the diameter of blood vessels, thus increasing the vascular space. ACE inhibitors are especially useful in the treatment of congestive heart failure. They work by blocking angiotensin converting enzyme (ACE), which reduces fluid retention and thus blood pressure	Prazosin, enalapril
Diuretics	Increase urine output, thus removing excess fluid in ascites and oedema	Furosemide
Xanthine derivatives	Act on heart muscle to strengthen contractions	Theophylline
Inodilators	Used in the treatment of congestive heart failure, a vasodilator and acts on heart muscle	Pimobendan

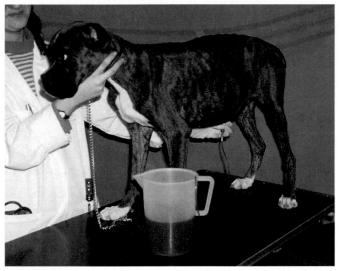

Fig. 20.9 Draining ascitic fluid from a dog

diet with a low sodium content must be fed (see Ch. 7)

- **Weight control** – obesity puts unnecessary overload on the heart. If obese, the patient must lose weight and then maintain a constant weight
- **Exercise** – should be regular and not excessive. Patients must maintain a constant exercise regime in terms of both frequency and amount. It is important to avoid sudden bouts of exercise, as this will put an unexpected overload on the heart. Owners must be warned against 'weekend exercise' when they may take their dog for longer walks than on weekdays.

Cardiac arrest

A 'heart attack' is a failure in cardiac output and is uncommon in dogs and cats. It results mainly from a sudden increase in demand, such as sudden exercise, excitement or an underlying deterioration of an existing medical disease or condition.

Signs of cardiac arrest include:

- No heart beat
- No peripheral pulse/weak or absence of main pulse
- Cyanotic mucous membranes
- Dilated pupils
- Respiratory arrest or apnoea
- Prolonged capillary refill time.

Treatment

This is an emergency and first-aid rules apply (see Ch. 19). These include:

- Establish a patent airway, e.g. using an endotracheal tube, tracheostomy, extend the neck to lengthen airway, extend the tongue and check for anything blocking the pharynx and trachea
- Breathe for the animal – artificial respiration via endotracheal tube or tracheostomy tube or directly into the animal's mouth and nose
- Cardiac massage
- Administration of cardiostimulant drugs
- Electrical stimulation to restart the heart.

Methods of diagnosis of heart disease

Auscultation

Auscultation of the thorax using a stethoscope will identify heart sounds, the heart rate and its rhythm. The optimum area for auscultation is between the third and sixth ribs on the mid-ventral thoracic wall usually on the left side:

- Heart sounds will be muffled if hydrothorax or neoplasia is present
- The area for satisfactory auscultation will be displaced in cases of cardiac neoplasia
- The rate and rhythm of the heart should be noted, as changes to this may indicate heart disease
- A heart murmur is a vibration due to the turbulence of blood flow through the cavity of the heart. Heart murmurs are usually systolic and diastolic murmurs are uncommon. Heart murmurs are graded according to their intensity (Table 20.9)
- Other chest sounds are also heard on auscultation, e.g. respiratory noise, the presence of fluid.

Table 20.9 Gradation of heart murmurs

Heart murmur	Definition
Grade 1	Faint heart murmur that is not immediately heard on auscultation
Grade 2	Faint heart murmur heard within a few seconds
Grade 3	Murmur heard immediately and widespread
Grade 4	A loud heart murmur that is heard with the stethoscope not quite in full contact with the chest wall
Grade 5	Very loud murmur that is heard with the stethoscope slightly withdrawn from the chest wall

Table 20.10 Laboratory tests that may aid the diagnosis of cardiac disease

Laboratory test	Abnormality may indicate heart disease
Leukocytosis	Congestive heart failure
Neutrophilia	Endocarditis
Urea	Congestive heart failure
High liver enzyme levels	Congestive and right-sided heart failure
Low globulin (and other plasma proteins)	Heart failure
High muscle enzymes	Myocardial disease

Radiography

Radiography (see Ch. 30) is used to diagnose changes to heart size, heart chamber enlargement, congenital abnormalities, pleural effusions and dilated blood vessels. A plain radiograph is taken initially, centring over the heart, which is level with the caudal border of the scapula. A dorsoventral view will define the outline of the heart. A lateral view will enable an approximate measurement of the heart within the thoracic cavity to be made. The normal size of the heart should span 2.5–3.5 rib spaces; on a dorsoventral radiograph the heart should fill less than three-quarters of the depth of the thorax.

Introduction of an iodine-based contrast agent such as Conray 420 intravenously to perform an angiogram will assist in diagnosing congenital cardiac defects. Fluoroscopy with angiography is used to diagnose congenital cardiac defects and pleural effusions. (Fluoroscopy converts X-rays into light, multiplies the intensity of the light and then converts it to photoelectrons. A 'moving radiograph' is then seen.)

Ultrasound

Commonly referred to as echocardiography, this uses ultrasonic sound waves to produce an image. As the image is in 'real time' it can be used to visualize the heart as it beats. Doppler ultrasound or ultrasound in M mode is used to examine the movement of blood through the chambers of the heart.

Electrocardiography

Electrocardiography (ECG) is the technique of recording the electrical activity of the heart and is used to investigate the heart rate and rhythm. Electrodes are attached to the forelimbs, a hind limb and the thoracic wall and lead to an amplifier and recording apparatus. To ensure good electrode contact with the skin, the hair should be clipped and surgical spirit applied to the area prior to connecting the electrodes. The patient's coat must be dry and an insulated table will aid contact.

Electrical signals received by the machine are converted to tracings on a screen or a paper strip and provide a permanent record. This ECG trace is then compared to that of a normal animal and is used to make a diagnosis. It must be remembered that an animal that is dying of heart failure will still have an ECG reading – an ECG does not measure cardiac output.

Laboratory tests

There are no specific laboratory tests used in the diagnosis of heart disease but some of the general tests will aid diagnosis (Table 20.10).

Haemopoietic system

Anaemia

Anaemia is a condition in which there is an abnormally low number of circulating red blood cells, which affects the oxygen-carrying capacity of the blood. Anaemia is a clinical sign of an underlying disease rather than a disease itself.

Clinical signs

These are all related to the lack of oxygen reaching the tissues and include:

- Lethargy
- Exercise intolerance
- Pale mucous membranes
- Possible heart murmur
- Tachycardia
- Tachypnoea
- Reduced packed cell volume (PCV).

Causes

Anaemia may be caused by:

- Acute haemorrhage – sudden and excessive loss of red blood cells which may be internal or external, e.g. trauma, surgery, rupture of an organ, clotting disorder, haemangiosarcoma, haemorrhagic gastroenteritis or warfarin poisoning
- Chronic haemorrhage – gradual but extensive loss of red blood cells which may internal or external, e.g.

haematuria, epistaxis, heavy ectoparasite or endoparasite burden, gastrointestinal bleeding
- Haemolysis – excessive destruction of red blood cells, e.g. autoimmune haemolytic anaemia, *Haemobartonella* infection
- Non-regenerative anaemia – insufficient production of replacement red blood cells, e.g. bone marrow hypoplasia, renal disease.

Laboratory tests

These are used to help confirm the diagnosis and to assess the degree of anaemia (see Ch. 29):

- Packed cell volume – measures the percentage of red blood cells within the blood. The normal parameters for the species and the time between onset of the condition and measurement of the PCV should be considered.
- Blood smear – examination of a smear will help to determine whether the anaemia is regenerative or non-regenerative:
  - Regenerative – presence of reticulocytes (immature red blood cells) which are produced to compensate for those being lost
  - Non-regenerative – little or no evidence of reticulocytes and there will be insufficient new red blood cells to compensate for the loss. Associated with bone marrow problems, chronic inflammation and renal disease.

Treatment

This should be aimed at the specific cause but very often the patient is treated symptomatically. The following are used:

- Corticosteroids – to reduce inflammatory processes
- Vitamin K$_1$ – involved in the formation of clotting factors in the liver
- Good-quality, high-protein diet provides the nutrients for the formation of body tissues
- Dietary supplements, e.g. vitamin B and iron
- Intravenous fluid therapy – blood transfusion or colloids where acute haemorrhage is present
- Stress-free environment and cage rest.

Lymphoma

Lymphoma is a neoplastic condition of the lymphocytes and is also known as lymphosarcoma. It is a relatively common disease in both dogs and cats. In cats lymphoma is associated with feline leukaemia virus (FeLV) infection; however, in dogs, lymphoma is a spontaneous condition. The most common form of the disease involves the infiltration of various organs (Table 20.11). Clinical signs relate to the system involved but may include enlargement of the affected organ, e.g. lymphadenopathy or enlargement of the lymph nodes (Fig. 20.10). In some cases the affected organ may fail, e.g. renal failure. Some lymphomas secrete a parathormone-like hormone, which induces hypocalcaemia.

Diagnosis of lymphoma is confirmed by taking a biopsy of the affected tissue. Some cases respond well to chemotherapy, e.g. thymic and multicentric lymphoma. It is very unusual for cases of lymphoma to recover.

Table 20.11 Types of lymphoma

Affected organ	Type of lymphoma
Lymph nodes	Multicentric lymphoma
Gastrointestinal tract	Alimentary lymphoma (Fig. 22.10)
Thymus	Thymic lymphoma
Kidneys	Renal lymphoma
Skin	Mycosis fungoides

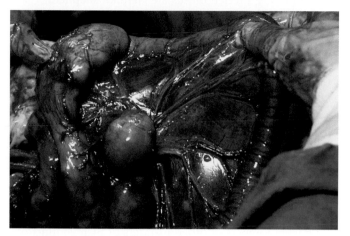

Fig. 20.10 Alimentary lymphoma

Leukaemia

Leukaemia is a special form of lymphoma in which there is an abnormally high number of white blood cells, in particular lymphocytes, in the peripheral circulation. This is a result of bone marrow neoplasia. Leukaemia is rare in dogs and cats and may present as a chronic or acute condition. Chronic lymphocytic leukaemia responds reasonably well to chemotherapy but the acute form has a poor prognosis. Leukaemia is diagnosed by haematology and confirmed by bone marrow biopsy.

Blood clotting and bleeding disorders

- **Rodenticide poisoning** – most commonly due to warfarin and related agents, which cause a disruption in blood clotting. Warfarin poisoning is more common in dogs. Treat with vitamin K$_1$ and supportive therapy
- **Thrombocytopenia** – this is a low platelet count due to an autoimmune destruction of platelets (autoimmune-mediated thrombocytopenia) or bone marrow suppression. Suppression of the bone marrow is caused by lymphoma or oestrogen toxicity, e.g. during the oestrus period in ferrets, Sertoli cell tumour and excessive oestrogen therapy
- **Von Willebrand's disease** – this is an inherited bleeding disorder affecting both males and females. The affected animal lacks the von Willebrand factor, which is an essential part of normal haemostasis. Some cases show spontaneous haemorrhage, while others have only abnormal bleeding following trauma

or surgery. Treat by the administration of a blood transfusion and supportive care. There is a breed disposition to von Willebrand's disease – Dobermans are commonly affected

- **Haemophilia** – this is a deficiency of factor VIII or factor IX in the clotting cascade. It is a sex-linked inherited disease seen in males and carried by the X chromosome. It is rare for females to be affected but they can carry the disease and pass it to their offspring. Unless the animal suffers trauma or requires surgery, haemophilia is unlikely to be identified until routine neutering is performed. Commonly affected breeds are German shepherd dogs and Dobermans.

Tests for clotting and bleeding disorders

Diagnosis is by:

- **Buccal mucosal bleeding time (BMBT)** – a reliable method of measuring platelet number and function. A commercially available kit is used to make a small incision in the lip and the lost blood is then blotted with filter paper. The time is measured from making the incision to when bleeding stops. The normal buccal mucosal bleeding time for a dog is 1.7–4.2 minutes; in the cat normal bleeding time is 1.4–2.4 minutes. A longer than normal buccal mucosal bleeding time indicates von Willebrand's disease, low platelet numbers or other disorders of platelet function
- **Activated clotting time (ACT)** – measured by collecting blood into an ACT tube, keeping at body temperature and after 60 seconds examining for clot formation. A clot should form within 90 seconds. A longer time than this indicates the possibility of a clotting disorder. Further clotting tests can be performed by commercial laboratories
- **Measurement of platelet numbers** by routine haematology tests
- **The von Willebrand antigen test** examines the genetic status of suspected individuals.

Nervous system

Epilepsy

Epilepsy is a disorder in which an irritable focus within the brain causes disorganized electrical activity resulting in convulsions or fits and a sudden loss of consciousness. It is a condition affecting dogs, rather than cats (see also Ch. 19). Convulsions are violent and uncoordinated contractions of muscles that occur when the animal has lost consciousness. The animal has periods of alternating relaxation and heightened muscular activity, which raises the body temperature. Box 20.2 shows the advice to be given to the owner of a dog during its convulsions.

Epilepsy is more common in some breeds, e.g. poodles, German shepherds, Cavalier King Charles spaniels. The cause is often unknown, i.e. idiopathic, but may be due to:

- Neoplasia of the brain
- Meningitis
- Hyperthermia
- Bacterial infection
- Viral infection
- Poisoning
- Renal disease
- Hypoglycaemia
- Hypocalcaemia
- Hydrocephalus.

Clinical signs

The convulsion is divided into three phases:

- **Pre-ictal phase** – the period of time just prior to the fit starting. Animals may be restless, anxious (described as an 'aura'), be asleep or appear normal with no noticeable signs
- **Ictal phase** – the animal collapses, falls on to its side, loses consciousness and moves its legs in a 'paddling' motion. Often the animal will involuntarily urinate and defecate and may chomp its jaws. Convulsions are very distressing for the owners to witness
- **Postictal phase** – the time immediately following the convulsion, when the animal may appear dazed or disorientated, gradually returning to its normal demeanour. The animal may appear to be exhausted and will sleep for several hours.

Status epilepticus is a series of repeated convulsions without the animal regaining consciousness, and is life-threatening. **Petit mal** is a short minor convulsion where slight muscle tremor is noticed but a full convulsion does not take place.

A convulsion is often witnessed by the owner and, since it only lasts for a few minutes, is rarely seen by veterinary staff. The advice given to owners whilst their dog is convulsing is shown in Box 20.2. The animal will appear perfectly normal on later clinical examination. It is important that a thorough and detailed history is taken from the owner and the person who saw the convulsion in order to be able to both determine the timing of the convulsion and its likely cause. In order to determine the exact cause of epilepsy, a number of tests may be performed, e.g. haematology, biochemistry, magnetic resonance imaging scan, urinalysis and cerebrospinal fluid tap.

Treatment

If it is known, removal of the underlying cause will prevent further attacks. In cases of idiopathic epilepsy, long-term anticonvulsive drug therapy is recommended. The animal will require a maintenance dose of an anticonvulsant, e.g. phenobarbital. Oral anticonvulsants are not used during a

---

Box 20.2 Advice to owners during convulsions

- Make a note of the time convulsions begin
- Monitor the animal and observe exactly what happens during the convulsion
- Remove any harmful objects from the animal's reach
- Maintain a darkened, quiet environment
- Do not move or handle the animal during convulsions
- Reassure the animal once convulsions cease
- Make an appointment at the veterinary surgery for a clinical examination once convulsions have ceased

convulsion but intravenous or rectal anticonvulsants may be administered.

Ataxia

Ataxia is defined as an irregular or unsteady gait caused by incoordination of the muscles. Causes of ataxia include muscle weakness, depression of the central nervous system, disease of the vestibular (balance) centre and spinal disease. A detailed clinical history will aid diagnosis. A detailed neurological examination must be carried out to determine the severity of ataxia and the presence of accompanying clinical signs.

Neurological examination

The patient will require a full neurological examination to assist in the diagnosis. Table 20.12 shows the neurological tests performed during a clinical examination.

Paralysis

Paralysis is the loss of voluntary muscle control resulting in either a partial or complete loss of movement in the affected body part (Fig. 20.11). Paralysis is due to nerve damage and is commonly a result of trauma to the brain or spinal cord. It may be further defined according to the extent of the paralysis:

- **Paraplegia** – paralysis of both hind limbs
- **Tetraplegia or quadriplegia** – paralysis of all four limbs
- **Hemiplegia** – paralysis of one side of the body.

Paresis is defined as muscular weakness and is often described as partial or incomplete paralysis.

A detailed neurological examination is performed to determine the extent of paresis or paralysis. The underlying cause must be treated or removed to gain long-term treatment.

Table 20.12 Neurological tests performed during a clinical examination

Body part	Examination
Consciousness	Fully conscious
	Depressed
	Stuporous
	Comatose
Posture	Presence of a head tilt
	Position of the head in relation to rest of the body
	Wheelbarrow reaction – hold animal's hind limbs and abdomen so all the weight is supported on the front limbs, 'walk' the animal forwards and backwards using a wheelbarrow motion – the normal animal is able to perform this
Spine	Visually examine the position of the spine for lordosis, scoliosis or kyphosis
	Spinal reflexes: • Patellar or quadriceps myotactic reflex, tested with a hammer • Flexor reflexes – skin between the toes is pinched, normal reflex is to withdraw the foot
Limbs	Increased or decreased muscle tone
	Limbs held in extension
	Normal stance or wide gait
	Presence of knuckling over of feet (proprioception)
	Proprioceptive positioning reaction – flex animal's foot until dorsal aspect is in contact with the floor – normal reaction is to replace foot correctly on floor
	Alternatively, place animal's foot on a piece of paper and withdraw the paper laterally in a sudden movement – normal reaction is to regain normal stance
Movement (examine standing still and during movement)	Presence of any involuntary movements
	Note the animal's gait
	Presence of muscular spasms
	Presence of muscular tremors
Skin	Panniculus reflex is tested by bilaterally pinching skin on flanks with a pair of forceps – normal reaction is a bilateral twitching of the panniculus muscle under the skin
Anus	Anal reflex is tested by stroking ring of anus with a solid object – winking of the anus should be seen

Nursing care

- Patients with paralysis are unable to walk unaided, urinate and defecate, and must be walking-assisted by the use of a long towel (see Chs 15 and 16) or walked with the aid of slings placed under the abdomen or hind limbs to support the patient's weight. In cases where the animal is unable to support any of its weight an indwelling urinary catheter and collection bag avoids urine scalding and maintains constant bladder drainage
- Soiled bedding must be changed immediately and any long hair around the perineum must be clipped to aid the passage of faeces and keep the anal area clean
- Monitoring of urine and faecal output is important and should be recorded on the hospital chart
- Soft bedding will alleviate decubitus ulcers on pressure points; for example, a plastic-covered deep foam mattress with a Vetbed covering will provide comfort and cushioning
- Turning the patient every 2–4 hours will prevent hypostatic pneumonia
- Provide support to position the animal in lateral or sternal recumbency, e.g. foam wedges and sand bags.
- Grooming the animal maintains patient interest and keeps the coat clean and free from matts
- Ensure food and water is within the patient's reach. Use hand feeding if necessary and syringe water into the mouth if the patient is unable to move the head and neck. Tube feeding will provide adequate nutrition in cases when the patient is unable to consume sufficient food (see Ch. 15)
- The paraplegic patient is not always able to maintain its body temperature because it is unable to move around.

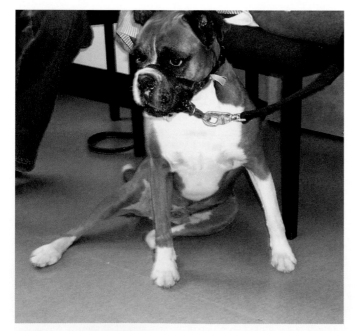

Fig. 20.11 A paralysed dog

- Monitoring and recording patient vital signs, including temperature, is important. Avoid hyperthermia by the use of fans
- Physiotherapy of the limbs and the use of coupage are required to stimulate the patient and aid healing of affected tissue.

Endocrine system

There are several endocrine diseases that affect both dogs and cats. Table 20.13 shows their cause and effects.

Diabetes mellitus

This is a disease caused by the degeneration of the beta cells within the islets of Langerhans of the pancreas, which fail to secret the hormone insulin (Table 20.13). Insulin lowers the blood glucose levels by enabling glucose to pass through the cell membranes into the cells, where it is used as source of energy and any excess glucose is stored in the liver as glycogen. Lack of insulin leads to hyperglycaemia, or raised blood glucose levels, and the clinical signs of diabetes mellitus are a result of this.

There are two types of diabetes mellitus:

- Insulin-resistant diabetes – most commonly seen in cats. Insulin is secreted but the tissues fail to respond
- Insulin-dependent diabetes – most common in dogs. The pancreas fails to produce insulin.

Clinical signs

Initially the patient is bright and shows polyuria, polydipsia and polyphagia. As the condition advances the patient may show anorexia, weakness, lethargy, vomiting and diarrhoea; some may develop cataracts. If left untreated, the body begins to utilize protein and fat as an energy source, resulting in metabolic acidosis and a build-up of ketones – ketoacidosis. This is an emergency and the patient will show signs of depression, leading to inappetence, vomiting and later coma. Insulin and intravenous fluid therapy are administered. Blood glucose levels are monitored hourly. Once ketoacidosis is reversed the patient then receives the usual treatment for diabetes mellitus.

Laboratory tests

These are used to confirm the diagnosis. Urinalysis will show the presence of glucose in the urine and in advanced cases may also show ketonuria. Blood tests will show a raised fasting blood glucose level.

Treatment

Treatment requires the owner to administer daily insulin injections balanced by a rigid regime of regular amounts of exercise and a constant amount of food given at the same time every day. Table 20.14 provides the details of the management of the condition.

Table 20.13 Endocrine disorders

Endocrine disease	Comments	Clinical signs	Diagnostic tests	Treatment
Diabetes insipidus (DI)	May be due to: 1) Pituitary gland fails to produce ADH (central diabetes insipidus) due to a pituitary tumour or trauma 2) Failure of kidneys to respond to ADH (nephrogenic diabetes insipidus)	Pronounced polydipsia and polyuria Production of very dilute urine	Urinalysis – low specific gravity Water deprivation test Slightly high PCV	Central diabetes insipidus – administer synthetic ADH, e.g. desmopressin in the form of nasal or eye drops Nephrogenic diabetes insipidus – guarded prognosis, drug therapy may reduce urine output but no long-term effective treatment is available
Hyperadrenocorticalism (Cushing's disease)	Common in dogs, rare in cats Excessive levels of cortisol are produced from the adrenal glands due to either: 1) An adrenal gland tumour or 2) A pituitary gland tumour – most common type – causes excess of adrenocorticotrophic hormone (ACTH), which stimulates adrenals to produce excess amounts of cortisol	Polyphagia Polydipsia Polyuria Bilateral alopecia on lateral flanks Muscle wastage 'Pot-bellied' appearance Possible change in coat colour Calcinosis cutis (calcium deposits in the skin)	ACTH stimulation test showing high post-stimulation cortisol levels Dexamethasone suppression test Increased blood alkaline phosphatase (ALP) Ultrasound to identify adrenal gland enlargement	If due to adrenal tumour – adrenalectomy (usually only one adrenal gland is affected so one remains intact) If due to pituitary tumour – drug therapy, e.g. oral mitotane or trilostane, suppresses adrenal function, maintenance dose for long-term use once condition is under control NB Health and safety note – gloves must be worn when handling mitotane
Hypothyroidism (Fig. 20.12)	Rare in cats Common in dogs aged 6–10 years Usually associated with autoimmune disease or thyroid gland atrophy	Cold and clammy skin Lethargy Weight gain Poor appetite Muscle weakness Bilateral alopecia of flanks Loss of temporal facial muscle to give a 'drawn' facial expression	Thyroxine (T_4) Thyroid stimulating hormone (TSH) test Raised liver enzymes High cholesterol levels	Oral thyroxine drug medication, long-term medication required NB Regular monitoring of thyroid hormone levels is necessary
Hyperthyroidism	Very rare in dogs Commonly seen in cats aged > 10 years Most are due to benign thyroid tumours causing excess production of thyroid hormone NB Most common endocrine disease in cats	Restlessness Aggression Polyphagia Tachycardia Weight loss Diarrhoea Poor coat Poor skin Mass palpable in thyroid gland (goitre)	T_4 Clinical examination: enlarged thyroid gland is palpable	Thyroidectomy of affected gland (preferred treatment) Radiotherapy using iodine-131 Carbimazole drug therapy but difficult to stabilize in long-term management NB Frequently, during surgical intervention, the parathyroid glands are damaged or removed inadvertently. This causes hypocalcaemia and the animal may show signs of muscle tremors and convulsions. Clinical signs indicate hypocalcaemia. Immediate treatment is necessary – calcium and vitamin D supplementation is essential. During the immediate postoperative period following thyroidectomy the patient is monitored for signs of low blood calcium levels. Calcium supplementation is sometimes only required for a few weeks postoperatively if the parathyroid glands are still intact and only disturbed during surgery

(Continued)

Table 20.13 Continued

Endocrine disease	Comments	Clinical signs	Diagnostic tests	Treatment
Diabetes mellitus (DM)	Commonly affects middle-aged entire bitches Also affects cats Due to a carbohydrate metabolism problem Blood sugar levels increase as cells do not take up glucose due to an insulin shortage. Glucose remains in the circulation and is eventually excreted in urine. NB In the normal animal, insulin is secreted by beta cells in the pancreas when blood glucose naturally rises, e.g. following a meal. Insulin lowers the blood glucose level by increasing the uptake of glucose into the cells and by storing glucose	Polydipsia Polyuria Polyphagia Obesity As the condition worsens: Anorexia Vomiting Diarrhoea Dehydration Lethargy	High blood glucose levels	Establish a strict daily routine: 1) Using urine dipstick, measure glucose in early morning free-flow urine sample 2) Follow a strict high-fibre diet; exact amounts at same time each day 3) Daily injections of insulin – either once a day or twice daily 4) Neuter entire females to maintain hormone stability 5) Treat underlying medical conditions/diseases
Hypoadrenocorticism (Addison's disease)	Affects mainly dogs Caused by atrophy of the adrenal cortex, resulting in decreased amounts of cortisol and mineralocorticoid production and a severe sodium and potassium imbalance Often an autoimmune disease	Vomiting Diarrhoea Anorexia Lethargy Collapse Signs of dehydration Bradycardia NB Clinical signs are often intermittent	Low blood sodium and high blood potassium levels ACTH stimulation test (showing low cortisol levels that do not rise following administration of ACTH)	Oral hormone replacement – synthetic mineralocorticoids, e.g. Florinef, and glucocorticoids, e.g. prednisolone
Insulinoma	A tumour of the beta cells in the Islets of Langerhans of the pancreas that produce insulin. An excess of insulin is produced	Signs of hypoglycaemia Collapse Convulsions	Low blood glucose levels Ultrasound to identify insulinoma	Surgical intervention to remove the insulinoma although the tumour is highly likely to metastatize, so successful treatment is not possible. Drug therapy, e.g. diazoxide or prednisolone, will manage the clinical signs but not provide a permanent solution

The standard treatment is to provide insulin in the form of regular injections. There are three main forms of insulin:

- Short-acting insulin – this is given intravenously or intramuscularly. It has a rapid effect and does not last for long and is used in hyperglycaemic emergencies. A patient is unlikely to be stabilized using this form of insulin
- Intermediate-acting insulin – may be given twice a day
- Long-acting insulin also called lente insulin – the activity of the insulin is slowed down by the addition of zinc. There are several forms of lente insulin and the timing of peak activity is related to the size of the

zinc insulin crystals. This is given subcutaneously and is the form used for most diabetic animals.

Injectable insulin is either derived from pork or beef and is available as a veterinary product only, or is available as human recombinant insulin.

At the start of treatment care is taken to identify which type of insulin suits the patient. Cats may be difficult to stabilize as they tend to suffer with stress hyperglycaemia which is exacerbated by such things as being in the hospital kennels and handling. Blood glucose curves may be used to assist in the initial stabilization of the patient or in the later stages, to help identify the reason for problems in stabilization. Regular blood glucose levels are plotted at hourly intervals on a graph. From these results it is possible to recognize

Table 20.14 **Management of diabetes mellitus**

Treatment	Details
Monitoring of urine sample for presence of glucose	Collection of a free-flow early morning urine sample. Measure glucose level using a urine dipstick that shows both glucose and ketone levels. Calculate the dose of insulin required according to the level of glucose present in the urine
Diet	Food must be given in relation to insulin administration; see below under Administration of insulin for details. A high-fibre diet allows weight control, slows gastric emptying, slows glucose absorption from the small intestine and prolongs the time during which glucose is absorbed The same diet must be fed at the same time each day to maintain the stability of this condition. No titbits are fed
Administration of insulin	The daily levels of glucose found in the urine determine the amount of insulin required. The insulin bottle is agitated to suspend the contents, an insulin syringe is used to withdraw the correct amount of insulin and is injected subcutaneously Insulin is either administered once or twice daily: • If administering once-daily insulin, one-third of the food is given with insulin and two-thirds of the food is given 8 h later • If administering twice-daily insulin, the food is divided into two equal meals, each meal given with the dose of insulin Insulin must be administered at the same time/s each day
Exercise	The same level of exercise at the same time each day and for the same amount of time. A change to the animal's exercise regime will increase the uptake of glucose and upset the stability of the animal's condition

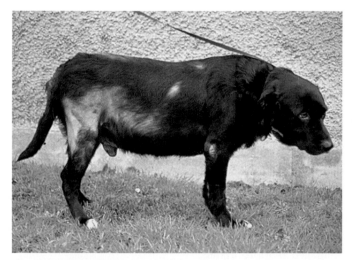

Fig. 20.12 Dog with hypothyroidism

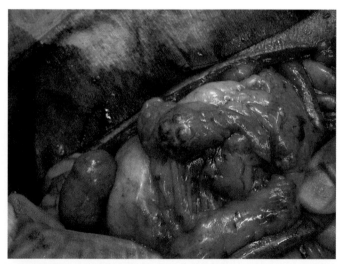

Fig. 20.13 Insulinoma in a dog

peaks and troughs in the blood glucose levels related to the activity of the insulin in use. The feeding times and periods of exercise are also plotted on the graph and will help to indicate any reasons as to why the patient is not stabilizing on the treatment.

Hypoglycaemia

Defined as an abnormally low blood glucose level, this is a common complication of the management of diabetes mellitus. It is often referred to as 'hypo'. The most likely cause

of hypoglycaemia is an overdose of insulin, either by injecting too much or because the animal has not eaten and the insulin has no glucose on which to act. An insulinoma (tumour of the pancreas) will also cause hypoglycaemia (Fig. 20.13).

Clinical signs

Present within 8 hours of insulin injection. The animal may shake and appear weak, lethargic and ataxic, and may collapse and go into a coma.

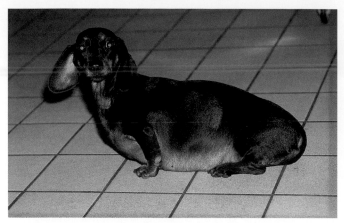

Fig. 20.14 Dog with Cushing's disease

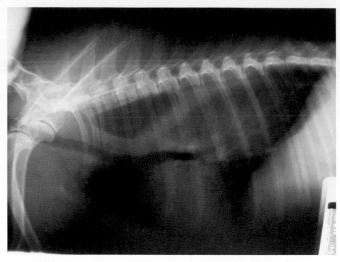

Fig. 20.15 Radiograph of a dog with megaoesophagus

Treatment

If the animal is conscious it should be offered sugary food, e.g. honey, chocolate, sweet biscuits, sugar or glucose solution; if unconscious the veterinary surgeon will administer intravenous glucose saline.

Cushing's disease

This is also called hyperadrenocorticalism and results from excessive levels of adrenal corticosteroids. Clinical signs of the condition are shown in Table 20.13. The diagnosis may be confirmed by the:

Adrenocorticotrophic hormone stimulation test – this is used to aid the diagnosis of Cushing's disease (Fig. 20.14) or of Addison's disease, which is hypoadrenocorticalism. Adrenocorticotrophic hormone (ACTH) is normally secreted by the pituitary gland to stimulate the secretion of cortisol from the adrenal cortex. A blood sample is taken and cortisol levels are measured. A synthetic ACTH, e.g. Synacthen, is then administered intravenously and blood cortisol levels are measured again within 60–90 minutes of the injection.

Dexamethasone suppression test – a high or low-dose dexamethasone test is used to aid diagnosis of Cushing's disease. A blood sample is taken and cortisol levels are measured. Intravenous dexamethasone is administered and blood cortisol levels are measured at 3 and 8 hours following injection. In the normal animal, dexamethasone suppresses adrenal function and an absence of cortisol is found in blood following administration of dexamethasone. In the animal with suspected Cushing's disease, a low-dose dexamethasone test will show incomplete suppression of cortisol production. A high-dose dexamethasone suppression test is used to distinguish between adrenal- and pituitary-dependent Cushing's disease.

Diabetes insipidus

This results from the failure in production of antidiuretic hormone (ADH) from the posterior pituitary gland or a failure of the kidneys to respond to ADH. The clinical signs are polyuria, polydipsia and the production of urine with a low specific gravity (SG) (Table 20.13). The diagnosis may be confirmed by performing the water deprivation test:

- The bladder is drained by catheterization and the SG of the urine is measured
- The animal's weight is recorded. Calculate 5% of the body weight
- Place the animal in a cage and withhold food and water
- Collect a urine sample every 1–2 hours – catheterization is often necessary.
- Measure the SG and weigh the animal
- Repeat until 5% of bodyweight is lost. At this point a normal animal will have concentrated its urine and SG should exceed 1.030. Animals with diabetes insipidus are unable to concentrate the urine and the SG will remain the same.

The water deprivation test must not be used in patients that display signs of dehydration or in cases where alternative causes of polydipsia and polyuria have not been investigated fully. Should the patient show any signs of dehydration during the test, it must be abandoned immediately. Constant monitoring of the patient undergoing a water deprivation test is vital as it is potentially harmful if managed inappropriately.

Digestive system

Regurgitation

Regurgitation is defined as the return of undigested material from the stomach via the mouth. The animal will show no abdominal effort in regurgitating and it occurs shortly after eating. It is vital that owners are able to distinguish whether their animal is vomiting or regurgitating. Causes include:

- Megaoesophagus (Fig. 20.15)
- Vascular ring anomaly/persistent right aortic arch

- Oesophageal stricture
- Oesophageal foreign body
- Oesophagitis.

Vomiting or emesis

Vomiting is defined as the violent expulsion of stomach contents via the mouth. Forceful abdominal contractions are required to eject the vomitus and it occurs several hours after eating. The vomit may be partly digested food from the intestines, bile or water. Severe cases of vomiting will lead to dehydration and a loss of electrolytes. Causes include:

- Gastritis
- Distension of the stomach following intestinal obstruction
- Gastric ulceration
- Gastric neoplasia
- Gastric foreign body
- Gastric dilatation
- Infection
- Systemic disease.

Blood tests may be used to monitor electrolyte levels and dehydration. Radiography will identify an obstruction or foreign body. Endoscopy will identify gastritis and gastric ulceration.

Treatment

Removal of the underlying cause of vomiting is essential. Intravenous fluid therapy is used to treat dehydration. Surgery is necessary to remove foreign bodies and repair gastric dilatation. Withholding food will allow the gastrointestinal tract time to recover from episodes of vomiting. Medical management of gastritis and ulceration may be needed.

Diarrhoea

Diarrhoea is defined as abnormally frequent emptying of the bowel, usually producing soft and watery faeces. Fluid and electrolytes are lost in diarrhoea resulting in dehydration and leading to metabolic acidosis (Fig. 20.16). Causes, some of which may be life-threatening, include:

- Colitis
- Enteritis
- Bacterial infection
- Viral infection
- Heavy intestinal parasite burden
- Stress
- Secondary to systemic disease
- Neoplasia of the gastrointestinal tract
- Dietary hypersensitivity
- Sudden dietary change
- Intestinal foreign body
- Malabsorption conditions
- Inflammatory bowel disease.

A full clinical examination and client history will determine whether the diarrhoea is due to a problem in the

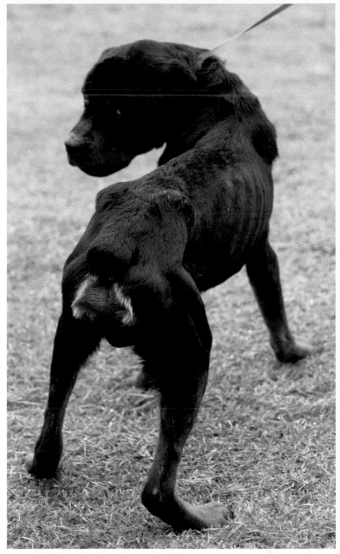

Fig. 20.16 A rottweiler with emaciation caused by prolonged diarrhoea

gastrointestinal system or whether a systemic disease, e.g. Addison's or pancreatic disease, is present. Some patients with diarrhoea appear bright and alert while others are lethargic and non-responsive. Less severe cases respond well to simple dietary management while more severe cases require aggressive fluid therapy and supportive treatment. It is useful to determine whether the diarrhoea is from the large or small intestine (Table 20.15).

Diagnosis of the cause of the diarrhoea is based on a range of tests including radiography, haematology, faecal tests, ultrasound, biopsies and endoscopy.

Management

- Identify and treat the underlying disease
- Fluid therapy to correct fluid, electrolyte loss and metabolic acidosis
- Antibiotics if bacterial infection present
- Parasiticides if parasite burden present
- Surgery to remove neoplasia or an obstruction
- Dietary tests to establish hypersensitivity

Table 20.15 Comparison between small intestinal and large intestinal diarrhoea

Small intestinal diarrhoea	Large intestinal diarrhoea
Large volume of diarrhoea	Small volume of diarrhoea
Very soft/liquid faeces	Soft faeces; fresh blood or mucus may be present
Diarrhoea passed less frequently: 3–5 times daily	Diarrhoea passed more frequently: 8–12 times daily

- Dietary management
- Drug therapy, e.g. in cases of chronic diarrhoea.

Constipation

Constipation is the failure to pass faeces in either the normal amount or normal frequency. Constipation is more common in elderly patients that have reduced exercise. Causes include:

- Dehydration – producing excessively dry faeces
- Low-residue diet
- Neoplasia of the intestinal tract
- Foreign body in the intestinal tract
- Prostatic disease – obstructing the rectum
- Pelvic fracture
- Spinal paralysis.

Constipation is often presented as faecal tenesmus, i.e. straining, and the animal will feel pain on defecation and will not be able to empty the rectum fully because of hard, impacted faeces. This is treated with an enema (see Ch.15). Surgical removal of an obstruction such as a foreign body or neoplasia will relieve constipation. Prevention of constipation includes feeding a high-fibre diet and encouraging the animal to take regular exercise and to defecate at regular times during the day.

Pancreatitis

Pancreatitis is defined as inflammation of the pancreas. It occurs in dogs and occasionally in cats. Table 20.16 describes the types of pancreatitis and their treatment.

Exocrine pancreatic insufficiency

Exocrine pancreatic insufficiency (EPI) is a result of the pancreas producing insufficient amounts of pancreatic enzymes, which means that the animal is unable to digest fat. EPI often occurs in dogs of 1–2 years of age, commonly German shepherd dogs. Affected animals initially develop well but then lose weight, have a ravenous appetite and produce pale, rancid faeces (steatorrhoea), with possible diarrhoea, and are coprophagic. Diagnosis is based on a serum trypsin-like immunoreactivity test (TLI). Treatment depends on the provision of pancreatic enzymes, usually given orally. Dietary management is also important and the dog should be given a low-fat but easily digestible diet.

Table 20.16 Types of pancreatitis

Type	Clinical signs/ diagnosis	Cause	Treatment
Acute pancreatitis			
Interstitial pancreatitis – more common in middle-aged bitches	Vomiting, lethargy, abdominal pain, melaena, haematemesis, high blood sugar	Often unknown, possibly due to high-fat diet, viral infection, e.g. parvovirus, corticosteroid therapy, inherited, *Toxoplasma gondii* infection in cats	Withhold food for 72 h and then introduce low-fat diet, fluid therapy, antibiotics, analgesia
Haemorrhagic – more common in male dogs	As above but more severe	As above	As above
Chronic pancreatitis			
May occur following episode of acute pancreatitis (dogs), low-grade constant inflammation of pancreas accompanying acute interstitial pancreatitis (cats)	Signs associated with diabetes mellitus, on palpation the pancreas feels hard	Idiopathic, biliary obstruction	Treatment of clinical signs, fluid therapy, dietary management (low-fat diet), analgesia

Liver disease

The liver has a huge capacity for regeneration and a substantial loss of hepatic tissue (around 70%) is present before any clinical signs of liver disease are seen. Clinical signs of liver disease are often non-specific because the liver is affected by many other metabolic diseases. Causes include:

- Infectious canine hepatitis
- Leptospirosis
- Poisons
- Drug overdose
- Hepatic trauma, e.g. following road traffic accident
- Primary neoplasia of liver or bile ducts (less common than secondary neoplasia)
- Bile duct obstruction
- Secondary neoplasia
- Storage diseases/enzyme deficiencies, e.g. copper toxicosis in Bedlington terriers
- Secondary to cardiac disease, diabetes mellitus, hyperadrenocorticalism, hypothyroidism.

Confirmation of liver disease is by blood biochemistry tests, e.g. ALT, serum alkaline phosphatase (SAP), bilirubin, plasma proteins, haematology (see Ch. 29). Radiography of the liver is used to determine size and position, ultrasound, biopsy to confirm a diagnosis and exploratory laparotomy. Management of liver disease involves the use of supportive therapy until a definitive diagnosis is made.

Splenic disease

An enlarged spleen is usually palpable on clinical examination but it must be remembered that general anaesthesia with some barbiturates causes a temporary enlargement of the spleen. Causes of splenic disease include:

- Neoplasia, e.g. lymphoma or haemangiosarcoma
- Viral or bacterial infection
- Splenic torsion
- Idiopathic
- Anaemia.

Radiography and ultrasound are used to confirm the diagnosis. Surgical intervention, i.e. splenectomy, is often the preferred treatment.

Jaundice

Jaundice, also known as icterus, is defined as staining of the tissues by the yellow bile pigment bilirubin, produced in the liver as a result of haemoglobin breakdown. Diagnosis is confirmed by measuring plasma bilirubin, routine haematology, analysis of blood liver enzymes and the presence of pale faeces.

Jaundice is treated by identifying and treating the underlying cause, which includes:

- Obstruction of the bile duct, e.g. gallstones
- Haemolysis (jaundice often occurs when the liver is overloaded with bilirubin)
- Blood transfusion reaction
- Leptospirosis
- Leishmaniasis
- Haemobartonellosis
- Babesiasis
- Hepatic jaundice – accompanies liver disease.

Portosystemic shunt

This is a vascular abnormality where the hepatic portal vein empties directly into the caudal vena cava, thus bypassing the liver (Fig. 20.17). A portosystemic shunt may be either congenital (most common) or acquired. Diagnosis is confirmed by analysing blood liver enzymes, radiography and ultrasound. Typically, affected animals have a small liver. Treatment is by surgical correction.

Reproductive system

Female

Many of the problems associated with the female reproductive tract are treated surgically; however, some, such as

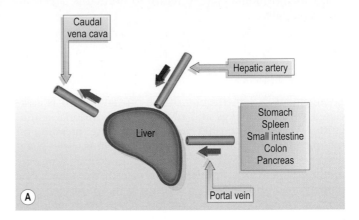

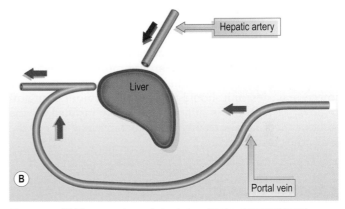

Fig. 20.17 (**A**) The normal portal circulation. (**B**) The abnormal portal circulation seen in cases of portosystemic shunt

pyometra, may be managed medically to stabilize the bitch before an ovariohysterectomy is performed.

False pregnancy (pseudocyesis or pseudopregnancy)

This condition is commonly associated with the bitch, although it may occur in the queen as a result of a sterile mating. Symptoms in the queen are simply a failure to return to oestrus.

False pregnancy may occur about 40–60 days after oestrus and is linked with high levels of circulating progesterone secreted by the corpus luteum. This is a normal part of the oestrous cycle but only a small percentage of bitches develop symptoms. Those that show signs in one oestrous cycle are likely to show them during subsequent cycles.

Clinical signs include maternal behaviour, e.g. nursing soft toys or slippers, nest-making, aggression to anyone who tries to remove the toy, mammary development and lactation. Some bitches may be more seriously ill, with vomiting and loss of appetite.

Before treatment is instigated, check that the bitch is not actually pregnant. Hormones to suppress lactation can be given, e.g. oestradiol benzoate or methyl testosterone over several days and in a reducing dose. A bitch that has repeated false pregnancies should be spayed during anoestrus. The idea that a bitch should be allowed to have a litter in order to get the hormonal cycle to return to normal is largely an old wives' tale.

Male

Prostatic disease

Enlargement or hypertrophy of the prostate gland is associated with older dogs and results from hormonal stimulation. The gland pushes upwards, causing pressure on the rectum and consequent faecal tenesmus. The gland may become infected by ascending infection from the urethra, which runs through the centre of the gland. The patient may show signs of cystitis and, in severe cases, pyrexia, anorexia and weight loss. Cysts and neoplasia may also develop inside the prostate gland. Diagnosis is confirmed by rectal palpation, radiography and the use of ultrasound.

Treatment usually includes castration, which will reduce the size of the gland. Chemical castration by the use of delmadinone acetate may give an indication as to whether surgical castration will produce a permanent response. If infection is present it should respond to antibiotics. Surgical removal of tumours is difficult and rarely justified, as the tumour metastasizes readily. Radiotherapy may relieve the symptoms for a time.

Sertoli cell tumour

This tumour of the Sertoli cells, which line the seminiferous tubules within the testis and secrete oestrogen, is usually associated with a retained testis. Clinical signs often seen in dogs over 6 years old include bilateral symmetrical alopecia over the flanks, enlargement of the mammary tissue and onset of attractiveness to male dogs. The unaffected testis may be atrophied. Diagnosis is based on clinical signs, and hormonal assay demonstrating high levels of oestrogen.

Treatment is by removal of the affected testis. Retained testis or cryptorchism is an inherited characteristic and an affected animal should be castrated to prevent the risk of developing a Sertoli cell tumour in later life.

Neoplasia

Neoplasia or the development of a tumour or cancer is an uncontrolled proliferation of a single type of cell. Neoplasia can affect most tissues of the body but the behaviour of the individual types of tumour in terms of growth rate and the method, degree and site of spread (metastasis) depend on the cell type.

Tumours can be classed as:

- **Benign** – grows slowly and do not often spread to other sites. Their size may cause symptoms by pressing on adjacent organs
- **Malignant** – locally invasive and metastasizes to other organs by means of the blood or lymphatic systems. This type is more likely to cause clinical signs.

Chemotherapy, giving cytotoxic drugs, is used in the treatment of neoplasia in both cats and dogs (Fig. 20.18). These highly potent drugs either destroy rapidly dividing neoplastic cells or inhibit their growth. They have a very narrow dose range so that the drug kills the neoplastic cells but causes minimal damage to surrounding body cells (Table 20.17). The calculation of the dose rate is based on the patient's surface area rather than body weight. This is because the blood supply to the liver and kidneys is related to body surface area rather than body weight.

Cytotoxic drugs are excreted via the liver and kidneys and must be used with extreme care in animals with compromised renal or liver function, since their excretion may be impaired and toxicity could occur.

Side effects from cytotoxic drugs are common and include vomiting, diarrhoea and anorexia but these may decline with prolonged use of the drug. The veterinary surgeon and owner will together decide on the best course of treatment and which clinical signs are to be tolerated in each individual patient.

Cytotoxic drugs are irritant and carcinogenic and extreme care must be taken in the handling of such drugs in veterinary practice (see Ch. 17). Local rules must be displayed in the practice area where cytotoxic drugs are used and all personnel must be made aware of the dangers (Box 20.3). Personnel are at risk during all stages of the procedure, i.e.

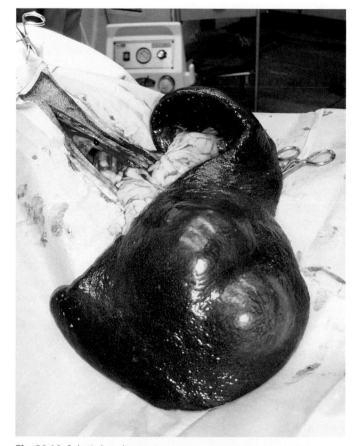

Fig. 20.18 Splenic lymphoma

Table 20.17 Drugs used in chemotherapy

Drug name	Comments
Cyclophosphamide	Used in treatment of lymphoma in dogs and cats. Available in tablet and injectable forms
Vincristine	Widely used in cats and dogs for treatment of leukaemias and lymphomas. Administered via intravenous route. Sometimes given in combination with other drugs. Perivascular injection causes sloughing, as drug is very irritant
Doxorubicin and epirubicin	Administered intravenously. Used in dogs for treatment of lymphoma
Cisplatin and carboplatin	Administered intravenously. Used in dogs for treatment of sarcoma, e.g. osteosarcoma following limb amputation

Box 20.3 Precautions to be taken to ensure safe handling of cytotoxic drugs

- Tablets must not be broken or crushed
- Disposable gloves must be worn when handling tablets
- Cytotoxic drugs must be dispensed in child-proof containers
- Cytotoxic drugs must be labelled with name of the drug and warnings regarding safe handling of the drug by owners
- Keep all cytotoxic drugs out of children's reach
- Wash hands after handling
- Wear gloves when administering tablets to patient
- Dispose of drugs by incineration
- Cytotoxic drugs must not be handled by pregnant women
- Wear protective personal equipment, e.g. gloves, long-sleeved gown, face mask, when reconstituting drugs
- Have eye-wash station and water available when reconstituting the drugs
- Do not inhale cytotoxic powders, e.g. when reconstituting drug
- Employ a good technique when handling cytotoxic drugs, e.g. care with pressure in vial of drug
- Label all cytotoxic drugs when in syringes
- Transport with care
- Administer via an intravenous catheter rather than a needle
- Restrain patient adequately for administration of drug
- Avoid skin contact with urine/faeces/vomit from patients undergoing cytotoxic drug therapy, since excreta will contain the drug
- All soiled bedding from treated animals must be incinerated as it will be contaminated with cytotoxic drug
- Dispose of used needles and syringes in the clinical waste
- Wash hard surfaces, e.g. floors, table tops, with plenty of water following contact with patients after administration of cytoxic drugs

when dispensing the drugs, reconstituting (when injectable forms are in powder form and require mixing with a fluid) and administering them, when disposing of them and when caring for the patient following its treatment with cytotoxic drugs.

Bibliography

Bowden, C., Masters, J., 2003. Textbook of Veterinary Medical Nursing. Butterworth-Heinemann, Oxford.

Concise Veterinary Dictionary, 1988. Oxford University Press, Oxford.

Lane, D.R., Cooper, B.C., Turner, L., 2007. Veterinary Nursing, 4th ed. Butterworth-Heinemann, Oxford.

Darke, P.G.G., 1986. Notes on Internal Canine Medicine. John Wright, Bristol.

Detweiler, D.K., Patterson, D.F., 1965. The prevalence and types of cardiovascular disease in dogs. Ann. N. Y. Acad. Sci. 127, 491.

Dobson, J.M., Gorman, N.T., 1993. Cancer Chemotherapy in Small Animal Practice. Blackwell Scientific, Oxford.

Simpson, J.W., Else, R.W., 1991. Digestive Disease in the Dog & Cat. Blackwell Scientific, Oxford.

Recommended reading

Bowden, C., Masters, J., 2003. Textbook of Veterinary Medical Nursing. Butterworth-Heinemann, Oxford.

Entire book devoted to all aspects of medical treatment.

Lane, D.R., Cooper, B.C., Turner, L, 2007. Veterinary Nursing, fourth ed. BSAVA, Gloucester.

General information for all levels of veterinary nursing.

Dobson, J.M., Gorman, N.T., 1993. Cancer Chemotherapy in Small Animal Practice. Blackwell Scientific, Oxford.

Provides detail of cancer treatment in animals.

Hotston-Moore, A., Rudd, S., 2008. BSAVA Manual of Canine and Feline Advanced Veterinary Nursing. BSAVA, Gloucester.

More detailed information suitable for diploma and degree nurses.

Hotston-Moore, P., Hughes, A., 2007. BSAVA Manual of Practical Animal Care. BSAVA, Gloucester.

General information for student veterinary nurses.

Mullinaeux, E., Jones, M., 2007. BSAVA Manual of Practical Veterinary Nursing. BSAVA, Gloucester.

General information for all levels of veterinary nursing.

Principles of surgical nursing

Julie Ouston

Shock

No matter how simple or complicated an animal's condition, one of the most important things veterinary clinical staff must do is to ensure that the patient is protected from or treated for shock. Untreated shock can rapidly lead to an animal's death so it is important that all nurses are able to recognize the early signs and know how to manage cases where shock is a potential risk (see also Ch. 18).

Shock is defined as a clinical syndrome in which the circulation progressively deteriorates and ultimately results in vital organs being deprived of a good blood flow, leading to widespread irreversible organ failure.

How does it develop?

Shock can develop in a number of ways:

- **Hypovolaemic shock** results from a fall in the circulating blood volume – either through blood loss or some form of dehydration
- **Endotoxic shock** is caused by the release of endotoxins from Gram-negative bacteria, which leads to vasodilation and consequently a fall in blood pressure and reduction in blood flow around the body
- **Neurogenic shock** is similar in that there is inappropriate vasodilation – in this instance it is caused by parasympathetic impulses from the brain
- **Cardiogenic shock** is due to a failure in the heart's ability to maintain the circulation.

In animals, hypovolaemic and endotoxic shock are seen quite commonly but cardiogenic shock is very rare.

Clinical signs

Since shock is a syndrome affecting the circulation it results in distinctive clinical signs no matter what the cause. The clinical signs are:

- Pale mucous membranes
- Increased capillary refill time (CRT)
- Tachycardia
- Weak, thready pulse
- Oliguria, progressing to anuria
- Gradual lack of consciousness
- Hypothermia
- In later stages petechial haemorrhages may develop on the gums or other mucous membranes as a result of disseminated intravascular coagulation (DIC). The blood flow at this point becomes so sluggish that it starts to clot and platelets and clotting factors are used up. The small defects that always occur in blood vessels cannot be sealed quickly and tiny pinpoint haemorrhages or petechiae start to develop.

Management of shock

Since an animal in shock, by definition, has poor circulation, the most important treatment is to provide intravenous fluid therapy. The type of fluid used varies depending on the initial cause but the provision of fluid is what makes the difference between life or death for the severely shocked patient.

In addition to fluids, body heat must be conserved, so warm the fluid prior to administration and keep the animal warm with Vetbed or blankets to prevent further heat loss.

Drugs may also be used, e.g. high doses of corticosteroids. These act to stabilize cell membranes and prevent cells on the borderline of survival from dying. However, steroids are only fully effective if they are given early, if they are given at a high enough dose rate and, most importantly, if the animal is already receiving intravenous fluids.

Patient monitoring

Patients suffering from shock must be monitored carefully. They may deteriorate quickly so initially these animals should be checked every 5 minutes. Temperature, pulse and respiration should all be assessed, as well as capillary refill time and mucous membrane colour. Urine output is also very important – until an animal is producing approximately 1 ml/kg/hour it can be considered to be oliguric and there is still a danger that the kidneys have been damaged irreversibly. Catheterization of the bladder is recommended and a collection bag should be used to allow accurate measurement of urine output (see also Ch. 15).

Urinary catheterization

Urinary catheters

Catheters are available in a variety of types and size. Traditionally these were made of nylon and polyvinyl chloride (PVC), but many are now available in other materials such as silicone. They are supplied in sterile packs of two polythene packets. All are measured using the French gauge unit, where 1 FG is 1/3 mm. The sizes refer to the external diameter of the catheter – thus a 3 FG catheter has an external diameter of 1 mm (Fig. 21.1).

Male dog catheters

These are very long catheters with a rounded tip, behind which are the two drainage holes or eyes. The end of the catheter that remains outside the animal is fitted with a Luer mount to which a syringe or three-way tap can be attached. If an indwelling catheter is required, zinc oxide tape can be used to make butterflies just behind the Luer fitting, which can then be sutured to the prepuce.

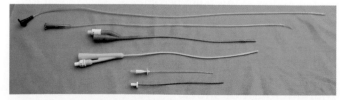

Fig. 21.1 Urinary catheters: from top – dog catheter, Tieman's catheter, Foley catheter (latex), Foley catheter (silicon), Jackson cat catheter, 'Slippery Sam' cat catheter

Bitch catheters

Tieman's catheter

Some vets use Tieman's catheter, although this is not specifically designed for bitches. It is similar to the dog catheter but has a curved bit of rigid plastic on the tip, which makes it easier to insert into the urethral opening in the bitch. These are human catheters and have several disadvantages:

- They are very long
- There are no small sizes available
- There is an increased risk of damage to the urethra and bladder because of the rigid tip.

Foley catheters

These are made of soft latex rubber or silicone and incorporate a balloon just behind the eyes. This is similar to the cuff of an endotracheal tube and, once the catheter has been inserted into the bladder, the balloon is inflated, usually with water, to prevent the catheter from coming out of the bladder.

Foley catheters are used as both temporary and indwelling catheters in the bitch as they are soft and cause relatively little trauma. However, because they are soft, a wire stylet or metal probe is inserted into the tip in order to place the catheter. This is removed once the catheter is in place.

Generally neither Foley catheters nor Tieman's catheters have Luer mounts – an adapter has to be fitted in most cases.

Cat catheters

Jackson cat catheters

These were initially developed to deal with cats with urethral obstruction caused by urinary calculi (Fig. 21.1). The catheter's features include:

- It has a wire stylet to stiffen it and help to unblock cats with urethral calculi
- Behind the Luer mount is a circular collar or flange with small holes to enable it to be sutured to the prepuce
- It is only 11 cm long so that its tip is just inside the bladder when the collar is sutured in position
- The eyes are closer to the tip of the catheter to prevent them becoming blocked by urethral crystals.

Catheters very similar to the Jackson cat catheter are also available in polytetrafluoroethylene (PTFE).

'Slippery Sam' tomcat catheters (Fig. 21.1)

This catheter has been developed more recently, and differs from the traditional Jackson catheter in a number of ways:

- It is made of PTFE and has a soft silicone hub. The PTFE is very smooth, and slides easily through the urethra
- It has an end hole rather than side holes to allow flushing or drainage of fluids
- They are available in two lengths – either 11 cm or 14 cm, and two widths (3.5 and 3 FG), which is suitable for smaller species such as ferrets.

Like the Jackson catheter, the hub of the catheter has small holes in it to allow it to be sutured to the prepuce, and requires a stiffening stylet for placement.

Specula

These are devices used to help catheterization, particularly in the bitch. They enable the urethral opening to be visualized by parting the vaginal walls. A number of different patterns and designs are available:

- Nasal speculum – this has two flat blades that can be separated by pressing the handles together. A small light source can be attached to one blade (Fig. 21.2).
- Rectal speculum – this is conical, with either a segment removed from the wall or a removable sliding panel, which allows the urethral opening to be seen (Fig. 21.3).

Specula are also available to fit on to auroscopes. These are similar to the ear speculum, except that a segment is missing from the wall.

Care of catheters

Most catheters are designed as single-use items and are therefore purchased pre-sterilized and disposed of after use. However, a few checks should be made prior to their use:

- Check basic cleanliness – there should be no obvious contamination
- Check for any signs of damage, e.g. splits or protruding fragments
- Check for signs of kinking.

Any damaged catheters should be discarded. To ensure that catheters are not damaged they should be stored flat and straight within their packets and out of sunlight. Avoid placing any weight on them.

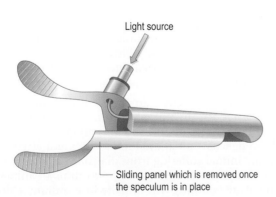

Fig. 21.2 Nasal speculum

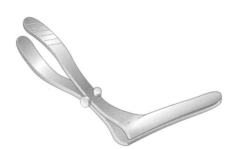

Light source

Sliding panel which is removed once the speculum is in place

Fig. 21.3 Rectal speculum

Technique for catheterization

General points:

- The animal must be well restrained – sedation or even a general anaesthetic may be required in some cases
- Local analgesic gel may be needed to desensitize the vagina or penis
- Good light is necessary
- Wear sterile disposable gloves to protect the catheter from contamination and protect yourself from urine contamination
- Use a sterile technique – do not allow the catheter to touch anything non-sterile. Ideally, it should be 'fed' out of the packet in which it has been sterilized
- Remove any discharge from the prepuce or vagina using a mild disinfectant (rinse well if urine is being collected for bacterial examination)
- Avoid lubricant if possible – it may not be sterile. If it is necessary, use a water-soluble lubricant rather than petroleum jelly (Vaseline), since this causes latex to perish
- Have a kidney dish and universal container handy to collect the urine
- Do not use force
- Once urine appears, do not feed any more catheter into the bladder, as it may cause the catheter to kink or even knot itself.

Male dog

1. The dog should be restrained either standing or in lateral recumbency. Cut the tip off the packet containing the catheter and feed out about 8–10 cm
2. Ask an assistant to hold this
3. Reflect the prepuce with the right hand and grasp the root of the penis with the left hand until the tip of the penis appears. The prepuce can then be reached with the fingers of the left hand and held. Any discharge should be removed
4. Introduce the catheter into the tip of the penis, holding the packet. Gently slide this back and gradually slide the catheter into the urethra
5. Never force the catheter – if it gets stuck, try gentle rotation and mild pressure
6. Once urine starts to flow, hold the catheter steady to prevent it slipping back out of the bladder.

Bitch

The bitch may be catheterized standing or in dorsal or sternal recumbency, depending on preference:

1. If the animal is standing the assistant should restrain the dog and hold the tail out of the way. The speculum should be introduced vertically up through the vulval lips and then turned to run horizontally
2. On the floor of the vestibule are two small indentations – the nearer one is the blind-ending clitoral fossa, the further one is the urethral opening set on the urethral papilla. The catheter tip should be carefully introduced through the urethral papilla
3. If the bitch is restrained on her back, then the hind legs should be drawn forwards until the catheter is in place in the urethra. The legs should be drawn forwards and

the catheter slid into the bladder using a no-touch technique, as for the dog.

Tomcat

This is normally performed under a general anaesthetic or heavy sedation, as there is a risk of damaging the narrow urethra:

1. The animal should be restrained in right lateral recumbency with the hind legs drawn forwards
2. The prepuce is retracted with the left hand to expose the tip of the penis and the catheter can be introduced as for the male dog.

Queen

This is also normally performed under a general anaesthetic.

1. The cat should be restrained in right lateral recumbency as for the tomcat
2. The vulval lips should be cleaned and pulled up gently towards the anus
3. The tip of the catheter is introduced along the vaginal floor and into the urethral opening.

Note For all the above descriptions, left-handed people should replace 'right' with 'left' and vice versa.

Fluid therapy

To appreciate fluid therapy and its uses it is important to remind yourself of the fluid situation in the healthy animal (see also Ch. 4).

Water in and out

The animal takes in water through eating and drinking and water is also created in many chemical reactions taking place within the tissues, e.g. the breakdown of glucose to release energy:

$$Glucose \rightarrow CO_2 + H_2O + Energy$$

Water (H_2O) produced in chemical reactions is referred to as metabolic water and usually makes up about 10% of an animal's fluid requirements. The remainder of the animal's fluid need is met through eating and drinking. The proportion of water acquired from each varies considerably with the type of food being fed.

Normal water loss occurs in a number of ways, including urine, faeces, sweat and respiration. In addition, animals suffering from disease lose fluid by vomiting, haemorrhage, burns or diarrhoea.

Estimations of normal fluid losses are usually as follows:

- Urine – 20 ml/kg/24 h
- Faeces – Up to 20 ml/kg/24 h
- Respiration – 20 ml/kg/24 h
- Sweat – Usually considered to be negligible
- **Total loss – 50–60 ml/kg/24 h.**

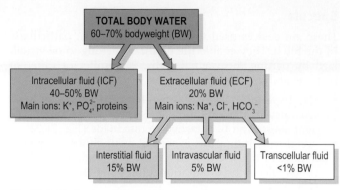

Fig. 21.4 Distribution of fluid within the body

Fluid in the body

Fluid is found in a number of different compartments within the body and its composition is different depending on its location. Figure 21.4 shows the major fluid compartments and the important electrolytes found in each.

The function of the body fluids is to maintain homeostasis and this relies on the body fluids remaining in the correct volumes within the fluid compartments, their electrolyte balance and osmotic pressure being normal and their pH remaining around 7.4. If any of these factors change, the animal will begin to show clinical signs and some form of treatment must be instigated.

It is useful to understand three terms used in fluid therapy that describe a fluid in relation to the osmotic pressure of plasma and affect the movement of the fluid through the fluid compartments:

- Isotonic – the fluid has the same osmotic pressure as that of plasma
- Hypotonic – the fluid has a lower osmotic pressure than that of plasma
- Hypertonic – the fluid has a higher osmotic pressure than that of plasma.

Most fluid therapy involves the use of isotonic fluids.

Dehydration

Dehydration may result from any situation in which an animal's fluid output exceeds the input. While urine concentration can be altered to conserve water in difficult conditions, faecal losses and respiratory losses cannot be controlled, so there is always a minimum rate of fluid loss that must be balanced. Dehydration results in hypovolaemia and rapidly leads to severe shock, so any situation in which fluid balance is compromised is potentially life-threatening.

Fluid deficits can be divided into primary fluid deficits or mixed deficits:

- Primary water deficits – an animal loses water but not electrolytes, e.g. an animal shut in a hot car suffering from heat stroke; an unconscious animal
- Mixed deficits – an animal loses water and electrolytes, e.g. an animal suffering from diarrhoea is likely to have lost bicarbonate, sodium and potassium; an animal with acute vomiting will initially lose sodium, chloride and hydrogen ions.

Assessing dehydration

There are three main ways in which dehydration can be assessed:

Clinical examination

This is the simplest method. Table 21.1 indicates the loss in terms of the percentage of an animal's body weight and the clinical signs linked with the degree of dehydration.

These figures can be used as shown in Box 21.1.

Clinical history

This method is most applicable for the animal that has not been eating or drinking.

We can also consider cases where there are pathological deficits. These are a little more difficult to estimate but provide a start point for deciding how much replacement fluid to administer.

Vomiting losses have been found to be between 1 and 4 ml/kg/vomit. Diarrhoeic losses can either be judged in a

similar way or can be considered as a multiple of normal faecal losses (see Boxes 21.2, 21.3).

As you can see from the examples in the boxes, for both the clinical examination and history techniques, there is some subjectivity. Each of us might make a different judgement about the animal's clinical state or decide to make

Table 21.1 Clinical assessment of dehydration

Degree of dehydration as % of bodyweight	Clinical signs
<4	Not detectable
5–6	Dry mouth
	Subtle loss of skin elasticity
7–8	Definite loss of skin elasticity
	Increased capillary refill time
	Cold extremities
	Sunken eyes
	i.e. signs of early shock
10–11	Cold legs and mouth
	Weak, recumbent
	Tented skin stays in place
12	Moribund, severe shock
14	Death

Box 21.1

A 5 kg cat appears to be 8% dehydrated.
In order to calculate its fluid deficit, first calculate the weight lost:

$= 8 \div 100 \times 5$
$= 0.4\,kg$

However, 1 l of water weighs exactly 1 kg, so a cat that has lost 0.4 kg has lost 0.4 l of water. This can be converted into millilitres by multiplying the litres by 1000:

$= 0.4 \times 1000$
$= 400\,ml$

Thus the cat in this example has lost 400 ml of fluid.

Box 21.2

A 4 kg cat has been shut in a shed for 2 days. It has had no history of renal problems and during this time it passed faeces once
Consider each of the normal losses in turn and what has been happening to the cat over the course of the 2 days

Respiration: It has been breathing the whole time and has consequently lost fluid as water vapour
We have to allow the full 20 ml/kg/day
$= 20 \times 4 \times 2$
$= 160\,ml$

Urination: There is no history of renal disease, so the cat should have been able to concentrate its urine
Probably over the 2 days it would have passed 1 normal day's worth
$= 20 \times 4 \times 1$
$= 80\,ml$

Faeces: We have been told that the cat has passed faeces once, so allow 1 day's worth
$= 20 \times 4 \times 1$
$= 80\,ml$

There have been no other reported fluid losses, so the total deficit
$= 320\,ml$.

Box 21.3

A 20 kg dog has been unwell for 1 day and has vomited 5 times and passed diarrhoea twice. It has not eaten or drunk anything since the previous day.
As for Box 21.2, we need to consider each of the possible areas of loss separately:

Respiration: 1 day's loss
$= 20 \times 20 \times 1$
$= 400\,ml$

Urination: 1 day's loss
$= 20 \times 20 \times 1$
$= 400\,ml$

Faeces: Here we need to consider the additional loss due to diarrhoea, say twice normal
$= 20 \times 20 \times 1 \times 2$
$= 800\,ml$

Vomiting: Five episodes of vomiting at, on average, 2 ml/kg/vomit
$= 2 \times 20 \times 5$
$= 200\,ml$

Therefore, the total deficit for this dog can be estimated as
$= 1800\,ml$

slightly different allowances for losses. However, each decision may be valid and since we monitor our patients carefully we shall be able to make the appropriate revisions to the fluid treatment as time goes on.

Packed cell volume

As an animal becomes dehydrated, the amount of plasma is reduced and the packed cell volume (PCV) gradually increases (see also Ch. 31). An estimate of fluid loss can therefore be made based on how high the PCV is compared with normal. The allowance used is 10 ml/kg/% increase.

We are not usually in the fortunate position of knowing each animal's normal PCV and often we need to estimate a normal value. For cats this is usually taken as 35% and for dogs 45%. This estimation decreases the accuracy of this method but, if used in conjunction with clinical examination or history techniques, it can be helpful (Box 21.4).

Please note that if there has been recent blood loss, this method cannot be used, as blood cells have been lost as well as fluid and the PCV will be lower than normal.

Fluid replacement therapy

Having established that our patient is dehydrated, or in danger of becoming dehydrated, it is now time to consider replacing the fluid loss.

Fluids may be given to a patient by several routes and each has advantages and disadvantages (Table 21.2).

Oral fluid therapy is the safest method, since the intestines selectively absorb what the animal actually needs and there is less danger of overinfusion, which can be life-threatening if not identified and treated quickly. In practice the main method used for supplying fluids to patients is via an intravenous drip. For surgical cases this is often helpful, since it can be continued both prior to and during any operation when normally animals would not be able to take any oral fluids. Postoperatively, animals are often anorexic for a short time and this technique ensures that they do not continue to lose fluids.

Choice of veins

- Cephalic vein – runs down the dorsal aspect of the lower forelimb and is the most commonly used
- Lateral saphenous vein – runs over the lateral aspect of the hock and may be used if both cephalic veins are damaged through repeated catheterization
- Jugular vein – less commonly used but can be very useful in patients that are critically dehydrated as it is a large vein that allows higher flow rates. It also should be used if central venous pressure (CVP) is to be measured. CVP provides a useful method of determining the effectiveness of the fluid therapy.

Box 21.4

The PCV from an 8 kg dog has gone up from 42% to 47% due to dehydration.
Its fluid deficit is therefore
(ml/kg) (kg) (% increase)

$\quad 10 \quad \times \quad 8 \quad \times \quad 5$

= 400 ml

Table 21.2 Routes for administration of fluid therapy

Route of administration	Advantages	Disadvantages
Oral (per os, p.o.)	Simple and cheap Painless Safe as the intestine selectively absorbs the fluid and electrolytes needed and excess is excreted Can be done at home	Absorption is slow Limited range of suitable fluids No use if the animal is vomiting or gastrointestinal tract is obstructed Time-consuming
Subcutaneous (s.c.)	Simple	Slow absorption, especially if the animal is dehydrated and circulation is poor Can only give small volumes at a time Painful Risk of infection
Intraperitoneal (i.p.)	Not too difficult Larger area over which to absorb fluid compared with s.c. fluids	Poor absorption in dehydration or shock Risk of puncturing an abdominal organ Strict asepsis necessary
Intravenous (i.v.)	Fluid can be given rapidly Good for animals with circulatory collapse Wide range of fluids can be used Only way in which hypertonic solutions can be given	Strict asepsis needed, or risk of thrombophlebitis and septicaemia Constant monitoring needed to prevent overhydration Specialized equipment needed Cold fluids may lead to hypothermia
Intraosseous (i/o)	Useful means of giving fluid in animals in which a vein cannot be catheterized, e.g. small exotic species Can be followed by intravenous fluids once circulation is improved	Specialized equipment required Needle placed directly into the bone, so cannot be left in place once animal starts to recover Aseptic technique required or risk of infection, e.g. osteomyelitis

Choice of fluid

There are a number of fluids available for intravenous (or intraosseous) infusion and these fall into three classes:

- Blood, plasma and Oxyglobin
- Colloids or plasma expanders
- Crystalloids.

The aim of fluid therapy is to replace the type of fluid lost with as close a substitute as possible.

Blood, plasma and Oxyglobin

- Whole blood can be used in cases of severe haemorrhage or in cases where specific blood factors are missing. Ideally, the patient and donor should both have the same blood type, or the blood should be cross-matched as there is a risk of a blood transfusion reaction developing
- Plasma is useful for less serious blood losses or where the missing blood factor is a plasma factor rather than a specific blood cell type. Plasma can be collected and stored by freezing. However, precipitates may occur within the fluid and this too can cause reactions in some patients. Plasma is therefore less commonly used
- Oxyglobin is a commercial product that contains large molecules of oxyglobin, which act in a similar way to haemoglobin molecules, i.e. combine with oxygen or carbon dioxide. This is not antigenic and therefore does not require cross-matching prior to use. It is expensive but does provide a useful alternative to whole blood if the problem the animal is suffering from is lack of oxygen-carrying capacity.

Colloids or plasma expanders

Colloids contain large molecules of inert substances that are too big to diffuse through the capillary walls into the interstitial spaces and so remain within the circulation. The molecules exert an osmotic effect, which also helps maintain the circulation by drawing water into the capillaries. Colloids do not remain in the circulation indefinitely – the molecules are gradually broken down but, by the time they have been removed from the blood stream, other fluids will have been given and circulatory balance should have improved considerably.

There are several different colloids available. In the UK colloids either contain gelatines such as Haemaccel and Gelofusine, or starch complexes such as hetastarch and pentastarch.

The situations in which colloids should be used rather than crystalloids are:

- Severe shock
- Haemorrhage where PCV is less than 20% but not so severe as to require whole blood or Oxyglobin
- Plasma protein levels of less than 35 g/l, leading to oedema and ascites
- Severe dehydration.

Crystalloids

Crystalloid solutions are simply water containing dissolved glucose and/or electrolytes. There are a range of solutions available designed to meet a variety of requirements (Table 21.3). Most crystalloids are isotonic and therefore will not affect fluid movement into or out of cells. The water is able to move freely between the different fluid compartments, so when giving a crystalloid it is important to appreciate that it does not stay within the circulation but spreads out between all the different areas of the body.

Choice of giving sets

A giving set is the piece of equipment used to deliver the fluid into the circulation. The choice of giving set depends on the individual case:

- **A standard giving set** usually delivers 15 or 20 drops/ml and is used for larger patients being given crystalloids or colloids
- **A paediatric giving set** is better for use in small patients. This often incorporates a burette so that the total amount of fluid the patient receives is limited (Fig. 21.5)
- **A blood administration set** has a filter incorporated into the chamber to prevent any small clots entering

Table 21.3 Crystalloids and their uses

Crystalloid	Contents	Uses	Comments
Hartmann's solution	Na, K, Ca, Cl, lactate	Diarrhoea Prolonged anorexia Pyometra Prolonged vomiting	Lactate is converted into bicarbonate NB do not add bicarbonate – will precipitate out chalk!
0.9% sodium chloride	Na, Cl	Vomiting	
5% glucose	Glucose	Hyperthermia Water deprivation Hypoglycaemia	5% glucose is equivalent to isotonic water
0.18% sodium chloride + 4% dextrose	Na, Cl, dextrose	Maintenance fluid Occasionally primary water deficits	Potassium supplementation will be needed for long-term maintenance
Ringer's solution	Na, Cl, Ca, K	Pyometra Severe vomiting	This is the same as Hartmann's without the lactate; bicarbonate should therefore not be added to this either

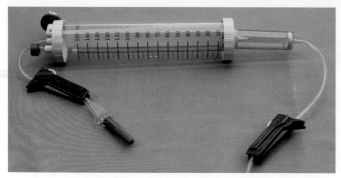

Fig. 21.5 Burette suitable for small-animal fluid therapy

the circulation. This type of giving set should also be used for plasma or serum
- **Flowline balloon infusers** may be used for very small patients, such as exotics, where only a few millilitres of fluid is required. These deliver fluid at a rate specified on the flow line that links the balloon and the catheter, and may be bandaged to the patient during the period of fluid therapy.

Many practices also use infusion pumps to help ensure that the correct volume is given at the appropriate rate for the individual.

Administration of intravenous fluid

Setting up the drip

1. Select the equipment required
2. Wear sterile gloves if possible
3. Check all equipment is in date and undamaged
4. Warm the fluid to blood temperature
5. Open the sterile packet containing the fluids and twist off the sterile plastic cover to the giving set port
6. Place bag in a position ready for the giving set to be positioned (can be on a bench or on a drip stand)
7. Open the sterile packet containing the drip line
8. Extend the drip line, taking care to ensure that the two ends do not come into contact with anything, and check that there are no kinks
9. Turn off the controller
10. Remove the protective cover from the spiked end and carefully introduce this end of the giving set into the port using a twisting motion and then hang the bag on to the drip stand
11. Give the chamber a gentle squeeze to fill it about one-third to half full
12. *Gently* open the flow controller and allow fluid through the giving set at a slow and steady rate
13. Try not to lose any fluid but make sure there are no bubbles within the line
14. Make sure that the cap is on the end of the line and hook this up over the drip stand ready to be used.

Preparation of the patient

The skin must be prepared as for surgery to avoid the risk of thrombophlebitis. The fur should be clipped and the skin prepared, using some type of antiseptic solution. Some practices prefer to use just chlorhexidine or povidone-iodine solutions whereas others use surgical spirit. Either method is appropriate so long as care is taken to ensure that the skin is as clean as possible.

Catheterization of the vein

A 'no touch' technique must be employed to prevent the introduction of infection.

Equipment required

For catheterization of the cephalic vein most veterinary surgeons use 'over the needle' **catheters** but for jugular vein catheterization longer catheters are needed. It is important that whichever vessel is chosen for the delivery of fluid the largest possible catheter is used to reduce the chance of blockage.

In addition to the catheter, other equipment needed includes **tape** to secure the catheter in place, **a bung or three-way tap** if the giving set is not to be connected immediately, and **bandaging material** to protect the site and hold the tubing in place. On larger patients some people prefer to use either the end of a hypodermic needle or a scalpel blade to make a small nick in the skin to ease the access of the catheter. A syringe containing 1 ml of **heparin saline** is also useful to check patency and ensure that clots do not form within the catheter.

Procedure for administration of fluids via the cephalic vein

1. Prepare the site aseptically and ask an assistant to restrain the animal and raise the vein (see Ch. 10)
2. Make a small incision in the skin over the point of entry for the catheter (may not always be necessary)
3. Push the tip of the catheter through the hole in the skin at an angle of approximately 45°
4. Watch for blood in the 'flashback' chamber of the catheter
5. Once blood appears, withdraw needle a few millimetres so that the point is protected by the catheter
6. Slide the catheter off the needle and into the vein
7. Withdraw the needle
8. Secure the catheter with tape
9. Flush with heparin saline to ensure that it is in place
10. Connect the giving set to the end of the catheter and start administration of fluids
11. Bandage the tubing in place and pack with swabs for comfort.

Calculating the drip rate

Once the fluid deficit has been calculated, the drip rate can be determined. There are different ideas as to how much of a given deficit should be replaced over a period of time and it is also important that ongoing losses are taken into consideration. Fluid rates should therefore be reviewed regularly based on the patient's clinical condition (see Box 21.5).

An animal requires 1800 ml over 24 h. Using a standard giving set, which delivers 20 drops/ml, the drip rate can be calculated as follows: 1800 ml to be given in 24 h

$= 1800 \div 24$ ml to be given in 1 h

$= 75$ ml/h

Then divide by 60 to give ml/min

$= 75 \div 60 = 1.25$ ml/min

Now convert the number of millilitres into drops. The giving set delivers 20 drops/ml, so the number of drops per minute is calculated as follows:

$= 1.25 \times 20$ drops/ml

$= 25$ drops/min

To calculate how many seconds it takes for each drop to fall, simply divide 60 by this number.

$= 60 \div 25$

$= 2.4$ s

Therefore, in this case, the drip rate is 1 drop every 2.4 s.

Monitoring the patient

Patients being given intravenous or intraosseous fluid therapy must be monitored carefully. It is obviously important that the fluid is delivered at the rate asked for by the veterinary surgeon, but it is also important to continually assess the patient to ensure that it is making the desired improvement.

Critical care cases may need to be checked as frequently as an anaesthetic case, with temperature, pulse and respiration being recorded every 5 minutes. As the case becomes less critical, observations should still be made at regular intervals, with particular reference to the fluids.

A fluid chart is helpful so that all parameters can be recorded. This includes fluid input and rate of administration, temperature, pulse and respiration and any urine output. Urine output should be quantified – the patient should be catheterized and the catheter connected to a urine collection bag. These are graduated so it is possible to get an estimate of the quantity of urine passed over a given time period. Remember that, if fluid therapy is successful, the kidneys should produce a minimum of 1 ml/kg of urine per hour.

CVP also provides a means of assessing the hydration state of a patient. Normally CVP should be between 3 and 7 cmH$_2$O, but in severely dehydrated patients it may be considerably below this. CVP can only be measured if a jugular catheter is placed in such a way that the end of the catheter is close to the right atrium of the heart.

As many practices do not use this technique it is very important that other regular clinical checks are made on patients, assessing temperature, pulse, respiration, capillary refill time, colour of the mucous membranes, skin turgor and general demeanour.

Overinfusion

It is possible to overinfuse patients, particularly small dogs, cats and exotics, and to avoid this burettes, flowline systems or infusion pumps should be used.

Signs of overinfusion vary, depending on the type of fluid being used:

- **Colloids** remain within the circulation, so overinfusion results in circulatory overload. The heart cannot cope (particularly the weaker right side) and the veins leading back to the heart become congested. Eventually the blood dams back into the capillaries and the pressure causes fluid to leak into the interstitial spaces. This will be seen as oedema of the tissues or ascites in the abdomen
- **Crystalloids** build up of fluid in all parts of the body and the tissues become 'waterlogged' if overinfusion occurs. This includes the brain, and the animal may appear to be more 'spaced out' and unresponsive to normal stimuli. If the lungs are affected, the patient's breathing may become compromised, and ultimately the fluid within the lungs will prevent adequate oxygenation of the blood and the animal will die.

Wounds and wound management

Classification

A wound can be defined as an injury in which there is a forcible break in the continuity of the soft tissues. This includes both open wounds, in which the skin or mucous membrane surface is broken, and closed wounds, in which the damage is below the surface.

Wounds are divided into different groups based on their cause and the resulting type of damage (Table 21.4). Wounds may also be categorized on the basis of the degree of contamination (Table 21.5).

Operating order is always dictated by the cleanliness of the surgery. Clean surgery should be carried out first, followed by clean-contaminated conditions. Contaminated surgery should be carried out last. Dirty procedures should not be carried out in theatre but in another area of the practice.

Wound healing

Wound healing occurs in three phases:

Haemorrhage, inflammation and primary wound contraction

Primary haemorrhage occurs at the time of injury. This then clots and forms a scab, which protects the wound from external contamination. Inflammation follows, encouraging white blood cells to the site. In the first few hours there is primary wound contraction as fibroblasts contract and the size of the wound decreases.

Granulation

After 12 hours, epithelial proliferation starts. New cells are produced and slide over the surface of the wound. This occurs at a rate of up to 2 mm per day if the wound is kept moist. After 36 hours, fibroblasts and new capillaries are produced, forming granulation tissue. This is usually bright red and firm but is quite easily damaged.

Table 21.4 Wound classification

Wound type	Possible cause	Type of damage
Incised	Sharp knife/scalpel Glass Tin	Clean cut with little damage to surrounding tissues Wound edges usually gape and bleed freely
Puncture	Nail Thorn Fish hooks Teeth (especially cats')	Small external wound but may be deep Little obvious sign on the surface Infection is a potential problem as bacteria or foreign material are carried deep into the tissues
Lacerated	Dog fight Road accident Barbed wire	Large irregular wound with considerable damage to the skin and superficial tissues The severity varies with the size and depth of the wound and the degree of damage to other tissues, such as muscles, nerves and blood vessels Infection is common and necrosis of the edges of the wound is likely
Abrasion	Friction	The epidermis is removed to expose the dermis. These are not full-thickness wounds and, although they are painful, are not usually serious
Avulsion	Dog fights	An avulsion wound occurs where there is forcible separation of a tissue from its attachments
Degloving	Road traffic accidents	Degloving injuries occur in a similar way or through damage to the blood supply such that an area of tissue dies and sloughs away over a period of time These are often heavily contaminated with dirt and bacteria
Shear	Road traffic accidents	These occur in the same way as degloving injuries, although as well as the removal of skin there is damage to the underlying bones and/or joints These are heavily contaminated and are often very serious
Contusion	Blunt trauma	Blood vessels rupture under the skin The blood seeps into the tissues and eventually clots Breakdown of the red blood cells and haemoglobin results in the discoloration of the skin that appears as the contusion heals
Haematoma	Blunt trauma Excessive head-shaking	Greater blood loss occurs than with a contusion and a pocket of blood develops under the skin The blood eventually clots and scar tissue is generated, which contracts with time Most usually associated with the ear, where the scar contraction can lead to a 'cauliflower ear'

Table 21.5 Wounds classified by degree of contamination

Wound type	Description
Clean	There is no break in sterility An incision is made into a tissue that has been surgically prepared and no contaminated body systems are entered
Clean-contaminated	A contaminated area (such as the gastrointestinal, urogenital or respiratory tract) is entered but there is no spillage or spread of contamination Clean-contaminated wounds also include fresh, open wounds after careful lavage and debridement
Contaminated	Wounds in which there is either spillage from a contaminated area or severe inflammation, but without infection Fresh, open wounds are also included in this category
Dirty	Wounds in which there is leakage from a pus-filled organ or there is pus or infection present within the wound Dirty wounds also include traumatic wounds with devitalized tissue or those containing foreign bodies

Scar formation

During epidermal growth new collagen is laid down. This is continually remodelled up to 2 years after the original incident. Once the wound cavity is filled, the wound undergoes secondary wound contraction and the size of the scar is reduced.

Open wounds can take weeks or even months to heal, depending on the severity of the initial injury. These wounds are described as healing by second intention. Wounds that are closed surgically with good apposition of the skin edges heal by first intention. This process is usually far quicker, as very little granulation tissue forms and the skin edges simply join together.

Inflammation

It is important to appreciate that inflammation is the reaction of normal tissue to injury and is part of the body's natural defence mechanisms. When cells are damaged, chemicals such as histamine and prostaglandins are released and these stimulate the inflammatory response. There is dilation of local vessels, and white blood cells and proteins are attracted to the site. This is all needed to start the healing process. Administration of anti-inflammatory drugs will reduce healing in the early phases, so generally should not be used. However, protracted inflammation may cause problems and this is where the use of drugs such as the corticosteroids or non-steroidal anti-inflammatory drugs (NSAIDs) might be indicated.

Factors affecting wound healing

Wound healing is a delicate process and many factors can delay the rate of healing. These include:

- Movement
- Infection
- Tension – e.g. sutures placed too tightly will produce cell death
- Interference with blood supply – e.g. bandages that are too tight, or heavily contused wounds
- Persistent irritation and self-trauma
- Tumour cells invading a wound
- Presence of foreign material.

These are all factors that relate specifically to the wound but there are also some general factors that will also influence the way in which wounds heal:

- Age – youngsters will heal faster than older animals
- Region of the body
- Malnutrition or specific deficiency of vitamins A, B and C
- Corticosteroids can decrease wound healing; anabolic steroids and the use of antibiotic creams/ointments can increase the rate of wound healing
- Other concurrent diseases.

Management of wounds

Wound management can be summarized as follows:

1. First clean the wound thoroughly and remove any devitalized tissue
2. The wound should then be repaired surgically or left as an open wound
3. Dressings should be applied as indicated by the type of wound
4. Follow-up checks should be carried out.

Cleaning and debridement

Wounds should always be cleaned carefully before any further management is undertaken. A heavily contaminated wound should be flushed thoroughly using warmed sterile Hartmann's solution. A large syringe and needle can be used to provide greater pressure where there is ingrained dirt. Dilute disinfectant solutions may also be used, but care must be taken as they can be toxic to fibroblasts if the concentration is too great. If the wound edges are damaged, the edge of the wound should be debrided. This can either be achieved through surgery, or the use of appropriate dressing regimes.

Wound closure

Wounds usually heal more quickly if they can be closed surgically, so this is done wherever possible. Wounds can be closed using a number of methods:

- Suturing – commonly used and generally well tolerated. However, most patients require general anaesthesia for both restraint and analgesia
- Staples – can be very quick and carried out in the conscious patient
- Tissue adhesive – glues are available suitable for skin closure.

Wound closure can be carried out at different stages depending on the type of wound and the degree of contamination:

- **Primary closure**: the wound is closed immediately after presentation once cleaned and debrided
- **Delayed primary closure**: this is carried out 3–5 days after the initial injury. The delay allows removal of contamination or any exudate that would compromise healing. At this stage granulation tissue has not yet started to form
- **Secondary closure**: this is similar to delayed primary closure, except that it has taken longer to remove any infection and therefore some granulation tissue has started to form. This usually is carried out after 5–7 days.

Dressings and bandages

Not all wounds are amenable to closure and some wounds are best left to heal by second intention. This is particularly the case where there is a large skin deficit, and such wounds will require some type of bandage to facilitate wound healing.

Bandages can help to:

- Protect a wound from bacterial contamination
- Provide comfort
- Support an area with a wound and reduce movement of the skin edges
- Reduce the development of swelling and oedema
- Absorb any exudates
- Provide a cosmetic appearance for the owner.

Whenever bandages are used it is very important that clients are given clear instructions about when they should return to the surgery for a check up and about any signs that could indicate a problem.

A bandage should consist of three layers:

- **Primary or contact layer** –this touches the wound and must be sterile
- **Secondary or intermediate layer** – padding, usually added for comfort or absorption
- **Tertiary or protective layer** – applied over the other layers to hold them in place, prevent interference and minimize contamination from the environment.

There are several types of skin dressing available for the management of open wounds (Table 21.6A). The dressing materials chosen depend on the stage of wound healing and the degree of contamination or necrosis. Topical treatments may also be helpful (Table 21.6B)

Drains

In some wound cases, drains can be very valuable. A drain is a device that allows fluid or air to pass from a wound or body

Table 21.6A Dressing materials

Dressing type	Use
Adherent contact layer	
Dry-to-dry dressing	Dry swabs are directly applied to the wound so that debris and necrotic tissue adheres to the swabs and is pulled away when the dressing is changed. This is an effective but painful way of debriding wounds
Wet-to-dry dressing	Sterile swabs soaked in Hartmann's solution are placed close to the wound. The dressing dries out and, when removed, takes with it any exudate and debris. These dressings should be changed every 12–24 h and are usually less painful than the dry-to-dry dressings
Non-adherent contact layer	
Gauze impregnated with petroleum jelly	Little used nowadays except occasionally for skin grafts
Silicone mesh, e.g. Mepitel	Very good as a dressing over skin grafts
Perforated film dressing, e.g. Melolin	Usually used for surgical wounds with little exudate. Provides a clean, dry environment for wound healing
Foam dressing, e.g. Allevyn	Very good for absorbing fluid from wounds where there is likely to be heavy exudate
Hydrogels, e.g. IntraSite, Biodres	Hydrogels are commonly used in practice and have the advantage of reducing bacterial contamination of wounds, as well as providing an excellent moist environment that promotes wound healing and some natural debridement. However, they are not suitable for infected wounds
Hydrocolloids, e.g. Tegasorb, Granuflex	Initially these are impermeable to water and help to rehydrate wounds and encourage debridement. Later, the structure becomes more gelatinous and fluid is able to escape from the wound site
Alginates, e.g. Kaltostat, AlgiSite	These are derived from seaweed and are usually presented as a soft, woven dressing. They react with sodium ions and a gel is formed that holds a considerable amount of fluid and ensures excellent moist wound-healing conditions.
Semi-permeable film dressing, e.g. OpSite, Tegaderm, Bioclusive	These are used in situations with very little exudate since there is minimal absorption by these dressings. However, they do provide a good moist wound-healing environment

Table 21.6B Topical wound treatments

Topical wound treatment	Description
Aloe vera	Can be used to activate macrophages within the wound site and promote debridement. Also useful for promoting granulation. However, it is important that medical grade *Aloe vera* is used, which can be expensive
Maggots	Very effective at debriding wounds. Sterile stage 1 larvae must be purchased, and placed in contact with the wound. At this stage the larvae do not have chewing mouthparts and do not cause further damage. They must, however, be removed before they reach stage 2, which are able to chew
Silver, e.g. Acticoat, Aquacel AG	Silver has very good antimicrobial properties, and has been shown to have activity against bacteria such as MRSA and *Pseudomonas*. There are a number of creams and dressings that contain silver. Care must be taken to follow directions with these products, as they are quite specific in some cases
Sugar paste & honey, e.g. Manukacare 18+, Activon	This can be used as a debridement dressing. It draws fluid from the wound, and lowers pH so therefore should not be used on granulating tissue. Care must be taken that the mix is free from bacterial contamination, so sterile medical-grade honey must be used. There are also commerically available dressings which incorporate honey

cavity to the surface. Several situations may benefit from the use of a drain, including the management of contaminated wounds, deep abscesses, and in seromas to prevent the accumulation of fluid in the dead space in surgical wounds. While seromas do not usually cause serious problems, they are unsightly and may delay the wound-healing process.

Drains can be described as either active or passive:

- **Passive drains** – rely on pressure and gravity to allow the fluid to drain. In order to be effective they should

be placed so that the opening is in a dependent position, i.e. below the level of the area from which the fluid is to be drained. The most common drain is a soft flexible tube known as the Penrose drain. Fluid follows the external surface of the drain. This type of drain should be left in place until such time as fluid production is minimal and the risk of dead space development has been removed. They can be made of either soft latex rubber or silicone.

Other types of passive drain that are occasionally used are corrugated drains, tube drains and sump drains.

- **Active drains** – require some source of suction to work. Suction devices include small compressible plastic containers, syringes or evacuated blood tubes. For continuous, low-level suction these must be permanently attached to a drainage tube and bandaged in place. Alternatively, intermittent suction can be used, e.g. a syringe used in conjunction with a three-way tap to ensure that air does not flow back into the area. Tube drains are usually used in these situations.

Monitoring – while in situ, any drain should be checked regularly to ensure that it is still in place and to assess the healing process. There should be no odour associated with the drain and the wound should appear clean, without excessive inflammation. Any fluid emerging should be almost clear, or possibly slightly blood-tinged, but not purulent.

Animals should not be allowed to interfere with drains. Active drains are usually covered with bandage but passive drains need to be left open to function. An Elizabethan collar may be needed to prevent the patient worrying at the end of the drain.

Removal – when drains are removed, it is usually quite a simple matter of cutting the sutures that hold the drain in place and then withdrawing the tube. Check that the drain is intact and that no material has been left behind. This could act as a foreign body and induce a marked tissue reaction.

Thoracic drains are more specialized and require the use of a fenestrated tube drain and a trocar. Insertion is carried out either under general anaesthesia, e.g. at the time of chest surgery, or under local anaesthesia. For drain placement in a closed thorax a skin incision is made between the 9th and 12th ribs and a subcutaneous tunnel made through to the level of the 7th or 8th intercostal spaces. The drain is pushed through the intercostal muscles at this site. Once in place the tube must be sealed to prevent air entering the thorax. This procedure must be carried out under aseptic conditions. Mechanical suction can then be performed as necessary. Suction should always be applied via a one-way valve such as a Heimlich valve or water trap, which also prevents excessive suction being applied. Alternatively, a syringe can be used, either attached directly to the chest drain or via a three-way tap. With any thoracic drain it is essential that air is not allowed to enter the thoracic cavity as the drain is checked or the suction device is attached.

Reconstructive surgical techniques

Where there is extensive tissue loss, standard surgical closures may not be possible but the site may still be amenable to surgical techniques to replace the missing tissue. These include skin grafts and skin flaps.

If the skin of an animal is tented it is possible to see that there is considerable slack in some areas of the body while the skin is quite tight in other areas. This means that it is possible to remove flaps of skin from one of the 'slack' areas and still close the remaining hole. With skin grafts, the skin is usually totally removed from the donor area. However, with skin flaps, the skin is usually left partially attached to the original site so that its blood supply is maintained. The flap is then rotated or slid in order to cover the recipient site:

- **Skin flaps** are becoming more widely used as these conserve the natural blood supply to the tissue. There are many different flaps possible, based on the position of major vessels, and careful planning is needed to ensure that the best site is used to get the desired result
- **Skin grafts** can be defined as full or partial thickness, depending on the depth of skin taken. Full-thickness grafts include the epidermis and dermis, whereas split-thickness grafts only include part of the dermis. These are more fragile than full-thickness grafts but tend to take more easily. However, hair growth is poor and they are more difficult to collect, and because of this split-thickness grafts are less commonly used in small animal practice.

Skin grafts can also be described according to the amount of tissue used. Sheet grafts are designed to fully cover the deficit, whereas pinch grafts, punch grafts or strip grafts are designed to break up the deficit and provide a start point for epithelialization.

As well as careful collection of the graft, the recipient site also needs to be well prepared. The site should be free of contamination and a good layer of well-vascularized granulation tissue should be present so that the graft has a good chance of 'taking'. Alternatively, fresh surgical wounds or clean wounds that have been thoroughly debrided can be suitable sites. The grafts are then placed in situ. Sheet grafts are usually carefully sutured in place, whereas small pinch or punch grafts are simply embedded into the granulation tissue.

Postoperative care is essential in these cases and careful bandaging is required. The bandage should have a non-adherent dressing in contact with the graft such as silicone mesh, which is then covered by a second dressing, padding and an external protective layer. Splints may be used to prevent movement at the site. The bandage must be maintained carefully – it must not be allowed to get wet, or to be interfered with by the patient. The graft should be checked every 24–48 hours and each time the dressing is changed great care should be taken to avoid disturbing the graft.

Wound complications

Wound dehiscence

Wound dehiscence is defined as the breakdown of a surgical wound. There are a number of reasons why this might occur:

- Insufficient debridement – such that the wound edges start to become necrotic
- Poor local blood supply
- Suture reaction – in some cases sutures act as a focus for a reaction
- Movement of wound edges.

In all cases the signs include redness, swelling, discharge, separation of the wound edges, irritation and the animal may start to appear unwell.

To manage these cases, the underlying problem must first be identified so that steps can be taken to avoid repetition.

Then the wound should be cleaned and debrided again. Where possible surgical closure should still be carried out but occasionally it is necessary to keep the wound open and treat it as an open wound.

Wound infection

Wound infection is a major concern when dealing with any type of wound. If the wound has been lavaged thoroughly and debrided fully the chances of infection are minimal. However, it is still very important that general hygiene is maintained so that the risk from environmental contamination is minimized, and, of course, animals with reduced immune function are more at risk.

If a wound becomes infected then the animal may show systemic changes, becoming anorexic, lethargic and pyrexic. The wound site will also show changes – the area will be red, swollen and uncomfortable and there may be an abnormal discharge.

Treatment is similar to that for wound dehiscence and the wound must be cleaned thoroughly and debrided again. If possible, it should then be managed as an open wound, as sutures may act as a focus for any residual infection. Swabs should also be taken and cultured so that appropriate antibiotics can be used. Systemic antibiotics must be used, but topical treatments may include the use of ointments or dressings contining silver. Topical antibiotics are not very useful as they tend to be absorbed by the dressing rather than going into the tissues.

Seroma formation

This is the accumulation of serous fluid under the skin. It usually forms where the surgery has involved the removal of subcutaneous tissue, or the skin is particularly loose or mobile, creating an empty or 'dead space'. In most cases seromata do not cause problems but may appear unsightly. However, they may delay wound healing and are particularly worrying where skin grafts or flaps have been carried out. Most cases, however, do not actually require treatment as the fluid will be reabsorbed gradually over time.

Surgical conditions

In general practice much of our time is spent dealing with animals requiring surgery. The cases range from relatively routine elective procedures to emergency life-saving operations. In all cases nursing staff carry out a vital role, ensuring that the animals are given the necessary care and support and also helping owners to understand both the surgery and the aftercare needed.

General cutaneous conditions

Abscess

An abscess is a localized collection of pus. Pus is tissue debris, dead and degenerating neutrophils and is usually cream or green in colour. An abscess usually contains pyogenic (pus-forming) organisms, but may be sterile. The wall of the abscess is lined with granulation and fibrous tissue.

Note that abscesses can be found in any tissue, e.g. skin, muscle, bone, organs and brain.

Most abscesses will give rise to the signs of pain, local swelling and reduced function of the area. In time, the abscess is likely to come to a head and may rupture on to a surface. For subcutaneous abscesses this usually helps, because the pressure is reduced and drainage is established. Deep abscesses are more of a problem as, if these rupture, the pus will leak into the abdominal cavity and peritonitis may develop, which can be life-threatening. It can also be serious if the pus enters the blood stream – the animal will develop pyaemia and toxaemia.

Treatment of abscesses always involves the same basic principles no matter where the abscess is located:

- **Establish drainage** – superficial abscesses can be lanced and flushed with saline, Hartmann's solution or weak disinfectant solutions. Hydrogen peroxide should not be used as this is extremely tissue-toxic. Hydrogels may be used to pack the abscess site. Deep abscesses require surgery and drains are usually required in order to allow sufficient ongoing drainage
- **Maintain drainage** – superficial wounds should be kept open through regular bathing and flushing with mild solutions. Deeper abscesses also require flushing via the drain
- **Treat with appropriate antibiotics** – only of benefit if drainage has been established. Without drainage the abscess will reduce in size but it is unlikely that all the bacteria within it will be killed, and once antibiotics are stopped it is likely to recur.

In most cases the protocol described above will allow the abscess to settle down but, if there is insufficient drainage or if there is any foreign material within the abscess cavity, then further treatment will be needed.

There are some occasions where the type or location of the abscess makes it more amenable to complete surgical excision. Providing this is done without spillage it can result in complete removal of the problem. However, dead space will be created so drains are often placed to prevent the accumulation of any serum within the operation site. Excision is often the treatment of choice in rabbits, even for superficial abscesses, as the prognosis is considerably better than when using local drainage.

Ulcers

An ulcer is defined as the loss of the epithelial surface of a tissue, usually skin or mucous membrane, leaving a raw area, which is often slow to heal. Examples include oral ulceration, pressure sores (decubitus ulcers) and corneal ulcers.

Treatment involves the removal of the primary cause, keeping the surface clean and dressing the wound if possible. This will avoid further aggravation of the ulcer. Any secondary infection should be treated with antibiotics.

Fistula

This is a channel that passes from one mucous membrane to a second mucous membrane or the skin, i.e. it passes from one epithelial surface to another. The fistula itself is also lined with epithelium. In general, these should be repaired surgically but the specific treatment will vary with the location of the individual fistula:

- **Anal sac fistula** – an opening forms between the anal sac and the external skin, usually as a result of chronic infection. This will probably require surgical excision of the anal sacs and the overlying skin
- **Rectovaginal fistula** – usually a congenital abnormality where an opening remains between the rectum and the vagina lying ventral to it. This is uncommon but may be corrected surgically. The condition is also likely to be inherited and affected animals should not be bred from
- **Oronasal fistula** – may occur after extraction of the canine teeth, which have extremely long roots, which leave a channel between the oral and nasal chambers. The hole should be closed surgically or food will lodge in the site, which may lead to chronic nasal infection.

Sinus

This is an opening or canal running from deeper tissues to the skin or mucous membrane. It is not lined with epithelium and is blind-ending. It is often associated with infection:

- **Foreign body tract** – grass seeds commonly cause problems in animals by penetrating the skin and tracking through the subcutaneous tissues. Bacteria are carried deep into the tissues and there is marked tissue reaction to both the foreign body and the infection. Treatment involves careful surgical exploration of the site and removal of the foreign body.
- **Anal furunculosis** – a deep pyoderma leading to many sinus tracts forming within the tissues. It can be very debilitating and painful and a number of treatment options are available, including radical surgical excision of the affected tissue, cryosurgery or the use of immunosuppressive drugs such as cyclosporins or topical tacrolimus.

Hernias and ruptures

These are similar, since in both cases abdominal contents come to rest in an abnormal position through an opening in the muscular wall. The difference between them is that in a hernia, the opening in the abdominal wall is natural – such as the umbilicus or inguinal ring. In a rupture there is a tear in the muscle wall that allows the abdominal contents to migrate through.

In all cases, the contents of the hernia/rupture should be replaced in their normal position. This is sometimes quite simple and can be done through gentle manipulation. Such hernias are described as **reducible.** However, the condition is likely to recur, so surgery is usually needed to close or reduce the size of the opening. With ruptures, adhesions may develop between the contents of the rupture and the wall, and they may then be **irreducible.**

In some cases the blood flow to the contents becomes compromised. Initially the venous flow is affected, as the vessels are relatively thin-walled and more easily compressed, and blood is able to enter the area but not to leave it. Very quickly the tissues become engorged and then even the arterial vessels are affected. The hernia is then said to be strangulated and the tissue trapped in the sac will very quickly become devitalized. These cases are emergencies and require emergency surgery to prevent the animal's condition deteriorating. The surgery for each type of hernia is different in each case (Table 21.7).

Diaphragmatic rupture

Although often referred to as a hernia, this is usually a rupture caused by trauma forcing the diaphragm to tear. This allows abdominal contents to move through into the thorax and compromise respiratory function.

Affected patients need careful handling to prevent the situation deteriorating, and treatment of shock is the primary concern. Surgery should be attempted only after the animal has been stabilized. During this time the animal should be encouraged to remain in sternal recumbency with its head and thorax propped up such that they are higher than the abdomen. This allows the abdominal contents to slide back

Table 21.7 Hernias – causes and treatments

Type of hernia/ rupture	Description	Treatment and prognosis
Umbilical hernia	Protrusion of abdominal contents through an enlarged umbilical opening	Surgical repair of the linea alba Rarely any complications
Inguinal hernia	Abdominal contents migrate through the inguinal canal to the groin region More common in bitches and rabbits	Surgery to draw abdominal contents back into the abdomen and to reduce the size of the hole in the abdominal muscle layers Can be serious if tissues have become devitalized, particularly if the bladder is involved
Perineal hernia	Muscle layers around the anal sphincter gradually break down and allow the rectal wall to stretch and form a diverticulum This results in constipation and impaction Most common in intact male dogs	Muscle reconstruction of the perineal area is possible Castration is also recommended, since the condition is hormone-related Prognosis remains guarded because of possible long-term difficulty in passing faeces or incontinence There is a risk of the other side developing the same condition – particularly if the dog is left intact

towards the abdomen under gravity rather than migrating forward into the thorax. These patients should not be given anything to eat – food encourages stomach contractions and this may also work the stomach cranially. Strict rest is essential as any activity increases the oxygen demand by the tissues. Additional oxygen can be helpful, providing this can be given without causing the animal any stress.

During surgery, the animal is usually placed in dorsal recumbency and the approach is via a cranial laparotomy incision. As the thoracic cavity is approached, the lungs tend to collapse, so there must be strict attention to the patient's respiration. Respiratory augmentation is often used to assist the animal. This can be achieved by gently squeezing the respiratory reservoir bag on the circuit at the same time as the animal's own respiratory movements. Thus the amount of air the animal takes in with each breath is increased and oxygenation is improved.

Postoperatively, a chest drain is usually placed, and as much trapped air as possible is withdrawn from the thoracic cavity to encourage the lungs to re-expand before the animal is allowed to recover, and the patient must be monitored closely to ensure that respiratory function is adequate. It may still be necessary to place the patient in an oxygen-rich environment during the recovery phase, and to aspirate the drain every 1–4 hours. Once the patient's breathing has returned to normal, and no more air is obtained from the drain, it can be removed.

Tumours

The words tumour and neoplasia refer to any abnormal new growth occurring in the body. These growths are either benign, with no tendency to spread, or malignant, which infiltrate extensively into local tissues and can spread throughout the body.

Benign growths

These usually have well-developed capsules and remain in the one site. They include:

- **Lipoma** – adipose tissue tumour
- **Fibroma** – superficial tumour of the skin and occasionally the mouth
- **Adenoma** – benign tumour of glandular tissue, e.g. anal adenoma, adenoma of the thyroid gland
- **Papilloma** – 'warty' growths found on the skin and occasionally in the bladder arising from epithelial tissues
- **Melanoma** – tumour of the melanocytes in the skin; although named as if they are benign, such tumours are usually malignant.

Malignant growths

Poorly differentiated tumours with indistinct edges. They tend to spread both into local tissues and systemically. They include:

- **Carcinoma** – produced from epithelium. Examples include squamous cell carcinomas (often seen affecting the ear tips of white cats) and mammary tumours, which are usually adenocarcinomas, i.e. affecting glandular epithelium
- **Sarcoma** – produced from mesodermal (connective) tissues. Examples include osteosarcoma and fibrosarcoma
- **Malignant melanoma** also comes into this category. Strictly this should be called melanocarcinoma and therefore fits with other epithelial cell tumours.

Malignant tumours often show ulceration, local infiltration and metastasis, i.e. they spread to sites distant from the original tumour site.

Carcinomas tend to spread to local lymph nodes via the lymphatic system, whereas sarcomas tend to spread via the blood stream and lodge in tissues where the blood passes through capillary networks, such as the lungs.

Haematological tumours – involve the lymphoid and myeloid tissues and can be solid or circulating: e.g. lymphosarcoma (solid) and leukaemia (circulating).

Common sites for tumours

Tumours can occur at any site in the body and in all species. The risk of developing some type of tumour increases as an animal gets older, since cellular repair mechanisms become less effective with age.

Complications of tumours

Tumours cause a number of problems within the body. Local effects include pain and ulceration leading to secondary infection. The physical presence of the tumour can also cause problems such as restriction of movement or prevention of the normal flow of ingesta through the intestines.

Metastases

These are secondary tumours that usually develop as small clumps of cells break away from the primary tumour and enter the circulation. When they encounter a mesh-like filter such as the capillaries in the spleen or lungs or the reticular structure within lymph nodes they are caught and start to multiply or metastasize at that site.

Metastases can occur in almost any site but the lymph nodes, lungs, liver and spleen are the most common. All metastases will produce loss of function at the affected site, which adds to the problems that may be developing at the primary site. The clinical signs will depend on the area affected.

Hormone production

Secretory tumours can overproduce normal hormones and affect the body's metabolism. Common endocrine tumours include thyroid adenomas, insulinomas, pituitary gland tumours and adrenal gland tumours.

Tumours affecting non-glandular tissues can also secrete substances that may behave like hormones: e.g. lymphomas and bone tumours can produce a substance that behaves like parathyroid hormone and causes hypercalcaemia; insulin-like hormones are produced by some tumours, leading to hyperglycaemia.

Haematological complications

These may also develop as a result of invasion of bone marrow by the tumour or changes in production of blood cells, platelets and clotting factors.

Causes of tumours

There is a considerable amount of research into why and how tumours develop and, although not all the answers are known, the following are thought to contribute:

- **Mutations** – random events leading to uncontrolled proliferation of mutated cells. There may be an inherited component as to why these occur in some breeds more than others
- **Viruses** – including feline leukaemia virus and papillomaviruses
- **Carcinogens** – chemicals that induce mutations in the DNA such as those released through smoking, solvents such as benzene and even such apparently benign substances as caramel, which in large enough quantities has been implicated in causing cancer
- **Chronic inflammation** – there is some evidence that sites of chronic inflammation may increase the chance of developing tumours in animals. This is well documented in human medicine, but studies relating to veterinary cases are still ongoing
- **Other causes** – irradiation, parasites and hormones are also being studied to determine the significance of these factors in the development of tumours in animals.

Tumour diagnosis

Diagnosis is usually confirmed by means of a sample of tissue, which is examined histologically to determine both the cell type and the degree of malignancy. The results will give an indication of the prognosis and the most appropriate treatment.

Wedge biopsy

A section of the tumour is taken after surgical excision. This is the best method as it provides cells from the centre and the edge of the tumour. The sample should then be fixed in formol-saline.

Tru-Cut needle biopsy

A specialized needle is used to take tiny samples from parenchymal tissues (Fig. 21.6). The needle has a small notch cut out of its barrel and a cover that is slid down so that a small quantity of tissue is caught between the notch and the cover. This can then be fixed and examined histologically.

A Tru-Cut needle can be used to obtain tissue from organs such as the liver and kidney. Biopsy of the kidney can even be performed percutaneously. However, it is not as good as the wedge biopsy, as you only get a small sliver of tissue for analysis and could miss the area where the cancerous cells are located.

Needle aspirate

This technique is commonly used for lymphomas and may also be used to differentiate between abscesses and other cutaneous swellings.

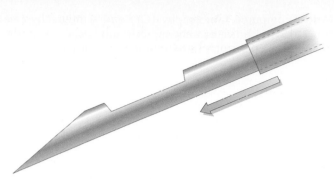

Fig. 21.6 Simplified diagram of a Tru-Cut needle

Method:

1. Introduce a 1 inch × 23 G needle into the mass
2. Move the needle to and fro within the mass, changing the direction
3. Withdraw
4. Connect an air-filled syringe
5. Depress the plunger of the syringe sharply, and blow out the cells on to a slide
6. Make a smear from the cells, stain and examine under the microscope.

It is also possible to obtain samples by suction, i.e. by having the syringe already attached, and drawing back on the plunger to collect the cells. However, lymphoma cells are fragile, and if this is suspected, the needle-only method may give better results. Examination of the stained smear may give sufficient information to start treatment. However, in other cases it may prove non-diagnostic.

Exfoliative cytology

Cells taken from the surface of the tumour are collected and analysed. This method is only used if other diagnostic techniques are not possible, as it is the least reliable. It can be carried out in several different ways, depending on the accessibility of the tumour:

- Tissue scraping – a scalpel blade is used to collect cells from the surface of a mass
- Impression smears – a glass slide is touched onto the surface of the lesion, which has been cleaned prior to collecting the sample
- Exudate is collected and then examined
- Sterile saline is flushed over the surface of the suspect tissue and then collected. Any cellular matter is then examined. Flushes can be used to examine the nasal cavity, bronchi and trachea and prostate gland.

If tumour cells are found, then the technique is diagnostic; if none are identified, it might simply mean that the tumour cells were not collected.

Tumour imaging

Diagnostic imaging techniques may also be very important in the initial diagnosis of the tumour, checking for evidence of metastases, and monitoring the progress of the patient. Several imaging techniques are now available, including radiography, ultrasonography, magnetic resonance imaging

(MRI), computed tomography (CT) and scintigraphy (see Ch. 29). The choice of imaging technique depends on the nature of the particular tumour under investigation.

Treatment

Surgery

This is generally the treatment of choice as, by complete removal of the tumour, the animal may be cured of that particular cancer. Operations should be carried out as soon as possible to decrease the risk of further growth of the tumour and to minimize the risk of metastasis.

Care should be taken when preparing the site for surgery. Wide excisions are needed to ensure that all the tumour cells are removed, but different tumours require different margins (Table 21.8). The area clipped and prepared for surgery must therefore be sufficient for the particular tumour type. The site should also be cleaned quite gently; if the site is scrubbed too hard there is possibly an increased risk of the tumour metastasizing.

In some cases it is not possible to remove the tumour completely and debulking surgery may be performed. This is indicated if it will either improve the animal's quality of life or reduce the amount of tumour sufficiently for follow-up treatments using radiation or chemotherapy to be more successful.

Radiation therapy

Radiation damages rapidly dividing cells and can cause chromosomal damage, thereby preventing them from dividing further. This is usually the reason why we avoid exposure to radiation during radiography. However, since tumour cells are dividing uncontrollably, they are often more sensitive to the effects of radiation than other cells. Radiation can be applied from an external source such as X-ray or gamma-ray machines (teletherapy) or from an implanted source such as radioactive iodine or iridium wires (brachytherapy). If an external source is used, it is usual for a dose to be given weekly for 4–5 weeks. On each occasion the beam is positioned slightly differently to minimize damage to unaffected tissues.

The technique is most commonly used for oral and nasal tumours that are not amenable to surgical resection. The prognosis is, however, still guarded and many tumours recur 6–9 months after treatment. Side effects, such as erythema of exposed skin and mucous membranes, alopecia, skin thickening and abnormal hair coloration, may also occur. Owners must therefore be given careful advice before embarking on a treatment programme so that they are fully aware of the possible outcomes.

Chemotherapy

This is the treatment of tumours using cytotoxic drugs and is most commonly used for tumours that have spread systemically or those affecting the bone marrow or lymphatic system.

There are a number of different drugs available for use as chemotherapeutic agents and different protocols involving combinations of these products have been developed for different types of cancer (Table 21.9). These are obviously very potent drugs and care is required whenever they are handled. During preparation of the product, care must be taken to avoid inhalation, so ideally this should be done in a biological safety cabinet, or somewhere away from where there are a lot of people, and away from any windows or draughts. Heavy-duty latex gloves are essential and hands should always be washed both before and after handling these products. If the drug is to be given intravenously it should always be given through a catheter to ensure accurate delivery.

However, it is not just during the preparation and administration of the products that care is needed, as body waste may also contain traces of the drugs so gloves and

Table 21.8 Excision margins for different tumours

Tumour type	Recommended margin
Squamous cell carcinoma	1 cm
Mast cell tumour	2–3 cm
Osteosarcoma	Limb amputation (or radical resection of the bone)

Table 21.9 Cytotoxic drugs used to treat tumours

Drug name	Tumours treated	Route of administration
Vincristine (Oncovin)	Lymphoma Transmissible venereal tumour Sarcomas Mast cell tumours	Intravenous
Cyclophosphamide (Endoxana)	Lymphoma Leukaemia Mammary tumours	Oral Intravenous
Doxorubicin (Adriamycin)	Lymphoma Adenocarcinoma Osteosarcoma Urogenital tumours	Slow intravenous infusion with 0.9% saline
Cis-platinum (Cisplatin)	Osteosarcoma Some carcinomas Urogenital tumours	Intravenous Toxic in cats
Carboplatin (Paraplatin)	Osteosarcoma Some carcinomas Urogenital tumours	Slow intravenous infusion with 0.9% saline
Cytosine arabinoside (Cytarabine)	Leukaemia Lymphoma	Intravenous
Chlorambucil (Leukeran)	Chronic leukaemia Lymphoma Mast cell tumours	Oral
Methotrexate (Methotrexate, Matrex)	Lymphoma Transmissible venereal tumour	Oral Intravenous Intramuscular Subcutaneous

protective aprons should be worn when handling faeces or urine from treated animals and owners should be advised accordingly.

Cryotherapy

This is the controlled destruction of tissues by freezing. In the past this has been used to manage some tumours which are difficult to excise. However, cryotherapy is now used predominantly in specialized ophthalmic surgery.

Surgical procedures by region of the body

The veterinary nurse has a number of very important roles to play in the management of surgical cases. This includes preoperative, intraoperative and postoperative care.

Preoperative procedures – on admission the necessary paperwork for the animal should have been completed fully and the client should have been made aware of what will happen during the surgery. Checks should be made as to when the animal last ate or drank to ensure it is ready for an anaesthetic.

The animal should then be weighed and any premedication drawn up ready for administration. This can be then given under veterinary direction. Analgesics are often given preoperatively as evidence has shown that their effectiveness is greater when given before a painful stimulus rather than afterwards. The theatre should be prepared ready for the procedure and all the appropriate instruments should be made ready.

When the premedication is fully effective anaesthesia should be induced (see Ch. 25). This should be done in the preparation area and the animal should then be clipped up ready to be taken through into theatre. The final skin preparation should be applied once the patient is in theatre.

Operative procedures – during the operation the veterinary nurse should provide assistance to the surgeon. This may mean that the nurse scrubs up and works alongside the surgeon, passing instruments, swabbing the site and cutting sutures as indicated. Alternatively, the nurse may remain non-sterile but be responsible for opening sterile packs for the surgeon, or monitoring the condition of the patient.

Postoperative procedures – the operation site should be gently cleaned before the animal starts to come round from the anaesthetic, and any dressings should be applied at this time. The patient should then be monitored carefully during recovery to ensure adequate respiration and return of the laryngeal reflexes. Patients should also be kept warm and the operation site should be checked regularly prior to discharge.

Nurses may also be involved at discharge and it is important that any nurse discharging a patient is fully aware of the procedures that have taken place. For example, if an animal has had dental treatment, the nurse must know whether extractions were required and, if so, how many and which teeth required removal.

The nurse must advise the client about postoperative care for the animal, including details about any medication that needs to be given, when and what to feed, any special instructions relating to the operation, when to make the next appointment at the surgery and what possible problems to watch for.

The ear

Aural haematoma

Cause

Aural haematomata usually develop on the ear pinna as a result of self-trauma secondary to either an ear infection or a foreign body within the ear canal. More rarely it can be due to direct trauma. It is most commonly seen in dogs.

Clinical signs

The ear pinna is swollen and on palpation the swelling is fluid-filled and warm to the touch. If there is otitis or a foreign body within the ear canal, the animal may resent examination of the ear, so care should be taken to ensure that no one is bitten.

Treatment

The ear should be examined carefully to determine the primary cause. This often needs to be carried out under general anaesthesia. If there is evidence of infection, the ear canal should be cleaned thoroughly using saline and the tympanic membrane checked prior to using any other solutions. If the tympanic membrane is damaged, then disinfectants or otolytic solutions should be avoided since these will cause problems within the middle ear.

The pinna should be clipped and prepared for surgery. An incision is made on the inside of the ear to allow the blood to drain. Compression is then applied across the pinna to prevent the dead-space between the skin and cartilage from refilling with blood. This is usually achieved by using a number of mattress sutures. To prevent the suture cutting into the tissue, something may be used to help spread the compression. Some veterinary surgeons use commercial products, whereas others improvise using materials such as X-ray film, pieces of drip tubing or buttons to do this. Whichever is used, consideration should be given to the animal's recovery as, if the materials used are too heavy, they will cause the animal discomfort and its attempts to scratch or shake the ear may make things worse. Alternatively, after surgery, the ear may be compressed using bandaging techniques, which will also help absorb any seepage from the wound.

In some cases, if the aural haematoma is very small, it may be possible just to drain the haematoma and then use an injection of long-acting steroids to reduce the inflammation and the likelihood of further bleeding under the skin. This method, while less invasive, does not always work and may need to be followed with surgical treatment.

Postoperative care

These cases require analgesia and antibiotics and will often need an Elizabethan collar to prevent self-trauma. It is usual to leave the sutures in place for slightly longer than a normal surgical wound just to make sure that the haematoma does not immediately re-form.

Lateral wall resection (Zepp's procedure)

This procedure is used in some cases of chronic ear infection in which the vertical canal has become chronically inflamed and narrowed. In this situation it is important that owners do not believe that this will provide a miracle cure for their animal – usually it just makes treatment of the underlying condition easier and allows air to circulate in the ear canal. Another indication for this surgery is an animal with polyps or a tumour affecting just the vertical canal. It is more commonly carried out in dogs than cats, particularly animals with 'floppy' ears where air circulation is reduced and infection more likely, e.g. labradors and spaniels.

Preoperative preparation

The ear canal should be cleaned thoroughly and the area ventral to the external opening of the ear canal should be clipped and prepared for surgery. One of the most common reasons for wound breakdown postoperatively is infection, so it is helpful if the animal has already been on treatment for any otitis prior to the surgery.

Procedure

The lateral wall of the vertical ear canal is resected and reflected such that when the operation is complete the medial wall of the vertical canal is exposed, as is the entrance to the horizontal canal.

Postoperative care

This is a painful procedure so analgesics are needed as well as antibiotics. An Elizabethan collar is used to prevent the animal trying to scratch or rub the affected ear.

There is often a considerable discharge from the ear due to underlying infection so it is important that the operation site is kept clean in the postoperative period. Not all patients will tolerate this so it may be necessary for the dog to come back to the surgery for sedation, enabling the ear to be cleaned and checked.

Sutures should remain in place until the wound edges have obviously healed – this may take longer than most other surgical wounds and to avoid the need for suture removal some surgeons prefer to use absorbable sutures.

Total ear canal ablation (TECA)

If the infection or tumours within the ear are very severe, then a complete aural ablation may be necessary, in which the horizontal and vertical canals of the ear are excised. After this operation, the cosmetic result is actually better than after the lateral wall resection, since the skin is closed beneath the ear and a small hole is left that leads directly to the tympanic membrane.

Preoperative preparation

This is almost identical to the preparation required for the lateral wall resection.

Procedure

An incision is made overlying the vertical canal and the skin edges are reflected to expose the cartilage of the vertical canal. The canal is then carefully dissected away from the underlying tissues right down to the tympanic bulla.

A **bulla osteotomy** is also usually needed to prevent recurrent problems with infection. This involves opening the tympanic bulla in order to release any infection from within the middle ear. This does result in deafness in the affected ear but in most cases requiring this type of surgery the animal is already unable to hear on that side.

Postoperative care

This is the same as for the lateral wall resection.

The eye

Prolapse of the eyeball (proptosis)

This is an emergency and is one of the few situations where an animal must be brought down to the surgery as soon as possible. It usually affects the brachycephalic breeds of dog such as pugs and pekes but can also affect other species such as hamsters and guinea pigs, which also have protruding eyes. In cases of severe trauma, it can affect any breed or species.

Cause

The prolapse has usually been caused by some type of trauma, e.g. road traffic accidents, in which case it may be accompanied by severe trauma to other parts of the body, and shock. Prolapse may also result from a fight or poor handling in the case of exotic species.

Clinical signs

People often imagine that a prolapsed eye will be hanging from the socket but in reality this is not often the case unless there has been severe head trauma. The eye may simply appear more bulbous than usual and the conjunctiva is more apparent and quite congested.

First-aid treatment

The most important action is to prevent the eye from drying out. Saline, ophthalmic ointment or even a water-soluble jelly should be used to prevent this. The animal should also be stopped from traumatizing the eye further by applying an Elizabethan collar. Any signs of shock should be assessed and treated as described earlier in this chapter.

Preparation

There may be relatively little time for extensive preoperative preparation but the surface of the eye should be irrigated thoroughly with sterile saline or false tear solutions prior to replacement. If a canthotomy is likely (incising the lateral canthus of the eye socket to widen it), the fur around the eye should be clipped carefully and the area should be prepared using dilute povidone–iodine solution (0.1%). The surface of the cornea should be protected with water-soluble jelly, which can then be rinsed off, taking with it any hair that might otherwise have become stuck to the surface of the eye.

Surgery

The eye should be replaced as soon as possible, which usually requires general anaesthesia. It may require a lateral canthotomy to open the eyelids sufficiently to allow the eye to be replaced. To prevent immediate recurrence, the eyelids are often sutured together for a short while to allow the bruised and swollen conjunctiva to heal and the eye to settle back into its normal position. If it is not replaced quickly, the eye may become permanently damaged and the animal may lose its sight. If this occurs or there is extensive damage to the eye enucleation may be necessary.

Postoperative care

An Elizabethan collar may be needed for a few days postoperatively to prevent the animal from rubbing the eye. However, once the eye has been in place for 1–2 weeks it should be safe to remove the sutures and collar. Topical antibiotics should be used as well as systemic antibiotics and anti-inflammatories.

Corneal damage

The most common type of corneal damage seen in general practice is a corneal ulcer.

Clinical signs

The eye is very painful and the animal usually holds the eyelids closed – described as **blepharospasm**. There is increased flow of lacrimal fluid due to the pain and irritation and this results in tear overflow or **epiphora**. Depending on the initial cause of the ulcer there may also be infection present, leading to a purulent ocular discharge.

Treatment

The eye should be examined carefully to see if the cause of the ulceration is still present. Small pieces of debris or bedding materials may be caught behind the third eyelid, which may have caused considerable damage to the corneal surface. Local anaesthetic drops such as amethocaine may be needed to aid the examination. Medical treatments are often tried first and antibiotic ointments may be sufficient in some cases. The lack of direct blood supply to the cornea does mean, however, that the healing process is very slow compared with that of other tissues. To provide additional protection for the cornea, corneal bandages, similar to contact lenses, can be used.

Surgery

In other cases the surgical approach is preferred. The simplest surgery is the third eyelid flap, known as a **tarsorrhaphy**. In this procedure the third eyelid is sutured in the closed position so that it does not move across the surface of the ulcer and irritate it further. Prior to this being carried out, the ulcer should be debrided using a dry cotton bud, and it may be necessary to actually excoriate the surface of the ulcer to stimulate healing. This can either be done using caustic chemicals such as phenol, or a hypodermic needle. This may seem to be the exact opposite of what is required, but often stimulates healing in an area that had become quite dormant.

More refined surgery for deep ulcers involves the use of conjunctival grafts. Pedicles of conjunctiva are sutured to the cornea to cover the ulcer. Rather like the use of skin flaps, these still have their vascular supply intact to allow nutrients to reach the ulcerated site more easily. After a few weeks the flap is freed from its origin and trimmed to leave just a small area covering the defect. With time this remodels and becomes less obvious.

Tissue glue has also been used in the repair of small ulcers which are quite deep. After debriding the ulcer and allowing the surface of the cornea to dry the glue is very carefully applied to the area it is needed. This is then be left in place until the ulcer is healed, and then either removed with forceps under local anaesthesia or allowed to slough away gradually.

Postoperative care

The most important thing is that the animal itself does not interfere with healing and aggravate the wound or injury still further, and it may be necessary for the animal to be fitted with an Elizabethan collar. Antibiotic ointments are continued even while the third eyelid flaps or conjunctival flaps are in place. The sutures holding third eyelid flaps are usually removed after 2–3 weeks (depending on the severity of the ulcer) and the ulcer is checked carefully.

Enucleation

This is indicated if the eye is too damaged to save, which may be due to any of the following conditions:

- Gross trauma
- Panophthalmitis (massive inflammation of the whole eye)
- Neoplasia – of the eye or behind the eye (retrobulbar)
- Untreatable glaucoma, which has led to blindness in the affected eye
- Irreducible prolapse or recurrent prolapse
- Retrobulbar abscess
- Any other conditions leading to blindness and pain.

Preparation

Before surgery, owners are often very concerned about the procedure and the likely postoperative appearance of their animal. It may be helpful if the practice has some photographs of animals who have undergone enucleation so that worried owners can see that the cosmetic effect in small animals is often not as bad as they had feared. The animals themselves tolerate enucleation very well!

The skin around the eyelids should be clipped and prepared using a dilute povidone-iodine solution as described previously.

Surgery

If the eye itself is the only problem the eyeball is removed, but the muscles can be left in place so that the skin does not fall so far back into the socket. If, however, enucleation is due to a retrobulbar tumour or chronic abscess in that region, more tissues will need to be removed. It is possible for prostheses to be used to avoid the sunken appearance but these are not commonly used in general practice. The eye is carefully dissected from the surrounding tissues, the third eyelid is removed and a strip of tissue is removed from the edge of each eyelid so that these can be sutured together.

Postoperative care

Some veterinary surgeons bandage the site, which helps to prevent seroma formation within the orbit and is perhaps is helpful for the owners in the initial postoperative period. This can be removed after 2–3 days and the wound can then be left open. To prevent the animal from rubbing the area an Elizabethan collar may be used.

Systemic antibiotics are necessary for a few days postoperatively but should only be continued for any length of time in cases where there was gross infection within the orbit area prior to surgery. Analgesics are not often required beyond the perioperative period, as in most cases the removal of the damaged eye provides sufficient pain relief.

Cataracts

A cataract is an increase in the opacity of the lens and in a true cataract is due to deposition of material within either the capsule, the cortex or the nucleus of the lens. The changes seen in the eyes of old dogs with increased lens opacity are not true cataracts. The lens is continually growing and increases in density so that gradually less and less light is able to pass through. This is called senile nuclear sclerosis and is a natural ageing change.

Surgery

True cortical or capsular cataracts can be removed using surgical techniques by eye specialists. This most commonly involves the use of phaecoemulsification techniques, which break up the cataract deposits.

For nuclear sclerosis, the only treatment available is lentectomy (surgical removal of the lens). The animal will have some vision restored, in that light will reach the retina again, but it will have lost the ability to focus, and there is a risk of developing glaucoma. As the majority of older animals have already learned to cope with the reduced vision due to the sclerosis, surgery is rarely carried out in these cases.

Entropion and ectropion

These are conditions of the eyelids. In entropion the eyelid rolls inwards, causing the eyelashes to irritate the cornea; in ectropion the eyelid bags open, exposing the conjunctiva. Occasionally, entropion and ectropion are found in the same eye. This is particularly the case in animals with so-called diamond eyes, such as the St Bernard.

Clinical signs

Entropion leads to excess tear production and epiphora. The animal shows signs of pain and blepharospasm. Conjunctivitis is usually present and without treatment corneal ulcers are a common consequence. Ectropion may also lead to conjunctivitis, as bacteria can easily gain access to the eye through the exposed area of conjunctiva.

Treatment

For both conditions this involves surgery of the eyelids. Small slivers of skin are removed to turn the eyelid out, or take up the slack of an oversized eyelid (Figs 21.7, 21.8).

It is essential that an assessment of the amount of tissue to be removed is made while the animal is conscious and before the animal has had any premedication – the use of aceromazine will make even a good eye appear like an ectropion!

Distichiasis and ectopic cilia

These are extra eyelashes. Ectopic cilia are just one or two abnormally positioned eyelashes, whereas distichiasis involves a whole row of extra eyelashes inside the normal lashes.

Clinical signs

These are very similar to entropion. Animals present with epiphora, conjunctivitis, blepharospasm and corneal ulcers.

Treatment

The extra eyelashes can be dealt with in a number of ways, of which the simplest is simply to pluck them. However, this only provides a temporary solution, since they will regrow. Electrolysis can also be used, which gives longer-lasting results but is also not necessarily permanent. Surgery can be used to remove the roots of the lashes but this is very delicate surgery and requires specialized ophthalmic instruments. Cryotherapy is another alternative. Neither of these methods is commonly used in general practice.

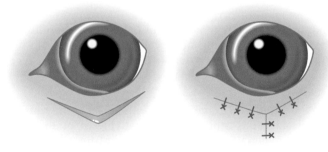

Fig. 21.7 V-Y plasty for ectropion management

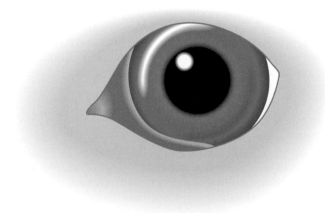

Fig. 21.8 Crescent-shaped sliver removal for entropion

Gastrointestinal tract

Gastrotomy

The surgical technique involving the opening up of the stomach may be used as treatment for the following conditions:

Foreign bodies

These are very common and very varied in type. Throughout your time in practice you will undoubtedly see a number of items removed from the gastrointestinal tract of animals and will certainly gain experience in dealing with this type of case.

Clinical signs

These vary depending on the type of foreign body. Sharp foreign bodies produce recurrent vomiting, often with blood, described as haematemesis, whereas others produce no obvious signs and might only be found when the animal is being investigated for something else.

Diagnosis

The most common method of confirming a diagnosis is radiography (see Ch. 30). Plain studies will be sufficient for some types but contrast studies may be needed to locate radiolucent objects such as plastic bags or pairs of tights.

Surgery

These patients usually require a laparotomy and gastrotomy for removal of the object. If the problem has been present for some while, consideration will need to be given to the hydration status of the patient and it may be necessary to provide preoperative intravenous fluids to rehydrate the animal before giving it a general anaesthetic.

During the procedure it is important to minimize the risk of spillage of gastric contents into the abdomen; large swabs may be needed to pack off the stomach from the abdomen as it is exteriorized. If gastric contents do leak into the peritoneal cavity, it should be lavaged with copious amounts of warmed, sterile saline.

Postoperative care

Initially small amounts of bland liquidized food should be given several times per day, and then a more solid version of the same can be used. Using this regime helps to prevent the development of gut stasis, which may develop if food is withheld for 24 hours. The animal's normal food should then be reintroduced gradually over a period of days. Antibiotics are often used for a few days after surgery, though not all surgeons agree with this procedure. Analgesics should be used to meet the animal's requirements. Careful monitoring is essential and any signs of vomiting, depression or pyrexia should be noted and the veterinary surgeon informed.

Gastric dilation and torsion (gastric dilation and volvulus, GDV)

This condition can be seen in any dog, but most commonly affects deep-chested breeds, e.g. greyhounds, pointers and German shepherds. The classic history for these cases is that the animal has been fed, often on dry foods, and then exercised. The dog becomes depressed and may start to salivate or attempt to vomit. Gradually the abdomen becomes distended and the animal may 'flank watch' as it tries to determine why it is feeling so uncomfortable. As time progresses the abdominal swelling becomes more obvious and the mucous membranes become a deep purple colour.

Pathogenesis

Initially the stomach dilates due to an accumulation of gas or fluid. The dilation may progress to torsion if the stomach starts to rotate about the oesophagus. The distal oesophagus and duodenum become twisted preventing ingesta leaving the stomach in either direction. The stomach continues to distend, which puts pressure on the hepatic portal vein and caudal vena cava and decreases venous return. This leads to hypovolaemic shock as blood is not returned to the heart and is not available to be re-oxygenated and delivered to the tissues. Without rapid treatment, this condition is fatal. In addition, the blood supply to the stomach is also compromised, leading to necrosis of the stomach wall. Toxins are able to leak into the blood stream, which leads to endotoxaemia.

Management

- **Gastric decompression** – the first thing to do is to attempt to pass a stomach tube to relieve the pressure in the stomach. The tube should be measured against the animal in order to determine the correct length and then gently passed through the oropharynx. If it will enter the stomach, then the stomach contents can be evacuated and the stomach can be flushed with warm saline (gastric lavage).
  If the twist in the oesophagus makes it impossible to pass the tube, then the best way to relieve the pressure is to introduce a 16 G needle into the right flank wall just behind the ribs. This will pierce the stomach and allow pent-up gas to escape. It should not be undertaken lightly and the advice of a veterinary surgeon should always be sought before this method is used. The stomach tube may then be passed and gastric lavage performed
- **Treat shock** – these patients are in hypovolaemic shock, so once the pressure in the stomach is relieved intravenous fluids will be needed to restore the circulating blood pressure
- **Surgery** – in cases where dilation is the main symptom, passing the stomach tube may be sufficient treatment, after which the animal should be monitored. However, cases also involving a torsion will require surgery to relieve the torsion and reposition the organs. A **gastropexy** may also be performed in which the stomach is sutured to the abdominal wall to prevent recurrence. In some cases, when the stomach rotates, the spleen is taken with it and a **splenectomy** may be needed, especially if the spleen has been caught in the twist for any length of time.

Postoperative care

Intravenous fluids are needed initially, and patients are usually starved about 12 hours before starting oral fluids. Providing the patient does not vomit, then small amounts of food can be offered. This should be bland, easily digestible food, and the patient should be fed 3–4 times per day.

Close monitoring of these patients is essential, especially in the first 48 hours, as toxins trapped in the blood supply of the stomach are released into the circulation as the stomach is untwisted. It is possible for animals apparently doing well after surgery to suddenly relapse and die from endotoxic shock, so the prognosis should still be considered guarded.

Long-term management of these patients involves looking at their normal feeding and exercise regimes. Studies have found that patients have a reduced risk of dilation and torsion if they are fed at least twice a day rather than once a day. Owners should also exercise their animals before feeding rather than the other way round.

Enterotomy and enterectomy

- **Enterotomy** – a surgical technique involving the opening up of the intestine
- **Enterectomy** – the removal of a length of intestine.

These techniques may be used as treatment in the following conditions:

Foreign bodies

The clinical signs seen with intestinal foreign bodies vary but in most cases the animals vomit and become depressed and anorexic, leading to dehydration and shock. To treat these cases an enterotomy is usually carried out.

An incision is made in the wall of the intestine, the object is removed and the incision is closed immediately. Omentum or mesentery may be sutured over the point of entry to reduce the risk of leakage. If, however, the intestine is badly damaged, an enterectomy may be carried out. The damaged portion is removed and the two cut ends of the intestine are sutured together. This is referred to as an **end-to-end anastomosis.**

Intussusception

This describes the telescoping of a piece of intestine inside itself. It is most often seen in young animals, especially if they have had diarrhoea, as the peristaltic contractions are exaggerated compared with usual movements.

Clinically, the animals are subdued, with a depressed appetite. They may try to vomit or may pass small amounts of diarrhoea and on examination the intussusception may be palpable within the abdomen.

Management usually requires a laparotomy to reveal the extent of the problem. In mild cases, it may be possible for the intussusception to be reduced by simply teasing the intestine apart. However, if the blood supply has been severely compromised, an enterectomy will be needed.

Postoperative care

All animals undergoing intestinal surgery should be carefully monitored post-operatively, and analgesia provided. Water can usually be provided within the first 12 hours, though intravenous fluids are also usually given. Bland, easily digestible food can be introduced providing the animal does not vomit, and after a few days, the patient can gradually switch back to its normal diet. If the patient does not improve after the first couple of days, it should be checked thoroughly again, as the possibility of wound dehiscence cannot be ignored.

Rectum and anus

Surgery to the rectal and anal areas may be indicated for a number of reasons, including perineal hernias as well as those detailed here:

Neoplasia and polyps

Growths within the colon are quite common and may cause problems with defecation. The owners may simply notice that the animal is having difficulty passing faeces (**dyschezia**), or is straining more than usual (**tenesmus**). There may also be fresh blood on the faeces.

To investigate problems in the terminal alimentary canal, plain radiographs and contrast studies are often used. Digital palpation of the rectum can also be useful and in many cases endoscopy is used to visualize the internal wall of the colon and rectum.

Some tumours and polyps are amenable to surgery and simple excision may be possible. Other cases require more radical surgery, in which the terminal part of the colon and rectum is removed. In all cases, postoperative care involves ensuring that the animal is able to pass faeces relatively comfortably, so the use of mild laxatives or hydrophilic compounds such as Peridale granules given orally may assist in keeping the faeces soft. Antibiotics are usually given.

Anal furunculosis

This is a painful condition. A deep pyoderma develops in the perianal tissues and is characterized by the formation of deep sinus tracts. It is most often seen in German shepherd dogs, especially those with a low tail carriage.

Clinical signs

These animals are in considerable pain and consequently show dyschezia, faecal tenesmus and anal irritation.

Treatment

A number of different treatments have been tried, including surgery in which the sinus tracts are fully debrided, leaving open wounds that are left to heal by second intention. It may be combined with the use of cryotherapy to remove tissue that was not easy to remove with a scalpel.

Postoperative care

The wounds should be kept clean by gentle washing of the area with warmed saline or Hartmann's solution. Antibiotics are also needed to reduce the risk of further infection and the patient must be closely monitored to ensure that it is able to defecate normally. More recently, immunosuppressive drugs such as cyclosporin or topical tacrolimus have been found to be useful.

Impaction and infection of the anal sacs

Impaction of the anal sacs is common, leading to anal irritation seen as bottom-rubbing, 'scooting' and biting at the rear end. Simple impaction can be managed by manual expression. However, if impaction becomes frequent or abscesses develop, the sacs should be removed by surgical excision.

Treatment

Prior to surgery the anal area must be prepared. The anal sacs should be evacuated fully and then flushed or cleaned using saline or very dilute Savlon solution. The perianal area should be clipped up and prepared for surgery. Some surgeons may fill the sacs with anal sac gel or wax to aid their location during removal, but there is a risk that this material may leak into the surrounding tissues, leading to chronic reactions. Others may simply use a probe in the duct to help locate the sac. To prevent faecal contamination of the operation site, some veterinary surgeons use a purse string suture around the anus, or a cotton wool plug. If this method is used, it should be noted, so that it can be removed at the end of the operation.

Postoperative care

Keep the area clean and ensure that the animal is able to pass faeces. Antibiotic cover is needed. Note that in some cases there is temporary faecal incontinence due to bruising of the anal sphincter tissues but this should settle down with time.

Reproductive tract

The most common elective surgery carried out in practice is the neutering of pets. This surgery, while considered 'routine', is not risk free and it is always worth reminding owners of this when discussing the procedure. However, if appropriate care is taken the risks are small and we should encourage owners to be responsible and not breed animals indiscriminately.

Ovariohysterectomy (spay)

In most cases animals are spayed in order to control oestrous cycles and to prevent unwanted litters. In addition, an ovariohysterectomy may be carried out to prevent an animal developing mammary tumours, to treat a pyometra or to manage an animal that has recurrent false pregnancies.

The timing of the surgery in the bitch is quite important and she can either be spayed prior to her first oestrus or during anoestrus – usually 2–4 months after the bitch has been in season or 6–8 weeks after giving birth.

The queen, during the breeding season, comes into oestrus every 3 weeks and it may be difficult to find a time when she is not in season. As a result, a veterinary surgeon will usually perform the operation any time after the onset of sexual maturity at around 5 months of age.

Surgery

In the bitch, surgery is usually carried out via a midline linea alba incision, whereas in the queen it is more usually done through a sublumbar incision in the left flank. In both cases the ovaries, uterine horns and uterine body are removed (Fig. 21.9).

During the procedure it is common for the animal to breathe more erratically as the surgeon exteriorizes the ovary, but this usually settles down once the vessels have been ligated and the ovary has been freed from its attachments.

Postoperative care

The animal should be kept quiet for the first couple of days and, in the case of a bitch, restricted to lead exercise only until the sutures are removed. Cats should be kept indoors until the wound has started to heal properly. If there is any interference with the sutures or any seepage from the wound, the animal should be brought back to the surgery for a check.

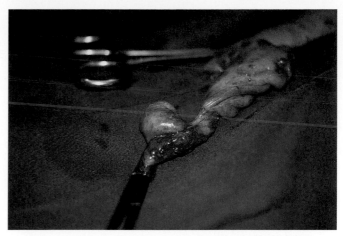

Fig. 21.9 Exteriorized ovary and uterine horn during a bitch spay

Complications

These include the risk of haemorrhage from either the ovarian or uterine vessels. Internal haemorrhage may be recognized by pallor of the mucous membranes, rapid heart rate, increased respiratory rate and lethargy, possibly combined with abdominal swelling or leakage from the operation site. These animals should be checked carefully by a veterinary surgeon, as it may be necessary to reoperate in some cases. In others the use of a compression bandage to increase back-pressure may be sufficient.

Long-term problems reported in some bitches include urinary incontinence. This can usually be managed with the use of phenylpropanolamine (Propalin). In others the coat may change in texture and become coarser. This seems to be particularly true for certain breeds such as cocker spaniels and retrievers. Obesity is also considered to be a problem as most spayed bitches do not need as much food as previously, so owners should be advised to monitor their pet's weight carefully and reduce the quantity of food given at each meal.

Hysterotomy (caesarean section)

There are a number of reasons why a caesarean section may be needed in a pregnant animal. These include:

- Primary or secondary uterine inertia
- Fetal oversize or a fetal monster
- Fetal malpresentation that cannot be reduced
- Obstructions of the birth canal such as pelvic deformities or vaginal polyps
- Neglected dystocias, especially if the fetal fluids have already been lost or a fetus has already died
- Elective reasons, particularly if the animal has had a history of problems previously, or is a breed that is prone to dystocia.

In all cases the aim of the surgery is to remove the young from the uterus to ensure that as many as possible survive, while also keeping the reproductive tract intact.

Preparation

Both the dam and her neonates must be considered, ensuring that suitable facilities are available to support all their needs. Additional nursing staff may be helpful, particularly if a number of young are predicted and may require resuscitation. Towels should be at the ready and somewhere warm ready for the young to recover in – an incubator or a box containing a covered hot water bottle may be suitable.

Surgery

The anaesthetic regime should be chosen so that it has minimum effect on the respiration and cardiovascular function of the neonates. Rapidly acting agents such as propofol (Rapinovet) are usually used without any premedicant. Once the neonates are removed, they should be stimulated to breathe by rubbing vigorously with a towel and clearing any mucus from the oral cavity. Doxapram (Dopram) may be necessary to stimulate respiration of any individuals that are reluctant to breathe.

Postoperative care

As soon as the dam has recovered from the anaesthetic, the young should be placed with her and watched closely to ensure that they are allowed to feed. It is essential that they receive the colostrum needed to provide them with both energy and antibodies. The dam may be reluctant to take the neonates initially but in most cases she can be persuaded to look after them. In very rare instances the young require hand-rearing or fostering because of maternal rejection.

Orchidectomy (castration)

Castration involves the surgical removal of both testes and ligation of the deferent duct on each side. It is often a more straightforward procedure than spaying, as the testes are more accessible. However, retained testes should be removed and these can prove more difficult to find within the abdominal cavity. Some owners think that castration in animals is simply a vasectomy, in which the deferent duct is ligated and transected but the testes are left in place. This should be clarified with the owner before the surgery is carried out.

The indications for castration are varied. It may be to prevent breeding or roaming, or to prevent male behaviour traits such as spraying in tomcats, or aggression. It will also prevent the development of testicular tumours (particularly important if the testes are retained) and reduce the risk of prostate problems and anal adenomas.

Surgery

The procedure is slightly different in different species:

- Dogs – the incision is usually made just in front of the scrotum and the testes are each removed through this incision before it is closed
- Cat – incisions are made through each scrotal sac to reach the testis on each side and these are usually left open
- Rabbits – have particularly large inguinal rings and are able to retract their testes (often seen when clipping up the site in preparation for surgery). However, this also means that when the testes are removed, there is a greater chance of inguinal hernias, so many veterinary surgeons reduce the size of the inguinal ring or take other measures to reduce the risk of this occurring postoperatively.

Castration can be carried out using either a closed or an open technique. In **closed** castrations, the tunica vaginalis is not cut to expose the testes: the testes and covering are dissected away from the overlying skin and the whole spermatic cord is ligated and transected. **Open** castrations allow visualization of the individual testicular vessels and these may then be ligated separately from the deferent duct. In both methods the tunica vaginalis is cut during the surgery. This tissue is simply an extension of the peritoneum, meaning that the procedure actually involves entry into a body cavity and should not be carried out by anyone other than a veterinary surgeon.

Postoperative care

The animal should be monitored for signs of haemorrhage or swelling at the operation site. Dogs should be discouraged from licking, as this can cause complications, and it may be necessary to use an Elizabethan collar to prevent this. Since cats do not have any external sutures they may not need to return to the surgery, but most other species will require suture removal after about 10 days.

Urinary tract

Bladder

- **Cystotomy** – opening up the bladder through the wall.

Surgery on the bladder is quite common, for example to remove calculi or bladder tumours or to repair a ruptured bladder (Figs 21.10–21.12). Animals with calculi or tumours may not be particularly ill but may have shown signs of urinary tenesmus or haematuria that alerted their owners to the problem. Animals with ruptured bladders are more likely to have been involved in some kind of trauma and, unless the bladder is repaired quickly, the animal will rapidly become uraemic as the urea is reabsorbed via the peritoneum from the urine within the peritoneal cavity. It also will develop peritonitis unless the abdomen is lavaged

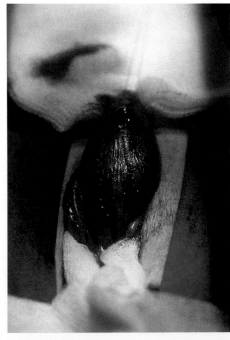

Fig. 21.10 Exteriorizing the bladder and packing it off from the abdomen

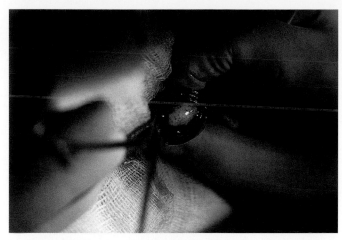

Fig. 21.11 Careful removal of urinary calculi from the bladder

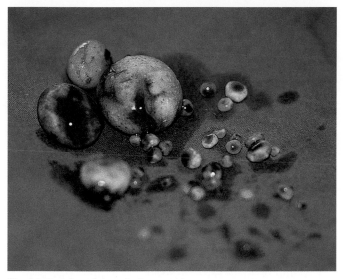

Fig. 21.12 A few of the calculi removed

thoroughly and quickly. Left untreated, both uraemia and peritonitis can be fatal.

Surgery

The bladder is usually approached via a ventral midline incision and should then be exteriorized and packed off from the rest of the abdomen with swabs to minimize the risk of contamination (Fig. 21.10). If there is any spillage of urine or the bladder has already ruptured, the abdomen should be flushed thoroughly with warmed saline.

Postoperative care

The animal should be monitored carefully. It is essential that the patient is able to urinate normally. Trauma cases may need catheterization initially, but no case should be sent home without having passed urine normally. If blood urea levels were high prior to surgery, then intravenous fluids may also be needed to induce diuresis and flush out the urea.

Urethra

- **Urethrotomy** – the temporary opening of the urethra
- **Urethrostomy** – creation of a permanent opening in the urethra.

The most common surgical condition involving the urethra is urethral obstruction. This is seen predominantly in the male animal, where the urethra is much narrower than in the female. Signs of obstruction include urinary tenesmus, haematuria, lethargy and abdominal discomfort.

Treatment

Collection of urine by means of a needle placed through the abdominal and bladder walls (cystocentesis) is often carried out first to relieve the pressure on the bladder and make the animal more comfortable. This allows time to get ready for other procedures.

The next step is to carefully catheterize the urethra and then flush it using saline. Placing the catheter will dislodge some of the calculi causing the obstruction and flushing may alleviate the immediate problem. Note that this procedure may be quite painful for the animal, so sedation or a general anaesthetic may be necessary.

If this has been successful, the animal is usually hospitalized and started on dietary management before returning home. However, if there are other larger calculi within the bladder it may be necessary to perform a cystotomy.

Surgery

If the condition recurs or the blockage cannot be removed, a urethrotomy or permanent urethrostomy is needed. The urethrotomy involves simply entering the urethra surgically, removing the obstruction and closing the wound. However, postoperative strictures are quite common, so this procedure is not done very frequently and it is more usual for surgeons to decide to leave a permanent opening or urethrostomy.

In the dog, obstruction usually occurs at the base of the os penis, so a low penile urethrostomy can be used. The incision is made just in front of the scrotum in this procedure. Alternatively a scrotal urethrostomy is carried out. For this technique castration and scrotal ablation are essential.

In the cat obstruction is usually higher and a high urethrostomy is needed where the incision is made in the perineal area. In the cat the distal penis is usually amputated at the same time.

Postoperative care

Most cases are hospitalized for several days after surgery to allow close monitoring, since it is essential that the animal is able to pass urine freely. An indwelling catheter is usually placed during the early stages. This allows urine to be passed easily and also ensures that the operation site does not contract down too much, preventing the urethrostomy site from working adequately. It is also important that the animal is given fluids or encouraged to drink in order to diurese the patient and prevent the recurrence of any calculi. An Elizabethan collar may be needed to prevent interference with the wound once the catheter is removed, particularly as the animal may feel urine dribbling from the site and wish to clean the area. It will take some training, particularly in dogs, for them to get used to the fact that urine emerges from a different site and owners may need to use petroleum jelly around the area to prevent urine scald and keep the area clean.

With cats, shredded paper should be used instead of cat litter in the litter tray to avoid this becoming stuck to the surgical wound and causing discomfort.

Any calculi removed should be sent for analysis, so that appropriate dietary management can be introduced to prevent recurrence.

Respiratory tract

Tracheostomy

This is the creation of an opening in the wall of the trachea. This may be required as an emergency procedure to enable the animal to breathe and if necessary can be carried out under local anaesthetic.

Technique

1. The animal is restrained on its back with its neck extended over a sandbag.
2. A small incision is made in the ventral midline of the neck. The best area is over the 5th and 6th tracheal rings since this is away from both the larynx and the thoracic inlet and so there is least risk of the tracheostomy site being obstructed through normal neck movements.
3. Under the skin are paired longitudinal neck muscles that must be separated so that a cut can be made between the tracheal rings (about one-third of the way round the trachea) and a tracheostomy tube inserted.
4. The tube should then be secured in place.

Care of the tracheostomy

The tube must be cleaned at least every 2 hours as it quickly becomes blocked with mucus. The best types of tubes have a separate inner sleeve that can be removed for cleaning. Animals with tracheostomy tubes are critical care patients and should be monitored around the clock.

Pneumothorax

This is the presence of air within the pleural cavity. A pneumothorax may be due to a number of causes, including trauma or following surgery, e.g. for ruptured diaphragm. Whatever the cause, the aim of treatment is to encourage reinflation of the lung on the affected side so that full aeration of the lungs can take place again.

If the pneumothorax is small it may be managed conservatively. Air is gradually reabsorbed from the pleural cavity and the lung should eventually reinflate. This takes time and the animal's colour and respiratory function should be monitored closely during its recovery.

In more serious cases, it may be necessary for the air to be removed. This can be done with the patient conscious if it is suffering severe respiratory problems but it is preferable for the animal to be under general anaesthesia, particularly if a drain is to be placed. Air can be removed in one of two ways:

- Butterfly needle or over-the-needle catheter and three-way tap attached to a syringe – this is the simplest technique and the air is removed by suction. The needle cannot be left in place and the technique is usually used when it is likely that the procedure will only be carried out once
- Place a chest drain – between the ribs, usually at the level of the 7th or 8th intercostal space. The drain should actually emerge from the skin further caudally reducing the risk of air leakage around the drain. The drain should be connected to a three-way tap or a Heimlich valve so that air is unable to get back into the thoracic cavity. Air is removed by continuous or intermittent suction.

During treatment the animal may require supplementary oxygen. For small patients, oxygen can be pumped into incubators to provide an oxygen-rich environment, or a kennel may be adapted using plastic sheeting over the front. Other methods of oxygen administration include via a mask, though many patients do not tolerate this well, or via a nasal catheter. Close monitoring will be essential to check that the animal's colour, temperature, pulse and respiration all gradually return to normal as the lung regains its function.

Thoracotomy

This is entry into the chest via the thoracic wall and it may be required for several reasons, e.g. an oesophageal foreign body, repair of a cardiac condition such as patent ductus arteriosus or persistent right aortic arch, or even lung surgery.

Thoracotomy is usually performed with the animal in lateral recumbency. The incision is made through an intercostal space and the ribs are then retracted using a self-retaining retractor (see Ch. 22). In some referral centres a median sternotomy ('sternal split') is carried out. For this procedure, the animal is positioned in dorsal recumbency and access to the thorax is via a midline incision through the middle of the sternum. With this technique the sternum must be repaired postoperatively using stainless steel wires, whereas with the other method no bones are actually cut or damaged. Splitting the sternum provides better access to the thoracic cavity for major surgery.

After completion, the thoracic cavity must be properly sealed and any air or fluid in the chest drawn off. This can either be done using a chest drain attached to a three-way tap and syringe, or other suction device. Postoperative monitoring is essential, checking temperature, pulse, respiration and colour regularly. Analgesics will also be needed as well as appropriate antibiotic treatment depending on the type of procedure performed.

Musculo-skeletal system

Fractures

Types of fracture

Fractures can be classified in a number of different ways (Table 21.10).

Clinical signs of fractures

In most cases the clinical signs of a fracture are similar. The animal shows signs of pain, there may be swelling or deformity at the site and on palpation there may also be crepitus

Table 21.10 Fracture types

Method of classification	Type of fracture	Description
Direction and location of the fracture line	Transverse Longitudinal Oblique Spiral	The fracture is at right angles to the long axis of the bone The fracture is parallel to the long axis of the bone The fracture is diagonal to the long axis of the bone The fracture line spirals around the long axis of the bone
Extent of fracture damage	Complete Incomplete (greenstick) Fissure	The bone is completely broken into two or more fragments The cortex is broken, but the periosteum remains intact on one side of the bone There is a crack in the cortex, but no displacement of any fragments
Extent of soft-tissue damage	Closed Open Complicated	There is no wound over the surface of the fractured bone There is a wound over the fracture site, such that the fracture is open to the environment There is damage to other important tissues as well as the bone, such as nerves or major blood vessels
Number of fracture lines	Comminuted Multiple	There is one fracture site, but more than two fragments are produced There is more than one fracture site and several fragments are produced
Position of the bone fragments	Depressed Over-riding Impacted Distracted	The fracture fragments are pushed inwards to reduce the size of a cavity The two fracture fragments slide over each other to result in shortening of the area The two fracture fragments are driven into each other to result in shortening of the area The two fracture fragments are pulled apart by muscle activity
Position of the fracture	Avulsion Physeal Condylar Intercondylar	A fracture at the site of insertion of a tendon A fracture through a growth plate A fracture in which a condyle of a bone is separated from the rest of the bone A Y-shaped fracture which involves two condyles being separated and fractured
Stability of the fracture	Stable Unstable	There is little tendency of the fracture fragments to move relative to each other The fracture fragments are quite free to move relative to each other

(grating of the fracture fragments against each other). As a result, the animal will not be able to use the affected area normally.

First-aid treatment

It is rare that fractures are a priority in first-aid management; therefore basic checks should cover the whole animal and ensure that there is nothing life-threatening that requires attention before the fracture itself is treated (see Ch. 18).

The following protocol should always be carried out:

- Check the animal's ABC – Airway, Breathing and Circulation
- Control any haemorrhage and treat shock with intravenous fluids, oxygen and warmth
- Antibiotics and analgesics should be given in accordance with the veterinary surgeon's instructions.

Only once the animal has been checked and supportive treatment given should the fracture be treated.

The aim of first-aid management of fractures is to minimize the movement of the fracture fragments so the bone should be handled as little as possible. In unconscious patients it may be appropriate to provide support for the fracture using either support bandages or splints. However, most conscious patients protect fracture sites by holding them in the way that hurts least. Attempting to bandage these might make the situation worse, particularly if the animal struggles.

Fracture repair

There are three basic principles that are often followed in fracture repair:

- Reduce the fracture – i.e. bring the fragments back together
- Align the fragments – ensure that the contours of the bones fit
- Immobilize the fragments.

Of these, the most important is that the fragments are immobilized. This will allow initial bone healing to occur more rapidly, and the patient is able to return to mobility sooner. This in turn promotes the gradual increase in strength of the healed fracture site.

However, there are different approaches to individual cases and the type and location of the fracture can make a significant difference as to which method of repair or treatment is chosen.

Note that in all cases the patient is likely to take reduced exercise, so it is important that its diet is considered. The healing process requires the provision of a good-quality diet but enforced inactivity reduces the energy requirement.

Conservative treatment

This is the simplest option in which no actual surgery or fixation is carried out. The animal is confined so that movement of the affected area is restricted and bone healing will take place. This can be used for stable fractures where there is unlikely to be movement of the fracture fragments, e.g.

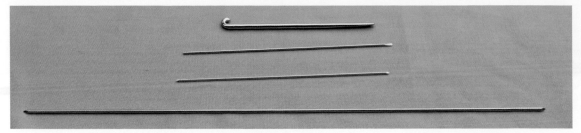

Fig. 21.13A Top to bottom: Rush pin, Kirschner wire, Arthrodesis wire, Steinmann pin

some pelvic fractures, scapular fractures and impacted fractures. Careful rehabilitation may be needed after the cage rest period to allow the fracture site to strengthen, and this may mean that the total convalescent time is longer than if some type of surgical treatment had been carried out.

External fixation

Available methods include casts and splints. They provide a cheap method of fracture repair and have the advantage of being relatively easy to apply and do not run the risk of introducing infection into the fracture. However, they are only suitable for a limited number of fractures, i.e. only fractures that are stable and distal to the elbow or stifle.

There are a number of different materials available for casting. The traditional material, plaster of Paris, has now been superseded, since this was messy, irritant, radiopaque and took a long time to reach full weight-bearing strength. Newer materials, often based on polyurethane resin on some type of bandage, are activated by immersion in warm or hot water, set within approximately 10 minutes and are fully weight-bearing after about 30 minutes. They are also radiolucent, so follow-up radiography can be carried out without actually removing the cast. There are some disadvantages though – they are more expensive than plaster of Paris and some are irritant, so it is essential that the patient has a protective bandage layer under the cast and that gloves are worn during its application.

Aftercare of casts and splints is also important. Casts must not be allowed to get wet and must be regularly checked for sores. Cotton wool underneath casts may bunch up into hard lumps, whereas synthetic orthopaedic wool does not tend to do this and dries more easily should the animal start to sweat under the bandaging. The patient must be prevented from interfering with the cast and kept on minimal exercise.

There is a danger that the cast may loosen as the muscle atrophies through disuse, so regular check-ups must be made. Sometimes casts need to be replaced during the time the fracture is healing and sedation or anaesthesia will be required to replace them. As a result this treatment method can be more expensive than was originally thought. 'Fracture disease' can occur in which tissues, including the bone, become weaker rather than stronger as a result of prolonged immobilization.

However, used appropriately on the right kinds of fractures, casts and splints can work very well.

Internal fixation

A wider range of fractures can be treated using internal fixation techniques and, as the fixation is stable, normal activity

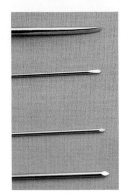

Fig. 21.13B The same pins as Fig. 21.13A – tips close up

can resume more quickly. The fixation device cannot be touched by the animal, so interference should be minimal. Aftercare is also reduced, providing that the surgery has been performed well.

There are some potential problems:

- In most cases open reduction is required, which increases the risk of infection and soft-tissue damage, particularly if the surgeon is inexperienced
- The initial cost is higher and greater skill is required to perform the procedures well
- It is possible that the implants may move after they are positioned
- The animal may develop a reaction leading to hygroma formation (a fluid-filled 'blister' over the implant).

In most cases internal fixation provides good bone healing and can provide the equivalent of primary wound healing in soft tissues.

Types of orthopaedic implant

There are a number of different types of implant that can be used to repair fractures:

Intramedullary pins

These are metal rods inserted into the medullary cavity of a bone to immobilize a fracture (Fig. 21.13). Providing that it is the right type of fracture and the pin fits snugly in the medullary cavity, a pin can be very effective. A pin will cause problems if it is loose or used incorrectly. There are several different types of pin used in practice (Table 21.11).

Screws

These can be used as the sole method for fracture repair or can be used in conjunction with other techniques such as

Table 21.11 Orthopaedic pins

Type of pin	Description
Steinmann pin (Fig. 21.13)	May have a trocar point on one or both ends
Kirschner drill wire (also referred to as K-wires; Fig. 21.13)	Small, thin pins with flattened spatulated ends described as bayonet ends
Arthodesis wire (Fig. 21.13)	Smaller versions of the Steinmann pin, designed to be used across joints
Rush pin (Fig. 21.13)	The Rush pin has a pointed 'sledge-runner' tip at one end and a hook at the other. These are often used in pairs for physeal fractures, since they do not interfere with the growth of the long bone

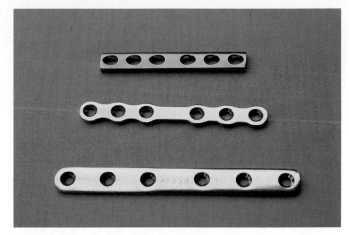

Fig. 21.15 Top to bottom: dynamic compression plate, Sherman plate, Venables plate

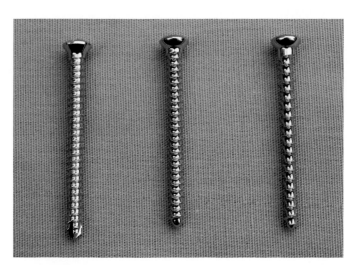

Fig. 21.14A Left to right: traditional screw, ASIF cortical screw, ASIF cancellous screw

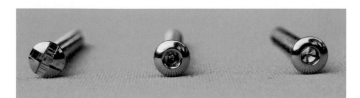

Fig. 21.14B Left to right: close up of heads of traditional screw, ASIF cortical screw, ASIF cancellous screw

plates or wires. Used alone, they can be placed using a lag screw technique providing compression across the fracture site. It is usually wise to also use some kind of splint or external support in these cases.

There are three different types of screw currently used (Fig. 21.14):

- Traditional self-tapping screw
- ASIF/AO cortical screw
- ASIF/AO cancellous screw (ASIF – Association for the Study of Internal Fixation).

As the screw's name suggests, the traditional screw cuts its own path into the bone as it is inserted but the ASIF screw requires that a tap is used prior to its insertion into the bone to precut the thread for the screw. This improves the holding power compared with the traditional screw.

Orthopaedic wire

This is made of braided or monofilament stainless steel. Monofilament wire is more usually used as it is easier to tighten. It is used around fracture fragments and tightened in order to bring them closer together.

Bone plates

Bone plates are available in a number of different designs. Traditional plates are used with self-tapping screws. The two most commonly used are the Sherman plate and the Venables plate (Fig. 21.15).

More modern plates include the ASIF/AO plates (Fig. 21.15). The main plate in this system is the dynamic compression plate or DCP. This is available in several sizes and the holes are shaped such that the screws can be placed either in a neutral position or a loaded position. With appropriate placement of the screws, compression across the fracture site is achieved as the screws are tightened.

Postoperative care

The operation site should be checked regularly for any signs of swelling or discharge. Analgesics are usually needed in the initial postoperative period but as the animal starts to recover these should no longer be required. Rest is essential for the first few weeks – this includes in the garden and house, and stairs should certainly be out of bounds! Exercise can be gradually increased under the veterinary surgeon's direction as the patient improves. Generally, fractures take between 4 and 6 weeks to heal depending on the factors listed below.

External fixator (Kirschner–Ehmer device)

The external fixator is useful in a number of situations where other methods of fracture fixation are not appropriate, e.g. open or infected fractures, since the pins can be placed away from the actual fracture site so that there is no implant device actually at the wound site. Access to the fracture site is also good and for infected sites this can aid treatment and recovery.

The device can also be used in cases of comminuted or unstable fractures, since the external bars of the fixator are able to take the animal's weight and hold the fracture fragments apart, preventing them from collapsing inwards. The fracture heals in the same way as a wound with tissue loss, i.e. by second intention. External fixation may also be used on a range of species. Avian fractures on both limbs and wings have been successfully managed this way and it also lends itself to use in other regions of the body such as pelvic fractures or mandibular fractures. In all cases it is essential that the surgeon has an accurate knowledge of the anatomy of the area so that the pins are not impinging on any vital structures. With care this repair method can be very successful.

The appearance of the device can be quite off-putting to start with but usually, with help from the practice, owners will appreciate the way in which the device works. There may be some discharge from the pin sites and these should be checked regularly to ensure that they are not becoming infected. Rods and clamps should be covered with protective bandage material to prevent any trauma from the metal, either to the animal or the owner.

Once bone healing is complete, the rods and pins are all removed under general anaesthesia. The pin entry wounds are left to heal by second intention and usually heal very quickly.

Fracture healing

Fracture healing, like wound healing, is affected by a number of different factors. This includes factors specific to the injury, such as the stability of the fracture, the proximity of the fragment, the type of fracture and its location and blood supply. More general factors relating to the overall health of the animal, such as its age and species, also have an effect. Many of the exotic species, including birds, heal more quickly than cats and dogs, although with reptiles healing may take considerably longer.

Complications of fracture healing

Unfortunately, not all fractures heal smoothly and it is important to be aware of the potential problems, so that the risks can be minimized:

- Fracture disease – the bone weakens as the repair device takes the weight. Gradually muscle atrophy, osteoporosis, joint stiffness and tissue adhesions develop. It may even result in a non-union
- Malunion – healing takes place but the alignment of the bones is altered from normal. Functionally this can have quite serious effects on the animal depending on the site of the fracture
- Delayed union – the bone fails to heal within the expected normal time. This is usually due to the presence of a gap at the fracture site that takes longer to bridge. Occasionally the fracture does not heal at all, producing a non-union
- Non-union – the bone fragments fail to heal properly. In some cases a fibrous connection may develop between the bones but in others there is no healing at all
- Osteomyelitis – inflammation of the bone and bone marrow. It is usually the result of infection introduced

at the time of surgery. It may be an uncontrolled virulent infection, or it may be more localized and controlled.

Treatment of osteomyelitis – first establish local drainage and remove any foreign materials, including any implants or sutures. This may mean that the original repair device has to be replaced with an alternative one. External fixators have been used with success in some of these cases. Antibiotics should be given systemically for 4–6 weeks based on culture and sensitivity tests on the bacteria found at the site.

Luxations and subluxations

- **Luxation or dislocation** – the persistent displacement of bones forming a joint
- **Subluxation or partial dislocation** – the bones are disturbed from their normal position but remain in contact.

Luxations can be divided into two types:

- Acquired luxations – caused by trauma. Hip and elbow joints are most commonly affected but the phalanges and the hocks may also be damaged
- Congenital luxations – due to anatomical abnormalities present from birth.

First-aid treatment

This follows the same basic pattern as for fractures as it is rare that a luxation is life-threatening:

1. Check A, B, C
2. Treat shock and control haemorrhage
3. In most cases, movement of the dislocated joint should be minimized to prevent further damage and pain.

Treatment

The use of general anaesthesia is recommended for analgesia and because it relaxes the muscles, which eases replacement. In many cases radiography is essential to confirm the diagnosis, to ensure that there are no fractures and to make sure that the bones are replaced accurately. Many luxations can be reduced in a closed fashion, i.e. by manipulating the bones back into position. This is best done as soon as possible after the trauma, since blood clots and muscle contraction can lead to difficulties in replacing luxations left for some time.

If after relocation the joint is still very unstable, an open reduction is needed and surgical measures are needed to stabilize the joint, e.g. in luxation of the carpus where the collateral ligaments are disrupted.

Congenital dislocations are not uncommon and replacement of the bones is not usually sufficient. Surgical intervention is required to correct or modify the anatomical deformity. Patellar luxations can be repaired using one or more techniques depending on the severity of the anatomical deformity. The simplest method is to perform a lateral imbrication, where the joint capsule overlying the patella is tightened. A trochleoplasty involves deepening the trochlear groove in the femur and is carried out in cases of patellar luxation, i.e. where the patella easily slips out of the groove.

In some cases, the distortion of the limb is such that the tibial crest migrates medially, in which case a tibial crest transplant may be needed in addition to the other repair techniques.

Postoperative care

Avoid forces that could produce a recurrence of the luxation; for example, with hip luxations it may be necessary to use an Ehmer sling (figure-of-eight bandage) to prevent use of the limb for 5–7 days. This should be followed by rest for 3–4 weeks, in the same way as for a fracture.

Possible complications

Recurrence is the main complication and this is true especially of luxations reduced by closed techniques. A recurrent luxation will require surgery to provide adequate stability, e.g. hip luxations may require surgery to the hip involving the creation of a synthetic round ligament.

Bibliography

Aspinall, V., 2008. Clinical Procedures in Veterinary Nursing, second ed. Elsevier, Oxford.

Bowden, C., Masters, J. (Eds.), 2003. Textbook of Veterinary Medical Nursing. Butterworth-Heinemann, Oxford.

Brinker, P., Brinker, F., 1997. Handbook of Small Animal Orthopedics and Fracture Treatment, third ed. W B Saunders, Philadelphia, PA.

Brockman, D.J., Holt, D.E. (Eds.), 2005. BSAVA Manual of Canine and Feline Head, Neck and Thoracic Surgery. British Small Animal Veterinary Association, Cheltenham.

Busch, S.J., 2006. Small Animal Surgical Nursing Skills and Concepts. Mosby, St Louis, MO.

Cooper, B., Lane, D.R. (Eds.), 2007. BSAVA Textbook of Veterinary Nursing, fourth ed. British Small Animal Veterinary Association, Cheltenham.

Coughlan, A., Miller, A. (Eds.), 2006. BSAVA Manual of Small Animal Fracture Repair and Management. British Small Animal Veterinary Association, Cheltenham.

Dobson, J.M., Lascelles, B.D.X. (Eds.), 2003. BSAVA Manual of Canine and Feline Oncology, second ed. British Small Animal Veterinary Association, Cheltenham.

Fowler, D., Williams, J.M. (Eds.), 1999. Manual of Canine and Feline Wound Management and Reconstruction. British Small Animal Veterinary Association, Cheltenham.

Hoad, J., 2006. Minor Veterinary Surgery. A Handbook for Veterinary Nurses. Elsevier, Oxford.

Hotston Moore, P., 2004. Fluid Therapy for Veterinary Nurses and Technicians. Butterworth-Heinemann, Oxford.

Houlton, J.E.F., Taylor, P.M., 1987. Trauma Management in the Dog and Cat. John Wright, Bristol.

Tracey, D., 2003. Surgical Nursing, third ed. Mosby, St Louis, MO.

Turner, S., 2005. Veterinary Ophthalmology. A Manual for Nurses And Technicians. Elsevier, Oxford.

Williams, J.M., Niles, J.D. (Eds.), 2005. BSAVA Manual of Canine and Feline Abdominal Surgery. British Small Animal Veterinary Association, Cheltenham.

Recommended reading

Busch, S.J., 2006. Small Animal Surgical Nursing Skills and Concepts. Mosby, St Louis, MO.

This provides an excellent overview of all aspects of surgical nursing, with review questions at the end of each chapter.

Fowler, D., Williams, J.M. (Eds.), 1999. Manual of Canine and Feline Wound Management and Reconstruction. British Small Animal Veterinary Association, Cheltenham.

This is an excellent text for anyone wishing to develop their knowledge of wound management. There are very good chapters on graft techniques and reconstructive flaps.

Hoad, J., 2006. Minor Veterinary Surgery. A Handbook for Veterinary Nurses. Elsevier, Oxford.

An informative and detailed text covering all areas of surgery nurses may legally undertake as part of their role within the Veterinary Surgeons Act 1966 (Schedule 3 amendment)

Hotston Moore, M.P., 2004. Fluid Therapy for Veterinary Nurses and Technicians. Butterworth-Heinemann, Oxford.

This handy-sized book explains clearly the rationale for fluid therapy and the techniques used in practice.

CHAPTER 22

Theatre practice

Emma Brooks

Key Points

- Correct design and layout of the surgical unit is essential to provide an environment that is conducive to both effective surgical treatment and care of the patient and in which high standards of asepsis can be maintained.
- In getting ready for surgical procedures the role of the veterinary nurse includes preparation of the operating theatre, instruments and other equipment and of the surgical gowns, gloves and drapes. It may also include acting as scrubbed or a circulating nurse, both of which have their own specific role in the procedure.
- An understanding of the design, use and care of the standard surgical instruments is essential.
- The veterinary nurse should be able to understand how to prepare a patient for surgery, the basic principles behind the surgical procedure to be performed and the aftercare of the patient.
- Every veterinary practice should develop a strictly adhered to, rigid routine for the maintenance of asepsis at all stages of surgery. This includes disinfection and sterilization of anything that comes into contact with the surgical site.

Introduction

The care and maintenance of the theatre suite, instruments and equipment is very important for the smooth running of any surgical procedure performed in the operating environment. Whatever type of surgical suite you have, there are basic rules that must be followed. This chapter will cover the preparation of the operating suite and the patient, care and maintenance of instruments and equipment. It will also cover preoperative, intraoperative and postoperative care of the patient.

The surgical unit

It is unlikely that the layout and design of the surgical unit is the responsibility of the veterinary nurse. However, it is important to have an idea of suitable requirements and features of a theatre suite, so that the best can be made of existing facilities. In an ideal world a surgical unit should consist of:

- Operating theatre
- Anaesthetic preparation area
- An area for washing and sterilizing equipment
- Sterile equipment store
- Scrub area
- Changing rooms
- Recovery room.

Operating theatre

Many practices only have one operating theatre, which is used for all surgery. Some, usually the larger hospitals, have several theatres, which are used for particular types of surgery, e.g. orthopaedic surgery, general surgery, dirty surgery, e.g. dental work. The size of the theatre will depend on the use for which it was intended. If it is predominately for orthopaedic work then it should be fairly large to accommodate the amount of equipment needed. If the theatre is too small, working conditions are compromised and it becomes difficult to maintain asepsis. Overall, the theatre has to be large enough to accommodate the patient and table, the anaesthetic equipment, the surgical instruments and trolley, any other equipment and the surgical team.

There are several other requirements that are desirable, if not essential:

- The theatre should be an end room, not a thoroughfare to other rooms
- It should be easily cleaned. The walls and floors should be made of impervious material. Walls and ceilings should be painted with a light, waterproof paint and corners and edges of walls should be coved for ease of cleaning. Drains should be avoided if possible
- There should be as little shelving and furniture as possible, as it will harbour dust
- Good lighting is essential. If possible, natural light should be used. Avoid clear glass windows to the outside, as they cause distraction. They must not open, as this will threaten asepsis. Any light fittings should be flush with the ceiling and walls. There should be an overhead theatre light

- There should be an adequate supply of waterproof electric sockets recessed into the wall
- An ambient temperature of 15–20°C should be maintained, as anaesthetized animals cannot regulate their body temperature. Panel heaters are ideal, but expensive. Fan heaters should be avoided as they cause air and dust to move and risk breaking asepsis
- Air conditioning and ventilation is necessary under the Control of Substances Hazardous to Health (COSHH) regulations.

There must be:

- A scavenging system for waste anaesthetic gases
- An air supply for power tools. This should be piped in from cylinders outside the theatre. Anaesthetic gases should also be delivered in the same way
- An X-ray viewer flush to the wall
- A clock to monitor the anaesthetic and time of surgery
- A dry wipe board for recording details such as number of swabs used, suture materials used, blood loss, etc.
- There should be double swing doors that are kept closed
- The operating table should be adjustable to suit the height of the surgeon and the position of the patient
- All equipment should be able to be cleaned easily.

Anaesthetic preparation area

This should be a separate area where induction and preoperative procedures take place. It should lead directly to the theatre. The clippers and vacuum cleaner to remove hair should be positioned near the preparation table. It is sensible to have an anaesthetic emergency box within this area.

Area for washing and sterilizing equipment

This should be a specific room where dirty equipment and instruments are washed and sterilized. It should be close to the theatre but away from the sterile store area. It should contain a washing machine for drapes and gowns only, a tumble dryer, sterilization equipment and an ultrasonic cleaner.

Sterile store area

Sterile packs should be stored in a closed cupboard near to the theatre. This room should be large enough to lay out instrument trolleys before surgery. It should have an entrance directly into the theatre.

Scrub area

This should be a separate scrub area within the theatre suite but not in the theatre. It should lead into the sterile store area, then the theatre. Swing doors should separate the rooms.

Changing rooms

These should be situated at the entrance to the theatre. A line marked on the floor should delineate the sterile area of this room. Theatre footwear should be kept at the entrance to the theatre beyond the line. A one-way traffic system should be in place to maintain asepsis.

Recovery room

This should be close to the theatre in case of an emergency. It should be quiet, warm and contain emergency equipment, e.g. oxygen, crash box, etc.

Theatre maintenance

Routine cleaning of the theatre suite is essential if asepsis is to be kept at a high standard:

- **Daily damp dusting** – at the start of each day, all furniture, surfaces and equipment must be damp dusted with a dilute disinfectant. Dry dusting is pointless, as it just moves the dust around the room
- **Between operative procedures** – the theatre suite should be cleaned as soon as the patient is removed from the operating theatre and before the next one arrives. All dirty instruments should be removed for cleaning and re-sterilization. All surfaces should be wiped over with a suitable disinfectant. The floor should be cleaned if necessary, and then the instruments and equipment can be prepared for the next patient
- **At the end of each day** – floors should be cleaned with a vacuum cleaner to remove debris. They should be washed with disinfectant solution. All waste should be removed and disposed of correctly. All surfaces, including the scrub sink, should be washed with a disinfectant solution
- **Weekly cleaning** – once a week a thorough clean should be performed. All equipment should be removed and walls and floors should be scrubbed. Any excess solution should be removed and then the surfaces should be allowed to dry, not rinsed off. This ensures a longer residual activity time for the disinfectant.

All cleaning equipment for the theatre should be kept separate from other cleaning equipment and should be rinsed and dried after each use. Where possible, mop heads should be laundered each day. Any cleaning equipment must be stored away from the sterile store area.

Preparation for surgery

The operating list

This should be planned so that 'clean' surgery, such as abdominal or orthopaedic surgery, is done first, followed by 'dirty' surgery, such as pyometritis, oral and anal operations.

Preparation of diathermy equipment

There are two types of diathermy equipment – monopolar and bipolar. If monopolar diathermy is to be used, the patient must be 'earthed' by a contact plate placed in a suitable position between the patient and the table. Contact gel is applied to the plate. For bipolar diathermy there is no contact plate.

Preparation of other equipment

1. Check and turn on the anaesthetic equipment
2. Connect the scavenging systems and anaesthetic circuit
3. Lay out scrub solutions, brushes, towel, gowns and gloves for the surgical team
4. Put out skin preparation materials ready for the patient
5. Lay out the instrument trolley, adding any spare instruments, drapes, sutures and swabs that may be required (Box 22.1).

Surgical attire

Theatre clothing should be worn in the theatre. This usually consists of a two-piece scrub suit. A clean scrub suit should be worn every day.

- **Footwear** – antistatic footwear, e.g. white clogs or wellingtons, is essential to prevent explosions caused by sparks when inflammable anaesthetic gases are used. They should be cleaned frequently and only worn in theatre
- **Headgear** – a theatre cap should be worn; these are usually made of cloth or paper
- **Facemasks** – these are used to filter expired air from the nose and mouth; they are only effective for a short time and should be changed between operations.

Scrubbing-up procedure*

As it is not possible to sterilize skin, the aim of scrubbing up is to destroy as many microorganisms as possible before putting on a sterile gown and gloves. There are many different scrub routines. Your practice should adopt a tried and tested routine and adhere to it (Box 22.2).

Gowning procedure*

The aim of a surgical gown is to provide a barrier preventing the transmission of microorganisms. There are two types of gown available – those that tie at the back and those that wrap around and tie at the side:

> **Box 22.1** Laying out the instrument trolley
>
> 1. Make sure that the trolley is clean.
> 2. Cover the base of the trolley with a sterile, water-resistant layer to help prevent a bacterial strike if the trolley becomes wet.
> 3. On top of this put a double layer of sterile linen drapes.
> 4. Lay out the instruments in a logical order – usually from left to right in the order that they will be used.
> 5. Sterile extras may be added such as suture materials and swabs.
> 6. Place a sterile cover over the top of the trolley until it is ready for use.

*These procedures are illustrated on the website.

1. Take the sterile gown from the pack and hold at the shoulders, allowing it to fall open
2. Place a hand into each sleeve. Do not try to adjust the gown or pull over your shoulders, as this can lead to contamination. An unscrubbed assistant will pull the gown over the shoulders by only touching the inside of the gown, and tie the ties at the back (Fig. 22.1)
3. Hands stay inside the sleeves and the waist ties are picked up and held out to the sides. The unscrubbed assistant takes the ties and secures them at the back. The back of the gown is now unsterile.

Gloving procedure*

Gloves are worn as a barrier between the surgeon's hands and the tissues of the patient. They should fit snugly but not too tightly. Sterile gloves should be worn for all surgical procedures.

> **Box 22.2** Scrub routine
>
> 1. Remove watch and jewellery.
> 2. Ensure finger nails are short and nail varnish is removed.
> 3. Regulate the hot and cold taps.
> 4. Wash hands with soap and clean under nails with a nail pick.
> 5. Once hands are washed, wash arms to elbows. Keep hands higher than elbows so that the water runs down the unscrubbed arms.
> 6. Rinse to remove all soap and lather by allowing water to flow down hands and off elbows.
> 7. Using a sterile scrubbing brush and surgical scrub, scrub palms, wrist and the four surfaces of each finger. (Remember to scrub under nails and knuckles.) Scrub arms last. Use a circular motion and scrub for 5 minutes by the clock. It is not recommended to scrub the backs of your hands and arms, as this can lead to excoriation, which predisposes to infection.
> 8. Discard brush and rinse well, once again allowing the water to flow over hands and down arms.
> 9. Dry hands and arms using a sterile towel. Use a different part for each hand and arm. Work from your wrist to your elbow.

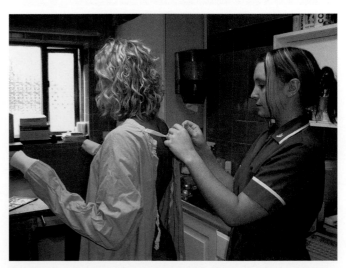

Fig. 22.1 An unscrubbed nurse ties the ties of the sterile surgical gown

There are three methods for gloving up – closed, open and plunge methods.

Closed method

1. Hands stay inside the gown sleeves. This minimizes contamination. The glove packet is opened and turned so that the fingers are pointing at the body. (The right glove will be on the left and vice versa)
2. Pick up glove at the rim of the cuff of the glove.
3. Turn hand over so that the glove is on the palm surface with fingers pointing at the body
4. Pick rim up with opposite hand and pull over finger and the dorsal surface of wrist
5. The glove is pulled on as the fingers are pushed forwards.

Open method (Fig. 22.2)

1. The hands are out of the gown's sleeves in this technique. With the left hand, pick up the right glove by holding the inner surface of the turned down cuff
2. Pull on to right hand. Do not unfold the cuff

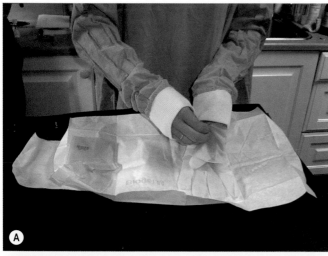

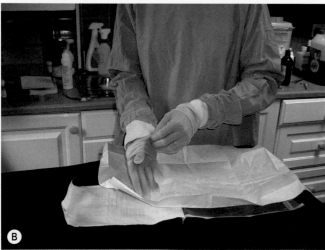

Fig. 22.2 (A, B) Open method of gloving procedure

3. Repeat steps 1 and 2 for left hand
4. Put gloved finger under cuff of opposite hand and pull on firmly
5. The rim of the glove is hooked over the thumb while the cuff of the gown is adjusted, then the cuff of the glove is pulled over the cuff of the gown using the opposite hand. Repeat for other hand.

Plunge method

A sterile glove is held open by a scrubbed assistant and the hand is inserted into the glove. This method is not used often, as there is a high risk of contamination.

Role of the theatre nurse

In veterinary practice the nurse may take one of two roles within the theatre – either a scrubbed nurse or a circulating nurse.

Scrubbed nurse

This is an important role and an understanding of the surgery to be performed is essential so that the needs of the veterinary surgeon can be anticipated:

- The instrument trolley should be prepared just before it is needed, i.e. just before the patient arrives in theatre. It is essential to know what and where the instruments are on the trolley at the start and during surgery
- Swabs, needles and sutures should be counted at the beginning and at the end before the incision is closed
- The surgeon must be watched to anticipate his/her needs
- Pass instruments so that they are ready to use and not upside down. They should be put back on the trolley in the same place so that you know where they are. Do not leave instruments at the operation site in case they fall on the floor or into the surgical site
- Instruments should be wiped over with a dry swab before replacing them on the trolley
- Only one swab at a time should be given. There should be a constant check on the number of swabs
- Swabs should be firmly applied to bleeding, without wiping, as this can destroy any clot formation
- Handle tissues, especially viscera, carefully to avoid unnecessary trauma
- You may have to irrigate tissues with warm saline to prevent desiccation, especially during long operations
- At the end check that all instruments, needles and swabs are on the trolley. Dispose of needles and blades in a sharps container.

Circulating nurse

The circulating nurse is there to assist with all non-sterile procedures:

- Help prepare the instrument trolley for surgery
- Tie surgical gowns

- Position the patient on the operating table
- Prepare the surgical site
- Connect apparatus, e.g. suction, diathermy, etc.
- Open packs of swabs, suture material, etc.
- Count swabs with the scrub nurse
- Be in theatre when surgery is in progress
- Assist anaesthetist
- Prepare postoperative dressings
- Clear theatre at the end of surgery.

Health and Safety within the theatre

The COSHH regulations are designed to ensure safety at work, including in the operating theatre (see Ch. 3):

- **Equipment** – it is very important that all nursing staff are told how to use and maintain new equipment. All equipment should be serviced regularly and tested for electrical safety
- **Pollution from gas** – all staff should be aware of the danger associated with inhaling anaesthetic gases. A scavenging system must be fitted and used
- **Disposal of needles/sharp instruments** – all blades, needles, stylets, etc., must be disposed of in commercially produced sharps containers. When full they must be sealed, labelled as clinical waste and removed by a licensed contractor, who will incinerate them
- **Clinical and pathological waste** – it is a requirement of COSHH that all clinical and pathological waste is separated from ordinary refuse with colour-coded bags:
  - **Clinical waste** – anything contaminated by blood or bodily fluids. Yellow bags. When full, seal and label with biohazard tape
  - **Pathological waste** – all tissues. Red bags. When full, seal and label with biohazard tape
- **Chemicals** – if chemicals are used, protective clothing must be worn, e.g. mask, gloves, apron.

Instrumentation

Good-quality instruments are very expensive but they will last for years if properly looked after. Stainless steel is the best choice as it combines high resistance to corrosion with great strength. Tungsten carbide is sometimes added to the tips of stainless steel instruments if used for cutting or gripping, e.g. scissors and needle holders. It is hard and resistant to wear but very costly. Instruments with tungsten carbide added are usually indicated by gold handles. Instruments made from chromium-plated carbon steel are the most common in veterinary practice as they are cheaper than stainless steel. However, they will rust, pit and blister in contact with chemicals and saline, and tend to blunt more quickly.

Maintenance of instruments

Instruments should always be handled carefully. Do not drop on to trolleys and into sinks. Any sharp edges should be cared for. New instruments are supplied without lubrication so you should wash, dry and lubricate them before use.

Cleaning instruments after use

COSHH states that protective clothing and gloves should be worn if dealing with surgical instruments:

1. Sharp items, i.e. blades and needles, should be removed from the trolley first
2. Delicate instruments should be separated and cleaned separately
3. Instruments should be cleaned as soon as possible after surgery to prevent blood and saline from drying on and causing corrosion
4. Open all the joints and soak in cold water or a chemical cleaning solution designed for instruments
5. Clean under warm running water with a scrubbing brush. Pay attention to ratchets, joints and serrations. Abrasive agents should not be used as they will damage the surface of the instrument. Ordinary soap causes an insoluble alkali film on the surface, trapping bacteria and protecting them from sterilization
6. After washing, rinse and dry carefully.

Ultrasonic cleaners

Bench-top cleaners are suitable for use in veterinary practice. They are effective at removing debris in areas inaccessible to brushes, e.g. box joints. Ultrasonic cleaners work by producing sinusoidal energy waves at a high frequency. After an initial soaking in cold water, place the instruments in the wire basket of the cleaner with their joints open. The unit is then filled with water and ultrasonic cleaning solution and the basket is placed in the solution. The lid is closed and the cleaner is switched on. Usually, 15 minutes is sufficient. When finished, remove the basket and rinse each instrument under warm running water. Dry carefully, as water trapped in areas such as joints may lead to corrosion.

Lubrication

This should be done on a regular basis, especially if using an ultrasonic cleaner. There are several antimicrobial water-soluble lubricants available. The instruments are usually dipped in the solution for a short time, then removed and dried. There is no need to rinse.

Specialized-instrument care

Compressed-air machines

These machines must never be immersed in water. All detachable parts should be cleaned in the normal way. Instruments should be detached from the air hose and then wiped with disinfectant. Pay attention to triggers and couplings. Rinse without immersing. The air hose can be cleaned in the same way. Lubricate after drying with the manufacturer's recommended lubricant before packaging for sterilization.

Motorized equipment

Care of these machines is very similar to that of compressed-air machines. The manufacturer's instructions should always be followed, as they can seize up after repeated autoclaving.

Dental instruments

Dental instruments must be maintained to a high degree if good dental work is to be performed (see Ch. 24). There are two types of dental instrument:

- **Hand held** – these include scalers, picks, luxators and curettes. They have delicate tips and should be washed and dried carefully. These instruments will then

require sharpening with an Arkansas stone and oil. Autoclaving can then be carried out in the normal manner, remembering to protect the delicate points and tips

- **Mechanical** – these include ultrasonic scalers and polishers. Always follow the manufacturer's instructions for each piece of equipment.

Surgical instruments

There are many different types of instrument available (Fig. 22.3). It is not necessary to know every single one, but a broad knowledge of the more common ones is essential (Table 22.1).

Table 22.1 General surgical instruments (see also Fig. 22.3)

Name	Type	Use	Comment
Scalpel		Divide tissues with minimal trauma	Size 3 handle used for small animal surgery. Use 10, 11, 12 and 15 blade Size 4 handle for large animal work. Use 20, 21, or 22 blade A small (beaver) handle is available with a very small blade. Good for ophthalmic work
Dissecting forceps (thumb forceps)	Plain Rat-toothed	Holding tissue Plain ends hold delicate tissue Rat-toothed hold dense tissue	Hold like a pencil
Scissors	Mayo dissecting Metzenbaum Carless Paynes	Routine surgery Delicate surgery Suture cutting Removing sutures	Hold with ring finger and thumb inserted into ring of the scissors Index finger is placed on shaft to guide scissors
Haemostatic artery forceps	Spencer Wells Dunhill Criles Cairns Kelly Halstead/mosquito	Clamping blood vessels to stop bleeding	Many different lengths and shapes. Most have transverse striations to help hold tissue. Mosquito forceps are the smallest and are used for fine blood vessels. Hold as for scissors
Towel clips	Backhaus Gray's cross-action	Attach drapes to patients and instruments to operating site	
Needle holders	Gillies Olsen–Hegar Mayo–Hegar McPhail's	Hold suture needles during suturing and knot tying	Gillies – have scissor action for cutting suture ends. No ratchet so must hold needle tightly Olsen–Hegar – have cutting edge and ratchet to hold needle securely. Very easy to cut suture material Mayo- Hegar – like long-handled artery forceps. Have ratchet but no cutting edge McPhail's – usually have copper or tungsten carbide insert in tip. Have spring ratchet so that squeezing jaws together opens holder and releases needle
Retractors	Hand-held: Langenbeck Senn Czerny Self-retaining: Gelpi West's Travers Gusset Balfour Finochietto	Expose operating field	Can be hand-held or self-retaining Gelpi, West's and Travers for muscle or joints Gusset and Balfour for abdominal surgery Finochietto for thoracic surgery

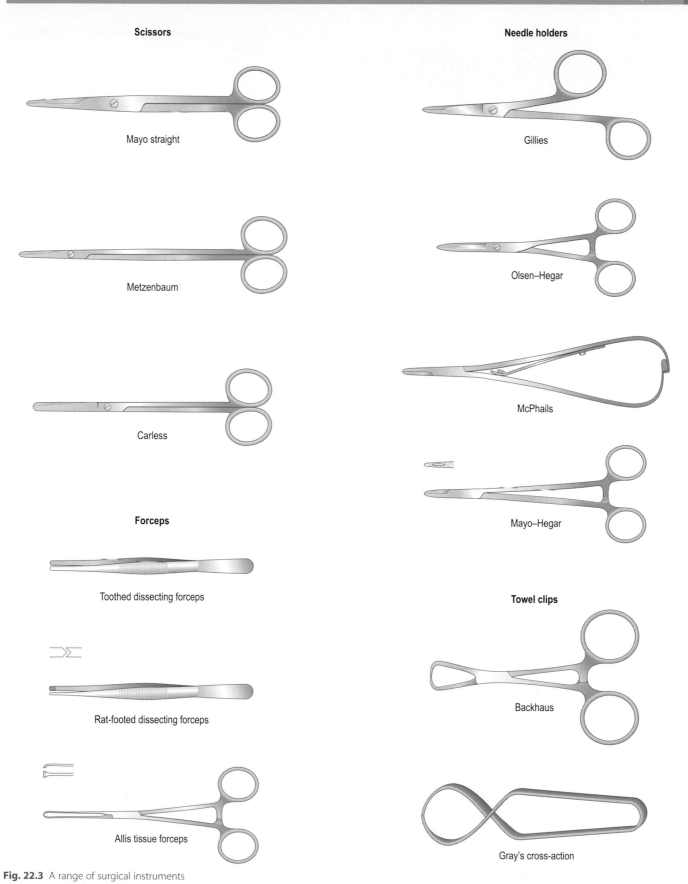

Fig. 22.3 A range of surgical instruments

(Continued)

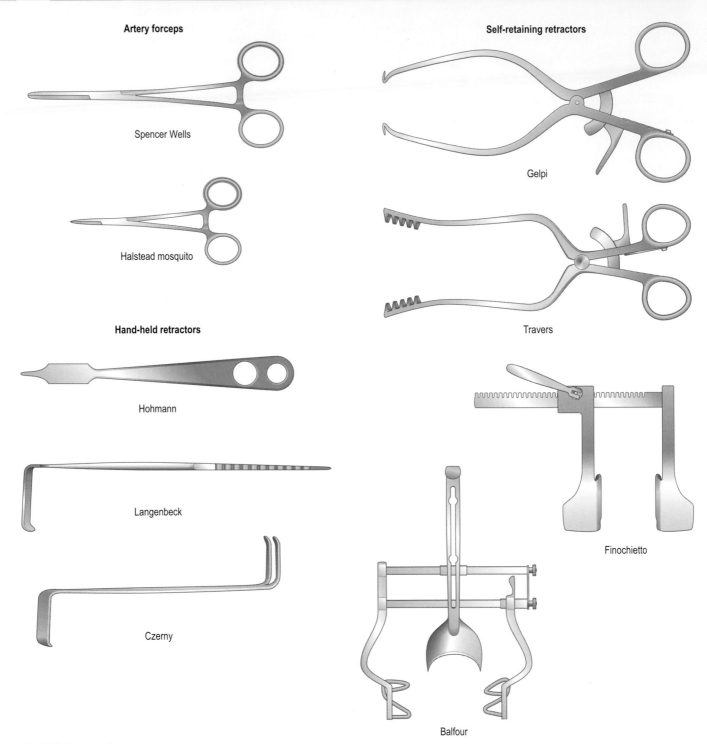

Artery forceps

Spencer Wells

Halstead mosquito

Hand-held retractors

Hohmann

Langenbeck

Czerny

Self-retaining retractors

Gelpi

Travers

Finochietto

Balfour

Fig. 22.3 Continued

Orthopaedic instruments

Common types are described in Table 22.2 and Figure 22.4. Other instruments may be needed, depending on the technique and the surgeon. These include Steinmann pins, orthopaedic wire, bone plates, screws and external fixator apparatus (see Ch. 21).

Packing surgical kits

Instruments are often packed together with swabs, drapes, suction tubing, etc. The pack is usually wrapped so that the outer layers will cover the instrument trolley when unwrapped. Ideally, a metal or plastic tray is lined with a linen sheet and the instruments are then laid out in a specific

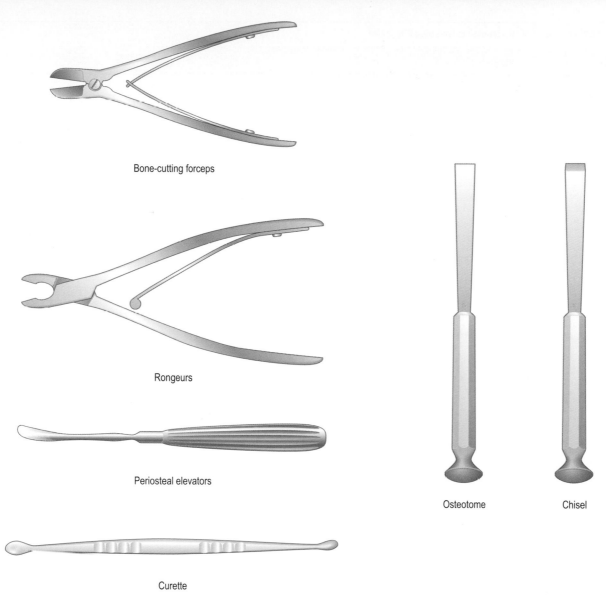

Bone-cutting forceps

Rongeurs

Periosteal elevators

Osteotome   Chisel

Curette

Fig. 22.4 Orthopaedic instruments

order (usually the order of use). Swabs, drapes, etc., are then added. A water-resistant drape is laid over the top followed by two layers of linen sheet. The pack is then wrapped and secured with Bowie Dick tape. It must be labelled and dated before sterilization.

Instrument sets

These collections of specific instruments are made up to suit the technique and the needs of the individual practice. Some practices have sets for specific operations, e.g. bitch spay kit. Others have standard sets that are used for all operations but have extra instruments that can be added depending on the procedure. It is important that each standard kit contains the same number and type of instruments so that the surgical team know what is there and can check at the end of the procedure that all instruments are present. Guidelines for types of kit are shown in Table 22.3.

Sutures

Suture materials

The choice of suture materials used within the veterinary practice depends on:

- Type of tissue to be repaired
- Risk of contamination
- Length of healing time, i.e. how long the suture material must remain effective within the tissue.
- Personal preference

There are two categories of suture material – non-absorbable and absorbable. Each category can be subdivided into:

- Natural or synthetic
- Monofilament or multifilament
- Coated or uncoated.

Table 22.2 Orthopaedic instruments (see also Fig. 22.4)

Name	Use	Comment
Osteotome	Cutting and shaping bone	Tapered on both sides
Chisel	Cutting and shaping bone	Tapered on one side only
Gouge	Cutting and shaping bone	U-shaped edge to remove larger pieces of bone or cartilage
Curette	Scoop surface of dense tissue to remove loose or degenerate tissue	The cup has a sharp cutting edge. Available in many sizes
Periosteal elevators	Lift periosteum and soft tissue from bone surface	Many sizes available
Bone-holding forceps	Grip bone fragments while reducing or aligning fractures	
Bone cutters	Cutting large pieces of bone	
Bone rasps	Remove sharp edges following arthroplasty	
Bone rongeurs	Cutting small pieces of dense tissue, bone or cartilage	
Drills	Hand drills are used around delicate structures where minimal drilling is required. Most surgery will require the use of a battery or air drill	Battery drills are slower and more cumbersome but less expensive than air drills
Saws and burrs	May be driven by air or electricity. Take care when connecting	
	Do not switch on until all the couplings are assembled	
Wire forceps	Used to apply cerclage wire and when stabilizing bones with wire	Various types available
Gigli wire and handles	Saw through bone with cheese wire effect	

Table 22.3 Suggested contents of different types of surgical kit

Type of kit	Contents	Type of kit	Contents
General surgical kit	Scalpel handle no. 3 Dissecting forceps (plain and rat-toothed) Scissors (Mayo and Metzenbaum) Artery forceps ×8 Allis tissue forceps ×2	Abdominal kit	General kit Self-retaining retractors Long-handled artery forceps ×6 Long dissecting forceps ×2 Bowel clamps ×4
	Retractors (Gelpi and Langenbeck) Backhaus towel clips ×4 Needle holders Suture scissors	Thoracic kit	General kit + periosteal elevator Rib cutters Rib retractors Long-handled artery forceps ×6 Long dissecting forceps ×2 Lobectomy clamps
General eye kit	Eyelid speculum Small scalpel handle (beaver) Fine dissecting forceps Fine scissors Corneal scissors Capsular forceps Irrigating cannula Vectis Iris repository Castroviejo needle holders	Orthopaedic kit	General kit + periosteal elevator Osteotome Chisel Mallet Curette Hohmann retractor ×2 Rongeurs Bone-cutting forceps

Tables 22.4 and 22.5 describe the most commonly used suture materials and their properties.

Alternatives to sutures

Today there are an increasing number of alternatives to suture materials (see also Ch. 21). These include:

- **Staples** – there are several different types of metal staple available. The most common type is skin staples but specialized staples are available for intestinal anastomoses and ligation. Staples are usually packed in a gun-type applicator
- **Tissue glue** – used for skin closure. It is designed for rapid healing and is most commonly used on small superficial wounds
- **Adhesive tape** – mainly used in human skin closure. They do not adhere well to animal skin and are therefore not widely used in veterinary medicine.

Suture needles

There are several types of suture needle and they are available with the suture material swaged on to them or with eyes through which the suture material is threaded. Choice is dependent on the type of wound to be sutured, the type of tissue and the characteristics of the needle.

The needle shape may be:

- **Curved** – the entire length of the needle is curved into an arc. Various degrees of curvature are available – half circle is most common
- **Half-curved** – the sharp end of needle is curved but the eye end is straight
- **Straight** – the entire needle is straight.

The cross-sectional design may vary according to the tissue that is being sutured (Table 22.6).

Common suture patterns

As qualified veterinary nurses are legally allowed to perform minor acts of surgery under the Veterinary Surgeons Act 1966 (Schedule 3 amendment), including suturing, it is important that you are familiar with basic suturing techniques. However, remember always to seek practical instruction from a veterinary surgeon beforehand.

Surgical knots

A surgical knot has three components:

- The loop – the part of suture material within the opposed or ligated tissue
- The knot – made from a number of throws
- The ears – the cut end of the suture that prevents the knot from being untied.

Knots can be hand-tied or instrument-tied. The basic surgical knot is a reef knot or square knot. A surgeon's knot has an initial double throw not a single throw. This reduces the risk of the first throw loosening while the second throw is being placed (Fig. 22.5). Hand tying will help prevent loosening and slippage of the first throw, as tension can be placed on both ends of the suture. It is, however, very wasteful of suture material.

Table 22.4 Non-absorbable suture materials

Suture material	Trade name	Mono or multifilament	Synthetic or natural	Coated	Knot security	Duration	Comments
Polyamide (nylon)	Ethilon (Ethicon)	Monofilament	Synthetic	No	Fair	Permanent	Causes minimal tissue reaction and has little tissue drag
Polybutylester	Novafil (Davis & Geck)	Monofilament	Synthetic	No	Fair	Permanent	Similar to polyamide with similar properties
Polypropylene	Prolene (Ethicon)	Monofilament	Synthetic	No	Fair – can produce bulky knots that untie easily	Permanent	Very inert. Produces minimal tissue reaction. Very strong but very springy. Little tissue drag
Braided silk	Mersilk (Ethicon)	Multifilament	Natural	Wax coat	Excellent	May eventually fragment and break down	Good handling properties, but high tissue reactivity. Do not use in infected sites
Braided polyamide	Supramid or Nuralon (Ethicon)	Multifilament	Synthetic	Encased in outer sheath	Good	Outer sheath can be broken	Better handling than monofilament polyamide. Can be used in skin but not as a buried suture
Surgical stainless steel wire		Available as monofilament or multifilament	Synthetic	No	Excellent, although knots are difficult to untie	Permanent	Not commonly used now, but is useful in bones or tendon. Difficult to handle

Table 22.5 Absorbable suture materials

Suture material	Trade name	Mono or multifilament	Synthetic or natural	Coated	Duration of strength	Absorption	Comments and uses
Polyglactin 910	Vicryl (Ethicon)	Multifilament	Synthetic	Yes – calcium stearate	Retains 50% of tensile strength at 14 days and 20% at 21 days	Absorbed by 60–90 days by hydrolysis	Dyed or undyed. Low tissue reactivity. Uses: in subcuticular layer, muscle, eyes and hollow viscera
Polyglactin 910	Vicryl Rapide (Ethicon)	Multifilament	Synthetic	Yes -calcium stearate	Retains only 50% of tensile strength at 5 days. Provides wound support for 10 days	Absorption complete by about 42 days. Absorbed by hydrolysis	Although the same as Vicryl it is manufactured to make it loose tensile strength and be fully absorbed much faster
Polydioxanone	PDS II (Ethicon)	Monofilament	Synthetic	No	Retains 70% tensile strength at 14 days and 14% at 56 days	Only minimal absorption by 90 days. Absorbed by 180 days, by hydrolysis	Good for infected sites as monofilament. Very strong but springy. Minimal tissue reaction. Uses: in subcuticular muscle, sometimes eyes
Polyglycolic acid	Dexon (Davis & Geck)	Multifilament	Synthetic	Can be coated with polysamer	Retains 20% at 14 days	Complete absorption by 100–120 days. Absorbed by hydrolysis	Similar to polyglactin but has considerable tissue drag. Uses: as for polyglactin
Polyglecaprone 25	Monocryl (Ethicon)	Monofilament	Synthetic	No	Retains about 60% at 7 days, 30% at 14 days. Wound support maintained for 20 days	Complete absorption between 90 and 120 days. Absorbed by hydrolysis	Less springy than other monofilament absorbables with minimal tissue drag. Available dyed or undyed
Polyglyconate	Maxon (Davis & Geck)	Monofilament	Synthetic	No	Retains 70% at 14 days	Complete absorption by 60 days. Absorbed by hydrolysis	Similar to polydioxanone but easy to handle. Uses: similar to polydioxanone
Chromic catgut		Essentially monofilament	Natural (made from purified animal intestines)	Coated with chromium salts	Retains tensile strength for approximately 28 days	Absorbed by enzymatic degradation and phagocytosis	Always causes a moderate inflammatory response
Plain catgut		Essentially monofilament	Natural (made from purified animal intestines)	No	Retains tensile strength for approximately 14 days	Absorbed by enzymatic degradation and phagocytosis	Also causes a moderate inflammatory response and rapidly loses tensile strength

Table 22.6 Cross-sectional design of suture needles

Cross-sectional design	Features	Uses
Cutting	Triangular in cross-section with apex on inside of curve. Point and sides of needle have cutting edges, which are very sharp	Skin and other dense tissue
Reverse cutting	Triangular in cross-section with apex on outside of curve. Point and sides of needle have cutting edges, which are very sharp	Skin and other dense tissue
Round-bodied	Round in cross-section. No sharp edges	Delicate tissues, e.g. fat, viscera
Taper point	Becomes round-bodied as needle widens. Similar to cutting needle at tip	Dense tissues other than skin, e.g. fascia, thick-walled viscera, mucous membranes

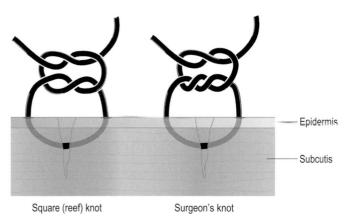

Square (reef) knot   Surgeon's knot

Fig. 22.5 Surgical knots

The knots of skin sutures should be pulled to one side of the incision. The suture loop should be loose. Sutures that are placed tightly will compromise the vascular supply and delay healing. They will also cause irritation and cause the patient to interfere with the wound.

Interrupted sutures

Each suture is tied individually and cut distal to the knot (Fig. 22.6). The main advantage of interrupted sutures is the ability to maintain strength and tissue apposition if one part of the suture line fails. The disadvantages are the amount of suture material required and the length of time it takes to place the sutures.

Continuous sutures

A continuous line of sutures is placed and only knotted and cut at the beginning and end of the suture line (Fig. 22.6). The advantages are the ease of application and removal and the fact that less suture material is used. The main disadvantage is that slippage of the knot at either end of the suture line will cause the entire suture line to break down.

Various patterns of sutures may be used depending on the site and the purpose of the suture line. They are shown in Figure 22.6, and include:

- Simple interrupted
- Simple continuous
- Ford interlocking
- Interrupted vertical mattress
- Interrupted horizontal mattress
- Cruciate mattress.

Sutures should be placed at least 5 mm from the wound edge and placed squarely across the wound. Rat-toothed forceps should be used to handle the skin and the wound edges should be apposed or slightly everted, with no gaping or overlapping.

Patient care

Preoperative care

On admission all relevant details about the patient should be recorded:

- The reason for admission must be checked
- Ensure that the owner understands what is to be done
- Check that the patient is in good general health or that the symptoms have not changed since last seen
- Make sure a contact number is taken and the general anaesthetic consent form is signed
- Check the patient has been starved – usually food is withheld for 12 hours prior to surgery to prevent regurgitation under anaesthesia
- Ideally, the patient should be bathed before surgery to minimize contamination of the surgical site
- The patient should have been given the opportunity to urinate and defecate before surgery; in some cases an enema may be required
- The patient should be weighed and any medication given, e.g. antibiotics, analgesia and premedication.

Preparation of the patient for a surgical procedure

Some form of premedication or sedation is given intramuscularly or subcutaneously 15–30 minutes before the induction of anaesthesia. Antibiotics and analgesics are usually given at the same time.

Clipping

This is necessary for most surgical procedures. It can be done before or under general anaesthesia. A large area around the surgical site should be clipped. It should be neat, as this is usually what the owner notices. Before starting, ensure that the clipper blades are in good working order, as nicks in the

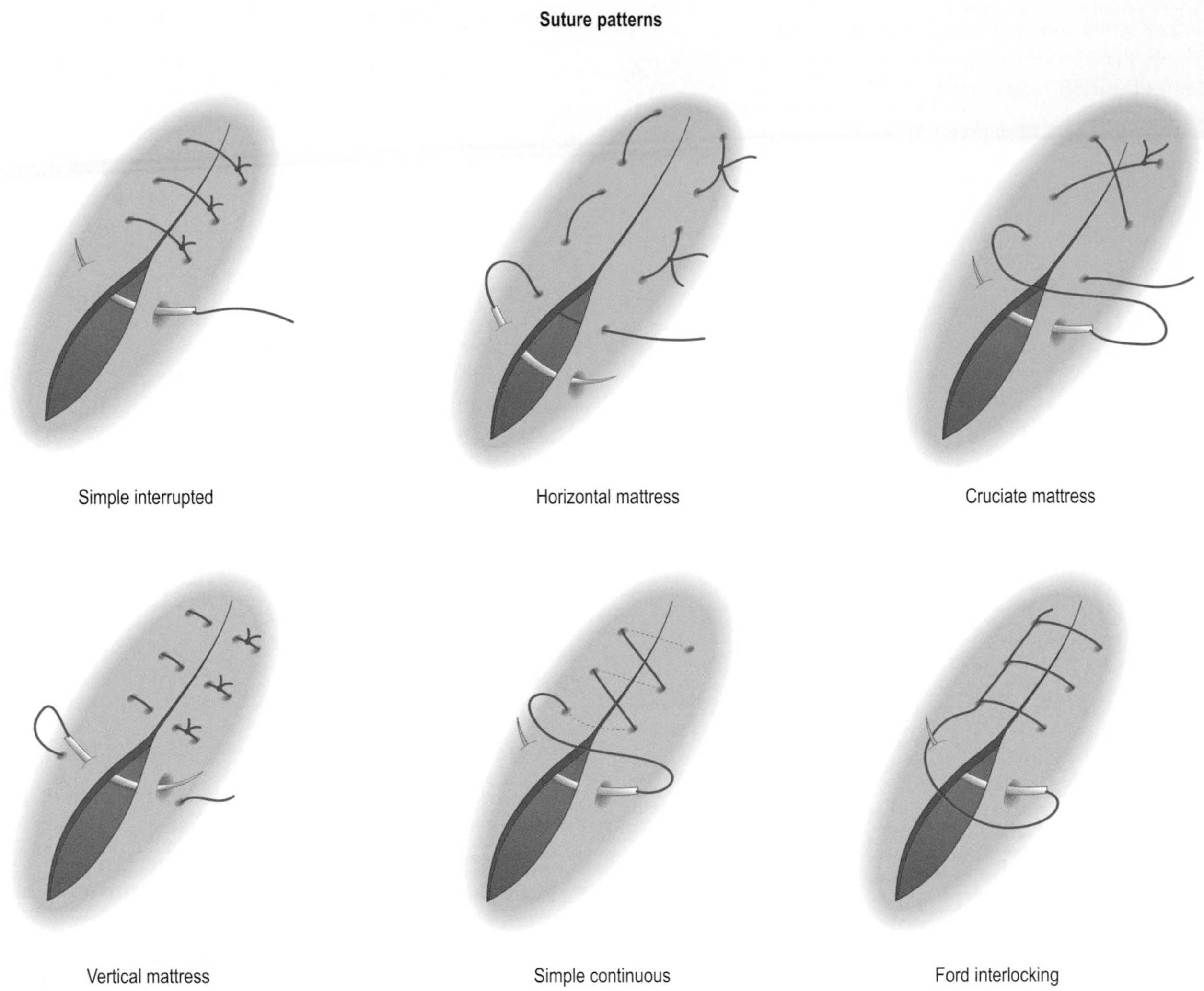

Suture patterns

Simple interrupted   Horizontal mattress   Cruciate mattress

Vertical mattress   Simple continuous   Ford interlocking

Fig. 22.6 Common suture patterns

skin will cause irritation and excessive licking postoperatively. All clipping should be done away from the theatre to minimize contamination.

Skin preparation

As it is not possible to remove all bacteria from the skin, the aim is to significantly reduce the number of organisms without damaging the skin itself. Antiseptic and detergent properties are needed in a skin cleansing agent and surgical scrub preparations such as chlorhexidine or povidone-iodine are ideal. There are various methods of skin preparation; the one outlined below is commonly used:

a. Wear surgical gloves to prevent contamination of the patient's skin by the nurse's hands
b. Use lint-free swabs to wash the site with surgical scrub and a little water. Begin at the operating site and work out to the edges of the clipped area. At the edge of the clipped area discard the swab and use a new one. Continue until the skin is clean, i.e. no discoloration on swab
c. A small amount of alcohol solution can be sprayed over the site to remove any remaining

detergent. Do not use on mucous membranes or open wounds
d. Move patient to theatre and position for surgery. The site will be contaminated now, so clean once again in the same fashion but using sterile swabs and gloves
e. The final-stage scrub is done by the surgical team, with an antiseptic solution using sterile swabs on sterile Rampley sponge-holding forceps.

Preparation of eyes and mucous membranes

Most skin preparations are irritating to the eye and mucous membranes. Dilute solutions of povidone-iodine (0.1%) can be used to irrigate the eye and oral cavity. Alcohol solutions must not be used. The skin around the eye is very thin and sensitive, so minimal clipping is required.

Draping the surgical site

This is done to maintain asepsis by preventing contamination of the surgical site by hair and the immediate environment. Drapes should be large enough to cover the entire patient, leaving only the surgical site exposed.

Plain drapes

Four rectangular drapes are used to create a window for the surgical site (Fig. 22.7). The first drape is placed between the surgeon and the nearest side of the patient. The second drape is placed on the opposite side of the patient. The remaining two drapes are placed at each end of the patient. They are then secured with towel clips.

Fenestrated drapes

These achieve the same effect as plain drapes but the 'window' is already formed within a single drape. The drape must be large enough to cover the entire patient. Such drapes are commonly used for cat and bitch spays.

Adhesive drapes

These are sterile, clear, adhesive plastic sheets. They are placed over the entire site. Standard drapes are then placed over the top in the usual fashion. An incision is made through the adhesive material.

Draping limbs

There are many ways to drape a limb. Most commonly the lower limb is bandaged and tied to an upright pole such as a drip stand – this keeps the limb out of the way while a

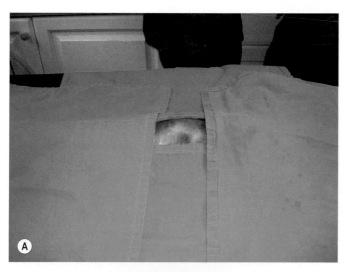

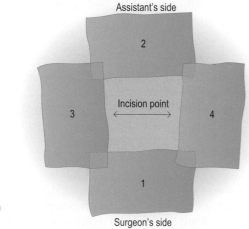

Fig. 22.7 Draping the patient. (**A**) Plain drapes placed on the patient ready for surgery. (**B**) Order of placing plain drapes on the patient

sterile drape is placed on the table top underneath. A sterile drape is then secured to the limb and the tie is released to lower the limb on to the drape on the table top. The surgical site is then draped in the usual manner.

Intraoperative care

You must always remember that underneath the drapes is a live patient. Towel clips must be positioned to avoid delicate structures. Hypothermia is common, particularly in small animals, and heat loss must be prevented. Use heat pads, hot water bottles, insulating wrap (bubble wrap) and warmed intravenous and irrigating fluids. The patient should be carefully positioned on the table to avoid any postoperative complications. If required, prepare yourself for surgery by scrubbing, gowning and gloving, as described earlier, to perform the duties of the scrub nurse.

Controlling haemorrhage

Haemorrhage can be controlled by using swabs, instruments (e.g. Spencer Wells or Halstead mosquito artery forceps, Fig. 22.3), ligatures or diathermy. If using swabs, blot the haemorrhaging area as opposed to wiping it, as wiping will disrupt any clot formation.

Postoperative care

- The patient should not be left unattended until conscious and sitting up
- The endotracheal tube should be removed as the cough reflex returns (in cats the tube is removed just before it returns) and the patient must be watched closely to ensure that an adequate airway is maintained. The colour of the mucous membranes and the presence or absence of respiratory noise are good indicators of effective ventilation
- Body temperature should be monitored and maintained
- The heart and pulse rate should also be monitored and any changes noted
- Dressings should be done before the patient regains consciousness. Any purse-string sutures and swabs should be removed
- The patient should be placed in a warm, comfortable and quiet recovery kennel
- Turn the patient regularly if it is unable to do this for itself
- Administer any analgesic drugs prescribed by the veterinary surgeon (Table 22.7). If you observe any signs of pain, inform the veterinary surgeon (see also Chapter 25)
- When fully recovered allow the patient to urinate and defecate
- Provide food and water if appropriate for the case, especially to very old or young patients.

Intubation

The advantages of intubation are:

- It provides a secure airway and protects it from saliva and other secretions such as water during dental procedures

Table 22.7 Analgesic drugs used intraoperatively and postoperatively

Chemical name	Trade name
Carprofen	Rimadyl
Meloxicam	Metacam
Morphine	–
Buprenorphine	Vetergesic
Pethidine	–
Fentanyl	–
Butorphanol	Torbugesic

- It allows intermittent positive pressure ventilation (IPPV) (see Ch. 25)
- It reduces anatomical dead space
- It allows the maintenance of anaesthesia and provides a means of supplying oxygen (see Ch. 25)
- It reduces pollution from waste anaesthetic gases.

Disadvantages include:

- The endotracheal tube may kink during positioning
- Overinflation of the cuff may occlude the tube and cause damage to the trachea
- A tube that is too small may increase the resistance to breathing
- Traumatic laryngitis may develop as a result of poor technique or oversized tubes – particularly in cats.

Method of intubation

Dogs

1. Place the anaesthetized patient in lateral recumbency
2. The assistant holds the head up, supporting the base of the neck with the left hand and holding the maxilla and nose with the right hand
3. Gently ease the tongue out of the mouth and pull it down to lower the mandible. This enables the larynx to be viewed
4. Using a correct-sized lubricated tube, insert it into the mouth towards the soft palate
5. Insert the tube over the epiglottis and between the vocal folds.

Cats

1. Place the anaesthetized patient in lateral recumbency
2. The assistant holds the head up, supporting the base of the neck with the left hand and holding the maxilla and nose with the right hand. Keep fingers out of the mouth
3. Gently ease the tongue out of the mouth and pull it down to lower the mandible. This enables the larynx to be viewed
4. If using a laryngoscope, hold the tongue with your thumb and forefinger and hold the laryngoscope with the same hand. Use the blade of the laryngoscope to push the tongue down, not the epiglottis, enabling the larynx to be viewed
5. To prevent the occurrence of laryngeal spasm, spray the larynx with local anaesthetic to desensitize it. Wait 60–90 seconds
6. Insert a correct-sized lubricated tube into the mouth and between the laryngeal folds during inspiration. The laryngeal folds can be seen moving in and out as the cat breathes.

Removing the endotracheal tube (extubation)

In dogs the tube should be removed when the swallowing/gag reflex returns; in cats it should be removed before the reflex returns. Leave the cuff inflated until removal. On removal, deflate the cuff and carefully pull the tube out in a downward direction to avoid damage to the trachea and larynx.

Immediate/short-term postoperative complications

Haemorrhage

Control any external haemorrhage with digital pressure or pressure bandages. Internal haemorrhage is more complicated. Usually, the patient will have to be re-anaesthetized and the incision opened up to control the haemorrhage with instruments and ligatures. Prepare warm intravenous fluids.

Laryngospasm

Keep the endotracheal tube in place if you have not already removed it. Steroid treatment may help or, in severe cases, a tracheostomy may have to be performed (see Ch. 21).

Shock

Monitor all vital parameters, i.e. heart and pulse rate, mucous membrane colour, capillary refill time and respiration rate. Prepare warm intravenous fluids. Keep the patient warm using blankets or bubble wrap. Do not apply direct heat using heat pads. Administer antidote to the anaesthetic agent, if appropriate (see Ch. 25).

Hypothermia

Keep the patient warm using blankets, bubble wrap and heat mats. Maintain room temperature between 21°C and 23°C. Monitor rectal temperature every 10 minutes. Give warmed intravenous fluids.

Vomiting

Stay with the patient at all times. Hold the head and neck down, or hang over the side of the table with the body raised so that the head and neck are in a downwards position. Keep in this position until the patient regains consciousness. Administer any antiemetic drugs that the veterinary surgeon has prescribed.

Long-term postoperative complications

These are listed in Table 22.8.

Asepsis and sterilization

Principles of sterilization

The saying 'Prevention is better than cure' is very true. Infection of clean surgical wounds is a concern across the world. Antibiotics should not be relied upon as a means of protection against infection because of poor aseptic technique. Every veterinary organization should have a routine that is adhered to, from correct theatre attire and scrubbing-up techniques to the cleaning of instruments and the practice environment. Box 22.3 provides some useful terminology.

Box 22.3 Definitions of common terms	

- **Sepsis** – presence of pathogens in the blood or tissues, i.e. infection
- **Asepsis** – freedom from infection
- **Antisepsis** – prevention of sepsis by destruction of pathogens
- **Sterilization** – destruction of all microorganisms, including bacterial spores
- **Disinfection** – destruction of all microorganisms except bacterial spores
- **Disinfectant** – a chemical agent that destroys microorganisms

Spread of infection

Contamination usually comes from four sources – the operating theatre and its environment, the equipment used, the personnel and the patient:

- **Operating theatre and its environment** – many microorganisms are airborne. Any movement within the theatre will cause them to disperse. Good ventilation is necessary, as hot humid conditions are also a threat to asepsis. Cleaner procedures should be done first, as organisms from the contaminated site will remain in the air. The operating room should be easily cleaned and contain little furniture
- **Equipment** – all equipment, e.g. instruments, must be sterile and a new set must be used for each operation
- **Personnel** – the more people there are in the theatre the greater the risk of infection. Correct theatre clothing should be worn, those in the surgical team must prepare their hands aseptically and sterile gowns and gloves should be worn
- **Patient** – the patient is the greatest source of contamination. Microorganisms are either:
  - Endogenous – within the body of the patient or
  - Exogenous – outside the body on the skin and coat of the patient.

Wounds may be classified as either clean, clean contaminated, contaminated or dirty and a wound does not necessarily have to be obviously infected for microorganisms to be present. There are also other factors, such as the virulence of the organism, the resistance of the patient and the duration of the surgery. The infection rate doubles for every hour of surgery, and surgical technique can also increase the risk of contamination, especially if there is excessive trauma and damage to the vascular supply. Impaired host resistance, the

Table 22.8 Complications associated with the postoperative period

Complication	Signs	Treatment
Shock	Tachycardia Weak rapid pulse Pale or cyanotic mucous membranes Slow capillary refill times Cold extremities Shallow breathing Tachypnoea	Monitor all vital parameters including heart and pulse rate, mucous membrane colour, capillary refill time, respiration rate and pattern – measure every 5 min Prepare and give warmed intravenous fluids Keep the patient warm with blankets and bubble wrap, but not direct heat. Administer any antidote to the anaesthetic agent
Decubitus ulcers	Bed sores on bony prominences Possible ulceration and bleeding Patient may show signs of restlessness and pain	Clean and dry the areas with skin disinfectant. Use extra padding and bedding. Turn the patient frequently
Coughing	Harsh coughing Grunting noises Wheezing Patient is restless and agitated Patient refuses to eat when offered food	Always differentiate the cough from kennel cough Give any drugs prescribed by the veterinary surgeon Feed soft mushy food. Hand-feed if necessary
Hypostatic pneumonia	Shallow rapid respiration Signs of restlessness and discomfort Pale or cyanotic mucous membranes Slow capillary refill time	Monitor all vital parameters, including heart and pulse rate, mucous membrane colour, capillary refill time and respiration rate and pattern – measure every 5 min Turn the patient every 2 hours Position the patient in sternal recumbency using foam wedges or bedding

use of drugs, nutritional problems and underlying disease will contribute to wound contamination.

Sterilization

All instruments and equipment must be sterilized before use. There are several methods of sterilization available and the choice, which must be both safe and economical, depends on:

- Amount and type of equipment to be sterilized
- Cost
- Available space within the practice.

There are two types of sterilization: cold sterilization and heat sterilization.

Cold sterilization

Ethylene oxide

This is a highly penetrating and effective method of sterilization but it is toxic, irritant to tissues and a flammable gas. COSHH regulations may make it impractical to use within a veterinary surgery. Ethylene oxide works by inactivating the DNA of cells and stops cell reproduction. It is effective against vegetative bacteria, fungi, viruses and spores. Several factors influence the ability of ethylene oxide to destroy microorganisms, including temperature, pressure concentration, humidity and time of exposure.

An ethylene oxide sterilizer is a plastic container fitted with a ventilation system to prevent gas from entering the workplace. It must be used in a clean, well-ventilated area away from any work areas. The temperature of the room must be at least 20°C during the cycle. Items are placed in a polythene liner bag with a gas ampoule and the bag is sealed with a metal twist tie and placed in the sterilizing unit. The top of the vial is snapped from outside the liner bag to release the gas. The sterilizer door is then closed and locked, the ventilator is turned on and the items are left to sterilize. This is usually done overnight, as it is a 12-hour process. At the end of the period a pump is switched on to ventilate the container and the door may be opened 2 hours later. Items must be left for a further 24 hours to allow the ethylene oxide to dissipate.

Suitable items to be sterilized include anything that might be damaged by heat, e.g. fibreoptic equipment (endoscopes), plastic catheters, anaesthetic tubing, plastic syringes, optical equipment, high-speed drills, burrs and battery-operated drills. Most things can be sterilized but the limiting factors are the size of the container, the duration of the cycle and the toxicity. Equipment containing polyvinyl chloride (PVC) cannot be sterilized in this way, as PVC may react with the ethylene oxide gas.

All materials must be clean and dry. The presence of protein and grease slows sterilization and reduces its effectiveness. Bungs, caps and stylets must be removed to allow the gas to penetrate freely. Items can be packaged, as ethylene oxide penetrates more easily than steam, but do not use nylon film bags. To monitor the effectiveness of the process, indicator tape can be used that has yellow stripes that turn red; however, this does not guarantee sterility as the stripes change colour after only a short exposure to the gas. Chemical indicators placed in the centre of the pack will change colour when exposed for the correct length of time. Spore strips can be added to the load. These can later be added to a culture medium and incubated for 72 hours. They are useful for checking the efficiency of the system but they are not an indicator of sterility.

Formaldehyde

This is used in a similar way to ethylene oxide, but COSHH regulations now restrict its use.

Chemical solutions

These are not very effective sterilants and are really only a means of disinfection. Some manufacturers guarantee sterilization if immersed for a long time – usually 24 hours. This method is useful for equipment that cannot be sterilized by any other means, e.g. endoscopic equipment.

Glutaraldehyde

Widely used but very irritant, so items must be washed with sterile water just before use. Gloves and masks should be worn. Glutaraldehyde is supplied as an acid solution that is activated by the addition of powder at the time of use.

Chlorhexidine-based solutions

Can only be used as disinfectants as chlorhexidine has poor activity against spores, fungi and viruses.

Irradiation

Gamma irradiation can only be used in a controlled environment. Prepackaged items such as needles and syringes are sterilized in this way.

Heat sterilization

Dry heat – hot air oven

Dry heat will kill microorganisms by oxidative destruction of the bacterial protoplasm. Microorganisms are more resistant to this method than if heated with moisture, so higher temperatures are required – about 150–180°C. If the temperature is below 140°C then it will not destroy spores in less than 4–5 hours.

Hot air ovens are usually small and economical to run. The oven is heated by electrical elements. The door is usually fitted with a device to prevent opening before it is cool. Any items sterilized must have a long cooling period before they can be used. It is important not to overload the oven, to allow the free flow of air.

Spore strip tests and Browne's tubes can be used to test the sterility in the oven.

Items that can be sterilized by this method include glass syringes, cutting instruments, ophthalmic drill bits, powder and oils that cannot be sterilized with moisture. Fabric, rubber and plastic cannot be sterilized by hot air as they are destroyed by the high temperatures.

Hot air ovens are not recommended, for health and safety reasons.

Steam under pressure – autoclave

This is a common and efficient method of sterilization. Instruments, drapes, gowns, swabs, most rubber products, glassware and some plastic can be sterilized in this way.

However, fibreoptics, lenses and plastics are usually heat-sensitive and are thus easily damaged.

There are three types of autoclave:

- **Vertical pressure cooker** – this is the simplest of autoclaves. It works by boiling water in a closed container. There is an air vent at the top that is closed after the air is evacuated from the container, and the pressure is then allowed to build up to 15 psi. The biggest disadvantage of this system is that the air vent is at the top, so some air may remain trapped underneath the steam; the temperature in that area is lower and sterility cannot therefore be guaranteed. It is also manually operated, so there is room for human error.
- **Horizontal/vertical downward displacement autoclave** – this is a larger and completely automatic autoclave. It uses an electrically operated boiler that is also a source of steam. The air outlet is at the bottom, so the air is driven out more effectively by downward displacement. Usually there is a choice of programmes with varying temperatures. This autoclave is designed for sterilization of loose instruments rather than packs, as the drying cycle is insufficient. Damp packs will allow microorganisms to penetrate the pack during the storage period.
- **Vacuum-assisted autoclaves** – this autoclave works on the same principle as the other two, but there is a high-power vacuum pump to evacuate the air from the chamber at the beginning of the cycle. Steam penetration happens quickly and sterilization is faster. A second vacuum cycle takes the moisture out after sterilization and dries the load. There is a choice of cycles with different temperatures and pressures. It is suitable for all instruments, drapes and equipment and is fully automatic, with fail-safe mechanisms.

Use of the autoclave

Autoclaves differ but the principle remains the same. Water boils at 100°C and converts into steam and the temperature of the water therefore remains the same however long the water is heated.

Many bacteria and bacterial spores are resistant to high temperatures no matter how long they are exposed; however, if the pressure is increased the temperature of the steam rises and the bacteria and spores will be killed. It is the increased temperature, not the increased pressure, that destroys the microorganisms, and the higher the temperature the shorter the time needed for sterilization.

The central sterilizing chamber of the autoclave is surrounded by a jacket of steam. When the pressure in the jacket is raised, steam enters the chamber, displacing the air downwards. When all the air is evacuated, the vents close and steam continues to enter the chamber until the desired pressure is reached. The steam condenses on the colder surfaces of the contents of the chamber, producing heat, which penetrates to the innermost layers of the pack – it is the moisture that increases the penetrability of the heat. After a certain time the steam is evacuated and the temperature and pressure drop to normal.

Effective sterilization relies on loading the packs correctly. There must be adequate space to allow the steam to circulate freely. You must not overload the autoclave or block the inlet and exhaust valves. Instruments must be free of grease and protein material to allow effective penetration of the steam. The autoclave itself should be regularly serviced by a qualified engineer to comply with health and safety regulations and to ensure that effective sterilization takes place.

Monitoring sterilization

- **Chemical indicator strips** (TST strips) – these change colour when the correct temperature, pressure and time have been reached. The strips should be placed inside the pack. It is important that the appropriate strip is used for each different time/pressure/temperature cycle or a false result may occur.
- **Browne's tubes** – these change colour when the correct temperature, pressure and time have been reached. They are small glass tubes partly filled with an orange/brown liquid that changes to green when certain temperatures have been maintained for a set length of time. It is essential that the correct tube is used for the selected cycle.
- **Bowie Dick tape** – this is usually used to seal an instrument or drape pack. It is beige-coloured tape impregnated with a chemical strip that turns dark brown when a temperature of 121°C has been reached. The tape is limited in value, as it does not ensure that the temperature has been maintained for the set time.
- **Spore tests** – these are strips of paper impregnated with dried spores. The paper is placed in a load and on completion of sterilization it is placed in the culture medium provided and incubated at room temperature for 72 hours. If sterilization is effective there will be no growth. These tests are more accurate than chemical indicator strips but the delay in results is a major disadvantage.
- **Thermocouples** – these are electrical leads with temperature-sensitive tips. They are placed in various parts of the sterilization chamber with the leads passed out of an aperture to a recording device. The temperature of the chamber is constantly checked and recorded throughout the cycle.

Packing supplies for sterilization

There are many packing materials and containers available, all with advantages and disadvantages (Table 22.9). Your choice will depend on several factors:

- Size of autoclave
- Packing material must be resistant to damage
- Steam or gas must be able to penetrate wrapping for sterilization to occur and must easily exhaust when sterilization is complete
- Microorganisms must not be able to penetrate from the outside of the wrapping
- Cost

Table 22.9 Advantages and disadvantages of packing materials used for sterilization of surgical equipment

	Advantages	Disadvantages
Nylon film (usually sealed with Bowie Dick tape)	Variety of sizes available Reusable	Becomes brittle after repeated use and develops tiny holes, leading to contamination Difficult to remove sterile item without contaminating it on the edges of the bag
Seal and peel pack	Variety of sizes available Can be used with ethylene oxide of autoclave Risk of contamination is small	Paper backing tears easily
Paper	Elastic and conforming	Water-repellent therefore ideal as an outer layer
Textiles (usually linen)	Conforming Strong Reusable	Permeable to moisture
Metal drums	Last for years Use for instruments, gowns and drapes	Expensive Contamination risk every time lid is opened
Boxes/cartons	Inexpensive Reusable	Can only use in autoclave

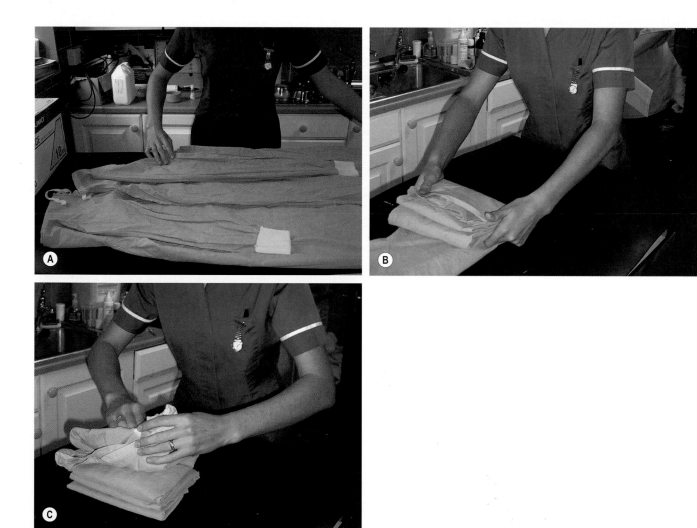

Fig. 22.8 Folding a gown. (**A**) The gown is laid out flat and the sides are folded into the middle (**B**). Then concertina it lengthways (**C**) to achieve a flat pack

- Time taken to reach sterility
- Personal preference.

Equipment care and sterilization

Gowns and drapes

Wash, dry and inspect for damage. They should be folded correctly (Figs 22.8, 22.9) to achieve flat packs and to allow penetration during sterilization. The outside of the gown should be on the inside so that the surgeon can put it on in an aseptic fashion. Drapes should be folded in a concertina fashion to allow free flow of steam during sterilization. These procedures are illustrated on the website.

Both gowns and drapes can be sterilized with ethylene oxide but it is very uneconomical because the sterilizer is small and the cycle is long. Autoclave sterilization is much quicker and more efficient. A hot air oven cannot be used as it will burn the material. Gowns and drapes can be sterilized in drums, boxes, bags or packs. Hand towels can be placed with the gowns and drapes in the instrument pack.

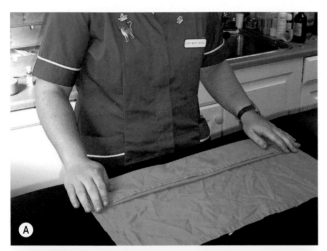

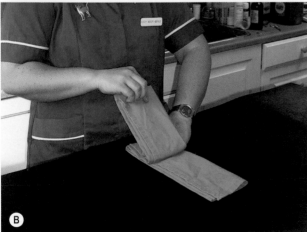

Fig. 22.9 Folding surgical drapes. (**A**) Concertina the cloth widthways. (**B**) Then concertina lengthways to achieve a flat pack

Swabs

These can be bought pre-sterilized, but this is expensive. Non-sterile swabs are packed into bundles of five or ten – the number of swabs is not important as long as it is consistent and all the staff are aware of the number. Swabs may be incorporated into the instrument pack or packaged alone. They can be sterilized in boxes, bags or drums.

Urinary catheters

These are designed for single use but can usually be re-sterilized once – a Foley catheter cannot be reused. After use, urinary catheters should be washed, dried and packed in the appropriate size of bag without coiling. They can be sterilized in an autoclave but some brands can be damaged by heat. Ethylene oxide can be used successfully for all types of catheter but it is essential that they are aired for the required amount of time before use.

Syringes

Plastic syringes are designed to be disposable and it is rarely economical to re-sterilize them. However, it is possible to reuse 30 ml or 50 ml syringes, which should be washed, dried, disassembled and packed individually ready for sterilization. Some brands can be autoclaved, but most will be damaged by the heat. Ethylene oxide can be used successfully. Glass syringes can be sterilized in a hot air oven, autoclave or ethylene oxide.

Liquids

These are usually bought pre-sterilized but some of the more sophisticated autoclaves have a cycle for sterilizing liquids. The risk of breakage is high and it is far more economical to buy fluids commercially prepared.

Power tools

Air drills, saws and mechanical burrs can be autoclaved, but follow the manufacturer's instructions. Autoclaving can cause motors to jam. Ethylene oxide can be used for all air-driven tools. Battery drills usually have a plastic casing that melts in the autoclave, but they can also be sterilized by ethylene oxide. Alternatively, an un-sterile drill can be placed in a sterile sleeve with a sterile chuck attached.

Storage after sterilization

There should be a separate dry, dust-free, well-ventilated area in the surgical unit for storing sterile packs. A closed cupboard is ideal. Handle the packs as little as possible to minimize damage, and pack loosely on the shelves so that the bags are not damaged. The length of time that sterile packs can be stored is debatable and all packs should carry the date of sterilization. A sealed pack should remain sterile for a limitless period but it can become contaminated by handling, damage to the pack or moisture and it is recommended that packs are repacked and sterilized every 6–8 weeks.

Bibliography

Aspinall, V., 2003. Clinical Procedures in Veterinary Nursing. Butterworth-Heinemann, Oxford.

College of Animal Welfare, 2000. Veterinary Surgical Instruments – An Illustrated Guide. Butterworth-Heinemann, Oxford.

Cooper, B., Lane, D.R., 2003. Veterinary Nursing. Butterworth-Heinemann, Oxford.

Moore, M. (Ed.), 1999. Manual of Veterinary Nursing. British Small Animal Veterinary Association, Cheltenham.

Recommended reading

Aspinall, V., 2007. Clinical Procedures in Veterinary Nursing, second ed. Butterworth-Heinemann, Oxford.

All tasks performed in the preparation of the surgical environment are described in a step-by-step format with explanations as to why you do it.

Moore, M. (Ed.), 1999. Manual of Veterinary Nursing. British Small Animal Veterinary Association, Cheltenham.

Includes several useful chapters on surgical procedures and theatre practice.

CHAPTER 23

High-dependency nursing

Claire Cave

Key Points

- A high-dependency unit (HDU) may be a dedicated department or a small room set aside for the care of critically ill patients, but both require expensive, highly technical equipment and dedicated nurses to ensure a high standard of care.
- Patient observation and monitoring are essential and this will be needed around the clock if the patient is to survive.
- Much of the expense of setting up an HDU comes from the wide range of monitoring equipment.
- Many of the procedures carried out in the HDU are similar to those performed on any patient but the difference is that the equipment and the drugs used are more specialized and the veterinary nursing team will only work within the HDU and provide hands-on 24 hours cover – each case may be allocated its own particular nurse.

Introduction

Nursing the critical care patient within a high-dependency unit (HDU) requires a detailed understanding of the complex techniques that must be carried out if the patient is to survive. Many of these techniques are rarely seen within the day-to-day workings of a veterinary practice. However, it is still important to remember that, for all the highly skilled techniques we may employ and for all the equipment used, the veterinary nurse and his/her ability to observe and care for the animal is still the major contributing factor to a quick recovery and prolonged survival time. Never forget that the animal needs home comforts, comfortable bedding, a stimulating environment (unless contraindicated) and huge amounts of 'TLC'. Relationships that develop between the nurse, patient and owner can be rewarding and satisfying and the sense of achievement at seeing one of your patients recovered and going home can be immense.

Designing a high-dependency unit

It is not always possible in a veterinary practice to have a designated room just for high-dependency cases, but an appropriate level of care can still be implemented. Space limitations may result in shorter equipment lists.

The following points may be helpful when setting up a unit:

- Although not essential, it is preferable to have a separate cat and dog ward
- The HDU should be light, airy and quiet. HDU patients require quiet and rest and this will not be achieved if they are next to a busy dog ward, particularly if they are cats
- The unit may be located either away from all noise and activity so that disturbance is reduced or, if the room is not attended at all times, it may be better to have it in a position that staff regularly walk past – patients are observed more closely and there are plenty of people on hand in the event of an emergency
- It should be possible to darken the room to reduce stimulation for seizuring patients and promote normal sleep patterns
- Room temperature must be able to be regulated, e.g. with air conditioning; fans are a cheaper but less effective alternative
- A sink and disinfectant should be available for hand washing
- There must be facilities for equipment storage. Consumables should be stored in cupboards to reduce the build up of dust and for effective cleaning (Box 23.1)
- Cleaning protocols should be carried out daily, weekly and monthly. Cleaning equipment must be used exclusively in the HDU
- Emergency equipment should be labelled, readily available and in a consistent location to ensure that all staff can find it (Box 23.2)
- Protocols for all treatment procedures should be available to ensure consistency
- It is preferable to have nurses who are dedicated to the HDU to ensure continuity of care and rapid recognition of deterioration. Owners also appreciate consistent care. A strong and rewarding relationship can develop between owners and patients and the nurse.

Box 23.1 Equipping the high-dependency unit (Equipment in **bold type** should be considered essential)

Consumables	**Syringes:**	**Insulin syringes, 1 ml, 2 ml, 5 ml, 10 ml, 20 or 30 ml, 50 ml**
	Needles:	**25 FG, 23 FG, 21 FG, 20 FG, 18 FG, 16 FG, 14 FG**
	Intravenous catheters:	**Peripheral vein – 16 FG, 18 FG, 20 FG, 22 FG, 24 FG**
		Central vein – peel-away, Seldinger, or through the needle
	Intraosseous needles	
	Intravenous bungs, T connectors	
	Giving sets, paediatric burette sets, blood giving sets, extension sets	
	Chest drains	
Fluid therapy	**Syringe drivers, infusion pumps**	
	Heparinized saline	
Bedding	**Large Vetbeds, blankets, thick foam mattresses**	
	Bair huggers, heated waterbeds	
Dressings	**Routine dressings**	
	Antibiotic impregnated dressings	
Monitoring equipment	**PCV tubes, glucometer, urine dipsticks, refractometer**	
	Practice facilities for measuring electrolytes and serum biochemistry	
	Blood gas analyser	
	Electrocardiograph	
	Pulse oximeter	
	Blood pressure monitoring (invasive or non-invasive)	
Miscellaneous	**Thermometer, stethoscope, clippers, scissors**	
	Clock (with second hand)	
	Surgical scrub and spirit, sterile gloves	
	Defibrillator	

Box 23.2 Equipping the crash trolley

The crash kit may be kept on a purpose-built trolley or kept in something as simple as a fishing tackle box. It must be kept in a consistent place at all times to avoid confusion in an emergency. Items should be clearly labelled and restocked at the beginning of each day or after use. The kit should contain:

Pharmaceutical

- Atropine
- Adrenaline (epinephrine)
- 2% lidocaine (without adrenaline)
- Sodium bicarbonate
- Glucose
- Calcium chloride or gluconate
- Dexamethasone
- Mannitol
- Potassium chloride

Airway access

- Endotracheal tubes – wide selection
- Laryngoscope and blades
- Tracheostomy tubes – wide selection
- Gauze tie
- Sterile lubricating jelly

Intravenous access

- Intravenous catheters – full selection
- Giving sets
- Butterfly catheters – wide selection
- Intraosseous needles

Fluid therapy

- Crystalloids – lactated Ringer's solution, 0.9% saline, 5% dextrose
- Colloids (Haemacel or Gelofusine)
- Starches (hetastarch)
- Haemoglobin-based oxygen-carrying solution, e.g. Oxyglobin

Miscellaneous

- Syringes – full selection
- Hypodermic needles – full selection
- Clippers
- Surgical scrub and spirit
- Various tapes and bandages
- Surgical gloves –range of sizes
- Surgical kit
- Scalpel blades
- Stethoscope
- Suction equipment
- Gel if defibrillator present
- External and internal paddles for defibrillator
- Spare leads for electrocardiograph
- Stopwatch
- Thermometer

If available, the following items should also be on the crash trolley or kept close to hand:

- Electrocardiograph
- Dinamap blood pressure monitor
- Pulse oximeter
- Defibrillator

The crash trolley must be checked regularly to ensure that drugs are in date, and that such things as the cuffs on endotracheal tubes are working. ECGs and defibrillators should be kept fully charged and surgical packs should be sterilized regularly.

Record-keeping

All observations must be recorded in a legible and accessible form. A daily summary sheet should be on each cage door recording patient and owner details, a problem list, a drug list and administration times, a monitoring list and times, and resuscitation orders. Resuscitation orders should have been discussed with the owner and recorded, e.g. Do Not Resuscitate or, if measures are to be carried out, to what level (closed or open chest). HDU patients may also need records of other aspects of their care, including fluid therapy, nutrition, and care of chest drains or tracheostomy tubes.

Patient monitoring and observation

Basic monitoring of temperature, pulse, and respiratory rates (TPR) is essential in the HDU as it is for any other patient, although there are many types of extra monitoring equipment that can also be used.

Temperature

Metabolic rate is closely linked to temperature regulation and this is especially true in shocked patients or those that are anaesthetized or comatose. Hypothermia may affect the mechanics of respiration, cardiac function and the patient's coagulation state.

Body temperature is usually taken rectally using either a mercury or digital thermometer. However, in poorly perfused animals, the rectal temperature may not truly reflect the core temperature. Thermometers should be placed carefully against the mucosa to avoid measuring faecal temperature. Core temperature can also be taken aurally (currently an expensive piece of equipment) or via the oesophagus in unconscious patients.

In a critical care patient pyrexia or hyperthermia may indicate:

- Pain
- Infection
- Sepsis
- Convulsion activity.

There are a variety of ways to cool an animal down but, in a critically ill animal, some methods may not be suitable. For example, fluids can be administered at room temperature, but not chilled; a crushed ice enema may work in extreme situations where temperatures are approaching 41–42°C. Total body cooling is best accomplished by immersing the body in cool but not cold water; if the water is too cold, peripheral vasoconstriction may occur, which slows the heat loss process.

Hypothermia may indicate:

- Shock
- Hypovolaemia/circulatory collapse
- Moribund patient.

It is vitally important to try and warm these patients as quickly as possible. When the temperature starts to dip below 36°C, the patient must be actively warmed from the core. Administering fluids at a temperature of no more than 40°C intravenously may help. Fluids can be warmed in warm water prior to administration or by running part of the drip line through a bowl of warm water as the fluids are being administered.

The bladder may also be used to administer fluids – a urinary catheter is placed aseptically into the bladder and boluses of sterile saline no warmer than 38–40°C can then be administered. Optimal effect will be seen if the fluid is left in place for at least 30 minutes, removed and another bolus administered. You can see temperature increases of up to a degree at a time with this method.

In a patient that is in hypovolaemic shock, direct heat is contraindicated, because vasodilation will occur, encouraging blood flow to non-essential parts of the circulatory system such as cutaneous vessels. The body does not consider these to be important in times of circulatory crisis.

Pulse

The pulse rate can be felt at any place where an artery runs close to the surface of the body and is commonly felt at the femoral artery in the dog and cat (Figs 23.1, 23.2). If a critically ill animal is in hypovolaemic shock, the peripheral pulses will be the first to be affected. In these situations, palpating and reading the peripheral pulses can be a good indicator of circulatory state or response to any fluid therapy that may have been initiated.

A slow pulse rate may indicate:

- Hypothermia/low body temperature
- Circulatory failure
- Hyperkalaemia.

A rapid pulse rate may indicate:

- Pain
- Pyrexia
- Sepsis
- Disease process
- Shock
- Ventricular tachycardia.

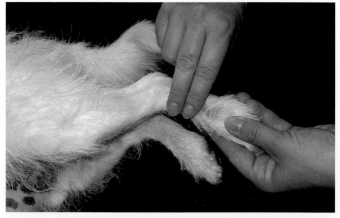

Fig. 23.1 Palpating the dorsal pedal pulse in a dog

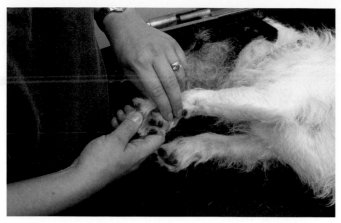

Fig. 23.2 Palpating the digital pulse in a dog

Sinus arrhythmia

This occurs in relation to the respiratory pattern of the animal. During inspiration the pulse rate will increase, and during expiration it will decease. This is a normal sequence of events.

Pulse deficit

This occurs when the pulse rate is slower or absent in relation to the corresponding heart sound. This indicates that, although the heart is pumping the blood through the chambers it is not able to pump it around the rest of the circulatory system. It is a good idea to get into the habit of palpating a pulse at the same time as listening to the heart rate with a stethoscope.

Pulse volume

Pulse volume should be part of the assessment of the pulse and it is essential that you recognize what the normal volume of a pulse should feel like. The pulse wave should be felt over three fingers.

Pulse volume is also called pulse quality:

- An abnormally strong pulse can be described as **hyperkinetic, bounding or a water-hammer pulse** and can sometimes only be felt across one finger width
- An abnormally weak pulse is called a **hypokinetic pulse** and almost flutters across your fingers.

Hyperkinetic pulse/bounding pulse is found in:

- Anaemia
- Fever
- Sepsis
- Cardiac disease
- Hyperthyroidism.

Hypokinetic pulse/weak pulse is found in:

- Hypovolaemic shock
- Dehydration
- Cardiac tamponade
- Left-sided heart failure.

Table 23.1 Classification of respiratory sounds

Respiratory sound	Description
Breath sounds	The normal airway and lung sounds that are audible during normal respiration
Stertor	Noise generated from the nasal passages
Stridor	High-pitched inspiratory sound generated from turbulent airflow in the extrathoracic airways
Rhonchus	Low-pitched, continuous inspiratory or expiratory sound associated with rapid airflow through the larger airways
Wheeze	High-pitched, continuous inspiratory or expiratory sound associated with narrowing of the airways
Crackle (coarse or fine)	High-pitched, discontinuous inspiratory sound associated with reopening of airways that closed during expiration

Respiratory rate

When assessing respiration it is important to count the rate, assess the pattern and depth and note any sounds associated with each breath:

- **Paradoxical respiration** – normally the chest wall expands during inspiration and returns to normal during expiration. Paradoxical respiration is usually seen when there is a flail chest present and happens because of a change in the intrapleural pressure, usually as a result of trauma. We see the fractured segment moving inwards during inspiration and outwards during expiration.
- **Abdominal respiration** – occurs when the animal uses its abdominal muscles to try and improve respiration and is a sign of respiratory distress. (Other signs of respiratory distress are listed below under Oxygen therapy.)
- **Respiratory sounds** – these are made during inspiration or expiration. A normal animal will breathe almost silently, so any sound may be abnormal and should be classified (Table 23.1) and reported to the veterinary surgeon.

Mucous membranes

Whenever basic monitoring is carried out, it is important to also check the mucous membranes. Check the colour, feel or texture of the membranes and the capillary refill time.

Colour

Cyanosis

This is generally recognized as a 'bluish' tone but the colour can range from a deep red-purple colour to a pale or dusky blue and is caused by excessive amounts of desaturated haemoglobin in the capillary blood. In cases where the mucous membranes are pigmented it will be necessary to look at other, non-pigmented, areas, e.g. vagina or prepuce. There may also be a difference in the appearance of the mucous membranes under natural or artificial light, especially under fluorescent lights. If the animal is found with cyanosed mucous membranes, supply with oxygen before calling the veterinary surgeon.

Hyperaemic (injected)

Membranes are a deep brick red and look 'injected'. This change is most commonly seen in hyperthermia, sepsis and polycythemia. In hyperthermia, it occurs because of the massive vasodilation needed for heat loss so there is a huge amount of blood present at places such as the peripheral membranes. In a septic patient, there is pooling of blood due to the loss of vascular tone, giving a dark, brick-coloured appearance.

Icteric (jaundiced)

This occurs when there is a build up of bilirubin in the plasma and tissues (hyperbilirubinaemia) which causes a yellow discoloration of the skin, mucous membranes and also the sclera of the eye.

Pale

Varies from a pale pink to grey/white. It may indicate that the animal has a low packed cell volume (PCV) or that the animal has circulatory shut down.

Texture

When the mucous membranes are touched, they should feel slightly moist. If they are dry or sticky to the touch, this could be an indicator of dehydration – described as 'tacky'.

Capillary refill time

Using a finger, put a little pressure on to the mucous membranes of the gum. This reduces the capillary blood flow and causes blanching of the mucous membranes. Lift up your finger and the capillaries will refill. In a normal animal, capillary refill time (CRT) should be no more than 1–1.5 seconds. If it is slower than this it could be an indicator of heart failure, hypovolaemic shock or severe vasoconstriction. Sometimes, it may appear that no blanching occurs or that the CRT is extremely rapid. This may be due to severe vasoconstriction, e.g. in septic shock or pyrexia. When digital pressure is applied, there is nowhere for the blood to flow to, so no blanching occurs.

Monitoring equipment

Equipment used in the HDU includes direct and indirect arterial blood pressure measurement, electrocardiograms, capnographs for the monitoring of carbon dioxide and oxygen-monitoring equipment such as pulse oximeters (see also Ch. 25). The measurement of central venous pressure can also be invaluable in the HDU.

A multichannel monitor incorporates all the following pieces of equipment in one big bedside monitor, which makes life easier if space is limited (Fig. 23.3).

Central venous pressure

Central venous pressure (CVP) is an essential part of monitoring the effects of fluid therapy in critical patients. It is

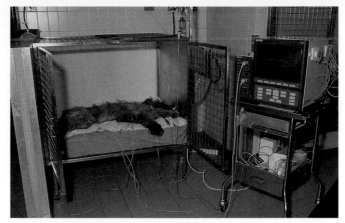

Fig. 23.3 A critically ill dog connected to a bedside monitor

sometimes necessary to challenge animals with fluid boluses and, in patients that may have cardiac disease, it is important to know how the heart responds.

Method

A jugular catheter is placed into the jugular vein. The tip of the catheter should ideally reach the right atrium but often it is positioned at the junction of the right atrium and the cranial vena cava. The measurement that is obtained still reflects change within the right atrium and so it is a reliable estimate:

- The catheter is attached to a three-way tap via some extension tubing
- An intravenous giving set and a bag of fluids are attached to the opposite side of the three-way tap and a water manometer is attached to the upright opening of the tap. The zero of the manometer measure must be level with the sternum (approximate level of right atrium)
- The manometer must be filled with fluid from the bag (always make sure that the whole system is filled with fluids before the tap is turned on to the catheter) and will reach an equal pressure to the right atrium when the tap is turned on to the catheter. If correctly set up, the meniscus in the manometer will rise and fall with each breath that is taken
- When not in use the tap can be turned off to the manometer and on to the fluids
- When a measurement is required, the tap is turned off to the fluids and on between the catheter and the manometer. A measurement can then be read from the manometer measure
- A series of three readings should be taken initially to ensure consistency and accuracy. A reading is taken in centimetres of water (cmH_2O):
  The normal range for CVP is 0–10 cmH_2O but the optimal range is 3–8 cmH_2O:
  - A low CVP is usually the result of hypovolaemia: a series of low readings would indicate that fluid rates could safely be increased
  - A high CVP might indicate a volume overload or right-sided heart failure. If there is no other evidence to support this, the patency of the catheter should be checked. An occluded jugular

catheter will give consistently high CVP readings and so regular flushing of the catheter will be necessary.

Blood pressure monitoring

Blood pressure can be measured directly and indirectly using invasive or non-invasive methods and blood pressure monitoring is regularly used within the HDU for animals that are in shock, have renal or cardiac failure, or may be suffering from diseases such as hyperthyroidism or hyper-adrenocorticism, where blood pressure may deviate from normal levels. Direct measurement is the most accurate way of monitoring blood pressure but special equipment (a transducer and monitor) is required, together with the placement of an arterial catheter, making it costly. (For more detail see Ch. 25.)

Electrocardiography

The electrocardiograph (ECG) records the electrical potential of the heart muscle and is an invaluable piece of equipment to have in the HDU. Its uses range from determining arrest rhythm during cardiopulmonary resuscitation (CPR) to monitoring cardiac arrhythmias caused by toxicity or poisoning. There is usually an audible sound linked to each heartbeat, and this can be very useful if the nurse is looking after several animals at once. A change in tone or speed will automatically alert you to a change in the patient's condition.

Capnography

This is used to record end-tidal carbon dioxide concentration. It is commonly used in the anaesthetized patient but can be used for animals that are being mechanically ventilated within the HDU. A detector is placed between the endotracheal tube and the anaesthetic machine and connected via tubing to the monitor.

Oxygen therapy

Oxygen therapy should be implemented at the very first signs of hypoxia. If an animal in the HDU is showing signs of respiratory distress (Fig. 23.4), oxygen should be given and the veterinary surgeon should be called straight away. Oxygen delivery via a mask, an oxygen cage or 'flow by', i.e. a gas tube that opens close to the patient's nose, would be the preferred methods of delivery in the first instance.

Signs of respiratory distress include:

- Abdominal effort
- Cyanosis
- Open-mouth breathing
- Flared nostrils
- Abducted elbows
- Extended neck
- Anxiety
- Tachypnoea
- Respiratory noise
- Irregular chest wall movement.

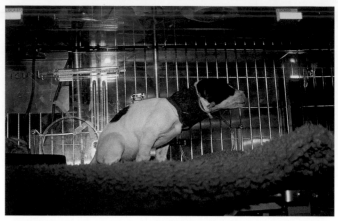

Fig. 23.4 A 4-month-old puppy showing classic signs of respiratory distress. Note the extended neck, abducted elbows and open-mouth breathing

Oxygen is one of the most commonly used drugs in the HDU. Supplementation of oxygen increases the oxygen content of the blood, increases the partial pressure of oxygen in the capillary system and improves tissue perfusion.

When oxygen therapy begins, ensure that as high a fraction of inspired oxygen (FiO_2) as possible is delivered:

- In room air FiO_2 is 21% or 0.21
- In a patient intubated with a cuffed endotracheal tube on 100% oxygen, the FiO_2 would be 100% or 1.

In the methods of oxygen delivery listed in Table 23.2 it is only possible to reach an adequate FiO_2 by using appropriate levels of oxygen.

Oxygen toxicity

Oxygen toxicity arises when too much oxygen is given. This situation can arise if an FiO_2 of 0.6 is sustained for longer than 24 hours, but if a patient already has lung disease it may occur at an earlier stage with a lower FiO_2. Toxicity occurs when the mitochondrial and non-mitochondrial metabolism of oxygen is saturated and clearance is limited. There will then be an accumulation of toxic oxygen intermediates.

During normal metabolism, oxygen radicals are produced at a low level and these are removed by normal defence

Table 23.2 Fraction of inspired oxygen (FiO_2) achieved by the different methods of delivering oxygen

Delivery method	FiO_2	O_2 flow rate (l/min)
Flow-by	0.24–0.45	6–8
Face mask	0.35–0.55	6–10
Nasal catheter	0.30–0.50	1–6
Oxygen cage	0.40–0.50	Variable
Oxygen collar	0.30–0.40	0.2–0.5
Ventilation	0.21–1.00	10–15
Intratracheal catheter	0.40–0.60	50 ml/kg/min

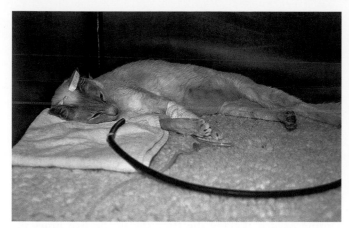

Fig. 23.5 A Siamese cat receiving oxygen therapy using the flow-by method. Note the lack of distress with this method

mechanisms. However, in a state of hyperoxia these defence mechanisms are overwhelmed and toxicity occurs. The lungs are particularly sensitive and signs of pulmonary damage will be the most obvious. This is a rare occurrence in practice but should be noted as a side effect of excess oxygen supplementation.

Oxygen delivery

There are various methods of delivering oxygen to the patient and they all have their advantages and disadvantages. When deciding which method to use the most important factor is patient tolerance, FiO_2 achievement and the equipment available.

1. Flow-by oxygen

This is mainly used in an emergency situation. It causes little interference and stress while enabling the clinician to stabilize the patient. The oxygen line is placed 1–3 cm away from the animal's nose and mouth and oxygen is administered at a rate of 5–8 l/min (Fig. 23.5).

The disadvantages of this method are that it requires an assistant to be present at all times. It also requires a high flow rate of oxygen, which is wasteful, and some patients can be distressed by the sound and the rapid airflow of the oxygen, which may cause them to avoid it.

2. Face mask

This is a quick method of delivering oxygen to a patient in an emergency situation. A mask is placed over the mouth and nose of the cat or dog and oxygen is administered at a rate of 3–10 l/min. A transparent mask seems to cause less distress to animals and makes it possible to observe the colour of the oral mucous membranes without removing the mask. Disadvantages include poor patient tolerance, leakage around the mask if it is poorly fitting and little or no removal of carbon dioxide.

3. Nasal catheter

For long-term use, this method produces good oxygenation with relatively low gas flow. The patient can also be exam-

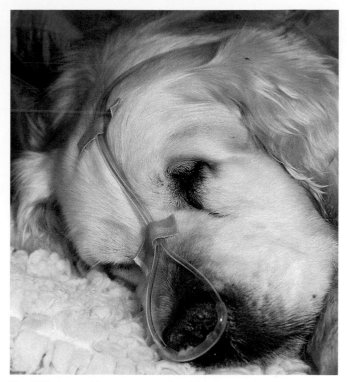

Fig. 23.6 A dog with nasal prongs placed for oxygen therapy

ined without disturbance of the oxygen flow. Measure a 5–10 French gauge catheter (usually a nasal feeding tube) from the nostril to the medial canthus of the eye and mark accordingly. A small amount of local anaesthetic gel/cream can be applied to the end of the catheter and also to the external nares that is to be used. Carefully introduce the catheter in a ventromedial fashion up the nasal chamber until the mark is reached. Fix the catheter on to the skin at the nares using glue, suture or staple. A second attachment can be made on the top of the head. Connect the catheter to a source of humidified oxygen using an adaptor. It may be necessary to fit an Elizabethan collar to prevent patient interference.

As the oxygen is going directly into the nasal passages it must be used with a humidifier. Humidification should be carried out using sterile saline at room temperature, which should be changed daily if long-term use is expected.

If using a unilateral catheter the site should be changed every 48 hours to reduce the risk of damage to the mucosa. It is also possible to buy nasal prongs made of very soft silicone, which originate from human oxygen therapy (Fig. 23.6). The disadvantages of this method include poor patient tolerance, jet damage to the mucosa and increased expense.

4. Oxygen cage

This is a non-invasive method providing a sealed and enclosed environment for emergency or prolonged use. It causes very little stress to the animal and is well tolerated. The newer models enable the control of humidity, temperature and FiO_2 and there is adequate removal of carbon dioxide. The patient can be observed at all times and there are ports for intravenous lines and monitoring leads.

Disadvantages include the fact that the patient is completely isolated from staff, it is expensive and a high flow rate is needed to enrich the cage adequately. There is also a danger of the patient decompensating whenever the cage door is opened and the oxygen-rich environment is lost. It takes a large amount of oxygen to resume adequate oxygen levels, which can be expensive and wasteful. The temperature within the cage must also be closely observed and adjusted accordingly.

5. Oxygen collar

This is very effective way of delivering oxygen in an emergency situation or for temporary use. An Elizabethan collar is placed on the patient and clear cellophane is then used to cover two-thirds of the front and is taped to the sides. The opening acts as a vent for removal of carbon dioxide and any excess oxygen. The size of the opening will determine the oxygen percentage. The temperature of the patient and the temperature and humidity within the collar must be monitored. Oxygen can dry the mucous membranes and it is necessary to lubricate the eyes with an appropriate ointment such as Lacri-Lube (Allergan) or Viscotears (Novartis Ophthalmics). Disadvantages include poor patient tolerance in some instances, hyperthermia, oxygen leakage and high humidity.

6. Intratracheal catheter

This method works by bypassing the anatomical dead space, i.e. the nasal chambers, pharynx, larynx and trachea, and allows continuous oxygen delivery at low flow rates. These catheters are placed between the fourth and fifth cartilaginous rings following full surgical preparation. A hole is made that is slightly larger than the catheter to be used. Select a large-bore, long, soft, preferably silicone catheter – it is preferable to fenestrate the end before application, which reduces the risk of jet damage. Place the needle of the catheter between the two cartilaginous rings in dogs and through the cricothyroid ligament in cats and small dogs. Feed the catheter through to the level of the fifth intercostal space. Withdraw the needle and, if appropriate, cover it with a needle guard and secure it to the animal's neck with a bandage. Connect the end of the catheter to a humidified oxygen source. This is a cheaper method of delivering oxygen as low flow rates are used. It is generally well tolerated by patients and allows easy access by the clinician or nurse.

The disadvantages include a risk of the catheter kinking at the site of insertion, subcutaneous emphysema, jet damage to the airways, tracheitis, bronchospasm, infection at the insertion site and possible airway obstruction.

Some animals may need sedating to carry out this procedure.

Monitoring oxygen therapy

Simple observation of patients may determine how well they are responding to oxygen therapy. Signs of improvement include decrease in respiratory effort and rate, an improved mucous membrane colour and reduced anxiety and stress. Cats will vocalize less. There are also pieces of equipment that indicate whether the oxygen therapy is sufficient.

Blood gas analysis

Blood gas analysis will measure the amount of oxygen (PaO_2) and carbon dioxide ($PaCO_2$) in the arterial blood.

Blood may be collected from the femoral artery or the dorsal metatarsal artery into a heparinized syringe, and it is then analysed by the appropriate machine. The results should be relayed to the veterinary surgeon, who will make an informed decision on the need for further oxygen therapy.

As a general rule:

- $PaO_2 < 70$ mmHg and/or $PaCO_2 > 45$ mmHg = need for supplemental oxygen
- $PaO_2 < 60$ mmHg and/or $PaCO_2 > 50$ mmHg = respiratory failure and need for ventilatory support.

During oxygen therapy the PaO_2 should be five times the FiO_2, e.g. FiO_2 of 40% = PaO_2 of 200 mmHg. If it is less than this, there could be a problem with gas exchange and the veterinary surgeon should be informed at once.

A blood gas analyser is a vital piece of equipment in a busy HDU, but they are expensive and not all critically ill animals will tolerate samples being taken frequently. For this reason it can be preferable to place an arterial catheter.

Pulse oximetry

This is a simple non-invasive method for monitoring oxygen saturation (SaO_2). It works by calculating the saturation of haemoglobin using the principle of spectrophotometry, i.e. an oxygenated haemoglobin molecule (oxyhaemoglobin) and a reduced or deoxygenated haemoglobin molecule (deoxyhaemoglobin) absorb different lights at different rates. The pulse oximeter shines red light and infrared light through an arterial bed and the microprocessor computes the difference (see also Ch. 25). If the SaO_2 falls to 93% or less, it signals the need for oxygen therapy. This is a less expensive piece of equipment than many others and the probes are well tolerated by the patient. However, the accuracy cannot always be relied upon and, as with blood gas analysis, should be noted in relation to the clinical observations.

Humidification

Where oxygen is supplied directly into the animal's airway, it must be humidified because the animal's own methods of warming and moistening the oxygen, i.e. within the nasal chambers, have been bypassed. Commercial bubble humidifiers (Fig. 23.7) are relatively cheap, but it is also possible to make one:

1. Take two lengths of piping
2. Take a plastic bottle, sterilize it and half fill it with sterile saline
3. Attach one length of tubing to the oxygen source. This should be long enough to go through the top of the bottle and into the saline
4. Attach the other tube to the animal – it should be out of the saline at all times.

Intravenous access

Intravenous access is required for fluid therapy, drug administration, blood sampling, monitoring, i.e. central venous pressure, and in some cases nutrition. Equipment, i.e. needles and catheters, must be carefully placed and be maintained and monitored to a high standard to prevent catheter infection and/or thrombophlebitis. There are various types of catheter and familiarity with them will ensure that they are used in the appropriate situation.

Intravenous catheters are usually classified by their method of application (see also Ch. 21). Specialist catheters used particularly in the critical care patient include jugular catheters, double/triple-lumen catheters and intraosseous catheters. The most appropriate sites (see also Ch. 10) are:

- **Cephalic vein** – this is the most common site in the dog and cat, as it is the most accessible. The catheter should be placed as low as possible if you can foresee multiple catheter placements – you can then go further up the foreleg if necessary
- **Lateral saphenous vein** – this site on the lateral hind leg can take an over-the-needle catheter or a longer central catheter in dogs and cats. The central catheter is most commonly placed using the Seldinger or Peel-Away (Cook UK) technique and gives easy access for fluid therapy, drug administration or peripheral parenteral nutrition (PPN) (Fig. 23.8)

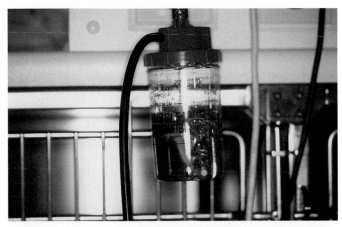

Fig. 23.7 A commercially available bubble humidifier

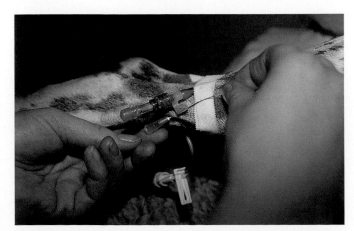

Fig. 23.8 A long catheter has been placed in the saphenous vein of a dog using the Seldinger technique. The catheter has been secured with tape and tissue glue, and sutures are being used to secure it further

- **Medial saphenous vein** – useful in cats and an excellent site to place a longer catheter for larger volumes of fluid and drug administration. It is not the best site for administration of PPN as it is not visible without disturbing the cat and it is more likely to become soiled. It is possible to reach the caudal vena cava via this vein if the catheter is long enough, to facilitate the delivery of hypertonic solutions such as 50% glucose, and for a very rough estimation of central venous pressure
- **Jugular vein** – this is a large vein that can take longer, large-bore catheters. The jugular vein is the only vein where an accurate measurement can be taken of CVP. The catheter must be long enough so that the tip reaches the junction of the cranial vena cava and the right atrium. (The theory behind this is discussed later.) Central lines can also be placed in dogs and cats for frequent blood sampling, e.g. for glucose curves, total parenteral nutrition (TPN), drug administration and fluid therapy
- **Marginal ear vein** – may be used in long-eared breeds such as basset hounds and in rabbits.

Placement of central lines

There are a variety of techniques for introducing central lines including through-the-needle, Peel-Away sheath and the Seldinger technique. Central lines that are placed into the jugular vein must be placed using an aseptic technique and must be checked regularly for signs of infection. If a patient has multiple catheters they should be labelled to avoid any confusion as to the purpose of the line.

Before beginning the task, ensure that all equipment is ready and that you have enough help to perform the procedure. A wide area over the jugular vein should be clipped. The point of insertion will be somewhere between the thoracic inlet and the angle of the jaw, depending on the length of the catheter and the size of the patient.

Central lines may be single-, double-, triple- or quadruple-lumen, which is of great assistance when numerous fluids or drugs are needed. Multilumen catheters have separate entry and exit ports, so there is no need to worry about drug or fluid incompatibility. (Note: when walking these animals around, a lead or harness should be placed around the shoulders rather using than a choke collar around the site of the jugular catheter. This decreases the risk of disturbing the catheter and prevents discomfort around the insertion site.) Complications of this procedure include infection, thromboembolism and haemorrhage.

Equipment required:

- Clippers
- Items for surgical scrub
- Drape
- Surgical gloves
- Blade
- Central line kit containing – hypodermic needle, guide wire, dilator, polyurethane intravenous catheter
- Sterile swabs
- T-connector
- Injection cap/bung
- Antibiotic dressing or ointment – may be needed

- Suture material and tissue/superglue for stabilizing
- Dressings.

Percutaneous vascular catheterization – Seldinger technique (1953)

Local anaesthetic cream can be topically applied before surgical preparation:

1. The clipped area is surgically scrubbed
2. A stab incision is made into the skin over the proposed entry site, using a No. 11 scalpel blade
3. Introduce the percutaneous entry needle into the vessel until blood flows
4. Introduce the guide wire down through the needle and advance it into the vessel, ensuring that the length of wire advanced is longer than the needle
5. Leaving the wire in place, remove the needle. A sterile swab should be placed over the hole with pressure to prevent haematoma formation
6. Pass the dilator over the wire and into the vessel to enlarge the entry hole
7. Withdraw the dilator and advance the catheter over the wire. You will need to use a twisting motion in some cases
8. Remove the guide wire
9. Flush the catheter with sterile heparin saline and cap it with a bung or T-connector
10. Suture the catheter in place in such a way that it cannot kink. Superglue or tissue glue can be used for extra security
11. Some people place triple antibiotic cream at the site of insertion. Another option is to cover the site with sterile transparent dressing for easy observation with minimal disturbance
12. Dress the neck in an appropriate fashion.

It is advisable to have a T-connector attached to the end of the catheter, which ensures that there is minimal contact with the actual catheter and that dressings can remain in place while drugs are introduced.

Sheathed needle technique

This technique involves the use of a Peel-Away sheathed needle system. The list of equipment is similar to that for the Seldinger technique with the addition of a Peel-Away catheter kit (Cook UK).

1. The insertion site is surgically scrubbed
2. A stab incision is made into the skin using a No.11 blade
3. Place the sheathed needle distally into the vessel and advance slightly
4. Remove the needle from the sheath and discard. A finger should be placed over the end of the sheath to minimize the risk of air embolization
5. Introduce the catheter through the sheath and into the vessel. The catheter should then be advanced further into the vein
6. Remove the sheath by pulling outwards and upwards on the two small knobs at either side of the sheath

7. Flush the catheter with heparinized saline, then cap it and secure to the neck of the animal with sutures or superglue/tissue glue
8. Dress the area as in the Seldinger technique.

Through-the-needle technique

This technique uses equipment that leaves the needle (in a protective case) attached to the animal.

1. The area of insertion is clipped and aseptically prepared
2. Introduce the needle in a distal direction into the vein and, once blood is seen at the hub of the needle, advance it further to ensure adequate placement
3. Advance the catheter through the needle into the vein until the hub of the catheter reaches the hub of the needle
4. The needle can now be withdrawn from the vein and clipped into the protective case
5. Flush the catheter with heparinized saline and attach a bung or T-connector
6. Cover the site of insertion with a clear, sterile dressing and dress the neck appropriately.

Arterial catheterization

In some critical cases, it may be necessary to place an arterial catheter, e.g. for blood pressure monitoring or for frequent blood gas analysis. Complications include infection, thrombosis and haemorrhage.

Sites include:

- **Dorsal metatarsal artery** – the most common site in the dog and cat. It runs along the mediodorsal aspect of the hind foot. Strict asepsis must be maintained while introducing the catheter
- **Femoral artery** – this is far more mobile and the veterinary surgeon may need to use a hand to steady the artery before attempting catheterization of the vessel. This artery should be avoided in animals with a coagulopathy because significant haemorrhage can occur if the catheter becomes dislodged.

Equipment required:

- Clippers
- Surgical scrub and spirit
- Surgical gloves
- Suitable catheter (arterial catheter or a 20–22-g 3-cm long over-the-needle catheter)
- T-connector and bung
- Sterile heparin saline
- No.11 blade or 21-g needle
- Tape
- Dressing material.

Local anaesthetic cream or gel may applied to the site of the artery before you start to place the catheter, to minimize arterial spasm during catheterization:

1. The site of insertion should be clipped and surgically scrubbed
2. If necessary, make a small nick in the skin with a needle or a blade

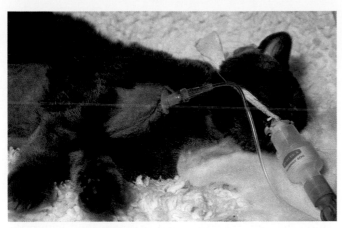

Fig. 23.9 A 6-month-old kitten with an intraosseous needle in position

3. Gently palpate the pulse in the artery and feel the course of the artery
4. Introduce the needle in a firm, stabbing manner and advance it until blood appears in the hub
5. Advance the catheter off the needle and into the lumen of the artery
6. Secure the catheter using tape
7. Remove the needle and attach the catheter to a bung or T-connector
8. Flush the catheter using heparinized saline.

The catheter site must be bandaged securely to avoid knocks or self-trauma. If a patient with an arterial catheter manages to bite through the connections it could suffer severe blood loss, so close observation must be undertaken at all times.

If the catheter is to be left in for regular monitoring, it should be flushed with sterile heparinized saline every 30–60 minutes.When removing the catheter from the artery, place pressure over the site for at least 5 minutes to minimize the risk of a haematoma formation.

Intraosseous catheterization

In some critical care patients it may not be possible to place an intravenous catheter, so an alternative is to administer fluids or drugs via an intraosseous catheter into the cavity of a bone. Commercial intraosseous needles are available but it is possible to use a spinal or hypodermic needle in an emergency situation. An over-the-needle intravenous catheter can be used in young animals because of the relative softness of their bones (Fig. 23.9).

Sites for placement include:

- The cranial aspect of the diaphysis of the ulna
- The cranial aspect of the greater tubercle of the humerus
- The trochanteric fossa of the proximal femur
- The flat medial aspect of the proximal tibia (at a site that is distal to the tibial tuberosity and the proximal tibial growth plate).

The last two sites are the most common in dogs and cats. (For sites in exotic species see Ch. 12.)

1. Clip and aseptically scrub the area of insertion
2. Inject a small amount of local anaesthetic agent into the skin and periosteum

3. While an assistant stabilizes the limb, make a small stab incision
4. Insert the needle in a distal direction. Use a firm and rotating action until the needle enters the cortex. If it is fully engaged in the cortex, the whole leg will move with the needle when it is rocked from side to side
5. Remove the stylet and flush the needle with sterile heparinized saline
6. Attach a T-connector or a fluid infusion set and secure the needle hub.

Commercially available needles have a 'butterfly' on the top for suturing to the skin. A bandage can be applied for extra stability and security. Aspiration of bone marrow will confirm correct positioning, as will the use of radiography. The needle should be flushed every 4–6 hours when not in use and should be removed 72 hours after placement. The same bone can be used again at a different site but you must wait at least 36 hours before introducing another needle.

The absorption of drugs through an intraosseous needle is similar to the absorption if placed centrally. Fluid rates should not exceed 11 ml/min infusing manually and 24 ml/min if using a pressurized infusion pump. Complications include infection, growth plate damage, fat embolism and leakage of fluid into the tissues if placement is incorrect.

Maintenance of catheters

All catheters should be introduced in an aseptic manner, but particularly in an HDU patient. Sterile gloves should be worn when introducing catheters into a vein, and gloves should be worn when checking catheters or when attending to connections with drug administration or blood sampling.

Peripheral and central lines should be checked thoroughly every 4 hours and glanced at whenever you are passing:

- The dressing should be checked for cleanliness and dryness. You should check that the bandage has not become too tight (especially around the neck) and that there are no signs of self-trauma. Any wet dressings should be removed and a new one applied as soon as the catheter site has been checked
- The catheter site should be checked without touching the actual point of insertion. You are looking for movement of the catheter, discharge or pus, leakage of fluid around the site and any signs of inflammation
- You should look above the catheter site to check for signs of extravascular leakage and phlebitis. Phlebitis is the inflammation of a vessel caused by infection and will manifest itself with redness and swelling. If the skin is palpated around and above the site of insertion it will feel hot. The vein itself, when palpated under the skin, will feel very hard and the patient may show signs of distress and pain
- The catheter should be flushed every 4 hours with heparinized saline (1 unit heparin/ml 0.9% saline) to check the patency of the catheter. This may not be necessary if there is a continuous intravenous drip running
- Drip rates should be checked more often than every 4 hours but, while checking the catheter, it is a good

idea to also check the rate of fluid infusion on the pump or in the drip chamber

- Check all connections. If there is an extension set or a T-connector attached, you need to make sure that the patient has not managed to chew through or ingest any of the catches.

During your other regular checks you must monitor the temperature and general demeanour of the patient. If there is unexplained pyrexia, catheter sites should be checked and if there is any doubt the catheter should be removed. If the catheter is removed aseptically, it can be sent away for culture and sensitivity.

It has been suggested that catheters should be removed and replaced every 72 hours; however, studies have shown that, unless the catheter is showing clinical signs of causing thrombophlebitis, it is not necessary to remove it. It is far better to place it properly and maintain it for the longest possible time, particularly in HDU patients, when veins may be at a premium.

Arterial catheters need similar checks but should not be used for drug or fluid administration, which minimizes the risk of infection. These catheters are used for monitoring purposes only so usually stay in for hours rather than days. They will need flushing every 30–60 minutes and the patient must be kept under close observation to avoid the risk of exsanguination during catheter dislodgement.

Fluid therapy in the high-dependency unit patient

There are several types of fluid that are essential to have on the shelf if you are dealing with critical patients – crystalloids, colloids and oxygen-carrying fluids (see also Ch. 21).

Crystalloids

Crystalloids can be hypertonic, isotonic or hypotonic. The most frequently used fluid is isotonic but, in an HDU, some clinicians may choose to use a hypertonic solution to resuscitate a shocked animal.

Hypertonic saline

This causes a rapid expansion of plasma volume, by an immediate shift of water into plasma from the interstitium by osmosis. The effect is transient because sodium and chloride ions will rapidly redistribute, like any other crystalloid, and isotonic fluids may need to be administered later. Indications for hypertonic crystalloids include haemorrhagic shock, traumatic shock, septic shock, gastric dilation and volvulus and severe burns.

Some clinicians consider that hypertonic saline may be particularly useful in patients that have suffered brain or lung trauma. Hypertonic saline may limit oedema in these organs, compared to an isotonic solution, but there is limited evidence to support this (DiBartola 1992).

Any saline solution that is more than 0.9% NaCl is hypertonic; the most usual formulation used is 7.2%.

It is extremely important that it is administered very slowly, at a rate not exceeding 1 ml/kg/min, to avoid bradycardia.

Usual doses are 2–8 ml/kg in total. Rapid administration of hypertonic fluid is contraindicated in dehydrated and cardiac patients. This fluid must only be given intravenously and never subcutaneously.

A total dose of 4–7 ml/kg (dogs) and 2–4 ml/kg (cats) can be given over 2–5 minutes and will have a similar effect to giving a dog or cat 60–90 ml/kg of isotonic fluid.

Artificial colloids

Within the vascular system of a healthy, normovolaemic animal there are naturally occurring colloids in the form of plasma proteins such as albumin. They are responsible for maintaining vascular volume because of their ability to stay within the capillary system and maintain fluid within the circulation by osmosis. During times of fluid disturbance and/or disease, these proteins may be depleted in numbers and so colloid osmotic pressure (COP) must be maintained artificially. A loss of COP will result in tissue oedema and low circulating volume because it is no longer possible for fluid to be kept within the vascular system.

The three most commonly used artificial colloids in veterinary medicine are gelatines, hydroxyethyl starches and dextrans. The basis of their use over crystalloids is their ability to stay in the intravascular space for longer and so help to maintain intravascular volume.

Gelatines

These are produced from cattle-bone gelatin. Solutions used in the UK are Haemaccel and Gelofusine. The average molecular weight is 30 000 and the half-life is 2.5 hours.

Indications: rapid intravascular volume replacement; hypotensive resuscitation; ongoing haemorrhage.

Hydroxyethyl starches

These are made from a waxy species of maize or sorghum. The most commonly used starches are pentastarch (average molecular weight 264 000) and hetastarch (average molecular weight 450 000). The half-life is about 2.5 hours for pentastarch and 25 hours for hetastarch.

Indications for hetastarch: rapid intravascular volume replacement; hypotensive resuscitation; ongoing haemorrhage; small volume resuscitation; systemic inflammatory response syndrome (SIRS); hypoproteinaemia.

Dextrans

Dextrans are produced by the enzyme dextran sucrase during the growth of various strains of bacteria of the genus *Leuconostoc* in media containing sucrose. There are two types of dextran – 40 and 70. The average molecular weight of dextran 40 is 40 000 and of dextran 70 is 70 000. The half-life of dextran 40 is 2.5 hours, and of dextran 70 is 25 hours.

Indications for dextran 70: rapid intravascular volume replacement; hypotensive resuscitation; ongoing haemorrhage.

Monitoring colloid administration

Artificial or synthetic colloids are the most efficient fluids for expanding intravascular volume but, because they are able to stay in the intravascular space for long periods of time, it

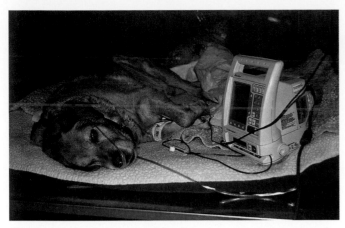

Fig. 23.10 A dog receiving Oxyglobin. Note the extremely dark colour of the fluid

Table 23.3 Suggested rates of administration for Oxyglobin

	Euvolaemic (ml/kg/h)	Hypovolaemic (ml/kg/h)
Dogs	3	3–10
Cats (not licensed)	0.5	1–2

is essential that patients are closely observed and monitored for volume overload.

Dose rates of colloids

A general dose for the administration of colloids is 20 ml/kg/24 hours. This rate will differ dramatically depending on the clinician, the breed of animal and the reason for administration.

Oxygen-carrying fluids

Oxyglobin

Oxyglobin (haemoglobin glutamer-200 (bovine)) is polymerized purified haemoglobin in a modified lactated Ringer's solution and is the most frequently used oxygen-carrying fluid. It is licensed for single use in dogs but has not been licensed for use in cats. It is used as an alternative to blood transfusion for a variety of conditions, including haemolytic anaemia, traumatic blood loss, hypovolaemia and other conditions that result in poor tissue perfusion.

An oxyglobin molecule is 1/1000th the size of a red blood corpuscle and is able to circulate freely in the plasma, enabling it to perfuse tissue that may not be reached by red blood cells.

Patients should be observed closely when receiving Oxyglobin as volume overload and pulmonary oedema can develop if the rate or dose is excessive. Mucous membranes may appear jaundiced in colour during administration because of the colour of Oxyglobin, but this is a relatively common finding and is not a cause for alarm (Fig. 23.10).

Oxyglobin must be used within 24 hour of the outer wrapper being opened and should be kept at room temperature or in the refrigerator. It must never be frozen and should be warmed gently if removed from a refrigerator. It can be administered via a normal giving set.

Dose rates

Table 23.3 shows suggested rates of administration but they should only be used as a guideline. Total doses should not exceed 30 ml/kg/24 hour (dogs), although enough should be given to maintain haemoglobin levels of at least 6 g/dl.

Blood

A large proportion of patients who pass through the HDU will eventually receive whole blood or a blood component as a transfusion. In the UK there are restrictions regarding the use and storage of whole animal blood and blood components. Table 23.4 summarizes the uses of blood components.

Blood types

- Feline – A, B, AB
- Canine – DEA 1.1, 1.2, 3, 4, 5, 6, 7, 8.

Blood type cards for use in practice use are available for A, B and AB feline types, but are only available for identifying DEA 1.1-positive dogs.

Whole blood

This is known as fresh whole blood (FWB) for up to 8 hours following collection from the donor. It contains red blood cells, white blood cells, platelets, plasma proteins and coagulation factors. Once the whole blood has been taken it should be given to a patient, separated into components or stored in a refrigerator at 1–6°C within 6 hours. After 24 hours of storage at this temperature, platelet function is lost and the concentration of coagulation factors decreases.

Whole blood becomes stored whole blood (SWB) after 8 hours and can be kept in the refrigerator for 4 weeks if a suitable anticoagulant such as acid citrate dextrose (ACD) or citrate phosphate dextrose adenine (CPD) has been used.

When administering blood to a patient it should be warmed gently in a warm water bath to a temperature of no more than 37°C. Never use a microwave, as this will 'cook' the cells and cause haemolysis and bacterial proliferation.

Packed red cells

Whole blood can be centrifuged and the plasma removed, leaving the red blood cells. Because the haematocrit will be around 70–80%, it is necessary to add sterile saline in order to decrease the viscosity. Packed red cells (PRCs) will have the same oxygen-carrying capacity as whole blood but with less volume.

Fresh frozen plasma and stored frozen plasma

Fresh frozen plasma (FFP) contains plasma, albumin and all coagulation factors. If taken and frozen within 8 hours

Table 23.4 Indications for the use of different blood components

Blood component	Indications	Shelf life
Fresh whole blood (FWB)	Acute massive blood loss	<8 h after collection
	Coagulopathy with blood loss	
	Thrombocytopenia with blood loss	
	Majority of disseminated intravascular coagulation cases	
	Hypovolaemic shock	
Stored whole blood (SWB)	Anaemias	Up to 35 days when ACD or CPD used
	Hypovolaemic shock	Refrigerate at 1–6°C
Packed red cells (PRCs)	Normovolaemic anaemia	Up to 35 days Refrigerate at 1–6°C
Fresh frozen plasma (FFP)	Coagulation disorders	12 months at −18°C or below
	Hypoalbuminaemia	
	Anticoagulant rodenticide toxicity	
Stored frozen plasma (SFP)	Coagulation disorders	5 years at −20°C or below
	Hypoalbuminaemia	
Platelet concentrate	Thrombocytopenia	5 days at 22°C
	Thrombocytopathy	
Cryoprecipitate (Cryo)	Haemophilia	12 months at −18°C or below
	Von Willebrand's disease	
	Hypofibrinogenaemia	

ACD, acid citrate dextrose; CPD, citrate phosphate dextrose adenine.

of collection it is stable for 12 months at a temperature of −18°C. After 12 months, it should be relabelled stored frozen plasma (SFP) and can then be kept for 4 years. These two products are virtually identical in their function but in SFP some of the coagulation factors will not be stable. Platelets are not functional in either product.

Platelet concentrate

Platelets can be separated from whole blood within 8 hours of donation. The whole blood must not be cooled below the temperature of 20°C and once harvested, the platelet concentrate must not be frozen or refrigerated. Platelets do not retain function or viability if kept below room temperature, and can be kept for 5 days with frequent agitation of the concentrate.

Cryoprecipitate

This is the cold, insoluble part of plasma that is left when FFP has been thawed slowly at 1–6°C. Once it has been collected from the plasma, cryoprecipitate (Cryo) can be frozen at −18°C or colder and stored for 12 months from the original blood donation date. It contains fibrinogen, fibronectin, factor VIII:C and a concentrated amount of von Willebrand factor.

Blood transfusions

Transfusion reactions are rare but any patient receiving whole blood or blood components must be carefully mon-

itored throughout the transfusion process. It is advisable to take the animal out to urinate and defecate and for TPR to be taken as a baseline before the transfusion commences. TPR should be taken every 10–15 minutes to begin with and continued throughout the transfusion. If there is no evidence of a reaction, TPR can be decreased to once an hour and then further reduced if the animal is still showing no signs of distress. Clinical signs of a transfusion reaction include:

- Vomiting
- Muscle tremors and weakness
- Tachycardia
- Tachypnoea
- Pyrexia
- Vocalization
- Urticaria.

All of these could indicate that the patient is suffering from:

- Haemolysis
- Bacterial contamination
- Anaphylaxis
- Circulatory overload
- Too rapid administration
- Hypercalcaemia due to anticoagulant overdose.

If any of the clinical signs develop, the transfusion should be stopped and the veterinary surgeon should be informed.

Blood products should be given through a filtered giving set that is specifically designed for the delivery of blood (see

Ch. 21). The filter reduces the risk of microagglutinates travelling into the circulation, especially if the blood has been stored. It is possible for the animal to have a delayed transfusion reaction (in days rather than hours) and this is usually caused by an immune response to an antigen of a different blood group to which the animal was previously sensitized.

Dose rates

- The dose rate depends on the animal's condition but a rate of 5–10 ml/kg/hour is most commonly used
- A rate of 20 ml/kg/hour can be used in animals with acute blood loss or hypovolaemia
- It is often a good idea to start at a rate of 2 ml/kg/hour for the first 15–30 minutes so that any reactions are identified early on. Some veterinary surgeons may choose to administer antihistamines before starting the transfusion, but this could mask early signs of reaction.

Analgesia

(See also Chapters 17 and 25.)

The usual signs of pain include vocalization, increased heart and respiratory rate, abnormal posture, inappetence, aggression, depression, restlessness, trembling, facial expressions, anxiety, insomnia and temperament change. However, in an already debilitated or recumbent animal the signs may not be as obvious.

If the following signs are observed with no other apparent reason, pain should be assumed and the appropriate analgesic agent should be given:

- Increase in heart or respiratory rate
- Increase in blood pressure
- Increase in temperature
- Inability to rest or sleep
- Trembling
- Inappetence.

In general, if the condition or procedure is known or assumed to cause pain, then appropriate analgesia should be prescribed.

Before analgesics are administered every effort should be made to ensure that the patient's other needs are being tended to. Some apparent signs of pain can also indicate the need for urination, defecation or comfort. The animal may be thirsty, stressed or anxious and these needs must be met before pharmacological comforts are given.

Drugs used in the HDU are similar to the analgesics described in Chapter 25, and the opioids are probably the most commonly used group. Techniques used within the HDU include continuous rate infusion and analgesia via an epidural catheter.

Epidural catheterization

Epidural analgesia usually uses single doses of opioids or local anaesthesia or a combination of both. The most commonly used drugs are morphine and bupivacaine; these can be administered as single doses or as a continuous rate infusion through a specialist epidural catheter.

Contraindications and complications

There are numerous contraindications; these include coagulopathies, bacteraemia, severe systemic infection, thoracolumbar neurological deficits, lumbosacral fractures or dislocations and an inexperienced operator. Complications can arise, such as infection, spinal damage and site haemorrhage.

Indications for use include peritonitis, severe pancreatitis, trauma (caudal) and animals undergoing caudal surgery. An epidural catheter should not be placed unless sterility and appropriate maintenance of the catheter can be ensured. Maintenance of the catheter includes regular checks for possible migration, patient interference and cleanliness.

Nutritional support

When simple starvation occurs in healthy animals, metabolic adaptations ensure that energy expenditure is decreased. Proteins are conserved and fat usage is increased, which will ultimately prolong survival. However, during stress starvation, these mechanisms are not triggered and the animal undergoes a state of hypermetabolism. If animals cannot or will not eat, they rapidly deteriorate into a state of malnutrition.

Providing the correct nutritional support to the critical patient will improve immune function, wound repair and response to medical therapy. It will shorten recovery time and prolong survival.

Enteral feeding

Whenever possible, it is preferable to use a method that makes use of the gastrointestinal tract, i.e. using the enteral route. It is very important to maintain the health of the intestinal mucosa and the function of peristalsis within the gastrointestinal tract to prevent destruction of the lining and malabsorption of food.

There are several different types of feeding tube available that deliver food to the gastrointestinal tract when the patient is unable to ingest food normally (Table 23.5). The choice of tube will depend on the disease process or injury, the expected duration of assisted feeding, the food type to be used, and sometimes cost.

Other methods include force-feeding and drug-induced stimulation such as diazepam (Valium)and cyproheptadine hydrochloride (Periactin); however, in patients that may already be depressed and stressed, force-feeding may prove detrimental and drug intervention rarely encourages the animal to ingest enough to reach its basal energy requirement (see Chs 7 and 8).

Parenteral feeding

This method is used when the gastrointestinal tract cannot be used or it is better that it is rested (see Ch. 15). Parenteral nutrition can be administered in two ways:

- Total parenteral nutrition (TPN) – nutrition given via a central vein, e.g. the jugular
- Peripheral parenteral nutrition (PPN) – nutrition given via a peripheral vein, e.g. the saphenous.

Table 23.5 Types of tube used for enteral feeding

Tube type and use	Location	Duration of placement	Comments	Contraindications
Naso-oesophageal Short-term nutrition where upper gastrointestinal tract is functioning normally	Distal oesophagus via the nose	Short term, <7 days	Simple and non-invasive to place Reasonably well tolerated Inexpensive Can be maintained at home	Long-term nutritional support Trauma or disease to head, neck, nasal cavity, oesophagus Comatose and recumbent patients Abnormal gag reflex Vomiting; functional or mechanical gastrointestinal obstruction
Oesophagostomy Facial trauma, injury or disease involving the mouth and pharynx	Distal oesophagus via surgical placement into the cranial oesophagus through the skin	Short and long term (months)	Well tolerated Wide bore, so more selection of diets Can be maintained at home	Oesophageal disorder Vomiting Comatose or recumbent patients Following oesophageal surgery
Gastrostomy/PEG tube Injuries or surgery to oral cavity, larynx, pharynx or oesophagus	The stomach via surgical laparotomy or endoscopically through the ventrolateral abdominal wall (left side)	Mid to long term (months to years)	Well tolerated More invasive procedure to place Can be maintained at home Wide bore, so more selection of diets	Primary gastric disease (ulceration or neoplasia) Intractable vomiting Peritonitis
Enterostomy (duodenostomy or jejunostomy) When stomach or duodenum must be bypassed Pancreatic disease or surgery Biliary system disease	The small intestine via surgical laparotomy through the abdominal wall or endoscopically via gastric tube and through the pylorus	Long term (weeks to months) but term limited because of need for hospitalization	Well tolerated Invasive procedure Not possible to maintain at home Very narrow bore	Patients must be stable enough for anaesthesia and surgery Dysfunction of the small intestine

PEG, percutaneous endoscopically placed gastrostomy.

Indications include complete mechanical intestinal obstruction, ileus or hypomobility, intractable vomiting or diarrhoea, patients that are unconscious or have severe neurological deficits, which increase the risk of aspiration, and those with acute pancreatitis or hepatitis. Patients that have had massive small bowel resection and those that are severely malnourished with a non-functional gastrointestinal tract also benefit from TPN. It is beyond the scope of this section to fully discuss parenteral nutrition and so the following is a brief overview.

Venous access

Parenteral nutrition can be administered centrally (TPN) or peripherally (PPN; Fig. 23.11). The catheter must be placed in strict aseptic conditions and must be dedicated to the purpose, because the nutrient-rich solution is an excellent bacterial medium. Once the catheter has been placed and the line has been connected, there should be minimal disconnection of lines.

The final osmolarity of the solution dictates whether to use a central or peripheral vein:

- A solution that is hyperosmolar will increase the risk of thrombophlebitis, so if the osmolarity of the solution is in excess of 800–900 mosmol/l, the cranial vena cava must be used. The cranial vena cava has a high flow rate and can therefore tolerate such solutions.

- If it is contraindicated or not possible to place a jugular line, a peripheral vein (usually the saphenous) can be used; however, the solution must be more dilute, i.e. <800 mosmol/l, so fewer calories and proteins are provided per unit volume. The patient must also be observed for volume overload if fluids are being administered at the same time.

Solutions used for parenteral nutrition

The three basic components to any parenteral nutrition solution are amino acids, lipids and dextrose:

- **Amino acid solutions** contain all the essential amino acids for dogs and cats (with the exception of taurine). They help to maintain nitrogen balance and can replenish lean tissue in cachectic animals. Solutions are available in concentrations of 3–15%
- **Lipid emulsions** provide a source of fatty acids and fat calories and are available in 10% and 20% emulsions
- **Dextrose** provides carbohydrates and is available in concentrations of 5–70%.

Vitamin B complex solutions and potassium phosphate must also be added. Calcium and magnesium sulphate can also be included.

The various products should be added in a particular order to prevent precipitation occurring and this order can be remembered by working alphabetically – amino acids, dex-

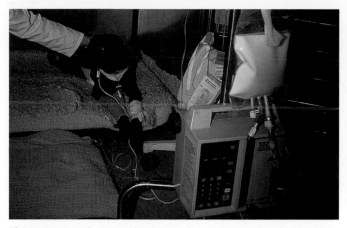

Fig. 23.11 A total parenteral nutrition solution connected to the dog and being infused via an infusion pump

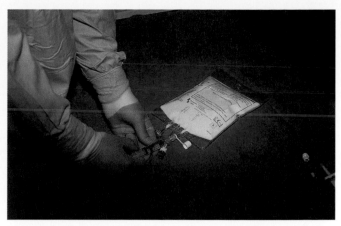

Fig. 23.12 Total parenteral nutrition solution being made up for the next 24-hour period. Note the aseptic conditions under which this is done

trose and lipid solution. The solution must be made up under aseptic conditions. Special compounding bags and equipment can be bought or evacuated glass bottles can be used (Fig. 23.12). The solution must be changed every 24 hours, although enough solution for 2–4 days can be made up and stored in the refrigerator.

Monitoring the patient on total parenteral nutrition

The patient on TPN must be kept under close 24-hour observation. This is not only to ensure line patency but also to ensure that any complications are noted at an early stage. A complete haematological and biochemical blood analysis should be carried out before TPN commences and at weekly intervals. Further assessments should include daily checks of plasma proteins, blood and urine glucose concentrations, and regular TPR. Some clinicians also include daily checks on electrolytes, blood urea nitrogen, creatinine and calcium. Hydration status, body weight, attitude/demeanour and respiratory rate should be noted frequently.

Complications of the procedure include sepsis, thrombophlebitis, electrolyte disturbances, hyperlipidaemia, hyperglycaemia and azotaemia. The most common complication is thrombophlebitis and the most severe is sepsis. The risk of both of these complications can be decreased by correct placement of the catheter and strict maintenance and observation in the following days. Frequent assessment of blood will also ensure that metabolic disturbances are noted at an early stage and corrected accordingly.

Bibliography

Battaglia, A.M., 2001. Pain assessment and treatment. In: Battaglia, A.M. (Ed.), Small Animal Emergency and Critical Care: a Manual for the Veterinary Technician. W B Saunders, Philadelphia, PA, pp. 108–123.

DiBartola, S.D., 1992. Introduction to fluid therapy. In: DiBartola, S.D. (Ed.), Fluid Therapy in Small Animal Practice. W B Saunders, Philadelphia, PA, pp. 321–340.

Hansenn, B., 2000. Epidural analgesia. In: Bonagura, J.D. (Ed.), Kirk's Current Veterinary Therapy XIII: Small Animal Practice. W B Saunders, Philadelphia, PA, pp. 126–131.

Harrel, K.A., Kristensen, A.T., 1995. Canine transfusion reactions and their management. Vet. Clin. North Am. Small Anim. Pract. 25, 1333–1361.

Harty, W.B., 2003. Providing nutritional support to critical care patients. Vet. Tech. June, 376–387.

Hohenhaus, A.E., 2000. Blood banking and transfusion medicine. In: Ettinger, S.J., Feldman, C.E. (Eds.), Textbook of Veterinary Internal Medicine. fifth ed. W B Saunders, Philadelphia, PA, pp. 348–356.

Kirby, R., Rudloff, E., 2000. Fluid therapy, electrolytes, and acid-base control. In: Ettinger, S.J., Feldman, C.E. (Eds.), Textbook of Veterinary Internal Medicine.

fifth ed. W B Saunders, Philadelphia, PA, pp. 325–347.

Kirk, C.A., 1992. Nutritional management of metabolic stress. In: Kirk, C.A. (Ed.), Enteral Nutrition: Its Importance in Recovery. Harmon Smith, Kansas City, KA, pp. 7–14.

Matthews, K.A., Brooks, M.J., Vallient, A.E., 1996. A prospective study of intravenous catheter contamination. J. Vet. Emerg. Crit. Care 6, 33–43.

Rudloff, E., Kirby, R., 2000. Colloids: current recommendations. In: Bonagura, J.D. (Ed.), Kirk's Current Veterinary Therapy XIII: Small Animal Practice. W B Saunders, Philadelphia, PA, pp. 131–135.

Recommended reading

Kirby, R., Rudloff, E., 2000. Fluid and electrolyte therapy. In: Ettinger, S.J., Feldman, C.E. (Eds.), Textbook of Veterinary Internal Medicine. fifth ed. W B Saunders, Philadelphia, PA, pp. 338–339.

Excellent coverage of blood transfusion medicine and fluid therapy. Also provides a comprehensive table on colloid administration.

CHAPTER 24

Dentistry

Cecilia Gorrel

Key Points

- The veterinary nurse is an essential part of the primary dental care team and must be prepared to be both dental nurse and hygienist.
- Primary care dentistry requires the use of a range of specialized instruments, which should be clean and preferably sterilized for each patient.
- Oral examination and all dental procedures require general anaesthesia and close attention must be given to preventing debris from entering the larynx and trachea and to monitoring the patient during the procedure and during recovery.
- All oral examinations and treatments should be recorded and the use of specific dental charts is recommended.
- Professional periodontal therapy performed by the veterinary nurse includes supragingival and closed subgingival scaling and root planing.
- Home care carried out by the owner and based on regular tooth brushing is the most effective way to maintain oral hygiene. The veterinary nurse can play a major part in educating and training the owner in these techniques.

Introduction

In human dentistry the team that supplies primary oral care consists of the dentist, the dental nurse, the dental hygienist and the dental technician. Each of these individuals has a clearly defined role: i.e. the dentist is responsible for oral diagnosis and treatment; the dental nurse assists the dentist in these duties; the dental hygienist performs dental hygiene instruction and treatment as requested by the dentist; and the dental technician manufactures appliances as requested by the dentist. In addition to this primary care team, there are specialists in the various dental disciplines (periodontics, orthodontics, endodontics, oral surgery, prosthodontics, etc.). The specialists provide treatment that is outside the scope of the general dental practitioner.

The veterinary primary oral care team is not as easy to define. Despite the fact that oral conditions are common in our domestic pets, education in veterinary dentistry and oral surgery is not a big part of the undergraduate veterinary curriculum. Consequently, many veterinary surgeons are not comfortable with diagnosing oral conditions or with performing dental and oral surgery procedures. Moreover, dentistry is often not considered 'important' and is often delegated to nurses, who have even less knowledge of the discipline. In fact, oral health and disease is often not covered at all in the nursing training programmes. This is an unfortunate situation and does not benefit the oral health and general welfare of our domestic pets. There is today an urgent need to provide education in dentistry and oral surgery for veterinary surgeons as well as for nurses. Moreover, the legal role of the veterinary nurse in the dental care team needs to be clearly defined. In the UK, veterinary nurses may do the things specified in paragraphs 6 (applies to listed veterinary nurses) and 7 (applies to student veterinary nurses) of Schedule 3 to the Veterinary Surgeons Act 1966, as amended by the Veterinary Surgeons Act 1966 (Schedule 3 Amendment) Order 2002, SI 2002/1479, with effect from 10 June 2002.

Veterinary oral care should be structured similarly to human oral care – i.e. the veterinary surgeon is responsible for diagnosis and treatment; the veterinary nurse assists the veterinary surgeon in these duties, and also performs dental hygiene instruction and treatment as requested by the veterinary surgeon. In other words, the veterinary nurse takes on the duties of both 'dental nurse' and 'dental hygienist'.

The nurse can only perform these duties if specifically requested to do so by the veterinary surgeon and then only under their direct supervision. Moreover, the veterinary surgeon is accountable for the adequacy of any procedures performed by the veterinary nurse. In other words, the veterinary surgeon is ultimately responsible.

In addition to the veterinary surgeon in general practice, there are now veterinary surgeons who are specialists in dentistry. They provide treatment that is outside the scope of the general dental practitioner, e.g. complicated extractions and other surgical procedures, endodontics, prosthodontics, etc.

The veterinary nurse is an essential member of an effective oral care team. The trained veterinary nurse should be able to carry out the following procedures:

- Care for and maintain instrumentation and equipment

- Perform an oral examination
- Record findings on a dental chart
- Take dental radiographs
- Perform routine professional periodontal therapy
- Perform oral/dental hygiene instruction.

Instrumentation and equipment for primary care dentistry

Primary care dentistry includes, but is not limited to:

- Oral examination and recording of findings
- Periodontal therapy
- Extraction
- Minor oral surgery.

Clean and preferably sterilized instruments should be available for each patient. Ideally, several pre-packed kits containing the required instruments for the different procedures, e.g. examination, periodontal therapy and extraction, should be available.

Power equipment requires regular maintenance (daily and weekly) in the practice and regular servicing by the supplier. Checklists should be drawn up for these chores. Maintenance and servicing requirements need to be decided with the supplier.

Instrumentation for oral examination

The details of how to perform an oral examination are covered later in this chapter.

The instrumentation required is shown in Figure 24.1.

The **periodontal probe** is a rounded, narrow or flat, blunt-ended, graduated instrument. Its blunt end can be inserted into the gingival sulcus without causing trauma.

The periodontal probe is used to:

- Measure periodontal probing depth
- Determine degree of gingival inflammation
- Evaluate furcation lesions
- Evaluate extent of tooth mobility.

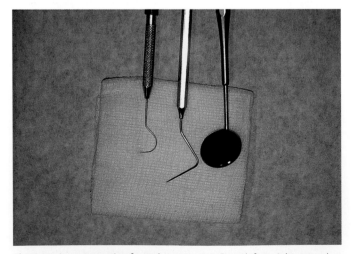

Fig. 24.1 Instrumentation for oral examination. From left to right: curved dental explorer, a periodontal probe and a dental mirror

The **dental explorer**, a sharp-ended instrument, is used to:

- Determine the presence of caries
- Explore other enamel and dentine defects, e.g. fracture, resorptive lesions.

The explorer is also useful for tactile examination of the subgingival tooth surfaces. Subgingival calculus and resorptive lesions may be identified in this way. Dental explorers are either straight or curved. They are also either single-ended or double-ended, usually combined with a periodontal probe, i.e. one end is an explorer and the other end is a periodontal probe.

A **dental mirror** is a vital, but traditionally rarely used, tool in veterinary dentistry. It allows the operator to visualize palatal/lingual surfaces while maintaining posture. The dental mirror can also be used to reflect light on to areas of interest and to retract and protect soft tissue.

Equipment and instrumentation for professional periodontal therapy

Professional periodontal therapy includes scaling, root planing and crown polishing. The procedure is detailed later in this chapter.

Scaling describes the process whereby dental deposits, i.e. plaque, but mainly calculus, are removed from the supra- and subgingival surfaces of the teeth. Scaling may be performed using a combination of mechanical (powered) instruments, e.g. ultrasonic or sonic scalers, and hand instruments, i.e. scalers and curettes. Hand instruments should be used to remove large, bulky supragingival deposits before going on to powered scalers. Hand instruments are also required to remove subgingival dental deposits.

Hand scaling instruments

Scalers and curettes are used to remove dental deposits from the tooth surfaces. Each has a handle, a shank and a working end or tip. They require frequent sharpening to maintain their cutting edges. The working end refers to that part of the instrument that is used to carry out the function of the instrument. The working end of a sharpened instrument is called the blade. It is made up of the following components:

- Face
- Lateral surfaces
- Back
- Cutting edge(s).

The cutting edge is the line where the face and a lateral surface meet to form a sharp cutting edge. A blade designed with a pointed tip is called a scaler. A blade that ends with a rounded toe is classified as a curette. Figure 24.2 demonstrates the differences between a scaler and a curette:

- **Scalers** – are used for the supragingival removal of calculus. As a scaler has a sharp, pointed tip it should only be used supragingivally. If a scaler is used subgingivally, the pointed tip will lacerate the gingival margin. A scaler should generally be pulled away from the gingiva towards the tip of the crown or the occlusal surface
- **Curettes** – are used for the subgingival removal of dental deposits and for root planing. They can also be

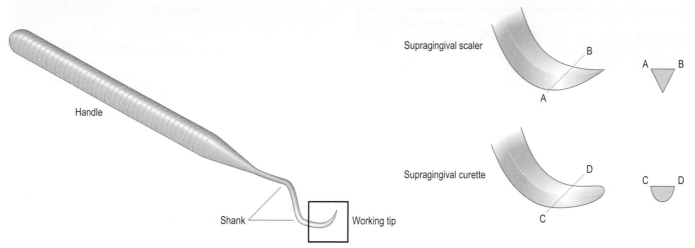

Fig. 24.2 Scaler and curette design. Each has a handle, a shank and a working tip. The working tip of a scaler is more robust than that of a curette. Also, the working tip of the scaler is pointed, while the curette has a rounded tip. A scaler is thus designed for supragingival work, while a curette can be used both supra- and subgingivally

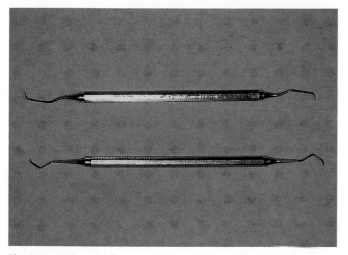

Fig. 24.3 A selection of curettes is required for periodontal therapy

used supragingivally. There are basically two types of curette, namely universal and area-specific, e.g. Gracey. The working end of a curette is more slender than that of a scaler and the back and tip are rounded to minimize gingival trauma. A selection of curettes (Fig. 24.3) is required for periodontal therapy. A separate scaler is not strictly required, as curettes can be used both above and below the gingiva while scalers are limited to supragingival use.

Mechanical scaling instruments

Mechanical scalers enable fast and easy removal of calculus. However, they have a great potential for iatrogenic damage (overheating a tooth may cause irreversible pulp pathology) if used incorrectly. There are three types of mechanical scaler:

- **Sonic scalers** are driven by compressed air, so they require a compressed-air-driven dental unit for operation. The tip oscillates at a sonic frequency. Sonic scalers are generally less effective than ultrasonic scalers but generate less heat and are thus less likely to cause iatrogenic injuries and safer to use. Depending upon

the design of the tip of the scaler, these instruments may be used for supra- and subgingival scaling. An insert with a thin pointed tip, sometimes called a perio, sickle or universal insert, is recommended

- **Ultrasonic scalers** are commonly used in veterinary practice. The tip oscillates at ultrasonic frequencies. They are driven by a micromotor rather than compressed air. The tip vibration is generated either by a magnetostrictive mechanism or a piezoelectric mechanism in the handpiece. The ultrasonic oscillation of the tip causes cavitation of the coolant, which aids in the disruption of the calculus on the tooth surface. Ultrasonic scalers are generally designed for supragingival use, but tips designed for subgingival scaling are available. A thin, pointed insert is recommended for supragingival use. Inserts specifically designed for subgingival use are recommended for subgingival scaling

- **Rotary scalers** are best avoided but are included here for completeness. In this system, roto pro burs are inserted in the high-speed handpiece of a compressed-air-driven unit. They are so-called 'non-cutting' burs, which when applied to calculus cause it to disintegrate while the coolant flushes the debris away. In humans, the use of these burs to scale teeth is associated with significant postoperative pain. They are thus no longer used for scaling. In addition to postoperative pain, roto pro burs can cause extensive damage to tooth enamel. Their use in veterinary dentistry is not recommended.

Polishing units

Polishing removes plaque and restores the scaled tooth surfaces to smoothness. A polished tooth surface is less plaque-retentive. Scaled teeth must be polished using either prophy paste in a prophy cup or in a brush in a slow-speed contra-angle handpiece, or by means of air polishing (particle blasting):

- **Prophy paste** in a cup or brush in a slow-speed contra-angle handpiece – the speed of rotation of the

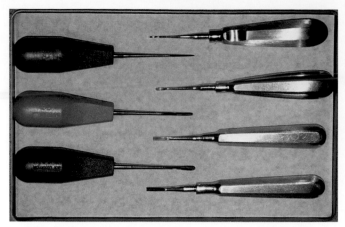

Fig. 24.4 Luxators and elevators. The three instruments with coloured handles are Svensk luxators. The remaining instruments are elevators

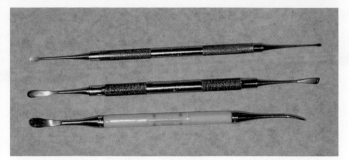

Fig. 24.5 Periosteal elevators. From top to bottom: Fine P24GSP, the Howard P9H and the Molt P9 (ceramic handle)

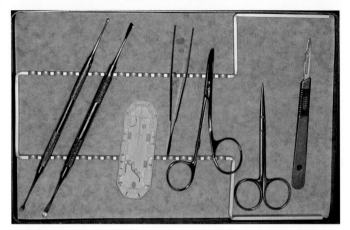

Fig. 24.6 Minor surgical kit for tooth extraction. A suture kit with small ophthalmic instruments and two periosteal elevators (the Fine P24GSP and the Howard P9H)

cup or brush can be regulated. To minimize the amount of heat generated, the prophy cup or brush should not rotate faster than 1000 revolutions per minute. Each patient should receive a new polishing cup or brush. Prophy paste is available in bulk containers and individual patient tubs. The latter are inexpensive and should be used to prevent contamination and iatrogenic transmission of pathogens

- **Air polishing (particle blasting)** – this technique, based on the sandblasting principle, is used to polish the supragingival parts of the teeth. The particles used, e.g. bicarbonate of soda, will polish the tooth surface without causing damage to the enamel, if used properly. It is essential to protect the soft tissues, i.e. gingivae and oral mucosa, during air polishing.

A simple way of protecting the soft tissues is to cover them with a piece of gauze.

Instrumentation and equipment for extraction

Tooth extraction requires hand instruments and power equipment.

Hand instruments

Hand instruments required for tooth extraction include luxators, elevators, periosteal elevators, possibly extraction forceps and a small surgical kit including a scalpel blade, forceps, suturing instruments and suturing material.

Luxators and elevators

Luxators and elevators are used to cut or break down the periodontal ligament, which holds the tooth in the alveolus. A selection of dental luxators and elevators of varying sizes are required (Fig. 24.4), so that an appropriate range for each size of root can be selected.

Periosteal elevator

A periosteal elevator (Fig. 24.5) is required for open or surgical extractions to expose the alveolar bone by raising a mucoperiosteal flap.

Extraction forceps

Although forceps can be used to aid ligament breakdown by rotational force on the tooth, it is easy to snap the crown off by using excessive force. Dental forceps are not essential but if they are to be used, a selection of sizes, to fit the root anatomy of the tooth being extracted, are required.

Scalpel blade

The use of a scalpel blade to free the gingival attachment to the tooth is recommended for both closed and open extraction technique. A size 15 or 11 blade, used in the handle, is ideal.

Suture kit and suture material

A suture kit with small ophthalmic instruments should be available (Fig. 24.6). Monofilament, absorbable suture material should be used in the oral cavity.

Power equipment

Power equipment is required to perform dentistry and oral surgery. Regular maintenance is essential to avoid problems with equipment failure.

Micromotor unit

A micromotor unit can be used for polishing teeth as well as for sectioning teeth, when the micromotor should be set at maximum speed. Micromotor units do not generally

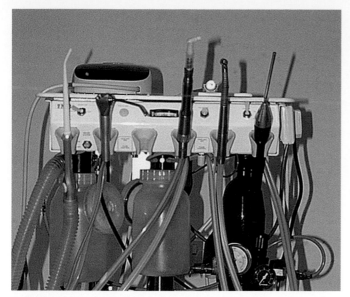

Fig. 24.7 A compressed-air-driven unit. This unit (IM3, Veterinary Instrumentation Ltd) has two high-speed outlets, one slow-speed outlet, a curing light, three-way syringe and suction

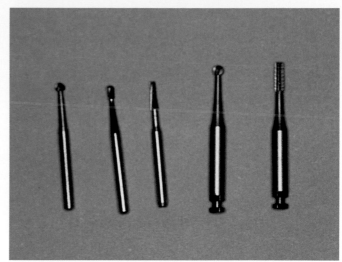

Fig. 24.8 A selection of tungsten carbide burs. From the left: round, pear-shaped and tapered fissure high-speed handpiece burs. Round and crosscutting straight fissure burs for the slow-speed handpiece are shown on the right

include water-cooling of the bur and an external source, e.g. an assistant applying coolant continuously to the tissues, is required to prevent thermal damage to teeth and alveolar bone.

Compressed-air-driven unit

The basic compressed-air-driven unit consists of a high-speed outlet, which accepts a high-speed handpiece, a slow-speed outlet, which accepts a slow-speed handpiece, and a combination air/water syringe. The high-speed outlet is fitted with water cooling. The slow-speed outlet may be fitted with water cooling but often this feature is absent. Some compressed-air-driven units have suction (Fig. 24.7). This is a real bonus.

Burs

Dental burs are made of a variety of materials, including stainless steel, tungsten carbide steel and 'diamond'. There is a wide selection of burs available to fit both the slow- and the high-speed handpiece (Fig. 24.8). The high-speed handpiece will only accept friction grip burs, while a slow-speed handpiece may accept either friction grip or latch key burs. A selection of round, pear-shaped, tapered fissure and straight fissure burs will be required for sectioning of teeth and removal of alveolar bone. 'Diamond' burs abrade rather than cut and may be safer for the inexperienced user. Blunted burs should be discarded.

Care and maintenance of instrumentation and equipment

The care and maintenance of dental equipment and instrumentation is the responsibility of the veterinary nurse.

Sharpening of hand instruments

Instruments must be sharp if they are to work efficiently yet with minimal trauma to the gingival tissues. Scalers and curettes, luxators and elevators all require regular sharpening. The basic goals of sharpening are to conserve a sharp cutting edge and to preserve the original shape of the instrument. Sharpening is usually performed after cleaning and prior to sterilization. Heat sterilization will result in blunting, so a clean sharpening stone should be available for sharpening during the procedure. Alternatively, sharpening can be performed after cleaning and sterilization. Dental instrument sharpening kits, i.e. stones and oil with instructions, are available through veterinary wholesalers. Attending a course to learn how to sharpen instruments is strongly recommended.

Cleaning and sterilization of hand instruments

Each patient should receive a clean and preferably sterile set of hand instruments. They are cleaned and sterilized by chemicals or heat in the same fashion as other surgical instruments.

Care and maintenance of power equipment

Power equipment also requires care and maintenance. The manufacturer and/or supplier of power equipment must supply you with detailed information of how to care for and maintain the unit you have purchased. An annual service contract should be part of the purchase agreement. There are similarities and differences in the care and maintenance of different units and you need to check with your supplier exactly how your unit should be looked after. The following is a general guideline.

Cleaning and sterilizing the ultrasonic scaler

The body of the ultrasonic scaler should not be cleaned in an ultrasonic bath. Instead, it can be cleaned using a cotton swab soaked in alcohol. Following cleaning, the handpiece should be sterilized (autoclave at 134 °C at 2 bar (200 kPa) for 20 minutes). The procedure is as follows:

1. Separate the handpiece from the cord and remove the scaler tip
2. Put the handpiece in the sterilizable cloth or bag if required
3. Take the handpiece out of the autoclave as soon at the sterilization is complete
4. Carefully dry the electrical contacts and the cord connector before use.

Cleaning and sterilizing handpieces

Handpieces need to be lubricated before and after sterilization or the bearings will fail.

After removing the bur, a brush is used to remove foreign particles from the handpiece. It is then wiped clean with a moist cloth. For the high-speed handpiece, a fine wire is provided for cleaning the water spray hole. Instructions should come with each unit as to how to dismantle handpieces.

Lubricate the handpiece. This can be achieved by inserting two or three drops of oil lubricant via a lubricant nozzle into the air supply tube. If a spray lubricant is used, it should be activated for 3 seconds. Operate the handpiece with a bur installed for 15–20 seconds. Remove the bur from the handpiece and disconnect the handpiece from the unit. The handpiece is now ready for autoclaving. Follow manufacturer's directions. After autoclaving is complete, and the handpiece has returned to room temperature, it needs to be lubricated again prior to use.

Precautions:

- Never autoclave handpiece with a bur in place
- Never operate handpiece without a bur inserted
- Do not forget 'before and after sterilization' lubrication procedures
- Dry heat sterilization is not allowed under any circumstances.

General maintenance

Table 24.1 indicates general maintenance, which must be carried out by the user. The high-speed handpiece requires clean air, and water that accumulates in the compressor must be removed daily. Refer to the handbook for details of how to empty the compressor.

Table 24.1 General maintenance of compressed-air-driven units

Operation	Daily	Weekly	Annually
Drain air receiver	*		
Drain filter/regulator	*		
Check oil level		*	
Change oil			*
Change air intake filter			*
Change line filter			*
Check electrical connections and all pipe fittings			*

Anaesthesia for dental procedures

General considerations

Oral examination and all oral/dental procedures require general anaesthesia. The procedures are often lengthy and close attention to life support is needed. Some general principles of anaesthesia for the patient undergoing dental or oral surgery are as follows:

Airway security

During dental surgery, the airway must be secured by endotracheal intubation to prevent aspiration pneumonia, which may occur if debris such as irrigation fluid and blood from the oral cavity enters unprotected airways.

Endotracheal tubes

Endotracheal tubes must be checked for defective cuffs and obstructed lumens before use. Any defective tubes should be discarded. Lightweight circuits are recommended.

To reduce apparatus dead space and the risk of endo-bronchial intubation, the tubing should be cut to fit the patient from mid neck to the level of the incisor teeth. Excessively long tubes that protrude from the oral cavity are prone to kinking, which may lead to pulmonary oedema as the patient inspires against an obstructed airway. The use of guarded endotracheal tubes should be considered for patients at high risk of tube kinking. Moreover, excessively long tubes are difficult to secure to the jaw with gauze bandage, which increases the risk of accidental extubation. Knots should be tied around the adaptor and not around the endotracheal tube itself. The cuff should be carefully inflated to a point where there is no air leaking around it. Be careful not to inflate the cuff excessively, as this can cause tracheal injury. The status of the endotracheal tube and integrity of the cuff should be monitored continuously. The operator will usually change the animal's position during surgery or while taking radiographs and this may cause tube displacement and/or kinking.

Pharyngeal packing

Pharyngeal packing should be used for greater airway security. Commonly used pharyngeal packs include surgical swabs, sponges and gauze bandage. A simple way to pack the pharynx is to insert a length of damp gauze bandage around the endotracheal tube, with the free end left visible for easy removal. It is important not to pack too tightly, as this impedes venous return and results in swelling of the tongue. Packs will become saturated with liquid during procedures and will then no longer offer adequate protection and should be replaced as required. It is imperative to remove any packing prior to extubation.

Eye protection

The eyes should be protected from desiccation by applying a lubricant eye ointment as required during the procedure.

Mouth gags

Mouth gags should be used with caution. Keeping the jaws wide open for prolonged periods may result in neuropraxia and inability to close the jaws (Robins 1976). The condition is self-limiting but may take several weeks to resolve. Mouth gags should be released and the jaws closed every 10–15 minutes. Keeping a record of how long the mouth gag has been in place ensures that the jaws are not inadvertently kept wide open for more than 15 minutes.

Suction

It is recommended to have suction available to protect the airways from saliva, irrigation fluids and other debris if required. In addition, blood loss can also be estimated by measuring the volume of blood in the suction jar.

Hypothermia

Hypothermia is a complication of lengthy anaesthesia and the use of cool irrigation fluids. Body temperature should be monitored regularly, e.g. every 20–30 minutes, and the development of hypothermia should be prevented by supplying external heat by blankets and warmed intravenous and irrigation fluids. Patients should be insulated with towels or bubble pack to prevent thermal injuries due to 'hot spots', which may occur with electrical heating mats. Circulating warm water mats may be safer.

Hyperthermia

Hyperthermia can occasionally occur in large, heavy-coated dogs connected to rebreathing circuits for long periods. By monitoring body temperature every 20–30 minutes, the development of hyperthermia can be identified and active cooling by fans, cooling pads, etc., can be initiated before damage occurs to vital organs.

Haemorrhage

Periodontal and other dental treatment rarely results in extensive haemorrhage unless the patient has an underlying disorder, e.g. coagulopathy, septicaemia.

A full haematological examination and clotting profile should be performed prior to any potentially haemorrhagic procedure, e.g. major oral surgery such as a maxillectomy. The patient should also be cross-matched with a healthy donor prior to any such procedure. An alternative to cross-matching is autologous transfusion.

During the procedure, blood loss should be estimated either by weighing blood-soaked swabs or by measuring the amount of blood collected in a suction jar. As a rough guide a saturated 3 × 3 inch swab contains 7 ml of blood and a saturated 4 × 4 inch swab contains 10 ml of blood.

Patient monitoring

All patients should be monitored continuously. Careful monitoring should enable the detection of problems before they become severe, so that they can be treated appropriately and crises can be avoided. Continuous anaesthetic monitoring is associated with reduced mortality (Dyson et al 1998). It is impossible to both monitor anaesthesia and perform the procedure. Moreover, with some procedures a surgical assistant is required. The surgical assistant needs to be a different person from the one monitoring the anaesthesia.

Routine anaesthetic monitoring includes:

- Inspecting respiratory function
- Assessing the colour of the mucous membranes
- Checking capillary refill time
- Listening to the sound of breathing
- Palpating the peripheral pulse.

All findings should be recorded on an anaesthetic chart at regular intervals, e.g. every 5 or 10 minutes, for the duration of anaesthesia. Also record current oxygen, nitrous oxide (if used) and volatile agent level at each check. Any changes in the anaesthetic regimen, e.g. altering flow rate or concentration of volatile agent, should be recorded on the chart.

This basic monitoring can be augmented with mechanical aids, which give additional information and allow a more precise picture of the patient's status. This allows closer control over the course of the anaesthetic. The disadvantage of mechanical monitoring devices is that they in turn must be monitored to ensure that the information they are giving is accurate. Unexpected readings should be verified by examination of the patient before they are acted on, i.e. monitor the patient, not the equipment.

Anaesthetic recovery

Anaesthesia should be lightened towards the end of the procedure. The oral cavity must be cleaned out, the pharyngeal pack removed and the cuff of the endotracheal tube deflated before recovery is allowed to proceed. Use of the three-way syringe (air–water spray) on the dental unit is recommended for removing debris from the tongue and gums. A dry swab can be used to remove any large blood clots. Ensure that there is no debris in the oropharynx before removing the pharyngeal pack and deflating the cuff of the endotracheal tube. The coat around the mouth and head should be cleaned and dried using a towel or hairdryer. The endotracheal tube is usually not removed until the animal has a swallowing reflex.

Anaesthetic recovery should be monitored closely and recorded. It should always occur in a warm environment. Animals that have had surgical procedures using flap techniques and suturing, e.g. open or surgical extractions or oronasal fistula repair, must be prevented from pawing at their mouths or rubbing their faces. In some animals, an Elizabethan collar may be used. If the surgical procedure has resulted in blood in the nasal cavity, e.g. oronasal fistula repair, it is wise to recover these patients in sternal recumbency with the head placed lower than the rest of the body to encourage drainage. Sneezing fits commonly occur in these patients on recovery.

Immediate postoperative care

Optimal immediate postoperative management involves appropriate analgesia and nursing. Sound nursing measures also have a profound impact on reducing the level of postoperative discomfort and pain. Giving the animal attention at regular intervals helps reduce the distress associated with pain and the unfamiliar environment, otherwise a cycle of pain/distress/sleeplessness can develop.

The provision of a comfortable bed in a warm, but not too hot, environment is beneficial. Food and water should be offered as early as possible in the postoperative period. Pain and inflammation increase the basic metabolic rate and a high level of nutrition is required to promote healing. Offering food as early as possible not only speeds recovery but can also have a soothing effect.

Oral examination and recording

Oral examination in a conscious animal will only give limited information. Definitive oral examination can only be performed under general anaesthesia. All detected abnormalities should be recorded. It saves time if one person performs the examination and another individual takes the notes and enters the findings on the dental record.

Conscious examination

Oral examination of a conscious animal is limited to visual inspection and some digital palpation. Gentle technique is essential. Examination involves assessing not only the oral cavity but also palpation of:

- Face – facial bones and zygomatic arch
- Temporomandibular joint
- Salivary glands – mandibular/sublingual; the parotids are usually only palpable if enlarged
- Lymph nodes – mandibular, cervical chain
- Having looked at the entire face, the mouth is first examined by gently holding the jaws closed and retracting the lips (do not pull on the fur to retract lips) to look at the soft tissues and buccal aspects of the teeth. This is the optimal time to evaluate occlusion.

After evaluating the occlusion the animal is encouraged to open its mouth. One method of achieving this in the dog is to place a thumb and finger on the margin of the alveolar bone caudal to the canine teeth of the upper and lower jaw on one side and with gentle pressure encouraging the animal to open its jaws. Another method, useful for both dogs and cats, is to approach the animal from the side, place one hand over the muzzle and press the lips gently into the oral cavity while tilting the head slightly upwards. A finger from the other hand is placed on the lower incisors and gentle pressure is exerted. Do not use the fur under the mandible to try to pull the jaw down. Most animals allow at least a cursory inspection of the oral cavity once the jaws have been opened. The mucous membranes of the oral cavity should be examined as well as the teeth. Apart from colour and texture of the mucous membranes, look for evidence of a potential bleeding problem, e.g. petechiation, purpura, ecchymoses. In addition, look for vesicle formation, ulceration, which could indicate a vesiculo-bullous disorder, e.g. pemphigus, pemphigoid. Obvious pathology, e.g. tooth fracture, gingival recession, advanced furcation exposure relating to the teeth, can be identified. Assess the oropharynx (soft palate,

palatoglossal arch, tonsillary crypts, tonsils and fauces) if possible. It is useful to identify any potential problems that may occur with endotracheal intubation prior to inducing anaesthesia.

Examination under general anaesthesia

The oropharynx should be examined prior to endotracheal intubation. Normal anatomical features of the oral cavity should be identified and inspected. Refreshing your memory on these features from an anatomy textbook is highly recommended. It is only with knowledge of the normal that abnormalities can be identified.

The periodontium of each tooth needs to be assessed. Examination of the periodontium is not routinely performed in veterinary practice. It is essential to perform a thorough periodontal examination in order to identify disease and plan treatment. The following indices and criteria should be evaluated for each tooth:

1. Gingivitis and gingival index
2. Periodontal probing depth (PPD)
3. Gingival recession
4. Furcation involvement
5. Mobility
6. Periodontal (clinical) attachment level.

In animals with large accumulations of dental deposits (plaque and calculus) on the teeth, it may be necessary to remove these to assess periodontal status accurately.

The purpose of the meticulous periodontal examination is to:

- Identify the presence of periodontal disease, i.e. gingivitis and periodontitis
- Differentiate between gingivitis – inflammation of the gingiva – and periodontitis – inflammation of the periodontal tissues, resulting in loss of attachment and eventually tooth loss
- Identify the precise location of disease processes
- Assess the extent of tissue destruction where there is periodontitis.

Periodontal probing depth, gingival recession, furcation involvement and mobility quantify the tissue destruction in periodontitis. Radiography to visualize the extent and type of alveolar bone destruction is mandatory if clinical evidence of periodontitis is found. In many cases, measuring or calculating the periodontal or clinical attachment level (PAL/CAL) is also useful.

1. Gingivitis and gingival index

The presence and degree of gingivitis (Fig. 24.9) is assessed based on a combination of redness and swelling, as well as presence or absence of bleeding on gentle probing of the gingival sulcus. Various indices can be used to give a numerical value to the degree of gingival inflammation present. In the clinical situation, a simple bleeding index is the most useful. Using this method, a periodontal probe is gently inserted into the gingival sulcus at several locations around the whole circumference of each tooth; and the tooth is given a score of 0 if there is no bleeding and a score of 1 if the probing elicits bleeding.

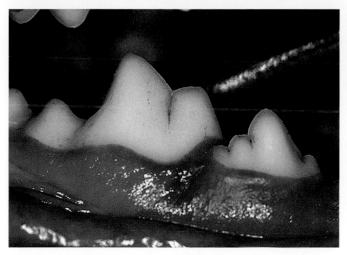

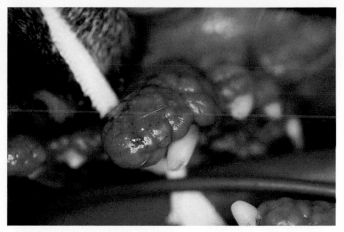

Fig. 24.11 Gingival hyperplasia

Fig. 24.9 Gingivitis is inflammation of the gingiva, which manifests as reddening, swelling and often bleeding of the gingival margin

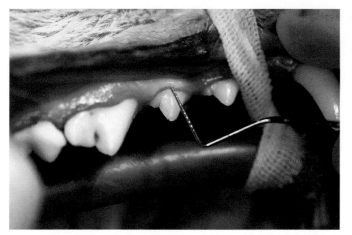

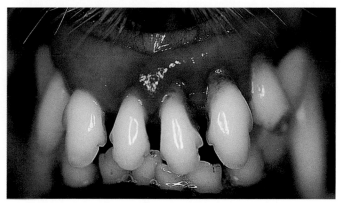

Fig. 24.12 Gingival recession is measured from the cemento-enamel junction to the free gingival margin using a periodontal probe. In this photograph of the upper incisors, the right second incisor has a normal gingival contour, while the right first incisor and the left first and second incisor all have gingival recession of varying degrees

Fig. 24.10 Periodontal probing depth

2. Periodontal probing depth

The depth of the sulcus can be assessed by gently inserting a graduated periodontal probe until resistance is encountered at the base of the sulcus. The depth from the free gingival margin to the base of the sulcus is measured in millimetres at several locations around the whole circumference of the tooth (Fig. 24.10). The probe is moved gently horizontally, walking along the floor of the sulcus. The gingival sulcus is 1–3 mm deep in the dog and 0.5–1 mm in the cat. Measurements in excess of these values usually indicate the presence of periodontitis: the periodontal ligament has been destroyed and alveolar bone resorbed, thus allowing the probe to be inserted to a greater depth. The term used to describe this situation is periodontal pocketing. All sites with periodontal pocketing should be accurately recorded. Gingival inflammation resulting in swelling or hyperplasia of the free gingiva (Fig. 24.11) will, of course, also result in sulcus depths in excess of normal values. In these situations, the term pseudo-pocketing is used, as the periodontal ligament and bone are intact, i.e. there is no evidence of periodontitis and the increase in PPD is due to swelling or hyperplasia of the gingiva.

3. Gingival recession

Gingival recession is also measured using a periodontal probe (Fig. 24.12). It is the distance (in millimetres) from the cemento-enamel junction to the free gingival margin. At sites with gingival recession, PPD may be within normal values despite loss of alveolar bone due to periodontitis.

4. Furcation involvement

Furcation involvement refers to the situation where the bone between the roots of multirooted teeth is destroyed by periodontitis (Fig. 24.13). The furcation sites of multirooted teeth should be examined with a periodontal probe. The grading of furcation involvement is listed in Table 24.2.

5. Tooth mobility

The extent of tooth mobility should be assessed using a suitable instrument, e.g. the blunt end of the handle of a dental mirror or probe. It should not be assessed using fingers directly, since the yield of the soft tissues of the fingers will mask the extent of tooth mobility. The grading of mobility is listed in Table 24.3.

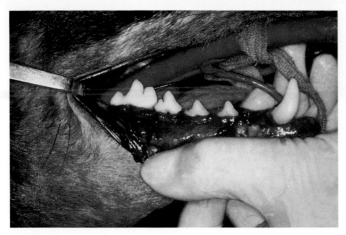

Fig. 24.13 Furcation involvement. The left maxillary second and third premolars have grade 2 furcation involvement and the fourth premolar has a grade 1 lesion

Table 24.2 Grading of furcation involvement

Grade 0	No furcation involvement
Grade 1	The furcation can be felt with the probe but horizontal tissue destruction is less than one-third of the horizontal width of the furcation
Grade 2	It is possible to explore the furcation but the probe cannot be passed through it from buccal to palatal/lingual. Horizontal tissue destruction is more than one-third of the horizontal width of the furcation
Grade 3	The probe can be passed through the furcation from buccal to palatal/lingual

Table 24.3 Grading of tooth mobility

Grade 0	No mobility
Grade 1	Horizontal movement of 1 mm or less
Grade 2	Horizontal movement of more than 1 mm*
Grade 3	Vertical as well as horizontal movement is possible

*Note that multirooted teeth are scored more severely and a horizontal mobility in excess of 1 mm is usually considered a grade 3 even in the absence of vertical movement.

6. Periodontal/clinical attachment level

Periodontal probing depth is not necessarily correlated with severity of attachment loss. As already mentioned, gingival hyperplasia may contribute to a deep pocket or a pseudo-pocket if there is no attachment loss, while gingival recession may result in the absence of a pocket but also minimal remaining attachment. Periodontal attachment level records the distance from the cemento-enamel junction or from a fixed point on the tooth to the base or apical extension of the pathological pocket. It is thus a more accurate assessment of tissue loss in periodontitis. PAL is either directly measured with a periodontal probe or it is calculated, e.g. PPD + gingival recession.

Recording findings

The information resulting from the examination and any treatment performed must be recorded. A basic dental record consists of written notes and a completed dental chart. Additional diagnostic tests and radiographs are included as indicated.

A dental chart is a diagrammatic representation of the dentition, where information (findings and treatment) can be entered in a pictorial and/or notational form. A dental chart needs to be supplemented by clinical notes, radiographs, etc., to make a complete dental record.

A copy of dog and cat dental record sheets used in our practice is depicted in Figure 24.14. The front is used to record clinical findings and the back is used to enter diagnosis, draw up a treatment plan and record treatment performed. The nurse who performs the clinical examination completes the front page. The veterinary surgeon checks the clinical findings and interprets any radiographs taken, and then fills in the back page of the chart.

Radiography

Radiography is a vital tool in veterinary dentistry. Pathological radiographic changes are usually discrete and therefore clarity and detail are essential. For a dental radiograph to be diagnostic, it should be an accurate representation of the size and shape of the tooth without superimposition of adjacent structures. Intraoral radiographic techniques are therefore required; a parallel technique for the mandibular premolars and molars, and a bisecting angle technique for all other teeth. (For intraoral radiographic techniques see Ch. 30.) Attending a practical course is strongly recommended. While a trained nurse can take radiographs, the interpretation of the films is the duty of the veterinary surgeon.

Periodontal therapy

The management of periodontal disease is aimed at controlling the cause of the inflammation, i.e. dental plaque. Conservative or cause-related periodontal therapy consists of removal of plaque and calculus, and any other remedial procedures required, under general anaesthesia, in combination with daily maintenance of oral hygiene. In other words, the treatment of periodontal disease has two components:

* Professional periodontal therapy
* Maintenance of oral hygiene.

Professional periodontal therapy is performed under general anaesthesia and includes:

* Supra- and subgingival scaling
* Root planing
* Tooth crown polishing
* Subgingival lavage.

Maintenance of oral hygiene is performed by the owner and is often called home care. Its effectiveness depends on the motivation and technical ability of the owner and the cooperation of the animal. If no home care is instituted, then plaque will rapidly reform after a professional periodontal therapy procedure and the disease will progress. Before any treatment is instituted, the owner must be made aware that

DENTAL RECORD: DOG

Client: .... Date: ....

Animal: .... Clinician: ....

Comp no: .... Student: ....

	OCCLUSAL EVALUATION	EXTRAORAL FINDINGS	ORAL SOFT TISSUES	OTHER RELEVANT FEATURES
Incisor occlusion:	....	....	....	....
Canine occlusion:	....	....	....	....
Premolar alignment:	....	....	....	....
Distal P/M occlusion:	....	....	....	....
Head symmetry:	....	....	....	....
Individual teeth:	....	....	....	....
Other:	....	....	....	....

PLAQUE

RP/M	RI/M	LI/M	LP/M

CALCULUS

RP/M	RI/M	LI/M	LP/M

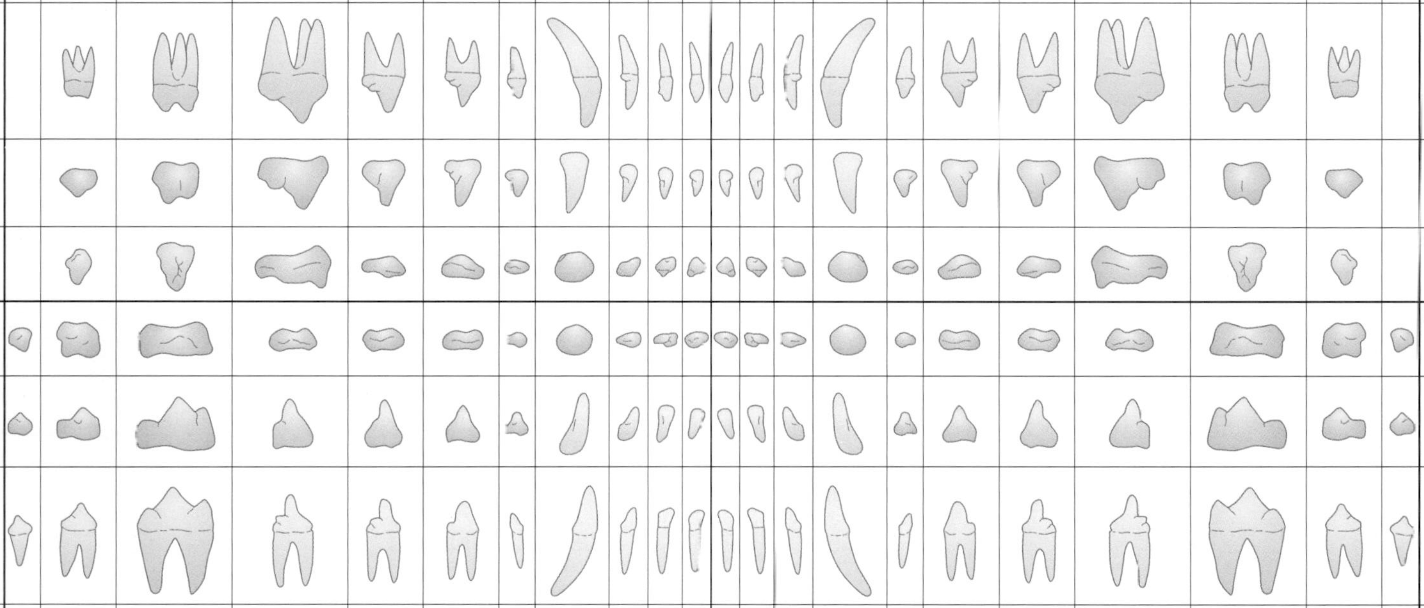

Furcation																							Furcation
Gingivitis																							Gingivitis
Mobility																							Mobility
RIGHT	M3	M2	M1	P4	P3	P2	P1	C	I3	I2	I1	I1	I2	I3	C	P1	P2	P3	P4	M1	M2	M3	LEFT
Buccal aspect																							Buccal aspect
Palatal aspect																							Palatal aspect
Occlusal: buccal palatel																							Occlusal: buccal palatel
Occlusal: lingual buccal																							Occlusal: lingual buccal
Lingual aspect																							Lingual aspect
Buccal aspect																							Buccal aspect
RIGHT	M3	M2	M1	P4	P3	P2	P1	C	I3	I2	I1	I1	I2	I3	C	P1	P2	P3	P4	M1	M2	M3	LEFT
Mobility																							Mobility
Gingivitis																							Gingivitis
Furcation																							Furcation

Fig. 24.14A Dog dental record sheet – the front is used to record clinical findings and the back is used to enter diagnosis, draw up treatment plan and record treatment performed

ORAL PROBLEM LIST

....
....
....

PERIODONTICS

☐ Sonic scaling   ☐ Ultrasonic scaling
☐ Subgingival curettage ☐ Periodontal debridement
☐ Pumice-polishing   ☐ Air-polishing
☐ Periodontal surgery..........

....
....
....

OTHER DENTAL PROCEDURES

....
....
....

THERAPEUTIC PLAN

....
....

ORAL SURGERY (Note sites on graph - X)

☐ Simple extraction(s)..........
☐ Surgical extraction(s)..........
☐ Incisional biopsy   ☐ Excisional biopsy
☐ Other/comments..........

....
....

COMPLICATIONS/COMMENTS

....
....
....

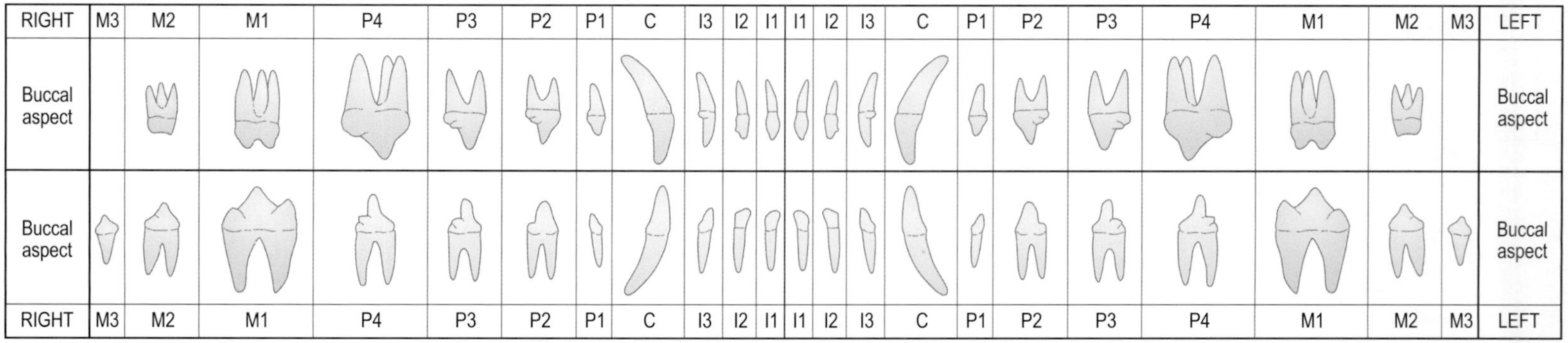

RIGHT	M3	M2	M1	P4	P3	P2	P1	C	I3	I2	I1	I1	I2	I3	C	P1	P2	P3	P4	M1	M2	M3	LEFT
Buccal aspect																							Buccal aspect
Buccal aspect																							Buccal aspect
RIGHT	M3	M2	M1	P4	P3	P2	P1	C	I3	I2	I1	I1	I2	I3	C	P1	P2	P3	P4	M1	M2	M3	LEFT

Fig. 24.14A Continued

DENTAL RECORD: CAT

Client: ....

Animal: ....

Comp no: ....

Date: ....

Clinician: ....

Student: ....

OCCLUSAL EVALUATION

Incisor occlusion: ....

Canine occlusion: ....

Premolar alignment: ....

Distal P/M occlusion: ....

Head symmetry: ....

Individual teeth: ....

Other: ....

EXTRAORAL FINDINGS

ORAL SOFT TISSUES

OTHER RELEVANT FEATURES

PLAQUE	RP/M	RI/M	LI/M	LP/M

CALCULUS	RP/M	RI/M	LI/M	LP/M

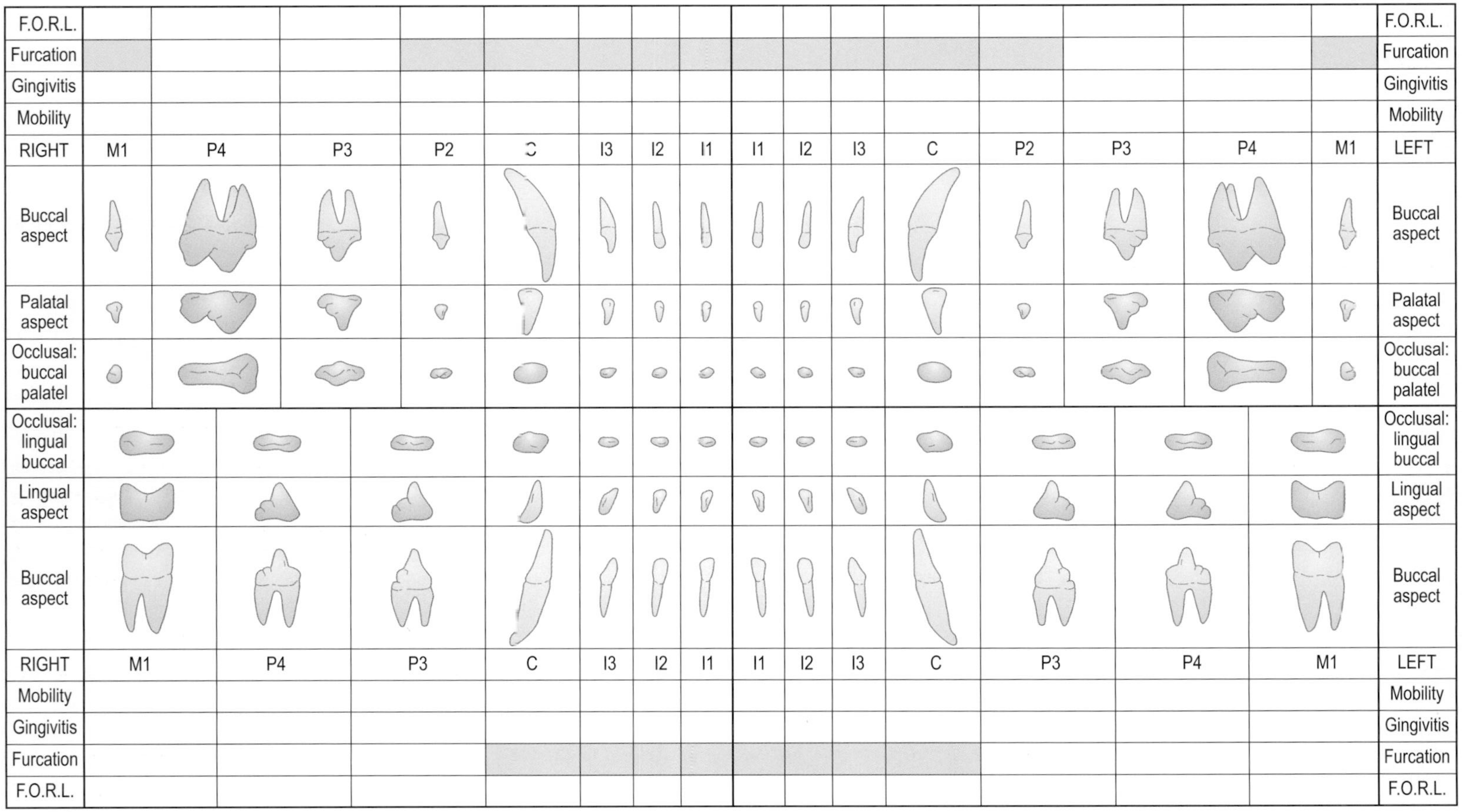

RIGHT: F.O.R.L. / Furcation / Gingivitis / Mobility / RIGHT M1 P4 P3 P2 C I3 I2 I1 / Buccal aspect / Palatal aspect / Occlusal: buccal palatel / Occlusal: lingual buccal / Lingual aspect / Buccal aspect / RIGHT M1 P4 P3 C I3 I2 I1 / Mobility / Gingivitis / Furcation / F.O.R.L.

LEFT: F.O.R.L. / Furcation / Gingivitis / Mobility / LEFT M1 P4 P3 P2 C I3 I2 I1 / Buccal aspect / Palatal aspect / Occlusal: buccal palatel / Occlusal: lingual buccal / Lingual aspect / Buccal aspect / LEFT M1 P4 P3 C I3 I2 I1 / Mobility / Gingivitis / Furcation / F.O.R.L.

Fig. 24.14B Cat dental record sheet

ORAL PROBLEM LIST

THERAPEUTIC PLAN

PERIODONTICS
- ☐ Sonic scaling
- ☐ Subgingival curettage
- ☐ Pumice-polishing
- ☐ Periodontal surgery
- ☐ Ultrasonic scaling
- ☐ Periodontal debridement
- ☐ Air-polishing

ORAL SURGERY (Note sites on graph - X)
- ☐ Simple extraction(s):
- ☐ Surgical extraction(s):
- ☐ Incisional biopsy
- ☐ Excisional biopsy
- ☐ Other/comments

OTHER DENTAL PROCEDURES

COMPLICATIONS/COMMENTS

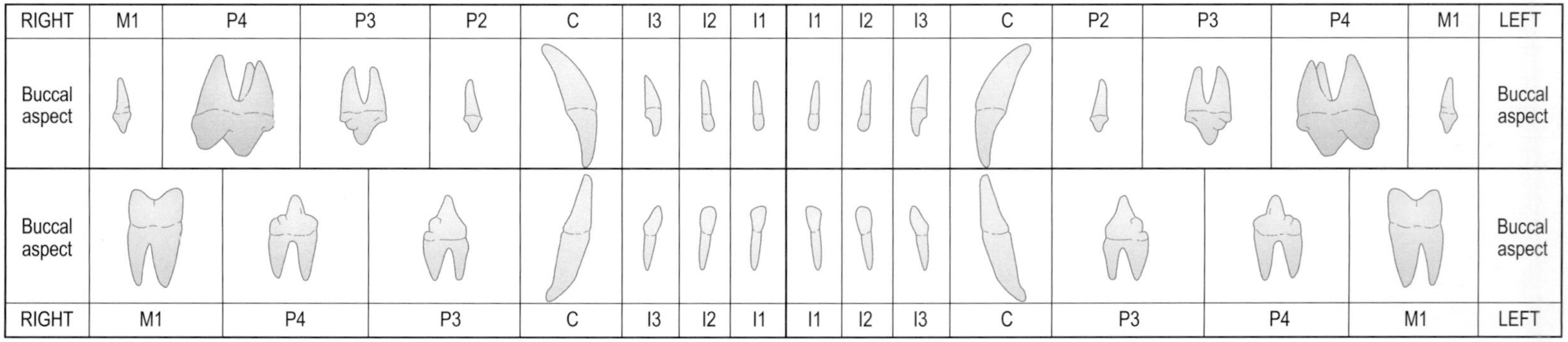

RIGHT	M1	P4	P3	P2	C	I3	I2	I1	I1	I2	I3	C	P2	P3	P4	M1	LEFT
Buccal aspect																	Buccal aspect
Buccal aspect					C	I3	I2	I1	I1	I2	I3	C	P2	P3	P4	M1	Buccal aspect
RIGHT	M1	P4	P3		C	I3	I2	I1	I1	I2	I3	C	P2	P3	P4	M1	LEFT

Fig. 24.14B Continued

home care is the most essential component in both preventing and treating periodontal disease. Whenever possible, it is useful to institute a home-care programme before any professional periodontal therapy is performed. The veterinary nurse has an important role to play in instituting and maintaining home care.

The aim of treatment differs whether the patient has gingivitis only or if there is also periodontitis.

Gingivitis

Gingivitis is by definition reversible (Fig. 24.9). Removal or adequate reduction of plaque will restore inflamed gingivae to health. Once clinically healthy gingivae have been achieved these can be maintained by daily removal or reduction of the accumulation of plaque. In short, the treatment of gingivitis is to restore the inflamed tissues to clinical health and then to maintain clinically healthy gingivae, thus preventing periodontitis (Fig. 24.15). The purpose of the professional periodontal therapy in the gingivitis patient is removal of dental deposits, mainly calculus (which is not removed by tooth-brushing). Once the teeth have been cleaned, it remains up to the owner to remove the plaque that reaccumulates on a daily basis.

Periodontitis

Untreated gingivitis may progress to periodontitis. Periodontitis is irreversible. It is important to remember that periodontitis is a site-specific disease, i.e. it may affect one or more sites of one or several teeth (Fig. 24.16). The aim of treatment is to prevent development of new lesions at other sites and to prevent further tissue destruction at sites that are already affected.

Professional periodontal therapy removes dental deposits above and below the gingival margin. It then rests with the owner to ensure that plaque does not reaccumulate. Meticulous supragingival plaque control, by means of daily tooth-brushing and adjunctive antiseptics when indicated, will prevent migration of the plaque below the gingival margin. If the subgingival tooth surfaces are kept clean, the sulcular epithelium will reattach.

Professional periodontal therapy

Professional periodontal therapy must be performed under general anaesthesia. To master the technical skills required for dentistry and oral surgery, attending practical courses is recommended.

Supragingival scaling

This is the removal of plaque and calculus above the gingival margin. It can be performed using hand instruments alone or a combination of hand instruments and mechanical scalers.

The recommended procedure is as follows:

1. Remove gross dental deposits – plaque-covered calculus – using rongeurs, extraction forceps or calculus-removing forceps (Fig. 24.17)
2. Remove residual supragingival dental deposits with sharp hand instruments, either a sickle-shaped scaler or a curette, as shown in Figure 24.18

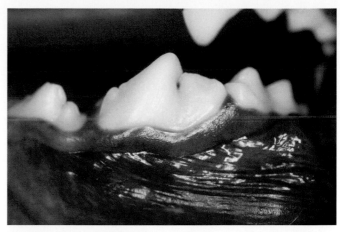

Fig. 24.15 Clinically healthy gingivae. This is the term used to describe gingiva that shows no clinical evidence of inflammation. There is no reddening, swelling or bleeding. The gingival margin is firmly adapted to the tooth surface

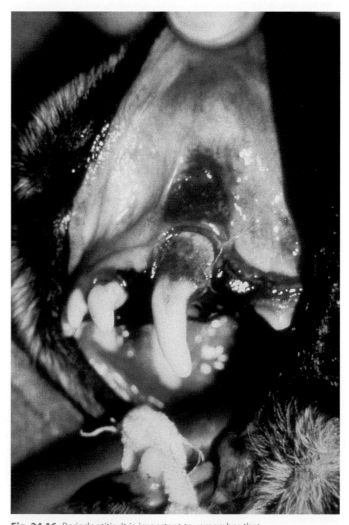

Fig. 24.16 Periodontitis. It is important to remember that periodontitis is a site-specific disease. Depicted is a lower first molar with periodontitis (destruction of periodontal ligament, bone loss and gingival recession) affecting the buccal surface of the distal root. The rest of the tooth shows no evidence of periodontitis (normal PPD and no gingival recession)

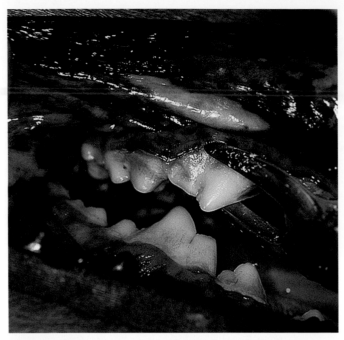

Fig. 24.17 Removing gross supragingival dental deposits with extraction forceps. Avoid traumatizing the gingival margin with the forceps

3. A mechanical scaler, either ultrasonic or sonic, is then used to remove residual dental deposits (Fig. 24.19).

Mechanical scalers generate heat and have the potential to cause iatrogenic damage if not used properly. Overheating a tooth will cause desiccation of the dentine and consequent damage to the underlying pulp tissue. Pulp damage may be a reversible pulpitis but it can become severe enough to cause pulp necrosis, which would necessitate extraction or endodontic treatment of the affected tooth.

An ultrasonic or sonic scaler should be used by gently stroking the tooth with the side of the tip and with continuous movement over the tooth surface. A plentiful supply of water is essential to cool the oscillating tip and flush away debris. Using the tip of the instrument or applying excessive pressure will cause gouging of the tooth surface as well as generating excessive heat. As an arbitrary rule, it is suggested that no more than 15 seconds of continuous scaling should be performed on any one tooth. If the tooth is not clean in that period of time, then return to it after scaling a few other teeth. This will allow the original tooth time to cool down.

Both sonic and ultrasonic scalers should be used with an insert that has a thin, pointed tip, sometimes called a perio, sickle or universal insert. An insert with a large (wide) tip is not recommended. A fine tip will remove dental deposits more accurately, with less likelihood of damage to the tooth enamel.

Subgingival scaling and root planing

This is the removal of plaque, calculus and other debris from the tooth surface below the gingival margin, i.e. within the gingival sulcus or periodontal pocket. There is no need to perform extensive subgingival scaling if there is no calculus below the gingival margin. However, the presence of

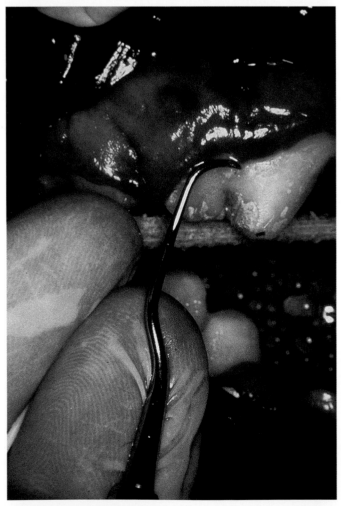

Fig. 24.18 Removing residual dental deposits with hand instruments. Here a universal scaler is being used to remove calculus

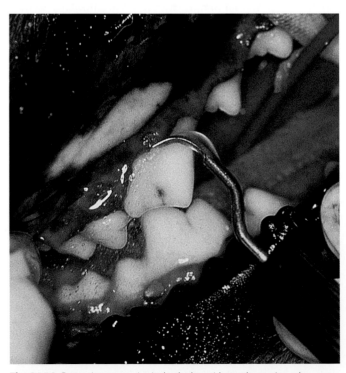

Fig. 24.19 Removing supragingival calculus with an ultrasonic scaler

subgingival deposits should always be investigated with a dental explorer and if any are identified they should be removed.

Root planing is the removal of the superficial layer of toxin-laden cementum from the root surfaces. Root planing produces a smooth root surface that is less likely to accumulate plaque and more likely to permit epithelial reattachment. Excessive root planing may damage the root surface (expose root dentine to the periodontal ligament) and predispose to further periodontal destruction. So, while a clean and smooth root surface should be obtained, overzealous root planing should be avoided.

Scaling and planing are achieved simultaneously using a curette. The procedure can be performed using either a closed (without raising an access flap) or open (raising an access flap) technique. An open technique is recommended for pockets deeper than 4 mm as it is difficult even for a skilled operator to ensure that all subgingival deposits have been removed without raising a gingival flap for direct access and visualization. However, an open technique is only indicated in patients with proven sufficient home care, i.e. it is not first-line treatment. The open technique is not a routine hygiene procedure. It is classified as periodontal surgery and should be performed by a veterinary surgeon with expertise in veterinary dentistry.

Ultrasonic and sonic scalers are designed for supragingival work. Once inserted into the gingival sulcus or pathological pocket, the water will no longer reach to cool the tip. The result is thermal damage of both hard and soft tissues. Quick subgingival excursions are permissible only if the gingiva is oedematous, or held mechanically out of the way to allow the water to reach the tip. Scalers with specially designed working tips where the water exits at the very end are safer to use under the gingival margin, but the removal of established subgingival deposits can only be adequately performed with meticulous use of sharp curettes.

The procedure for closed subgingival debridement is shown in Figure 24.20. It is often a lengthy procedure. It must be emphasized that removing subgingival plaque, calculus and debris as well as the superficial layer of toxin-laden cementum and restoring the root surfaces to smoothness is a most important step. Removing only the supragingival debris at a periodontitis site does not have any therapeutic benefit.

It will not prevent disease progression, as the cause of the disease – subgingival plaque – is still present.

Polishing

Scaling, even when done correctly, will cause minor scratches of the tooth. A rough surface will facilitate plaque retention. Polishing smoothes this roughness and helps remove any remaining plaque and stained pellicle.

Polishing is performed by applying a mildly abrasive prophylaxis paste to the tooth surface with a prophylaxis cup/brush mounted in a slowly rotating slow-speed handpiece (Fig. 24.21). The handpiece should be running at less than 1000 rpm to avoid generating excessive heat by friction. The amount of heat that can easily result from incorrect polishing can cause severe pulpal pathology. A surplus of paste is applied to the tooth surface, using light force. If a rubber cup is used, the force should be just enough to cause

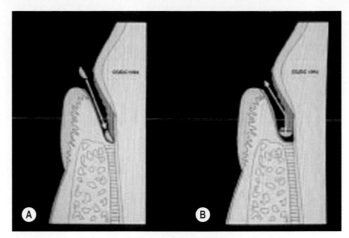

Fig. 24.20 Procedure for closed subgingival debridement. (**A**) The curette is inserted to the bottom of the gingival sulcus or pocket. (**B**) The cutting edges of the curette are engaged by turning the handle of the instrument, against the root surface and pulling out of the sulcus or pocket in this position. The instrument is worked in this way around the whole circumference of the tooth, using overlapping strokes. Mainly vertical, but also oblique and horizontal strokes are used

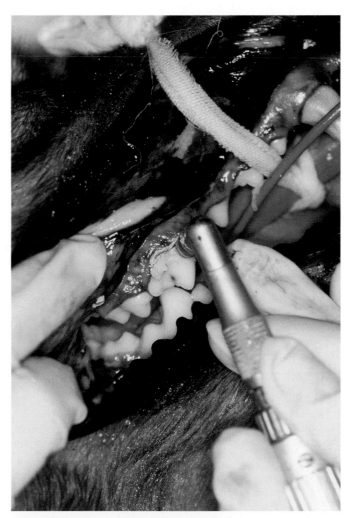

Fig. 24.21 Tooth crown polishing with a prophylaxis cup in a slow-speed handpiece

the cup to flare out on the tooth surface. The prophylaxis cup is kept moving over the entire tooth surface for a few seconds per tooth. The flared edge of the prophylaxis cup can be used to polish slightly subgingivally, taking care to avoid causing any further gingival damage. It is useful to check that all tooth surfaces are clean by using a plaque-disclosing solution after polishing. Any residual plaque is thus visualized and can be removed with further polishing.

Sulcular lavage

This involves gently flushing the gingival sulcus and pathological pockets with saline or dilute chlorhexidine to remove any free-floating debris. This step is particularly important in a deep pathological pocket as free floating debris may occlude the orifice of the pocket and lead to the formation of a lateral periodontal abscess.

Maintenance of oral hygiene (home care)

The benefit of any professional periodontal therapy is short-lived unless maintained by effective home care. In fact, if no home care is instituted after professional periodontal therapy, then plaque will rapidly reform and disease will progress. It has been shown that 3 months after periodontal therapy, gingivitis scores are equivalent to those recorded prior to therapy if no home care is instituted (Gorrel & Bierer 1999).

The cause (dental plaque) and effects (discomfort, pain, chronic focus of infection, loss of teeth and possibility of systemic complications) of periodontal disease must be thoroughly explained to the pet owner. The owner must be made aware that home care is the most essential component in both preventing and treating periodontal disease. The responsibility of maintaining oral hygiene, i.e. keeping plaque accumulation to a level compatible with periodontal health, rests with the owner of the pet. Once instituted, home care regimens need continuous monitoring and reinforcement.

The veterinary nurse can play a vital role in educating clients, checking compliance and reinforcing the need for home care. It is strongly recommended that the trained veterinary nurse takes on the responsibility of educating and training pet owners to perform optimal home care by setting up preventive care clinics.

Tooth-brushing is known to be the single most effective means of removing plaque – studies have shown that in dogs with both experimentally induced gingivitis (Tromp et al 1986) and naturally occurring gingivitis (Gorrel & Rawlings 1996), daily tooth-brushing is effective in returning the gingivae to health. In a 4-year study using the beagle dog (Lindhe et al 1975) it was shown that with no oral hygiene plaque accumulated rapidly along the gingival margin, with gingivitis developing within a few weeks. Dogs that were fed an identical diet under identical conditions but were subjected to daily tooth-brushing developed no clinical signs of gingivitis. In the group that were not receiving daily tooth-brushing, gingivitis progressed to periodontitis in most individuals.

Tooth-brushing is the gold standard for plaque control – every effort should be made to get every pet owner to commit to brushing their pet's teeth on a daily basis. The success of tooth-brushing depends on pet cooperation and owner motivation and technical ability. Tooth-brushing should be introduced gradually and as early in the animal's life as possible. Adult cats are generally less amenable to the introduction of tooth-brushing than adult dogs, but with patience and persistence, many will accept some degree of home care. In contrast, kittens often accept tooth-brushing more readily than puppies.

Bibliography

Dyson, D.H., Maxie, M.G., Schnurr, D., 1998. Morbidity and mortality associated with anaesthetic management in small animal veterinary practice in Ontario. J. Am. Anim. Hosp. Assoc. 34, 461–471.

Gorrel, C., Bierer, T., 1999. Long-term effects of a dental hygiene chew on the periodontal health of dogs. J. Vet. Dent. 16, 109–113.

Gorrel, C., Rawlings, J.M., 1996. The role of tooth brushing and diet in the maintenance of periodontal health in dogs. J. Vet. Dent. 13, 139–143.

Lindhe, J., Hamp, S.-E., Löe, H., 1975. Plaque induced periodontal disease in Beagle dogs. A 4-year clinical, roentgenographical and histometrical study. J. Periodontal Res. 10, 243–255.

Robins, G.N., 1976. Dropped jaw – mandibular neurapraxia in the dog. J. Small Anim. Pract. 17, 753.

Tromp, J.A., van Rijn, L.J., Jansen, J., 1986. Experimental gingivitis and frequency of tooth-brushing in the Beagle dog model. Clinical findings. J. Clin. Periodontol. 13, 190–194.

Recommended reading

Aspinall, V., 2007. Clinical Procedures in Veterinary Nursing, second ed. Butterworth-Heinemann, Oxford.
Within the chapter on Surgical Nursing Procedures there is a step-by-step guide to scaling and polishing teeth.

Gorrel, C., 2004. Veterinary Dentistry for the General Practitioner. W B Saunders, Edinburgh.

Gorrel, C., Derbyshire, S., 2005. Veterinary Dentistry for the Nurse and Technician. Butterworth-Heinemann, Edinburgh.

Holmstrom, S.E., 1999. Veterinary Dentistry for the Technician and Office Staff. W B Saunders, Philadelphia, PA.

CHAPTER 25

Principles of anaesthesia and analgesia

Michael Stevenson

Introduction

Anaesthesia is described as the reversible production of insensibility to pain. Pain is the conscious perception of a noxious stimulus. These definitions allow us to subdivide anaesthesia into:

- **Hypnosis** – reversible unconsciousness: the sleep induced by anaesthetic drugs
- **Analgesia** – the reduction or abolition of the perception of pain
- **Muscle relaxation** – flaccid paralysis of the skeletal muscles, which facilitates surgery and which tends to increase with dose of the anaesthetic agent. This is drug-specific, e.g. ketamine causes no relaxation. Neuromuscular blocking agents that cause complete muscular relaxation are not anaesthetic agents, as they do not affect consciousness.

The anaesthetist's aim is to achieve all the above without endangering the patient or the personnel administering the anaesthetic. The current methods available achieve this by careful choice of a variety of drugs in order to reduce the side effects of each.

Anaesthesia may be used for two main reasons:

- To perform a surgical procedure
- To restrain the patient for a diagnostic procedure.

All anaesthesia carries with it a considerable risk to the patient, so prior to the procedure a cost–benefit assessment should be carried out by veterinary staff and this should be discussed with the client before inducing the anaesthetic. In a recent study, anaesthetic death rates were 1 in 2055 for dogs and 1 in 736 in cats. In humans, the anaesthetic death rate is 1 in 10 000 (Broadbelt 2003). As veterinary knowledge improves, these rates should drop.

The veterinary nurse's role in the anaesthetic process is vital. The nurse will assess the animal preoperatively, administer any premedication, assist with induction and intubation and monitor the patient for the duration of the anaesthetic. Recovery is usually entirely the responsibility of the nurse, so a deep and firm understanding of the techniques, the drugs used and the consequences of anaesthesia is essential. In order to understand this most technically demanding area of nursing, the nurse must have a good understanding of anatomy, physiology and the pathological conditions that can influence anaesthesia.

Pre-anaesthetic assessment

This is usually performed by the veterinary surgeon prior to admission for a procedure but the nurse should be aware of the factors likely to affect the anaesthetic. Animals can be loosely divided into four risk groups:

1. **Normal healthy animals for routine procedures**, e.g. neutering – most likely to be admitted by a nurse and may not be seen by a vet. A full pre-anaesthetic examination should be carried out and should include a detailed history and a physical examination. The nurse should watch out for any conditions requiring further investigation, e.g. polydipsia may require blood tests and urine samples
2. **Healthy animals admitted for diagnostic procedures** – these may be quite well but have an underlying

medical condition, e.g. metabolic or cardiovascular disease. The vet will take this into consideration when preparing the anaesthetic

3. **Sick animals** – these have an increased anaesthetic risk and require increased care, increased supportive therapy and increased preparation, e.g. blood tests electrocardiogram (ECG), urine sample
4. **Emergency cases** – there is often little time for a full pre-anaesthetic assessment but maximum support and monitoring are essential.

Taking the history

The following are significant factors:

- **Age** – neonates and geriatrics may require different anaesthetic drugs from adult animals as they have different metabolisms
- **Weight** – every animal should be weighed to enable doses of anaesthetic agents and fluid therapy requirement to be calculated accurately. If an animal is underweight for its breed it may indicate metabolic problems, e.g. hyperthyroidism. Obesity may increase the anaesthetic risk by reducing respiratory capacity
- **Sex** – male animals tend to be more aggressive and have a lower percentage of body fat. Female animals may have sex-related conditions, e.g. pyometritis
- **Breed** – this is particularly significant in dogs, with their huge range of shapes and sizes. For example, boxers have an increased susceptibility to acetylpromazine; greyhounds/sighthounds are prone to poor redistribution of thiobarbiturates; brachycephalic breeds are adapted to chronic hypoxia and inspiratory stridor
- **Previous medical problems** – may be on medication, e.g. non-steroidal anti-inflammatory drugs (NSAIDs), which affect renal blood flow and clotting; cardiovascular drugs; insulin – patient may require glucose saline drip; polydipsia may indicate many underlying medical conditions.

Owner preparation

The owner should be asked to starve the patient for 12 hours prior to admission in order to ensure an empty stomach. This will reduce the risk of reflux of stomach contents into the mouth and possible aspiration into the lungs, which can cause respiratory obstruction or even pneumonia. Starvation may be undesirable in some cases; for example, neonates may become hypoglycaemic if starved. Also check that:

- The owner knows why the animal is coming in and the associated risks of the anaesthetic
- A consent form has been signed
- Contact details been left with the practice.

Physical examination

The following factors are significant:

- **Temperature** – 38.5°C. If pyrexia is present the animal may be toxaemic, the cardiovascular system may be compromised and oxygen consumption will be raised. Hypothermia reduces anaesthetic drug requirements

- **Pulse rate** – 80–120 beats/min in dogs and 120–180 beats/min in cats. Check quality – weak pulse may indicate cardiac problems or hypovolaemia. Does pulse rate correspond to heart rate?
- **Respiratory rate** – 8–12 breaths/min. Tachypnoea, e.g. more than 20–30 breaths/min, may be due to reduced lung volume, e.g. pleural fluid, thoracic mass, anaemia, pulmonary oedema, chronic pulmonary disease or pain. These may result in reduced oxygen transportation and uptake of volatile anaesthetic gas
- **Colour of mucous membranes** – may be:
  - White – anaemia: preoperative haematology required
  - Red – polycythaemia, i.e. too many red blood cells
  - Purple – cyanosis: reduced oxygen tension in blood
  - Dirty pink – toxaemia
  - Ecchymotic haemorrhages – clotting disorder, disseminated intravascular coagulation (DIC)
  - Grey – circulatory collapse.
- **Heart auscultation** – check the rate and rhythm and listen for murmurs, which may indicate valvular disease. If the heart rate and the pulse rate are different, this indicates an electrical problem with the heart and a pre-anaesthetic ECG is required
- **Lung auscultation** – rasping, wheezing or crackling sounds may indicate pulmonary disease or oedema; hyporesonance may indicate fluid build up in chest cavity or solid masses; hyperresonance may indicate pneumothorax
- **Hydration status** – check for skin turgor and texture of mucous membranes. Any pre-existing dehydration should be corrected prior to anaesthesia
- **Mentation** – evidence of normal central nervous system (CNS) function. Reduced CNS function can dramatically alter the anaesthetic requirements and may be due to brain tumours, hypothyroidism, reduced brain perfusion or toxaemia. Increased mentation may be due to hyperthyroidism, aggression or panic and will increase requirements.

A happy, active and calm dog is a better anaesthetic risk than either a dull, lethargic one or a nervous one.

Pre-anaesthetic blood tests

If there is anything suspicious in the animal's history or physical examination then further tests should be carried out. It is very common to offer a standard pre-anaesthetic blood test, which consists of six biochemical tests:

- **Alanine amino transferase (ALT)** – raised values indicate acute hepatic cell damage
- **Alkaline phosphatase (ALKP)** – raised values indicate biliary stasis but can also indicate intestinal or bone disease or raised steroid levels in the body
- **Blood urea nitrogen (BUN)** – raised in cases of advanced renal disease, dehydration, high protein meals or intestinal haemorrhage
- **Creatinine** – raised in cases of severe renal disease or dehydration
- **Glucose** – raised in diabetes mellitus and in 'stressed' cats but reduced in insulinomas, some liver tumours and starved neonates.

- **Total protein** – raised values may be due to dehydration or high globulin levels; reduced in protein losing diseases or severe liver disease.

Biochemical tests can be helpful but three other tests should be performed to provide a guide to diagnosis along with the clinical signs:

- **Packed cell volume (PCV)** – raised levels indicate dehydration; lowered levels indicate anaemia.
- **Urine specific gravity** – using a refractometer (see Ch. 29). This will show if an animal is drinking excessively, well before renal disease is indicated by raised creatinine levels. If an animal with renal insufficiency undergoes prolonged hypotension due to an anaesthetic this may precipitate renal failure
- **Urinalysis by dipstick examination** – covers a range of parameters that will reinforce the other test results.

Summary

A full history has been taken and the patient has had a physical examination. Food and water have been withheld prior to admission. A consent form has been completed and the owner's contact details have been taken. Appropriate pre-anaesthetic tests have been performed and the animal has been admitted to a warm, calm environment. Now the anaesthetic process can begin.

Premedication

The use of premedicant drugs can be reduced by a calm, reassuring environment. A happy, relaxed dog given reassurance by a caring veterinary nurse will gladly present its cephalic vein for catheterization without a large release of adrenaline (epinephrine). A fractious cat scruffed and held flat on a table for intravenous induction will be tachycardic, probably hypoxic, and have high levels of circulating adrenaline – leading to the risk of cardiac arrhythmias and possible cardiac arrest when a bolus of a cardiodepressant induction agent hits its myocardium.

The aim of premedication is to:

- Calm the animal, allowing for a smooth induction using a small dose of induction agent
- Enable easy handling of the animal by the veterinary staff.

The drugs used may continue to exert an effect during and after anaesthesia, resulting in a calm induction and maintenance period, reduced levels of anaesthetic agents, an uneventful recovery and intra- and postoperative analgesia. No one drug is able to achieve all these things, so mixtures of different drugs are used.

Chemical restraint using sedatives rarely comes without side effects and it is a commonly held misconception that using a sedative to perform a minor procedure holds fewer risks than a using a general anaesthetic. During the latter you have intravenous access, a direct supply of 100% oxygen, the ability to intubate and also close veterinary nurse monitoring. By contrast, when a sedative is given, the animal is often left in its kennel while the drugs take effect and monitoring is, at best, intermittent. During this period it may experience cardiovascular collapse, dyspnoea, regurgitation, etc. Thus a

Table 25.1 Standard neuroleptanalgesic doses

Drug	Canine dose rate	Feline dose rate
Acetylpromazine plus buprenorphine	0.03–0.05 mg/kg ACP plus 0.01 mg/kg buprenorphine	0.03–0.05 mg/kg ACP plus 0.01 mg/kg buprenorphine
Acetylpromazine plus pethidine	0.03–0.05 mg/kg ACP plus 2–4 mg/kg pethidine	0.03–0.05 mg/kg ACP plus 2 mg/kg pethidine
Acetylpromazine plus morphine	0.03 mg/kg ACP plus 0.3 mg/kg morphine	0.03 mg/kg ACP plus 0.2 mg/kg morphine

ACP, acetylpromazine.

premedicant sedative should really be regarded as the initial phase of the anaesthetic monitoring period and maximum care should be taken.

Each premedication must be tailored to the individual animal and based not only on body mass but also on the variables previously discussed. Routine premedication tends to follow individual practice protocols and is often reserved for routine surgical cases. Table 25.1 suggests some useful drug combinations.

Drugs used for premedication are sedatives and analgesics. The ideal combination should have few side effects, be predictable, fast acting and safe and be easy to administer, i.e. work well if given subcutaneously.

Sedatives

These drugs calm the animal, improve induction and recovery and reduce the quantity of anaesthetic agent required. They include the phenothiazines, butyrophenones, benzodiazepines and alpha-2 agonists.

Phenothiazines

Anxiolytic sedatives. This group includes acetylpromazine, chlorpromazine, promethazine and methotrimeprazine.

- **Acetylpromazine (ACP)** – the most common. It is a yellow solution at a concentration of 2 mg/ml for small animal use. It can be given subcutaneously (s.c.), intramuscularly (i.m.) or intravenously (i.v.) in order of increasing speed of action. Its effects are shown in Table 25.2.

Efficacy:

- 65% are sedated
- 30% are very sedated
- 5% are not sedated or may be stimulated.

ACP is safe to use in normal animals because increasing the dose increases the duration of the effect rather than increasing the effect; in high doses it produces a cataleptic state.

Butyrophenones

Similar to phenothiazines. The one most frequently used in practice is fluanisone as part of a commercial mixture with fentanyl.

Table 25.2 Effects of acetylpromazine

Advantages	Disadvantages
Synergizes with opiates	Hypotension due to vasodilation
Anti-arrhythmic in sensitized myocardium	– can cause severe problems in hypovolaemic or hypotensive
Anti-emetic	animals leading to cardiovascular
Anti-histamine (useful in mast cell tumour surgery)	collapse
Spasmolytic	Unpredictable – stimulated animals can fight against its
Long acting which smoothes recovery	effects
	Long lasting – day cases may be still sedated when sent home
	Hypothermia – reduces thermoregulation and cutaneous vasodilation
	Breed sensitivity – boxers are very sensitive to the effects

Table 25.3 Effects of alpha-2 agonists

Body system	Effect
Central nervous system	Profound sedation dependent on dose
	Excellent visceral analgesia
	Moderate somatic analgesia
Cardiovascular system	Profound bradycardia and bradyarrhythmias
	Very reduced respiratory rate
	Peripheral vasoconstriction, which causes initial hypertension, followed by peripheral vasodilation with marked hypotension and hypothermia
Gastrointestinal system	Initial emesis
	Intestinal relaxation
Uterus	Ecbolic, may cause abortion
Kidney	Inhibition of ADH causes diuresis
	Hyperglycaemia may also cause glycosuria

Benzodiazepines

The main benzodiazepines used are diazepam and midazolam. This class of drug is widely used and abused in human practice but its use is increasing in small animal anaesthesia.

Benzodiazepines are anxiolytic, hypnotic, muscle-relaxant and anticonvulsant. In healthy animals they cause little sedation but reduce inhibitions, which makes the animal less easy to control! In sick animals the sedative effect is much greater and the cardiovascular side effects are minimal, providing safe premedication or sedation even in severely compromised animals. They are useful in reducing the dose of anaesthetic required. There is a specific antagonist, flumazenil, which may be used for rapid reversal of the effect in critical cases or for day cases:

- **Diazepam** – available in two preparations – an oil-based form given i.v. or i.m., which may cause some phlebitis and pain on injection, and a milky white emulsion given i.v. only, which is less irritant
- **Midazolam** – water-soluble, given by i.v. or i.m injection. This is more potent than diazepam but lasts half as long.

Alpha-2 agonists

These drugs – **xylazine, medetomidine** – have had a huge impact on veterinary anaesthesia because of their predictability and reversibility. They act on the alpha-2 noradrenaline (norepinephrine) and adrenaline (epinephrine) receptors centrally and peripherally and have many effects (Table 25.3). **Dexmedetomidine** is a new alpha-2 agonist which is licensed in Britain as Dexdomitor 0.5 mg/ml for intravenous and intramuscular use in dogs and intramuscular use in cats. Its dose rate is based on body surface area and conversion tables are provided by the manufacturer. Its effects are as for other alpha-2 agonists. They are all very powerful sedatives, capable of producing states very close to general anaesthesia. As premedicants they reduce the amount of induction and maintenance agents required. They can be given s.c., i.m., i.v. and orally.

There is a specific antagonist – **atipamezole**. One of the main benefits of alpha-2 agonists is that you can easily reverse the sedation, recovery occurs in 5–10 minutes after i.m injection and day cases can be returned to their owners straight away. However, although the animal appears awake and ambulant, the cardiovascular effects are still present and sedation may reoccur. The owner should be warned and advised that the animal should be kept warm and under observation. (**Note:** the bradycardia seen with alpha-2 agonists should not be reversed with atropine. This will increase the initial hypertension, potentially causing ocular or CNS damage.)

Analgesics

These drugs, which are used to relieve pain, are used in a premedicant combination to synergize with the sedatives, increase the depth of sedation and provide a baseline of intraoperative analgesia. Premedication with a sedative combined with an opioid is termed **neuroleptanalgesia**. The degree of sedation achieved is much greater than with either a sedative or opioid alone. Ideally, the mixture should be combined with a preoperative dose of an NSAID if the animal is a suitable candidate for this class of drug.

Analgesics and their provision will be covered in this section as well as their use for premedication. Veterinary nurses should be acutely aware of the need for analgesia, as they are the ones who will be monitoring the anaesthetic and postanaesthetic period and will be the primary assessor of pain in their patients.

Pain is a protective reflex, as it is part of the 'fight or flight' reflex. Pain is the conscious perception of a noxious stimulus, so upper CNS function is involved. Pain is also subjective, so what may be a minor pain to one individual may be intolerable to another. Animals cannot understand why they are in pain and do not have the capacity to understand that the pain will go away, so adequate provision of analgesia in animals is important at a physiological and emotional level.

Table 25.4 Drug groups used for pre-emptive and balanced analgesia

Sites at which pain stimuli act and the response produced	Drugs used to reduce pain	Site of action
Cerebral cortex – conscious perception of pain leads to vocalization, aggression, etc.	Non-steroidal anti-inflammatory drugs/glucocorticoids	Peripherally (some central effects)
	Local anaesthetics	Peripherally
Hypothalamus – induces fear, flight response, i.e. raised heart rate, raised blood pressure, etc.	Benzodiazepines Alpha-2 agonists	Spinal cord Spinal cord/central nervous system
Medulla – raised heart rate, blood pressure and respiratory rate	Opioids	Spinal cord/central nervous system
Spinal cord – withdrawal reflex	General anaesthetics	Central nervous system

Nociception is perhaps just as important to the anaesthetist. This is the unconscious perception of pain by receptors classed as nociceptors, e.g. chemoreceptors and baroreceptors. Their stimulation may result in reflex activity such as altered blood pressure, increased respiratory rate, increased heart rate and withdrawal of part of the body from a painful stimulus, which may ultimately change the physiology of the patient (Table 25.4). Thus the prevention of pain and nociception are extremely important prior to, during and after an anaesthetic and analgesia can be provided by acting at one or more of these sites.

Using these drugs prior to the noxious stimulus being applied is termed **pre-emptive analgesia** and this method is believed to increase the analgesic's efficacy. Blocking the pain impulses at several sites using different drugs is termed **balanced analgesia**.

Non-steroidal anti-inflammatory drugs/glucocorticoids

These reduce peripheral inflammation and some also have CNS effects. Inflammation of a tissue results in vasodilation, oedema and heat at the site, which are due to the release of cyclooxygenase and lipoxygenase. NSAIDs block cyclooxygenase and glucocorticoids block cyclooxygenase and lipoxygenase. If these drugs are given preoperatively before inflammation develops they have a much greater effect. Commonly used NSAIDs include carprofen, meloxicam, firocoxib, tepoxalin, tolfenamic acid, aspirin and phenylbutazone (Table 25.5).

Side effects of NSAIDs can be a problem in some animals, so care should always be taken. In the kidney they block prostaglandin production and compromise renal blood flow, so in patients with hypotension they can cause renal ischaemia. This can be more of a problem in animals with pre-existing or subclinical renal disease.

NSAIDs, especially the older formulations, may also cause gastrointestinal ulceration and increase the clotting time. Most remain active for some time and provide adequate analgesia once the patient has gone home. This can be prolonged by continued administration of tablets by the owner.

Corticosteroids

These are not normally used perioperatively for analgesia as they reduce the rate of healing. However, they are still useful in controlling oedema and inflammation in respiratory tract surgery and, more controversially, in spinal surgery.

Local anaesthetics

These are underused in small animal surgery despite their widespread use and efficacy in large animals. They are extremely useful in patients with cardiovascular or metabolic problems where general anaesthesia would be dangerous.

Drugs used as local anaesthetics are weak acids that act on the nerve fibres and prevent them from transmitting impulses to the CNS. The pain fibres in a nerve are more sensitive than the rest of the fibres to these drugs, so local analgesia is theoretically possible without causing complete loss of motor function. In reality, all the nerve fibres tend to be blocked and a degree of loss of function of the anaesthetized area should be expected. Inflamed areas are less responsive to these drugs because local acidosis reduces their availability to the tissues.

Local anaesthetic drugs include:

- **Lignocaine (lidocaine)** – the most widely used drug. It comes as a gel, topical cream, aerosol, sterile injectable solution and a solution with preservative ± adrenaline (epinephrine). This is added to cause local vasoconstriction, which keeps the anaesthetic at the site and prolongs its actions. Care must be exercised in using such solutions in poorly vascularized areas where ischaemia could result. Lignocaine has a rapid onset of about 5 minutes and lasts 50–90 minutes without adrenaline or 80 minutes with adrenaline: 1% and 2% solutions are available and there may be some local tissue reaction and stinging on infiltration; however, they spread well in the tissues. If accidentally given intravenously, lignocaine can cause cardiac arrest or syncope. The toxic threshold of 10 mg/kg is easily reached in cats so 2 ml of a 2% solution is the maximum dose in a 4 kg cat.
- **Procaine** – an old-fashioned drug but still available combined with adrenaline (epinephrine). Slower onset and shorter-acting
- **Amethocaine** – used topically as 1% solution for desensitizing the cornea for ophthalmic procedures
- **Bupivacaine** – four times as potent as lignocaine. Available as 0.5% and 2% solutions with a similar rate of onset and depth of effect as lignocaine but much longer-acting – up to 8 hours. It is well tolerated by the tissues ± adrenaline (epinephrine) but accidental intravenous injection will cause cardiac arrest, as it is severely myocardiotoxic
- **Cinchocaine** – very powerful, only low doses are required. It is severely myocardiotoxic and is now mostly used in combination with quinalbarbitone for intravenous euthanasia.

461

Table 25.5 Dose rates of commonly used NSAIDs

Drug	Canine dose	Feline dose	Comments
Aspirin	10–20 mg/kg p.o. t.i.d.	10 mg/kg p.o. e.o.d.	Gastric irritant Prolonged metabolism in cats
Carprofen (Rimadyl)	2–4 mg/kg s.c., i.v., p.o. b.i.d.	2 mg/kg s.c. s.i.d.	Less renal and gastric toxicity, chronic use in dogs
Flunixin (Finadyne)	1 mg/kg s.c p.o. s.i.d.	1 mg/kg s.c. sid	Renal and gastric toxicity Powerful analgesic and anti-endotoxin effect
Firocoxib (Previcox)	5 mg/ kg s.i.d.	Not used in cats	Given 2 h prior to surgery and for 3 days after
Ketoprofen (Ketofen)	1–2 mg/kg s.c. p.o. b.i.d.	1–2 mg/kg s.c. p.o. b.i.d.	Renal and gastric toxicity
Meloxicam (Metacam)	0.2 mg/kg s.c. i.v. p.o. s.i.d.	0.2 mg/kg s.c. p.o. s.i.d.	Fewer gastric and renal problems, chronic use possible
Paracetamol	25–30 mg/kg p.o. q.i.d.	Toxic	Less gastric irritation
Phenylbutazone	10 mg/kg p.o. b.i.d.		Gastric irritation
Tepoxalin	10 mg/kg p.o. s.i.d.		
Tolfenamic acid	4 mg/kg s.c., i.m., p.o.	4 mg/kg s.c., p.o.	Not preoperatively

Clinical use of local anaesthesia

- **Topical** – superficial desensitization of an area:
  - *Local anaesthetic cream* applied to the skin prior to catheter placement
  - *Proxymetacaine drops* – used in ophthalmology to allow minor corneal procedures
  - *Laryngeal sprays* – applied to the larynxes of cats to enable intubation without reflex spasm
  - *Intrapleural* – bupivacaine can be instilled over the pleural surfaces to reduce postoperative pain after thoracotomy
  - *Intradermal* – injection with a fine needle to create a desensitized weal in the skin, allowing placement of large-bore catheters, needles, etc.
- **Local infiltration of tissues**, e.g. skin or muscle. Use a fine-bore needle for the initial injection, which creates a desensitized area and subsequent injections pass through the site to minimize further injection pain. An incision line can be made using this method but local anaesthetic alone can cause vasodilation and increased haemorrhage at the site. If adrenaline-augmented solutions are used, vasoconstriction at the site can delay healing
- **Field block** – e.g. on the chest wall or flank. Here the pattern of innervation allows infiltration of local anaesthetic far away from the site of surgery so analgesia is complete but wound healing is not compromised
- **Ring block** – e.g. around a distal limb or digit. Three-hundred and sixty degree injections desensitize the distal area but ischaemia could be a problem
- **Intrasynovial** – only used to help identify painful bursae or joints in lame animals.

Regional nerve block

A small dose of local anaesthetic is administered around a nerve – described as being perineural, so desensitizing the whole area it supplies. This is a greatly underused and very effective technique but requires a detailed knowledge of nerve anatomy:

- **Intercostal block**. – the intercostal nerves lie caudal to each rib next to the artery and vein: 0.5 ml of lignocaine will desensitize each nerve and three or four nerve blocks will provide excellent analgesia for a thoracotomy site. This makes postoperative recovery essentially pain-free and a great deal safer because deeper respiration will ensure better oxygenation
- **Inferior alveolar nerve** – perineural lignocaine injected where the nerve exits the mental foramen will desensitize the rostral mandible, e.g. for fracture fixation or tumour resection
- **Optical block** – infiltration of the palpebral branch of the facial nerve and auriculotemporal nerve desensitizes the orbital fissure, i.e. the orbit, conjunctiva, eyelids and eyebrows.

Intravenous regional anaesthesia

This is used for surgery on distal limbs. The arterial and venous blood supply is occluded by a tourniquet, preferably after application of an Esmarch bandage to exsanguinate the limb, and lignocaine is injected intravenously. This provides excellent anaesthesia in 10–15 minutes and lasts as long as the tourniquet remains in place, so operative times of up to 45 minutes are easily achieved.

Spinal and epidural block

- **Epidural** – commonly used in large-animal anaesthesia as it is technically easy and is useful for perineal, anal, tail and pelvic limb surgery. The site must be prepared aseptically and a spinal needle should be introduced between vertebrae L7 and S1. The drug is injected into the epidural space between the dura mater and the periosteum of the spinal canal to block the nerves as they leave the spinal cord.
  Choice of drug depends on what effect is needed: e.g. local anaesthetics produce excellent analgesia and

paralysis of muscles; opiates provide analgesia alone. Dose and volume will determine how far cranially these effects occur. For prolonged analgesia, catheters may be placed epidurally to allow top-up doses. Vasodilation and consequent hypotension may occur in some tissues, so intravenous fluid therapy is required. To avoid respiratory paralysis the maximum dose is 1 ml/5 kg of 0.5% bupivacaine or 2% lignocaine.

- **Spinal anaesthesia** – rarely used and involves introduction of drug doses of half those used for epidural injection between L5 and L6 into the cerebrospinal fluid surrounding the spinal cord.

Opioids

These are the most widely used group of analgesic drugs. They were originally derived from opium – the dried latex from unripe Himalayan poppy seed heads (*Papaver somniferum*). As the plant's name suggests, they also cause a variable degree of sedation. Opiates are now synthetically manufactured but the term opioids will be used here to cover both natural and synthetic forms. They all act by receptor mediation and there are four main receptor types in the brain and spinal cord – mu and kappa receptors, which are the main ones targeted by the clinically used opioids, and sigma and delta receptors.

As opioids are subject to recreational abuse by humans, the use of opioids is controlled by the Misuse of Drugs Act 1971 and the drugs are grouped into Schedules CD 1, 2 and 3. Only Schedule 2 and 3 drugs are used in veterinary medicine (see Chapter 17).

Opioid drugs have many useful effects and many disadvantages depending on the individual drug. They may cause profound analgesia and variable sedation, with little effect on the cardiovascular system. They will synergize with anaesthetic drugs, lowering the requirement of the latter, and also induce a sense of euphoria and well-being in the patient. However, other forms of the drug may cause dysphoria and anxiety. They may also cause increased cerebral blood pressure, urinary retention, gastrointestinal effects such as constipation and vomiting, and in some cases respiratory depression. It should be emphasized that not all these side effects are caused by all opioids; they are dependent on the individual form of the drug and the action of the receptors that are stimulated by it.

Administration

Opioids can be administered in many ways (Table 25.6). The drug dose depends on the degree of pain present and a lower dose can be used as part of premedication to achieve pre-emptive analgesia. In severe pain much higher doses can be used without unwanted side effects, so if a patient has been given a standard dose but still appears to be in pain then incrementally higher doses may be given until the pain is controlled.

Examples of opioid drugs and their specific uses are shown in Table 25.7. Premedicating with opioids before surgery will reduce the quantity of drugs required to induce and maintain anaesthesia and will reduce the levels of pain intra- and postoperatively. Opioids given prior to a painful stimulus will reduce subsequent doses required to keep the animal

Table 25.6 Administration of opioids

Route	Comments
Intravenous	Not pethidine
Intramuscular	Pethidine stings
Subcutaneous	Variable uptake
Oral	Metabolism affects efficacy
Sublingual	Technically difficult in animals
Rectal	Suppositories
Epidural	Sterility required
Transdermal	Fentanyl patches

pain-free. Higher doses will be required if pain is already present.

Naloxone is a specific opioid antagonist that reverses the effects of mu-binding opioids, so can be used in cases of overdose. It has a short action, so repeat doses may be required.

Anticholinergics

In the past, anticholinergic drugs have been given as part of the premedication but there is little general indication for them now. Atropine was used to dry the secretions stimulated by the use of ether as an inhaled anaesthetic, as it is a respiratory irritant. As modern anaesthetic gases do not cause such irritation there is no need for atropine, and in fact it can jeopardize the anaesthetic by stimulating tachycardia during a period of hypoxia prior to intubation. It is still a valuable drug where indicated and is best kept for specific purposes, e.g. reversal of severe bradycardia.

Summary

Premedication aims to ease the induction of anaesthesia, reduce the quantity of anaesthetic drugs required and provide pre-emptive baseline analgesia. A combination of ACP, an opioid and an NSAID is ideal in healthy animals. Other drugs may be specifically indicated for premedication, e.g. antibiotics, histamine blockers in mast-cell tumour surgery.

Anaesthesia

Anaesthesia can be considered to take place in two stages:

- **Induction** – administration of drugs that bring about a state of unconsciousness
- **Maintenance** – process by which a state of unconsciousness is continued until such time as the patient is allowed to regain consciousness.

Injectable anaesthetic drugs

In small animal practice most anaesthesia is induced by means of injection and maintenance is controlled by inhalation agents. However, injectable agents can also be used to

Table 25.7 Examples of opioids used in veterinary practice

Drug name/action/schedule	Dose rate and route of administration	Comments
Morphine/mu agonist/2	0.1–0.4 mg/kg s.c., i.m., i.v., epidural, rectal	Not licensed in cats and dogs. Very powerful and predictable. Lasts for 3–4 h. Sedative effect except in high doses in cats, where it may cause excitement. Slower elimination in cats because of lack of liver glucuronidation
Pethidine/mu agonist/2	2–4 mg/kg i.m., **not** i.v. as it causes histamine release	Lasts for 2 h. Ten per cent of the strength of morphine. Has vagolytic effects. Can be used to provide additional analgesia to supplement that provided by drugs that are mixed agonists. Excellent for gastrointestinal surgery and pancreatitis
Papaveretum/mu agonist/2	0.1–0.4 mg/kg i.m.	Not licensed for cats and dogs. Less potent than morphine. Lasts for 2 h. Excellent sedative, especially if combined with acetylpromazine
Methadone/mu agonist/2	0.1–0.4 mg/kg i.m. or i.v.	Moderate analgesia. Less sedation and more dysphoria
Fentanyl/mu agonist/2	1–10 µg/kg i.v.	Rapid onset. 50 times as potent as morphine. Lasts for 20–30 min, so used during an operation. Can cause respiratory depression so IPPV may be needed. Combined with fluanisone as a neuroleptic anaesthetic
Alfentanil/mu agonist/2	10–25 µg/kg i.v. and by infusion, as it is rapidly metabolized	Not licensed in cats and dogs. 12 times as potent as morphine. Very rapid effect. Apnoea may occur with clinical dose – use in combination with an anticholinergic drug. Used as part of balanced induction in high-risk patients
Etorphine/mu agonist/2	–	No longer licensed. Extremely potent and long-lasting. Marked respiratory depression. Dangerous to handle. Specific reversal agent – diprenorphine
Buprenorphine/partial agonist/3	3–10 µg/kg i.m. i.v. s.c.	Takes 45 min to have an effect. Lasts for 6–8 h in dogs and 12 h in cats. Useful for postoperative pain. Can be used to reverse respiratory depression caused by overdose of mu agonists without abolishing analgesia
Butorphanol/partial agonist/3	0.05–0.3 mg/kg i.m. i.v.	Very poor analgesia somatically; moderate visceral analgesia. Excellent antitussive – good for bronchoscopy. Excellent sedation in combination with alpha-2 agonists. Should not be used as sole means of analgesia.

Pure agonist – affects only one type of receptor. Partial agonist – affects both mu and kappa receptors, being either an agonist or an antagonist at mu and an agonist at kappa receptors. Dose rate is critical – if the maximum dose is given and the patient is still in pain, increasing the dose further may reduce the analgesic effect

IPPV, intermittent positive pressure ventilation

maintain anaesthesia, either alone if their length of activity is adequate or by infusing them intravenously at set rates. If this technique is used for safety reasons, an airway must be maintained and oxygen must be supplied. Most induction agents are given intravenously to produce an immediate response, but some can be given intramuscularly.

Intravenous injection

Placing an indwelling intravenous catheter into the cephalic vein prior to induction is cheap and technically easy. The site should be aseptically prepared and an 'over the needle' catheter should be secured with adhesive tape. A suitable giving port should be attached to it, e.g. three-way tap. This allows for safer induction and for administration of other drugs during the anaesthetic. If an anaesthetic emergency occurs it could mean the difference between life and death. Indwelling catheters should be changed on the third day after placement to prevent ascending thrombophlebitis.

Mode of action

These drugs act directly on the CNS, which receives at least 25% of cardiac output so as the drug is injected, the CNS is immediately bathed in it. Once a critical level of drug has reached the CNS, unconsciousness occurs. As the drug concentration drops in the systemic circulation, so the drug is redistributed away from the CNS, allowing consciousness to resume.

Systemic drug concentration depends on redistribution of the drug to less-well-perfused tissues, e.g. muscle and fat, and then metabolism of the drug by the liver, kidneys and other organs. Duration of action of the induction agent depends on individual drug properties and on individual animal characteristics, e.g. thin, poorly muscled animals, have less tissue so redistribution is slower, prolonging unconsciousness. Metabolic problems, e.g. liver or renal disease, will also reduce metabolism of the drugs, so increasing the duration of drug action.

Drug types

Barbiturates

Examples include thiopentone (thiopental), methohexitone (methohexital), pentobarbitone (pentobarbital) and phenobarbitone (phenobarbital). These drugs all cause unconsciousness and muscle relaxation but provide very little analgesia. They cause a degree of dose-related cardiorespiratory depression and, as they are strongly alkaline sodium salts, they are very irritant to the tissues if not administered intravenously.

Thiopentone sodium (thiopental) has been the most widely used induction agent in veterinary medicine in Britain but at present there are no manufacturers of this compound.

This situation may be remedied in the future, so the notes on its use will continue to be included in this textbook. It is made up by reconstituting a sulphur yellow powder with water to achieve a 5% or 2.5% solution. Only 2.5% or less concentrated solution should be used in small animals because of the severe tissue necrosis associated with perivascular injection of 5% solutions. If a perivascular injection does occur, copious amounts of sterile saline or 2% lignocaine should be infused into the affected tissues:

- **Dose rate**: 5–20 mg/kg (average 10 mg/kg) given i.v. High doses should be avoided because the drug is only slowly metabolized by the body, resulting in prolonged recovery. The induction dose and the risk of cardiovascular depression can be substantially reduced by combining induction with intravenous diazepam
- **Contraindications:** thiopentone (thiopental) may cause hypotension, reduced cardiac output and transient respiratory depression. It binds to proteins, so care should be taken in hypoalbuminaemic animals. It redistributes rapidly to the muscles and fat and is metabolized by the liver but it may still last for several hours in the body. Care should be exercised in cases of renal disease, cardiovascular disease and liver disease. Use in pregnancy is not advised as it will cause respiratory depression in the neonates.

Special breed sensitivity has been reported in sight hounds e.g. greyhounds, Afghan hounds, whippets, borzois, and salukis, where it causes prolonged recovery.

Methohexitone (Methohexital) is an ultra-short-acting barbiturate prepared from dry powder before use. Causes apnoea on induction lasting about a minute so intermittent positive pressure ventilation (IPPV) may initially be required. It is rapidly redistributed and metabolized. Recovery is rapid and may be violent, so premedication with ACP and an opioid is desirable:

- **Dose rate**: 4–6 mg/kg as a 1% solution given i.v.

Pentobarbitone (pentobarbital) is associated with relatively slow induction and recovery. It is mainly used for controlling status epilepticus, as is **phenobarbitone** (pentobarbital) solution:

- **Dose rate**: 25–30 mg/kg i.v. No longer available as a sterile solution so now used only for euthanasia.

Phenol anaesthetics

The only phenol anaesthetic in veterinary use is propofol. It is insoluble in water so is either dissolved in or comes as a nano–droplet formulation, which produces its characteristic white milky appearance. It is non-irritant to tissues but intravenous injection of a room temperature solution can cause pain. It does not contain a preservative, so once a vial is opened it should be used that day. Propofol produces rapid dose-dependent induction of anaesthesia but apnoea is a common problem unless it is administered very slowly. Occasionally, muscle activity and twitching is seen upon induction, but this generally resolves once gaseous maintenance is stabilized.

- **Dose rate**:
  - **Induction** – Dogs – up to 6.5 mg/kg (0.65 ml/kg) body weight. The dose should be titrated against the response of the patient and may be administered over a period of 30–60 seconds. The use of premedicants may significantly reduce the propofol requirements.
    Cats – up to 8.0 mg/kg (0.80 ml/kg) body weight. The dose should be titrated against the patient's response and may be administered over a period of 30–60 seconds. The use of premedicants may significantly reduce the propofol requirements.
  - **Maintenance** – can be used in dogs because it is not cumulative: dose 0.3–0.5 mg/kg/min but provides no analgesia
- **Contraindications**: in dogs, propofol is rapidly metabolized in the liver and lung, so recovery is rapid. However, the cat liver is not capable of detoxifying phenols quickly, so recovery time is similar to that of thiopental. It is the drug of choice for use in dogs with liver disease but it is contraindicated in cats with liver disease. It is a potent venodilator and can cause profound hypotension. It binds strongly to proteins, so care must be taken in cases of hypoalbumnaemia, in renal disease and in geriatric patients.

Propofol has a rapid rate of clearance in dogs, so often the early part of the anaesthetic is more unstable than with thiopental. The depth of anaesthesia must be closely monitored for the first 10 minutes because the dog may suddenly seem to become very light as the effects of the propofol are lost and at that time an insufficient level of anaesthetic gas may have been inhaled.

PropoClear is a unique nano-droplet microemulsion that results in an essentially clear and colourless presentation versus all the other available propofol 'milky' formulations. Unlike other formulations, PropoClear includes preservatives which confer a 28-day broached shelf-life. This allows larger presentations (50 ml or 100 ml) depending on practice requirements. It is also licensed for use with premedicants such as acepromazine.

Steroid anaesthetics

Alfaxalone (Alfaxan) is the only one now in use in veterinary medicine. It is a 10 mg/ml aqueous solution of alfaxalone and it can be used in cats and dogs. Alfaxan is solubilized in cyclodextrin, which does not cause histamine release unlike the Cremaphor EL used in the previously licensed product Saffan. In dogs induction is achieved using 2 mg/kg iv and in cats it is used at 5 mg/kg. Induction is smooth but apnoea can be a problem especially in dogs and may last 1–2 minutes. IPPV may be initially required. Anaesthesia may also be maintained using alfaxalone in intermittent boluses or by constant rate infusion as it has no cumulative kinetics and is metabolized by the liver and excreted via the kidneys. Alfaxalone has a very high therapeutic index so slight overdose is seldom dangerous, it has only minor effects on the cardiac index and it is non-irritant if given perivascularly. It has no analgesic properties but gives good muscle relaxation and an uneventful recovery. It use is increasing as thiopentone becomes less widely available

Dissociative anaesthetics

Ketamine is widely used in veterinary medicine. It produces a unique state of anaesthesia in which unconsciousness is achieved while airway reflexes and some cranial nerve reflexes are intact, the eyes remain open and pupils dilate. Salivation occurs and skeletal muscle tone is maintained but changes to the cardiovascular system are minimal and blood pressure is maintained.

Ketamine has moderate analgesic properties and a high therapeutic index. It may be given intravenously or intramuscularly but, as it is acidic, it stings on intramuscular injection. It is usually combined with a sedative with good muscle-relaxant properties, e.g. a benzodiazepine or an alpha-2 agonist:

- **Dose rate**: wide range as it is never used by itself so dose rate depends on the other components
- **Duration**: anaesthesia lasts 20–40 minutes but effects may be seen for up to 10 hours
- **Contraindications**: Ketamine is excreted via the kidneys so should not be used in cats with renal disease. Dogs metabolize it in the liver, so it should not be used in liver disease. It raises intracranial pressure and should not be used in head trauma.

Diazepam plus ketamine – this combination is excellent for providing 5–10 minutes of light general anaesthesia in cardiovascularly compromised patients.

Alpha-2 agonist plus ketamine – a commonly used combination, especially in cats, where the intramuscular route is useful in fractious patients. This can provide light chemical restraint up to full general anaesthesia depending on the dose, for example:

- ketamine 5 mg/kg + medetomidine 0.05 mg/kg i.m. provides adequate anaesthesia for minor procedures
- ketamine 5–10 mg/kg + medetomidine 0.05–0.08 mg/kg + buprenorphine 0.01 mg/kg provides adequate anaesthesia for routine neutering.

Dexmedetomidine – this product has recently been released for use in the UK. It is a purer form of the alpha-2 agonist medetomidine and is marketed as Dexdomitor (Pfizer Animal Health) as a sterile solution of 0.5 mg/ml.

- Very small doses are required so the dose is based on body surface area with smaller doses per m^2 being required for larger animals. It can be administered i.m. or i.v. in dogs and i.m. in cats.
- It may be used as a sedative or as a premedicant and can be used in conjunction with ketamine in the same syringe for general anaesthesia or with opiates for more profound sedation and analgesia
- The effects are the same as for other alpha-2 agonists. The peak effect occurs 15 minutes after an i.v. injection and 30 minutes after i.m. injection.
- As with other alpha-2-agonists the effects may be reversed with atipamezole.

Note: Dissociative anaesthetics are widely abused by humans so they should be kept in a locked drugs cabinet and it is recommended that records of its use are kept in the dangerous drugs book.

Induction of critically ill animals

Induction of anaesthesia in critically ill animals can precipitate catastrophic cardiovascular depression because they are often physiologically on a 'knife edge' and even a minor alteration in cardiac output or oxygenation can prove fatal. The induction period must be rapid, stress-free, cause minimal physiological changes and be followed by intubation and a supply of 100% oxygen. Preoxygenation and fluid therapy are essential and all parameters must be closely monitored. The use of a benzodiazepine with a powerful opioid and minimal dose of an induction agent such as ketamine alfaxalone or propofol is recommended., e.g. diazepam 0.2 mg/kg + fentanyl 0.05 mg/kg 2–3 mg/kg + propofol i.v.

Inhalational agents

These agents are volatile liquids, i.e. they evaporate easily at room temperature to form a gas that is inhaled. They can be used to induce, or more commonly to maintain, anaesthesia. They are carried into the body via the respiratory tract by a carrier gas, which is usually oxygen ± nitrous oxide. The chemicals dissolve in the blood and cross the blood–brain barrier to affect the CNS, causing unconsciousness.

Halothane and isoflurane are the principal volatile agents used in animals but sevoflurane and desflurane may also be seen in practice. Diethyl ether, chloroform and methoxyflurane no longer have a role in modern veterinary practice.

Carrier gases

Oxygen – O_2

Oxygen is essential for normal aerobic metabolism. It makes up 20% of atmospheric air but is used at a minimum of 33% in anaesthesia. The normal PaO_2 in dogs is 85–105 mmHg; the normal PaO_2 in cats is 100–115 mmHg. Oxygen is supplied in black cylinders with a white collar.

The haemoglobin in red blood cells is usually about 95% saturated when breathing room air. This should rise to 100% on inspiration of enriched oxygen, assuming that there is no cardiovascular or respiratory depression. Only a small change in haemoglobin saturation is possible but, as O_2 is a very soluble gas, total oxygen saturation of whole blood can increase and the PaO_2 can reach 500 mmHg. A rule of thumb is that the PaO_2 should be five times the inspired concentration. If it is not, there may be a perfusion ventilation problem.

Respiration is normally controlled by the carbon dioxide (CO_2) concentration in the arterial blood, which is normally 30–40 mmHg. If the concentration rises the chemoreceptors in the brain and vascular system stimulate increased respiration. However if PaO_2 drops to 60 mmHg – hypoxaemia – it becomes the driving force for respiration independent of the $PaCO_2$. Hypoxaemia or low blood oxygen is an extremely serious situation, as it can cause irreparable brain damage, cardiac arrhythmias and arrest, and kidney damage. If an animal's PaO_2 drops to about 85 mmHg it should be ventilated and if it reaches 60 mmHg it should be treated as an emergency.

Hypoxaemia may be due to:

- Poor O_2 uptake, e.g. lung disease – tumours, infections, pulmonary oedema – or cardiac disease – lung perfusion problems. In lateral recumbency more blood perfuses the lower lung and more gas enters the uppermost lung, causing a ventilation–perfusion mismatch. This not only reduces oxygen uptake but also reduces uptake of the volatile agent, so altering the depth of anaesthesia. Thus prolonged anaesthesia in one position is not recommended

- Hypoventilation – very common in anaesthesia because of the respiratory depressant effects of the drugs.

In cases of hypoxaemia, increasing the oxygen supply to the animal may not be adequate to correct the problem and actively ventilating the patient is often even more important. Even in a normal stable anaesthetic where the animal appears to be breathing satisfactorily, the anaesthetist should periodically 'sigh' the patient's lungs, i.e. provide a supramaximal tidal excursion to fully expand the alveoli, which may be undergoing progressive atelectasis, i.e. collapse.

Note: Oxygen toxicity is often mentioned but is seldom important. A dog would need to be on 100% O_2 for 3 days before it died. There is a risk of fire and explosions when using oxygen in pressurized containers.

Nitrous oxide – N_2O

Nitrous oxide is odourless, non-irritant and non-flammable but will support combustion. It is available in blue cylinders as a liquid at 40 atm pressure, which means that a pressure gauge will always read full until most of the liquid is gone (be careful!). It is insoluble in blood, so it rapidly enters and leaves the blood stream, which can be beneficial in inducing anaesthesia because it increases the rate of uptake of the volatile agent. It also diffuses into gas-filled areas of the body, e.g. gas-dilated intestine, so should not be used in cases of gastric tympany, intestinal obstruction or pneumothorax. Once anaesthesia is terminated there can be a sudden release of large quantities of N_2O into the alveoli, reducing the alveolar oxygen concentration and causing diffusion hypoxia. To avoid this, oxygen should be supplied at 100% for 10–15 minutes following cessation of N_2O.

The main use of N_2O in veterinary practice is as a carrier gas but it also has marked analgesic properties and is useful in reducing the amount of volatile agent needed. For example, N_2O at 66% will reduce halothane requirements by 25%. It is not metabolized and helps to support cardiac output, respiratory rate and blood pressure. It can be used in all circuits but care must be taken in low-flow rebreathing systems, where it can build up, so reducing oxygen tension. N_2O is not absorbed by charcoal canisters so active scavenging is essential.

Note: Prolonged exposure of theatre staff to N_2O can lead to bone marrow toxicity because of vitamin B_{12} oxidation, and it is also an abortifacient.

Mode of action of the volatile agents

These volatile agents are liquids which evaporate at room temperature to form a gas. The solubility of a gas in blood determines the rate at which changes in anaesthesia occur. If a gas is very soluble then large amounts will dissolve, so changes will occur slowly, e.g. methoxyflurane; if a gas is insoluble, then rapid uptake and elimination from the blood occurs and changes take place rapidly, e.g. sevoflurane. The technical term for this effect is the **blood/gas solubility coefficient** – the smaller the coefficient the faster the changes occur (Table 25.8). As changes occur more quickly with insoluble agents, overdosing and underdosing may happen easily so careful monitoring is required.

The potency of these drugs also varies, and is measured as the alveolar concentration of the drug that will anaesthetize

Table 25.8 Blood/gas solubility coefficient for common volatile anaesthetic agents

Agent	Coefficient
Desflurane	0.42
Nitrous oxide	0.47
Sevoflurane	0.6
Isoflurane	1.39
Enflurane	1.8
Halothane	2.4
Methoxyflurane	12

Table 25.9 Minimum alveolar concentration for common volatile agents

Volatile agent	Minimum alveolar concentration (%)	Potency
Methoxyflurane	0.23	Most potent
Halothane	0.8	
Isoflurane	1.3	
Sevoflurane	2	
Enflurane	2.2	
Desflurane	6.8	
Nitrous oxide	188–220	Least potent

50% of a certain type of animal. This is expressed as the **minimum alveolar concentration (MAC)** and varies for each drug and for each species. The lower the MAC the more potent the gas (Table 25.9). MAC is also altered by the type of premedication given, the induction agent and the carrier gas used.

When an animal inhales volatile gas it is initially all absorbed by the body so the induction phase requires a higher inspired percentage of gas. As the body reaches saturation the percentage of gas required drops as more gas starts to be exhaled by the animal. The maintenance phase is reached when only the proportion exhaled has to be replaced by the incoming gas.

Volatile agents

Examples of volatile agents include the following:

Diethyl ether

Still available and may be seen in practice but it is very old-fashioned and cannot be recommended. It is extremely flammable, irritant to respiratory mucosae and causes slow recovery because of its high fat solubility. It causes good muscle relaxation and is analgesic. It is heavier than air so its fumes gather on the floor, where static electricity can cause explosions.

Chloroform

Chloroform is occasionally used but it is very toxic and dangerous to administer.

Halothane

Widely used since the 1950s. It is non-irritant and non-explosive but as it is a chlorofluorocarbon (CFC) it causes environmental pollution. It is decomposed by ultraviolet light so must be stored in dark glass bottles. It contains thymol as a preservative, which can build up in the vaporizer, affecting its function.

Induction is achieved at concentrations of 2–4% and is relatively fast; maintenance is achieved at 0.8–2%. Halothane is 60 times as soluble in fat as in other body tissues, so uptake by the CNS in relation to uptake by the blood is 2.5:1. Total body clearance of halothane can take a long time as it is slowly released from the fat and up to 25% of it is then metabolized by the liver. Some breakdown products are slightly toxic:

- **Contraindications:** halothane-associated hepatitis can occur in humans after repeated exposure to the gas, so careful scavenging is important. Malignant hyperthermia is a genetically based disease seen in pigs, dogs, cats and humans. It can be triggered by halothane exposure and is fatal but extremely rare. Analgesia is poor even when deeply anaesthetized and muscle relaxation is moderate. Halothane reduces cardiac output and predisposes the heart to arrhythmias by sensitizing the myocardium to adrenaline (epinephrine) and by causing hypercapnia secondary to mild respiratory depression. Postoperative shivering is common even in normothermic animals, which can cause increased oxygen demand during recovery, when oxygen tension may be low.

Enflurane

Enflurane has similar properties to halothane. It is also a CFC and is widely used in humans but seldom in animals. It is rapid in onset and recovery and causes a dose-dependent reduction in cardiac output but less hypotension than halothane. Muscle relaxation is good. Very little is metabolized. Induction is achieved at concentrations of 4–6% and maintenance at 1–3%.

Methoxyflurane

This is a non-explosive halogenated ether. It is extremely potent but not very volatile so 3% is the maximum concentration achievable at room temperature. Methoxyflurane is very soluble in blood so induction and recovery are very slow. It provides excellent muscle relaxation and analgesia, which can last up to 24 hours, making it useful in orthopaedics. It is a cardiorespiratory depressant and is extensively metabolized, releasing fluoride and oxalate ions, which can damage the kidneys.

Induction at concentrations of 1.5–2.5%; maintenance at 0.2–1.25%.

Isoflurane

Isoflurane is a halogenated ether with an unpleasant smell and is slightly irritant to respiratory mucosae. It is non-explosive, very potent and has a low blood gas solubility so induction, changes in depth and recovery are very rapid even after prolonged anaesthesia. Very little is metabolized so it is non-toxic.

Induction at 2–3%; maintenance at 1.5–2.5%.

- **Contraindications:** heart rate is maintained but there is a dose-dependent hypotension due to vasodilation. It is not arrhythmogenic. Muscle relaxation is good but respiratory depression is more marked so supplementary ventilation may be required.

Sevoflurane

This is a modern anaesthetic that, because of its insolubility, produces a rapid induction and recovery and is widely used for day-case anaesthesia in humans. It has similar cardiorespiratory effects to isoflurane. It reacts with soda lime so cannot be used in rebreathing circuits, and is expensive to use.

Desflurane

Desflurane is a halogenated ether that is very insoluble in blood and causes some airway irritation. Its cardiorespiratory effects are similar to isoflurane. It requires a special vaporizer, which is heated and pressurized to achieve the high concentrations for its MAC. Its main advantage is its extremely rapid induction and recovery times.

Vaporization

All volatile liquid anaesthetic agents must evaporate to form gas, which must be delivered in accurate doses to the animal. This is achieved by the use of a calibrated vaporizer (Fig. 25.1). There are many types available but only the more modern models are accurate at all times and under all conditions of use. Temperature, gas flow rate, back pressure, volume of liquid in the chamber, etc., can all affect accuracy, so the concentration of inspired gas may not be what is indicated on the machine.

The most common vaporizer design, as seen in the Fluotec or Isotec, involves a vaporizing chamber and a bypass channel. The gas inflow divides into two streams and most gas passes straight through the machine and into the animal. The smaller flow passes through the chamber containing the volatile liquid, which becomes saturated and is introduced back into the main gas flow, giving a set concentration.

Both high and low flow rates can cause problems in accuracy. High flow rates cause cooling of the liquid, so progressively less liquid is vaporized, but modern vaporizers have a temperature-controlled valve to increase the flow into the chamber. Vaporizers are very heavy because they are made of copper to allow for a fast transfer of heat from the room air to the chamber. Modern vaporizers, e.g. Fluotec 3 and 4, can be relied on to be accurate down to 500–1000 ml/min flow rates.

Anaesthetic circuits

Anaesthetic circuits can be divided into two categories:

- Rebreathing
- Non-rebreathing.

Rebreathing circuits

These circuits allow for a proportion of the expired gases to be reinhaled. The fresh inhaled gas mixture contains only carrier gas plus volatile liquid anaesthetic evaporated into a

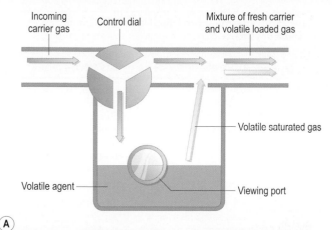

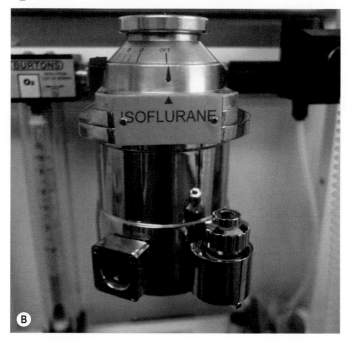

Fig. 25.1 Plenum vaporizer. (**A**) Schematic diagram. (**B**) Vaporizer attached to anaesthetic machine

Soda lime dust is particularly dangerous; if inhaled by staff or through the circuit by the animal it can cause respiratory tract damage and bronchiolitis. A full soda lime canister should contain only 50% granules; the remaining 50% is the space between the granules. There should be enough space to accommodate at least twice the animal's tidal volume to allow for efficient absorption. If the canister is insufficiently filled, a gap will develop between the soda lime and the canister wall and a process known as 'channelling' will occur. Here the exhaled gases pass through the canister without having mingled with the soda lime, resulting in a build-up of carbon dioxide in the system, which leads to hypercapnia and raised carbon dioxide levels in the breath.

Nitrous oxide can be used in rebreathing circuits but, as oxygen is used by the patient and carbon dioxide is removed by the soda lime, nitrous oxide can build up. Thus, in low-flow use, 50% is the maximum amount that can be used without using an inspired gas analyser. In higher-flow use, i.e. over 30 ml/kg/min, the influx of fresh gas will prevent a build-up.

When an animal is freshly anaesthetized it breathes out all the nitrogen dissolved in its blood. This is called denitrogenation and can be a problem in rebreathing circuits. The nitrogen may build up in the rebreathing circuit if there is a low inflowing rate of fresh gas. To avoid this, when the animal is first connected to a rebreathing circuit a high inflow rate of fresh gas, e.g. 100 ml/kg/min, is used for the first 10 minutes.

Types of rebreathing circuit

The circle system

This is the most common type seen in practice but is the most complex. It relies on a one-way valve system to direct the gas flow and can malfunction. These circuits are bulky and expensive but carbon dioxide management is very good because of a clever canister design (Fig. 25.2). The canister is distant from the patient so dust and breathing resistance is reduced and IPPV can be administered if necessary. The circuit cannot be used in animals under 10 kg unless it is specifically designed for paediatric use.

To-and-fro system

In the to-and-system (Fig. 25.3), the patient breathes in fresh gas from the inlet pipe and exhales it into the closely positioned Waters' canister, where carbon dioxide is removed by soda lime. The 'scrubbed' gas is then rebreathed along with the fresh gas inflow. As the fresh gas inflow pipe is close to the patient, concentration of volatile gas can be measured accurately.

The disadvantages of the circuit are mainly due to the position and design of the canister. As it lies close to the endotracheal tube, its weight may predispose to extubation as the animal is moved around. Soda lime dust may be inhaled more easily and the soda lime in the canister tends to settle, leaving a channelling gap at the top. The soda lime tends to become exhausted at the patient end of the canister first so that the dead space in the circuit increases as time passes and more carbon dioxide is rebreathed. IPPV is difficult because of the positioning of the expiratory valve.

Advantages of the circle and to-and-fro systems are shown in Table 25.10.

gas. The exhaled gas contains carrier gas, volatile gas, carbon dioxide, water vapour and heat. If this can be reinhaled, less carrier gas and volatile gas is required and heat and moisture are conserved. To avoid a build-up of exhaled carbon dioxide a soda lime scrubbing system is used.

Soda lime is a granular compound consisting of 80% sodium hydroxide (NaOH) and 18% calcium hydroxide (CaOH). The remainder consists of silicates and a pH indicator. It is an alkaline, irritant reactive material and care must be exercised when handling it. Different companies make different colours of soda lime and the colour changes as the reactivity of the compound runs out. It is therefore important to know which colour indicates fresh and which exhausted soda lime. Using exhausted soda lime, i.e. saturated with carbon dioxide, would be disastrous for the animal, as it will no longer absorb carbon dioxide. As the soda lime reacts with carbon dioxide in the exhaled gases, the soft, soapy soda lime is replaced by hard brittle carbonates and heat is produced, which can help in preventing hypothermia.

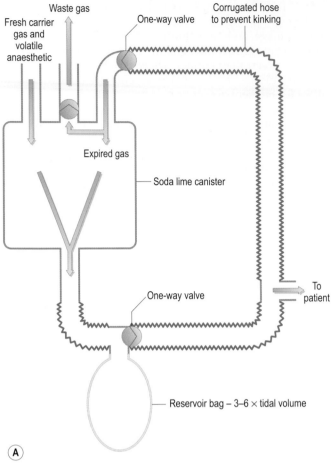

Labels in figure:
Waste gas
Fresh carrier gas and volatile anaesthetic
One-way valve
Corrugated hose to prevent kinking
Expired gas
Soda lime canister
One-way valve
To patient
Reservoir bag – 3–6 × tidal volume
(A)

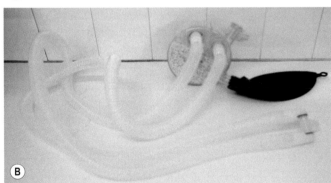
(B)

Fig. 25.2 (**A, B**) The circle system

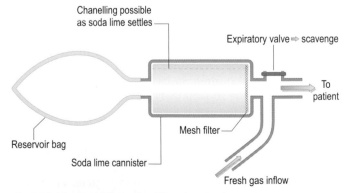

Labels in figure:
Chanelling possible as soda lime settles
Expiratory valve ⇒ scavenge
To patient
Mesh filter
Reservoir bag
Soda lime cannister
Fresh gas inflow

Fig. 25.3 The to-and-fro system (Waters' canister)

Table 25.10 Advantages and disadvantages of the circle and to-and-fro systems

	Advantages	Disadvantages
Circle system	High gas efficiency Constant dead space Low resistance Reduced risk of bronchiolitis IPPV possible	Complex, so malfunctions more likely Cumbersome but distant to patient Expensive 10 kg and over Difficult to clean Difficult to sterilize
To-and-fro system	High gas efficiency Good heat conservation Low resistance Denitrogenation is quick Simple Good control of gas concentration Easy to clean and sterilize	Heavy and too close to the patient No IPPV Increasing dead space with time Channelling Bronchiolitis Hyperthermia may occur

IPPV, intermittent positive pressure ventilation

Non-rebreathing circuits

Non-rebreathing circuits rely on the flushing out of the exhaled volatile gas and carbon dioxide produced within the circuit by the fresh gas inflow. The circuits are less economical in their use of carrier gas and anaesthetic agent. The flow rate required varies from circuit to circuit and heat and moisture are not conserved. Although these circuits can be used in animals of very low body weight they may lead to loss of heat and moisture, which may be a problem in types of animal that are already prone to hypothermia and dehydration. Non-rebreathing circuits are all simple and relatively cheap, they are easily sterilized, they allow accurate control of inspired gases and soda lime is not required.

Types of non-rebreathing circuit

Ayre's T piece

The original Ayre's T piece does not have a reservoir bag so it is unlikely to be used in practice as it wastes anaesthetic gases. The Jackson–Rees modification includes a reservoir bag added to the expiratory tubing (Fig. 25.4). This is the circuit of choice for all animals under 10 kg. It has very low resistance and IPPV is easily achieved. Nitrous oxide can be safely used. Flow rates are shown in Table 25.11. The range of flow rates depends on body size, metabolic rate, respiratory disease, etc.

As the waste gases vent from the open end of the reservoir bag, scavenging can be a problem. In some cases attachments can twist and occlude gas flow, so some T pieces have an expiratory valve added just before the bag, and tubing to the scavenging unit is attached to it (Fig. 25.5). This has a greater resistance to expiration and is used in 5–10 kg animals.

Bain circuit

This circuit is similar to the T piece but uses coaxial tubing (Fig. 25.6). The coaxial system involves placing one part of the tubing within another so that heat from exhaled gases can be transferred to the incoming fresh gas. Scavenging is

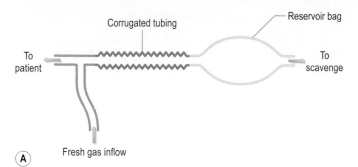

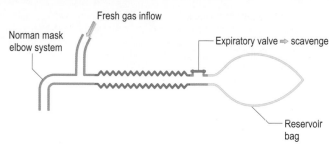

Fig. 25.5 Modified Ayre's T piece with variation in the scavenging valve, which provides greater assistance with expiration and can therefore be used in animals of 5–10 kg

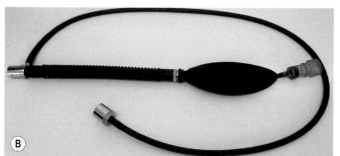

Fig. 25.4 (**A, B**) Jackson–Rees modified Ayre's T piece

Table 25.11 Flow rates for non-rebreathing circuits

Type of circuit	Flow rate
Jackson–Rees modified Ayre's T piece	2.5–3.5 (average 3) × minute volume = flow rate in l/min, e.g. for a 5 kg animal – 3 × 300 ml × 5 kg = 4.5 l/min for a 10 kg animal – 3 × 250 ml × 10 kg = 7.5 l/min
Bain	2.5–3.5 (average 3) × minute volume
Magill	0.8–1 × minute volume
Lack	1–1.5 × minute volume
Parallel	Lack 1–1.5 × minute volume

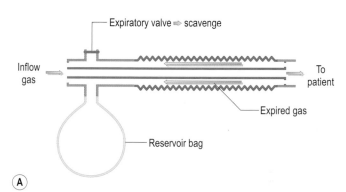

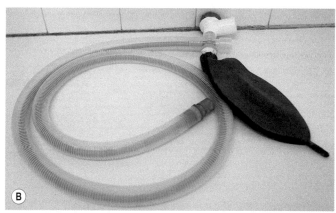

Fig. 25.6 (**A, B**) The Bain circuit

achieved by attaching tubing to the expiratory valve; expired gases are then conducted along the outer tubing and out through the valve. The reduced diameter of the expiratory tubing and the expiratory valve creates a higher resistance than a T piece.

The Bain is useful in patients of 10–20 kg. Flow rates are shown in Table 25.11. It is good for administering IPPV. The tubing should be checked before use to ensure that the inner tube has not become disconnected.

A modified Bain circuit can be used but as it does not use coaxial tubing the incoming gas is not warmed by the expired gases (Fig. 25.7). However, resistance is reduced by having a larger diameter of expiratory tube.

Magill circuit

The Magill circuit is very simple and takes the animal's anatomical dead space into account, reducing the fresh gas requirements (Fig. 25.8). The dead space gas has the same composition as the inflow gas so it can be used again without causing carbon dioxide build-up. The circuit is cheap, simple to clean and sterilize and can be used in animals over 10 kg.

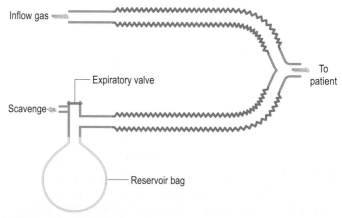

Fig. 25.7 The modified Bain circuit

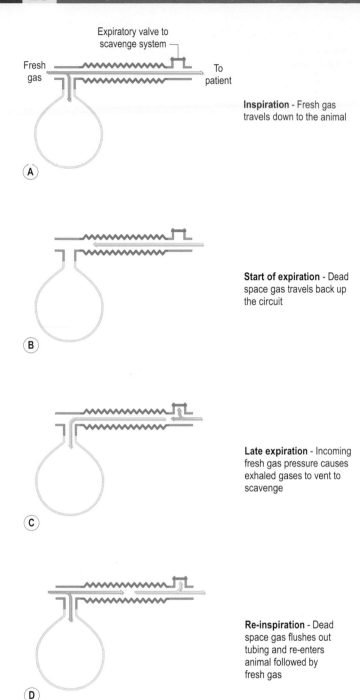

Fig. 25.8 (**A–D**) Movement of gas within the Magill circuit

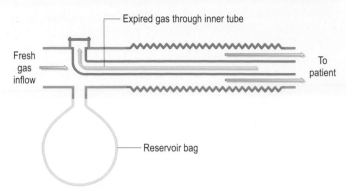

Fig. 25.9 The Lack circuit

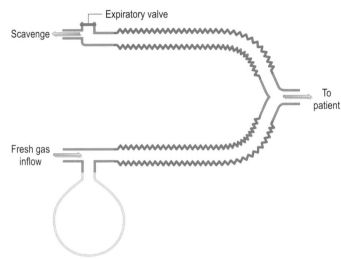

Fig. 25.10 The parallel Lack circuit

Flow rates are shown in Table 25.11. If IPPV is used, the flow rate should be increased to 1.5 × minute volume. However, a Magill circuit is not ideal for IPPV because of the position of the expiratory valve.

Lack circuit

This is essentially a coaxial Magill circuit (Fig. 25.9). The inflow gas comes down the exterior tubing and the expired gases leaves through the interior pipe and out of the expiratory valve. There is a risk that the inner tube may become disconnected but there is no easy way to check for this before use. IPPV is easier than in the Magill circuit. Flow rates are shown in Table 25.11.

The parallel Lack circuit is a non-coaxial system that was designed to make maintenance and inner tube safety better (Fig. 25.10). It has a lower resistance, so paediatric versions can be used on animals of 5 kg upwards. It has the same flow rate as a Lack circuit but does not warm incoming gas.

The Humphrey ADE breathing system

This recent innovation is a system that has a switchable soda lime canister so it can be used either as a rebreathing or a non-rebreathing system (Fig. 25.11). It is expensive to buy and cannot be used with N_2O. Its advantages are that in its semi-closed mode it can be used for small animals under 10 kg and in rebreathing mode it is very economical. It provides one system for all animals and is gaining in popularity.

Management of the patient's airway

Useful respiratory measurements are provided in Box 25.1. During gaseous anaesthesia the patient must have a steady supply of carrier gas and anaesthetic agent delivered to its lungs. Anaesthesia removes the protective reflexes of the pharynx and larynx that normally keep the airway functioning so, ideally, all animals should be intubated, using an **endotracheal tube** that connects the anaesthetic circuit directly to the respiratory tract. This prevents gas leaving via

Box 25.1 Definitions of respiratory measurements

- **Tidal volume** – volume of gas inspired at each breath. 15–20 ml/kg. Higher values in smaller animals.
- **Respiratory rate** – number of breaths per minute. Usually 10–15 breaths per minute.
- **Minute volume** – tidal volume × respiratory rate. Approximately 200–300 ml/kg/min.
- **Dead space** – area where gaseous exchange does not take place. May be anatomical, i.e. trachea, bronchi and bronchioles, or mechanical, i.e. endotracheal tube and exhausted area of soda lime in canister.
- **Airway resistance** – resistance to the flow of gas through the airway. Depends on the viscosity of the gas and the diameter and length of the circuit tubing.

Table 25.12 Endotracheal intubation

Advantages	Disadvantages
Airway protection	Increased resistance to breathing
Direct connection to incoming gases	Iatrogenic damage to larynx or trachea
Cuffed tube protects inhalation of oral material	Kinking. Blockage may cause respiratory obstruction
Cuffed tube prevents breathing round the tube and anaesthetic gas escaping into the theatre environment	Endobronchial or intra-oesophageal intubation possible
IPPV possible	
Reduced mechanical dead space	

IPPV, intermittent positive pressure ventilation

Table 25.13 Endotracheal tube type comparison

Rubber	PVC
Stiff – easier to intubate	Softer
Poor resistance to kinking	Moulds itself to the local anatomy at body temperature
Thick walls	Can be armoured
	Vapour from respiration may help to indicate that tube is in the trachea

the animal's mouth and prevents the inhalation of foreign material, e.g. regurgitated stomach contents. Table 25.12 shows the advantages and disadvantages of intubation.

Tube types and selection

The Magill tube is the typical red rubber tube seen in most practices. It may also be made from PVC (Fig. 25.12). The distal end is bevelled to allow easier separation of the arytenoid cartilages. The cuff is also at the distal end and is inflated via a pilot tube and balloon system. The cuff seals the gap between the tube and the tracheal mucosa, providing an airtight seal. This prevents inhalation of debris and the animal breathing around the tube, but if overinflated it can cause damage to the tracheal rings and mucosa and may also occlude the main lumen of the tube.

The size printed on the tube relates to the internal diameter, and this affects the resistance to breathing. For example, a thick-walled rubber tube used in a small cat would result in the cat having to generate a huge negative pressure to ensure adequate respiration. Anaesthetics tend to reduce respiratory effort, so hypoventilation is a risk. Some tubes have armoured walls – wires embedded in the plastic – and these are useful where kinking may occur, e.g. head surgery, cisternal puncture positioning (Table 25.13).

Intubation

Veterinary nurses should be proficient at intubating any animal. Establishing an airway in an emergency could save a life.

Before use, make the following checks of the endotracheal tube:

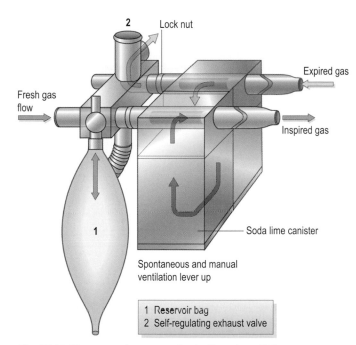

Fig. 25.11 Diagram to show set-up for the Humphrey ADE system

Lock nut

2

Expired gas

Fresh gas flow

Inspired gas

Soda lime canister

Spontaneous and manual ventilation lever up

| 1 | Reservoir bag |
| 2 | Self-regulating exhaust valve |

1

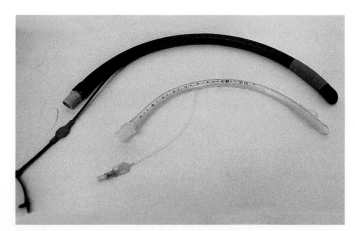

Fig. 25.12 Red rubber and PVC endotracheal tubes

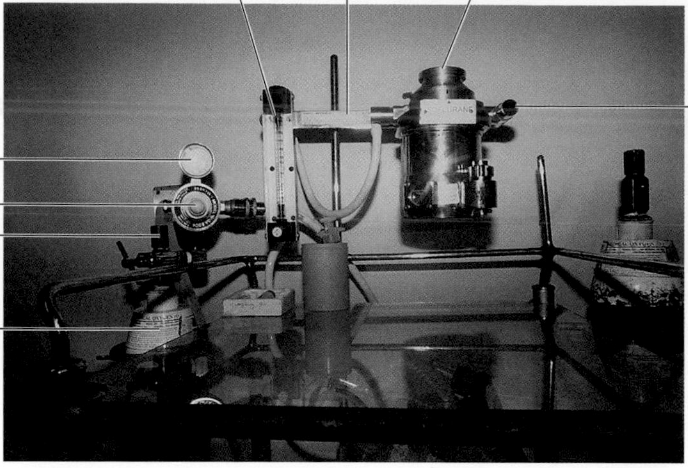

Pressure gauge — Regulator — Pillar valve — Oxygen cylinder —
Oxygen flow meter — Back bar — Plenum vaporizer
Fresh gas outflow

Fig. 25.13 A basic anaesthetic machine

1. **Correct size** – have at least three different sizes available in case of unexpected narrowness of the trachea or intrapharyngeal obstructions
2. **Check patency** – blow through it before use to remove any dried mucus or blood from previous patients
3. **Check cleanliness** – no debris should be left on the tube as it may enter the lungs. Ensure that any cleaning agents have been thoroughly rinsed off, as they may cause sloughing of the tracheal mucosa
4. **Check that the cuff** and balloon are functioning
5. **Ensure adequate lubrication** to avoid mucosal trauma.

Intubation is performed once the airway reflexes have been suppressed by the induction agent. Select a tube of the correct diameter and of a length that reaches to the level of the scapula. The tube is passed between the arytenoids. In cats the arytenoids should be anaesthetized with a lignocaine spray to avoid laryngospasm. The tube should not protrude beyond the tip of the nose, to reduce mechanical dead space. It should be secured to the maxilla or mandible using a length of soft bandage to prevent accidental extubation during patient manipulation. The animal should be connected to the circuit and 100% oxygen supplied until you can see that the animal is breathing satisfactorily. The cuff should be inflated.

Anaesthetic masks

These may seem old-fashioned and are often overlooked but they can be extremely useful in certain circumstances. There are two main types – malleable black rubber or a clear plastic cone with a black rubber seal.

A mask can be used to:

- Provide oxygen pre- and postoperatively
- Provide oxygen intraoperatively in short procedures when ketamine has been used to provide anaesthesia
- Allow for gaseous induction, e.g. in neonates or when inducing intravenously using a very low dose of drug in severely compromised patients
- Provide maintenance in short procedures.

The disadvantages of masks are that IPPV is almost impossible, there is an increased mechanical dead space and gas

Table 25.14 Compressed gases used in anaesthesia

Cylinder	Shoulder of cylinder	Gas
Black	White	Oxygen
Grey	Black and white	Air
Grey	Grey	Carbon dioxide
Blue	Blue	Nitrous oxide

flow rates must be high to ensure an adequate provision, which means that the risk of atmospheric pollution is also high.

The anaesthetic machine

Anaesthetic machines come in a wide variety of shapes and sizes with varying degrees of complexity; however, the basic concept is the same (Fig. 25.13). Carrier gas is passed through the machine via a calibrated flow meter to the vaporizer. The anaesthetic mixture is then passed to an outlet port, to which the anaesthetic circuit attaches. There is an oxygen bypass circuit from the supply to the outlet, which is used to provide oxygen in an emergency.

Gas supply

Sterile carrier gases are supplied in a variety of cylinders. These are high-pressure systems so that large volumes of gas can be stored and used locally. The cylinders are made of molybdenum steel and are colour-coded to help identify the contents (Table 25.14). They all have pillar valves, which should be rotated anticlockwise to allow the gas out. These pillar valves connect to the anaesthetic machine or on to connector hosing. There is a pattern of holes in the pillar valve that interconnect with a set of pins in the valve seat. This ensures that only the gas assigned to that port will fit. In a case where a large cylinder is used that does not connect directly on to the anaesthetic machine, the hose connector is also designed to accept only the valve of a particular gas.

Table 25.15 Commonly used sizes and volumes of oxygen cylinders

Size	Volume (litres)
E	680
F	1340
G	3400
J	6800

Cylinder size ranges from AA to J (Table 25.15). The E-sized cylinder with 680 litres of oxygen at 1 atmosphere contains enough oxygen to supply a 20 kg dog for 3 hours. G-sized cylinders tend to be used as part of the supply for a piped gas system, where hoses from the anaesthetic machine plug into gas-supplying wall sockets. These systems are more expensive to set up but are more economical to run because the gas supplied in large cylinders is cheaper per unit volume. Pressurized gas cylinders are potentially very dangerous. Accidental damage to a cylinder can result in explosion of compressed gas. In cases of fire, oxygen and nitrous oxide will both intensify the flames.

Cylinders should be stored upright, held against a solid wall by chains or metal hoops in a dedicated safe area, in a quiet part of the practice where access is only available to trained staff. Most of the larger anaesthetic machines will have valve blocks for two cylinders each of oxygen and nitrous oxide. This allows for immediate access to a reserve cylinder when one runs out. To avoid an accidental shortfall in gas supply, place tags marked 'in use' and 'in reserve' around the necks of the cylinders and make sure that the system is used by all staff.

When a cylinder is replaced, the plastic seal should be removed and the pillar valve examined for damage or debris. Some gas should be vented to blow any dust away from the orifice. The sealing O ring on the valve block should be checked for debris or damage.

If the supplying cylinder is being changed, the animal should be disconnected from the circuit and left to breath room air for a short period. The nearly empty cylinder valve should be shut and the new cylinder turned on. The animal is then reconnected. Leaving the original cylinder's valve open can result in cylinder-to-cylinder transfer and adiabatic heating which could prove dangerous. Some gas should be left in the empty cylinder to prevent ingress of moisture, which can cause rust inside the cylinder.

The pressure gauge and regulator

The pressure gauge allows the anaesthetist to know how much gas remains in the cylinder and may be part of the anaesthetic machine or attached to a connecting hose. The gauge is usually a curved tube that straightens out at high pressures, known as a Bourdon gauge.

When assessing the fullness of cylinders of most gases, you can assume that if the pressure reading is half then the cylinder is half full. However, measurement of the amount of nitrous oxide in a cylinder is difficult to assess because it exists as a liquid under pressure. To calculate the volume of

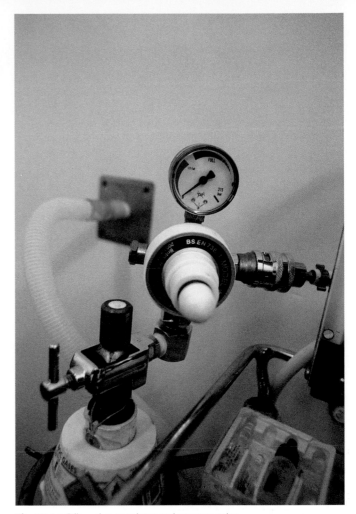

Fig. 25.14 Pillar valve, regulator and pressure valve

gas in a nitrous oxide cylinder you need to weigh it and apply this formula:

Full weight of cylinder (kg) − empty cylinder (kg) × 534
= volume of gas

Once the gas enters the anaesthetic machine it encounters a pressure reduction valve or regulator (Fig. 25.14), which reduces the cylinder pressure to a working pressure of generally about 4 atmospheres.

The flow meter

The flow meter (Fig. 25.15) controls the supply of gas entering the vaporizer and circuit. There are two main types, the bobbin and the ball bearing, which are suspended by the gas flow within a tapering glass tube calibrated in litres per minute – one for each gas. Readings are taken from the top of the floating bobbin or the equator of the ball-bearing system.

The flow meters are attached to a structure called the back bar to which the vaporizer is also attached. The vaporizer may be directly connected into the circuit tubing or it may attach to a specially designed manifold, e.g. Selectatec. This allows for a variety of type 3 and 4 Tecs, and hence

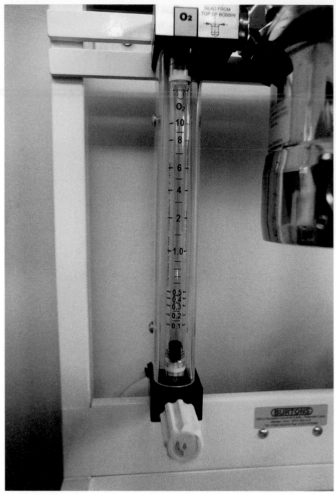

Fig. 25.15 A bobbin-type oxygen flow meter

Table 25.16 Current maximum exposure per 8-hour period

Anaesthetic gas	Maximum exposure (parts per million)
Nitrous oxide	100
Halothane	10
Enflurane	50
Isoflurane	50
Ether	400

anaesthetic gases, to be used on the same anaesthetic machine. At the end of the back bar is the common gas outlet, to which the circuit attaches.

Safety devices

The number of these depends on the design of the machine:

- **Oxygen failure warning device** – the 'bosun's whistle'. As the oxygen pressure fails, a valve opens, allowing gas to escape through a whistle. In some machines where nitrous oxide is in use the gas enters the whistle if oxygen pressure falls
- **Nitrous oxide cut-out** – if the oxygen runs out, some machines will cause the nitrous oxide supply to be cut off, which stops the animal breathing 100% nitrous oxide, which would result in hypoxia.
- **Over pressure valve** – any blockage to gas flow beyond the common gas outlet will cause an alarm to sound and the gas to escape out of the valve
- **Oxygen flush or purge valve** – takes oxygen directly from the regulator, bypassing the flow meters and vaporizers. It provides oxygen in emergencies and can be used to flush the circuitry out at the end of the anaesthetic process

- **Check valves** – these prevent backflow of gas from full cylinders to empty ones.

Waste gas management

Once the anaesthetic and carrier gases have passed back out of the animal, they must be safely removed from the working environment by a process known as **scavenging**. Health and Safety legislation specifically relating to anaesthesia is incorporated in a set of recommendations known as the Anaesthetic Agents: Controlling Exposure under the Control of Substances Hazardous to Health Regulations 1994. Chronic inhalation of waste gases by theatre staff has been linked to headaches, irritability, bone marrow toxicity, hepatopathies, infertility, abortions and teratogenesis, so adequate scavenging of volatile gases and nitrous oxide is mandatory (Table 25.16).

Scavenging can be provided in three ways:

- **Active** – the method of choice. The waste gas pipe conveys the gases through an air gap by which a suction system removes them from the building and out into the open air. The air gap is designed to prevent the suction system from removing gas from the anaesthetic circuit
- **Semipassive** – waste gases pass down a wide-bore tube to a ventilation system, which expels the gas to the outside air
- **Passive** – waste gas passes down a wide-bore tube and into a canister that contains activated charcoal and reacts with hydrocarbon volatile gases, e.g. halothane, ether. These canisters do not remove nitrous oxide. They must be weighed frequently to determine when they have become saturated and inactive.

Theatre pollution monitoring should be carried out routinely and the following steps should be taken to reduce pollution:

- Fill the vaporizer in a well-ventilated room
- Clean up spillages of volatile agents immediately and increase room ventilation
- Flush the anaesthetic system with oxygen at the end of use
- Allow recovery of animals in a well-ventilated room as they can continue to excrete volatile agents for many hours, especially in the case of halothane
- Use a cuffed endotracheal tube to prevent the escape of anaesthetic mixtures
- Avoid induction by mask or anaesthetic chambers.

Monitoring the anaesthetized patient

Once anaesthetized, the patient's critical parameters must be continually assessed by the anaesthetist and in small animal practice this tends to be entirely the responsibility of the nurse. The nurse must know the normal values of these parameters in order to pick up any variations or trends and make changes to the anaesthetic as appropriate. Although there is now an increasing use of anaesthetic monitoring equipment, a well-trained and alert nurse is still the best way of monitoring and controlling an anaesthetic. Anaesthesia is all about the correct balance between unconsciousness, analgesia and physiological stability.

Monitoring should begin once the premedication has been given and it should cease once the animal is fit to be sent home.

The following parameters must be measured:

- Central nervous system depression – depth of anaesthesia
- Cardiovascular function – heart rate, pulse rate and quality, mucous membrane colour, respiratory depth and effectiveness
- Body temperature.

The following parameters should be measured if possible:

- Blood pressure
- ECG
- Exhaled carbon dioxide
- Urine output
- Fluid acid–base balance
- Loss of blood during surgery.

Central nervous system depression

The depth of anaesthesia required depends on the procedure being undertaken: e.g. a dog anaesthetized for radiography only needs to be immobilized and have adequate muscle relaxation as there will be no noxious stimuli applied to it, while a fracture fixation will require a deeper plane of unconsciousness, excellent muscle relaxation and analgesia.

Descriptions of the depth of anaesthesia are classically related to the four stages of anaesthesia noted in human anaesthesia:

1. Voluntary excitement, fear, apprehension, disorientation
2. Start of unconsciousness until respiration stabilizes
3. Surgical anaesthesia – subdivided into four planes
4. Overdose, including respiratory paralysis and pale mucous membranes.

This is not directly relevant to veterinary anaesthesia but the phases can be recognized in animal patients.

Stages 1 and 2 are often not observed because of the rapid smooth induction achieved with intravenous agents.

In stage 3 – surgical anaesthesia – the four planes refer to increasing depth with reducing neurological signs and increasing cardiovascular depression. If the anaesthetic reaches overdose there is severe cardiovascular depression and no neurological reflexes, leading to death. Recovery involves the reverse of the three stages.

CNS depression is mostly monitored by cranial nerve reflexes, although the withdrawal or pedal reflex (toe web pinch) is still useful.

Cranial nerve reflexes

- **Palpebral reflex** – touch the medial canthus of the eye to stimulate a blink. This is present in light planes of anaesthesia. It can be reduced by repetition. It should be very sluggish or absent for adequate surgical anaesthesia
- **Corneal reflex** – not very useful. It may be present even in very deep anaesthesia and its absence is best used to ascertain brain death
- **Eye position** – as the depth of unconsciousness increases the eye moves to a ventromedial position and then returns to a central position. This can prove confusing because the eye may be central if the animal is too light or too deep, but in the latter case there will be no palpebral reflex. In ketamine anaesthesia the eye may remain central at all times
- **Pupil diameter** – as anaesthesia deepens, the pupil will dilate but should still be responsive to light. This can also be influenced by drugs used, e.g. atropine and ketamine
- **Jaw tone** – in the initial phases of anaesthesia there is strong jaw tone and the animal will often make masticatory movements. These should be absent in surgical anaesthesia
- **Pharyngeal/laryngeal reflexes** – should be absent. Ketamine anaesthesia preserves these reflexes
- **Lacrimation** – present in light anaesthesia but absent in deeper planes. Ocular lubricants should be used to protect the cornea during prolonged procedures
- **Salivation** – can be excessive in light planes or as a result of using ketamine.

In the rest of the body, muscle tone should be abolished and pinching the web of the toe should not evoke a withdrawal reflex.

The surgical planes of anaesthesia should be exhibited by:

- Poor or absent palpebral reflex
- Ventromedial or slightly rising eye position
- No jaw tone
- No pedal skin pinch withdrawal
- No muscle tone
- Constricted pupil.

Cardiovascular parameters

Increasing the amount of gaseous anaesthetic to achieve surgical anaesthesia can cause detrimental effects on the physiology of the heart and lungs. The depth of anaesthesia must be moderated by considerations for cardiovascular function. The anaesthetic agent is not the only influence on this system, as surgical stimulation, haemorrhage, etc., also alter its function.

Technology has produced many aids to cardiovascular monitoring. However, the nurse must not rely on these and must continue to make the following basic checks:

Heart rate

Rate depends on species, physical state, disease state, breed, size, level of fitness, etc. Examples of normal values are the cat – 120–180 bpm; small, overweight dog – 100–160 bpm; large, fit dog – 70–120 bpm (Table 25.17).

Table 25.17 Normal clinical parameters used to monitor anaesthesia

Clinical parameter	Dog	Cat
Body temperature (°C)	38.3–38.7	38.0–38.5
Pulse or heart rate (bpm)	70–120	120–180
Respiratory rate (bpm)	10–30	20–30
Capillary refill time (s)	1–2	1–2
Mean arterial blood pressure (mmHg)	60–120	60–120
Central venous pressure (cmH₂O)	3–7.5	3–7.5
Normal pH of blood	7.31–7.41	7.24–7.40
Oxygen saturation (%)	99	99
Pa_{O_2} – room air (mmHg) – 100% O₂ (mmHg)	85–105 500	100–115 500
Pa_{CO_2} (mmHg)	29–42	29–42
End-tidal CO₂ (mmHg)	35–54	32–35
Urinary output (ml/kg/h)	1–2	1–2

Table 25.18 Mucous membrane monitoring

Mucous membrane colour	Condition
Pink	Good perfusion and oxygenation
Brick red	Hypercapnia
White	Anaemia, vasoconstriction, hypotension
Blue/purple	Hypoxia – difficult to assess if anaemic
Yellow	Jaundice
Congested brown/red	Toxaemia
Grey	No cardiac output

Monitoring the heart rate can be done using a stethoscope in three simple ways:

- Palpation of the apex beat
- Precordial auscultation – this allows good assessment of rate and rhythm but draping or operative positioning may preclude its use
- Oesophageal auscultation – using an oesophageal stethoscope. This can be good for non-oral surgery as the nurse can remain remote from the animal. Positioning is critical and there is an increased risk of oesophageal stricture.

Heart rhythm

This should be regular or showing sinus arrhythmia, i.e. accelerating on expiration and decelerating on inspiration. If an irregular heart rhythm is detected, an ECG should be performed immediately.

Pulse

Pulse is described as the difference between systolic and diastolic arterial pressure. It is generated by left ventricular contraction combined with elastic recoil of the arterial system. Digital palpation of a peripheral artery should be carried out every 5 minutes to ascertain pulse rate and quality. Pulse rate should be the same as heart rate. Any discrepancy indicates cardiac electrical problems, so an ECG should be carried out. Pulse quality is a subjective assessment and can only be learned with time but it gives a general indication of cardiac output and therefore tissue perfusion. If the patient is suffering from hypotension then peripheral pulses are likely to be absent or weak; if the pulse is hyperdynamic then it is described as bounding; if there is only a small difference between systolic and diastolic pressures, i.e. poor cardiac function, it is described as being thready. Normal values are shown in Table 25.17.

Mucous membrane colour and capillary refill time

This is easy to assess in animals with non-pigmented gums and is useful in assessing tissue perfusion and oxygenation (Table 25.18). Capillary refill time is an indicator of perfusion but it can be misleading – dead animals may still have a refill.

Monitoring equipment

Most practices will now have some form of anaesthetic monitoring equipment. The most common is the pulse oximeter, but real-time ECGs, capnographs and arterial blood pressure monitors may be available.

Pulse oximeters

These are very popular because they are relatively cheap, easy to apply, non-invasive and easy to interpret. They measure the arterial oxygen saturation of haemoglobin by comparing the absorption of red and infrared light through the epithelium. They then give a read out of oxygen saturation in the arteries (Sa_{O_2}), expressed as a percentage. They also give a pulse rate. An audible 'beep' at every pulse can be very useful in alerting any change of pulse rate between standard manual counts. They should not be solely relied upon because, if the Sa_{O_2} does fall when the animal is already breathing oxygen-enriched gas, then this means other parameters are probably already badly deranged, e.g. poor cardiac output, hypercapnia, etc.

If Sa_{O_2} falls to 90% it means that Pa_{O_2} is only 60 mmHg; if Sa_{O_2} falls to 75% then there is inadequate ventilation and remedial action is required. On 100% oxygen even a poorly ventilated animal will have 95% saturation, so 75% shows the presence of severe cardiovascular compromise. The poor ventilation indicated will also mean that carbon dioxide levels will have built up, which should have stimulated increased ventilation. The absence of respiratory drive indicates that CNS depression is too great, so anaesthesia should be lightened. The hypercapnia may also lead to tachycardia or tachydysrhythmia, so worsening the cardiac output. In anaemic animals haemoglobin saturation may be 100% but overall oxygen carriage may be significantly reduced. This will not be revealed by pulse oximetry.

The pulse oximeter is at its most useful during recovery, when the patient has been taken off the oxygen and monitoring intensity has often been reduced. Any hypoxia when the animal is physiologically stressed by recovery may result in myocardial arrhythmias and cardiac arrest.

The most common reason for alteration in reading is artefactual. Probes may be placed on the tongue, lip, pinna, vulval labia, prepuce and toe web. As the probe compresses the skin it reduces its perfusion, so reducing pulses detected and local oxygenation. The more expensive oesophageal probes do not suffer from this problem.

Electrocardiography

Electrocardiography records the electrical activity of the heart muscle, but this may not reflect the mechanical activity of the heart. Electromechanical dissociation is a condition, often seen during cardiac arrest, where the electrical trace is normal but there is no cardiac contraction. ECGs are primarily for the detection of dysrhythmias, which could affect cardiac performance or lead to cardiac arrest. Any critically ill animal should have leads attached prior to induction and for the duration of the anaesthetic.

Arrhythmias may be caused by many things, e.g. catecholamines, anaesthetic agents, hypoxia, hypercapnia, electrolyte disturbances, myocardial disease or myocardial trauma. Some arrhythmias are important and should be acted upon, e.g. runs of ventricular premature complexes; others have little significance, e.g. sinus arrhythmia.

Blood pressure

Blood pressure is an extremely useful parameter to monitor but is underused due to the technical difficulty of measuring it accurately in small animals. The importance of having adequate blood pressure is obvious because pressure determines tissue perfusion. If it is inadequate then the tissues become hypoxic, hypercapnic and acidotic, which leads to cellular failure. If the mean arterial pressure drops below 60 mmHg, then certain pathological signs may be apparent postoperatively, e.g. blindness in cats, renal failure.

A rise in blood pressure may be due to anaesthetic drugs; for example, alpha-2 agonists cause initial hypertension due to massive peripheral vasoconstriction, or to pain because of inadequate analgesia causing catecholamine release. A fall in blood pressure may be due to reduced cardiac output because of myocardial depression or to inadequate circulating blood volume, i.e. lack of blood or widespread vasodilation.

There are two methods of measurement:

- **Direct** – this is achieved by placement of an indwelling catheter in a peripheral artery, e.g. dorsal metatarsal artery. This is connected directly to either a pressure transducer, which gives a reading for systolic, diastolic and mean arterial pressure, or an aneroid manometer, which only displays mean arterial pressure. This technique is easy to perform but it is invasive and time-consuming to set up and maintain. It is extremely useful in critical cases
- **Indirect** – using:
  - a. **Oscillometric sphygmomanometry** – relies on arterial occlusion by a cuff that is inflated above systolic pressure to occlude the artery. The cuff is then slowly deflated until either the cuff detects systolic pulsations or Korotkoff sounds are auscultated by the operator. The cuff is then further deflated until the pulsation or Korotkoff sounds decrease which gives diastolic pressure. Automatic monitoring machines, e.g. Dinamap, Kritikon, can be programmed to repeatedly cycle these inflations and produce a read-out of systolic, diastolic and mean pressure and pulse rate. The disadvantage of these machines is that they are unreliable. They are reasonably good in large dogs, where a wide cuff can be applied to a distal limb, but in small dogs and cats where only a narrow cuff can be used the readings are less accurate, especially if the animal is hypotensive
  - b. **Doppler flow detection** – a cuff is used to occlude arterial flow and the pulsations are detected by a Doppler ultrasound probe. This is a cheap method and still effective in hypotensive patients, but is rather clumsy to use.

If hypotension is detected then remedial measures should be taken:

- Reduce the depth of anaesthesia
- Administer fluid therapy – rapid infusions of crystalloid or colloid fluids
- Cardiac stimulation – in severe cases drugs such as dobutamine may be required.

Central venous pressure

Central venous pressure (CVP) measures the blood pressure in the intrathoracic cranial vena cava and represents the adequacy of circulating blood volume. Each animal may have a slightly different CVP, so actual values are not as important as the trend, i.e. pressure changes. For example, if CVP starts as 5–10 cmH$_2$O but later drops, this may indicate hypovolaemia. Measurement of CVP also enables the response to fluid therapy to be monitored accurately.

CVP is measured by introducing a catheter via the jugular vein and passing it down into the vena cava. This is connected to a manometer or to a fluid bag, where the distance between the catheter tip and the fluid level equals the CVP.

Body temperature

Anaesthesia disrupts the body's ability to thermoregulate. It depresses CNS reflexes to temperature changes and the body's ability to initiate action to increase heat production by shivering and muscular movement. Core body temperature may drop markedly (hypothermia) and very small animals, metabolically compromised animals and those with poor or wet coats are particularly at risk (Table 25.19).

The effects of hypothermia are:

- Reduced CNS activity, thus increasing depth of anaesthesia – hypothermic animals need less anaesthetic agent
- Reduced cardiac output
- Increased chance of arrhythmias
- Increased blood viscosity.

Table 25.19 Causes of heat loss during anaesthesia

Cause of heat loss	Method of reducing heat loss
Large body surface to body weight ratio. Problem in small animals	Be aware of the problem. Minimize hair clipping. Wrap body in 'bubble wrap' or 'space blankets'
Evaporation from fluids on surface of animal	Avoid excessive wetting of skin and use of surgical spirit to sterilize surgical site
Non-rebreathing circuits with high oxygen flow	Limit anaesthetic time. Use heat exchange circuits
Open body cavities: expose serosal surfaces to room air	Limit exposure of viscera to the air. Warm intravenous fluids
Conduction of body heat from cold surface of operating table	Avoid use of stainless steel table tops. Use insulated or heated surface
Radiation – direct heat exchange between patient's body and room environment	Warm room temperature – even to the point of discomfort for staff

As none of these are desirable, efforts should be made to maintain normothermia.

Core temperature is measured with an oesophageal thermometer; peripheral temperature is measured by a rectal thermometer. Measurement of core temperature is the more significant because in shocked animals with peripheral shutdown the rectal temperature may be very low yet the core temperature remains adequate.

Upon recovery from anaesthesia the animal should be kept in a warm environment and kept well insulated, e.g. 'bubble wrapped', but it should not be wrapped up in blankets. Their ventilatory capacity is very poor and once extubated respiration may become inadequate so any constrictive pressure on the thoracic wall will exacerbate this, leading to hypoxia, hypercapnia and their sequelae.

Respiration

The entire body needs to be well oxygenated during anaesthesia and this is usually easily achieved by providing an oxygen-enriched carrier gas for the volatile anaesthetic agent. However, adequate respiration must also ensure adequate carbon dioxide removal and normal blood pH.

An adequate respiratory rate is not an indication of adequate respiration. Respiratory rate monitors are of very little use because a respiratory rate of 10–12 breaths per minute is recognized as normal but if the depth of respiration is insufficient the patient may in fact be hypoventilating. A visual assessment of depth of respiration can be made by watching the effect of chest movements on the reservoir bag. Shallow breathing may lead to poor gas exchange and insufficient uptake of volatile agent, so destabilizing the anaesthetic.

Mechanical respiration monitors

Capnographs

These are excellent for monitoring the adequacy of ventilation. The probes are connected between the endotracheal tube and the anaesthetic circuit and they measure the respiratory rate and carbon dioxide levels per breath. This gives accurate information on the efficiency of gas exchange. High carbon dioxide levels may indicate hypercapnia or acidosis, which leads to increased expiration of carbon dioxide. More advanced machines may also have monitors for inspired and expired oxygen content and levels of volatile agents. The final carbon dioxide content of tidal air (end-tidal CO_2) approximates to $PaCO_2$.

Blood gas analysis

This is widely used in human and equine anaesthesia but it is rarely seen in small animal practice due to the cost. Blood samples are taken directly from a peripheral artery so $PaCO_2$, PaO_2 and pH, base excess, HCO_3, K, Na and other electrolytes can all be accurately assessed. Thus adequacy of ventilation, adequacy of oxygen supply, and respiratory or metabolic acid–base imbalances can be detected and corrected.

Urinary output

Hypotension can reduce renal blood supply and renal function so reducing urine production. In severe hypotension, hypoxia of renal tubular cells can cause renal failure. Catheterizing a bladder is cheap and easy. If the catheter is attached to a collecting bag then the volume of urine produced per unit time can be assessed. It should be greater than 1 ml/kg/hour. If it is not then fluid therapy is required. If blood tests indicate acute renal failure then furosemide or mannitol may be required.

Muscle relaxation

In veterinary practice the muscle-relaxant properties of the anaesthetic agents provide adequate relaxation for most procedures. Specific muscle-relaxant drugs cause complete neuromuscular blockage in skeletal muscle but have no effect on smooth muscle or cardiac muscle. They do not affect the CNS so have no effect on the level of consciousness; the anaesthetist must therefore still ensure that adequate hypnosis and analgesia is present before surgery begins. Assessing the level of unconsciousness is much harder under the influence of muscle relaxants because the normal signs used to assess it, i.e. movement, vocalization, eye position and the cranial nerve reflexes, are abolished. In addition, because the muscles of respiration are paralysed, IPPV must be instituted.

There are two types of neuromuscular blocking agent:

- **Depolarizing agents** e.g. succinylcholine (suxamethonium) – similar to acetylcholine and binds to the postsynaptic receptors. This lasts for 3–5 minutes in cats and 20 minutes in dogs. It cannot be reversed and is only really used clinically to aid intubation in cats. It can cause muscle pain postoperatively and hyperkalaemia intraoperatively so its use cannot be recommended

- **Non-depolarizing agents** – more widely used as they are reversible and can be topped up. There are many available and they act by competing with acetylcholine to block the postsynaptic receptors (Table 25.20). They do not cause hyperkalaemia or muscle pain.

Non-depolarizing agents can be reversed by administering anticholinesterases, which block the breakdown of acetylcholine, increasing its concentration at the neuromuscular end plate and out-competing the relaxant drug. Too much acetylcholine can cause side effects, so antimuscarinic agents, e.g. neostigmine or edrophonium plus atropine or glycopyrrolate, are given at the same time.

The action of neuromuscular blocking agents is monitored by stimulating a peripheral nerve with a small electrical stimulator. The number and degree of muscle twitches are used to assess the depth of blockade.

Muscle relaxation is used in the following cases:

- Thoracic procedures, e.g. thoracotomies, diaphragm repairs – IPPV can be accurately controlled
- Oesophageal foreign bodies can cause marked spasm of the surrounding muscles and neuromuscular relaxation may aid their removal without recourse to surgery
- Surgery requiring total immobility of the patient, e.g. ophthalmic or neurological procedures
- Orthopaedic procedures or laparotomies in large muscular dogs to increase access to the operative site.

Intermittent positive pressure ventilation (IPPV)

IPPV is the act of ventilating a patient by squeezing the reservoir bag at regular intervals and its use may be indicated during thoracic surgery, diaphragmatic surgery or in cases of poor spontaneous ventilation. IPPV can be achieved in small animals by mechanical or manual compression of the bag without recourse to neuromuscular blockade.

In most practices IPPV involves the nurse squeezing the reservoir bag within a suitable circuit, e.g. T piece, Bain or circle system, causing a normal or slightly supranormal chest excursion. This is carried out 10–12 times per minute and in most cases will provide adequate oxygenation, removal of carbon dioxide and provision of anaesthetic gas. There is a slight risk of overventilation, resulting in mild hypocapnia and slightly deeper anaesthesia than is required, so the concentration dial on the vaporizer may need to be set slightly lower than for spontaneous ventilation. At the end of anaesthesia, reducing the number of chest excursions while keeping the patient on 100% oxygen will allow the carbon dioxide levels to rise again and stimulate a normal respiratory pattern.

Note: It is good practice in spontaneously ventilating animals periodically to generate a supramaximal tidal excursion (sighing) to re-expand the lungs, which will spontaneously collapse with time. It also allows assessment of lung compliance; for example, increased resistance will occur if pneumothorax is present.

Forcing gas into a patient's lungs is not a natural process, so it does have some negative physiological effects:

- Reduced venous return – normally negative intrathoracic pressure aids the flow of blood back to the heart. In IPPV there is positive intrathoracic pressure, which reduces venous return and cardiac output
- Carbon dioxide tension is altered, with consequent pH imbalance.

Inadequate IPPV results in hypercapnia, respiratory acidosis, arrhythmias, increased intracranial pressure, increased tissue perfusion and increased haemorrhage at the operation site.

Excessive IPPV results in hypocapnia, hypotension, reduced tissue perfusion, especially in the CNS, and loss of the stimulus to breathe.

Mechanical ventilators

These perform IPPV mechanically, avoiding the need for the nurse to squeeze the bag at regular intervals, and there are a great many on the market. Some rely on dividing the fresh gas inflow into breaths, while others essentially squeeze a reservoir bag with a predetermined volume of gas. They can be set to administer the gas at a safe pressure, i.e. less than 20 cmH$_2$O, to avoid pulmonary barotrauma. Manual IPPV relies on experience to avoid trauma.

Anaesthetic emergencies

When the patient is anaesthetized it has no protective mechanisms and is entirely dependent on the anaesthetist to provide adequate cardiorespiratory function. Problems may arise within the patient or in the delivery of the anaesthetic. Many small problems may coalesce into major life-threatening situations.

The most frequent time for emergencies to occur is during recovery, when hypotension, lack of a protected airway, shivering to rewarm and relapsing into unconsciousness are all common. Most problems involve:

- Cardiovascular compromise
- Respiratory compromise
- Thermoregulatory compromise
- Delayed recovery to full consciousness.

Cardiac arrest

If the heart stops beating the circulation fails and the main organs will start dying within 3 minutes. An effective circulation must be restored within 1–2 minutes to avoid brain damage. If resuscitation takes longer than this the future

Table 25.20 Muscle relaxants

Drug	Duration	Comments
Pancuronium	Lasts 40 min	Some hypertension and tachycardia
Vecuronium	Lasts 30 min	Better cardiovascular stability
		Breakdown is not dependent on liver function
Atracurium	Lasts 40 min	Histamine release possible

ability of the animal to function properly will be reduced by brain damage.

Cardiac arrest is usually the result of several factors but if only a single cause is present the chances of a successful resuscitation are greater. Causative factors include:

- Hypoxia
- Hypercapnia
- Arrhythmias
- Hypothermia
- Toxaemia
- Drug overdose
- Hyperkalaemia
- Acidosis.

Signs of cardiac arrest

- Absence of heart sounds and pulse
- Mucous membranes grey or very pale in colour
- Absence of haemorrhage
- Gasping ventilation or apnoea
- Eye position centralizes
- Dilated pupils
- Absence of cranial nerve reflexes.

Treatment

An emergency protocol should be established in the practice so that everyone knows what role they should play (see also Ch. 18). A fully equipped and regularly maintained emergency kit should be close to hand and cardiopulmonary resuscitation should be started, following the ABCDEF rule:

A Airway

Ensure it is patent. Clear the throat and intubate.

B Breathing

Supply 100% oxygen and commence supramaximal chest excursions every 5 seconds.

C Circulation

Support circulation by either:

- *External thoracic massage* – compress the chest wall in an area immediately caudodorsal to the heart in medium/large dogs or directly over the heart in small dogs or cats
- *Direct compression of the exposed heart* through a thoracotomy incision. This is a much more effective method of providing circulation and it allows you to see the myocardium for the administration of intracardiac drugs and diagnosis of fibrillation or asystole.

The hind limbs should be raised above the level of the heart to improve venous return and the abdomen should be compressed with a tight dressing. If the treatment is having an effect, a pulse should be palpable, the pupils should constrict and mucous membrane colour should improve.

D Drugs

A wide variety of drugs may be required, which depend on the patient's requirements (Table 25.21). It is unlikely that in a serious situation a diagnosis will be made of the cause of cardiac arrest, so resuscitation depends on two principal drugs – adrenaline (epinephrine) and atropine. Administration of these drugs may be made more difficult by the collapse of the patient's circulation.

Routes of administration:

- **Peripheral vein** – drugs may not reach the heart in sufficient concentration

Table 25.21 Drugs for cardiopulmonary resuscitation

Drug	Indication	Dose	Route
Adrenaline (epinephrine)	Asystole, bradycardia, myocardial depression Anaphylaxis	0.1–0.2 mg/kg 0.2–0.4 mg/kg	Intravenous Intrathoracic
Atropine	Asystole, sinus bradycardia	0.02–0.04 mg/kg 0.4 mg/kg	Intravenous Intrathoracic
Calcium gluconate	Myocardial depression, hyperkalaemia, hypocalcaemia	10 mg/kg	Intravenous
Dobutamine	Myocardial failure	Dog 2–20 µg/kg/min Cat 4 µg/kg/min	Intravenous Intravenous
Dexamethasone	Blood pressure support, reduction of cerebral oedema	2 mg/kg	Intravenous
Furosemide	Cerebral oedema, pulmonary oedema, acute renal failure	Dog 2–4 mg/kg Cat 1–2 mg/kg	Intravenous
Lignocaine (Lidocaine)	Ventricular tachycardia, Ventricular fibrillation	Dog 2–4 mg/kg Cat 0.5–1 mg/kg	Intravenous bolus
Mannitol	Cerebral oedema, acute renal failure	1–2 g/kg	Intravenous
Methyl prednisolone; sodium succinate	Cerebral oedema	30 mg/kg q12 h	Intravenous
Naloxone	Opioid reversal	0.04–1 mg/kg	Intravenous
Sodium bicarbonate	Electromechanical dissociation, acidosis	0.5–1 mEq/kg	Intravenous

- **Jugular vein** – intravenous injection is easy and more effective, especially if a long intravenous catheter can be introduced
- **Intratracheal** – the drug must be diluted in saline at twice the normal dose and is injected via a urinary catheter passed down the trachea. Forced inflation of the lungs aids absorption
- **Intracardiac injection** – this can be dangerous and the heart must be surgically exposed first. If not, the drug could be injected into the myocardium, causing irreparable damage, or a coronary artery could be lacerated. However, it does place the drug where it is needed, so can be very effective.

If the heart re-establishes a rhythm, the follow-up drug and treatment regime can be very complex and time-consuming. These animals can be very ill for a considerable time period and will certainly require 24 hour care in the early stages.

E Electrical defibrillation

The use of an electric current to convert ventricular fibrillation into sinus rhythm. It will not work for asystolic hearts. The defibrillator can be applied externally via gel-coated paddles at 1–5 J/kg. It can also be used internally after a thoracotomy at 0.1–0.5 J/kg, with saline-soaked swabs covering the heart.

F Follow-up

- **Ventilation** – continue on 100% oxygen until a normal respiratory pattern is established. Capnography is useful to detect acidosis due to anaerobic metabolism or hypocapnia due to excessive mechanical ventilation
- **Fluid therapy** – use a crystalloid solution initially to support blood pressure and improve perfusion which helps to correct metabolic acidosis. Take care in cases with cerebral oedema as this may exacerbate it
- **Cardiac function** – positive inotropes may be required, e.g. dobutamine infusion, to support cardiac output and blood pressure
- **Renal function** – monitor urine output – should be over 1 ml/kg/hour
- **CNS support** – hypoxic damage to the CNS tends to cause cerebral oedema, which may cause pressure to build up in the skull in a self-perpetuating manner. It should be treated aggressively. Reperfusion of the damaged areas leads to a worsening of the situation. Corticosteroids may help reduce oedema and may reduce the effects of free radicals liberated during reperfusion. The head should be positioned slightly elevated and hyperventilation will reduce cerebral blood flow, so reducing intracranial pressure
- **Body temperature** – patients tend to be hypothermic so need rewarming slowly. This should be very slow in cases of cerebral oedema because a return to normothermia may increase the damage.

Respiratory emergencies

These can be broadly divided into apnoea and respiratory obstruction.

Apnoea and hypoventilation

- Apnoea is the cessation of breathing
- Hypoventilation is a reduction in the amount of air entering the pulmonary alveoli.

Both result in hypoxia and hypercapnia, which rapidly result in cardiac arrest. Respiratory arrest will often appear to occur concurrently with cardiac arrest.

Causes

- **CNS depression:**
  - Properties of the anaesthetic agent or overdose, e.g. propofol given as a bolus causes apnoea
  - Raised intracranial pressure
  - Hypothermia
- **Thoracic-wall dysfunction:**
  - Pneumothorax
  - Mechanical restriction – heavy blankets, tight bandages
  - Pain after thoracic surgery
- **Pulmonary disease:**
  - Oedema
  - Diaphragmatic hernia
  - Intrapulmonary haemorrhage
- **Tachypnoea:**
  - Panting under anaesthesia so the inspired gas does not reach the alveoli
  - Inadequate anaesthesia
  - Pyrexia.

Signs of apnoea

No respiratory movements, cyanosis of mucous membranes.

Treatment

- Check airway is patent and intubate if necessary
- IPPV with 100% oxygen every 5–10 seconds, ensuring good chest excursions. Failure to cause chest wall movement needs investigation and might be due to pneumothorax or thoracic effusion
- Assess level of unconsciousness and alter accordingly
- Analeptics may be required but, as they are general analeptics, other conditions may be exacerbated
- Doxapram 1–2 mg/kg i.v. or sublingually is the most specific respiratory stimulant but it may cause a very violent recovery from anaesthesia.

Respiratory obstruction

This could occur at any time from premedication to recovery. It is most frequently seen postoperatively when the semiconscious animal has to support its own airway, and may especially be a problem if the patient's anatomy is abnormal, e.g. brachycephalic breeds or after pharyngeal/laryngeal surgery.

Obstruction may be due to: soft-tissue obstruction of the larynx, such as by the soft palate or tongue; foreign bodies such as regurgitated vomit, tooth fragments, blood or mucus; laryngeal spasm; oedema; or bronchospasm.

Intra-anaesthetic obstruction should not occur but poor circuit management may cause endotracheal tube kinking, mucus build-up in the endotracheal tube and closure of the expiratory valve resulting in overdistension of the reservoir bag.

Signs of obstruction

- **Intraoperatively** – extreme respiratory movements with no movement of the reservoir bag, leading to cessation of respiratory movement and bradycardia
- **Pre- or postoperatively** – dyspnoea, snoring sounds, increased respiratory efforts, gasping, cyanosis.

Treatment

- **Intraoperatively** – disconnect from the circuit; if no gas movement, extubate and reintubate

with a fresh endotracheal tube. Ventilate with 100% oxygen
- **Pre- or postoperatively** – if vomiting or regurgitating, place head downwards and lavage mouth or apply suction to the pharynx. If soft tissues are obstructing the larynx, extend the head and neck and pull the tongue forwards.

If severe obstruction continues then reintubate or, if this is impossible, perform a tracheostomy.

Bibliography

Abrams-Ogg, A., 2000. Practical blood transfusion. In: Day, M.J., Mackin, A., Littlewood, J.D. (Eds.), BSAVA Manual of Canine and Feline Haematology and Transfusion Medicine. British Small Animal Veterinary Association, Quedgeley, Gloucestershire, pp. 263–303.

Broadbelt, D., 2003. Anaesthesia: perioperative fatalities. Vet. Rev. 86, 28–29.

Hall, L.W., Clarke, K.W., Trim, C.M., 2001. Veterinary Anaesthesia, tenth ed. W B Saunders, London.

Short, C.E., 1987. Principles and Practice of Veterinary Anaesthesia. Williams & Wilkins, Baltimore.

Tennant, B., 2005. Small Animal Formulary, fifth ed. British Small Animal Veterinary Association, Quedgeley, Gloucestershire.

Welsh, E., 2003. Anaesthesia for Veterinary Nurses. Blackwell, Oxford.

Recommended reading

Aspinall, V., 2008. Clinical Procedures in Veterinary Nursing, second ed. Butterworth-Heinemann, Oxford.
Dedicated chapter describes the practical aspects of setting up circuits and monitoring the anaesthetic in small animal practice.

Cooper, B., Lane, D.R., Turner, L. (Eds.), 2007. Veterinary Nursing, fourth ed. BSAVA, Gloucester.
Detailed chapter closely follows veterinary nursing syllabus.

Welsh, E., 2003. Anaesthesia for Veterinary Nurses. Blackwell, Oxford.
Entire book devoted to the subject of anaesthesia and written for veterinary nurses rather than veterinary surgeons.

Equine anaesthesia

Anja Walker

Introduction

Anaesthesia in equids incorporates general anaesthesia, standing sedation and local anaesthetic techniques and is carried out to perform painful or difficult procedures, to position the animal in dorsal or lateral recumbency, as a method of restraint for fractious or unhandled animals and as a diagnostic tool. General anaesthesia or standing chemical restraint of horses allows maintenance of a clean or sterile operating area, calm handling of large or difficult animals and a concomitant increase in safety for both patient and attendants. Modern sedative drugs available for use in equine practice, often combined with local anaesthetic techniques, allow many procedures to be performed standing that might previously have required a general anaesthetic, e.g. cheek tooth removal. Local anaesthesia, e.g. perineural and intra-articular anaesthesia (nerve or joint 'blocks'), has a major role to play in diagnosis, particularly of lameness.

Preoperative care

Client instructions for presentation of animal for anaesthesia

Clients should be aware of the procedure to be performed when making an appointment for anaesthesia of their horse. Anaesthetics, either field- or clinic-based, should not be booked in at short notice, so that all parties can be adequately prepared.

The owner may or may not be asked to have the horse's shoes removed before admission for general anaesthesia. It is preferable for elective procedures to admit the horse to the clinic the night before a general anaesthetic, to minimize the stresses associated with travelling and immediate introduction to a new environment. If the horse must be kept at home the night before the anaesthetic, the owner should be given careful instructions to remove food at least 12 hours before surgery and to ensure that the horse is stabled on an unpalatable bed. Water should not be removed until approximately 1 hour prior to surgery, or when the premedicant is administered. On admission to the clinic (and increasingly in cases of field anaesthesia), it is essential that the client be asked to sign an anaesthetic consent. This is to safeguard the practice in a legal situation and gives the veterinary nurse the opportunity to inform the client of the risks of anaesthesia and to answer or redirect any questions or concerns before anaesthesia is performed. Box 26.1 provides a pre-anaesthetic checklist.

Patient assessment and recording of animal details

Pre-anaesthetic records and assessment of patients for elective procedures should at least consist of the following:

- Patient name, age, sex, breed and colour – basic markings should be recorded if several similar animals are present in the hospital at the same time
- Owner name, address and telephone number, including number for contact during or after surgery
- Record of any drug allergies known, tetanus vaccination status, feed requirements and any other relevant history; record what equipment is left with the horse

- Quotes for the surgery may or may not be recorded in writing on the admission form
- Anaesthetic consent forms should contain a written statement of the risks of anaesthesia and must be read, understood and signed. If a responsible party cannot attend, the form may be completed over the phone and faxed for signing
- Record a full pre-anaesthetic clinical examination, including temperature, heart rate and rhythm, respiratory rate and auscultation of lung sounds, mucous membrane colour and capillary refill time
- Weight measured as accurately as possible, using calibrated scales or a weigh tape
- Any previously obtained relevant laboratory results. (At present, routine pre-anaesthetic blood sampling is only occasionally performed in equine practice.)

In addition to the above, especially in the case of emergency procedures, further information such as history of circumstances leading up to surgery and other diagnostic procedures used, e.g. joint or peritoneal fluid analysis, packed cell volume and total protein or radiographs, should be included in the records of the case.

Classes of risk according to physical status

Statistics show that routine general anaesthesia in horses carries an inherently higher risk than in other companion animals. This increased risk is related to their large size and temperament as well as to their anatomy. Awareness and careful assessment of these risks and the laying down of routine protocols to be carried out before, during and after all general anaesthetics are therefore of great importance.

The Confidential Enquiry into Perioperative Equine Fatalities (CEPEF) study (Johnston et al 2002) identified risk factors in equine anaesthesia and found that animals could be categorized according to several factors. Emergency colic surgery carries the highest risk of intra- or perioperative death, with mares in the last trimester of pregnancy and foals less than 1 month of age also in the high-risk category. Surgical conditions, such as dorsal recumbency, surgery performed out of normal work hours and anaesthesia administered without premedication, all carry a higher risk of perioperative death. The study concluded that the rate of perioperative death in equine anaesthesia is 1 in every 100.

Pre-anaesthetic assessment of risk for each individual should include the clinical parameters summarized above, as well as a careful evaluation of the type, age, reason for anaesthesia and physiological condition, e.g. pregnant, shocked, exhausted or frightened. These findings must be taken into account when preparing the animal for and performing general anaesthesia.

Factors determining choice of anaesthetic agent

Drug choice in equine anaesthesia is usually determined by the following:

- **Type and duration of operation** – these have a bearing on drug choice; for example, muscle relaxants may be avoided in orthopaedic and short-duration surgery, as ataxia during recovery would increase the risk of injury
- **Type and condition of patient** – pre-anaesthetic protocol may alter in a fractious or unhandled animal to improve induction conditions for the animal and the handlers. Drugs may be altered in anaesthetizing a horse in a state of hypovolaemic shock in order to minimize the depressive effects of anaesthesia
- **Normal facilities used for surgery** – surgery routinely performed in an operating theatre on a table will usually have gaseous methods of anaesthetic maintenance, whereas, for field anaesthesia and anaesthesia performed on a cushioned floor, total intravenous anaesthesia may be more practical
- **Anaesthetist familiarity** – frequent use of certain drug combinations will improve anaesthetic technique as the anaesthetist becomes familiar with the reactions of a variety of patients to a known drug protocol
- **Cost** – this is a factor in most establishments and may restrict, for example, the acquisition of more than one vaporizer, restricting use of more than one type of volatile agent. Newer generations of anaesthetic gases are usually more expensive than the older drugs.

Premedication

Premedication is the use of a drug or combination of drugs given prior to or concurrently with administration of the drugs to induce general anaesthesia (Table 26.1). Premedication is used, as in other species, to create a relaxed and sleepy patient and in order to reduce stress and anxiety during the anaesthetic procedure for both the patient and its attendants. Lack of anxiety lowers the risk of complications that may occur as a result of adrenaline (epinephrine) release, e.g. cardiac arrhythmia. Judicious choice of drug combinations given prior to anaesthesia can allow a 50–75% reduction of the dosage of anaesthetic agents required to both induce and maintain anaesthesia, helping to minimize the depressant effects that these drugs have on circulatory and respiratory functions. In the horse, the use of premedication often aids or enables the control of unhandled, fractious or temperamental animals. Drugs may be included in premedication protocols for their physiologically beneficial effects, e.g. analgesia and myocardial protection.

Preparation of drugs

The dosage of anaesthetic and premedicant drugs should be calculated as accurately as possible by accurate assessment of the weight of the animal. Once the premedication and

Table 26.1 Drugs used in premedication

Group	Drug	Classification	Form	Route/effect	Pharmacology
Alpha-2 agonists (sedatives)	Romifidine	POM-V	Injection, 10 mg/ml	i.v., quick predictable action Maximum effect 5 min after injection i.m., slow onset, less reliable, higher doses required Detomidine can be given by sublingual route in extreme cases; very slow onset of action	Combination with opioids increases depth and reliability of sedation Side effect of hyperglycaemia and polyuria; possible hypotension Sedative potency: detomidine > romifidine > xylazine Analgesic potency: detomidine > xylazine > romifidine All are muscle relaxants Romifidine produces least ataxia and is a common premedication Horses can still kick! Sedivet (romifidine) has a 6-day meat withdrawal. Xylazine and detomidine not for use in horses for human consumption
	Detomidine	POM-V	Injection, 10 mg/ml		
	Xylazine	POM-V	Injection, 20 mg/ml or 100 mg/ml		
Phenothiazines (neuroleptics)	Acepromazine	POM-V	Injection, 10 mg/ml Paste, various concentrations	i.v. or i.m. most reliable route Oral, more reliable than tablets Slow onset of action	Mild–moderate sedation with no analgesic properties Good anxiolytic (useful for shoeing, travelling, premedication) Given i.v., peak effect is in about 5 min, duration of action 4–24 h Orally, onset takes approximately 1 h, duration of action 4–24 h Contraindicated in hypotensive animals Not for use in breeding stallions/pregnant mares Not for use in horses intended for human consumption
			Tablets, 10 mg or 25 mg	Oral, unpredictable sedation Slow onset	
Benzodiazepines (sedative)	Diazepam	Human drug not licensed for veterinary use	Injection 5 mg/ml in 2 ml Tablets 2 mg, 5 mg or 10 mg	Slow i.v. (do not give alone to adult horses)	Highly effective anxiolytics, low toxicity, short duration of action Useful for control of seizures in foals and pre-myelography Possible excitation in normal healthy animals if given i.v. Ataxia and panic in conscious horses due to muscle relaxing effect Not for use in horses intended for human consumption
Opioids (opioid analgesics)	Butorphanol	POM-V	Injection, 10 mg/ml	i.v.	Extremely potent analgesia (far greater than NSAIDs) Deepens and prolongs sedation when used in combination with alpha-2 agonists Morphine may cause excitement and box walking in pain-free horses Torbugesic (butorphanol) has a meat withdrawal of 0 days Pethidine is not for use in horses intended for human consumption
	Morphine	CD (S2) Human drug	Injection, 10 mg/ml or 60 mg/ml, vials	i.m., i.v., epidural or intra-articular	
	Pethidine	CD (S2)	Injection	i.m.	
Sedative–hypnotic	Chloral hydrate	POM-V	Crystalline powder	i.v. or oral	No longer in wide use May be useful to sedate untouchable horses by adding to water (nasty taste)

CD, controlled drug; NSAID, non-steroidal anti-inflammatory drug; POM-V prescription-only medicine – veterinarian; S2, Schedule 2 controlled drug

anaesthetic protocol have been decided upon, dosages of the required drugs should be calculated and the drugs should be prepared and clearly labelled for use during premedication and induction of anaesthesia. Drugs should be ready for use either in syringes with needles appropriate for the route of administration, in drip bags or bottles with the required giving set available, or in a suitable presentation for other routes of administration. Diazepam should not be drawn into plastic syringes until immediately prior to injection.

Analgesia

Analgesia is a state of insensitivity to pain even though the subject is fully conscious. It involves the abolition of pain alone while normal sensation is maintained; anaesthesia removes both pain and normal sensation and, in the case of general anaesthesia, removes consciousness.

The importance and benefits of analgesia

Analgesia in the equine patient is important not only on humane grounds to reduce suffering but also to reduce the undesirable effects of pain, e.g. violent rolling and self-trauma associated with colic or overload strain on a limb when resting the contralateral limb. Control of pain may improve temperament and aid handling. Perioperative pain control can reduce the amount of anaesthetic agent required and, by reducing the stimulus of pain, improve the quality of recovery.

Pain can be recognized in horses in many forms:

- Subdued attitude
- Loss of appetite
- Increased (or decreased) respiratory rate and effort
- Increased (or decreased) pulse rate
- Alteration in pupil diameter
- 'Flehmen' or curling of the upper lip
- Teeth-grinding
- Reluctance to move or 'guarding' of painful area
- Limb-resting and lameness
- Recumbency
- Posturing to urinate without passing urine
- Rolling
- Flank-watching
- Objection to palpation of painful area.

Monitoring anaesthesia

Anaesthetic drugs (Table 26.2) have a depressive effect on the cardiac and respiratory functions of the patient. This depressive effect can be life-threatening if careful and ongoing assessment of these functions is not performed and the appropriate actions taken.

Anaesthetic monitoring should be continuous and should be carried out by one dedicated anaesthetist throughout a procedure. Monitoring methods will depend on the conditions in which anaesthesia is being carried out – field conditions do not lend themselves to use of electrical monitors, which may take some time to set up and may prolong anaesthetic time for limited benefits. Whether in field or theatre conditions, the primary tool of anaesthesia should

---

> **Box 26.2** Patient monitoring routine
>
> - Clinical examination of horse at rest in the stable
> - Observation of response to premedication
> - Check vital signs after induction before lifting or positioning
> - Intra-operative monitoring using manual checks and monitors as appropriate
> - Periodic intra-operative checks on equipment
> - Manual monitoring should continue after the horse is placed in recovery and observation at a distance maintained until it stands up

---

be observation by the anaesthetist and electrical equipment should only be used to enhance careful monitoring. It is good practice to complete anaesthetic record charts but this again should not be done at the expense of careful patient monitoring. Familiarity with monitors should be gained through training during low-risk procedures. It can be argued that it is only useful to monitor things that you have the ability to alter. For example, it may not be useful to monitor blood oxygen without the facility for positive pressure ventilation.

Anaesthetic monitoring is most effective when a routine is established to reduce the likelihood that any areas are overlooked (Box 26.2). Equipment that should be checked prior to an operation includes:

- Oxygen cylinders
- Adequate supplies of anaesthetic drugs required
- Leak check on endotracheal tube cuff
- Mouth gag
- Soda lime
- Mats, etc., to position horse on floor or table
- Anaesthetic machine, including vaporizer fluid level
- Electrical monitor check
- Fill in patient information on anaesthetic chart.

Monitoring equipment – uses and limitations

Short routine procedures undertaken in a field or clinic environment are often monitored purely by observation, pulse palpation and use of a stethoscope (Table 26.3). All equine clinics undertaking surgery in a theatre on a regular basis should have, as a minimum, facilities for electrocardiography and blood pressure monitoring.

Stethoscope

Essential to auscultate heart and lungs, very portable, familiar piece of monitoring equipment. There is a limitation in auscultation of the heart in the unconscious horse as it can fall away from the body wall, leading to a false diagnosis of cardiac arrest.

Electrocardiography

ECG monitors show the heart rate and the pattern of activity in the heart. They are easily and quickly applied and provide easily visible, reassuring monitoring of cardiac activity. Heart rate is displayed on the screen and an alarm will sound on

Table 26.2 The main pharmacological properties of each of the commonly used analgesics

Group	Drug	Classification	Form	Route	Pharmacology (peculiar to individual drugs)
Non-steroidal anti-inflammatory drugs (NSAIDs)	Phenylbutazone (Equipalazone)	POM-V	Powder (1 g sachets) Paste (1 g per unit/6 g per tube)	Oral	Very commonly used because of low cost and convenient preparation Very irritant if injected outside the vein Greater analgesia achieved by the intravenous route
			Injectable solution (200 mg/ml)	i.v.	
	Flunixin (Finadyne)	POM-V	Powder (250 mg sachets) Paste (500 mg tube)	Oral	Commonly used NSAID licensed for use in horses intended for human consumption Meat withdrawal is 7 days from the last dose given
			Injectable solution (50 mg/ml)	i.v.	
	Ketoprofen (Ketofen)	POM-V	Injectable solution (10 mg/ml)	i.v.	
	Carprofen (Rimadyl)	POM-V	Injectable solution (50 mg/ml)	i.v.	The least damaging to gastrointestinal mucosa and hence the drug of choice for use in foals if the use of NSAIDs is unavoidable
			Granules (210 mg sachets)	Oral	
	Aspirin	P-GSL	Tablets (various formulations)	Oral	Not licensed for use in horses Occasionally indicated for treatment of thromboembolic disorders
	Meloxicam (Metacam)	POM-V	Injectable solution 20 mg/ml Oral suspension 15 mg/ml	i.v.	Licensed for use in horses intended for human consumption. 5 day meat withdrawal May be useful in foals
	Suxibuzone (Danilon Equidos)	POM-V	Granules (1.5 g sachets)	Oral	
Pharmacology pertaining to all of above			Effective in the relief of pain and swelling Act by inhibiting cyclo-oxygenase (COX), which acts to generate inflammatory mediators Highly bound to plasma protein; acute inflammation causes exudates rich in plasma protein, thus carrying high levels of the drug to the site Adverse side effects include gastrointestinal ulceration and nephrotoxicity Foals are particularly prone to gastric ulceration and NSAIDs should be used judiciously in the very young (see carprofen, above) Use of anti-inflammatory drugs is prohibited in competition, including racing: stop use at least 8 days prior to a race or competition With the exception of flunixin and meloxicam the use of NSAIDs is not licensed in horses intended for human consumption		

Opioid analgesics, see Table 26.1.

most machines if this drops. The displayed heart rate should be periodically checked manually, because, as monitors are adapted for human use, they occasionally count more than one beat for each 'PQRS' complex. It is sometimes possible to correct this by altering the lead position. ECG in the horse is limited to giving information on rate and rhythm. Other electrical equipment and physical movement or vibration, e.g. by clippers, affect the monitor display.

Blood pressure

This is most reliably measured by direct methods, i.e. arterial catheter placement. Arteries used for this procedure are the facial, transverse facial and dorsal metatarsal arteries (Fig. 26.1). The blood pressure monitor is often combined with the ECG monitor. A direct blood pressure trace will give information on cardiac output, and blood pressure values are an important guide to depth of anaesthesia, i.e. higher for 'light' planes of anaesthesia and lower as the patient becomes 'deeper'. It also indicates peripheral perfusion, which is important in the horse because of the association of poor perfusion of muscles with postoperative myopathies. Mean arterial blood pressure should be maintained above 65 mmHg to decrease the risk of myopathy. Desirable mean arterial blood pressure in anaesthetized horses is 65–85 mmHg.

The main limitation of direct blood pressure monitoring is that some skill must be learned in the placement of arterial catheters and use of the machine. Indirect methods involving pneumatic cuffs applied around the leg or tail are available but are unreliable in horses.

Table 26.3 Signs of anaesthetic depth for inhalation anaesthesia

Light anaesthesia	Medium anaesthesia	Deep anaesthesia	Anaesthetic overdose
Eye central (or caudal)	Eye medially rotated	Eye central	Eye central
Pupil moderate dilated	Pupil dilation slight	Pupil dilated	Pupil very dilated
Nystagmus brisk	Nystagmus slow/absent	No nystagmus	No nystagmus
Brisk palpebral reflex	Sluggish palpebral reflex	No palpebral reflex	No palpebral reflex
Brisk corneal reflex	Sluggish corneal reflex	Cornea very slow/absent	No corneal reflex
Eye wide open	Eye closing	Eye open	Eye wide open
Lacrimation ++	Lacrimation +	Lacrimation −	Dry eye
Head and limb movement possible (tension in tendon of m. sternocephalicus)*	Muscle relaxation (tendon of m. sternocephalicus relaxes)*	Total muscle relaxation*	Muscles flaccid*
Breath-holding or rapid breathing	Regular breathing pattern	Reduced respiration rate, often irregular	Cheyne–Stokes breathing or gasps
Anal reflex +++	Anal reflex ++	Anal reflex ±	Anal reflex −
High blood pressure		Low blood pressure	Very low blood pressure
Mucous membranes pink, CRT < 2 secs	Mucous membranes pink, CRT < 2 secs	Mucous membranes pale/blue, CRT ↑	Mucous membranes grey/blue
Pulse easily palpable	Pulse good to moderate	Weak pulse	Pulse not palpable

*Muscle relaxants (glyceryl guaiacolate ether) will increase muscle relaxation further; horses can often vary from the 'normal' in their responses to anaesthesia.
CRT, capillary refill time.

Respiration monitors

Monitoring of respiratory rate, depth, rhythm and pattern is extremely important but is best achieved by observation of the chest wall movement, excursion of the bag and sound of the valves during respiration. Breathing should be rhythmical and deep, with a normal rate of 6–10 breaths per minute in the horse. Shallow breathing may lead to poor lung ventilation; mucous membrane colour and capillary refill time should be monitored to check this.

Respiratory monitors are usually limited to measuring rate of respiration and do not indicate tidal volume or lung perfusion. The expense of acquiring a machine is unlikely to be justified.

Pulse oximeters

Non-invasive monitoring of the haemoglobin oxygen saturation of the blood (SaO_2) can be achieved by a clip attached to the tongue or the nasal septum. These machines usually measure pulse rate as well as oxygen saturation and will bleep with each heartbeat. Pulse oximeters may be useful in field conditions because they are easily portable, quickly connected and the audible pulse signal may be useful.

Pulse oximetry is poor at predicting problems and tends to indicate when a problem has occurred. Correcting low oxygen haemoglobin saturation in the horse, without means of positive pressure ventilation, is extremely difficult, and the value of these monitors without the availability of an artificial ventilator is doubtful.

Capnograph

Monitors are very useful and relatively inexpensive; they measure the CO_2 in expired air ($PaCO_2$). Elevated $PaCO_2$ can be addressed by increasing ventilation by compression of the rebreathing bag manually with the pressure relief valve closed. Capnography may be more useful in showing trends in $PaCO_2$ than in giving absolute values.

Blood gas machines

These are expensive pieces of equipment that require the ability to take arterial blood samples for immediate analysis in order to obtain accurate results. Correct sample handling is vital if accurate results are to be obtained. A blood gas machine will measure $PaCO_2$, PaO_2 and pH, which are of great benefit if severely compromised patients are routinely being anaesthetized and acid–base monitoring becomes increasingly important, e.g. colic surgery (see Chapter 25). Some hand-held blood electrolyte analysers are now available in the veterinary market and have the facility to measure blood gases.

General anaesthesia

General anaesthesia can be considered to take place in two stages:

- Induction – in which the animal becomes unconscious
- Maintenance – in which the animal is administered a continuous level of anaesthetic drug in order to keep it in a state of unconsciousness.

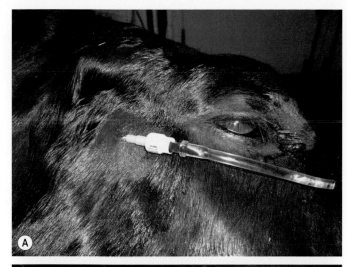

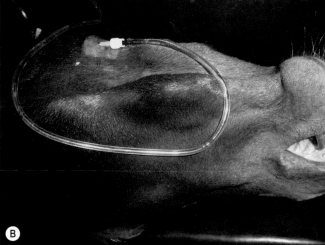

Fig. 26.1 (**A, B**) Position of the arteries used for direct blood pressure monitoring

be available to avoid mishaps and to deal with unexpected reactions on the part of the horse.

1. 'Free-fall' induction

The horse is positioned with the hindquarters in a corner and a handler on either side of the head to encourage the horse to drop its head and sink to the ground. This method does not require large numbers of personnel or special adaptations of the induction area.

2. 'Gate' technique

A padded gate is hung on one wall of the induction box and is used to restrain the horse against the parallel wall. One handler holds the head and another handler holds a rope that closes the gate by running the rope through a ring on the parallel wall in front of the horse, thereby controlling the fall and preventing the horse from moving forward. The alternative to this uses several handlers to replace the gate to push the horse against the wall as anaesthesia is induced; the effectiveness of this method is greatly improved if the handlers refrain from pushing against the horse until it starts to lose consciousness. If this does not happen the horse is likely to push against the handlers and increase the risk of injuring somebody or falling awkwardly.

3. Tilting operating table

The table is tilted to a vertical position and the sedated horse is restrained with straps against it, with a handler controlling the head. As consciousness is lost, the straps take the weight of the horse and the table is rotated into the horizontal position, the horse now being in lateral recumbency. Lifting may be necessary to alter the position or to place padding under the horse. Recovery may involve transfer to a recovery box or a reversal of the induction procedure.

Induction

Anaesthesia should be induced in an environment that is safe for both the horse and handlers and one that is quiet and conducive to relaxation on the part of the patient. Field anaesthesia in a fenced, clean field is a common place to perform anaesthesia outside an operating theatre. Account must be taken of the temperament and 'handle-ability' of the patient and frightened or unhandled patients should be sedated prior to being taken into an open space. It may be necessary to compromise, and a hay barn with a clean, soft floor and bales to protect the horse from colliding with hard or sharp obstacles may mean not losing the patient.

Induction boxes designed for equine anaesthesia should have padded floor and walls and, if possible, should not have any corners, e.g. hexagonal in shape. Doors should have padding that is thick enough to ensure that they are flush with the walls on either side. Viewing hatches are desirable but mirrors placed so that the horse can be observed during recovery also work quite well. Boxes should be large enough to induce a large horse safely but small enough to prevent the patient from building up any speed during recovery.

Techniques for induction vary between practices. For all techniques an adequate number of trained personnel should

Facilities required for anaesthesia

Field anaesthesia

Facilities required are as for induction but the area then becomes the operating site and positioning of the horse is facilitated by using bales, sandbags or similar.

The equipment required (Box 26.3) is similar to that for a theatre environment with some obvious changes. Intravenous catheterization is desirable to allow easy 'top-up' of the anaesthetic drugs and equipment to resuscitate the patient in an emergency is advisable. This includes a suitable endotracheal tube with an inflatable cuff and an oxygen supply with a demand valve or suitable tubing, and drugs to treat cardiac arrest. A pulse oximeter may be useful if available, as it is the most easily carried and quickly attached (non-invasive) piece of monitoring equipment.

Theatre anaesthesia

Anaesthesia in an induction box can be carried out as in the field, if it is to be carried out without lifting the horse, for short uncomplicated procedures. It is preferable to have facilities for gaseous maintenance as the anaesthetic machine doubles up as a means of ventilating the animal in an emergency situation.

For normal theatre anaesthesia, a machine for gaseous maintenance is necessary. A variety of sizes of endotracheal (ET) tubes, mouth gags and K-Y jelly to aid intubation, syringes to inflate ET tube cuffs, etc., should be available; a suitable scavenging system for the safe removal of waste gases from the area must be used. Spare oxygen canisters should be easily accessible if required during an anaesthetic.

Various table designs are available, including tables that sink into the induction box floor to conventional tables in an operating area separate from induction, onto which the horse must be lifted. An electronic or manual hoist is usually necessary for lifting and positioning and if so it is necessary to have either a generator or a manual backup hoist, in case of power failure. Hobbles used for lifting must be suitable for the hoist used and frequently checked for wear and tear.

Positioning of the horse and adequate padding are vital in a theatre, especially as the duration of the anaesthetic increases. Postoperative myopathies are distressing when a procedure has otherwise gone well. Horses may be positioned on purpose-made inflatable cushions or large foam rubber mats with waterproof covering. The induction box floor may be too hard for longer procedures and a cushion should be placed under the horse if surgery is to be carried out in that area. Attention must be paid to ensuring that there are no pressure points, particularly on the dependent muscles. In lateral recumbency, supports must be available to raise the legs slightly, so that upper and lower limbs are parallel with the ground, in order to reduce the pressure on the lower muscles and maximize venous return of blood from the limbs. Secure props or suspension from overhead supports can achieve this.

Facilities to measure ECG and blood pressure should be available and acquisition of equipment in addition to this may depend on practice finances. A 'crash box' should be available. All personnel should be trained so that, in the case of an emergency, reaction can be quick.

Intravenous induction agents

The most commonly used intravenous anaesthetic combinations are as follows:

Ketamine and diazepam

This combination is usually used after suitable sedation with an alpha-2 adrenoceptor agonist (Table 26.1). Ketamine alone can potentially cause excitement and induction quality is greatly improved by combination with a benzodiazepine. Ketamine (2 mg/kg) and diazepam (0.01–0.2 mg/kg) can be combined in the same syringe (diazepam reacts with plastic and should be drawn up immediately before administration); the combination is given as an intravenous bolus 5 minutes after the alpha-2 adrenoceptor agonist has been given. There may be a moment of ataxia before the horse sinks smoothly into sternal and then lateral recumbency, the horse should not be handled and no noise made until full relaxation is achieved, which may take up to 30 seconds. Voluntary eye movement and brisk reflexes usually remain initially, making accurate assessment of anaesthetic depth difficult. Ketamine gives minimal depression of cardiac and respiratory functions and is a good analgesic. Incremental top-up doses of ketamine can be used to prolong anaesthesia without significantly prolonging recovery time.

Ketamine/diazepam or thiopentone (thiopental) with glyceryl guaiacolate ether (GGE)

Thiopentone (thiopental) is becoming less available and hence its use in equine practice is becoming limited to 'tops-ups' during anaesthesia. Ketamine/diazepam can be used as an induction agent with GGE and should be combined with alpha-2 adrenoceptor agonist sedation. GGE is given by rapid intravenous bolus to effect (50–100 mg/kg). As the horse becomes ataxic, GGE infusion is stopped and ketamine/diazepam as above or thiopentone (5–6 mg/kg) is given by intravenous bolus. The horse should be adequately restrained to avoid panic as ataxia develops. GGE should never be given without an anaesthetic agent as inhumane conscious paralysis will result. Thiopentone is strongly irritant if injected perivascularly and should always be administered via a catheter at the lowest practical concentration – in larger horses a 10% solution is required to make the dose required a practical volume. Thiopentone produces transient depression of respiration and blood pressure and has no analgesic properties. Anaesthesia can be prolonged for short periods with thiopentone and GGE top-ups but, at higher total doses, this will prolong recovery and increase ataxia.

Propofol

The use of propofol for the induction of anaestheisa in foals is increasing, although the volumes required and concurrent cost prevent its use in adult horses in most commercial settings. Propofol is adminstered intravenously to effect to induce anaesthesia.

Table 26.4 Insertion of 'short-stay' and 'long-stay' catheters

Short-stay	Long-stay
Clip area over vein and clean skin	Large area over vein is clipped to ensure good sterility and the skin prepared as for surgery
A subcutaneous 'bleb' of local anaesthetic is injected and a small skin incision is made to reduce skin drag when inserting the catheter	Local anaesthetic is injected as for short-stay but skin incision is not normally made – improving the seal of the skin around the catheter and reducing the risk of infection
The vein is raised by applying digital pressure and the catheter is inserted with clean hands, taking normal intravenous injection precautions	The vein is raised as for short-stay and the catheter is inserted in a fully sterile manner using sterile gloving. The catheter should be primed with heparin saline before insertion
Placement with or against blood flow	Placement with blood flow
A three-way tap or injection cap is applied to the hub of the catheter and a small amount of heparin saline is injected to prevent clotting	A short length of purpose-made extension tubing with a valve or injection port is attached to the hub. All subsequent handling should be clean or preferably sterile
The catheter and port are sutured in place by a pre-placed skin suture, or skin glue can be used	The catheter is sutured in place as appropriate for its design
Short-stay catheters are normally over-the-needle design and less than 15 cm in length	Long-stay catheters can be over-the-needle or Seldinger type, placed over a guide wire. They are longer and softer than short-stay catheters

Total intravenous anaesthesia (TIVA)

This is a method of anaesthetic maintenance that is useful in a field situation but can also be used in a theatre in place of gaseous methods. Anaesthesia is induced with an alpha-2 adrenoceptor agonist/ketamine/diazepam protocol; GGE induction should be avoided to reduce the risk of GGE overdose. TIVA combinations can be made with xylazine or detomidine (romifidine is cheaper but requires higher drip rates, increasing the chance of GGE overdose), ketamine and GGE:

e.g. 1 g ketamine
10 mg detomidine or 500 mg xylazine
added to 500 ml ready-made 10% solution of GGE.

Infusion is usually at a rate of about 1 ml/kg/hour. This method should not be used for procedures longer than 90–120 minutes as the accumulated dose of GGE and ketamine will increase the risk of a prolonged and ataxic recovery. Intubation and oxygen supplementation is recommended for procedures lasting more than 20–30 minutes.

Placement of intravenous catheters

Intravenous catheterization of the horse is usually via the jugular vein. Cephalic and lateral thoracic veins can be used in cases where one or both jugular veins are occluded. Whether the catheter is placed with or against the direction of blood flow depends on the preference of the personnel involved. If large volumes of fluid are to be infused it is preferable to place the catheter with the blood flow; care must be taken as this position increases the possibility of air being drawn through the catheter and even a very small quantity of air in the circulation can cause a horse to collapse. Choice of catheter size depends on the size of the patient and the catheter's intended use.

Catheters for anaesthetic induction are usually designed for 'short-stay' and should be removed after recovery (Table 26.4). Catheters for use over several days are 'long-stay' and designed to be less irritant and more compliant to the lumen of the vessel, reducing the risk of thrombus formation within the vein. Preparation of the skin for 'long-stay' catheters is important and the site should be sterile to avoid the introduction of infection and the development of thrombophlebitis. This risk is even greater when treating an animal in a state of septicaemia.

Health and Safety issues

Accidental self-administration of injectable drugs used for premedication and induction is dangerous, and can occur by absorption through skin and mucous membranes:

- Spills on to skin during drawing-up and administration should immediately be washed off with large amounts of water
- Contamination of the atmosphere by volatile agents occurs during vaporizer filling and use. Vaporizers should be filled with purpose-made attachments and outside the operating area when possible. Volatile agent monitoring should be carried out at least annually to detect possible problems.
- Circuits should be regularly checked for leaks and scavenging systems should be used
- Emptying of the rebreathing bag should be done through the scavenging system by fully opening the pressure release valve, rather than by detachment of the bag from the cylinder
- Toxic effects on theatre personnel at the levels encountered during normal veterinary use have not been proved but COSHH and Health and Safety Executive regulations relating to the substances should be adhered to. Advice should be sought during pregnancy.

Table 26.5 Advantages and disadvantages of inhalational and total intravenous anaesthesia

Advantages	Disadvantages
Inhalational anaesthesia	
Effective, controllable and normally predictable maintenance of anaesthesia	High cost of initial set-up
Low running costs	Varying degrees of cardiovascular and respiratory depression
Concurrent oxygen delivery	Required gases are potentially flammable/explosive
Activity does not rely on metabolism by the body	Possible risk to personnel as a result of exposure to volatile agents
Duration of anaesthesia can be safely increased within a certain range	
The airway patency is maintained	
Total intravenous anaesthesia	
Minimal equipment required, convenient for field conditions	Drugs required are expensive
Endotracheal intubation may not be required	Drugs have a cumulative effect and rely on clearance by the animals' metabolism. This may lead to prolonged recovery
No reliance on respiratory function to deepen anaesthesia	Depth of anaesthesia can be easily increased but not decreased
No flammable or explosive gases or cylinders are required	Causes respiratory depression and oxygen may be needed

Storage

Anaesthetic drugs should be stored as other prescription-only medicines in a suitable, preferably locked, drug store. Controlled drugs, e.g. pethidine and morphine, should be kept in a separate, locked cupboard or safe and all records of purchase and dispensing should be written in a bound book. Although the law does not, at the moment, define ketamine as a dangerous drug it is recommended that it is kept in the locked drugs cupboard and records are kept of its use. Compressed gas cylinders should be kept away from extremes of temperature or open flames and should be stored, according to fire regulations, outside the building, away from entrances and secured in a lockable metal cage where they cannot fall over or be damaged.

Withdrawal periods

Horses are considered to be 'food-producing animals' under European legislation and should now have a signed passport declaration to say that the horse will not be used for human consumption before an anaesthetic is administered. If it is possible that the horse may enter the human food chain, products should be chosen that are licensed for use in food-producing animals (consult the Department for Environment, Food and Rural Affairs or the Veterinary Medicines Directorate for lists of licensed products). Drugs and their withdrawal periods should be recorded on the passports of animals that may enter the human food chain. Use of any product 'off-licence' should be carefully considered and should be justifiable on the 'cascade' system (see Ch. 17). Consequences of the use of drugs in this way are, first, that the manufacturer is unlikely to take responsibility for any adverse reaction and, second, that in the event of an adverse reaction, a successful legal prosecution might be mounted against the practitioner. The owner's informed consent should be obtained in cases where it is necessary to go 'off-licence'.

Maintenance of anaesthesia

In the horse, general anaesthesia may be maintained either by the inhalation of gases, or of liquids with sufficient vapour pressure to produce a gas, or by total intravenous anaesthesia, i.e. both induction and maintenance produced by intravenous agents. The advantages and disadvantages of both systems are shown in Table 26.5.

Inhalation of anaesthetic agents

The volatile anaesthetic agent most commonly used in equine anaesthesia is isoflurane. Halothane is still currently available but its use is decreasing. Some centres have the facility to use sevoflurane in foals and compromised adults, e.g. colic and caesarean operations.

Anaesthetic gases used are oxygen and nitrous oxide; carbon dioxide is rarely used in equine anaesthesia and nitrous oxide is less widely used in equine than in small animal practice. For moderate case loads oxygen is usually obtained in 'G'-sized cylinders for ease of use and most large animal anaesthetic machines have the facility for two cylinders to be attached at a time (see Ch. 25). Larger hospitals may have banks of large gas cylinders (O_2 and N_2O) stored outside the building and piped into the operating theatre via colour-coded pipes to which the anaesthetic machine can be attached. The properties of these volatile agents and gases have been described in Chapter 25.

Anaesthetic equipment

Once the animal is unconscious, gaseous agents are administered via ET tubes, nasotracheal intubation and facemasks attached to the appropriate type of anaesthetic circuit.

Endotracheal intubation

A range of sizes of ET tubes is required:

- 12–16 mm diameter tube is suitable for a thoroughbred foal (or smaller for a pony foal)
- 24–30 mm diameter for a 500 kg adult
- 34 mm or larger for adult heavy horse breeds.

The tube should be long enough to reach the middle to lower third of the cervical trachea.

Endotracheal intubation is used to maintain the airway and, by inflation of the cuff, to deliver a controlled mixture of gases to the lungs. Control of the airway is essential in anaesthetic emergencies so that oxygen supply can be artificially maintained. Intubation is usually via the mouth and a gag is inserted between the upper and lower incisors to aid insertion and to prevent the horse from biting on to the tube. In cases when mouth surgery is to be carried out, the tube may be inserted into the trachea via the nose. Nasotracheal intubation is achieved by the use of a smaller-diameter ET tube than that used for tubing via the mouth; for example, a 20 mm diameter tube would be suitable for the average thoroughbred. Intubation of the airway increases its resistance by reducing its diameter and, in the case of nasotracheal intubation, this increase is exacerbated by the use of a small tube.

Once intubation has been achieved, correct placement can be checked by connecting to the anaesthetic machine and squeezing the rebreathing bag to check that the chest rises, rather than compressing the chest to check for breath coming out of the tube. Care must be taken in inflation of the cuff, as overinflation can cause damage to the tracheal lining and can compress the tube, causing increased resistance or complete obstruction; underinflation leads to leakage of gases and uncontrolled anaesthesia.

Facemasks

Gas induction via a facemask is restricted to use in foals and the mask should be adequate to fit over the muzzle to form a seal around the nose without obstructing the nostrils. The advantages of this method are that it removes the need for repeated injections as well as reducing the number of anaesthetic drugs and their potential side effects, which is especially pertinent in the anaesthesia of sick foals. Disadvantages are that strong and healthy foals may struggle to resist the pungent smell of the gas and become stressed, and a transition has to be made to endotracheal intubation once induction has been achieved. The stress can be reduced by gradually increasing the volatile agent content of inspired gas.

Anaesthetic circuits

Circle and to-and-fro circuits are almost exclusively used in equine anaesthesia (Figs 26.2, 26.3). These are both rebreathing systems, i.e. the expired gas is reused after being passed through soda lime to remove CO_2 (see Ch. 25). Non-rebreathing systems, where the expired gases are pushed out of the circuit by providing a high flow of replacement gases to displace them, would be impractical and costly in large animal anaesthesia. The rebreathing circuit has advantages in its conservation of the warmth and humidity of the expired air, as well as its low gas-flow requirements, low volatile agent usage and hence low waste/pollution.

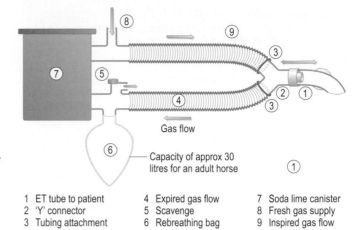

Gas flow

Capacity of approx 30 litres for an adult horse

1 ET tube to patient	4 Expired gas flow	7 Soda lime canister
2 'Y' connector	5 Scavenge	8 Fresh gas supply
3 Tubing attachment	6 Rebreathing bag	9 Inspired gas flow

Fig. 26.2 Large animal circle rebreathing circuit

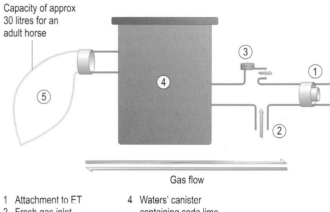

Capacity of approx 30 litres for an adult horse

Gas flow

1 Attachment to ET	4 Waters' canister containing soda lime
2 Fresh gas inlet	
3 Expiratory valve attached to scavenge	5 Rebreathing bag

Fig. 26.3 Large animal to-and-fro circuit or Waters' canister

The disadvantages of such systems are the initial expense, high resistance to breathing, size and relatively slow changes that are possible in levels of anaesthesia. Rebreathing circuits rely on soda lime to remove CO_2 from the circulating gas and this must be checked regularly and changed as soon as it becomes exhausted. Soda lime is manufactured with a colour indicator; some change from pink to white and some from white to lilac when exhausted. (This depends on the manufacturer, so make sure you know which you are using and never mix them.) Active soda lime will become hot during use which is another indicator that it is working. Soda lime status should be checked immediately after use, as it will regain its active colour to some extent when not in use, but may not become chemically active again.

Rebreathing circuits can be used as 'open', 'low-flow' and 'closed' systems:

- **Low-flow system** – most easily operated and requires the flow of oxygen to slightly exceed the requirements of the horse, allowing the excess gas to escape via the pressure release valve, which is left partly open
- **Open system** – one in which the pressure relief valve is left fully open, which would greatly reduce the efficiency of the circuit

- **Closed system** – one in which the gas flow replaces, without exceeding, the anaesthetic and oxygen used by the horse. The closed system is the most efficient but is more difficult to operate than a low-flow.

Nitrous oxide (N_2O) should not be used in rebreathing circuits in horses as it is used at a different rate from oxygen and may result in the gas mixture becoming relatively low in oxygen.

The to-and-fro system must be attached close to the horse to reduce the amount of dead space from the extra tubing. The fresh gas inflow is situated near the ET tube and the air is exhaled through the canister containing soda lime into the rebreathing bag and inhaled in the opposite direction via the same path; hence 'to-and-fro'. Care must be taken to avoid soda lime dust being inhaled. The advantages are that the system is simple and relatively portable for use in field conditions if necessary.

Foal anaesthesia

The major consideration in choosing a circuit for foal anaesthesia is the resistance of the circuit. The immature chest cavity of a foal is not able to generate sufficient pressure to overcome a circuit with high resistance. The most convenient system available for foals up to approximately 100 kg is an adult human circle, with a rebreathing bag of approximately 6 l capacity (Fig. 26.4). Magill or Lack circuits can be used for gaseous induction in foals as they allow greater control than induction with a circle system (see Ch. 25).

Premedication in very young and debilitated foals should be avoided where possible; the foal has an immature hepatic detoxifying system, rendering it less able to cope with drugs than adults. If necessary, small foals can be restrained with diazepam; older healthy foals tolerate the use of alpha-2 adrenoceptor agonists such as xylazine quite well.

When anaesthetizing foals it is important to keep them with the dam until the foal is unconscious. Sedation of the mare prior to handling the foal greatly reduces the stress in both animals. Romifidine is a good sedative in this case as the mare will be minimally ataxic when led back to the stable once the foal is fully anaesthetized. The mare can be returned before or after the foal is standing, depending on the system employed. The presence of the mare will stimulate the foal to stand but care must be taken to prevent the mare from stepping on it. The foal should be allowed to suckle up to and straight after anaesthesia. Because of their small size, foals are at risk of hypothermia during anaesthesia and steps should be taken from the outset to preserve body heat and to warm the foal if necessary.

Use of artificial ventilators

Intermittent positive pressure ventilation (IPPV) in its simplest form can be achieved by compression of the rebreathing bag having closed the pressure relief valve. This is a cumbersome procedure and is usually restricted to emergencies or for short periods.

Ventilators are available for use in equine anaesthesia and they are becoming more frequently used. Ideally, blood gases, especially CO_2, should be monitored during IPPV to enable 'fine-tuning' of the tidal volume and ventilation rate according to the requirements of the patient. Most horses ventilate quite adequately by spontaneous respiration during anaesthesia. Cases in which IPPV may be used include those in which the respiratory rate falls below 4 breaths per minute, in which case the horse may be inspiring inadequate volatile agent to maintain a level plane of anaesthesia, and cases where abdominal distension restricts normal respiration. IPPV is always required for intrathoracic surgery.

Recovery from anaesthesia

An ideal recovery involves the horse remaining calmly in lateral and then sternal recumbency until the effects of the anaesthetic drugs have worn off and it can stand without ataxia. Recovery time should be as short as possible within those limits.

A horse positioned in lateral recumbency during surgery should be placed on the same side in recovery; if the horse has been in dorsal recumbency it should be placed on its left side in recovery.

Turning a horse over from one side to the other from surgery to recovery will allow reperfusion of the formerly dependent muscles but results in atelectasis (partial collapse) of the newly dependent lung lobes. This can result in respiratory embarrassment as the lung lobes that have been dependent during surgery will already be in a state of atelectasis, which will not resolve quickly enough to allow adequate ventilation. Extubation can be carried out before the swallow reflex returns if the airway is clear. If a nasotracheal tube is to be placed for the full recovery, it should be secured in place to prevent it being pushed up the nose. (Wrapping adhesive bandage around the nasal end to form a 'ball' is quite effective.)

In some cases the horse can recover with the ET tube left in the mouth but this carries the inherent risk that the horse will obstruct its own airway by biting the tube, and a secure, safe mouth gag is needed.

Horses can be sedated for recovery if they are likely to stand too quickly because of their temperament, pain or distended bladder. Analgesia, bladder catheterization, etc., and then sedation, e.g. xylazine 0.1 mg/kg intravenously, can be used.

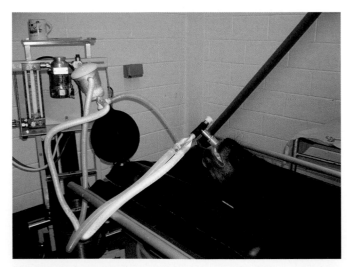

Fig. 26.4 Foal maintained on an adult human circle system

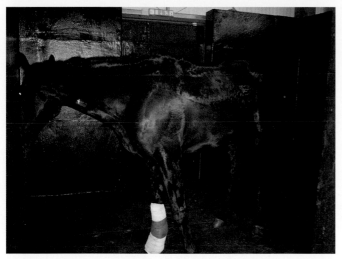

Fig. 26.5 Horse recovering from anaesthesia in a recovery box

Recovery boxes should be designed to achieve a good, safe recovery (Fig. 26.5). The box should be of a size that allows free movement but is too small for the recovering patient to gather speed. The walls and floor should be padded without protruding edges and the floor should provide good grip, even when wet. It should be possible to dim the lights and keep the area quiet while a horse is recovering.

Assistance during recovery may be required for foals to prevent injury and for adults in some cases of orthopaedic surgery. Assistance during recovery should only be given to adults by experienced teams and preferably with a method of restraint, such as ropes attached to the headcollar and tail running through rings on the wall to provide a secure anchor. Slings are poorly tolerated unless the horse has previously become acclimatized to them.

Complications and emergencies

Equipment and drugs required for emergency resuscitation

The larger pieces of equipment used for routine anaesthesia are also used for resuscitation and are therefore readily to hand in an emergency. A 'crash box' containing a selection of needles, including spinal needles for cardiac injection, syringes, fluid giving sets, intravenous cannulas and a stethoscope should be kept together with the drugs listed below.

Equipment required:

- Endotracheal tube to maintain airway
- Tracheostomy/laryngotomy tube
- Means for IPPV – anaesthetic circuit/ventilator/ (Hudson) demand valve
- Drugs for emergency resuscitation should be drawn up into capped syringes and labelled with the name of the drug and the appropriate weight of horse.

Drugs required:

- Adrenaline (epinephrine)
- Atropine
- Lignocaine (lidocaine)
- Doxapram.

Respiratory obstruction

Causes include:

- Kinking of the ET tube – do not overflex the neck; check the tube inside and outside the mouth where it may be prone to kinking during movement
- Overinflation of the cuff leading to compression of the tube or inflation of the cuff over the end of the tube – become familiar with the amount of air usually required to inflate the cuff and measure this by using a normal syringe
- Foreign material in the airway, e.g. blood – if it is suspected that blood or gastric reflux may enter the airway, leave the ET tube in position with the cuff inflated until the patient is able to swallow to clear the airway
- Oedema of the nasal passages when the head has been in a position that is lower than the body during anaesthesia – leave a suitable design of nasotracheal tube in place for the duration of recovery
- Dislocation of the soft palate – stimulate the larynx to make the horse swallow or pass an ET tube gently to open the airway
- Laryngeal spasm – place a tracheostomy tube in a laryngotomy wound prior to recovery and leave in place overnight after surgery.

Complete airway obstruction during anaesthesia is shown by the presence of chest and abdominal movements without excursion of the rebreathing bag. Partial airway obstruction is often audible, as air will be forced through a narrowed airway, e.g. snoring when the nasal passages are narrowed by oedema of the nasal lining. Signs of hypoxia (inadequate oxygen supply to tissues) or anoxia (total lack of oxygen supply) include grey or blue mucous membrane colour and reduced blood O_2 and elevated blood CO_2 observed if blood gas analysis or capnography are available.

Emergency treatment

- Aim is to restore oxygen supply to the tissues
- Establish cause of obstruction and remove or correct it if possible. If this is not possible, regain airway patency by passing a naso- or endotracheal tube or in the extreme case open the airway by tracheostomy
- Ventilate manually, making sure no further anaesthetic gas is given
- Monitor pulse and mucous membrane colour to check efficacy of ventilation.

Respiratory arrest

This is the cessation of breathing that results in apnoea. This frequently occurs transiently during induction, especially after placement of the ET tube. More serious causes of apnoea include respiratory obstruction, excessive resistance in the breathing circuit, central nervous depression during anaesthetic overdose, and cardiac arrest.

Breathing after induction can often be restarted by stimulation of the larynx or other reflexes, or a sharp compression of the chest wall. These methods, as well as surgical stimulation, may also be effective during anaesthesia. If breathing still does not begin, e.g. because of drug effects or other conditions causing central nervous depression, then IPPV should be initiated and should continue until spontaneous breathing resumes. Doxapram (0.5–1 mg/kg) may be used in severe circumstances but its efficacy relies on an effective circulation.

Cardiac arrest

Cardiac arrest usually results from the occurrence of several factors simultaneously, e.g. halothane overdose, hypoxia and hypercapnia (elevated blood CO_2). Vagal stimulation during head and neck surgery may cause cardiac arrest in horses with very little warning.

Clinical signs include loss of palpable peripheral pulse, loss of heart sounds (may also occur without cardiac arrest) and very pale mucous membranes.

Emergency treatment

This involves the use of cardiopulmonary resuscitation, which consists of the following steps:

- **Airway** – ensure it is clear; intubate if necessary
- **Breathing** – initiate IPPV or manual compression of rebreathing bag – use pure O_2 if possible
- **Circulation** – cardiac massage is difficult in the horse. If possible, place horse on a hard surface and give a sharp blow to the precordial chest region to attempt to stimulate heart contraction. If this fails, attempt external massage by exerting strong force over the chest with the knees or foot (about 30 compressions per minute). If all else fails, surgical exposure of the heart and internal massage can be performed
- **Drug treatment** should only be initiated when cardiac massage results in blood flow. IPPV and cardiac massage should be continued:
  - Adrenaline (epinephrine) given intravenously (0.3 ml per 100 kg) – if this is not possible, give directly into left ventricle of heart or into bronchial tree via ET tube
  - Atropine intravenously (1.6 ml per 100 kg of 0.6 mg/ml solution = 0.01 mg/kg)
  - Repeat adrenaline (0.5 ml per 100 kg)
  - For ventricular fibrillation use lignocaine (2.5 ml per 100 kg of 20 mg/l = 0.5 mg/kg).

Normal mucous membrane colour and a palpable pulse show that the circulation is returning to normal.

Other anaesthetic complications

- **Hypoxaemia** – inadequate oxygenation of blood: due to reduced ventilation, reduced oxygen content of inspired air or low cardiac output (effectively reduces circulation)
- **Hypercapnia** – excess of CO_2 in blood: due to reduced ventilation or circulation
- **Hypotension** – blood pressure below expected normal: due to deepening of anaesthetic plane, loss of circulating volume, dilation of peripheral vasculature or reduced cardiac output
- **Cardiac arrhythmias** – loss of normal heart rhythm: occur as a result of drug administration. Arrhythmias that have a significant effect on circulation are rare

- **Musculoskeletal injury** – usually long-bone fractures and head trauma: usually occur during unaided recovery as a result of attempts to stand before the drugs' effects have worn off or as a result of previous injury or pain
- **Postanaesthetic myopathy** – muscle damage as a result of failure of blood supply to the muscle during anaesthesia: caused by poor positioning, lying on firm surfaces, prolonged anaesthesia, prolonged periods of hypotension
- **Postanaesthetic neuropathy** – nerve damage as a result of trauma, pressure, stretching and failure of blood supply: caused by pressure of headcollar on facial nerve during induction, stretching of limbs for the duration of surgery, e.g. positioning for arthroscopy, or focal pressure causing blood flow to be occluded.

Local anaesthesia

Local anaesthetic is used to desensitize a restricted area to allow painful surgical procedures or paradoxically to abolish existing pain to prove its existence, e.g. diagnosis of some types of lameness. Local anaesthetic techniques usually aim to abolish pain and sensation, leaving motor functions intact, but occasionally are directed at motor nerves to abolish movement as in the auriculo-palpebral nerve block to stop blinking during eye examination. Local anaesthesia can be combined with sedation to allow surgery to be performed 'standing' or it can be used during general anaesthesia to reduce pain and the amount of maintenance drugs required.

Types of local anaesthesia

Topical anaesthesia

Topical anaesthesia can be achieved using creams designed for skin absorption. For example, creams containing lignocaine (lidocaine) are available for treatment of minor but painful skin abrasions; local anaesthetic eye drops, e.g. amethocaine, are used to desensitize the cornea to aid examination or minor surgery. Absorption through intact skin is slow and the use of topical anaesthesia prior to injection has limited use.

Regional anaesthesia

Regional anaesthesia involves desensitization of a specified area and includes several methods of administration:

- **Perineural infiltration of local anaesthetic**, i.e. infusion around a nerve whose precise position is known. This effectively prevents the transmission of impulses from beyond that point back to the brain and renders the structures supplied by that nerve insensitive. This is the principle used in lameness diagnosis
- **Infiltration of local anaesthetic into a wide area**, often of skin, blocks the nerves that supply the area, which is then desensitized. This technique is commonly used in suturing wounds
- **Intravenous anaesthesia** is useful for the desensitization of the distal limb. As the technique requires the occlusion of blood flow from the area, a

tourniquet is applied proximal to the area to be 'blocked' and local anaesthetic is injected distally into a prominent vein. This produces good anaesthesia in the area below the tourniquet while it is in position. This technique is rarely used in horses and in large animal practice is mainly restricted to bovine digit surgery

- **Epidural anaesthesia** is achieved by injection of local anaesthetic around a specific part of the spinal cord, blocking conduction in the spinal nerves of that area and sometimes the spinal cord itself. The structures supplied by the spinal nerves are then desensitized. A caudal block is the most commonly used in horses to allow surgery in the perineal region, e.g. to replace a rectal prolapse and prevent further straining. More cranial blocks carry the risk of desensitizing the hind limbs and inducing collapse. Xylazine and xylazine/local anaesthetic combinations are useful in the horse to provide anaesthesia without ataxia.

Intrasynovial anaesthesia

Intrasynovial anaesthesia is used in equine practice and, like perineural anaesthesia, is primarily for lameness diagnosis. Local anaesthetic is injected directly into joints and tendon sheaths and produces anaesthesia of a known, specific structure. A positive result is a good indication for medication or further investigation of the sheath or joint.

Application

Topical anaesthesia

- Place appropriate preparation on a dressing directly on to the skin for 1 hour

- Apply appropriate drops on to cornea or into conjunctival sac.

Perineural infiltration and infiltration into a wide area

- Clipping hair is optional
- Skin should be cleaned with spirit swab or chlorhexidine wash according to the level of dirt
- Smallest possible needle is used to minimize patient reaction
- Agent is injected into target site.

Intrasynovial and epidural anaesthesia

- Strict aseptic technique must be employed, i.e. clip hair, scrub, sterile gloving
- Place an intradermal skin bleb of local anaesthetic
- A suitable drug, volume and needle size is chosen
- Adequate restraint of the horse will be necessary, e.g. sedation or twitch
- Inject local anaesthetic through the bleb.

Drugs used for local anaesthesia

Local anaesthetic drugs are variably lipid-soluble; those that have good lipid solubility diffuse quickly through tissues and nerve trunks and have a quicker speed of onset of activity (Table 26.6). Other factors affecting speed of onset include the accuracy of the injection and the concentration rather than the volume of agent used.

Duration of action is affected by the volume and type of drug chosen and whether a vasoconstrictor, i.e. adrenaline (epinephrine), has been combined in the preparation. Vasoconstriction slows the diffusion of drug out of the target area

Table 26.6 Local anaesthetics used in equine practice

Local anaesthetic drug	Applications	Speed of onset	Duration of action
Lignocaine (Lignol)	Topical Infiltration Perineural Epidural (without adrenaline (epinephrine))	<5 min	30–40 min (doubled by adding adrenaline (epinephrine))
Prilocaine (Citanest)	Infusion Perineural Intrasynovial Epidural Intravenous	5–15 min	Approx. 1 hour
Mepivacaine (Intra-Epicaine)	Infusion Perineural Intrasynovial Epidural	10–20 min	Up to 2 hour
Bupivacaine (Marcaine)	Infiltration Perineural Intrasynovial	15–20 min	Up to 8 hour
Amethocaine	Mucous membrane (topical) Corneal (topical)	<1 min	10–15 min
Proxymetacaine (Ophthaine)	Corneal (topical)	<1 min	15 min

by reducing blood flow. Preparations containing adrenaline should be confined to perineural and infusion techniques. Care must be taken to avoid significant systemic uptake.

Humane destruction of *Equidae*

Indications for euthanasia

Euthanasia is usually carried out on grounds of welfare. This can range from severe inoperable injury resulting in intractable pain to ill or elderly animals that no longer have a 'good quality of life'. Euthanasia should be performed humanely and in the best interests of the animal. The British Equine Veterinary Association (BEVA) has issued guidelines for the decisions involved in the destruction of horses, with particular regard to insurance implications.

Current methods

The handling of the euthanasia of a horse is very important throughout the practice and lack of sympathy or failure to act correctly can cost clients (see Ch. 1). Consent must be obtained from the owner or keeper of the horse to be euthanased. If the animal is insured, then permission should be sought from the insurance company, if it is humanely possible to delay destruction of the animal. A euthanasia consent form should be signed prior to humane destruction of an animal and a description of the animal should be kept if necessary for insurance or other purposes. It may be necessary to perform a post-mortem examination and the whole carcass or the relevant part should be retained. It may be a good idea, if appropriate, to ask if the owner would like the shoes returned or a piece of mane or tail saved.

Methods available for the humane destruction of horses are as follows:

Gun

This is usually a single-shot 0.32 calibre free-bullet humane killer (weapons smaller than 0.31 calibre are not suitable and neither are captive bolt weapons considered appropriate for destruction of horses outside an abattoir situation, as death is induced by pithing, a process not aesthetically acceptable to the majority of horse owners).

Sedation is often used and assistance is required in the handling of the horse. It is vital that nurses/assistants are aware of people around the area. All humans and other animals should be removed from the area if possible, or at the least they should stand behind the person using the gun – including the assistant, even if they continue to hold the animal.

Lethal injection

This uses a high dose of pentobarbitone (pentobarbital) or Somnulose. Controlled drugs – lock up and record their use!

Somnulose (cinchocaine and quinalbarbitone)

- Preload correct dose (10 ml per 100 kg) into a single syringe
- A 14 FG intravenous catheter is placed
- The assistant restrains the horse, pulling its head down to encourage the horse to sink backwards
- The full amount of Somnulose is injected over about 15 seconds
- Collapse will occur 35–45 seconds after the start of injection, death within 2 minutes.

Pentobarbitone (pentobarbital)

- Pentobarbitone is preloaded into as many 50ml syringes as required (dose 200 mg/kg)
- A 14 FG intravenous catheter is placed
- Sedative may be used if required, usually an alpha-2 agonist at full sedative dose
- The assistant restrains the horse, being aware that sudden or violent movements may occur
- The full volume of pentobarbitone is injected as quickly as possible
- Collapse should occur 35–40 seconds and death 1.5–2.5 minutes after injection; gasping may occur.

Disposal of the carcass

Disposal of the animal should preferably be arranged prior to euthanasia and the preferred method of disposal discussed with the owner. Even though this may be difficult at the time, it may have a bearing on the method of euthanasia.

Common routes of disposal are:

Cremation/incineration:
- Expensive
- Method of euthanasia unimportant
- Ashes can often be returned if requested.

Carcass used for animal consumption by a hunt kennel or abattoir:
- Depends on personal wishes or opinions and may be distasteful to many horse owners
- Less expensive than incineration
- Horse cannot be euthanased with Somnulose or pentobarbitone.

Carcass used for human consumption:
- May retrieve 'meat' value of the animal, which gives some financial return
- Animal must be euthanased by gun
- Animal must not contain residues of any controlled drugs or substances and all medication must have been recorded in the passport under the passport scheme
- Horse will have to be transported alive to a registered abattoir.

Bibliography

Bishop, Y. (Ed.), 1996. The Veterinary Formulary, third ed. Royal Pharmaceutical Society of Great Britain/Pharmaceutical Press, London.

Hall, L.W., Clarke, K.W., Trim, C.M., 2001. Veterinary Anaesthesia, tenth ed. Butterworth-Heinemann, Oxford.

Johnston, G.M., Eastment, J.K., Wood, J.L.N., Taylor, P.M., 2002. The Confidential Enquiry into Perioperative Equine Fatalities (CEPEF): mortality results of phases 1 and 2. Vet. Anaesth. Analg. 29, 159–170.

Knottenbelt, D.C. (Ed.), 1997. Formulary of Equine Medicine. Liverpool University Press, Liverpool.

Taylor, P.M., Clarke, K.W., 1999. Handbook of Equine Anaesthesia. W B Saunders, Philadelphia, PA.

Recommended reading

Taylor, P.M., Clarke, K.W., 1999. Handbook of Equine Anaesthesia. W B Saunders, Philadelphia, PA.

This book is written for veterinary surgeons but provides useful information for the veterinary nurse.

Bibliography

Recommended reading

Parasitology

Maggie Fisher

Definitions

- **Parasite** – a eukaryotic organism that lives off another (the host) to the advantage of the parasite
- **Endoparasite** – a parasite that lives inside the host, e.g. a roundworm
- **Ectoparasite** – a parasite that lives on or in the skin of the host, e.g. a flea
- **Permanent parasite** – a parasite that lives for its entire life cycle on the host, e.g. a louse
- **Temporary parasite** – a parasite that lives for only part of its life on a host, e.g. a flea – the adult stage is entirely parasitic but the immature stages live in the environment. A mosquito is still more temporary – only the adult females are parasitic as they take a blood meal from a human or animal
- **Zoonoses** – animal infections that can infect humans

- **Host specificity** – refers to the range of hosts that a particular parasite can utilize; for example, lice are very host-specific as each species will only infect one specific host. Thus *Bovicola equi*, formerly *Damalinia equi*, the horse louse, will not infect dogs and *Linognathus setosus*, the sucking louse of dogs, will only survive on dogs. In contrast *Ctenocephalides felis*, the cat flea, has been recorded living successfully on cats, dogs, rabbits, ferrets, sheep, goats and calves
- **Final host** – only occurs in a life cycle involving more than one host. It refers to the host in which sexual reproduction of the parasite occurs, e.g. *Echinococcus granulosus* – this tapeworm occurs in dogs but the hydatid cyst, the immature stage, occurs in sheep, which are the **intermediate hosts**. These include:
  - *Paratenic hosts* – act as host for a parasite but little or no development of the parasite occurs within them; for example, infective *Toxocara canis* eggs eaten by a mouse hatch and the larva migrates into the mouse's tissue (the paratenic host), where it remains without further development until the mouse is eaten by a dog
  - *Transport host* – simply carries the parasite from one host to another
- **Vector** – is an arthropod responsible for the transmission of a parasite among vertebrate hosts. The arthropod may act as an intermediate host, a paratenic host or a transport host
- **Prepatent period** – the time between the ingestion of the infective stage, e.g. egg, and the production of eggs by the adults. A parasitic infection is said to be **patent** when eggs are found in the faeces
- **Direct life cycle** (refers to nematodes) – a life cycle which does not involve an intermediate host. Larvae may be directly transmitted from host to host or be free-living in the environment, e.g. pasture
- **Indirect life cycle** – a life cycle in which the larval stages pass through an intermediate host.

Nomenclature of parasites

It is normal to refer to a parasite by its genus and then species name, e.g. the canine worm, *Toxocara canis*: the genus is

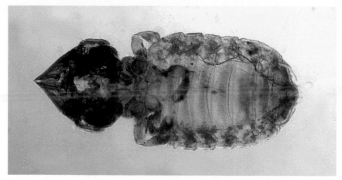

Fig. 27.1 *Felicola subrostratus*, the biting louse of the cat. Adult is 1–1.5 mm in length

Toxocara and the species *canis*. After the first use the genus name can be abbreviated to its initial, in this case becoming *T. canis*.

Ectoparasites

Ectoparasites include the arthropod species and certain species of fungus.

Most ectoparasitic arthropods belong either to the insect group, i.e. lice, fleas, mosquitoes, sand flies and *Culicoides* or the acari, a sub-group of the arachnids, i.e. mites and ticks. Adult arthropods have an exoskeleton (as opposed to the mammalian endoskeleton) and reproduce by laying eggs. The immature stages may be similar to the adult but smaller, e.g. lice or mites, or may be maggot-like and change to the adult form, e.g. flies and fleas during pupation.

Insects

Lice

Lice are small, wingless, permanently parasitic insects. They are dorsoventrally flattened and possess claws for clasping hairs or feathers. They are host-specific and there are many species of louse. However, rather than focusing on identifying the species, it is usually more important to identify whether lice are present and whether they are sucking or biting lice. 'Sucking' or 'biting' (also known as chewing) refers to the method of feeding: biting lice have mouthparts adapted to chewing the surface of the skin and sucking lice have narrow mouthparts for piercing skin and sucking blood. A heavy burden of the latter can result in anaemia. Cats have just one species of louse, the biting louse *Felicola subrostratus* (Fig. 27.1). Dogs in temperate climates have one species of biting louse, *Trichodectes canis* (Fig. 27.2), and one species of sucking louse, *Linognathus setosus* (Fig. 27.3). In horses, *Haematopinus asini* is the sucking louse and *Bovicola equi*, formely known as *Damalinia equi*, is the biting louse.

Life cycle: Female lice lay their eggs or nits on the host attached to hairs (Fig. 27.4) and these can give lousy animals a speckled appearance, depending on their hair colour. Immature lice emerge from the eggs and progress through a series of moults to become adults. The entire life cycle takes about 4–6 weeks.

Animals with clinical lousiness or pediculosis will rub and scratch themselves. A heavy burden may cause debility, par-

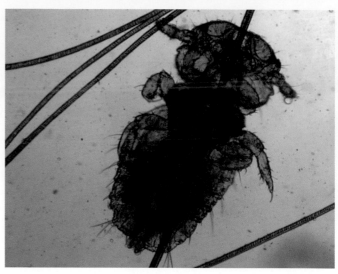

Fig. 27.2 *Trichodectes canis*, a biting louse of dogs. Adult is 1–2 mm in length

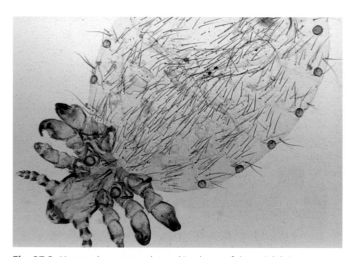

Fig. 27.3 *Linognathus setosus*, the sucking louse of dogs. Adult is approx. 2 mm in length

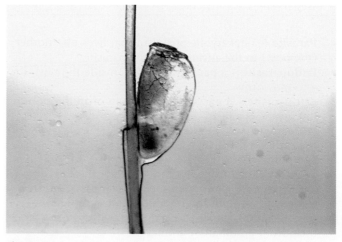

Fig. 27.4 Louse egg or nit on a hair shaft. Egg approx. 0.7 mm long

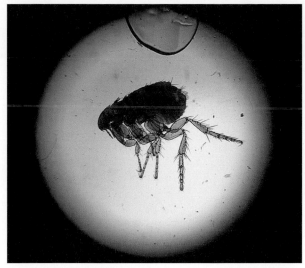

Fig. 27.5 Lateral view of an adult 'cat' flea, *Ctenocephalides felis*. Adult measures 1–2.5 mm in length

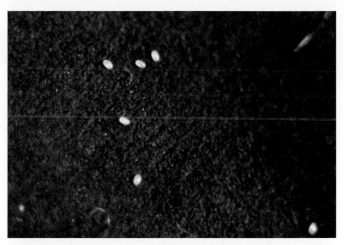

Fig. 27.6 Cat flea eggs are smooth and are laid by the adult female on the host but drop off into the environment. Egg is approx. 0.5 mm in length

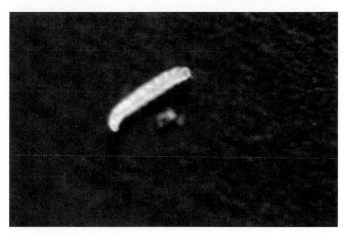

Fig. 27.7 Flea larvae go through two moults before pupating. Larvae measure approx. 0.5 cm

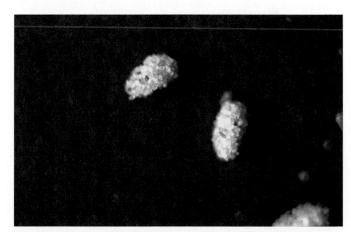

Fig. 27.8 Pupae are covered in sticky cocoons, which become coated in debris from the environment

ticularly if sucking lice are present. Infection is most common in young, old or debilitated animals. Infection is seen relatively rarely in cats and dogs in the UK but more often in horses. Louse burdens can build up in horses during the winter when they are stabled, with louse populations diminishing during the summer at pasture.

Infected animals can be treated with a suitable insecticide. Few insecticides penetrate the eggs, so unless a residual insecticide such as fipronil, selamectin or imidacloprid is used a repeat treatment may be necessary approximately 10 days after the first.

Fleas

Fleas (Fig. 27.5) are wingless, laterally flattened, dark brown insects capable of moving rapidly through a coat or jumping with their specialized legs. Their mouthparts are adapted for piercing skin and sucking blood. The details of the head, such as the presence of combs, are often characteristic of the species of flea and can be used for identification. One species, *Ctenocephalides felis*, more commonly referred to as *C. felis* or the cat flea, is the predominant species on cats and dogs in the UK and may also be found on ferrets and rabbits. The dog flea, *Ctenocephalides canis*, is more host-specific, is found on some dogs in the UK and is the most common flea on dogs in Ireland. Other species of fleas parasitize small mammals and birds.

Life cycle: Adult *C. felis* emerge from their pupal case in the environment and begin to seek a host. Once they have found a suitable host they begin to feed within 5 minutes. Female fleas begin to lay eggs approximately 24–48 hours after they begin to feed. The eggs (Fig. 27.6) are smooth and fall off into the environment, typically in the area where the animal rests. In ideal conditions the eggs hatch after about 2 days, although development is slower in cool conditions (Dryden & Rust 1994). Eggs and larvae require warmth and humidity to remain alive and develop – dry conditions and heat over about 35°C will kill them. Maggot-like larvae (Fig. 27.7) hatched from the eggs undergo two moults before pupating. The pupal case is sticky, so typically becomes camouflaged with environmental debris (Fig. 27.8). The life cycle can be completed in about 12 days in ideal conditions. Other species of flea, such as the bird flea *Ceratophyllus gallinae*, are nest-dwelling fleas, where the adults remain in the environment except when they find a host to feed.

Fleas suck blood and a moderately heavy burden can cause severe anaemia, particularly in small animals such as

Table 27.1 Flea control agents

Chemical group	Examples	Mode of action	Application to
Organochlorides	Lindane	Acts on the neuromuscular junction	Animal (broadly phased out now)
Organophosphates	Fenthion	Acts on the neuromuscular junction	Animal (broadly phased out now)
Carbamates	Carbaryl	Acts on the neuromuscular junction	Animal, particularly collars
Phenylpyrazole	Fipronil	Neurotransmitter inhibition	Animal
Pyrethrins and pyrethroids	Natural pyrethrin	Acts on the nervous system	Animal and environmental formulations available (NB. cats are susceptible to pyrethroid toxicity)
	Permethrin		
	Deltamethrin		
Macrocyclic lactones (insect growth regulators)	Selamectin	Neurotransmitter inhibition	Animal
	Lufenuron	Chitin synthesis inhibitor (prevents development of immature stages)	Animal, orally or by injection
	Methoprene	Juvenile hormone and analogues (prevents development of immature stages)	Animal or the environment
	Pyriproxyfen		

kittens. As fleas feed, saliva is injected, which contains antigens that provoke the development of an allergic response in some individuals. In cats and dogs this often manifests as a pruritic dermatitis or 'flea allergic dermatitis'. Fleas can transmit diseases and also act as the intermediate host for the tapeworm *Dipylidium caninum*. *C. felis* is zoonotic and will bite, although not live on, humans. Control of an existing problem can be achieved by treatment of affected dogs or cats with an insecticide that is active for just a few hours, or with sustained activity. Depending on the severity of the infestation, elimination may be accelerated by concomitant treatment of immature flea stages in the environment by insecticide or by insect development inhibitors that prevent maturation of eggs and larvae (Table 27.1). Fleas can be prevented by prophylactic use of insecticide or larval development inhibitors.

Flies

Some fly larvae are facultative parasites, i.e. they can, but do not have to, infest living animals, while some others are obligate parasites that cannot complete their life cycle without an animal host. Any animal can develop fly strike and the condition is seen occasionally in dogs and cats and more frequently in rabbits and sheep, particularly during the summer months.

Life cycle: Adult flies lay their eggs in moist conditions to which they have been attracted by odours, such as those of faeces. The larvae hatch rapidly and begin to feed on the surface of the animal and invade deeper tissues as they grow and moult (Fig. 27.9). Once fully developed the larva drops to the ground and pupates. Proteolytic enzymes secreted on to the animal to assist in tissue breakdown together with the breakdown products, have toxic effects on the host, which can rapidly become depressed and anorexic.

Careful husbandry is important during the summer months to prevent a build-up of faeces on the animal or, in the case of rabbits, in its pen so that flies are not attracted by the smell. Careful observation is needed so that if fly

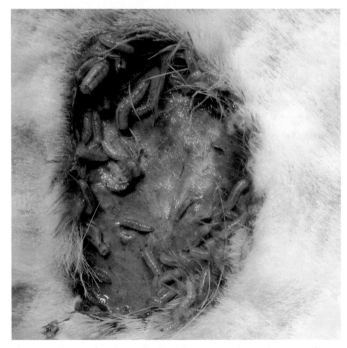

Fig. 27.9 Fly eggs hatch rapidly, then the maggots begin damaging the skin, which is often penetrated by the time the infestation is noticed (Courtesy of Steve Warren). Each maggot measures approx. 0.9 mm

strike does occur it can be dealt with rapidly. Development of larvae on rabbits can be prevented by application of the larval growth inhibitor cyromazine. When an animal becomes fly-blown the wound must be cleaned and the larvae removed. Prognosis is good if the infection is caught early but reduces as the larvae burrow deeper into tissues and enter body cavities. Supportive nursing and adjunctive therapy may also be necessary.

Various species of flies bite horses and feed off secretions around horses' eyes (Fig. 27.10). The flies can transmit infections, including *Habronema* spp. Horses may become

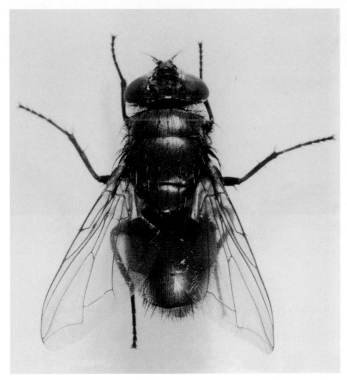

Fig. 27.10 Horses are worried in the summer by a number of species of flies that feed off eye secretions, etc. *(Courtesy of John McGarry)*

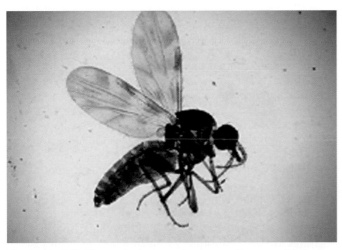

Fig. 27.11 *Culicoides* are also known as 'no-see-ums' because of their very small size *(Courtesy of John McGarry, © Liverpool School of Tropical Medicine).* Flies measure 1–4 mm

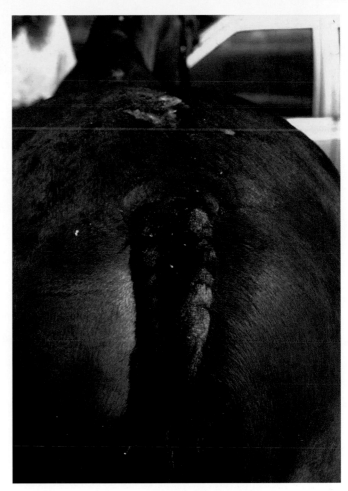

Fig. 27.12 'Sweet itch' is caused by *Culicoides* bites activating an inflammatory allergic response that is very pruritic, so the affected horse rubs affected areas, primarily the mane and tail *(Courtesy of Mark Craig)*

hypersensitive to fly bites, and hypersensitivity to the small biting midge *Culicoides* spp. (Fig. 27.11) can result in a severe pruritic dermatitis, known as sweet itch, during the summer months. The tail, head and mane are often the most affected areas (Fig. 27.12). Horses can be protected from flies and midges in a number of ways, including keeping them indoors and using proprietary insect repellents or head nets. Female mosquitoes and sandflies are temporary parasites, requiring a blood meal prior to egg laying. Mosquitoes are the vectors of heartworm caused by *Dirofilaria immitis* and sandflies are responsible for the transmission of *Leishmania* spp.

Acari

Ticks and mites appear as a single sac without the definition of head, thorax and abdomen that is seen in the insects. The mouthparts protrude anteriorly and nymphal and adult stages possess four pairs of legs.

Mites

Mites can be roughly grouped into surface dwellers (Table 27.2), which have long legs, and subsurface dwellers, which typically have short, stumpy legs. The entire life cycle of most parasitic mites occurs on the host, with transfer from host to host occurring through close contact or occasionally by acquisition of mites from the environment, since some mites can survive in the environment for some time in some of their stages. Other species of mites are temporary parasites, e.g. *Dermanyssus gallinae*, opportunistic parasites or, in the case of *Trombicula autumnalis* parasites, parasites during their larval stage only. Treatment of mite infections involves using an appropriate acaricide on single or repeated occasions. Symptoms of mite infection are collectively referred to as **mange**.

Surface mites

- *Otodectes cynotis*, the ear mite – normally inhabits the external ear canal, although it is occasionally found

Table 27.2 Summary of mite species

Mite species	Host species			
	Cat	Dog	Horse	Other pets
Surface mites				
Otodectes cynotis	Yes	Yes	–	Ferrets
Chorioptes equi	–	–	Yes	–
Psoroptes spp.	–	–	*Psoroptes equi*	*Psoroptes cuniculi* in rabbits
Cheyletiella spp.	Yes	Yes	–	Rabbits
Trombicula autumnalis	Yes	Yes	Yes	–
Subsurface mites				
Sarcoptes scabiei and related species	*Sarcoptes scabiei* rarely *Notoedres cati*	*Sarcoptes scabiei* var. *canis*	*Sarcoptes scabiei* rarely in the UK	*Sarcoptes* spp. can infect rabbits and hamsters *Notoedres* spp. in rats *Trixacarus caviae* in guinea pigs
Demodex spp.	Yes, rarely	Yes	Yes, rarely	Hamsters

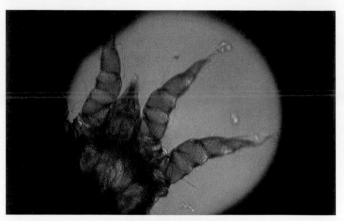

Fig. 27.14 *Psoroptes* spp. mites can be identified by the suckers on the end of jointed stalks or pedicels at the ends of the front pair of legs. Adult female is approx. 750 μm

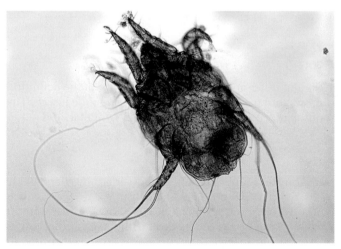

Fig. 27.13 The ear mite *Otodectes cynotis* can be recognized by the unjointed stalks or pedicels with suckers on the end that occur on the front two pairs of legs in all developmental stages. Adult mite approx. 300 μm

elsewhere on the host. Cats, dogs and, occasionally, ferrets can be infected. The mites have bell-shaped suckers on the end of unjointed stalks or pedicels (Fig. 27.13). The mites are off-white and can be clearly seen against the brown of ear wax when magnified with an auroscope. The entire life cycle occurs on the host and begins with the female mite laying eggs. Immature stages appear similar to those of adult mites and the life cycle is completed in about 3 weeks. Transfer from animal to animal probably occurs through close contact. Some animals tolerate the presence of ear mites without apparent discomfort, although the external ear canal may produce excessive wax, that appears like brown coffee grounds. Others, particularly dogs, will show pruritus and inflammation. Affected animals can be treated with an acaricidal product applied down the ear canal, or with a systemic product such as selamectin or imidacloprid/moxidectin (Curtis 2004)

- *Chorioptes equi* – similar in appearance to *O. cynotis* but has cup-shaped suckers on the end of unjointed pedicels. It is found on the surface of horses' skin, particularly on the feathered lower legs of heavy horses
- *Psoroptes cuniculi* (Fig. 27.14) – has trumpet-shaped suckers on the end of jointed pedicels or stalks and causes 'ear canker' in rabbits
- *Psoroptes equi* – identical in appearance to *P. cuniculi* and causes an itchy dermatitis in horses
- *Cheyletiella* spp. – are parasites of cats, dogs and rabbits, each host having its own species, although the individual species may not be entirely host-specific. The mites are large (about 0.5 mm in length) so can just about be seen with the naked eye. They possess large claws on their palps and comb-like appendages on the ends of their legs (Fig. 27.15). They typically cause a scurfy dermatitis, sometimes with erythema, and the condition is often referred to as 'walking dandruff'. There is evidence that mites are capable of surviving for some days in the environment, so cleaning of the environment is recommended, alongside acaricidal treatment of affected animals
- *Trombicula* or *Neotrombicula autumnalis* larvae (Fig. 27.16) parasitize animals for a short time in high summer. The mites are hairy and bright orange and can be seen as small orange spots formed by a cluster of larvae. Once they have fed, the larvae drop off into the environment and complete their life cycle. The larvae can cause pruritus and dermatitis.

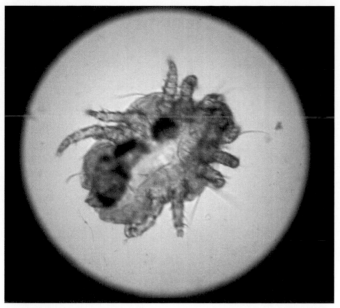

Fig. 27.15 *Cheyletiella* spp. mites are large surface mites with long legs. They have a characteristic waist, large palps at the anterior end each carrying a heavy claw and 'combs' on the ends of their legs

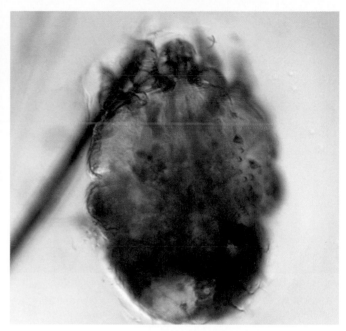

Fig. 27.17 *Sarcoptes* spp. mites are rotund with short legs. The back is covered in pegs and spines and the anus is terminal. Measures approx. 360 μm

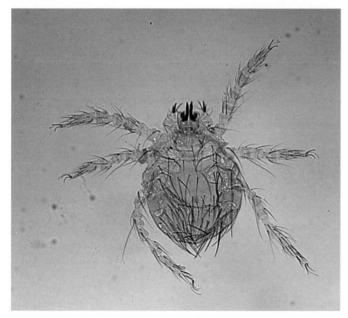

Fig. 27.16 The larvae of *Neotrombicula* or *Trombicula autumnalis* mites are hairy and have six legs. Measures approx. 200 μm

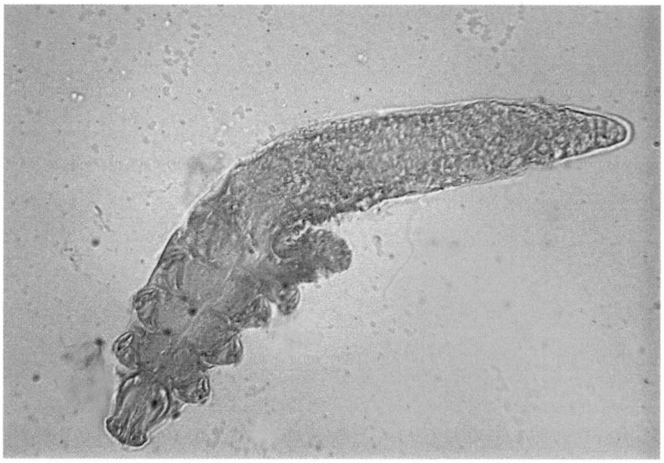

Fig. 27.18 *Demodex* spp. mites are often described as cigar-shaped. The legs are arranged in pairs at the front of the body. Measures approx. 0.2 mm

Subsurface mites

*   *Sarcoptes scabiei* (Fig. 27.17) – a parasite of foxes and dogs and occasionally horses, cats and rabbits. There appear to be different strains, referred to as, for example, *Sarcoptes scabiei* var. *canis*, relating to the host species. The mite has pegs and spines on its dorsal surface. Female mites burrow into the stratum corneum of the skin and lay eggs within the burrows. Immature mites hatch from the eggs, develop, then move to create burrows of their own. The infection typically begins in the pinna, elbow or hock area causing an erythematous, alopecic dermatitis that is extremely pruritic. Untreated, crusting lesions develop that can spread to cover much of the animal. A similar parasite of cats is *Notoedres cati*, which has a dorsal anus and concentric rings on its dorsum. It does not occur in the UK but is found in several European countries, as well as in other warmer parts of the world. Infection by *Notoedres* spp. also occurs in rats, where it can be associated with dermatitis. *Trixacarus caviae* is the burrowing mite that commonly occurs in guinea pigs and is similar in appearance to *Sarcoptes scabiei*.
*   *Demodex* spp. (Fig. 27.18) – cigar-shaped and believed to be normal inhabitants of hair follicles in many species. Occasionally in dogs and rarely in cats, host immunosuppression or immunomodulation allows the population of *Demodex* spp. to expand, and this is

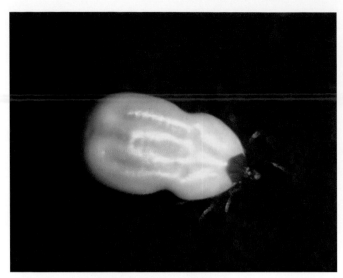

Fig. 27.19 *Ixodes* spp are the ticks commonly found all over the UK. All *Ixodes* spp. ticks have a groove that runs anterior to the anus. Female engorged tick measures approx. 1 cm

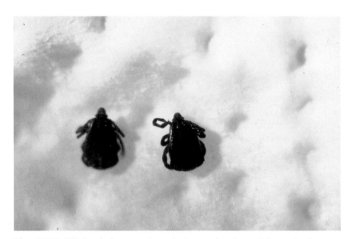

Fig. 27.20 *Rhipicephalus sanguineus* is the predominant tick species in southern Europe and is an important disease vector. Here a male and female are shown side by side; both are quite plain and brown, hence its other name, 'the brown dog tick'. Size varies from 1 to 12 mm

Table 27.3 Common tick species of dogs and cats in Europe

Tick species	Approximate geographical location	Main infections transmitted
Ixodes ricinus	Throughout Europe, including the UK	Lyme disease, tick-borne encephalitis (northern Europe)
Ixodes hexagonus	Throughout Europe, including the UK	May be involved in disease transmission but role less well defined than that of *I. ricinus*
Dermacentor reticulatus	Mainland Europe from Germany south	*Babesia canis*
Rhipicephalus sanguineus	Mainland Europe from southern France south (i.e. the Mediterranean area)	*Babesia canis, Ehrlichia canis, Hepatozoon canis*

Most ticks parasitizing dogs, cats, horses and other pets are 'hard' ticks and possess a scutum or shield on their dorsal surface (Figs 27.19, 27.20). In the female this covers just the anterior portion but male ticks are entirely covered by the scutum. There are a number of species of tick but relatively few that infest dogs and cats in the UK (Table 27.3).

Life cycle: All ticks spend part of their life cycle in the environment, as females lay their eggs on the ground in a suitably moist location before dying. Once hatched, larval ticks have to locate a host, attach and feed. Once they have fed for a few days, depending on the species, they may remain on the same host to develop to the nymphal stage or may drop off to continue their development in the environment.

Most ticks on cats or dogs drop off after both the larval and nymphal stages and, as they thus have to find a separate host to feed on at each stage, they are known as 'three-host' ticks.

As ticks suck blood, a heavy infection can cause anaemia but this occurs rarely in dogs and cats, and ticks are generally most important in these species as vectors of diseases, including Lyme disease and babesiosis. Ticks can also transmit infections to humans, although the source of the ticks is not normally directly from pets; rather, they are derived from wildlife reservoirs. Since the introduction of the PETS travel scheme (www.defra.gov.uk), ticks have become important as a source of non-endemic diseases such as *Babesia canis*. Compulsory acaricidal treatment of dogs and cats prior to their entry into the UK has been introduced, but this does not protect pets during their stay in Europe or elsewhere. It is therefore necessary to advise pet owners of the need for adequate tick control throughout their stay. The risk of tick infections can be reduced by avoiding tick-infested areas such as woodland, especially during spring, summer and autumn when ticks are most active. Whenever possible, pets should be checked daily and any ticks removed using, for example, a proprietary tick-removal device. Alternatively, or additionally, ticks can be repelled using pyrethroid-based products and pets can be protected by using a suitable acaricide.

associated with local or widespread areas of alopecia. The local form may be non-pruritic and may self-resolve but the generalized form is more severe and is very unlikely to clear without treatment. Affected dogs can be in considerable pain and secondary bacterial infection is not uncommon. Treatment should be carried out with a suitable acaricide, but a cure may not be achieved, particularly when it is not possible to identify or treat the underlying condition. Some animals improve with treatment but relapses require repeated treatment.

Ticks

Ticks look similar to mites but are the only parasites to possess a hypostome, part of the specialized mouthparts developed for piercing skin, attaching and removing blood from the host. Larval ticks may be only about 1 mm in length, while fully fed female ticks can reach up to 1 cm.

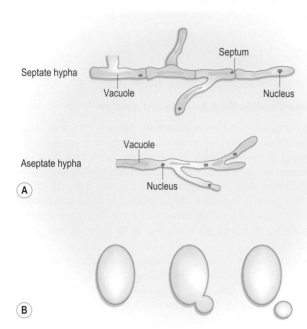

Fig. 27.21 Fungi appear as (**A**) mycelia or (**B**) yeast-like organisms

Septate hypha

Septum

Vacuole

Nucleus

Vacuole

Aseptate hypha

Nucleus

(A)

(B)

Fungi

Fungi exist as unicellular yeasts or multi-nuclear mycelia (Fig. 27.21) and most are non-parasitic. Several species of fungi are parasitic dermatophytes or ringworm-causing species and the yeasts *Candida albicans* and *Malassezia* spp. in particular.

Ringworm

Ringworm is caused by *Trichophyton* spp. or *Microsporum* spp. Spores are introduced on to abraded skin and then a mycelium begins to develop in hair or keratinized skin. Classically, an area of alopecia develops, which gradually becomes larger in diameter, with infection disappearing as a result of the inflammatory response in the centre, which heals as the infection spreads outwards. Some infections show signs of inflammation or pruritus while others do not (Fig. 27.22). Some species, e.g. *Microsporum canis* infection in cats, have adapted so well to the host that infection can remain inapparent. The simplest way to diagnose infection in cats and dogs is to expose suspect lesions to ultraviolet light, as about 50% of *Microsporum canis* lesions fluoresce under a Wood's lamp. However, where fluorescence does not occur it is necessary to collect hair and/or superficial skin samples and examine them directly or submit them for culturing. Samples for direct examination can be placed on a microscope slide, covered with water or Q-ink (which will preferentially stain fungal elements) and a coverslip and then examine for fungal hyphae or arthrospores (Fig. 27.23). The classic medium for dermatophyte culture is Sabouraud's agar but, as dermatophytes can be slow-growing, several media designed to show a rapid colour change in the presence of a dermatophyte have been developed, e.g. dermatophyte test medium (Quinn et al 1994).

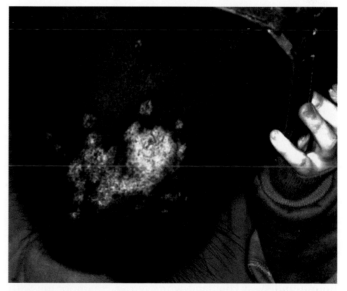

Fig. 27.22 Ringworm lesions may vary from a small area of alopecia to a severe thickened and pruritic lesion. Here lesions on the nose of a horse are caused by *Microsporum gypseum* (Courtesy of Mark Craig)

Candida albicans

Candida albicans is a normal commensal yeast but occasionally overgrows on mucous membranes or even on skin, usually in young or immunocompromised animals. Smears from affected areas show numerous yeasts that must be differentiated from *Malassezia* spp. organisms.

Malassezia

Malassezia spp. (Fig. 27.24) can be found on normal skin but the population may grow on some animals to cause an

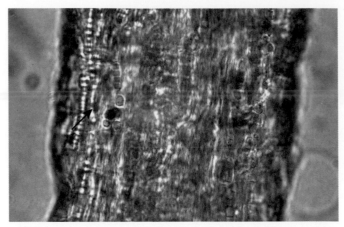

Fig. 27.23 Arthrospore formation (arrowed) in or on hairs that occurs with ringworm infection can be used diagnostically *(Courtesy of Mark Craig)*

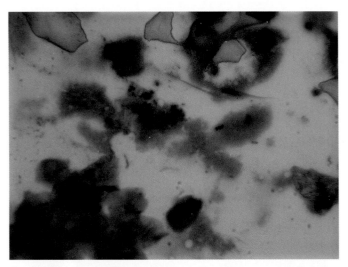

Fig. 27.24 *Malassezia* organisms are bottle-shaped yeasts, some of which may appear to be budding. This slide was stained with methylene blue. Each organism measures 3 μm in length

itchy, red dermatitis. The skin may appear greasy and the animal may smell rancid. Swabs or Sellotape strip samples can be collected, stained with Diff-Quik or equivalent and examined for *Malassezia* spp. organisms. Infection occurs more commonly in dogs than cats, and infection occurs more commonly in some breeds of dog, such as the basset hound and West Highland white terrier. Shampooing with a treatment effective against *Malassezia* spp. usually controls the condition (Scott et al 2001). (For further details see Ch. 29.)

Nematode-related dermatitis

In horses, *Habronema* spp. and *Draschia megastoma* are stomach worms that are transmitted by flies. Flies deposit infective larvae as they feed on secretions or wounds. If the larvae are close to the mouth they will be ingested by the horse and thus complete the life cycle. Elsewhere the larvae burrow into the skin and cause moist, weeping lesions that are slow to heal and are known as 'summer sores'. The larvae or microfilariae of another nematode, *Onchocerca*

cervicalis, can gather in the skin and may be associated with patches of dermatitis with alopecia and scaling, which may be itchy.

Diagnosis of ectoparasite infection

Specimen collection and examination

Surface parasites can be examined by placing coat brushings into a suitable container and examining with the aid of a magnifying lens or stereo microscope. Take care that any fleas present do not hop away at this stage! Evidence of flea infestation can also be obtained by brushing the coat of the dog or cat over damp absorbent paper. If fleas are present then any flea faeces will fall onto the paper. This then appears as a small black speck surrounded by a halo of red partly digested blood.

Burrowing mites can be collected from scrapings taken from the edge of lesions. Some people like to add a little liquid paraffin to the scalpel blade so that the material attaches to the blade. Alternatively, *Demodex* spp. can sometimes be collected by plucking hairs, since the mites can be found around the hair roots. Collected material is placed on to a microscope slide and more liquid paraffin, or a 10% potassium hydroxide (KOH) solution, is added (but the two should not be mixed). Liquid paraffin allows any mites to remain alive, so movement may be seen, while KOH preparations can be left or heated and this assists in removing keratin, making mites more readily visible. However, KOH solution will kill the mites, so movement will not be seen. The preparation should be covered with a coverslip and examined systematically. Alternatively, biopsy samples can be collected for histology, which is particularly useful where the parasites are found deep in the skin. There are additional tests such as blood and skin tests that can be used to help to confirm some parasite infestations including fleas and *Sarcoptes scabiei*. (For further details see Ch. 29.)

Endoparasites

The endoparasites that affect companion animals and horses in the UK are divided into four main groups:

- **Nematodes** – thread-like roundworms
- **Cestodes** – flattened tapeworms
- **Trematodes** – flukes or flat worms – rarely affect companion animals
- **Protozoa** – single-celled organisms.

Nematodes

Nematodes are commonly referred to as roundworms, as they are round in cross-section. Typically, they are cylindrical and featureless except that some species have features at their anterior and posterior ends (Fig. 27.25). The main intestinal nematodes found in dogs, cats and horses are shown in Table 27.4. Treatments for endoparasites are shown in Tables 27.5–27.7. More information can be obtained about each of the treatments by referring to the NOAH Compendium of Data Sheets for Animal Medicines. This provides a listing of anthelmintics and ectoparasiticides for each host species.

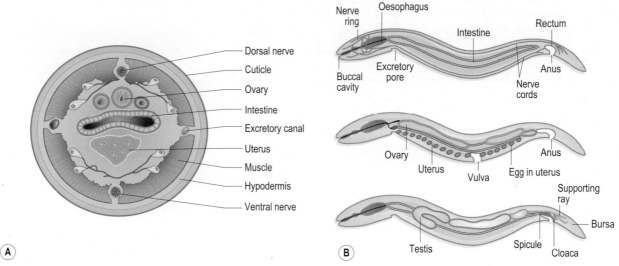

Fig. 27.25 Nematodes. (**A**) Cross-section through a typical nematode. (**B**) Longitudinal sections

Table 27.4 Major intestinal nematodes of dogs, cats and horses

Nematode group	Cat	Dog	Horse
Ascarids	*Toxocara cati*	*Toxocara canis*	*Parascaris equorum*
	Toxacaris leonina	*Toxascaris leonina*	
Hookworms	*Ancylostoma tubaeforme*	*Ancylostoma caninum*	
	Uncinaria stenocephala	*Uncinaria stenocephala*	
Whipworms		*Trichuris vulpis*	
Strongyles			Cyathostominae
			Large strongyles
Pinworms			*Oxyuris equi*

Ascarids

The ascarids are found in the small intestine and are the largest roundworms found in dogs, cats and horses.

Toxocara canis

Adult female *Toxocara canis* can measure up to 20 cm in length (Fig. 27.26), are off-white and possess cuticular enlargements at their anterior end known as cervical alae.

Life cycle: Eggs laid by adult female worms are passed in faeces and embryonate in the environment. This occurs in approximately 11 days in optimal conditions and more slowly in cooler weather (Lloyd 1993). The eggs are protected by a thick outer shell and can survive in the environment for extended periods. Survival for over a year has been recorded but this may be reduced by desiccation or exposure to ultraviolet light. Dogs become infected when they ingest eggs from the environment or eat prey that have themselves eaten eggs and are carrying infective larvae in their tissues. Depending on the route of infection (Fig. 27.27) the larvae migrate through the liver and lungs or remain in the intestine to develop into adult worms. Larvae that have migrated may return to the intestine or migrate into tissues, where they remain as somatic larvae. In a bitch, some somatic larvae are reactivated when pregnancy occurs and they migrate across the placenta to the pups from about the 42nd day of pregnancy or, particularly when infection has occurred late in pregnancy, across the mammary gland to infect pups in milk. As a result, pups can carry a large number of egg-laying worms from about 3 weeks of age. When a pup has had a heavy infection the worms are expelled as the pup grows older and subsequent infection will tend to result in somatic larvae and not intestinal infections. However, the factors that result in adult dogs acquiring patent intestinal infections are not clearly understood and it is estimated that about 10% of adult dogs carry infection.

A small number of intestinal worms are well tolerated by dogs, as are developing worms or somatic larvae. However, a heavy burden of migrating larvae in a pup can cause pneumonia as the worms pass through the lungs. Adult worms interfere with absorption of nutrients and a heavy burden can cause a pup to be cachectic, with an intestine distended by worms. Intestinal worms may cause acute emergencies such as intestinal obstruction or intussusception.

Zoonotic infection: Humans can be infected by accidentally ingesting embryonated eggs from the environment. Clinical signs are seen most commonly in children, although a larger proportion of the population is seropositive,

Table 27.5 The spectrum of activity offered by different canine antiparasitic products

Product	Spectrum of activity				
	Protozoa	Cestode	Nematode	Insect***	Acari***
Piperazine			■		
Pyrantel			■		
Dichlorophen		■			
Benzimidazoles	■	■	■		
Nitroscanate		■	■		
Praziquantel		■			
Pyrantel, febantel and praziquantel		■	■		
Pyrantel and febantel			■		
Selamectin			■	■	■
Lufenuron and milbemycin			■	■	
Milbemycin and praziquantel		■	■		
Moxidectin and imidacloprid			■	■	■
Oxantel, pyrantel and praziquantel		■	■		
Emodepside and praziquantel		■	■		

** *Giardia* spp. only
*** Some genera only – see individual data sheets for more information
Note: diagram is based on the data sheet claims for the products
Diagram first appeared in *Veterinary Review*

Table 27.6 Diagram of the spectrum of activity offered by different feline antiparasitic products

Product	Spectrum of activity				
	Protozoa	Cestode	Nematode	Insect***	Acari***
Piperazine			■		
Dichlorophen		■			
Benzimidazoles	■	■	■		
Praziquantel		■			
Pyrantel and praziquantel		■	■		
Selamectin			■	■	■
Milbemycin and praziquantel		■	■		
Emodepside and praziquantel		■	■		
Moxidectin and imidacloprid			■	■	■

*** Some genera only – see individual data sheets for more information
Note: diagram is based on the data sheet claims for the products
Diagram first appeared in *Veterinary Review*

indicating exposure without showing clinical signs. There are two classical disease entities: ocular larva migrans (OLM), associated with larval migration within the eye, and visceral larva migrans (VLM), associated with mass larval migration through, for example, the liver. There are also less obvious forms of infection associated, for example, with asthma-like symptoms.

It is very difficult to prevent dogs acquiring infection from the environment when they walk in public places such as parks. Control depends on the prevention of egg output by appropriate anthelmintic treatment of the dog. Treatments are focused on preweaned pups and their dams, as bitches can carry patent infections while they are lactating. Weaned pups and adult dogs can then be treated at appropriate

Table 27.7 The spectrum of activity offered by different equine antiparasitic products

Product	Spectrum of activity				
	Protozoa	**Cestode**	**Nematode**	**Insect**	**Acari**
Mebendazole			■		
Fenbendazole			■		
Pyrantel		■	■		
Ivermectin and praziquantel		■	■	■	■
Moxidectin			■	■	■
Ivermectin			■	■	■
Praziquantel		■			
Moxidectin and praziquantel		■	■	■	■

* At double the normal dose rate
** Bots only
Note: diagram is based on the data sheet claims for the products

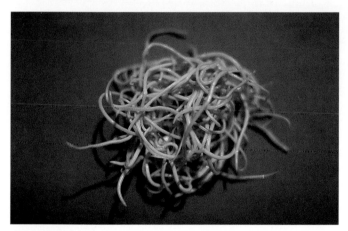

Fig. 27.26 Adult *Toxocara canis* are stout, off-white or pinkish worms when fresh (these are preserved specimens)

intervals. Dogs should be prevented from defecating in children's play areas and faeces should be picked up.

Toxocara cati

Toxocara cati are similar in appearance to *T. canis* but if they are examined under a stereo microscope it may be seen that the cuticular enlargements at the anterior end are like arrowheads. The life cycle of *T. cati* is similar to that of *T. canis* except that there is no prenatal migration of larvae across the placenta so kittens first acquire infection from the queen in milk (Fig. 27.28). This means that kittens are probably about 6 weeks old when they begin passing *T. cati* eggs in their faeces.

A small number of worms will be well tolerated by a cat, but a large number may interfere with intestinal function. A large number of larvae following a hepatotracheal migration may cause pneumonia or even death of young kittens. In the past, *T. cati* has not been regarded as as much a zoonotic risk as *T. canis*; however, there is increasing evidence that *T. cati* and *T. canis* should be regarded as equally important zoonoses (Fisher 2003). Cats may acquire infection through ingesting embryonated eggs from the environment or by eating infected paratenic hosts such as mice. Control is normally based on anthelmintic treatment, as prevention of infection is almost impossible unless the animals are maintained in specialized environments. As cats may carry patent infection at any age, anthelmintic treatment should be repeated at regular intervals.

Toxascaris leonina

Toxascaris leonina can infect both dogs and cats and has a life cycle similar to *T. canis*, but animals are only infected by ingesting eggs or paratenic hosts. Dogs and cats do not acquire a patent infection until they are about 3 months of age or older, because the prepatent period is about 8 weeks in dogs and 13 in cats. Infection is normally well-tolerated without clinical signs and, like the other ascarids in dogs and cats. *T. leonina* is regarded as a potential zoonosis.

Parascaris equorum

Parascaris equorum is the ascarid found in the small intestine of horses. It is a very large worm, with adults measuring up to 40 cm long.

Life cycle: Foals acquire infection from embryonated eggs in their environment. Once ingested the infective larvae hatch from the eggs and penetrate the intestinal wall to undergo a hepatotracheal migration before being coughed up and swallowed, thereby returning to the small intestine, where they mature to adult worms and begin egg-laying approximately 10–12 weeks after infection. Egg output by adult worms is high, so massive environmental contamination with eggs can occur. The eggs are sticky and thickly coated, so tend to remain in the horse's environment for extended periods, acting as a source of reinfection for the foal or a source of infection for foals in subsequent seasons.

As they become older, horses become more recalcitrant to infection, so patent infections are common in foals and yearlings but unusual in older horses. A few worms are well-tolerated but a heavy infection can cause signs of pneumonia as the larvae migrate through the lungs and a large number of adult worms can cause intestinal obstruction. Control is

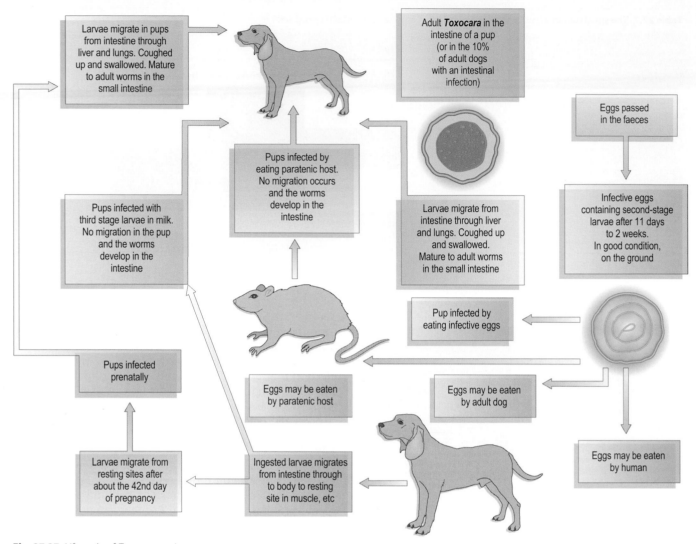

Fig. 27.27 Life cycle of *Toxocara canis*

Hookworms

Hookworms are so-called because the buccal capsule or mouth of the worm is set at an angle to the body of the worm, giving a slightly hooked appearance like a crochet hook. There are many species of hookworm that parasitize the small intestine in a wide range of host species. All have a direct life cycle, with eggs passed into the environment, where they develop into infective larvae. Three species that infect cats or dogs will be considered in more detail: *Uncinaria stenocephala*, *Ancylostoma caninum* and *Ancylostoma tubaeforme*. In each case the adult worm measures about 1.5 cm.

Uncinaria stenocephala

Uncinaria stenocephala is also known as the 'northern hookworm' and is the hookworm that occurs endemically in dogs in the UK. It has a typically large buccal capsule with two

cutting plates at the entrance. Dogs are infected when they ingest infective larvae from the environment and the prepatent period is about 3 weeks. The larvae can penetrate skin but in doing so only cause a local dermatitis, unlike other hookworm species where larvae are capable both of penetrating skin and migrating through the animal to culminate in an intestinal infection. Infection is most likely to occur in dogs in kennels such as greyhound or hunt kennels. Dogs carrying a heavy infection may have diarrhoea and there will be some intestinal protein loss. Cats may also carry infection, although they appear to be rarely infected in the UK.

Ancylostoma caninum

Ancylostoma caninum is endemic in continental Europe and has been recorded sporadically in the UK. The buccal capsule has two pairs each of three teeth at the entrance (Fig. 27.29). The larvae in the environment prefer a higher temperature to *U. stenocephala* larvae and so flourish best in warmer climates than the UK. It may be possible for infection to become established in the UK, either in a sheltered kennel environment or in southern England, and the infection may be imported in dogs that have lived in Europe. Dogs are

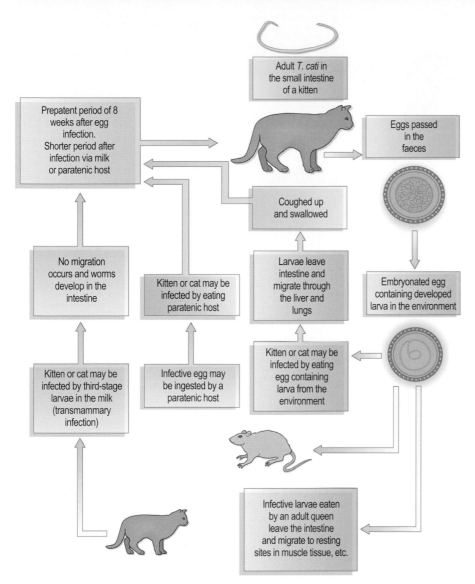

Fig. 27.28 Life cycle of *Toxocara cati*

Boxes in figure:

- Adult *T. cati* in the small intestine of a kitten
- Prepatent period of 8 weeks after egg infection. Shorter period after infection via milk or paratenic host
- Eggs passed in the faeces
- Coughed up and swallowed
- No migration occurs and worms develop in the intestine
- Kitten or cat may be infected by eating paratenic host
- Larvae leave intestine and migrate through the liver and lungs
- Embryonated egg containing developed larva in the environment
- Kitten or cat may be infected by third-stage larvae in the milk (transmammary infection)
- Infective egg may be ingested by a paratenic host
- Kitten or cat may be infected by eating egg containing larva from the environment
- Infective larvae eaten by an adult queen leave the intestine and migrate to resting sites in muscle tissue, etc.

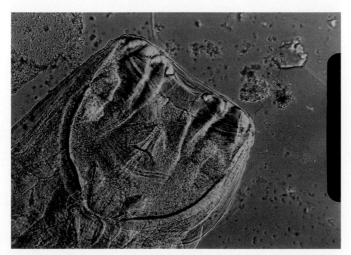

Fig. 27.29 Head end of *Ancylostoma caninum*. Like other hookworms it has a large buccal capsule. *A. caninum* has two pairs each of three teeth

infected by larval penetration through the skin or by ingesting infective larvae (Fig. 27.30). Some larvae fail to develop into adult worms in the intestine, instead remaining as larvae in tissues. Some of these larvae can transfer from the dam to pups in milk. In large numbers, milk-acquired larvae can cause the death of pups by 10 days of age, before the infection has had time to become patent. A low level of intestinal infection is well tolerated but the worms are voracious blood suckers, grasping the intestinal mucosa with their mouths and slashing with the teeth in their buccal capsule, so a heavy infection results in substantial blood loss and subsequent anaemia. Not all the blood is eaten by the worms and large amounts can pass in the faeces, appearing as bloody mucus or blackened blood, which is termed melaena. Over a long term, a smaller number of worms can cause anaemia due to chronic blood loss. Penetrating *A. caninum* can cause dermatitis in dogs and humans and *A. caninum* has caused eosinophilic enteritis in humans.

Ancylostoma tubaeforme

Ancylostoma tubaeforme is a hookworm of cats. It has a buccal capsule with two pairs of three teeth at the entrance to the

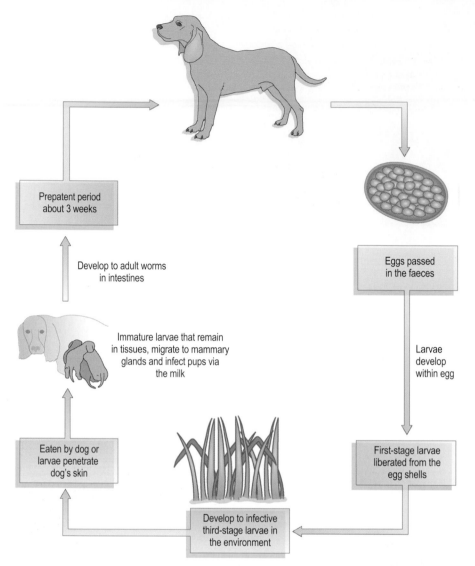

Fig. 27.30 Life cycle of *Ancylostoma caninum*

Prepatent period about 3 weeks

Develop to adult worms in intestines

Immature larvae that remain in tissues, migrate to mammary glands and infect pups via the milk

Eaten by dog or larvae penetrate dog's skin

Develop to infective third-stage larvae in the environment

Eggs passed in the faeces

Larvae develop within egg

First-stage larvae liberated from the egg shells

mouth. It does not appear to be prevalent in the UK but has been reported in cats in mainland Europe and so may be imported in cats entering the UK. *A. tubaeforme* is a blood sucker and can cause anaemia with either a heavy infection or a smaller chronic infection.

Whipworms

Trichuris vulpis

These are known as whipworms, as their anterior end is long and narrow like the lash of a whip and the posterior end broad like a whip handle (Fig. 27.31). The adult worms are found in the large intestine, where the anterior end is buried in the mucosa and the posterior end is free in the lumen. They are found occasionally in the UK, particularly in dogs in kennels. Infections are most likely in southern England, where the climate is most favourable for the development of the infective stages in the environment. Once passed in faeces, the eggs embryonate in the environment, with the larvae remaining within the shell once developed (Fig. 27.32). The larvae are thus protected from environmental conditions and can remain viable for up to 1 year in favourable conditions. This means that substantial infection can

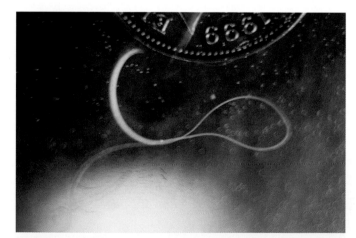

Fig. 27.31 *Trichuris vulpis*, the whipworm, next to a 1p coin to illustrate size

accumulate in the kennel or surroundings of infected dogs. A low-level infection is well tolerated but a heavy infection can result in diarrhoea and metabolic disturbance if untreated. Established infections can be treated using a suitable anthelmintic and thereafter repeat infections can be

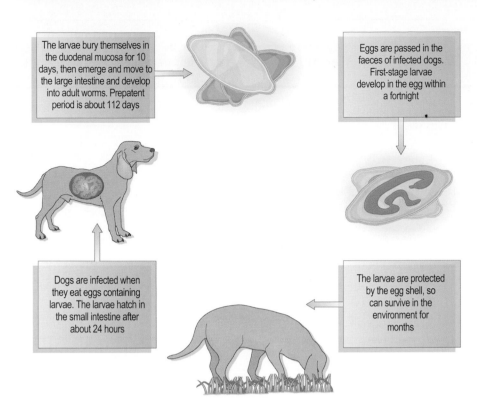

Fig. 27.32 Life cycle of *Trichuris vulpis*

The larvae bury themselves in the duodenal mucosa for 10 days, then emerge and move to the large intestine and develop into adult worms. Prepatent period is about 112 days

Eggs are passed in the faeces of infected dogs. First-stage larvae develop in the egg within a fortnight

Dogs are infected when they eat eggs containing larvae. The larvae hatch in the small intestine after about 24 hours

The larvae are protected by the egg shell, so can survive in the environment for months

prevented by moving the animals to uncontaminated surroundings and/or regular anthelmintic treatment. Repeat faecal sampling to monitor the success of any control programme is suggested.

Strongyloides species

Infection with *Strongyloides* spp. is typically seen in young animals. The worms are tiny and hair-like, characterized by an oesophagus that is approximately one-third of the length of the entire worm. *Strongyloides westeri* is an important infection in young foals from about 2 weeks of age. Larvae pass from the mare in the milk and develop in the foal's small intestine with a prepatent period of 8–14 days. Infection can be supplemented with larvae ingested directly from the environment and a heavy infection can cause diarrhoea. As foals become older, patent infections and associated clinical signs become less common. Occasionally dogs show diarrhoea associated with *Strongyloides* spp. infection.

Strongyles

Cyathostomes

Horses have a large number of species of nematodes that inhabit the large intestine, many of which are about 1 cm long (Fig. 27.33). There are more than 40 different species but they are grouped together as the cyathostomes, also known as the 'small strongyles' or trichonemes. The life cycle is direct, with horses acquiring infection by ingesting third-stage larvae off pasture. The young larvae burrow into the wall of the large intestine, where they may remain in a state of suspended development or hypobiosis for extended periods, or develop and emerge after a short period to develop into adults within the lumen of the intestine. The

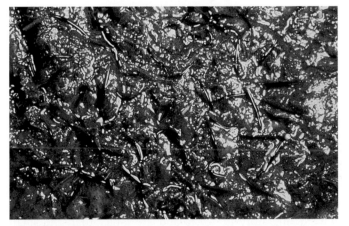

Fig. 27.33 The cyathostomes or small strongyles are small worms that can be present in enormous numbers in the large intestine of a horse (*Courtesy of Merial Animal Health*)

adults are found close to the wall of the intestine, where they feed on the superficial layers of the intestinal mucosa. Adult worms lay typical 'strongyle' eggs that are passed in faeces and develop on pasture.

Low levels of infection are well tolerated but contamination can build up substantially on pasture, and a heavy infection, especially in foals or yearlings, can cause poor condition, anaemia and diarrhoea. An acute syndrome may be seen in spring when thousands of hypobiotic larvae leave the mucosa simultaneously to continue their development. Many may be passed in the faeces and appear as a red layer on the surface of dung. Affected animals show profuse diarrhoea, weight loss and sometimes colic and death. Control depends on reducing the access of horses to larvae on pasture

Table 27.8 Summary of the large strongyles of horses

Species	Prepatent period (months)	Migratory route of larvae	Adult appearance	Adult length (cm)
Strongylus vulgaris	6–7	Migration up the cranial mesenteric artery and branches and back to the intestine where they form nodules in the intestinal wall	Two rounded teeth at the base of the buccal capsule	1.5–2.5
Strongylus equinus	8–9	Form nodules in the deep layers of the intestine and then migrate through the liver before returning to the intestine	Three teeth, one with two points, at the base of the buccal capsule	2.5–5.0
Strongylus edentatus	10–12	Migrate through the liver into the peritoneum where they develop into L5 before returning to the intestine	No teeth in buccal capsule	2.5–4.5

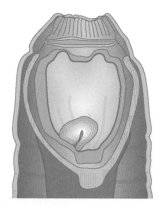

Fig. 27.34 Head of *Strongylus vulgaris*

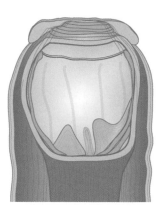

Fig. 27.35 Head of *Strongylus equinus*

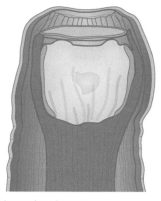

Fig. 27.36 Head of *Strongylus edentatus*

by measures such as avoiding heavily contaminated pasture and dung collection, together with anthelmintic treatment. Although it may be possible to rely on a combination of pasture management and monitoring of egg counts, normally control is a mixture of anthelmintic treatment and pasture management.

Large strongyles

Three species of nematode occur in the large intestine but have a migratory life cycle and are larger than the small strongyles, so are known as the large strongyles to differentiate them. The species are *Strongylus vulgaris*, *Strongylus equinus* and *Strongylus edentatus* and the features of each species are shown in Table 27.8 and Figures 27.34–27.36. Infection, particularly with *S. vulgaris* larvae, can cause severe clinical signs. *S. vulgaris* larvae in the cranial mesenteric artery cause considerable pathology, including clot formation and infarction caused by blockage of a branch of the artery and subsequent death of the area of intestine supplied by that artery. The adult worms cause small ulcers as they feed on the large intestinal mucosa. Control is based on pasture management and anthelmintic treatment as described for the cyathostomes.

Triodontophorus species

Triodontophorus spp. are a third group of strongyle nematodes that inhabit the large intestine of the horse. They are differentiated primarily by their feeding habit. They feed as a

large group, causing the formation of deep ulcers that may measure several centimetres in diameter.

Pinworms

Oxyuris equi

Oxyuris equi is the pinworm of horses, so called because the worms look like carpet tacks. The females measure up to 10 cm but the male worms measure only about 1 cm. The worms inhabit the large intestine but unusually the female worms leave the intestine to lay their eggs on the perineum around the anus of the horse. Larvae develop in the egg and horses are reinfected by ingesting eggs containing fully developed larvae. The prepatent period is 5 months. The activity of the female worms on the perineum and the presence of the eggs can cause severe irritation, seen as rubbing and alopecia over the tail head. Infection can be diagnosed by placing a piece of sticky tape across the perineum around the anus and examining it microscopically for eggs. Control is based on anthelmintic treatment, which can be supplemented in heavy infections by washing of the perineal area to remove eggs.

Lungworms

A number of species of nematode inhabit the lungs and upper respiratory tract. In the dog, *Oslerus osleri* is found around the area of the tracheal bifurcation, adult *Crenosoma vulpis* and *Capillaria (Eucoleus) aerophila* are found in the bronchi and *Filaroides hirthi* occur in the alveoli:

- *Oslerus osleri* has a direct life cycle, with first-stage larvae passed directly from dog to dog in saliva. An infected bitch may pass larvae to her pups within a few days of birth. Ingested larvae are swallowed and migrate from the intestine to the lungs, where they ascend the respiratory tree and grow to adults at the base of the trachea. The presence of the worm causes a granulomatous lesion to grow around it, so that the worms become completely enclosed. These nodules may be well tolerated but can be associated with exercise intolerance and coughing, particularly in dogs at exercise
- *Crenosoma vulpis* is known as the fox lungworm as it is endemic in the fox population. Slugs or snails act as intermediate hosts so dogs become infected by eating an infected slug or snail. A heavy infection may be associated with coughing or exercise intolerance
- *Capillaria (Eucoleus) aerophila* has a similar appearance to *T. vulpis*, but are smaller and are found embedded in the bronchial wall.

Most lungworm infections can be diagnosed by finding larvae in the faeces using the Baermann technique or in bronchoalveolar fluid. The exception is *C. aerophila*, which produces eggs that are not dissimilar to *T. vulpis* eggs, except the polar plugs are smaller and the outer surface is rough. *O. osleri* nodules can sometimes be seen as radio-opaque densities in the trachea. Adult *C. vulpis* may be found in bronchoalveolar fluid, where they appear like pieces of white thread:

- *Aleurostrogylus abstrusus* is the main lungworm in cats. This has an indirect life cycle with a slug or snail as intermediate host. Cats may be infected by eating slugs or snails or possibly small mammals that act as paratenic hosts. Infection may be well tolerated but some cats show respiratory signs, including coughing. Cats can also be infected with *C. aerophila*
- *Dictyocaulus arnfieldi* is the lung nematode that occurs in the horse. The life cycle is direct, with larvae passed in the faeces and developing to third-stage larvae on pasture. Ingested infective larvae leave the intestine and migrate to the lungs, where the slender adult worms are found in the smaller bronchi. The prepatent period

is about 2 months and the female adult worms lay eggs that have often hatched by the time they are coughed up. Infection in donkeys can be symptomless, while infection in horses can be associated with chronic coughing, sometimes in the absence of a patent infection.

Heartworms

There are two nematodes that inhabit the pulmonary artery and the right side of the heart in the dog – *Angiostrongylus vasorum* and *Dirofilaria immitis*.

- *Angiostrongylus vasorum* occurs in both dogs and foxes in the UK. The first reports in dogs about a decade ago were limited to Cornwall, South Wales and the southeast of England but it has now been reported in Scotland. The adult worms measure only about 2 cm in length, very different from the 30 cm of female *D. immitis*, so there is little problem in differentiating the two species. Dogs are infected when they ingest infected slugs or snails and the larvae leave the intestine and migrate to the pulmonary artery (Fig. 27.37). Female worms lay eggs that are swept into the lung circulation. These hatch and the larvae migrate into the alveoli and are eventually coughed up, swallowed and passed in faeces. A wide range of clinical signs may be seen with some, such as clotting disorders, being related to the presence of worms in the circulatory system and others caused by pulmonary damage. Infection can be diagnosed by finding the characteristic larvae in the faeces or in bronchoalveolar fluid
- *Dirofilaria immitis*, the true heartworm, does not occur in the UK unless a pet already carrying heartworm is imported. At present the northern extremity of the area endemic for heartworm is the south of Switzerland, although the endemic area does appear to be spreading. The adult worms are found in the right side of the heart and the pulmonary artery (Fig. 27.38). Female worms are long and slender, measuring up to 30 cm in length. Instead of eggs they lay larvae, known as microfilariae, which travel in the blood. Infection is transmitted by mosquitoes, which imbibe microfilariae as they feed on blood. The larvae develop to third stage in the mosquito and once mature they leave to infect another final host as the mosquito feeds. At first, the larvae develop in the area where they first penetrated the skin, later entering the circulation and travelling to the heart. The prepatent period for heartworm in dogs is about 6–7 months. Cats can also be infected but they are not such a good host: the prepatent period is extended to about 8 months and many infections never produce microfilariae.

A few heartworms in a dog may be well tolerated but a substantial burden can partially obstruct the pulmonary artery, causing right-sided heart failure.

In addition, dead worms may be swept into the lungs, where they form a focus for inflammatory reactions. Clinical signs associated with infection can be graded as mild, moderate and severe. A dog with severe disease might show low exercise tolerance, marked coughing, weight loss and ascites. Occasionally a large number of worms move suddenly from

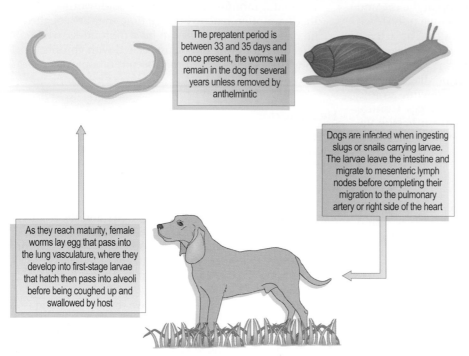

Fig. 27.37 Life cycle of *Angiostrongylus vasorum*

The prepatent period is between 33 and 35 days and once present, the worms will remain in the dog for several years unless removed by anthelmintic

Dogs are infected when ingesting slugs or snails carrying larvae. The larvae leave the intestine and migrate to mesenteric lymph nodes before completing their migration to the pulmonary artery or right side of the heart

As they reach maturity, female worms lay egg that pass into the lung vasculature, where they develop into first-stage larvae that hatch then pass into alveoli before being coughed up and swallowed by host

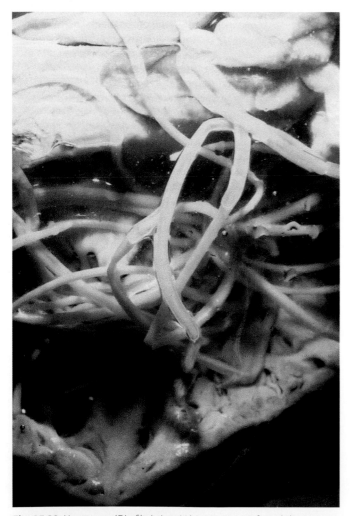

Fig. 27.38 Heartworm (*Dirofilaria immitis*) in situ in an infected dog
(Courtesy of John McGarry)

the pulmonary artery into the right side of the heart, causing an acute condition known as caval syndrome. Infected cats show more diverse signs, which include vomiting and even sudden death.

Adult heartworms may be removed surgically or by anthelmintic treatment but both methods can pose risks to the dog or cat. It is recommended that dogs or cats travelling to an area where heartworm is endemic are treated prophylactically with a macrocyclic lactone throughout the season of mosquito activity. These treatments are administered at monthly or 6-monthly intervals and are highly effective against third- and fourth-stage heartworm larvae, which are killed before they begin to migrate towards the heart.

Cestodes

Cestodes are flat tapeworms composed of a head or scolex and a chain or strobila of clearly defined segments or proglottids (Fig. 27.39). The adult tapeworm is found in the intestine attached to the intestinal wall by the scolex, which often bears hooks and suckers to assist in making a secure attachment. The segments are produced in a neck region behind the scolex and contain both male and female reproductive tracts, so a single tapeworm can reproduce without need of other tapeworms. As a segment becomes older, signified by its being pushed towards the end of the worm by the younger segments, the eggs inside it develop, until it is almost nothing more than a bag of eggs. Ultimately the attachment to the segment behind breaks down and the segment moves down the intestine with the other intestinal contents to pass through the rectum and into the environment. Segments have a primitive nervous system and are capable of some movement, so may make their own way out of the anus. In the environment the segment is broken down and the eggs are released.

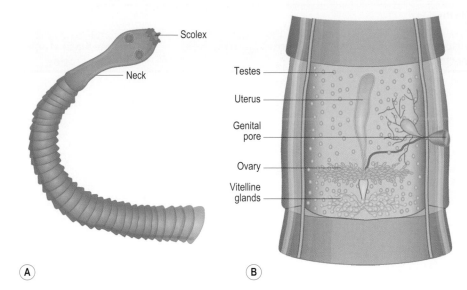

Fig. 27.39 Cestode. (**A**) Anterior end. (**B**) Mature segment or proglottid

All tapeworms have an intermediate stage of development called the metacestode, the appearance of which varies with tapeworm species. Normally the metacestode is found in a host of a different species from the final host in which the adult tapeworm occurs. The final host is infected when it eats the intermediate host carrying the metacestode. For example, the flea carries the immature cysticercoid stage of *Dipylidium caninum* and dogs and cats are infected when they eat an infected flea. Drugs with cestocidal action are shown in Tables 27.5–27.7.

Anoplocephala perfoliata

Anoplocephala perfoliata and its relation *Anoplocephala magna* are two squat, stumpy tapeworms typically found around the ileocaecal junction of a horse's intestine. The intermediate host is the oribatid mite, which can occur in large numbers on pasture. Horses are infected when they ingest the mites with grass. Large numbers of tapeworms are associated with an increased incidence of colic. Control is based on the use of anthelmintics with cestocidal action.

Dipylidium caninum

Dipylidium caninum is a tapeworm that occurs in dogs and cats (Fig. 27.40). It is delicate in appearance compared to *Taenia* spp., the other type of large tapeworm found in dogs and cats in the UK. The intermediate hosts are fleas or biting lice, and dogs or cats are infected when they ingest an infected louse or flea. The tapeworm causes little harm to the animal unless present in very high numbers, apart from anal irritation associated with segments crawling out of the anus. Occasionally, humans are infected with adult tapeworms. Control depends on anthelmintic treatment, together with flea or louse control to prevent reinfection.

Taenia species

Cats are normally infected with just one *Taenia* species, *Taenia taeniaeformis*. The metacestode stage occurs in rodents and the prepatent period in the cat is approximately 47 days. A number of species occur in dogs, with a variety of intermediate hosts, and they are listed in Table 27.9. Without

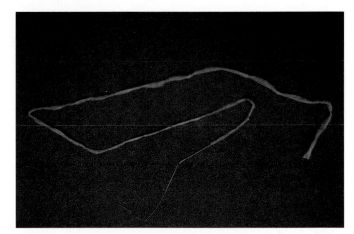

Fig. 27.40 *Dipylidium caninum.* May measure up to 50 cm long

detailed inspection of the shape of the hooks, all *Taenia* tapeworms look the same (Fig. 27.41), although there is some variation in length.

The presence of tapeworms is well tolerated by the host, apart from possibly some anal irritation caused by the presence of segments. Often, however, clinical signs of the metacestode are more severe – sheep with *Coenurus cerebralis* cysts in the brain develop nervous signs known as 'gid', and affected muscle may be devalued as meat. It is therefore important to control *Taenia* tapeworms because of their impact on the intermediate hosts. The eggs of *Taenia* spp. may be seen on faecal egg examination, but this is not a very sensitive technique for detection of cestode eggs. Alternatively, segments may be seen in faeces or on an animal's coat. It is also possible to assess whether a pet is likely to acquire a *Taenia* sp. infection. For example, if a cat lives entirely indoors, eats tinned food and the environment is mouse-free, it is not possible for the cat to become infected with *T. taeniaeformis*. Where there is evidence of tapeworm infection, or a likelihood of the animal acquiring infection, the dog or cat can be treated with an appropriate cestocide. It may be possible to prevent further infection by, for example,

Table 27.9 *Taenia* species of tapeworms found in the dog

Species	Final host	Approximate prepatent period (weeks)	Intermediate host	Intermediate stage – metacestode
Taenia pisiformis	Dog and fox	6–8	Rabbit	*Cysticercus pisiformis*
				Abdomen or liver
Taenia hydatigena	Dog and fox	7–10	Cattle, sheep	*Cysticercus tenuicollis*
				Abdomen or liver
Taenia multiceps	Dog	4–6	Sheep, cattle	*Coenurus cerebralis*
				Brain and spinal cord
Taenia ovis	Dog and fox	6–8	Sheep and goat	*Cysticercus ovis*
				Muscle
Taenia serialis	Dog	–	Rabbit	*Coenurus serialis*
				Connective tissue

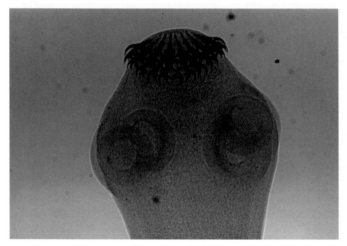

Fig. 27.41 Head of *Taenia* sp. tapeworm

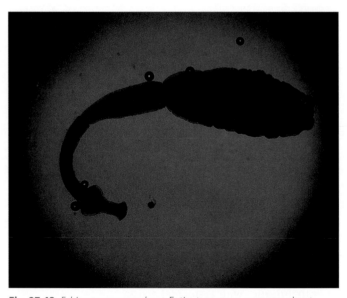

Fig. 27.42 *Echinococcus granulosus*. Entire tapeworm measures about 6 mm

preventing access to raw meat, but in some cases where an animal hunts it can be very difficult to prevent re-exposure.

Echinococcus granulosus

Echinococcus granulosus (Fig. 27.42) is a minute tapeworm found in the small intestine of dogs and foxes and is so small that a dog may carry hundreds or even thousands of worms without any external sign of infection. Each worm measures about 6 mm and consists of only about four segments. The terminal, gravid segment measures about half the length of the worm. The normal intermediate hosts are sheep, although the hydatid cyst, the metacestode stage, can develop in cattle. Infection is widespread across the world and only a few countries have managed to eliminate the disease completely – Iceland has done so and New Zealand and Tasmania are in a transition period before being declared free. There are two areas of infection in the UK: Wales, particularly the Powys area, and the Hebrides. An eradication programme was conducted in Powys in the 1980s but was not totally successful, as a proportion of lambs carried the metacestode stage in the

1990s after the eradication scheme had been scaled down to an educational programme. A new eradication campaign has recently been initiated by the Welsh Assembly. More details can be found on the Welsh Assembly website.

Infection by this cestode is an important zoonosis. If humans eat the eggs passed by a dog or fox then a hydatid cyst may develop in the person's liver, lungs or rarely elsewhere. The cyst can grow to 10 cm or more in diameter and causes pain and debility. Cysts are removed by surgery or anthelmintic treatment. Control depends on regular treatment of dogs in endemic areas with effective cestocides and preventing dogs from having access to sheep carcases or uncooked offal. There is a separate species, *Echinococcus equinus*, that has a dog-to-horse life cycle. It is not believed to be zoonotic.

Echinococcus multilocularis

Like *E. granulosus*, *Echinococcus multilocularis* is a very small tapeworm but the final segment comprises slightly less than half the length of the worm compared to *E. granulosus*. *E. multilocularis* does not occur in the UK but the infection is endemic throughout a large part of mainland Europe from eastern France to Germany in the north and across to Poland in the east. The southern boundary is the southern borders of Switzerland and Austria.

Foxes are the main hosts but dogs and, to a lesser extent, cats can act as final hosts, the normal intermediate host being small rodents. In the intermediate host a cystic structure develops that contains many protoscolices, each of which is an immature tapeworm. The cyst has an invasive nature and parts can break off and metastasize, particularly in aberrant final hosts such as humans. As *E. multilocularis* is an important zoonosis, it was the reason for the introduction of mandatory tapeworm treatment with an approved cestocide, i.e. praziquantel, prior to entry into the UK under the PETS scheme.

If humans ingest eggs, an alveolar cyst may develop in the liver and, as in rodents, it has an invasive nature and if untreated will lead to the death of the individual. Treatment is sometimes difficult in advanced cases but consists of surgery and/or anthelmintic treatment. Control in dogs and cats is based on regular anthelmintic treatment. Pet owners should be warned prior to travelling about the risk of their pet acquiring infection. As the prepatent period is approximately 1 month, if they are away for longer than this and the animal becomes infected it could begin passing segments prior to the cestode treatment on return.

Trematodes

Trematodes are the flukes, flat worms that parasitize a number of organs including the intestine, bile ducts, blood and lungs of domestic animals. In the UK we are familiar with the liver fluke, *Fasciola hepatica*, which is normally a parasite of sheep and cattle. Horses can be infected but clinical signs associated with infection are rare. Animals on wet ground with standing water are at risk, as these are often suitable locations for the intermediate host, a tiny snail called *Lymnea truncatula*. Eggs passed in the faeces of infected animals develop in the environment and the first stage, the miracidium, infects snails. Eventually, after two more developmental stages, cercariae leave the snail and encyst as metacercariae on grass, ready to infect a new mammalian host when they are ingested.

There are a number of fluke species that occur in cats and dogs but none are endemic in the UK pet population.

Protozoa

The protozoa are small, unicellular organisms, some of which are parasites of animals. A major group are the coccidian parasites, which produce oocysts as a result of sexual reproduction.

The coccidian protozoa

Isospora species

A number of *Isospora* (*Cytospora*) species are parasites of the intestine of dogs and cats, but only some, such as *Isospora* (*Cytospora*) *felis* in cats and *Isospora* (*Cytospora*) *canis* in dogs,

are considered pathogenic. The parasite goes through a complex series of reproductive stages in the dog or cat that terminate in sexual reproduction and the production of oocysts, which are passed in faeces. This is similar to that seen in *Eimeria* spp. (Fig. 27.43). *Isospora* spp. infection may be well tolerated or may result in diarrhoea, particularly in puppies and kittens. The life cycle is direct and hosts are infected when they ingest sporulated oocysts from the environment. Control depends on hygiene, particularly in between litters of pups or kittens, as oocysts are robust and will survive in the environment for long periods.

Horses and rabbits may be infected with *Eimeria* spp. (Fig. 27.43) and infection may result in diarrhoea. One species of *Eimeria* in rabbits affects the liver rather than the intestine.

Some coccidian parasites have a more complex life cycle, with the final host infected by eating an infected intermediate host. These include the agent of equine protozoal myeloencephalitis *Sarcocystis neurona* and other *Sarcocystis* species. The *Sarcocystis* species each have a two-host life cycle and typically for any particular species both hosts are defined, e.g. *Sarcocystis tenella* infects dogs and sheep. The dog is normally little affected by the presence of the intestinal stages but the stages in the sheep occur in muscle tissue and can cause severe illness and even death (Rommel 1985). Equine protozoal myeloencephalitis is a severe nervous disease of horses that is currently the focus of a great deal of research in the USA.

Toxoplasma gondii

Toxoplasma gondii has a complex life cycle consisting of asexual and sexual reproductive components (Fig. 27.44). The main host is the cat and both stages can occur in the cat, but the asexual reproductive stage can also take place in many other mammals.

Cats are infected by eating infected prey or by ingesting oocysts in faeces. Normally, following infection, sexual reproduction takes place, with the production of oocysts without clinical signs. Oocyst production continues for a period of days and then ceases and thereafter cats are believed not to become reinfected. Other mammals become infected when they ingest sporulated oocysts from a cat's faeces. In these hosts replication takes place in tissues, initially rapidly dividing tachyzoites are formed and then, under the influence of host immunity, slower-dividing bradyzoite cysts.

Like other mammals, humans can become infected. Immunocompromised people and foetuses are most at risk of developing severe disease. A proportion of the adult population are seropositive, i.e. show evidence of infection, but remain healthy. In immunocompromised individuals, including those whose immunity is suppressed during transplant surgery, the tissue cysts can multiply rapidly. Infection during pregnancy may result in abortion, an affected baby or an infected baby who does not show any clinical signs but may develop them later in life.

Steps to avoid human infection include:

- Wear gloves while gardening and wash hands thoroughly prior to eating
- Cover children's sandpits to prevent cats from using them as litter trays
- Wear gloves when cleaning the cat's litter tray and clean it out daily

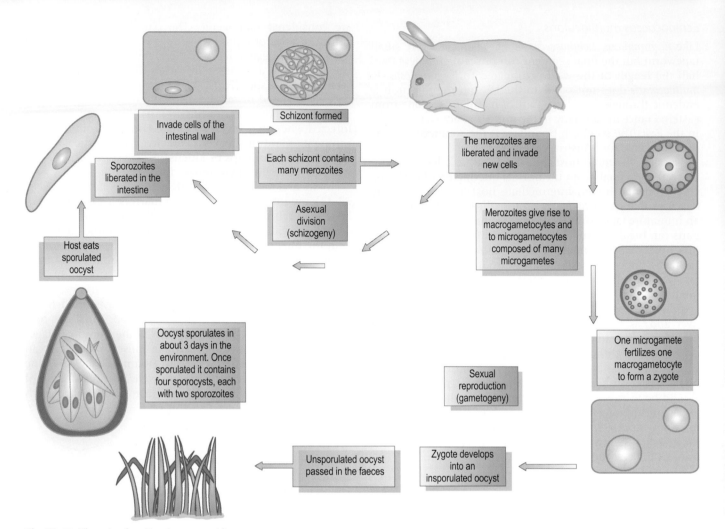

Fig. 27.43 Life cycle of an *Eimeria* spp. coccidium

- Wash fruit and vegetables prior to eating
- Chop meat separately from vegetables and wash hands after handling raw meat
- Avoid undercooked meat and unpasteurized milk and cheese.

The baby charity Tommys (www.tommys.org) provides advice, including leaflets about human infection and how to avoid it.

Neospora caninum

Neospora caninum was first identified about 30 years ago. It is closely related to *T. gondii* and shows similar tissue cysts associated with asexual reproduction, and sexual reproduction in the intestine of dogs that results in oocyst production. Cattle are the intermediate host and infection can cycle within the cattle population without passing through dogs, causing abortion when fetuses are affected. Occasionally, the tissue stages cause clinical signs in dogs, usually of an ascending paralysis and paresis, together with muscle wasting. Infection can be diagnosed in dogs on the basis of a high antibody titre. Infection in dogs can be treated with a combination of antiprotozoals and is most successful when commenced early in the infection.

Cryptosporidium spp.

Cryptosporidium spp. are small intestinal protozoan parasites that have a direct life cycle with oocysts passed in faeces. The host range includes a wide variety of mammalian species and genetic research is currently engaged in clarifying species relationships. Both dogs and cats can be infected and some individuals continue to be subclinical carriers after an initial infection. Diarrhoea associated with infection is most commonly seen in puppies and kittens. The infection may be zoonotic, so care should be taken to avoid transmission to humans, where diarrhoea may be severe particularly in the immunocompromised.

Giardia spp.

Giardia spp. are flagellate protozoa that infect the small intestine of many mammalian species, causing diarrhoea and increased frequency of defecation. Following infection some animals may remain as carriers and may act as a source of infection for others. Dogs and cats can both acquire infection, particularly puppies and kittens. The stage in the intestine, the trophozoite, multiplies by binary fission and environmentally resistant cysts are passed in faeces. The infection may be zoonotic, so care should be

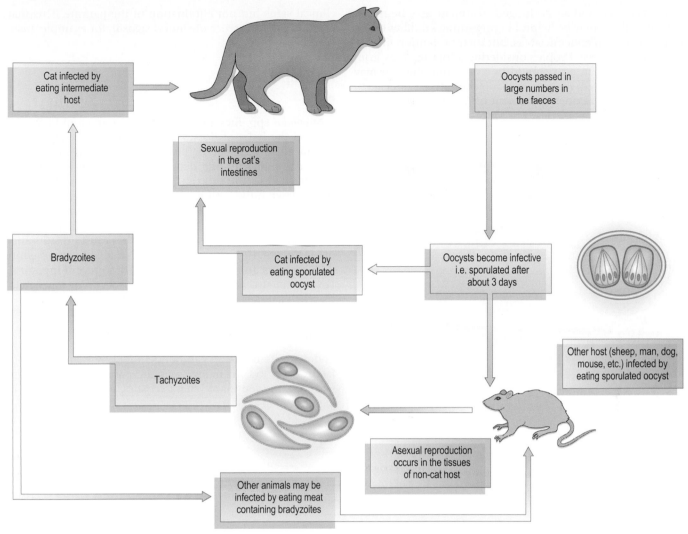

Fig. 27.44 Life cycle of *Toxoplasma gondii*

taken to ensure that humans are not exposed to infection. Infected dogs may be treated with fenbendazole. There is a vaccine available in the USA but it is not currently available in the UK.

Babesia spp.

Babesia spp. are parasites of red blood cells and the presence of the parasite in red blood cells causes breakdown of the cells. Infected animals show bouts of fever and then anaemia, which can be followed by death in some cases. Infection is tick-transmitted and the most prevalent species in Europe, *Babesia canis*, is transmitted by *Rhipicephalus sanguineus* and *Dermacentor* spp. ticks. It does not occur in the UK but there have been reports of dogs returning from Europe with babesiosis. Prompt treatment of clinically affected animals, normally with imidocarb, is essential. Pet owners planning to take their animals on holiday should be informed of the risks associated with tick infestation and how to avoid them. A babesiosis vaccine is available in some European countries. Cats can be infected with *Babesia* spp. but the main species infecting cats occur in Africa and the East but not in the Mediterranean. Cats appear to tolerate infection well until the anaemia becomes very severe,

and then they die rapidly. *Babesia equi* occurs in southern Europe and infects horses.

Leishmania spp.

Leishmania spp. are intracellular parasites of macrophages and the infection is endemic in many of the tropical and subtropical areas of the world, including the Mediterranean. Infection in southern Europe is transmitted by the sandfly, *Phlebotomus* spp. Dogs are the main species infected and clinical signs may occur 5 years after infection. Initial signs vary, but may consist of a skin wound that doesn't heal. Infected macrophages proliferate in a variety of different organs and clinical signs are related to the organ systems affected. Not every dog that acquires infection will develop disease but a proportion will do so. Presence of infection may be detected using antibody (IFAT) tests or polymerase chain reaction tests (PCR).

Dogs act as a reservoir for human infection, as leishmaniosis is an important zoonosis. The Mediterranean infection, normally referred to as *L. infantum*, is not as pathogenic in humans as some of the other species; nonetheless, the disease can be severe in the young and immunocompromised. Infected dogs can be treated but a parasitic cure is rarely achieved and so prolonged treatment may be necessary. Repellents may be helpful in preventing sandflies biting dogs and cats in endemic areas, but total prevention may be difficult to achieve. People considering adopting dogs from the Mediterranean area should be aware that the dog may already be infected. Frequency of infection in cats appears to be far less than in dogs. Treatment of leishmaniosis is difficult – most treatments lead, at best, to a resolution of the clinical signs but not elimination of the parasite. This may result in the recurrence of clinical signs if, for example, treatment is stopped.

Arthropods

Bots

Gastrophilus spp. flies are active in the summer and lay their eggs on the hairs of horses. Horses ingest the eggs as they groom and the larvae or bots develop in the stomach or proximal small intestine, depending on the species. The bots are attached to the mucosa (Fig. 27.45) but the following spring when fully developed they pass into the environment and pupate. The adult fly emerges in the summer to complete the life cycle. In the horse they cause some pathology and in addition, the presence of the flies causes disturbance or even panic in horses. The eggs are visible as small white dots on hairs and these can be cut off to prevent ingestion. Horses can also be treated with an ivermectin or other macrocyclic lactones, such as moxidectin, to eliminate bots.

Diagnosis of endoparasite infection

Endoparasite infection can be identified by examination of faeces or blood. In many cases the parasite produces eggs with certain identifiable characteristics, which are shown in Figures 27.46–27.48.

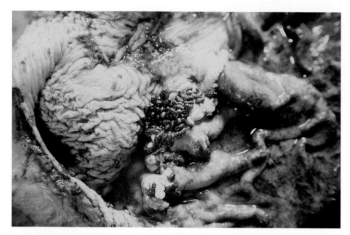

Fig. 27.45 The larvae of *Gastrophilus* sp. or bots attached to the stomach wall of a horse

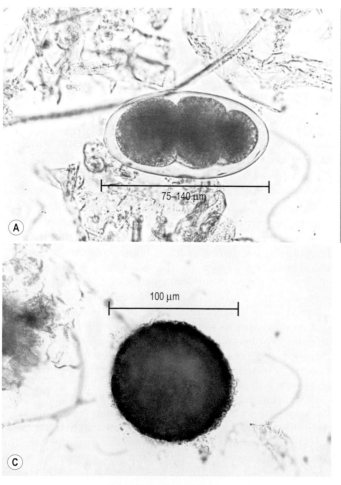

75–140 µm

(A)

100 µm

(C)

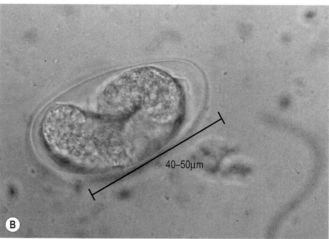

40–50µm

(B)

Fig. 27.46 Horse nematode eggs. (**A**) Strongyle egg. (**B**) *Strongyloides* sp. egg. (**C**) *Parascaris equorum* (*All courtesy of John McGarry*)

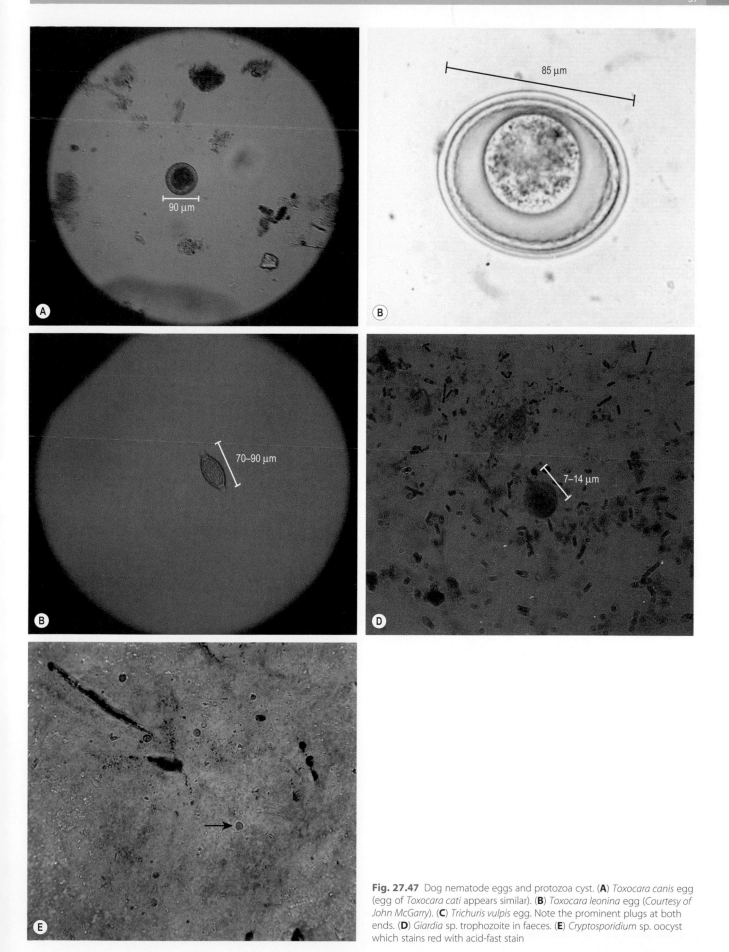

Fig. 27.47 Dog nematode eggs and protozoa cyst. (**A**) *Toxocara canis* egg (egg of *Toxocara cati* appears similar). (**B**) *Toxocara leonina* egg (*Courtesy of John McGarry*). (**C**) *Trichuris vulpis* egg. Note the prominent plugs at both ends. (**D**) *Giardia* sp. trophozoite in faeces. (**E**) *Cryptosporidium* sp. oocyst which stains red with acid-fast stain

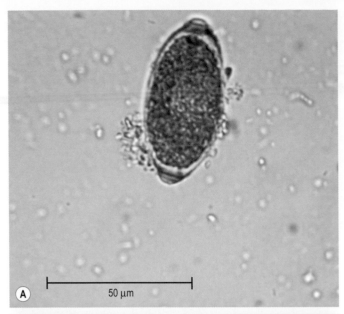

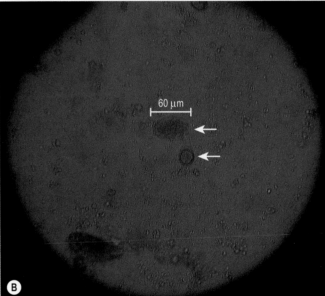

Fig. 27.48 Cat nematode eggs. (**A**) *Capillaria* sp. egg. (**B**) *Isospora felis* oocyst – this is the largest oocyst that occurs in cats. Also visible is an egg from *Ancylostoma tubaeforme*

Collection of samples

Faeces

Faecal samples should be collected from the animal's rectum or fresh off a cage floor. Old faecal samples from a kennel floor may be contaminated with free-living nematodes, which can confuse identification.

Laboratory analysis – examination of faeces for parasite eggs

The majority of endoparasites produce eggs or larvae which pass out in the host's faeces and there are a variety of techniques that can be used to examine the faeces:

- Where eggs are abundant, e.g. in ascarid infection, a small piece of faecal material can simply be added to some water on a microscope slide to form an emulsion.

The mixture is covered with a coverslip and examined systematically under a microscope
- Two methods, based on the use of fluid of a particular density to separate eggs by floating them from faecal debris, which sinks, are described below. Both use saturated sodium chloride solution as the flotation fluid. The density of 1.0 can be increased to >1.5 using saturated zinc sulphate, which will float both nematode and the heavier trematode eggs. Alternatively, trematode eggs can be sedimented by spinning them down in a centrifuge.

Modified McMaster (quantitative method)

- Place 3 g of faeces in 42 ml water in a beaker or jar, add several glass beads and shake to break up the faecal matter. Cat faeces are notoriously difficult to break up and using lukewarm water and leaving for a few hours in the water will help
- Pour the mixture through a tea strainer and catch the fluid in a bowl
- Discard the debris in the tea strainer
- Fill a 15 ml test tube with the filtrate and centrifuge for 5 minutes at 1500 rpm
- Discard the supernatant
- Add a small amount of saturated salt solution (NaCl) to the tube and mix to suspend the pellet from the bottom of the tube. Fill the tube to the 15 ml mark and mix again
- Remove an aliquot with a pipette and use this to fill one side of a McMaster chamber; repeat to fill the second side of the McMaster slide
- Dry any excess water off the McMaster slide. Place on to a microscope stage and examine under × 40 magnification
- Focus on the grid etched on to the upper surface of the slide and work methodically, examining each section of the grid systematically. Any eggs will be in focus at the same time as the grid lines, as will round, black circles, which are air bubbles
- Count all eggs (if different types of egg are present then each should be counted separately) found on one side of the slide. Repeat the count on the other side of the slide, add the totals together and multiply by 50 to get the number of eggs per gram of faeces.

Faecal flotation (semi-quantitative method)

- Place 3 g of faeces in 42 ml water in a beaker or jar, add several glass beads and shake to break up the faecal matter. Cat faeces are notoriously difficult to break up and using lukewarm water and leaving for a few hours in the water will help
- Pour the mixture through a tea strainer and catch the fluid in a bowl
- Discard the debris in the tea strainer
- Fill a 15 ml test tube with the filtrate and centrifuge for 5 min at 1500 rpm
- Discard the supernatant
- Add a small amount of saturated salt (NaCl) to the tube and mix to resuspend the pellet from the bottom of the tube. Fill the tube totally and place a coverslip on to the top of the tube – it should be held in place by the fluid beneath it

- Place into a centrifuge and spin at 1500 rpm for 2 minutes. Gently remove the tube from the centrifuge, pick off the coverslip with a vertical action and place on to a microscope slide
- Place the slide on to the microscope stage and examine under × 40 magnification
- Work methodically, examining each section of the coverslip systematically
- Count all eggs (if different types of egg are present then each should be counted separately) and the number counted equals the number of eggs per gram of faeces.

Baermann technique for detection of larvae in faeces

Equipment: a funnel, a metal clamp stand, a short piece of rubber tube, a clip, two strong wires, some muslin, a centrifuge tube, a slide and coverslip, and Lugol's iodine:

- Place the rubber tubing on to the end of the funnel and clamp the funnel into the stand. Place the clip across the end of the rubber tubing so that it forms a watertight seal
- Fill the funnel with lukewarm water up to about 1 cm of the rim
- Take a piece of muslin measuring about 15 cm^2 and thread the two wires through two sides. Place the muslin into the top of the funnel so that the wires are lying across the top of the funnel
- Place about 10 g of faeces gently on to the muslin, ensuring that it is well covered with water
- Leave the apparatus overnight and in the morning draw off a centrifuge tube full of fluid from the bottom of the apparatus by unclipping the clip across the rubber tube

- Allow the tube to stand for about 4 hours or centrifuge at 1500 rpm for 1 minute
- Remove the supernatant and place the sediment on a microscope slide with a coverslip on the top. A drop of Lugol's iodine can be added, which kills the larvae and stops them moving. It also stains them light brown, which can help to highlight features.

Blood

Blood samples should be collected into ethylenediaminetetraacetic acid (EDTA) as a anticoagulant for microscopic or PCR examination.

Laboratory analysis – examination of blood

A conventional blood smear can be prepared and stained with Giemsa to examine for blood parasites such as *Babesia* spp. or *Leishmania* spp.

Heartworm microfilariae can be identified in blood using the Knott's test:

- The process requires 1 ml blood and any excess blood should be conserved so that, if necessary, a sample can be sent to an expert for identification of microfilariae
- Add 1 ml of blood (heparinized or EDTA) to 9 ml 2% formaldehyde solution in a centrifuge tube. Mix thoroughly
- Centrifuge the tube at 1500 rpm for 5 minutes. Discard the supernatant
- Place the sediment on to a microscope slide, add a drop of methylene blue and mix well
- Place a coverslip over the preparation and examine systematically.

Bibliography

Acarus – The University of Bristol's dedicated laboratory for the PCR detection of arthropod-borne infectious diseases in companion animals. Available from: <www.bris.ac.uk/acarus/welcome.htm>.

American Heartworm Society, www.heartwormsociety.org

Curtis, C.F., 2004. Current trends in the treatment of *Sarcoptes*, *Cheyletiella* and *Otodectes* mite infestations in cats and dogs. Vet. Dermatol. 15, 108–114.

Department of Environment, Food and Rural Affairs, DACTARI – Dog and Cat Travel and Risk Information. Available from: <www.defra.gov.uk/animalh/diseases/veterinary/dactari/>.

Details of the Pet Travel Scheme, www.defra.gov.uk/animalh/quarantine/pets/index.htm

Dryden, M.W., Rust, M.K., 1994. The cat flea, biology, ecology and control. Vet. Parasitol. 52, 1–19.

Fisher, M., 2003. *Toxocara cati*: an underestimated zoonosis. Trends Parasitol. 19, 167–170.

Guidelines for parasite control, www.esc cap. org

Lloyd, S., 1993. *Toxocara canis*: the dog. In: Lewis, J.W., Maizels, R.M. (Eds.), *Toxocara* and Toxocariasis, Clinical, Epidemiological and Molecular Perspectives. British Society for Parasitology with the Institute of Biology, London.

Pet owner website about parasites and their control, www.petparasites.co.uk

Quinn, P.J., Carter, M.E., Markey, B.K., Carter, G.R., 1994. Clinical Veterinary Microbiology. Wolfe, London.

Rommel, M., 1985. *Sarcocystosis* of domestic animals and humans. In Pract. 7, 158–160.

Scott, D.W., Hillier, W.H., Griffin, C.E., 2001. Muller and Kirk's Small Animal Dermatology, sixth ed. W B Saunders, Philadelphia, PA.

TestAPet – Veterinary Parasitology Diagnostics, www.testapet.com

Recommended reading

Jacobs, D.E., 1986. A Colour Atlas of Equine Parasites. Gower Medical, London.

Provides numerous illustrations of the appearance and life cycles of an extensive range of horse parasites.

Macpherson, C.N.L., Meslin, F.X., Wandeler, A.I., 2000. Dogs, Zoonoses and Public Health. CABI Publishing, Wallingford.

Focuses on dog diseases from the perspective of the risk of human disease.

Noah Compendium of Data Sheets for Animal Medicines. National Office of Animal Health, London.

Provides data sheets of individual parasiticides.

Taylor, M.A., Coop, R.L., Wall, R.L., 2007. Veterinary Parasitology, third ed. Blackwell Publishing, Oxford.

A thick textbook on parasitology covering all the species. You may also want to the refer to the 2nd edition (1996) for a good basic textbook.

Trotz-Williams, L., Gradoni, L., 2003. Disease risks for the travelling pet: leishmaniasis. In Pract. 25, 190–197.

One of an In Practice series examining the infections that may enter the UK under PETS. The others in the series are also worth looking out for.

CHAPTER 28

Microbiology

Helen Moreton

Key Points

- Microorganisms are too small to be seen with the naked eye and include bacteria, viruses, fungi, algae and protozoa. The majority of microorganisms are non-pathogenic and are essential for life, e.g. in the breakdown and decay of dead matter.
- Before the symptoms of a disease develop, a pathogenic organism must invade the host, establish itself in the tissues and overcome the host's defence mechanisms.
- Bacteria vary in size and shape and are able to survive away from the host, provided that they do not dry out or encounter extremes of temperature.
- They may be visualized using a light microscope but it is easier to distinguish between different species if biological stains, e.g. Gram's stain, are used to highlight their morphological features.
- Bacterial replication occurs asexually by binary fission and by conjugation, which allows new characteristics to develop as a result of the transfer of genetic material.
- Bacteria can be grown in the laboratory in order to identify them but the culture must be provided with the correct balance of nutrients, water, pH, temperature and gaseous environment.
- Viruses are minute obligate intracellular parasites that can only be seen using an electron microscope.
- Each virus particle or virion consists of either RNA or DNA surrounded by a protein coat. Some viruses also have an envelope around the outside.
- Viral replication occurs inside the host cell and depends on the virus's ability to instruct the cell to start producing virus particles. The new virions burst out of the cell, invade other cells and clinical signs develop.

Introduction

Microbiology is the study of organisms, and other biologically important agents, that are too small to be seen by the naked eye, deriving its name from the Greek words *mikros* ('small'), *bios* ('life') and *logos* ('science'). The organisms are smaller than 1 mm in diameter and are mostly unicellular, i.e. consisting of only one cell, which carries out all the functions necessary for life. A few, such as some fungi, are multicellular.

Microorganisms include:

- **Bacteria** – including the very small forms *Rickettsia*, *Chlamydia* and *Mycoplasma* spp.
- **Viruses**
- **Fungi** – covered in Chapters 27 and 29
- **Algae** – no pathogenic forms affecting animals
- **Protozoa** – covered in Chapter 27.

Microorganisms vary in size from the relatively large protozoa to viruses that can only be seen with an electron microscope (Figs 28.1, 28.2). Viruses range in size from about 10–40 nm (nanometres) and differ from other microorganisms in that they have no cellular structure, although they have a wide variety of shapes (Table 28.1).

Microscopes

A light or optical microscope can magnify up to approximately 1500 times without losing resolution (image loses clarity), which means that objects smaller than 0.2 µm (micrometres) cannot be seen in clear detail. As suggested by the name, electron microscopes use an electron beam, which achieves much higher magnification and resolution than light microscopes and distinguishes objects as small as 0.2 nm (250 000 × magnification) (Table 28.2).

Over 10 000 species of bacteria are known, most being less than 10 µm in diameter, while virus particles, virions, range between 10 nm and 400 nm in diameter (Fig. 28.2).

Visualization of living bacteria is difficult using bright-field optical microscopy, as they are transparent and often colourless. Contrast-enhancing optical systems can help to elucidate the morphological characteristics of cells (shape, flagellae, etc.), but in order to learn more about their properties bacteria must be differentiated into specific groups for identification purposes. This can be done by the use of biological stains, selective culture media and biochemical tests, for example. Staining procedures involve applying dyes to bacterial smears, which are air-dried and heat-fixed. Gram stain to divide then into positive or negative depends on the thickness of the cell wall and also shows cell shape, and typical morphology of groups of cells.

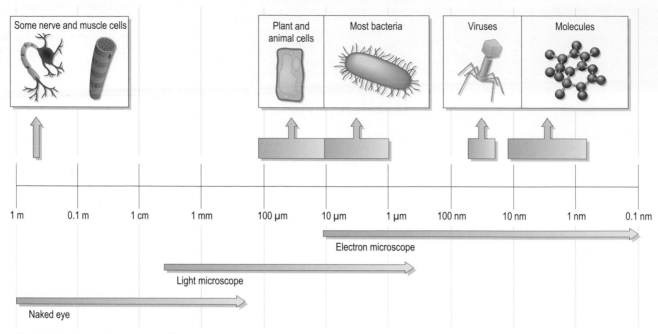

Fig. 28.1 Relative sizes of various types of structure

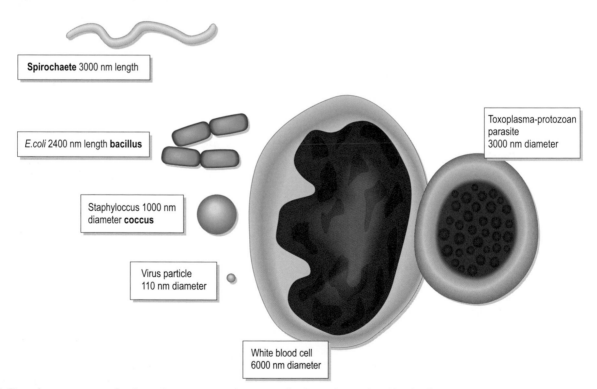

Fig. 28.2 Sizes of common types of pathogenic organism in relation to each other and to a white blood cell

Table 28.1 Comparison between the characteristics of mammalian cells and those of microorganisms

Characteristic	Mammals	Bacteria	Viruses	Fungi	Protozoa	Algae
Size	10–100 μm	0.5–<10 μm	200–300 nm	Yeasts 3.8 μm	10–200 μm	0.5–20 μm
Cell arrangement	Multicellular	Unicellular	Non-cellular	Uni- or multicellular	Unicellular	Uni- or multicellular
Cell wall	None	Mainly peptidoglycan	None	Mainly chitin	None	Mainly cellulose
Nucleus	Membrane-bound nucleus	No true membrane-bound nucleus	Absent	Membrane-bound nucleus	Membrane-bound nucleus	Membrane-bound nucleus
Nucleic acids	DNA and RNA	DNA and RNA	DNA or RNA	DNA and RNA	DNA and RNA	DNA and RNA
Reproduction	Cells in tissues asexual; new individuals sexual	Asexual – binary fission	Replicate only within living cell	Asexual and sexual by spores, budding in yeast	Asexual and sexual	Asexual and sexual
Nutrition	Heterotrophic	Mainly heterotrophic, can be saprophytic, parasitic, a few autotrophic	Obligate parasites	Heterotrophic, can be saprophytic or parasitic	Heterotrophic, can be saprophytic or parasitic	Autotrophic
Motility	Some cells are motile, whole individual motile	Some are motile	Non-motile	Non-motile except for certain spore forms	Motile	Some are motile
Toxin production	None	Some form toxins	Some form toxins	Some form toxins	Some form toxins	

Table 28.2 Units of measurement of microorganisms

1 millimetre (mm)	$= 10^{-3}$ metre (m)	$= 1/1000$ m
1 micrometre (μm)	$= 10^{-6}$ m	$= 1/1\,000\,000$ m
1 nanometre (nm)	$= 10^{-9}$ m	$= 1/1\,000\,000\,000$ m

Microorganisms

Microorganisms can be classified according to their method of nutrition:

- **Autotrophs** – manufacture their own food, often by photosynthesis with the aid of chlorophyll
- **Heterotrophs** – obtain their food from the environment. Most microorganisms are this type. They may be:
  - **Saprophytes** – feed on dead material. None are pathogenic
  - **Parasites** – feed on a living organism, which is referred to as the host.

There are three types of parasite:

- **Pathogens** – disease-causing organisms
- **Commensals** – live in or on the host but cause no harm and derive no benefit, e.g. *Staphylococcus intermedius*, which lives on the skin. May become pathogenic if the balance between the host and the organism is upset
- **Mutualistic or symbiotic organisms** – live in or on the host and both provide a benefit for the host and derive a benefit for themselves, e.g. microbial flora which colonize the caecum of the horse and rabbit, breaking down plant food material for digestion from which the microorganisms gain a source of energy.

When a microorganism invades a host and starts to multiply, it establishes an infection. If the host is susceptible to the infection then disease results.

In order to cause disease, a pathogen must:

- Gain entry into the host
- Establish itself and multiply in the host tissue
- Overcome the normal host body defences for a time
- Damage the host in some way.

Some microorganisms cause disease by secreting or releasing poisonous substances called **toxins** that disrupt specific physiological processes in the host while others invade tissue cells and damage or destroy them. Viruses, for example, cause cell damage because they interfere with the normal cell metabolism and many leave the host cell by rupture of the cell membrane. Once they have entered the tissues of the host, some microorganisms are localized and remain at the site of entry; for example, *Staphylococcus intermedius*, which causes skin disease, generally attacks in this way. Others spread through the body (systemic spread), usually via the lymphatic system and blood circulation. Once they have invaded the host, some microorganisms can grow and multiply in any tissues of the body but many are more selective and localize in a particular tissue or organ. If these more demanding organisms do not reach the particular cells in which they can live, they will not produce disease. Viruses in particular often have an affinity for a specific tissue or organ, which is known as **tissue trophism**. A virus is only able to attach to cells that carry a compatible receptor; for example, influenza viruses can only attach to ciliated epithelial cells in the respiratory tract.

Definitions

Infection is the invasion and multiplication of microorganisms in body tissues and may lead to cellular damage.

Table 28.3 Routes of infection

Source of infection	Susceptible organ system	First line of defence
Contaminated food and water	Digestive	Lysozymes in saliva, stomach acid and enzymes
Droplet infection	Respiratory	Mucus, cilia, macrophages
Sexual transmission	Reproductive and urinary	Mucus, acidic, urine flow
Direct contact	Skin	Acid, salty, oily skin. Rapid healing process
Vector organisms	Injected straight to blood	Bypasses the first line of defence

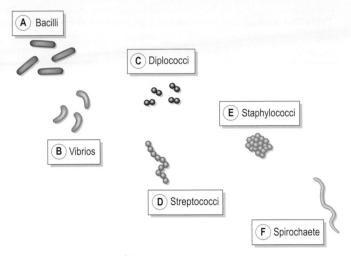

Fig. 28.3 (**A–F**) Shapes of bacteria

Damage may result from competitive metabolism, intracellular replication, the presence of toxins or by the action of the body's defence mechanisms, such as inflammation and antibody–antigen responses.

An infectious disease is one caused by, or capable of being communicated by, the process of infection. If the disease is capable of being transmitted from one animal to another it is described as being **contagious** or **transmissible**. Pathogens may invade the body in many ways but successful invasion, i.e. one that results in disease, depends on the pathogen avoiding the body's first lines of defence (Table 28.3). See also Chapter 19.

Bacteria

Classification and naming of bacteria

Bacteria are referred to by describing their basic shapes (Fig. 28.3):

- Cylindrical or rod-shaped cells are called **bacilli** (singular: bacillus)
- Some bacilli are curved and these are known as **vibrios**
- Spherical cells are called **cocci** (singular: coccus). Some cocci exist singly while others remain together in pairs after cell division and are called **diplococci**. Those that remain attached to form chains are called **streptococci** and if they divide randomly and form irregular grape-like clusters they are called **staphylococci**
- Spiral or helical cells are called **spirilla** (singular: spirillum) if they have a rigid cell wall or **spirochaetes** if the cell wall is flexible.

Bacterial cell structure

Bacteria vary in size, e.g. rickettsias, mycoplasmas and chlamydias, which are considerably smaller than a typical bacterium (Table 28.4). Both rickettsia and chlamydia possess a cell wall like other Gram-negative bacteria (Fig. 28.4) but both of these organisms must live inside other cells, i.e. they are obligate intracellular organisms. They are still considerably bigger than viruses, which are also obligate intracellular parasites.

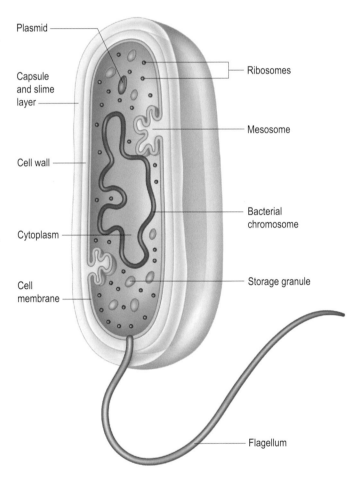

Fig. 28.4 Structure of a bacterial cell, using *Escherichia coli* as an example

The cell wall and its significance in drug therapy

Like plant cells, most bacteria have a cell wall, but this has a different biochemical structure from the polysaccharide (cellulose) cell wall of plants, being made mainly of a substance called peptidoglycan (sometimes called murein). It maintains cell shape and prevents the cell from bursting. Cell walls vary in thickness and in composition and it is

Table 28.4 Comparative characteristics of bacteria and viruses

	Bacteria			Viruses
	Typical bacterium	*Rickettsia/Chlamydia*	*Mycoplasma*	
Size	<5–10 μm	0.8–2 μm	±0.5 μm	10–400 nm
Intracellular parasite	–	+	+	+
Cell wall	+	+	–	–
Plasma membrane	+	+	+	–
Binary fission	+	+	+	–
Filterable through bacteriological filters	–	±	+	+
Possess both DNA and RNA	+	+	+	–
ATP-generating metabolism	+	±	+	–
Ribosomes	+	+	+	–
Sensitive to antibiotics	+	+	?	–
Sensitive to interferon	–	–	–	+

these differences which are a key aid to initial identification using Gram's stain.

The cell wall:

- Resembles a football, i.e. it is elastic but rigid
- Contains several amino acids not found in the proteins of plants and animals so chemotherapeutic agents such as antibiotics can be directed specifically against them without harming the host cell wall.

The peptidoglycan of Gram-negative cells has the same fundamental structure as that of Gram-positive cells but only one or two layers linked to the outer membrane by lipoprotein bridges, which anchor it. There are other biochemical differences in the outer layers of the two types of bacteria.

Chemicals that target these differences in cell structure, biochemical composition and metabolism between bacterial and plant or animal cells are frequently used as therapy against bacterial pathogens (see Ch. 17). A common example of this is the antibiotic penicillin, which disrupts the synthesis of new bacterial cell walls during binary fission and hence bursts or lyses the pathogen. Any antibacterial drug that affects the cell wall will be particularly suited to use against Gram-positive organisms.

Bacterial diseases

Examples of diseases in dogs and horses are shown in Tables 28.5 and 28.6.

Groups of very small bacteria are responsible for a number of diseases in animals, including:

- *Chlamydia* – various strains of *Chlamydia psittaci* are the cause of **psittacosis** in psittacine birds (parrots, parakeets) and mammals. Psittacosis is a zoonotic infection that humans can acquire by inhaling *Chlamydia* in the airborne dust or cage contents of infected birds. **Feline pneumonitis** is also caused by *Chlamydia psittaci* and the organism may be the cause of conjunctivitis in the cat. They are transmitted by inhalation of infectious dust and droplets and by ingestion. There is also evidence to suggest that vector-borne infection may occur.

- *Rickettsia* – transmitted by vectors such as the tick, louse, flea and mite from an infected individual; for example, *Haemobartonella felis* (*Mycoplasma haemofelis*) causes **infectious feline anaemia**. Another rickettsial infection is caused by *Ehrlichia* spp. A particularly pathogenic species is *Ehrlichia canis*, endemic in much of France and the Mediterranean basin.

Generally, the identification of *Rickettsia* and *Chlamydia* is more difficult and thus more specialized than that of most bacteria. Diagnosis of infection may be based on demonstration of the organisms themselves or on the demonstration of increased titres of antibodies in paired serum samples. The rickettsiae are smaller than most bacteria and are barely visible under the ordinary light microscope. They can only be cultivated in tissue culture or in the yolk sac of embryonated eggs. Typically, they are rod-shaped.

- *Mycoplasma* – tiny bacteria-like organisms. Unlike other bacteria they do not possess a cell wall. Mycoplasma species have been implicated in complicating respiratory tract infections in a number of species, notably calves and horses (especially young racehorses in training). They include *Mycoplasma felis*, a cause of chronic conjunctivitis in cats. Mycoplasma will grow on agar-based media but, as the bacteria are so fragile, isolation and identification are specialized skills.

Pathogenicity

Pathogenicity is the ability of an organism to enter the body, set up disease and cause symptoms. A pathogen is an organism capable of causing disease. A virulent pathogen readily sets up infection and produces severe symptoms.

Virulence may vary between different strains of the same bacterium. Disease is the result of the virulence of the pathogen versus the resistance (defence mechanisms) of the host. In some diseases, symptoms occur because of an overreaction of the host's own defence mechanisms. This can lead to cell damage or an allergic reaction.

Some pathogens will almost always cause serious disease, while others are less pathogenic and cause milder illnesses.

Table 28.5 Bacterial diseases of dogs

Bacterium	Disease caused	Gram stain	Shape	Aerobic
Salmonella spp.	Diarrhoea, etc.	Negative	Rod/bacillus	Yes
Campylobacter spp.	Diarrhoea, etc.	Negative	Curved rods	Yes (but prefer less oxygen than in the air)
Bordetella bronchiseptica	Kennel cough	Negative	Short rods/bacilli	Yes
Leptospira spp.	Leptospirosis	Negative	Helically coiled/spirochaete	Yes
Staphylococcus spp.	Pyoderma	Positive	Cocci	Yes
Clostridium tetani	Tetanus	Positive	Long rods/bacilli	No

Table 28.6 Bacterial diseases of horses

Disease	Bacterium	Tissue affected	Comment
Strangles	*Streptococcus equi*	Upper respiratory tract	Very infectious
Contagious equine metritis	*Taylorella equigenitalis*	Reproductive tract	Notifiable
Summer pneumonia	*Rhodococcus equi*	Lungs	Foals most susceptible
Lyme disease	*Borrelia burgdorferi*	Systemic, joints	Vector-borne – tick

Many produce toxic enzymes to assist in the process of invasion and tissue destruction; for example, the enzyme hyaluronidase helps the pathogen to penetrate the tissues of the host by breaking down the 'tissue cement' that holds the cells together. Another enzyme, lecithinase, lyses or disintegrates tissue cells, especially red blood cells.

Virulence is determined by factors such as:

- The ability of the parasite to invade particular cells and tissues and cause damage, i.e. its invasiveness
- Its ability to secrete toxins that disrupt physiological processes in the body, i.e. its toxigenicity
- Its ability to survive in unfavourable conditions.

Invasiveness

- May be assisted by enzymes (which are also toxins) secreted by the bacteria, e.g. collagenase secreted by *Clostridium*; coagulase secreted by *Staphylococcus aureus*; hyaluronidase and protease secreted by *Streptococcus*
- Most bacteria get into the body tissues but some get inside the cells as well, which may assist them in avoiding the immune mechanisms of the host. For example, *Salmonella* species are facultative intracellular parasites, i.e. they live between the cells but may also get inside them; *Rickettsia* are obligate intracellular parasites, i.e. they have to live inside the cells
- Some bacteria, e.g. *Bacillus anthracis*, have capsules that are antiphagocytic
- Some, e.g. *Escherichia coli*, adhere to the host cells by means of rod-like pili, which prevent them from being swept away by body fluids.

Toxigenicity

Toxins are poisonous substances that have a damaging effect on the cells of the host. The effects of the toxin are not only felt in the affected cells and tissues but also elsewhere in the body as the toxin is transported through the tissues.

Two types of toxin are recognized:

- **Exotoxins** are proteins produced mainly by Gram-positive bacteria during their metabolism. They are released into the surrounding environment as they are produced. This may be into the circulatory system and tissues of the host or, as in food poisoning, into food that is then ingested. Microbial toxins include many of the most potent poisons known to man and may prove lethal even in small quantities. Some examples include those toxins produced by the genus *Clostridium*, which includes *Clostridium tetani*, which causes tetanus, and *Clostridium botulinum*, which causes botulism. Nowadays Botox, a diluted form of the toxin, is used to paralyse the facial muscles to provide a youthful appearance.
  The body responds to the presence of exotoxins by producing antibodies called antitoxins that neutralize the toxins, rendering them harmless.
  As they are proteins, exotoxins are destroyed by heat and some chemicals. Chemicals such as formaldehyde are used to treat toxins so that they lose their toxicity but not their ability to elicit an immune response. These treated toxins are called **toxoids** and if they are injected into the body they will stimulate the production of antitoxins. For example, tetanus toxoid is used to provide immunity to tetanus
- **Endotoxins** are part of the cell wall of certain Gram-negative bacteria and are released only when the cells die and disintegrate. In Gram-negative cells the outer bilayer membrane has the typical phospholipids replaced by lipopolysaccharides, which comprise up to 40% of the surface structure and act as the major somatic antigen of these bacteria. Compared with exotoxins, they are less toxic, cannot be used to form toxoids and are able to withstand heat. Blood-borne endotoxins are responsible for a range of non-specific reactions in the body such as fever. They also make the walls of blood capillaries more permeable, causing blood to leak into the intercellular spaces, sometimes resulting in a serious drop in blood pressure, a condition commonly called endotoxic shock. They are

also responsible for the change in capillary blood flow in equine hooves that leads to laminitis.

Toxins are not made exclusively by bacteria. The saprophytic fungus *Aspergillus flavus* produces a toxin called **aflatoxin**. The fungus grows in warm, humid conditions and contaminates a variety of agricultural products such as peanuts, cereals, rice and beans. Aflatoxin has been implicated in the deaths of many farm animals that have been fed on mouldy hay, corn or on peanut meal.

Spore formation

To survive unfavourable conditions, such as when the supply of nutrients is inadequate, some species of bacteria produce spores or sporulate. These dormant forms are also called **endospores**. Spore formation is most common in the genus *Clostridium*, which contains the causative agents of tetanus and botulism, and in *Bacillus anthracis*, the causative agent of anthrax. These diseases are zoonotic, most commonly affecting domestic and farm animals. Species susceptibility to each varies; for example, dogs only infrequently suffer from tetanus, while horses are very susceptible and require routine vaccination, as do humans. It is important to note that spore formation is not a method of reproduction: one vegetative bacterial cell produces a single spore, which, after germination, is again just one vegetative cell (Fig. 28.5).

The spore develops within the cell and under the micro scope appears as a bright, round or oval structure. Many spore-forming bacteria are inhabitants of the soil but spores can exist almost everywhere, including in dust. They are extremely resistant structures that can remain viable for many years. Cattle have died from anthrax contracted by contact with spores that have remained in soil after the death of an animal there decades before. Spores can survive extremes of heat, pH, desiccation, ultraviolet radiation and exposure to toxic chemicals such as some disinfectants. The reason why spores are so resistant is not completely understood but heat resistance is thought to be due to the fact that a dehydration process occurs during spore formation, which expels most of the water from the spore.

The fact that spores are so hard to destroy is the principal reason for the various sterilization procedures that are carried out in veterinary practice. Common techniques employed to kill spores include the use of moist heat under pressure and dry heat for at least 2 hours (see Ch. 22).

Bacterial replication

Bacteria reproduce or replicate asexually by simply dividing into two identical daughter cells, a process known as **binary fission** (Fig. 28.6). If their environment is suitable, bacteria can grow and reproduce rapidly. The time interval between successive divisions is called the generation time. Even under optimum conditions the generation time varies:

- *Escherichia coli* – 20 minutes
- *Mycobacterium tuberculosis*, which causes tuberculosis – approximately 18 hours.

Given appropriate conditions, growth is exponential, i.e. one bacterium produces two, then two produce four, then eight, potentially reaching many millions within 24 hours.

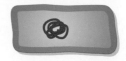
1. Bacterial cell

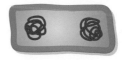
2. Chromosome replicates

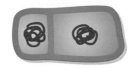
3. Septum forms and produces a forespore

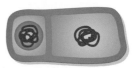
4. Spore coat forms around chromosome

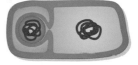
5. Further layers thicken the spore coat

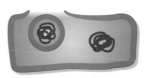
6. Spore is released by rupture of parent cell

Fig. 28.5 Sporulation

To enable cell replication, the chromosome, i.e. the genetic material, is copied first to form two identical chromosomes. As the parent cell enlarges, the chromosomes separate and the cell membrane grows inwards at the centre of the cell. At the same time, new cell wall material grows inwards to form the septum and this divides the cell into two daughter cells. In some species, e.g. streptococci and staphylococci, the daughter cells remain attached to each other to form the characteristic chains or clusters. In most species the new bacterial cells separate.

Conjugation

Conjugation is rare among Gram-positive bacteria but common among those that are Gram-negative. It is sometimes regarded as a primitive type of sexual reproduction but this is misleading because, unlike sexual reproduction in other organisms, it does not involve the fusion of two gametes to form a single cell. Frequently, plasmid DNA is

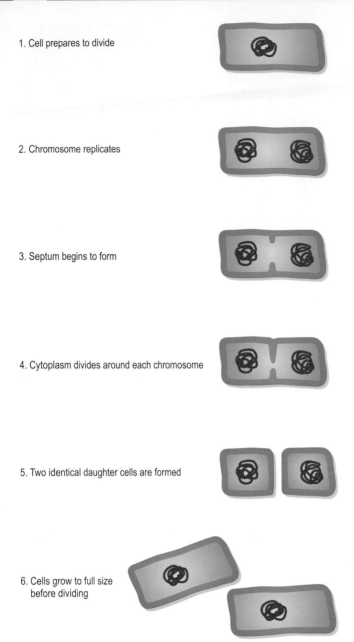

1. Cell prepares to divide

2. Chromosome replicates

3. Septum begins to form

4. Cytoplasm divides around each chromosome

5. Two identical daughter cells are formed

6. Cells grow to full size before dividing

Fig. 28.6 Bacterial replication by binary fission

transferred from the donor to the recipient but sometimes part of the donor cell chromosome, or even the whole chromosome, is transferred.

Conjugation is important because the recipient acquires new characteristics. For example, one plasmid, the R plasmid, carries genes for resistance to antibiotics, and is the mechanism by which some species can acquire resistance from a similar species. Enterobacteria such as *E. coli* and *Salmonella spp.* are thought to transfer resistance between serotypes in this way.

The process of conjugation involves the passage of DNA from one bacterial cell, the donor, to another, the recipient, while the two cells are in physical contact.(Fig. 28.7) The cells are pulled together by a sex pilus, which is formed by the donor cell. Once contact has been made, the pilus retracts so that the surfaces of the donor and recipient are very close

to each other. The cell membranes fuse, forming a channel between the two cells to enable transfer to take place.

Bacterial cultivation in the laboratory

It may be necessary to cultivate bacteria in the laboratory from a sample collected from a patient, e.g. faecal or skin swab, in order to identify the cause of an infection or to perform an antibiotic sensitivity test. Unlike viruses, bacteria are not dependent on the presence of host cells and can be cultured using artificial media.

The culture medium must provide the correct balance of:

- Water
- Essential nutrients – vary according to the needs of the individual species
- Correct pH – most mammalian pathogens require a pH of about 7.4
- Correct temperature – the optimum temperature for most pathogens is body temperature, i.e. 37°C–40°C and they are described as being normothermic
- Correct gaseous environment – bacteria may be classified according to their gaseous requirements:
  - **Obligate or strict aerobes** – must have oxygen for growth
  - **Obligate anaerobes** – will only grow in the absence of oxygen
  - **Facultative anaerobes** – may grow both in the presence or absence of oxygen
  - **Microaerophiles** – will only grow if the percentage of oxygen is lower than that of atmospheric air.

Culture media consist of two basic types:

- **Liquid broths** – particularly used for bacteria that will grow in fluid
- **Solid or jelly-like nutrient solutions** – based on agar, which is derived from seaweed. Agar can be purchased ready prepared in sterile flat-lidded Petri dishes or can be reconstituted in the lab. The agar provides no nutrients for the bacteria and these are added according to the needs of the species being cultivated.

Solid media can be classified as follows:

- **Simple or basal** – provide all that is needed for basic growth. Simple media are used for nutritionally undemanding species, e.g. *E. coli*
- **Enriched** – used for bacteria that need extra nutrients, e.g. blood agar used to detect haemolysis, chocolate agar (heated blood), serum, egg
- **Selective** – these will inhibit the growth of some bacteria while selecting for others, e.g. deoxycholate citrate is used for growing *Salmonella* spp.; McConkey's bile lactose agar contains bile salts that encourage the growth of enteric species such as *E. coli*; Sabouraud's medium is used for growing ringworm fungi
- **Biochemical** – used to distinguish between species of bacteria by detecting how they react biochemically, e.g. with different types of sugar or urea.

To produce a bacterial culture:

1. Label the Petri dish with the client's name, the case number or an appropriate lab code to avoid mixing up the samples

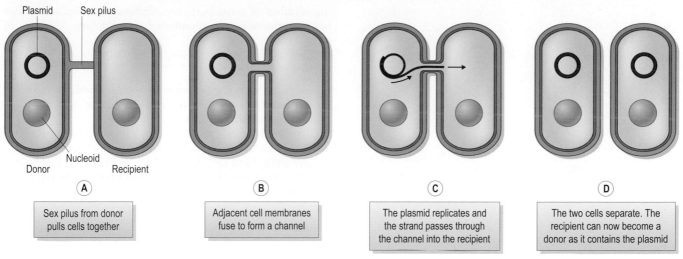

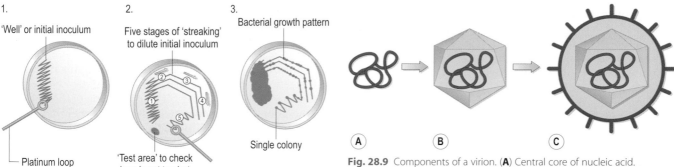

Fig. 28.7 (A–D) Conjugation

Fig. 28.8 Technique for the inoculation of an agar plate

Fig. 28.9 Components of a virion. (**A**) Central core of nucleic acid. (**B**) Surrounding protein coat. (**C**) Some viruses have an outer envelope

2. Heat a platinum loop in the flame of a Bunsen burner to sterilize it. Cool the loop in the air for few seconds. If it is too hot it will kill the bacterial cells, resulting in no growth
3. Dip the loop into the sample
4. Pick up the Petri dish containing the agar with the agar uppermost and smear the material on the loop over a small area to create a well or inoculum (Fig. 28.8)
5. Heat the loop in the flame and allow it to cool. Make three or four short streaks from the well, all in the same direction (Fig. 28.8). Be careful not to tear the agar
6. Continue to spread the sample over the agar
7. Place the lid on the Petri dish and put it into an incubator at 37°C for 18–24 hours
8. Remove the plate and examine for bacterial growth. If there is no growth reincubate for a further 18–24 hours.

Colonies of bacteria appear as rounded lumps, which are often raised and are distributed along the streak lines. Colonies of different species of bacteria may show individual characteristics, which will be helpful in their identification. To further identify a species of bacteria a smear is made on a glass microscope slide, stained with Gram's stain or methylene blue and examined under the microscope.

To identify the appropriate antibiotic with which to treat a patient it is often quicker and more effective to carry out an antibiotic sensitivity test. In this, discs impregnated with a range of antibiotics are placed on an agar plate that has been smeared with a colony selected from the original culture. The plate is incubated for 18–24 hours and the zones in which bacterial growth has been inhibited by the antibiotic are noted.

Virus

Viruses are subject to debate over whether they really are living organisms as they are incapable of reproduction without a host cell – described as obligate intracellular parasites. A virus particle or virion is little more than a package containing instructions for the recreation of further virus particles.

Each virus particle is composed of two parts:

- **Nucleic acid** – either RNA or DNA (never both), forming a central core
- **A capsid** (Fig. 28.9) – a protein coat

Together, these two parts form the nucleocapsid. For some viruses, this is all that comprises an individual virus particle.

Various shapes of virus nucleocapsid have been identified and are illustrated in Figure 28.10:

- Helical
- Icosahedral

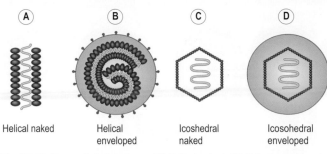

Helical naked   Helical enveloped   Icoshedral naked   Icosohedral enveloped

Fig. 28.10 Types of viral structure. (**A**) Helical naked. (**B**) Helical enveloped. (**C**) Icosohedral naked. (**D**) Icosohedral enveloped

- Complex
- Composite – some bacteriophages.

Some viruses have an additional envelope around the outside, often formed of the host cell membrane. Each of the helical or icosahedral shapes of the nucleocapsid could be enveloped or non-enveloped (Fig. 28.10), giving four possible basic shapes for viruses. In fact, there are no animal viruses (only plant viruses) that are helical and non-enveloped, so cat or dog viruses can be grouped by and large into the other three types. Viruses have been classified together on the basis of structural similarities; for example, the group of viruses causing true human flu make up the influenza viruses and horse flu is caused by equine influenza virus. Cat flu, unlike equine and human flu, is caused by two viruses, neither of which is an influenza virus.

Viruses are usually both host- and tissue-specific, so that each influenza virus is specific to the host species – an owner is not at risk of catching flu from their horse. There is a concern over avian flu (bird 'flu') as it seems to be able to transfer to humans that are in very close contact with infected poultry. Humans cannot at the moment transmit it to other humans but the possibility of avian flu merging with the human influenza virus in an infected human to produce a transmissible disease is of great concern because of the huge potential for a fatal pandemic as happened in the early part of the 20th century.

Viral replication

Replication of pathogenic viruses takes place inside the host cell, unlike pathogenic bacteria, where reproduction usually takes place outside the host's cells (Fig. 28.11). Enveloped viruses attach to a cell with a suitable receptor, and then the virus envelope merges with the host cell membrane. Alternatively, the host cell is stimulated to engulf the virus particle of a non-enveloped virus and take it into the cell. Once inside the cell, the virus is able to switch the cell's normal metabolism to replication of the virus.

Once a host animal has been infected with a small number of virus particles, there is a time lag before symptoms are seen; this is the incubation period. During this time, the virus reaches the cells with which it has an affinity and initially infects only a small number of cells to increase the number of virus particles. Clinical signs are seen once large numbers of virus particles infect a large number of cells.

There are two types of virus which differ in the period of latency of the infection:

- Replication in the cell may happen immediately, so the cell begins to produce the constituents of new virus particles within hours of infection
- Retroviral genetic material may join with the host cell's own nucleic acid for an extended period before making any changes to cell metabolism, as in the case of feline influenza virus (FIV), and human immunodeficiency virus (HIV).

Infection may not be apparent for many years after initial disease challenge. New virus particles are then assembled and released from the cell. Depending on the virus, this may leave the host cell intact or may cause its rupture and destruction.

Viral transmission

Viruses are transmitted from host to host either:

- Directly, e.g. by a cat licking feline calicivirus in nasal secretions off the face of another cat
- Indirectly, e.g. by a dog picking up virus particles from the floor of an inadequately cleaned kennel that has been occupied by a dog with parvovirus infection.

Different viruses have adapted their means of transmission according to their structure, which affects their ability to survive in the environment and their location in the host. So, for example, a respiratory tract virus is often transmitted by sneezing virus particles from one host into the air breathed in by another host. This is ideal for influenza virus, as these enveloped viruses are not very robust so do not survive for extended periods in the environment. An ability to survive in the environment for longer periods is beneficial for canine parvovirus. The virus must be licked up and ingested by another dog for infection of the gastrointestinal tract to occur (see Ch. 19).

Examples of viral diseases in the dog, cat and horse are listed in Tables 28.7–28.9.

Common disease terminology

Terms relating to disease organisms once they are within an animal are:

- **Bacteraemia** – the temporary presence of bacteria in the blood, usually precedes infections such as arthritis, meningitis, etc., without showing clinical signs
- **Viraemia** – viruses in the blood, either free, or associated with cells
- **Toxaemia** – a condition that can arise from the presence of bacterial toxins in the blood, or from metabolic disturbances
- **Septicaemia** – the presence of multiplying pathogens, such as bacteria and their toxins, in the blood, leading to systemic disease

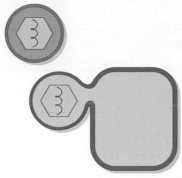

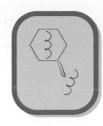

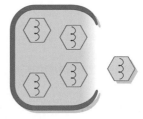

1. The virus attaches to the receptor sites on the host cell membrane and fuses with it

2. The virus enters the host cell and the protein coat (capsid) breaks down to release the viral nucleic acid

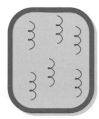

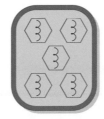

3. The viral nucleic acid replicates (either in the host cell cytoplasm or nucleus) and directs the host cell metabolism to make new virus material

4. The new viruses are assembled

5. They leave the host cell either by budding through or rupture of the cell membrane

Fig. 28.11 The process of replication in an enveloped virus

Table 28.7 Some canine viral diseases

Name of virus	Disease caused	Nucleic acid type	Shape of nucleocapsid	Enveloped
Parvovirus	Parvovirus	DNA	Icosahedral	No
Canine adenovirus 1 (CAV-1)	Infectious canine hepatitis	DNA	Icosahedral	No
Canine adenovirus 2 (CAV-2)	Infectious canine tracheobronchitis	DNA	Icosahedral	No
Canine distemper virus	Distemper	RNA	Helical	Yes
Canine parainfluenza virus	Part of kennel cough syndrome	RNA	Helical	Yes
Rabies virus	Rabies	RNA	Helical	Yes

- **Pyaemia** – multiple abscesses formed from secondary foci of infection related to septicaemia, resulting in pus in the blood.

Terms relating to disease patterns within a population of animals or man include:

- **Epidemiology** – the study of relationships of various factors determining the frequency and distribution of diseases in a community. In veterinary science it is how the specific causes of localized outbreaks of infection and other diseases are determined. It is used to monitor the number of cases of disease and to monitor the effectiveness of a control policy as was shown by the 2001 outbreak of foot and mouth disease (FMD) in the UK. It can also predict the likelihood of occurrence of a disease/accident by elucidating the risk factors for the disease associated with the population studied, e.g. the increased risk of heart disease if overweight.

- **Epidemic** (epizootic more specifically refers to an animal disease) – a pronounced increase in the level of infection. Recent examples of epidemics include FMD in the UK, parvovirus infection in dogs after its first appearance in the 1970s, and mumps during 2005 in the unvaccinated 16–24-year-old cohort of students in the UK.

- **Endemic** (enzootic refers to animal disease) – a situation in which a particular disease is present at a low level in a country or area, e.g. myxomatosis in wild rabbits in the UK. FMD is not endemic in the UK, but is in parts of sub-Saharan Africa and South America.

- **Pandemic** – an epidemic which occurs all over the world.

Table 28.8 Some feline viral diseases

Name of virus	Disease caused	Nucleic acid type	Shape of nucleocapsid	Enveloped
Feline parvovirus (panleukopenia)	Feline infectious enteritis	DNA	Icosahedral	No
Feline herpesvirus	Feline rhinotracheitis (cat flu)	DNA	Icosahedral	Yes
Feline calicivirus		RNA	Icosahedral	No
Feline coronavirus	Feline infectious peritonitis (FIP)	RNA	Helical	Yes
Feline leukaemia virus	Retrovirus causing feline leukaemia	RNA	Icosahedral	Yes
Feline immunodeficiency virus	Retrovirus	RNA	Icosahedral	Yes
Rabies virus	Rabies	RNA	Helical	Yes

Table 28.9 Some equine viral diseases

Name/type of virus	Site of infection	Disease caused	Nucleic acid type	Shape of nucleocapsid	Enveloped
Adenovirus	Gastrointestinal tract Respiratory tract	'Scours' Cold/snotty nose	DNA	Icosahedral	No
Rotavirus	Gastrointestinal tract	'Scours'	RNA	Icosahedral	No
Bovine papilloma virus	Skin	Sarcoids	DNA	Icosahedral	No
Arterivirus	Reproductive tract	Equine viral arteritis	RNA	Icosahedral	Yes
Lentivirus	Respiratory	Equine infectious anaemia	RNA	Helical	Yes
Influenza	Respiratory	Equine flu	RNA	Helical	Yes
Equine herpes virus	Several, depending on type	Coital exanthema Rhinopneumonitis Herpes paralysis	DNA	Icosahedral	Yes

- **Zoonosis** – a disease which can pass from animals to man, e.g. leptospirosis in dogs, cattle and rats; psittacosis in birds; ringworm in many animal species. Sensible routine hygiene precautions and awareness of the existence of such diseases will help to prevent them

- **Anthroponosis** – a disease which can be passed from man to animals, e.g. it is possible for gorillas and chimpanzees to become infected by measles.

Bibliography

Aspinall, V., 2003. Clinical Procedures in Veterinary Nursing. Butterworth-Heinemann, Oxford.

Cooper, B., Lane, D.R. (Eds), 2003. Veterinary Nursing, third ed. Butterworth-Heinemann, Oxford.

Jawetz, E., Melnick, J.L., Adelberg, E.A., 1991. Medical Microbiology, eighteenth ed. Prentice Hall, Canada.

Recommended reading

Aspinall, V., 2008. Clinical Procedures in Veterinary Nursing, second ed. Butterworth-Heinemann, Oxford.
Provides information about the practical aspects of bacteriology.

Ikram, M., Hill, E., 1991. Microbiology for Veterinary Technicians. American Veterinary Publication, Santa Barbara, CA.
Useful book which provides information at the right level.

CHAPTER 29

Laboratory diagnostic aids

Lorraine Allan

Key Points

- Laboratory tests are an invaluable aid to making an accurate diagnosis, assessing the severity of the condition and its response to treatment.
- Health and safety in the laboratory must be observed at all times.
- A wide range of equipment is used in the lab and the veterinary nurse must understand how and when it is used and must ensure that it is properly maintained.
- A variety of body tissues and fluids can be sampled to provide an insight into the current health status of the patient.
- The veterinary nurse must know how to collect and preserve the samples and if necessary to dispatch them to a distant laboratory.
- All laboratory tests must be performed correctly following a rigid protocol so that the results are both accurate and comparable to other tests of the same type.
- Accurate records must be kept and passed on to the appropriate veterinary surgeon.

Introduction

The majority of veterinary practices in the UK today are equipped with an 'in house' practice laboratory where a variety of procedures are undertaken, the range and complexity being dependent on various factors, including the equipment available, the expertise of the staff, time and financial constraints. However, some procedures are not within the scope of the average practice and commercial laboratories are used for these more sophisticated tests. The increased utilization of clinical pathology examinations has resulted in veterinary nurses becoming more involved in laboratory procedures. Their role may encompass taking the samples, performing the tests, recording the results and sending off samples to a commercial laboratory. Furthermore, an increased awareness of the significance of the results is expected, which can impact on the nursing care provided to the patient.

(More detailed information on parasitology and microbiology has been provided in Chapters 27 and 28.)

Laboratory diagnostic aids are an invaluable tool to the veterinary surgeon in four main ways:

- **As an aid to making an accurate diagnosis** – although a considerable amount of information can be gained from taking a detailed history and from performing a clinical examination, it might still not be possible to make a precise diagnosis. Further investigative procedures, including laboratory tests, may help clarify the situation, enabling a definitive diagnosis to be made
- **To assess the severity of a condition** – this could influence the choice of treatment and the subsequent recovery of the patient, e.g. monitoring blood glucose levels in patients suffering from diabetes mellitus
- **To assess response to treatment** – on occasion it can be difficult to determine if an animal is responding to treatment solely from its clinical condition. A valuable insight into the patient's progress can be obtained from laboratory tests, e.g. monitoring blood parameters in anaemia
- **To adjust treatment regimes** – monitoring drug levels can allow adjustment of therapeutic drug doses, e.g. the levels of barbiturate in the treatment of epilepsy.

Health and Safety in the laboratory

In common with the rest of a veterinary practice, the laboratory is subject to legislation that attempts to make the workplace as safe an environment as possible (Table 29.1).

Common hazards in the laboratory

A laboratory is potentially a dangerous place with many hazards, i.e. something with the potential to cause harm. The Control of Substances Hazardous to Health (COSHH) Regulations set out to identify hazards and to develop safe protocols to reduce the risks, i.e. something that is likely to cause harm, from these hazards to an absolute minimum and thus creating a safe working environment (see also Ch. 3).

The range of potential hazards in a practice laboratory include:

- Clinical material
- Biological agents

Table 29.1 Laboratory Health and Safety legislation

Legislation	Key points
Health and Safety at Work Act 1974	Applies to all businesses. Sets out specific duties of employer and employee to ensure a safe working environment. Provides protection against risks in the workplace and ensures that all equipment and substances used are handled, stored and transported safely
The Control of Substances Hazardous to Health (COSHH) Regulations 2002	The main legislation covering the control of risks to staff from exposure to harmful substances at work. Includes undertaking risk assessments, drawing up written standard operating procedures (SOPs), monitoring and controlling exposure to harmful substances, and staff training
Control of Pollution (Special Waste) Regulations 1988 Collection and Disposal of Waste Regulations 1992 Environmental Protection Act 1992	The principal regulations that control the correct handling, segregation, storage, transfer and disposal of products, including clinical waste and chemicals, minimizing damage to the environment and reducing risks to staff
Reporting of Injuries, Diseases and Dangerous Occurrences (RIDDOR) Regulations 1995	Describe the procedures that must take place if death, serious injury or work-related disease occurs in the workplace. Such occurrences must be reported to the Health and Safety Executive (HSE)
First Aid at Work Act	This regulates first-aid provision and the recording of accidents

- Chemicals, which may be toxic or corrosive
- Sharp objects
- Toxic fumes
- Eye contaminants
- Zoonoses
- Fire.

Hazard warning signs give clear indications of potential hazards in a variety of situations including the laboratory (see Ch. 3).

To ensure a safe working environment in the laboratory a code of conduct must be followed that encompasses both the local Health and Safety rules and the COSHH regulations:

- Ensure access is only to authorized personnel
- Provide adequate training and supervision of staff
- Fully buttoned protective laboratory coats must be worn
- Disposable gloves and, if necessary, eye glasses and masks must be worn when handling hazardous materials
- Long hair should always be tied back
- Smoking, eating, drinking, chewing gum and mouth pipetting are prohibited
- Hands should be washed when leaving the laboratory using an antibacterial soap and protective coats should be removed
- The laboratory should be kept clean, neat and tidy
- The work surfaces must be cleaned and disinfected after use
- Books and papers should be kept away from the work area and any other source of contamination
- Labelled containers of suitable disinfectant solutions should be provided for contaminated equipment disinfection
- Correct disposal of laboratory waste must be observed. Different types of clinical waste must be clearly segregated. Disposal containers should be clearly marked, preferably colour-coded, to prevent mistakes being made
- 'Sharps' containers must be provided
- Hazard warning signs must be displayed as appropriate
- Appropriate action should be taken in case of spillage and any spills should be contained and disposed of

safely. If an infectious agent is involved, thorough disinfection or sterilization may be required
- When performing bacteriological procedures, especial care must be taken not to contaminate the operative or the environment
- Bunsen burners must be placed on a heat-resistant mat, must not be left on a working flame in between stages of the procedure and must be turned off immediately when they are no longer required
- A well-stocked first-aid box must be provided and first-aid equipment, such as eyewash, must be readily available and in working condition. Ideally, a member of staff should be a trained first aider
- In case of accident, immediate remedial action should be taken. Medical attention should be sought if necessary. All accidents, no matter how trivial, must be reported to a responsible member of staff and recorded in the accident book, and if of a serious nature should be reported according to the RIDDOR regulations
- Fire fighting equipment should be available and an evacuation procedure displayed
- A senior member of staff should be consulted if any problems are encountered.

Disposal of laboratory waste

The disposal of laboratory waste is controlled by legislation; see Table 29.1 for the specific Acts. The regulations control the correct segregation, storage, transfer and destruction of waste products in the practice including the laboratory. All businesses have a duty of care to ensure that:

- All waste is stored and disposed of responsibly
- Waste is only handled or dealt with by those authorized to do so
- Appropriate records are kept of all waste that is transferred or received

Infectious waste (formally clinical waste)

The term 'Infectious Waste' constitutes any veterinary waste containing viable micro-organisms or their toxins which are known or reliably believed to cause disease in man or other living organisms. Much of the materials generated within the lab may be classed as infectious waste.

Following a veterinary assessment, waste deemed to be contaminated may include:

- Clinical items (for example swabs, masks and gloves)
- Animal bedding
- Blood, body parts and cadavers.

Disposal of infectious waste:

- This should be collected and stored in yellow-coloured plastic bags for high-temperature incineration only.
- However, infectious clinical items can be further segregated into orange containers for suitable alternative treatment (for example autoclaving) as best practice.
- It must be collected by a registered carrier in a designated vehicle, licensed specially for the transport of infectious waste and transferred to a licensed plant for incineration with a waste transfer note.

Contaminated 'sharps'

This comprises all sharps contaminated with animal blood or pharmaceuticals (other than cytotoxic or cytostatic). These may include partially and fully discharged sharps, hypodermic needles and other sharp instruments.

Disposal:

- All sharps can be segregated into yellow sharps containers for high-temperature incineration only
- Or, non-pharmaceutically contaminated sharps can be further segregated into orange-lidded bins for suitable alternative treatment (for example autoclaving) as best practice.
- Uncontaminated broken glass can be disposed of in a glass disposal container.

Contaminated microscope slides, coverslips and capillary tubes should be placed in the yellow sharps bins.

Chemical waste

There are specific legal requirements about the disposal of waste chemicals when they are discharged into public sewers. All chemical reagents used in the laboratory are subject to COSHH Regulations. Each chemical must be identified and the hazards and risks associated with its use assessed, including its disposal.

Domestic waste

This is non-hazardous waste and should be disposed of in black refuse bags. Any confidential paperwork should be shredded prior to disposal.

Routine laboratory equipment

Glassware

Glassware is used to measure and hold reagents and samples usually liquids. Borosilicate glass (Pyrex) is used as it is harder than ordinary glass and less easily broken.

It is important that all glassware is thoroughly cleaned to remove any contaminated material that might interfere with the accuracy of the tests. New glassware should always be washed before use.

Cleaning glassware

- Rubber gloves should be worn
- Contaminated glassware should be soaked in an approved disinfectant for 24 hours prior to cleaning
- Any residues should be removed with the aid of a soft bristle brush. The glassware should then be washed in commercial laboratory detergent, following the manufacturer's instructions, or in an ultrasonic bath
- The glassware should then be rinsed thoroughly two or three times in distilled/deionized water to remove all traces of the cleaning solution, which could affect the accuracy of results
- The glassware should be allowed to drain and then dried in a drying cabinet. Bottles should not be dried with their stoppers in place, as the water will not evaporate
- Once dry, the glassware should be stored in a cupboard or drawer to protect it from dust, grease and possible damage
- The same method should be adopted to clean plastic ware, although cooler water should be used. Organic solvents should be avoided as they could cause damage
- Microscope slides and coverslips are usually discarded, after soaking in an approved disinfectant for 24 hours, because of their relatively low cost
- Pipettes can prove difficult to clean, especially if left, but must be thoroughly cleaned.

Microscope

A microscope is an essential piece of equipment in any veterinary laboratory. It is advisable to use a monocular or binocular compound light microscope with an inbuilt light source (Fig. 29.1); some older microscopes utilize a mirror and external light source. Table 29.2 explains the function of the parts of the microscope.

A microscope is an expensive precision instrument and should be treated as such:

- In common with all electrical equipment it should be checked regularly for safety
- Do not site it near a window or sources of heat, moisture or vibration
- The microscope should be switched off and covered when not in use to avoid contamination from spills and dust
- The stage should be cleaned with disinfectant wipes
- The eyepieces and objective lenses should only be cleaned with special lens tissue
- The oil immersion lens should be cleaned after each use with lens tissue to ensure that the oil does not solidify and damage the lens
- When moving the microscope, carry it by the limb with one hand under the base
- If glasses are normally worn, remove them to prevent damage

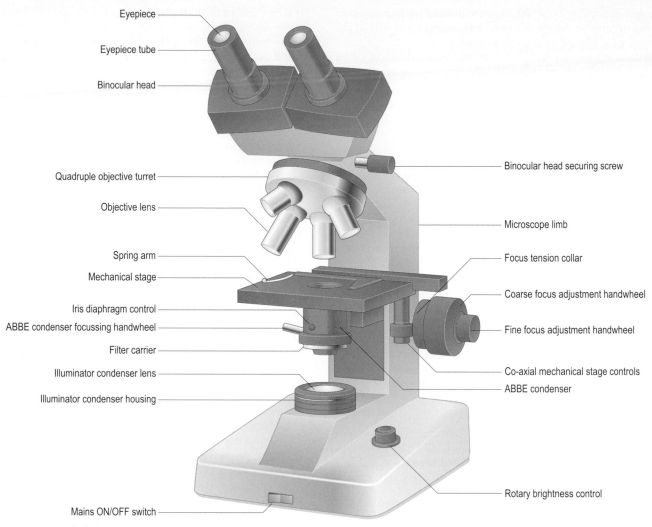

Eyepiece

Eyepiece tube

Binocular head

Binocular head securing screw

Quadruple objective turret

Objective lens

Microscope limb

Spring arm

Focus tension collar

Mechanical stage

Coarse focus adjustment handwheel

Iris diaphragm control

ABBE condenser focussing handwheel

Fine focus adjustment handwheel

Filter carrier

Illuminator condenser lens

Co-axial mechanical stage controls

Illuminator condenser housing

ABBE condenser

Rotary brightness control

Mains ON/OFF switch

Fig. 29.1 A binocular light microscope

- Never move the objective lens and slide towards each other while looking down the microscope, as this could result in breaking the slide and damage to the objective lens
- Keep spare light bulbs in stock. Do not handle the bulb when replacing it
- Ensure that the microscope is regularly serviced.

Examination of a blood smear on a microscope slide

- Switch on the microscope
- Move the stage approximately 5 cm below the objective lenses
- Rotate the nosepiece clockwise and click the ×10 objective lens into place
- Rack up the condenser until its top surface is as high as possible
- Looking from the side, not down the microscope, adjust the iris diaphragm control lever so that it at the middle position of its range of movement, i.e. approximately half-open. As the lens power is increased the aperture of the iris diaphragm should be increased to allow more light to be directed up the microscope
- Place the slide on the mechanical stage and secure it firmly in position

- Position the area to be viewed over the light source using the mechanical stage control knobs
- Looking from the side, move the stage towards the lens, by using both the coarse adjustment controls, until it is 4 mm away
- Looking down the microscope, very carefully and slowly move the stage away from the lens until the image comes into focus
- Then, adjusting the fine focus, obtain the sharpest possible image. Do not use the fine focus to excess – if you have to do this it means you are not near enough to focus with the coarse focus
- To view the specimen under ×40, move the stage away from the ×10 lens and click the ×40 lens clockwise into position
- Looking from the side, move the stage up towards the lens until the slide is almost touching it
- Looking down the microscope, focus the slide as previously described.
  Note: the slide will be much closer to the lens when in focus than when using the ×10 lens
- Next use the oil immersion lens ×100 by moving the stage away from the lens and rotating the nosepiece so that neither the ×40 or ×100 lens are in position

Table 29.2 Parts of the microscope

Part	Function
Stage	A flat square platform on which the specimen is placed. A hole in the centre allows light from the condenser to illuminate the specimen. The surface of the stage is covered with chemical resistant vulcanite and can be moved up and down by the coarse and fine adjustment control knobs to focus the specimen
Mechanical stage	This is attached to the stage holding the slide in place and also facilitating movement of the slide in east–west and north–south directions with accuracy
Vernier scales	These are located on both movements of the mechanical scales at right angles to each other and allow relocation of a particular point on the slide. Each scale consists of a main scale divided into millimetres and a Vernier plate with 10 divisions each of 0.9 mm. To read a Vernier scale, observe where the zero mark on the Vernier plate meets the main scale. If it falls between two divisions record the lower one. In Figure 29.2 the zero is between 55 and 56, so 55 is recorded. Next note which of the divisions on the Vernier plate is exactly opposite a division on the main scale. In the example, this is the mark 5. The complete reading is recorded as 55.5. If the zero mark had been exactly opposite 55 the reading would have been 55.0. It is essential that readings from both scales are taken and recorded
Body	This houses the focusing mechanism for the body tube
Body tube	A hollow metal tube that contains no lenses or other optical parts. An eyepiece fits into the upper part and a nosepiece into the lower end
Eyepiece	Contains two lenses: the one closest to the eye is known as the ocular lens and the more distal one is the field lens. Most have a magnifying power of ×10. Its purpose is to magnify the primary image formed by the objective lens. Binocular microscopes have two eyepieces
Nosepiece	Found at the lower end of the body tube with a rotating turret that holds the objective lenses and can be rotated to click a different objective lens into place. It should always be rotated in a clockwise direction so as to move from a lower power to a higher power
Objective lenses	Normally four lenses, each with a different magnification, are housed in the nosepiece. Usually ×4 (scanning), ×10 (low-power), ×40 (high dry) and ×100 (oil immersion)
Condenser	Fitted below the stage and is therefore sometimes called the substage condenser. It consists of two lenses that condense the light from the light source on to the specimen to make it brighter and the image sharper. The position of the condenser and the amount of light passing through the specimen can be adjusted. Remember that when viewed the image will be upside down and reversed
Iris diaphragm	Adjusting the aperture of the iris diaphragm with the iris diaphragm control can regulate the amount of light that passes through the condenser. Below the iris diaphragm there are often glass filters that can alter the wavelength of light passing through the condenser
Limb	This connects the base with the body and supports the stage and condenser. The base houses the light source and on/off switch. Some microscopes have a brightness control which can vary the intensity of light delivered

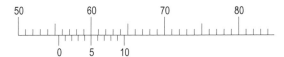

Fig. 29.2 The Vernier scale

- Place a small drop of immersion oil on the slide (Fig. 29.3)
- Click the ×100 lens in position
- Looking from the side, move the stage up towards the ×100 lens until the slide touches the lens
- Move the stage even closer to the slide; the oil will be seen to spread out from the lens
- Looking down the microscope, very carefully and slowly focus the slide
- When focused, the lens must be in the oil
- It is only practice that will make you proficient in the use of a microscope.

Tips

- Blood and bacterial smears should be examined under ×10, ×40 then ×100 with oil immersion
- Urine sediments and faeces should be examined under ×10 then ×40

- Parasite slides should be first examined with the naked eye. If macroscopic, examine under ×5 then ×10. If microscopic, examine under ×10 then ×40.

Centrifuge

This is an important piece of laboratory equipment and is used in many diagnostic tests, including:

- Separation of blood cells from plasma or serum
- Urine sedimentation
- Faecal analysis.

Modern centrifuges are very sophisticated, but all work on the same principle The samples are contained in special centrifuge tubes and subjected to centrifugal force, which results in the heavier constituents of the suspension settling to the bottom of the tube while the lighter ones settle at the top. This accelerates the process that would occur if the samples were left to settle under the influence of gravity alone.

Centrifuges contain a rotor or centrifuge head, drive shaft and motor enclosed in the guard bowl. Other features include a timer, speed control, break and safety lock.

Standard centrifuges are of two types according to the type of rotor head:

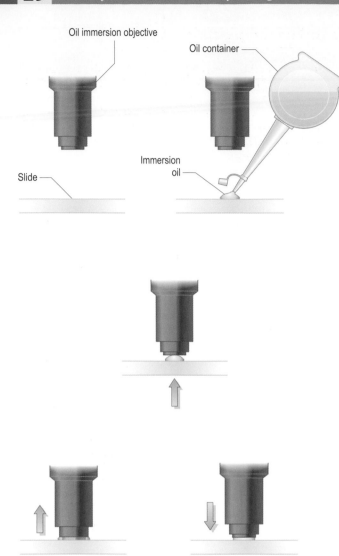

Oil immersion objective

Oil container

Slide

Immersion
oil

Fig. 29.3 Use of the oil immersion objective

- **Swing-out head with specimen buckets**, which contain rubber cushions to reduce damage to the centrifuge tubes, suspended vertically from the arms of the rotor. As the rotor turns, the buckets swing out into a horizontal position, falling back to the vertical when the rotor slows down and stops. The sediment is uniformly distributed, allowing the supernatant (liquid) to be easily removed by a pipette
- **Angle head**, where the tubes are held in a fixed position, usually 25–40° from vertical. The sediment forms at an angle, making the sediment difficult to remove. However, much higher centrifuge speeds can be achieved because of the aerodynamic shape of the rotor.

The **microhaematocrit centrifuge** is very specialized and is used to measure blood packed cell volume (PCV). It utilizes capillary tubes that are held horizontally on a grooved metal plate.

Care and cleaning of the centrifuge

- Never attempt to open the centrifuge until the head has completely stopped rotating

- Ensure that the samples are balanced in diametrically opposite buckets by weight, not volume
- If, with increasing revs, the machine develops excessive vibrations, stop the centrifuge and, when the head has finished rotating, examine the chamber, as the most likely cause is improperly balanced arms
- Follow the manufacturer's instructions to operate the centrifuge
- Regularly clean and disinfect the centrifuge
- Any spillages/breakages should be carefully cleaned away and the chamber disinfected while wearing disposable gloves
- When using a microhaematocrit centrifuge ensure that the safety plate is fastened over the samples to hold the capillary tubes safely in place. Regularly check the rubber gasket for wear and replace it if necessary
- Ensure regular servicing and cleaning.

Electronic analysers

Increasing numbers of veterinary practices are using electronic analysers to improve the diagnosis of many conditions. These include biochemistry, haematology, electrolyte and hormone analysers, the first two being the most commonly found in practice laboratories.

Care and maintenance

- To avoid damage, position away from vibrations, e.g. produced by centrifuges, or liquids
- Switch off and cover when not in use
- Use in accordance with the manufacturer's instructions
- Service regularly
- Quality control tests against known results should be regularly undertaken. These are in addition to the external quality control tests performed to ensure the accuracy and validity of all tests.

Biochemistry analysers

These are used to measure the levels of various biochemical substances in blood, e.g. glucose, total protein, blood urea nitrogen (BUN) and plasma enzymes.

Most are dry chemistry systems. The sample is placed on a series of slides that results in a colour change reflecting the amount of the substance being tested. The machine reads and interprets the colour change as the level of the substance that is present in the sample. Some biochemistry analysers utilize small wells of fluid rather than slides and are known as wet chemistry systems. Whatever the system, the results are compared with the normal reference range for each parameter measured, which gives valuable information about the clinical condition of the patient, facilitating diagnosis and monitoring. Such investigations are also being increasingly used to check the health status of patients prior to anaesthesia.

Haematology analysers

These are used to automatically determine total red and white blood cell counts, differential white blood cell counts, packed cell volume and platelet counts, among other parameters. They provide useful information regarding the blood picture of the patient.

Electrolyte analysers

Plasma electrolyte levels provide valuable information that can help in diagnosing diseases such as Addison's disease, monitoring changes caused by dehydration and acid–base balance and also in cases of hypocalcaemia and neoplasia. Parameters commonly measured include sodium, chloride, potassium, bicarbonate, calcium and phosphate.

Hormone analysers

Blood hormone levels that are regularly measured include thyroxine, cortisol, insulin and reproductive hormones. Most are measured at commercial laboratories. Hormone measurements are valuable in the diagnosis of endocrine disorders, e.g. Cushing's disease and hypothyroidism. They are also helpful in diagnosing reproductive disorders and assessing the stage of the reproductive cycle.

Commercial test kits

A number of in-house test kits are available that can be used to diagnose certain viral diseases, determine hormone levels in breeding animals, investigate allergic conditions and blood clotting.

Most utilize the enzyme-linked immunosorbent assay (ELISA) test (see also Ch. 19). The test detects the presence of specific antigens dependent on the test being undertaken. The test well is impregnated with appropriate antibodies for the test to be performed; the antibodies bind any viral antigens present in the sample and a dye is activated, producing a colour change that indicates a positive result.

Test kits in common use in practice include:

- **FeLV ELISA test** – detects viral antigens to feline leukaemia in blood. A coloured spot or line indicates a positive result
- **FIV ELISA test** – detects viral antigens to feline immunosuppression virus in blood
- **Parvovirus ELISA test** – detects viral antigens in faeces. Care must be taken in interpreting the results in dogs that have recently been vaccinated with live parvovirus as they can shed the virus for 5–12 days post-vaccination, resulting in a false-positive result
- **Premate test** – an ELISA test that measures progesterone levels in serum or plasma. It is used to determine the optimum time for mating in the bitch and utilizes the fact that blood progesterone levels rise at ovulation. Serial blood samples are taken before ovulation; the test shows a dark pink colour; increased progesterone is indicated by a colour change to pink
- **Allercept e-screen test** – an ELISA test that detects immunoglobin E (IgE) in blood. A serum or plasma sample is required. A positive test suggests that an allergic condition is likely, but further testing at a commercial laboratory will be necessary to determine the specific cause or causes of the allergic condition.

Recording sample details and test reports

This is probably the most important part of laboratory practice. It is vital that the sample can be correctly linked with the patient, the tests required linked with the sample and finally the results of the tests performed linked with those requested and the sample. Provided that each stage of the process is recorded accurately immediately upon completion, this should not be a problem.

Protocol

Immediately the sample has been collected and placed in a suitable container it should be labelled, either with the details of the owner's name and address and the patient's name or with a reference number that can be computerized. This identifies the sample for all time.

A laboratory request form should then be completed, even if the tests are to be performed 'in house'. A typical request form should include:

- Practice name and address. This can be omitted if an 'in-house' test is to be performed. Many commercial laboratories provide preprinted forms that include a practice reference number
- The name of the veterinary surgeon submitting the request
- Owner's name and address or reference number
- Species and breed of the patient. Its name can also be included
- Age and sex of the patient, including whether the patient is neutered
- A description of the sample(s)
- A clinical history and provisional diagnosis
- Details of any medication
- The tests required
- The date the sample was taken. Histology samples should be accompanied by a chart indicating the sample sites
- Any additional information that could help in the interpretation of the results, especially if the sample is sent to a commercial laboratory.

On receipt at the laboratory, even an internal one, the request sheet should be stapled to a laboratory report sheet. A serialized laboratory reference number should be put on the form and all apparatus, e.g. microscope slides, should be labelled with that number. This links the laboratory request and report forms with the sample, ensuring that no confusion arises, especially if tests are undertaken on multiple samples simultaneously.

On completion of the tests, the results, together with the date the results were obtained, should be entered on the report form. This form should then be returned to the presenting veterinary surgeon. Commercial laboratories also include an interpretation of the results, which may be faxed to the practice to decrease the turn-around time.

The results should be given to the veterinary surgeon concerned and any other appropriate members of staff and also recorded on the patient's records immediately on receipt. Communicating the results to the client is usually undertaken by the veterinary surgeon but a veterinary nurse, under the direction of a veterinary surgeon, can communicate uncomplicated results if the veterinary surgeon feels it is appropriate.

Dispatch of pathological material

In order for the test results to be accurate and meaningful it is essential that the samples sent to a distant laboratory should arrive in the same condition as when they were sampled, with minimal deterioration. Correct preservation, clearly labelled samples, accurately completed paperwork and correct packaging will ensure this is the case. It is vitally important to clearly label the samples and ensure that the accompanying paperwork is correct.

Samples must be preserved if any delay is expected between sampling and subsequent testing. If preservation is not performed correctly, spoilage of the sample will occur and the results obtained will not reflect the true disease status of the animal. For some tests, e.g. haematology, correct preservation is essential to allow the tests to be undertaken.

Causes of spoilage of samples include:

- Haemolysis of blood
- Clotting of blood – due to absence or insufficiency of anticoagulant or failure to mix the blood sufficiently with the anticoagulant
- Contamination of the sample – bacterial or gross contamination
- Death of bacteria – due to using inappropriate preservatives
- Insufficient volume – this can result from insufficient collection of the sample or leakage of the sample in transit
- Desiccation – usually of pus or faeces. This may occur if too little of the sample is collected or the sample is collected into a non-airtight container that allows evaporation, especially during hot weather. Plain swabs are especially susceptible
- Autolysis of tissue samples – digestion of tissue by its own enzymes. This may occur in portions of tissue despatched to a laboratory, especially if the time taken to reach their destination is increased, i.e. over weekends or holiday periods, or if the ambient temperature is increased. It may also occur if a piece of tissue is too large for the fixative solution to penetrate it completely. Post-mortem samples and cadavers should be properly packed to prevent leakage and sent as quickly as possible to distant laboratories to prevent autolysis rendering the results useless
- Fragmentation of preserved tissues – this can result from preserving them in containers that have a narrow neck, making their removal difficult.

It is equally important that the samples are correctly packaged to ensure they are not damaged during transit and that the containers do not break or leak. The containers should be leak-proof, robust, securely fastened and protected from breaking by padding. It should also be ensured that the risk of contamination of the paperwork, other samples, anyone handling the samples in transit or on receipt of the samples should be minimized. However, this should not make it impossible for the laboratory staff to extricate the samples from the packaging safely!

Samples are usually sent to commercial laboratories by post, although sometimes they are sent by courier service or taken directly if within a reasonable distance. In general the despatch of pathological samples is banned by the Post Office; however, there are special exemptions for such material being sent by veterinary surgeons to laboratories. Very highly infectious material, such as anthrax, and dangerous human pathogens are excluded from this exemption.

Pathological specimens pose a potential hazard to members of the public involved in their transport so it is vitally important that they are correctly packaged and correctly labelled according to Post Office regulations. The containers should also conform to United Nations Regulation 602. This protocol should also be followed if despatched by courier or if taken by hand:

- Faeces or liquid samples, such as blood, serum, urine, body fluids and tissue samples, should be placed in an appropriate sealed primary container. This container must not exceed 50 ml unless Post Office approved multispecimen packs are used
- Dry samples such as blood or bacterial smears should be placed in special slide-holding containers. Coat brushings and hair samples can be put into sealed plastic bags. Skin scrapings can be sent in a sealed container or on a slide in a slide-holding container
- The sample should then be wrapped in enough absorbent material to absorb all possible leakage in case of damage. This also protects the sample against damage in transit
- This should then be placed in a sealed leak-proof plastic bag
- The package must then be placed, along with the request form, into a secondary container: either a plastic clip-down container, a cylindrical lightweight metal container, a strong cardboard box with a full-depth lid or a two-piece polystyrene box with a special grooved join
- It is recommended that this complete package is then placed and securely sealed in a padded 'Jiffy' bag. This should be labelled on the outside with the words: PATHOLOGICAL SPECIMEN – FRAGILE WITH CARE and the name and address of the laboratory. The package must show the name, address and telephone number of the sender to be contacted in case of leakage, on the reverse side. A biohazard symbol can also be included.
- First class or data post should be used, not parcel post, if the parcel is to be delivered by the Post Office
- Other packaging systems must be approved by the Post Office
- Improperly packaged or labelled samples will not be handled by the postal services.

When sending samples by post it is essential that they reach the laboratory as quickly as possible to reduce deterioration of the samples, so send the samples by first class post, data post or courier. Avoid sending the samples over a weekend or a public holiday. Some samples deteriorate faster than others, even though they have been preserved, e.g. bacteriological samples. Also remember that deterioration will be accelerated by high ambient temperatures.

It cannot be emphasized enough how important the correct packaging and despatch is to ensure accurate results.

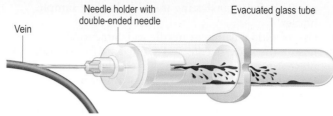

Fig. 29.4 A Vacutainer

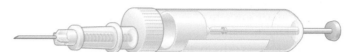

Fig. 29.5 S-Monovette blood collection system

Blood

Examination of blood samples can provide an invaluable insight into the health status of patients, aiding diagnosis, monitoring response to treatment and the severity of conditions.

Collection of blood

Collection of a blood sample is normally by venepuncture using a syringe and needle (see also Chs 10, 11 and 12). It is important that, before the sample is taken, the correct equipment is assembled. The correct gauge of needle should be selected. It should be the largest gauge possible to allow the sample to be taken quickly and reduce damage to the red blood cells. The syringe selected should be the smallest size possible, to reduce the pressure on the red blood cells while the sample is being taken and hence the risk of them rupturing. If 1 ml of blood is required then a 2 ml syringe is quite adequate for the procedure. Scissors, a spirit swab and a suitable blood collection bottle should be close at hand.

An alternative method is to use a Vacutainer kit (Fig. 29.4). A Vacutainer is an evacuated tube, i.e. one containing a vacuum. The small tubes have a 3 ml volume but only a 2 ml draw to reduce the pressure on the red blood cells. The tubes are made of glass and are sealed at one end with a rubber bung. The rest of the kit comprises a holder with a double-ended needle (Fig. 29.4). One end of the needle is inserted into the vein and the other end pierces the bung and the blood is drawn into the Vacutainer, available as plain tubes or containing different anticoagulants.

Syringes are available that have detachable barrels coated with anticoagulant, negating the necessity for sample bottles – these are sold as Monovette. Convertible syringe/evacuated tubes or S-Monovette are also available. These combine the best features of Vacutainers and blood-collecting syringes and can be used in either mode (Fig. 29.5).

Depending on the species and volume of blood required there are various sites available for venepuncture. The largest accessible vein should always be used (Table 29.3).

Technique

1. Handling and restraint for venepuncture varies with the species involved and the sampling site. Manual restraint

Table 29.3 Venepuncture sites

Species	Vein/site
Dog and cat	Jugular – ventral aspect of the neck
	Cephalic – cranial aspect of the radius
	Lateral saphenous – lateral aspect of the hock
Rabbit	Jugular
	Lateral marginal ear vein – base of pinna
	Lateral saphenous
Guinea pig	Jugular
	Lateral marginal ear vein
	Intracardiac under anaesthesia
Rat/mouse/gerbil	Lateral tail vein
	Intracardiac under anaesthesia
Hamster	Intracardiac under anaesthesia
Ferret	Jugular
	Cephalic
	Caudal – ventral aspect of tail
Bird	Jugular
	Brachial – medial aspect of the elbow
	Medial metatarsal in larger birds
	May require anaesthesia
Snakes	Jugular
	Ventral tail vein
	Palatine – roof of the mouth
	Intracardiac under anaesthesia
Lizard	Jugular
	Cephalic
	Ventral tail vein
Chelonians	Jugular
	Dorsal tail vein

    is usually adequate for restraining dogs and cats. However, if the patient is aggressive then a different protocol may be require, e.g. muzzles, wrapping in a towel. If necessary, sedation or anaesthesia may be required, especially with exotic species. It is usually less stressful and safer to anaesthetize most birds prior to blood sampling but large birds such as swans can be blood sampled from the metatarsal vein without causing distress. The application of local anaesthetic gel to the site when taking blood from the marginal ear vein can also make the procedure less stressful

2. Once suitably restrained by an assistant, the injection site should be clipped and swabbed with spirit to ensure asepsis

3. The assistant should then occlude the proximal part of the vein, which makes the vein easier to visualize and

also prevents the blood from returning to the heart – always known as 'raising the vein'.

4. The needle should be inserted at a shallow angle while tensing the skin over the site. Once in the vein the plunger is slowly pulled back to ensure the blood is not subjected to excessive pressure, which could damage the red blood cells and also to ensure the vein does not collapse

5. Once the required volume has been obtained the needle is carefully removed from the vein and the assistant should apply pressure on the injection site to prevent bleeding

6. The blood sample should then be transferred quickly to the previously selected sample bottle. The needle should be removed prior to filling the sample bottle to reduce damage to the red blood cells

7. If the sample is transferred to a sample bottle containing anticoagulant the blood should be gently squirted into the bottle and filled to the 'fill line' to ensure that the anticoagulant is diluted correctly; the bottle should then be inverted or rolled to mix the contents. Avoid violent shaking as this can damage the red blood cells. If a serum sample is required there is no need to mix the sample and there is no specified fill line

8. The sample must then be labelled with the date and some means of identification

9. Any waste should be disposed of appropriately.

Provided the correct protocol is followed the red blood cells will not be damaged and release their haemoglobin into the plasma. This process of rupture of the red blood cells is called haemolysis. If haemolysis has occurred the plasma or serum will be pink in colour. Haemolysis will ruin all the tests used in haematology except total white blood cell counts and haemoglobin levels, as the number of red blood cells will be diminished. The presence of free haemoglobin will also interfere with biochemical tests. Therefore, it is essential that haemolysis is avoided.

Tips to avoid haemolysis

- Excessive suction should be avoided when taking the sample
- The blood should only pass through the needle once to reduce the trauma to the red blood cells, so remove the needle before transferring the blood to the sample bottle
- Use as wide a gauge of needle as is practicable
- Ensure the skin, needle and syringe are free of water to prevent osmotic damage to the red blood cells
- Do not shake the sample bottle – roll or invert it to mix the sample
- The sample should be examined as soon as possible after sampling
- Store the sample at the correct temperature, cool (4°C) but not freezing
- Avoid direct sunlight.
- If sending the sample to an external laboratory, ensure it is packaged correctly to protect against careless handling and temperature variations. Ensure it is despatched as soon as possible.

Preservation of blood

Blood can be preserved in a number of ways depending on the investigations that are to be undertaken. These include:

- Preventing the blood clotting by using anticoagulants
- Leaving the blood whole and allowing it to clot naturally then removing the serum
- Making blood smears.

Anticoagulants

To perform haematology, the study of the physical characteristics and the number of cells per unit volume in blood, it is essential that the sample is not allowed to clot. To prevent the blood from clotting the inherent clotting process must be disabled by the addition of chemicals immediately on collection of the sample. The clotting process is a complex one that depends on the presence of calcium and a number of enzymes in addition to various clotting factors.

Anticoagulants fall into two categories:

- Those that block calcium – ethylenediaminetetraacetic acid (EDTA), oxalates, citrates and fluorides
- Those that interfere with the enzyme systems – heparin and fluorides.

All the anticoagulants listed in Table 29.4 are available commercially, as ready-prepared sample bottles and the majority as their equivalent Vacutainers.

Table 29.4 Anticoagulants

Anticoagulant	Test	Bottle colour	Vacutainer colour
Ethylenediaminetetraacetic acid (EDTA), also known as sequestrene	Routine haematology	Pink Some small bottles <0.5 ml may be red	Lilac
Sodium fluoride/potassium oxalate	Glucose estimation	Yellow	Grey
Lithium heparin	Biochemistry	Orange	Green/green orange
Sodium citrate	Coagulation profiles	Purple (solid) Green (liquid)	Black
Ammonium/potassium oxalate	Glucose estimation	Turquoise	None
No anticoagulant	Biochemistry	White	Red

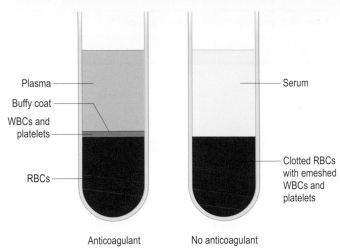

Plasma

Buffy coat

WBCs and platelets

RBCs

Serum

Clotted RBCs with emeshed WBCs and platelets

Anticoagulant

No anticoagulant

Fig. 29.6 The difference between blood being left to clot naturally or with an anticoagulant

No one anticoagulant is ideal for every test: each individual anticoagulant has properties that make it better suited for some tests than others. The preference for sodium fluoride/oxalate as the anticoagulant of choice for glucose estimation illustrates this point. It reduces the amount of glucose metabolized by the blood cells prior to the glucose estimation, more accurately representing the glucose levels present at the time of sampling.

Serum samples

Serum is plasma, the fluid in which the cellular components of blood are suspended, minus the clotting factors such as fibrinogen. In biochemical examination it is usually serum that is used, although plasma can be used for most tests except bile acids, insulin and a number of specific serological investigations. It is important that the difference between plasma and serum is appreciated.

If a blood sample is placed in a sample bottle containing an anticoagulant, e.g. EDTA, and allowed to stand, the red blood cells, being the heaviest components, will fall to the bottom of the sample tube. On top of these will lie the white blood cells and platelets forming the 'buffy coat', and above this layer will be the plasma. Inversion of the bottle will result in resuspension of the cellular components (Fig. 29.6). However, if the blood sample is placed in a sample tube that does not contain an anticoagulant and is left to stand, the red blood cells will clot, enmeshing both the white blood cells and platelets and a fluid will form above the clot, serum. In this case there will not be a distinct buffy coat and inversion of the sample will not result in resuspension of the sample, as the cellular components have clotted.

Serum collection can involve simply collecting the sample into a sample bottle containing no anticoagulant, then leaving the sample to clot, which may take up to 2 hours. The serum is then transferred to a sterile container. Centrifuging the sample may accelerate the process.

Alternatively the sample can be placed in special serum separation bottles. These contain a gel that, when the blood is introduced, allows the sample to clot but separates it from the serum, which lies above the gel. This prevents haemolysis from interfering with subsequent testing. Separated serum

Table 29.5 Changes in the colour of plasma/serum

Colour	Implication
Pink	Indicates haemolysis has occurred within the body or more usually through faulty collection
Milky appearance	Due to the presence of fat droplets, i.e. lipaemia. When found in fasted animals this suggests the existence of liver disease
Yellow	Due to the presence of bilirubin. Indicative of severe liver damage or obstruction of the bile duct

can be stored for a few days at 4°C; if testing is to be delayed longer than this, the sample can be frozen but must be thawed at room temperature and then thoroughly mixed before any tests are performed.

Normal canine and feline plasma and serum are clear and almost colourless to pale yellow in colour. The presence of various substances in the blood can alter this colour and provide valuable information as to the health status of the individual (Table 29.5). Lipaemia is normal in animals that have been fed within the previous 3 hours, so blood samples should be taken from fasted animals to reduce the risk of misinterpretation of results. Haemolysis interferes with haematological tests and lipaemia with biochemistry analysis.

Blood smears

Smearing blood on to a slide is a common method of preserving blood to examine it for its relative cellular contents, any cellular abnormalities, presence of blood parasites and a rough estimation of the number of platelets. The smear can be left to air-dry but if examination is to be delayed the smear is best fixed by immersing it in 100% methyl alcohol for 1 minute; staining can then be postponed for up to 3 days. Dried smears are very delicate and should be handled with care and carefully packaged if being despatched to an external laboratory.

Preparation of a blood smear

1. Gloves must be worn
2. Take a grease-free microscope slide. If it has been stored in alcohol, thoroughly wash it and dry with lint-free tissue
3. Label the slide with a chinagraph pencil to identify the sample. This should be done on the underside to prevent the labelling from being removed during staining
4. Place the slide on the bench, against a white background, with its long sides parallel to the edge of the bench
5. Draw a small sample of fresh or well-mixed EDTA-treated blood into a capillary tube
6. The description that follows is for a right-handed technician (Fig. 29.7). If you are left-handed the directions 'left' and 'right' should be reversed
7. Place a small drop of blood at the right-hand end of the slide about 1 cm from its edge
8. Take a 'spreader' in the right hand, holding the long sides between the thumb and index finger, with the

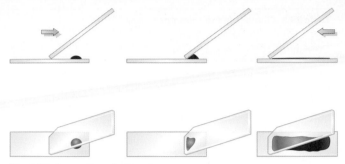

Fig. 29.7 Preparation of a blood smear

spreading edge, which is narrower than the microscope slide, directed downwards. The spreader can be made by cutting the corner off a microscope slide. The narrower edge to the spreader prevents the cells being pushed to the edge of the slide. Ensure that the spreader is not chipped nor has an irregular edge, as this could affect the quality of the smear. Always wipe the edge of the spreader between making smears, as dried blood will produce grooves in subsequent smears

9. With both elbows resting on the bench, place the spreader in contact with the slide, a little to the left of the drop of blood and parallel to the short side of the slide. Hold the spreader at an angle of 20° to the vertical. A wider angle will result in a thicker smear while a more acute angle produces a thinner smear. Draw the spreader to the right until it makes contact with the blood. Allow the blood to run along the whole edge of the spreader

10. Once this has occurred, immediately move the spreader to the left-hand end of the slide in a single rapid, smooth, firm action. The blood will be drawn along behind the spreader. Ensure that the edge of the spreader is in contact with the surface of the slide throughout. Never place the spreader to the right of the drop of blood and push the blood across the slide, as this will damage the cells

11. The faster the spreader is moved the thinner and more even will be the resulting smear. Ideally, the red blood cells should overlap slightly, becoming more separate at the tail. A smear that covers half to two-thirds of the slide is ideal. Usually there are three definable parts to a smear – the head, body and tail

12. Allow the smear to dry slowly without heating, keeping it horizontal. Heating will distort the cells, making the smear useless. Similarly, exposing the smear to water vapour while it is drying will render the smear of no diagnostic value as haemolysis may occur

13. It is always advisable to make at least two smears in case one is unsatisfactory

14. Remember, it takes practice to make a smear of diagnostic quality (Table 29.6).

Staining blood smears

To facilitate examination of the blood cells various stains are employed:

Table 29.6 Common faults in blood smears

Fault	Cause
Too thick	Too large a drop of blood
Too thin	Too small a drop of blood Spread too slowly
Transverse alternate thin and thick bands	Spreading done with a jerky motion, usually due to hesitation
Streaks throughout the length of the smear, especially at the tail	An irregular edge to the spreader Dried blood on the edge of the spreader Dust on the slide or in the blood
'Spots' where blood is absent	Grease on the slide
Very narrow, thick smear	Smear made before the blood has run along the spreading edge One surface of the spreader is lifted during spreading

- **Romanowsky stains**, e.g. Leishman's and Giemsa's stains and rapid stains such as Diff-Quik. This type of stain can be used to:
  - Detect changes in the size, shape and staining of the cells
  - Perform a differential white blood cell count
  - Detect the presence of blood parasites such as *Mycoplasma haemofelis* and *Babesia* spp.
  - Roughly estimate the number of platelets.
- **Supra-vital stains**, e.g. new methylene blue and brilliant cresyl blue. This type of stain can be used to:
  - Perform a reticulocyte count
  - Detect Heinz bodies.

These staining techniques are not routinely carried out in practice.

Technique for Leishman's stain

Always wear gloves as the stain is toxic by ingestion, inhalation and skin contact:

1. Place the labelled slide, smear side uppermost on to a staining rack over a staining bath
2. Place sufficient concentrated Leishman's stain on the slide to cover it
3. Leave for 2 minutes
4. Do not wash off the stain but add twice the stain's volume of buffered distilled water (pH 6.8) and mix well
5. Leave for 15 minutes
6. Tip the stain off the slide and wash it well, front and back, with buffered distilled water
7. Wipe the back of the slide, taking care not to wipe away the label. Prop upright and allow to dry.

Technique for Diff-Quik stain

This is a frequently used staining technique in practice, as it is easy, quick to perform and gives excellent results, comparable with May–Grünwald–Giemsa stain.

1. The staining set consists of three solutions: fixative solution, stain solution I and stain solution II. The blood smear is dipped in each in turn five times for a period of 1 second, i.e. 5 seconds in total

2. The slide is allowed to drain after each dip
3. Finally the slide is rinsed with distilled water and allowed to dry.
4. The whole procedure takes approximately 15 seconds
5. By varying the number of dips in the appropriate solution, different degrees of shading and colour intensity are easily obtained.

It is important that all staining procedures are conducted properly, otherwise the smear may be useless, as the cells cannot be identified with any accuracy nor any abnormalities detected with any certainty. The reasons for the problems will depend on the particular staining technique being used but might include incorrect timing, failure to wash the stain off correctly or using stains at the incorrect concentrations.

Microscopic examination of a blood smear

Blood smears should be examined under ×10, ×40 then ×100 with oil immersion (Fig. 29.3). The slide should be carefully examined and any abnormalities noted (Table 29.7). (For illustrations of individual blood cells see Chapter 4).

Blood smears can also be used for performing manual differential white blood cell counts. This determines the relative proportions of the different types of white blood cell and can give a valuable insight into the health status of the patient. However, it is time-consuming and requires a certain degree of expertise and experience to produce accurate results. The technique involves identifying and recording at least 200 white blood cells. The selection of a suitable area to count the cells can be problematic, as the distribution of the white blood cells is not uniform, with accumulation of the white blood cells at the edges and tail of the smear and a disproportionate number of monocytes and eosinophils, the larger blood cells, being found. In the past the 'four-field meander' method was used but this has been superseded with a strip count technique where all the white blood cells lying in one or more longitudinal strips running the complete length of the smear are classified (Fig. 29.8). The results are recorded on a tally chart and, by using a simple calculation, the percentage of each type of white blood cell is determined.

Many practices now carry out **quantitative analysis** of blood using electronic haematology machines, which if used correctly are more accurate and produce the results in a much shorter time frame. An **automated haematology analyser**, or a QBC (quantitative buffy coat) machine, can be used to assess both total and differential white blood cell counts and also total red blood cell counts. Whole blood is pipetted into a microhaematocrit tube and a special float is added. The sample is then spun in a microhaematocrit centrifuge, which separates the sample. The red blood cells sink to the bottom of the tube, with the white blood cells and platelets on top, and above this lies the plasma. The float

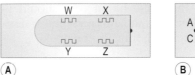
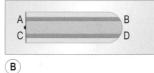

Fig. 29.8 Methods of performing a manual differential white blood cell count. (**A**) By the four-field meander method. (**B**) By the strip count method

Table 29.7 Blood cells

Cell	Description	% Dog	% Cat	Size	Function
Erythrocyte	Biconcave disc			Dog 7.0 μm Cat 4.5 μm	Carriage of oxygen
Lymphocyte (small)	Round with a large round purple nucleus which almost fills all the cell, with a pale blue rim of cytoplasm	12–30	20–55	8 μm	Immunity Production of antibodies
Lymphocyte (large)	Similar to small lymphocyte but more oval in shape of the lymphocytes	Variable, approximately 8%	Variable	12–14 μm	As above
Monocyte	Pleomorphic nucleus (slightly indented oval to horseshoe-shaped) with enlarged knob-like ends. Blue-staining cytoplasm which may contain vacuoles	3–10	1–4	20 μm	Chronic phagocyte
Neutrophil	Irregular lobed nucleus with pale bluish pink cytoplasm with diffuse indistinct pale granules	60–70	35–75	10–12 μm	Phagocyte
Immature, juvenile or band neutrophil	Nuclei horseshoe-shaped and not as darkly staining as mature neutrophils	Variable, 0–3	Variable, 0–3		
Eosinophil	Bilobed or segmented nucleus. Numerous reddish pink granules that are rod-shaped in the cat, round in the dog	2–10	2–12	12–14 μm	Increased numbers in parasitic and allergic conditions
Basophil	Segmented or irregular-shaped nucleus. Blue grey cytoplasm with dark, bluish granules	Very rare in both dog and cat	0–0.1	10–12 μm	Associated with the release of histamine and heparin

separates the buffy coat into its constituent cell layers, which are then measured in a special reading machine. Only a two-part differential count is produced, which gives a granulocyte count and a combined monocyte/lymphocyte count in addition to a red blood cell count.

Other more sophisticated machines are available, such as Coulter counters and Laser cell counters, which give a much wider range of result parameters.

Total red and white blood cell counts can also be performed manually using a **haemocytometer** but, even with practice, the accuracy obtained is not very high and the process is time-consuming. In this test the blood is diluted to a known concentration using special pipettes and the number of cells in a known volume is counted, under the microscope, on the grid etched on the haemocytometer. Different areas of the grid and different diluting fluids are used depending on whether a total red or white blood cell count is to be undertaken. Dacie's fluid is used for a red cell count and Turck's for a white blood cell count.

A **qualitative examination** of a blood smear should always be performed when an automated cell count is performed, as valuable information regarding the health status of the individual may be overlooked and also as part of the quality control protocol. The red blood cells should be examined for any abnormalities. The white blood cells should be checked for a 'shift to the left' and the presence of toxic neutrophils. Platelet clumping should also be noted.

Normal values are:

Total red blood cell count

- Dog – 5.5–8.5 × 10^{12}/l
- Cat – 5.0–10.0 × 10^{12}/l

Total white blood cell count

- Dog – 6–17 × 10^{9}/l
- Cat – 5.5–19.5 × 10^{9}/l

Abnormalities seen in blood smears

Erythrocyte abnormalities

These include:

a. **Size**
  - Anisocytosis – a variation in the size of the red blood cells that is greater than would normally be expected
  - Microcyte – an unusually small cell; may be indicative of a bone marrow defect
  - Macrocyte – a large cell; usually a juvenile cell.
b. **Shape**
  - Crenated – shrinkage of the cells giving a crinkled appearance; seen in old samples or if too high a concentration of anticoagulant has been used
  - 'Star' or 'Burr' cells – appear to have blunt processes protruding from their surface; seen in old samples
  - Spherocyte – do not have the normal biconcave shape; seen in autoimmune disease.
c. **Colour:**
  - Hypochromic – very pale in colour as a result of low levels of haemoglobin
  - Polychromasia – irregular areas of blue intermingled with the normal orange-pink colour; seen in immature cells.

d. **Inclusions** – these can be easily confused with stain debris:
  - Reticulocyte – presence of dark blue inclusions when stained with supra-vital stains such as new methylene blue stain. Immature red blood cell, still containing residual RNA; seen in increased numbers in anaemia
  - Heinz body – round, refractile, blue granular inclusions, again only seen when stained with a supra-vital stain. Formed due to the precipitation of denatured haemoglobin; common in cats. Can result from the action of drugs or infectious agents
  - Howell–Jolly body – can be seen with Romanowsky stains as spherical blue-black granules near to the periphery of the cell. These are the remains of the nucleus which is absent in mature erythrocytes. Increased numbers are seen in regenerative anaemias and following splenectomy.
e. **Red cell parasites:**
  - *Mycoplasma haemofelis* – the causal agent of feline infectious anaemia. Can usually be detected by Romanowsky stains but more easily seen with acridine orange stain. They are very small coccoid organisms that are found attached to the cell membrane, either singly or in short chains. Easily confused with stain debris. Fresh blood is best used as EDTA can detach the parasites from the cell surface
  - *Babesia* – several forms. *Babesia canis* is the commonest form in Europe. Transmitted by ticks. Can be detected by Romanowsky stains. As there are usually only a few organisms present, a peripheral sample is best taken. The organism is pear-shaped and usually occurs in pairs, with up to eight or more present. Increasing in incidence in the UK because of the introduction of the PETS travel scheme
  - Rouleaux formation is also often seen on blood smears. The red cells stack up behind one another, resembling a pile of Pringles! This occurs due to spreading the smear too slowly.

Leucocyte abnormalities

These include:

- A **'shift to the left'** describes an increase in the number of immature neutrophils and is indicative of an inflammatory condition
- **Toxic neutrophils** are seen in severe toxaemic conditions and are characterized by a bluish pink cytoplasm, which is often vacuolated, with dark blue round or angular shaped inclusions known as Döhle bodies.

Abnormal cell counts

Various clinical conditions can cause abnormal blood cell counts (Table 29.8):

- **Leucocytosis** – an increase in the number of white blood cells above the normal range. Possible causes include:
  - Presence of pathogenic organisms
  - Neoplasia
  - Haemorrhage

Table 29.8 Interpretation of differential leucocyte and platelet counts

Cell	Increased numbers	Decreased numbers
Neutrophil	Neutrophilia caused by inflammation, bacterial infection, stress, fear, excitement, canine pregnancy, regenerative anaemia, neoplasia, necrosis and corticosteroid therapy	Neutropaenia caused by overwhelming infections, virus infections, e.g. FIV, FeLV, poisons, toxaemia, aplastic anaemia, cytotoxic drugs
Lymphocyte	Lymphocytosis caused by stress, strong immune stimulation, lymphocytic leukaemia, transiently following vaccination. Young animals have a higher count than adults	Lymphopaenia caused by viraemias/toxaemias, stress, corticosteroid therapy, Cushing's disease and chylothorax
Eosinophil	Eosinophilia caused by parasitism, allergy, eosinophilic leukaemia, Addison's disease, eosinophilic myositis	Eosinopaenia caused by stress, Cushing's disease and corticosteroid therapy
Monocyte	Monocytosis caused by acute or chronic infection/inflammation involving necrosis, pus, cell debris, internal haemorrhage, haemolytic anaemia and immune-mediated disease	Not significant
Platelets	Thrombocytosis caused by infections, trauma, haemorrhage, splenectomy and some tumours	Thrombocytopaenia caused by autoimmune disease, disseminated intravascular coagulation, aplastic anaemia and chemotherapy

- ■ Steroid hormones
- ■ Degenerative non-inflammatory disease.
- • **Leucopenia** – a reduction in the number of white blood cells below the normal range. Usually the decrease is limited to one type of leucocyte and can give a useful insight into the health status of the patient. If all the leucocyte types are involved this is known as panleucopenia. Possible causes of leucopenia are:
  - ■ Bone marrow failure
  - ■ Overwhelming infections
  - ■ Viral diseases, e.g. feline viral panleucopenia
  - ■ Cushing's disease.

Packed cell volume or haematocrit

Packed cell volume (PCV) is the red blood cell to fluid ratio in the blood. It is expressed as a percentage or litres per litre. Normal ranges are:

- • Dog 37–55% (0.37–0.55 l/l)
- • Cat 24–45% (0.24–0.45 l/l).

Haemolysis and the use of a liquid coagulant will invalidate the results. Low PCVs are found in anaemia, sedation and anaesthesia and late canine pregnancy. High values are seen in dehydration, which results in a relative polycythaemia (increase in the number of red blood cells), splenic contraction, anabolic steroids, and hyperthyroidism in cats. The PCV is often normally elevated in athletic breeds of dog, e.g. greyhounds, where it may be at the top end of the range.

Measurement of packed cell volume

The most common procedure used in practice is the **microhaematocrit method**. This employs the use of capillary 'microhaematocrit' tubes, which are heparinized if fresh blood is used, to prevent clotting. Plain tubes are used with anticoagulated samples.

Using anticoagulated blood:

1. A well-mixed sample is allowed to three-quarters fill a 'haematocrit' tube by capillary action

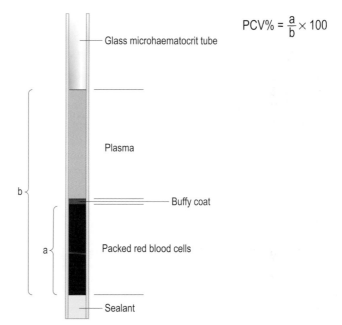

$$PCV\% = \frac{a}{b} \times 100$$

Glass microhaematocrit tube

Plasma

Buffy coat

Packed red blood cells

Sealant

Fig. 29.9 Packed cell volume

2. The outside of the tube is wiped clean and the unfilled end is sealed with a special filler, e.g. Cristaseal
3. The tube is then placed, sealed end outwards, into a special microhaematocrit centrifuge and spun for approximately 5 minutes at 10 000 rpm
4. The centrifuge must be balanced so a minimum of two samples are spun at the same time at diametrically opposite sides of the centrifuge
5. The centrifugal process results in the red blood cells concentrating at the bottom of the tube with the white blood cells and platelets – forming a grey/cream layer, the buffy coat – above them. The platelets tend to lie at the top of the buffy coat and can be seen as a thin, cream-coloured layer. The plasma is found above this layer. Gross examination of the plasma can indicate haemolysis, jaundice or lipaemia (Fig. 29.9)
6. The PCV is then read off on a special microhaematocrit reader. Different types of readers are available but all

work on a similar principle. The PCV is calculated by dividing the length of the column of red blood cells (a) by the combined length of the red blood cells, buffy coat and plasma (b) then multiplying by 100 to give the result as a percentage (Table 29.9).

The method is rapid, very accurate and relatively easy to perform. It also only requires only a small volume of blood.

Haemoglobin estimation

Haemoglobin, packed into the red blood cells, combines reversibly with oxygen and transports it around the body. In order for the body to function properly adequate amounts of haemoglobin are essential. Haemoglobin (Hb) levels are estimated by haematology analysers and are measured in grams per decilitre.

Normal ranges are:

- Dog 12–18 g/dl
- Cat 8–15 g/dl.

This test is not affected by haemolysis. Haemoglobin levels are decreased in cases of anaemia.

Further information calculable from these tests

'Corpuscular values' can be calculated from the total red blood cell counts, PCV and haemoglobin contents, or obtained more accurately from haematology analysers.

- **Mean corpuscular volume (MCV)** – indicates the average size of the red blood cells:

$$MCV (fl) = \frac{PCV (l/l) \times 1000}{Total\ red\ cells\ (10^{12}/l)}$$

(fl = femtolitre: 1 fl = 10^{-15} l).

- **Mean corpuscular haemoglobin concentration (MCHC)** – indicates the average concentration of haemoglobin per red blood cell:

$$MCHC (g/dl) = \frac{Total\ haemoglobin\ (g/dl)}{PCV\ (l/l)}$$

The MCV and MCHC are useful in the evaluation of anaemic conditions. The normal ranges of haematological values are listed in Table 29.9.

Blood biochemistry

Studying the biochemical parameters of normal substances in the blood can help in the diagnosis of many conditions (Table 29.10). It must be borne in mind that the normal ranges of values of the various determinations will show a degree of variation depending on the analytical system being used.

Blood urea nitrogen (BUN)

Urea is a nitrogenous waste product formed by the liver from the breakdown of amino acids. It is carried in the plasma to the kidneys, where it is excreted in the urine.

Table 29.9 Normal ranges of haematological values

Species	RBC (10^{12}/l)	WBC (10^9/l)	PCV (%)	Hb (g/dl)
Dog	5.5–8.5	6–17	37–55	12–18
Cat	5.0–10.0	5.5–19.5	24–45	8–15

Table 29.10 Common blood biochemistry estimations

Substance	Normal range*	Causes of elevated levels	Causes of depressed levels
Total serum protein	Dog 50–78 g/l Cat 60–82 g/l	Dehydration, chronic and immune-mediated disease, lactation, infection and neoplasia	Renal disease, haemorrhage, malnutrition, malabsorption, hepatic and pancreatic insufficiency. Lower in young animals because of minimal levels of immunoglobulins
Serum albumin	Dog 22–35 g/l Cat 25–39 g/l	Haemoconcentration secondary to dehydration	Chronic liver disease, ascites, tissue oedema, congestive heart failure and renal failure
Cholesterol	Dog 2.7–9.5 mmol/l Cat 1.5–6.0 mmol/l	Diabetes mellitus, hypothyroidism, hyperadrenocorticism, nephritic syndrome and post-feeding sampling	Maldigestion, malabsorption and severe hepatic insufficiency
Total bilirubin	Dog and cat 0–6.8 μmol/l	Haemolytic anaemia, hepatic jaundice, obstruction to bile flow and impaired liver function	Not applicable
Amylase	Dog and cat 400–2000 units/l	Acute pancreatitis but not specific, therefore it is advisable to cross-reference with lipase levels Renal failure and gastrointestinal problems	Not applicable
Calcium	Dog and cat 2.20–2.90 mmol/l	Dehydration, neoplasia, primary hyperparathyroidism, hypoadrenocorticism, renal failure and hypervitaminosis D	Primary hypoparathyroidism, eclampsia, acute pancreatitis, intestinal malabsorption and following bilateral thyroidectomy
Bile acids	Dog and cat 0–15 μmol/l†	Primary or secondary hepatic disease Biliary obstruction and portosystemic shunt	Intestinal obstruction and severe malabsorption

*May vary depending on analyser. †Normally a bile acid stimulation test is performed. This involves taking a preprandial (fasting) blood sample then feeding the patient with a fatty meal. A postprandial sample is then taken 2 h later and the change in the two samples is analysed.

There are two different measurements of urea concentration, which can lead to confusion as both are expressed as mg/100 ml. One is the quantity of urea per 100 ml, i.e. blood urea. The other is the quantity of urea nitrogen per 100 ml, i.e. BUN. It is important to be sure which is being used, as a urea molecule is heavier than the two nitrogen atoms it contains. Generally, it is the latter that is used to evaluate kidney function.

Normal range of BUN values:

- Dog – 3.0–9.0 mmol/l
- Cat – 5.0–10.0 mmol/l (some researchers give the upper value as 15 mmol/l).

Elevated BUN can be considered under three categories:

a. **Pre-renal**
   - Fever
   - Infection
   - Necrosis
   - Metabolic conditions
   - High-protein diet
   - Chronic heart failure
   - Corticosteroid administration
b. **Renal** – increased BUN levels are seen in renal failure but approximately 75% of the nephrons have to become non-functional before this occurs
c. **Postrenal**
   - Urethral obstruction
   - Ruptured bladder.

Decreased BUN can occur as a result of:

- Liver failure
- Anabolic steroids
- Portosystemic shunt
- Low-protein diet.

In addition to biochemical analysers, diptests are also available. However, these are not as accurate as the biochemical analysers.

Creatinine

This is a metabolite of creatine, which stores energy in muscles. It is freely filtered by the glomeruli of the kidney and the clearance of creatinine from the plasma can be used to provide an approximation of the glomerular filtration rate. Like BUN, it is not a very accurate indicator of kidney function, as approximately 75% of the kidney tissue must be non-functional before elevated levels are seen. The levels of creatinine are not influenced by a high-protein diet.

Normal range of values:

- Dog – up to 120 μmol/l. Greyhounds and other sight-hounds up to 150 μmol/l
- Cat – up to 180 mol/l.

An increase in plasma concentrations of urea nitrogen or creatinine, or both, is known as azotaemia.

Glucose

Glucose is the principal source of energy for all the cells of the body. Other sources can be utilized by some cells but glucose is essential for the survival of brain tissue.

Blood glucose concentrations are controlled in the main by two hormones:

- **Insulin** – produced by the beta cells of the islets of Langerhans of the pancreas. Facilitates the passage of glucose into cells, converts glucose into glycogen, which is stored in the liver, and promotes the synthesis of protein and fats. These actions have the effect of reducing blood glucose levels
- **Glucagon** – produced by the alpha cells and has the opposite effects.

Adrenaline (epinephrine) and cortisol also influence blood glucose levels. In the dog and cat glucose is actively reabsorbed in the renal tubules up to the renal threshold of 10–12 mmol/l. If the level of glucose exceeds the renal threshold, glucose will be excreted in the urine, i.e. glucosuria.

Normal ranges of fasting plasma glucose levels:

- Dog – 3.5–5.5 mmol/l
- Cat – 3.5–6.5 mmol/l

Elevated blood glucose levels (hyperglycaemia) may be seen in:

- Diabetes mellitus
- Post-feeding sampling
- Stress
- Cushing's disease
- Administration of corticosteroids
- Pancreatitis
- Administration of drugs, e.g. morphine.

Decreased blood glucose levels (hypoglycaemia) may be seen in:

- Neoplasia, e.g. insulinoma, hepatocellular carcinoma
- Hepatic insufficiency
- Hypoadrenocorticism
- Malabsorption
- Starvation
- Idiopathic in some toy breeds
- Insulin treatment.

Blood samples for glucose determination must be collected into fluoride oxalate tubes, as fluoride blocks glycolysis in the red blood cells ensuring that the glucose levels determined at sampling more accurately reflect the glucose levels at the time of testing. If the biochemical analyser requires the use of heparinized plasma, the sample must be separated immediately to prevent glycolysis occurring.

Reagent strips, e.g. BM-Test 1-44, can also be used but require whole blood. In general, these are less accurate at high glucose levels. Glucometers can also be used.

Many other blood biochemistry estimations can be made with biochemical analysers (Table 29.10).

Plasma enzymes

Within all cells are enzymes, which are essential for intracellular metabolism. Normally, low levels of these enzymes are found in the plasma but, if a cell dies or is badly damaged, increased amounts of its enzymes are detected. Cells of different tissues contain different enzymes so it would seem feasible to be able to identify the damaged cells by the enzymes found in the plasma. Unfortunately, it is not as simple as this, as one enzyme is seldom specific for one particular tissue, but it is usually possible to localize the damage by looking at a number of different enzymes or, to be more precise, by investigating the isoenzymes involved, which are often specific for a particular tissue.

Results are not expressed as concentrations but as 'activities'. This is a measure of how fast the enzyme can convert substrate to product under standardized assay conditions, and is measured in international units (IU). Reaction temperature can influence the results obtained and is now commonly standardized at 37°C, but results using different temperatures may still be encountered.

- **Alanine aminotransferase (ALT),** formerly serum glutamic-pyruvic transaminase (SGPT) – in dogs and cats, elevated levels are predominantly specific for hepatocellular damage Activities of more than 150–200 IU/l are of clinical significance. In very acute conditions, e.g. acute hepatitis, levels of 5000 IU/l are not uncommon. Levels will also increase in severe muscle damage. Mild increases in ALT are also seen in feline hyperthyroidism
- **Aspartate aminotransferase (AST),** formerly serum glutamic-oxaloacetic transaminase (SGOT) – this enzyme is widely distributed throughout the body in skeletal and cardiac muscle, liver and red blood cells. Elevated levels are indicative of muscle damage in dogs and cats. Normal levels are below 100 IU/l
- **Alkaline phosphatase (ALP),** formerly serum alkaline phosphatase (SAP) – this is one of the most widely distributed enzymes in the body and has several isoenzymes found in bone (osteoblasts), liver and the intestinal wall. The range of values is quite wide, up to 300 IU/l. It is higher in young animals because of bone development.

It is clear that a plasma enzyme activity result should not be considered in isolation in deciding on a diagnosis.

Hormones

Thyroid

The thyroid produces two important hormones, thyroxine (T_4) and tri-iodothyronine (T_3). These hormones have widespread physiological effects on the body, including controlling the metabolic rate. Abnormal fluctuations in the levels of these hormones can result in the development of various clinical signs and endocrine disorders. The secretion of these hormones is controlled by thyroid stimulating hormone (TSH) from the anterior pituitary and thyrotrophin releasing hormone (TRH), produced by the hypothalamus.

Diagnostically T_4 is used to assess thyroid function, as abnormalities show up more readily in this hormone. Normal ranges vary between laboratories but generally fall between 13 and 52 nmol/l.

Increased serum T_4 may be due to:

- Hyperthyroidism
- Young age
- Anti-T_4 antibodies
- Certain drugs
- Oestrus and pregnancy.

Decreased serum T_4 may be due to:

- Hypothyroidism

- Hyperadrenocorticism
- Chronic illness, known as sick euthyroid syndrome, such as renal, liver, or heart failure and diabetes mellitus
- Advanced age
- Drug therapy
- Iodine deficiency.

Serum samples are preferred for testing as this decreases the risk of fibrinogen interfering with the test. T_4 is stable in serum for up to 8 days at room temperature and is unaffected by haemolysis and lipaemia. Radioimmunoassay is the preferred laboratory method for determining serum T_4 and is undertaken at specialist laboratories. Modified human test kits are also employed.

Dynamic thyroid function tests – a range of these tests are used to confirm or refute a diagnosis of thyroid dysfunction. The TSH stimulation test is used to confirm hypothyroidism in dogs. Basal T_4 levels are measured, then the dog is injected with bovine TSH, and a second blood sample is taken after 6 hours. The TSH has little effect on the T_4 levels in hypothyroid dogs as there is little functional thyroid gland to stimulate. Dogs that have a low T_4 but are not hypothyroid, e.g. those suffering from sick euthyroid syndrome, will show a rise in T_4 following the TSH injection.

Adrenal cortex

The adrenal cortex produces approximately 30 different steroid hormones. The most common disorders affecting the adrenal cortex are hyperadrenocorticism (Cushing's disease) or hypoadrenocorticism (Addison's disease). The hormone involved in these conditions is cortisol. A basal plasma or serum cortisol level is not very helpful due to other causes which can affect the cortisol levels, e.g. stress. For this reason dynamic manipulation tests with ACTH or dexamethasone are used.

The ACTH stimulation test is used to:

- Screen for primary and secondary Cushing's disease
- Monitor mitotane therapy
- Diagnose primary Addison's disease.

An initial basal cortisol level is performed followed by an intravenous injection of a synthetic form of ACTH. This will stimulate the release of cortisol. A second sample is taken 2 hours later and the cortisol level is determined. High postinjection cortisol levels indicate Cushing's while low levels indicate Addison's disease.

Low-dose dexamethasone tests are used to screen for Cushing's. High-dose dexamethasone tests are used to distinguish between animals that have pituitary-dependent Cushing's disease and those that have non-pituitary-dependent Cushing's disease caused by a neoplasm in the adrenal cortex:

- **Low-dose dexamethasone test** – a basal cortisol level is determined. A low dose of dexamethasone (0.01 mg/kg) is then administered intravenously and a second sample is taken 8 hours later to assess the animal's response. In normal animals the release of ACTH will be suppressed by negative feedback and the cortisol levels will be reduced. In animals with Cushing's disease the dexamethasone will not be able to suppress the release of ACTH and the cortical levels will be higher

- **High-dose dexamethasone test** – a basal cortisol level is determined but on this occasion a high dose of dexamethasone (0.1 mg/kg) is administered intravenously. Subsequent blood samples are taken at 3- and 8-hourly intervals to assess the response:
  - Normal – both post-injection samples will be below the basal level
  - Pituitary-dependent – one of the post-injection samples will be below the basal level
  - Non-pituitary-dependent – very little suppression and both post-injection samples above the basal level.

Urine

The analysis of urine samples can give a rapid insight into the health status of a patient. It is generally held that the normal dog will produce within the range of 20–40 ml/kg and the cat 18–25 ml/kg of urine daily:

- **Polyuria** – production of excess urine
- **Oliguria** – reduction of the amount of urine produced
- **Anuria** – absence of urine production
- **Dysuria** – difficulty in passing urine.

Collection and preservation of urine samples

Urine is potentially a hazardous substance and protective disposable gloves should be worn during its collection and analysis. Ideally, a sterile sample should be used but this can only be obtained by catheterization.

Collection of urine can be achieved by:

- **Free flow** – a midstream overnight sample is best for routine urinalysis, as this is the best indicator of the true composition of urine. The first stream of urine is the best sample to collect for lesions low in the urethral tract, e.g. urethral plugs, uroliths and bacteria; however, this fraction is the most likely to be contaminated. End stream is the best to collect for examination for prostatic disease or for haemorrhage or sediment that might have collected on the floor of the bladder. However, the practicalities of obtaining the last two types of sample are difficult, to say the least! In the case of dogs, a well-cleaned container should be used to collect the sample, then it should be transferred to a sterile container. Commercial sterile collection kits are available, e.g. Uripet. Cats are more problematic but again commercial kits are available, which involve using a litter tray with an inert substrate from which the urine can be obtained.
- **Manual expression** – this is convenient provided the bladder contains sufficient urine to be isolated manually on palpation of the abdomen. However, if strong resistance is encountered care must be taken to prevent undue pressure rupturing the bladder. This is especially true when dealing with male cats with a potential urinary obstruction.
- **Catheterization** – involves the passage of a tube aseptically into the urethra to collect urine directly from the bladder (see Ch. 15). This will provide a sterile sample.

- **Cystocentesis** – involves the passage of a needle through the abdominal wall and into the bladder.

Preservation

Ideally, examination of the urine sample should be performed as soon as possible after collection, i.e. within an hour. If the sample is left, bacteria present in the sample will cause decomposition of the urea and the production of ammonia. This, being alkaline, will elevate the pH of the sample, which in turn will facilitate the precipitation of phosphates, which will interfere with subsequent testing. If testing is to be delayed, the sample should be refrigerated, not frozen.

Chemical preservatives can be used if refrigeration is not available, including formalin or thymol, but probably the only one commonly used in practice is boric acid. This will preserve and prevent the multiplication of bacteria for up to 4 days and will also preserve cells and urinary casts. It is commercially available in red-capped specimen containers.

Physical properties of urine

The physical properties should be observed initially, including colour, odour, turbidity, pH and specific gravity.

Colour

The pigment urochrome is responsible for the colour of normal urine. It is normally yellow and the depth of colour indicates the concentration of the urine. There may be considerable variation in the depth of colour from almost colourless to a darkish brown. This variation depends on numerous factors, including concentration, diet, species, breed and exercise regime.

Abnormal colours in dogs and cats can be due to:

- Presence of blood, haemoglobin or myoglobin – impart a red or pink colour to the urine
- Bile pigments – colour the urine orange
- Drugs
- Food.

Rabbit urine colour ranges from light yellow to orange and even red with brown coloration. Certain pigments may cause a reddish appearance and can be confused with haematuria.

Odour

Normal urine has a sourish odour. Ammonia can be detected in stale urine. Ammonia in freshly passed urine may be due to the presence of urease-producing bacteria, which are commonly involved in cystitis. Male animals, notably cats, produce very strong-smelling urine. This is important in territorial scent marking. Animals suffering from diabetes mellitus produce a sweet and fruity, pear-drop-smelling urine because of the presence of ketone bodies, e.g. acetone and acetoacetic acid. This can also be smelt on the breath of such ketoacidotic animals.

Turbidity (cloudiness)

Dog and cat urine is normally clear. However, if the urine is allowed to stand it will become turbid because of phosphate precipitation. Rabbit urine is normally turbid because of the presence of calcium carbonate. Abnormal turbidity can arise from the presence of mucus, pus and vaginal or prostatic secretions.

pH

This is the expression of the hydrogen ion concentration. A pH above 7.0 is alkaline while a pH below 7.0 is acidic. False results may occur if the sample is not kept cool and covered. Urine pH is affected by diet: carnivorous animals have acid urine while animals that eat a vegetarian diet have alkaline urine.

Normal pH:

- Dog pH 5.2–6.8
- Cat pH 6.0–7.0.

Acidic urine may be due to pyrexia, acidosis, high-protein diets, starvation, diabetes mellitus and muscle catabolism.

Alkaline urine may be due to urinary retention or infection, alkalosis, a high-vegetable-content diet or certain drugs.

The pH can be determined by pH papers, multireagent dip sticks or electrode pH meters, which are the most accurate and reliable.

Specific gravity

This is the density or weight of a known volume of a fluid, i.e. urine compared with an equal volume of distilled water. Distilled water has a specific gravity of 1.000.

Normal specific gravity:

- Dog – 1.015–1.045
- Cat – 1.020–1.040.

The specific gravity of urine varies considerably even in the same individual and a single measurement should not be taken as conclusive.

Elevated specific gravity may be due to dehydration, acute renal failure, diabetes mellitus or shock.

Lowered levels are seen in diabetes insipidus, chronic renal failure or various causes of polydipsia.

Measurement of specific gravity

An accurate measurement of specific gravity can be made by the use of a refractometer (Fig. 29.10). This is an optical instrument that assesses the refractive index of fluids: the higher the refractive index the higher the concentration of urine, i.e. the specific gravity. This method requires only a small volume of urine and is quick and easy to perform.

It is essential that the refractometer is initially calibrated with distilled water before the specific gravity reading is taken. A few drops of distilled water are placed on the face of the prism and the cover plate is gently closed. The refractometer is held up to the light and the scale is brought into focus by turning the eyepiece. If the boundary line does not coincide with the 1.000 line, adjustments are made with a small screwdriver to the scale adjustment knob until the boundary line does coincide with the 1.000 line.

The water is then cleaned away with a soft piece of tissue and a few drops of urine, at room temperature, are applied to the prism surface. The specific gravity is then read off on the appropriate scale. If the reading goes off the scale, this means that the urine is very concentrated; the sample should then be diluted with an equal volume of distilled water and the reading retaken. Multiplying the scale reading after the decimal point by 2 will give the correct final specific gravity of the sample. Different refractometers have different scale layouts displayed and the manufacturer's instructions should be consulted to ensure that the correct scale is read.

A refractometer can also be used to measure the refractive index of other liquids and enables the plasma protein level to be ascertained. Urine specific gravity can also be measured by dip-stick methods but most are designed for human use and are not very accurate.

Chemical tests

Many substances can interfere with the chemical testing of urine, giving rise to erroneous results, e.g. concurrent medication. It should also be borne in mind that the majority of commercial strips are designed for measuring human parameters. Test strips are available which test for varying numbers of chemical substances in the urine (Table 29.11). The BM-Test-8 can be used to test for nitrate, pH, protein, glucose, ketone bodies, urobilinogen, bilirubin and blood in urine.

Use urine that is fresh, uncentrifuged and thoroughly mixed. The test strip must be briefly (no longer than 1 second), dipped into the sample and any excess wiped off on the rim of the container. After 60 seconds the colour changes should be compared with the colour scales on the label and the results recorded. Different brands of reagent strips will have different arrangements of the scales and timings, so the manufacturer's instructions should always be followed.

To ensure that the most accurate results are obtained, the following points should be followed:

- Ensure the strips are in date and are stored at a temperature not exceeding 30°C
- Close the container with the desiccant stopper immediately after taking out a test strip
- Use only clean, well-rinsed containers to collect the urine, and preservatives should be avoided
- Do not expose the urine sample to sunlight as this induces oxidation of bilirubin and urobilinogen, which can lead to artificially low results for these two parameters

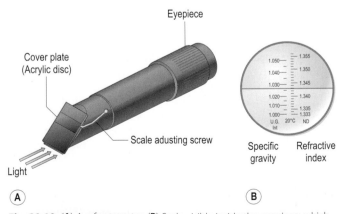

Fig. 29.10 (**A**) A refractometer. (**B**) Scale visible inside the eyepiece, which must be calibrated before use

Table 29.11 Urinary chemical tests

Substance	Test	Normal parameters	Causes of elevated values
Protein	Albustix	Commercial test strips in common use are more sensitive to albumin and may underestimate the presence of other proteins. These tests are not as sensitive as those for protein in blood so a negative result does not rule out the presence of haemoglobin or myoglobin in the urine	**Pre-renal**, e.g. haemolytic anaemia, azotaemia, multiple myeloma and congestive heart failure **Renal**, e.g. acute and chronic renal failure, pyelonephritis and amyloidosis **Post-renal**, e.g. cystitis, urolithiasis, prostatitis and vaginitis
	20% sulphosalicylic acid test, which is more sensitive to proteins other than albumen	A trace reading for protein, which equates to 0.3 g/l, is of no clinical significance	
Blood	Hemastix	Any positive result is significant other than a bitch in pro-oestrus	Cystitis, associated infection of the urinary tract, urolithiasis and acute nephritis
Glucose	Clinistix Clinitest not specific for glucose but will detect any reducing sugar, e.g. lactose, so always test first with Clinistix, which is specific for glucose	The presence of glucose in urine, glucosuria, is always significant	Diabetes mellitus, chronic liver damage, Cushing's disease and hyperthyroidism
Ketones	Ketostix	Any levels are significant	Diabetes mellitus, starvation and liver damage

- False positives for blood and glucose can result from residues of strongly oxidizing disinfectants in the collecting container
- Excessive amounts of ascorbic acid can also interfere with some of the tests, but this is unlikely to be encountered in dogs and cats.

Individual tests are available to detect chemical substances in urine but these also have limitations on their validity.

Blood and blood pigments

If dog or cat urine is coloured red it may be due to the presence of blood, haemoglobin or myoglobin:

- **Haematuria** is the presence of whole blood in the urine
- **Haemoglobinuria** is the presence of free haemoglobin in the urine and may result from haemolytic anaemia, leptospirosis, poisoning and autoimmune disease.

To differentiate between the two, microscopic examination or centrifugation of the sample should be undertaken.

- **Myoglobinuria** is the presence of myoglobin in the urine and is usually seen in muscle-wasting disease, e.g. myasthenia gravis.

Microscopic examination of urine

This provides useful information on various disease processes that might be present.

Preparation of a wet preparation

1. Place 5 ml of a well-mixed fresh urine sample into a centrifuge tube and spin at 1500 rpm for 5 minutes
2. Discard the supernatant liquid, leaving the sediment with a small amount of urine in the tube
3. Resuspend the sediment by flicking the bottom of the tube

4. An unstained wet preparation can be made, but usually a stain is added to facilitate examination of the sample. Stains such as 0.5% new methylene blue, or preferably Sedi-Stain, can be added to ease examination. Add 2 drops to the sample and mix well
5. Pipette a drop of the suspension on to a clean, labelled microscope slide and carefully place a coverslip on top of the sample using a mounted needle
6. Examine the slide systematically under low power, ×10 then ×40. Only a small amount of light is needed so the iris diaphragm should be partially closed
7. To make a dry preparation, all the supernatant is decanted and a small drop of the sediment is placed on a microscope slide, covered by a coverslip and examined.

Various microscopic components can be identified in a urinary sediment including the following:

Epithelial cells

Flat, irregular squamous cells. Small numbers are normally present

Transitional cells

Small, round polyhedral cells. Indicate cystitis or pyelonephritis. Higher numbers are detected in catheterized samples, because of trauma to the urethra and bladder

Tubular epithelial cells

Small, cuboidal epithelial cells. Indicative of renal tubule damage. Can be confused with white blood cells

Leucocytes

Usually neutrophils. The presence of large numbers is known as pyuria and suggests inflammation of the urogenital tract or pyelonephritis

Red blood cells

Large numbers are indicative of bleeding into the urogenital tract

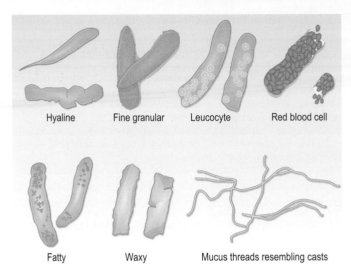

Hyaline   Fine granular   Leucocyte   Red blood cell

Fatty   Waxy   Mucus threads resembling casts

Fig. 29.11 Types of casts that may be found in urine

Casts

These are precipitated protein, which tend to form in the distal convoluted tubules and collecting ducts of the nephrons because of the acidic conditions in these regions (Fig. 29.11). All the casts have a basis of protein that is moulded into the shape of the tubules. They are short cylinders, usually with one rounded and one broken end, although on occasion both ends may be rounded.

Other materials may be incorporated into the basic protein matrix, resulting in different types of casts:

- **Hyaline casts** – clear, refractile, colourless and cylindrical in shape. An increase in numbers is found in mild inflammation of the tubules, poor circulation and pyrexia
- **Cellular casts** – a variety of cells may be incorporated into the casts:
  - Erythrocytes – indicative of haemorrhage into the tubules
  - Leucocytes – indicate an inflammatory reaction
  - Epithelial cells – indicate acute renal failure
- **Granular casts** – these are hyaline casts containing granules that are remnants of degenerating leucocytes or epithelial cells. The presence of large numbers of these casts are associated with renal failure, especially in the dog
- **Waxy casts** – these are more opaque and wider than hyaline casts, with square rather than rounded ends. They are found in chronic degenerative renal tubular damage.

Casts, being relatively large structures, tend to be found at the edges of the coverslip. They may be confused with hairs, fibres or mucus strands but these are thinner and longer than casts and are usually twisted strands. They are usually products of the lower urinary tract. They tend to dissolve in alkaline urine and easily break up on centrifugation.

Spermatozoa

Commonly found in urine samples from male dogs.

Bacteria, fungi and yeasts

May be found as contaminants and their presence is only significant if accompanied by large numbers of leucocytes.

Crystals

The presence of crystals can be associated with various clinical conditions, e.g. urolithiasis, cystitis and haematuria, but they can also be detected in apparently normal animals. Crystals are more likely to be found if freshly collected urine is allowed to stand.

The presence of increased numbers of crystals depends on the pH, concentration of the urine and the solubility of the salts in the urine. Various conditions can influence crystal production, including genetic predisposition, bacterial infection, diet, concurrent illnesses and breed, e.g. Dalmatians excrete uric acid in their urine, hence the relatively high incidence of uric acid crystals in their urine (Table 29.12). Other less common crystals include silica, xanthine, bilirubin and crystals caused by drugs.

Occasionally, urinary crystals clump together to form **calculi or stones**. Calculi in the bladder are known as **cystic calculi**. Those found in the urethra are known as **uroliths**. Chemical analysis of the calculi will identify the crystal and facilitate treatment and control of the condition, usually by adjusting the pH of the urine.

Skin and hair

Laboratory tests can prove invaluable in the diagnosis of many skin conditions. It is important, when handling animals with skin disease, to avoid transmission of the condition to humans (zoonosis) and cross-contamination of other patients. Examples of potential zoonoses include ringworm, *Cheyletiella* and *Sarcoptes*. To reduce the risk, gloves and aprons should be worn when handling suspect patients and samples.

The animal should be adequately restrained while the samples are taken, as few people as possible should handle the patient and care should be taken to avoid contact with other animals. The owner should also be made aware of the risks and precautions that need to be taken to reduce them.

Sampling techniques

It is important that the correct sampling protocol is employed when investigating skin problems. These techniques include:

Skin scrapings

This is an easy technique to perform and is routinely performed in practice to diagnose parasitic skin conditions. It is used to detect burrowing mites such as *Sarcoptes scabei*, *Notedres cati* and *Trixacarus caviae* (see Ch. 27). Deeper scrapings will reveal *Demodex* spp. Superficial scrapings may also detect *Malassezia* yeasts.

Technique

1. The area to be scraped should be selected carefully and several sites sampled. Any erythematous (reddened) papules or scaly areas should be investigated, especially the lateral aspect of the pinna, the elbows and the

Table 29.12 Common urinary crystals

Appearance	Name/composition	pH of urine in which crystals are deposited
Struvite	Magnesium ammonium phosphate. Also known as triple phosphate or struvite crystals. Coffin-lid-shaped	Alkaline, but can occur at any pH
Cystine	Cystine. Large, flat hexagonal crystals	Acidic, but can occur at any pH
Calcium oxalate	Calcium oxalate. Envelope-shaped, octahedral/pyramidal in shape	Acidic, but can occur at any pH

carpal region if *Sarcoptes* is suspected. *Notedres* is found mainly on the head of the cat, especially below the ears. *Demodex* tends in the early stages to be concentrated on the head but as the infestation progresses the whole body may be affected

2. The sample site should be clipped, as contaminating hair can make subsequent examination of the sample difficult. The area should be moistened by liquid paraffin, propylene glycol or 10% potassium hydroxide

3. The skin is stretched between the thumb and forefinger and gently scraped with a sterile scalpel blade until pinprick drops of blood are seen. This means that the full thickness of the epidermis has been sampled, as there are no capillaries in the epidermis and if capillary bleeding is observed then the dermis must have been exposed. A drop of mineral oil on the blade aids collection and prevents the skin scrapings from being blown away. The procedure is not usually very painful

Table 29.12 Continued

Appearance	Name/composition	pH of urine in which crystals are deposited
Uric acid	Uric acid. Diamond or rhomboidal in shape	Acidic
Ammonium urate	Ammonium urate. 'Thorn-apple'-shaped	Acidic
Calcium phosphate	Calcium phosphate	Alkaline, but occur at any pH

4. The material should be transferred to a clean, labelled microscope slide and a coverslip carefully applied using a mounted needle. Prior to this, a few drops of 10% potassium hydroxide can be applied to the slide, which is then heated. This will clear the sample, i.e. make it transparent, and facilitate subsequent examination. The sample should then be examined under the microscope under low power ×10 then higher magnification if

necessary. If there is to be a delay in examination then the sample can be stored in 10% potassium hydroxide

5. *Demodex* spp. require a more vigorous sampling method as they live deep within the hair follicles. The skin is squeezed between the thumb and forefinger to extrude material from the hair follicles. The area is scraped until capillary ooze appears, then the sample is transferred to a microscope slide, as previously

described. The pustular lesions of *Demodex* can be easily sampled by expressing the contents of a pustule directly on to a microscope slide.

6. When examining microscopic ectoparasites, e.g. *Sarcoptes* and *Demodex*, remember that they are transparent, not solid as depicted in idealized diagrams. In fact they look as if they have been etched on to the slide. This can cause confusion, as they may not look like what is expected.

Swabs

Swabs can be taken for the pustular form of *Demodex* or ear wax samples for evidence of *Otodectes* or *Malassezia*.

Tape impression

This technique can be used to detect superficial parasites, surface bacteria and fungi. It is very useful for the identification of *Cheyletiella* spp. and *Malassezia*. A strip of clear, colourless adhesive tape is placed on the sample site then pulled away and transferred to a microscope slide for subsequent microscopic examination.

Hair brushings

This technique is used to detect surface ectoparasites. The animal is placed on a white background and the coat is brushed through with a fine-toothed comb to collect superficial debris. This can then be examined with a hand lens or under the microscope for evidence of surface ectoparasites or their eggs.

Hair plucks

These can be used to identify parasitic eggs, e.g. lice, *Cheyletiella*, and ringworm.

The hair samples should be plucked with forceps, not clipped. They are then examined under the microscope and in the case of suspected ringworm they can also be cultured. (For identification of individual parasites see Chapter 27.)

Ringworm (dermatophytosis)

This is caused by a group of fungi known as dermatophytes. Those important in the dog and cat are:

- *Microsporum canis* – responsible for 70–80% of cases in the dog and 90% of cases in cats
- *Microsporum gypseum* – occasionally encountered in dogs and cats
- *Trichophyton mentagrophytes* – responsible for 20% of cases in dogs and occasionally seen in cats.

Ringworm is a zoonosis, so adequate precautions should be taken to reduce the risk of transmission of the disease to anyone handling the suspect patient and to other animals, including wearing protective clothing and gloves.

Presenting signs

The major sign is alopecia with crusting and scaling. In the dog typical circular lesions are seen, which may coalesce into larger lesions. In the cat the fungus invades the hair follicles and the lesions are more discrete. Sometimes only a few hairs or a claw may be infected. The head and extremities are often the sites of the lesions.

Diagnosis

Wood's lamp

This is an ultraviolet lamp that emits light of a wavelength of 365–366 nm. When the light is directed on to a hair or claw affected with *M. canis*, ideally in a darkened room, it will emit a characteristic yellowish green (apple green) fluorescence, similar to that seen on a luminous clock dial. This is due to the presence of a fluorescent metabolite produced by the fungus. However, it must be remembered that only 60% of cases of *M. canis* show this fluorescence, so the only significant result is a positive one. A negative result does not mean that the animal does not have ringworm, as it might have non-fluorescing *M. canis* or one of the other species that do not fluoresce.

It is important to warm up the Wood's lamp for 5–10 minutes before it is used, to ensure it is emitting the correct wavelength of light and also to allow sufficient time when viewing an area to allow the fluorescence to develop. The examination should be undertaken in a darkened room to aid recognition of the fluorescence. The animal should be screened thoroughly, including the nails. The eyes of the operator and the patient should not be exposed to ultraviolet light unnecessarily, as it can damage the eyes. Other substances, such as cotton fibres, skin scales and petroleum jelly, can also fluoresce and give false-positive results, but their fluorescence is bluish-white. It takes experience to be able to correctly diagnose *M. canis* infections by this technique.

Microscopic examination

Suspect hairs should be plucked, not clipped, from the edge of the lesion. If the animal is being examined under a Wood's lamp then select the fluorescing hairs. The hairs should be transferred to a clean microscope slide and 10% potassium hydroxide and 1–2 drops of lactophenol cotton blue stain added. A coverslip should be applied and the sample gently heated to clear it. The dye enhances the visibility of the spores. Some dermatologists simply suspend the hair samples in mineral oil.

The specimen is examined under low and then high power. It can be useful to examine a normal hair for comparison. Infected hairs appear broken and damaged. The cortex and cuticle are irregular and have a fuzzy outline because of the presence of the branching hyphae and arthroconidia (spores). The arthroconidia of *M. canis* are small, bead-like and form a dense mosaic pattern on the outside (ectothrix) of the hair shaft. Those of *T. mentagrophytes* are larger and occur as sparse chains (Fig. 29.12). Those of *M. gypseum* are much larger, less numerous and in chains. Care should be taken not to confuse the melanin pigment found within the hair shaft with the fungal growth. The microscopic characteristics of the arthroconidia can be used to identify the ringworm species.

This is probably the most reliable method of diagnosing a dermatophyte infection. Hair samples are plucked as described previously and placed directly on to Sabouraud's dextrose agar or on to dermatophyte test medium (DTM),

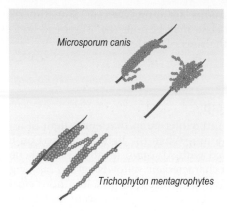

Microsporum canis

Trichophyton mentagrophytes

Fig. 29.12 Fungal spores or arthroconidia along a hair shaft

which contains an indicator system to detect dermatophyte species. In a positive culture the DTM changes colour from yellow to red; this should occur within 3–5 days. The colonies should be checked daily. Non-pathogenic fungi may produce false positives if the incubation period is prolonged. Samples on Sabouraud's dextrose agar should be incubated at room temperature (25–27°C) for 10–14 days, but on occasion this may take as long as 4 weeks.

Colony characteristics:

- *M. canis* – flat, with a white, silky centre and a bright yellow edge. The reverse side is yellow
- *M. gypseum* – flat brown, with a powdery irregular fringe. The reverse side is yellow brown
- *T. mentagrophytes* – flat, granular, tan-coloured or heaped, white, cottony appearance. Reverse side is yellow-red.

Microscopic examination of the arthroconidia will confirm the species identification. The easiest way of transferring the arthroconidia to a microscope slide is by attaching a short length of tape to the end of a spatula or swab and pressing it against the surface of the fungal colony, then applying the tape sticky side down to the surface of the slide. It can then be stained with lactophenol cotton blue stain and examined under the microscope. The arthroconidia of *M. canis* are thick-walled, boat-shaped and have spines at the terminal end that may resemble a knob. Those of *T. mentagrophytes* are cigar-shaped and thin-walled, and the accompanying hyphae are spiral.

Yeasts

The most common species to affect dogs and cats are:

- *Malassezia* **spp**. – can be cultured, by clipping the hair away from the sample site and pressing a culture plate containing a malt-extract-agar-based medium on to the skin for 10 seconds. The plates are then cultured at 32°C for 3 days, when white glistening colonies will be seen and a colony count per square centimetre of skin can be made
- *Candida albicans* – this is a Gram-positive, yeast-like fungus but is best stained with lactophenol cotton blue,

when it appears as oval cells showing replication by budding. It will grow on all routine bacteriological media. On blood agar at 37°C small grey colonies appear after 2–3 days. On Sabouraud's dextrose agar, large, cream-coloured colonies develop that have a yeasty odour.

Body tissues and fluids

Various fluids and tissues can be analysed to monitor the health of the patient.

Cerebrospinal fluid

Examination of cerebrospinal fluid (CSF) can be very useful in diagnosing some neurological conditions. In the dog and cat the normal sampling site is the cisterna magna at the articulation between the atlas and the occipital bone. This technique is similar to the one used for administering contrast material for myelography (see Ch. 30). Occasionally, the lumbosacral space is used.

Technique

1. The animal must be anaesthetized to prevent it moving during the procedure and placed in lateral recumbency with the neck flexed
2. Strict asepsis must be observed to prevent the introduction of bacteria and contamination of the sample
3. The site should be prepared as for a surgical procedure
4. A 20–22 FG spinal needle is carefully inserted and advanced into the subarachnoid space until a sudden decrease in resistance is felt and CSF wells up in the needle hub
5. CSF is allowed to drip into an EDTA and a plain container. The first few drops are discarded, as they often contain mild blood contamination. Suction should not be applied. It is possible to collect 1 ml/5 kg body weight safely.

Synovial fluid

This is collected by **arthrocentesis** from a joint to investigate any joint problems, including arthritis. Depending on the temperament and the degree of pain, a local or general anaesthetic may need to be administered. Aseptic procedures should be observed. Only a relatively small volume of fluid will be obtained and should be initially collected into a plain sample bottle.

Thoracic fluid

Normally the thoracic fluid only contains sufficient fluid to lubricate the thoracic organs and the parietal pleura. Certain clinical conditions can result in accumulation of fluid, of different types, in the thorax, e.g. hydrothorax, pyothorax, haemothorax. The collection of fluid from the thorax, thoracocentesis, can help to determine the nature of the fluid and aid in the diagnosis. Collection is performed aseptically into EDTA and plain tubes (see also Ch. 21).

Abdominal fluid

In certain clinical conditions, fluid accumulates in the abdomen, i.e. ascites, and can be collected by an abdominal paracentesis. Aseptic collection is usually performed at the most dependent part of the ventral midline of the abdomen in the standing animal. Some of the sample is transferred to an EDTA tube for cytology while the rest is placed in plain sample tubes for biochemistry or bacteriology.

Tissue samples, tumour and abdominal organ biopsy

A biopsy is a sample of tissue taken from a live animal for histopathological examination. Various techniques are available including excision, incision, punch, needle and endoscopic biopsies (see Ch. 21).

Preservation

It is important to preserve specimens, as the cells will rapidly undergo autolysis – the digestion of a tissue by its own enzymes.

Various preservatives are available:

- **10% formalin** – this is a 40% solution of formaldehyde gas
- **10% formol saline** – made by diluting formalin in a saline solution. It is the solution most commonly used
- **10% neutral buffered formalin** – also a 10% solution of formalin but buffered to protect against changes in pH and tends to be used in anatomical display specimens
- **Alcohol** – may be used but causes excessive shrinkage and hardness.

Formalin in its various formulations is a hazardous substance as it gives off formaldehyde, a gas that is irritant to the eyes and mucous membranes. It is important that Health and Safety and COSHH regulations are followed and protective clothing is used, including protective glasses, when handling these substances. Ensure any procedures are carried out in a well-ventilated room. Formalin is a strong antiseptic and disinfectant that will preserve tissues by 'fixing' or hardening them.

Important facts to consider when preserving tissues are:

- It takes a long time for formalin to penetrate tissues so ensure the tissue samples are thin wedges
- Use plenty of formalin, i.e. at least 10 times the volume of tissue to be fixed
- Try and take a sample from the junction between healthy and diseased tissue, especially with tumours and excision biopsies. The presence or absence of a capsule can help to determine if the tumour is benign or malignant, which will influence the prognosis
- Use wide-necked sample bottles that allow easy removal of the fixed sample
- Label the container to identify the specimen
- Ensure that the sample bottles are robust and not easily broken, and are sealable to prevent leakage
- Do not send whole organs but small representative samples

- Body fluids can be preserved by making a fixed smear or by adding a drop of formol saline to 1 ml of fluid. This will preserve the morphology of any cells present
- Samples should not be frozen, as this damages the cells.

Toxicological examination

Toxicological samples should be sent to a commercial laboratory for analysis. It is always advisable to ensure that the laboratory is able to perform the tests that are required and the precise nature of the samples required. Usually, from live animals these are blood, faeces, urine and vomit. Samples from dead animals should include blood, urine, stomach and intestinal contents, liver and kidney.

Protocol

- Specimens should be collected free from contaminants, e.g. bedding. If they are contaminated, then a sample of the contamination should be sent in a separate container
- Each sample should be placed in a separate sterile, labelled container
- Unless samples are to be examined histologically, samples should be frozen and despatched with ice
- The samples should be sealed and an identical unused container should be sent to the laboratory
- Preservatives should be avoided. If necessary, alcohol should be used and a sample from the same supply should be sent, as a control, in a separate container
- Accurate records must be kept, as evidence may be needed for possible litigation.

Virological samples

Obviously, the ideal method of virus identification is the isolation and growth of the virus in tissue culture. However, this is time-consuming, expensive and, as the number of viruses is so vast, only research institutes can offer this service. Some of the common viral diseases can now be diagnosed in practice by ELISA tests. These do not involve growing the virus but employ the reaction between an antibody and a specific antigen to indicate the presence of the virus.

It is important when sending virological samples to ascertain which particular type of sample the laboratory requires. These may be blood, nasopharyngeal aspirates, bronchoalveolar lavage samples, swabs, faeces, body fluids, organ smears and ocular discharges. The sample required will depend on the viral disease being investigated, as will the method of sampling and despatch (see also Ch. 29).

Normal equine physiological values

The majority of laboratory diagnostic procedures for horses are carried out using the same protocols as in small animals although consideration must be made regarding sample collection: for instance, the vein of choice for equine venepuncture is the jugular. Here is a brief outline of normal equine physiological values. Please refer to the texts listed in the Bibliography for more extensive details.

Haematological normal values

Total red blood cell count

- Hot-blooded breeds – 6.8–12.9×10^{12}/l
- Cold-blooded breeds – 5.5–9.5×10^{12}/l
- Foals can vary from an initial 8.2–11.0×10^{12}/l at birth, declining to 7.4–10.6 by 7 days of age, then rising to 8.9–12.7×10^{12}/l by the time they are 4 months of age.

Total white blood cell count

- Hot-blooded breeds – 5.4–14.3×10^{9}/l
- Cold-blooded breeds – 6.0–12.0×10^{9}/l
- Foals can vary from an initial 4.9–11.7×10^{9}/l at birth, rising to 6.3–11.6×10^{9}/l at 7 days, then to 6.2–14.2×10^{9}/l by the time they are 4 months of age.

PCV

- Hot-blooded breeds – 32–53%
- Cold-blooded breeds – 8–14%
- Foals – 32–46%.

Haemoglobin

- Hot-blooded breeds – 11–19 g/dl
- Cold-blooded breeds – 8–14 g/dl
- Foals – 12.0–16.66 g/dl at birth, declining to 10.7–15.8 at 7 days, then rising again to 11.6–17.2 by the time they are 4 months old.

Biochemical adult normal values

- Total serum protein – 5.8–7.7 g/dl
- Serum albumin – 2.3–3.6 g/dl
- Cholesterol – 1.94–3.88 mmol/l
- Total bilirubin – 0.5–2.3 μmol/l
- Glucose – 4.9–6.2 mmol/l
- Creatinine – 80–177 μmol/l
- Urea – 2 4.5 mmol/l
- Alkaline phosphatase – 86–285 IU/l
- Aspartate aminotransferase – 138–409 IU/l
- Creatine kinase – 119–287 IU/l.

The values in foals vary with age.

Normal urine parameters

Normal urine production

- Adults 1.24 ml/kg/h
- Foals 6.17 ml/kg/h.

Normal pH

- Adults 7.0–9.0
- Foals 5.5–8.0.

Normal specific gravity

- Adults 1.020–1.050
- Foals 1.004–1.008.

Urinary crystals

Calcium carbonate crystals are the most commonly seen, although struvite and calcium oxalate crystals can be found.

Bibliography

Bush, B.M., 1975. Veterinary Laboratory Manual. Heinemann, London.

Bush, B.M., 1991. Interpretation of Laboratory Results for Small Animal Clinicians. Blackwell Science, Oxford.

Corley, K., Stephen, J. (Eds.), 2008. The Equine Hospital Manual. Blackwell Publishing, Oxford.

Feldman, B.F., Zinkl, J.G., Jain, N.C. (Eds.), 2000. Schalm's Veterinary Hematology, fifth ed. Lippincott Williams and Wilkins, Baltimore.

Kerr, M.G., 2002. Veterinary Laboratory Medicine, second ed. Blackwell Science, Oxford.

Kramer J.W., 2000. Normal Hematology of the Horse. In: Feldman, B.F. et al. Schalm's Veterinary Hematology, 5th ed. Lippincott Williams and Wilkins, Baltimore.

Villiers, E., Blackwood, L. (Eds.), 2005. Manual of Canine and Feline Clinical Pathology, 2nd ed. BSAVA, Gloucester.

Recommended reading

BVA Poster, Good practice guide to handling veterinary waste. Available from: <www.bva.co.uk>.
Well worth a visit.

Papasouliotis, K., 2002. Atlas of Canine Haematology. Nova Professional Media, Oxford.
A super little book that describes normal blood cell morphology in the dog and includes many coloured photographs. It also includes normal ranges of values, haematological definitions and techniques. Other titles in the range cover feline and equine haematology. They are also quite reasonably priced.

Pratt, P.W. (Ed.), 1992. Laboratory Procedures for Veterinary Technicians, second ed. American Veterinary Publications, Santa Barbara, CA.
Although aimed at the American market, this is a very useful book. It describes a wide range of laboratory procedures in a simple descriptive manner and is well illustrated throughout. It also contains information on large animals, including horses.

Villiers, E., Blackwood, L. (Eds.), 2005. Manual of Canine and Feline Clinical Pathology, second ed. BSAVA, Gloucester.
This is a comprehensive guide to laboratory diagnostic practice which is beautifully illustrated throughout.

CHAPTER 30

Principles of diagnostic imaging

Suzanne Easton

Key Points

- The production of an image of an affected area of the body is a useful diagnostic tool and can be achieved by radiography, ultrasound, nuclear scintigraphy, computed tomography and magnetic resonance imaging.
- Radiography is the most common method and makes use of the fact that X-rays, which are part of the electromagnetic spectrum, will create a permanent image on radiographic film.
- X-rays are produced by an X-ray tube as a result of fast-moving electrons released from the cathode colliding with a tungsten anode or target.
- The exposure used to produce a diagnostic image is controlled by the milliamperage (mA), which affects the number of electrons produced from the cathode and thus the quantity of the X-rays produced, and the kilovoltage (kV), which affects the speed at which the electrons move from the cathode to the anode and thus the force with which they hit the anode. This affects the penetrating power or quality of the X-rays produced.
- The X-ray beam may be absorbed by the tissues of the patient, pass straight through to reach the film or be deflected in a different direction with a loss of energy. This deflected radiation is known as scatter.
- Scattered radiation is the main danger of radiography and can be reduced by the use of a grid, accurate collimation, reducing the thickness of the tissue and reducing the voltage as much as possible.
- The Ionizing Radiation Regulations 1999 detail all the measures that must be taken to reduce the dangers of radiation and ensure the safety of personnel within a veterinary practice.
- The latent image formed by the passage of X-rays through the patient to the film is made into a permanent radiographic image by the developing process. This may be achieved by using developing and fixing chemicals within developing tanks or within an automatic processor.
- Correct and accurate positioning of the patient will produce an image from which a diagnosis can be made.
- Contrast media, which may be either negative (i.e. gas) or positive (i.e. barium or iodine preparations), can be used to highlight soft tissues not otherwise visible on plain radiographs.
- Ultrasound uses high-frequency sound waves that are sent into the body by a transducer and, when reflected from interfaces between the tissues, are collected by the transducer and an image forms on a computer screen. It can be used to demonstrate soft tissues, which are not always clearly visible on radiographs, and is painless and non-invasive.
- Computed tomography and nuclear scintigraphy use radiation to create an image, which thus presents safety problems, while magnetic resonance imaging uses a combination of a strong magnetic field and radio waves, so safety is less of an issue.

Introduction

There is no doubt that diagnosis is made easier by the production of 'pictures' of the affected area within the body and nowadays we take it for granted that we are able to do this in several ways. Radiography has been available for many years and is the method used by the majority of veterinary practices.

In recent years, veterinary surgeons have become increasingly experienced in the use of ultrasound for both large and small animals and it has the advantage of being non-invasive and much safer for personnel involved in the process. Other less common techniques include computed tomography (CT) and magnetic resonance imaging (MRI) scans.

Each technique has its advantages and disadvantages, and in order for veterinary nurses to be able to make a contribution to the procedure it is important that they have a thorough understanding of the underpinning physical principles and the practical aspects involved in creating a useful diagnostic image.

Principles of radiography

Physics for radiography

All solids, liquids and gases are composed of elements, or materials that cannot be broken down into something else. The details of all elements known are recorded in the periodic table, which gives full details of every element.

Every element is made up of atoms (Fig. 30.1). These atoms contain a nucleus, composed of neutrons and protons, surrounded by orbiting electrons. Protons are always positively charged; neutrons are neutral and have no charge. The orbiting electrons are always negatively charged (Table 30.1). The electrons orbit the nucleus in shells. Each shell can hold a certain number of electrons. The shell nearest the nucleus will always fill first, working outwards until all the electrons are contained in a shell. If a shell is not completely full it will be the outermost shell and this will be where any interactions take place. For the atom to be stable the outermost shell should be full. The number of electrons should be equal to the number of protons. The number of protons is unique to each element.

In radiography the electrons are used in various ways in the production of X-rays and play an important role in the interactions of X-rays within the body.

The electromagnetic spectrum

X-rays are part of the electromagnetic spectrum. This is composed of energy waves. Contained within the electromagnetic spectrum are radio waves, ultraviolet light, visible light and cosmic rays, as well as X-rays and gamma rays (Fig. 30.2).

Every wave has a different wavelength and frequency. The wavelength is the distance from the peak of one wave to the peak of the next. The frequency is the number of peaks passing a set point every second. Frequency is measured in hertz (Hz). 1 Hz is equal to 1 cycle per second. X-rays have a short wavelength and high frequency.

When electromagnetic radiation is emitted, whether it is from the sun or an X-ray tube, the intensity will decrease as the distance from the source increases. This is known as the **inverse square law**. This is useful in radiation protection. The further away from the X-ray tube you can get, the lower the intensity of X-rays reaching the body and causing damage.

Electrical energy

The production of X-rays is dependent on the provision of electrical energy to the X-ray tube. An electric charge is produced as the electrons of an atom move from the outer shell of one atom to the outer shell of the adjacent atom. This can be done in three main ways:

- **Friction** – electrons build up as two objects are rubbed together
- **Contact** – if two suitable materials make contact, electrons will flow
- **Induction** – this uses the electrical field of a charged object to create a charge in a previously uncharged object.

Table 30.1 Details of the particles within an atom

Particle	Position	Charge	Symbol
Proton	In nucleus	Positive	+
Neutron	In nucleus	Neutral	0
Electron	Orbiting nucleus	Negative	–

An atom

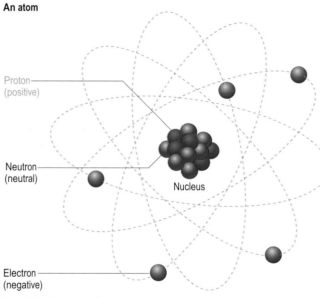

Proton (positive)

Neutron (neutral)

Nucleus

Electron (negative)

Fig. 30.1 Structure of an atom

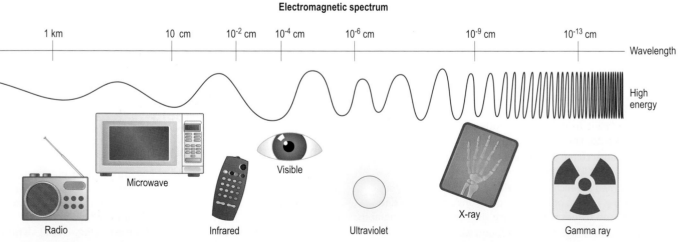

Electromagnetic spectrum

1 km   10 cm 10^{-2} cm 10^{-4} cm 10^{-6} cm 10^{-9} cm 10^{-13} cm   Wavelength

High energy

Radio   Microwave   Infrared   Visible   Ultraviolet   X-ray   Gamma ray

Fig. 30.2 The electromagnetic spectrum

An electric charge will always move from negative to positive. Like charges will repel each other, unlike charges will attract each other. If electrons are able to move easily through the atoms of a material then the material is a conductor. If the electrons cannot move freely or easily then the material is an insulator. All electrical charges have a potential energy and when released, and the electrons move through a material, the energy generated can be used. This electrical potential is measured in volts (V).

An electric current is formed when electrons flow through a conductor. If the electrons flow in one direction, then a direct current (DC) is generated. If the electrons go in alternating directions, then an alternating current (AC) is formed.

X-ray tube construction

Tube structure

The X-ray tube produces the X-rays and is composed of a Pyrex tube surrounding the anode and cathode (Fig. 30.3) The tube contains a vacuum to prevent unwanted interactions during the production of the X-rays. The anode and cathode both have a high-tension electrical supply, providing the direct current necessary to generate X-rays. The Pyrex tube is surrounded by oil to prevent the build-up of heat and lead to prevent X-rays from passing straight out of the tube. The entire structure is surrounded by a lead case, within which is a small window directly under the anode to allow the primary beam to exit the tube. The window has a small aluminium filter to remove any low-energy, undesirable X-rays from the primary beam, improving its quality.

The cathode

The cathode is the negative part of the X-ray tube (Fig. 30.3). The cathode is made up of the filament and focusing cup. The **filament** is a very small piece of wire and is heated to produce electrons in a similar way to the heating filament in a toaster. The filament is made of tungsten, which has a very high melting point. In dual-focus X-ray tubes the cathode has two filament wires. If broad focus is selected, the longer (0.4–1.3 mm) of the two wires will be used; if fine focus is selected the shorter (0.1–0.4 mm) wire will be selected.

The **focusing cup** surrounds the filament wire. The function of the focusing cup is to stream the electrons in a narrow band towards the anode when an exposure is made. The electrons are negatively charged, as is the focusing cup. The focusing cup will repel the electrons to the centre, ensuring that they flow in a narrow band and do not spread out. This ensures that the electrons fall within the target of the anode and do not extend beyond its boundaries.

The anode

The anode is the positive part of the X-ray tube (Fig. 30.3). The anode may be stationary or rotating, depending on whether it remains in one place or rotates during exposure. Stationary anodes are usually found in dental machines and smaller portable machines. In general machines the anode rotates. This allows for the production of high-quality X-rays in a very short period of time, with reduced damage when compared to stationary anodes using similar exposure factors.

The anode conducts electrons away from the tube to the generator, provides support for the target and removes excess heat from the tube. The process of X-ray production results in 99% heat and 1% actual X-rays. The heat must be removed to prevent the anode from melting.

The **target** is the area that the electrons strike. In a rotating tube this is a disc around the entire circle of the target disc. As the target rotates, so the area that the electrons strike changes, increasing the area that the electrons can strike and increasing the lifespan of the tube. If the anode is stationary the whole surface is the target.

The target is made of tungsten alloy embedded in a copper anode. In some tubes the target is supported on molybdenum or graphite to make tube rotation easier. The area actually hit by the electrons is called the **focal spot** and this is

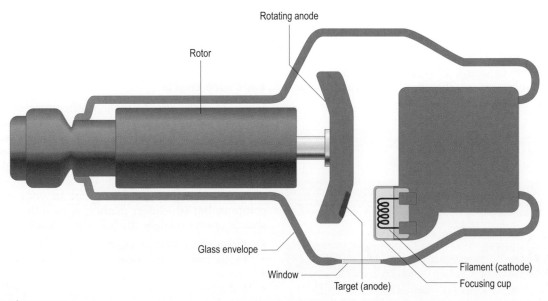

Fig. 30.3 X-ray tube structure

the source of the radiation emitted from the X-ray tube. The effective focal spot that is emitted from the tube will alter depending on the angle of the target. This angle is usually between 7° and 20° to the vertical. As the angle of the target increases, so the effective size of the focal spot increases.

X-ray production

The production of X-rays takes place as the exposure button is fully depressed. In two-stage exposure buttons, the first stage 'preps' the machine, heating the cathode and starting the rotation of the anode; the second stage produces the X-rays, enabling the exposure to be made (Fig. 30.4). The exposure will be terminated immediately if finger pressure on the button is released:

- During the **first stage** the filament at the cathode is heated and the milliamperage selected determines the amount of heating. The higher the milliamperage, the higher the heat and the more electrons produced. Heating releases electrons from the surface of the filament wire. The electrons collect in the focusing cup. These electrons contain electrical potential and, when a charge is applied, will flow from negative to positive (i.e. cathode to anode)
- During the **second stage**, a potential difference is applied between the cathode and anode, ensuring that the electrons flow to the anode. This is achieved by applying a kilovoltage selected when setting the exposure factors. The higher the kilovoltage selected, the faster the electrons will move towards the target, resulting in higher-energy X-rays. The electrons are accelerated from the cathode to the anode and as they strike the target they are stopped. This sudden braking results in the electrons changing into X-rays, which are then released from the X-ray tube through the window.

Exposure factors

The exposure factors selected will alter the resultant image dramatically. The factors that can be altered are the amperage (mA), time (seconds), voltage (kV) and distance.

Amperage

The amperage controls the amount of heat applied to the cathode and changes the quantity of X-rays produced, which affects the density or degree of blackening of the film. As the amperage increases, so the number of electrons and ultimately the number of X-rays produced increases. If the amperage is inadequate the film will appear grey, even in areas where there is no patient to penetrate. In some very large animals it may be necessary to increase the amperage, to produce enough X-rays to blacken the film, as well as the voltage, to ensure adequate penetration.

Time

When setting exposure factors, it is essential to determine a period of time (in seconds) over which to allow the production of X-rays to take place. In the ideal world the time should be as short as possible. This allows limited time for patient movement to occur as even breathing or heart movements can produce blurring on the radiographic image:

Milliamp seconds or mAs – in most machines the amperage and time are combined to provide one exposure factor known as the mAs. When setting the mAs, the time should be as low as possible and the amperage should be as high as possible, i.e. mA × time(s) = mAs.

Voltage

The voltage alters the speed at which the electrons accelerate across the tube and strike the target. The faster the electrons move the higher the energy or penetrating power of the resultant X-rays. The voltage of the beam affects the contrast of the image, i.e. the difference between black and white. If a patient is very small, a low voltage is needed so that the X-rays do not overpenetrate and cause the image to be very dark.

Distance

The focal distance of the film is the distance (usually measured in centimetres) from the target (or source of the X-rays) to the film, and changing it has an effect on the image created. It is usually around 100 cm and should remain constant, as altering it between patients will cause confusion. As the distance increases, so the intensity of the X-ray beam reaching the patient decreases, resulting in underexposed films. This is expressed as the inverse square law.

If a new table or X-ray tube support is purchased and the distance has to be altered, then the mAs must be adjusted to allow for the change. This can be calculated using the following equation:

$$\text{Old mAs} \times (\text{new distance}^2 / \text{old distance}^2) = \text{new mAs}.$$

Exposure charts

Exposure charts should be kept wherever possible. The use and provision of an exposure chart is outlined in the Ionizing Radiation Regulations 1999 (see Chapter 3) and by referring to it you should achieve accurate, reproducible exposures and reduce the need for repeat exposure because of incorrect exposure setting. The chart may be taken from a purpose-designed book or kept in your own preruled columns; but whichever method is used the exposure chart should always contain the following details:

- Patient breed/size/weight
- Projection, i.e. position
- Distance
- Voltage
- mAs

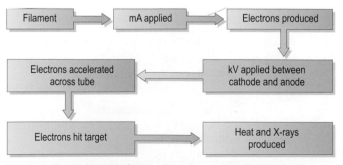

Fig. 30.4 The production of X-rays. Flow diagram from Easton 2002, page 44

- Film–screen combination
- Grid (if used).

If there is more than one X-ray tube or grid in use, then specific details should be given to avoid confusion. The exposure chart should be regularly updated. Patients vary in size and a 15 kg bulldog has different exposure needs from a 15 kg border collie. Consider the area of interest and the patient's conformation before automatically setting what has been listed in the exposure chart. If barium sulphate is used for an examination, the voltage must be increased to counteract the X-ray absorption by barium due to its high atomic number. If this is not done, the high contrast generated will provide a suboptimal image.

Effects of radiation

Properties of X-rays

X-rays are part of the electromagnetic spectrum and have a wide range of properties which may affect their use:

- **Direction of travel** – X-rays will always travel in straight lines, giving a true representation of the patient or objects they pass through. The only time they can change direction is if they collide with an atom, which may degrade the image
- **Ionization** – X-rays can interact with tissues and cause ionization, which occurs when atoms become positively charged through the loss of an electron in the outer shell. This fact is used to form the image on the film and is the effect that causes absorption of the X-rays within the body. However, ionization can cause damage to cells, including burns and the induction of cancer, and is the reason for the need for radiation protection
- **Penetration** – X-rays are able to pass through most types of solid matter and this is used in radiography to form an image on a film. If the amount of matter is increased, the X-rays will eventually be absorbed and stopped. The denser the object the more easily the X-rays will be stopped. This property is used in radiation protection
- **Divergence** – as the X-ray beam travels from the target it will lose intensity and will also spread out, following the inverse square law. This is used in radiation protection to reduce the risk and should be considered when setting the focal film distance, to ensure consistent radiographs
- **Absorption** – as the X-rays pass through the patient they may be stopped or slowed down by the tissues in the patient. If a tissue is very dense, e.g. bone, then the X-rays will be stopped – the tissue is described as being **radiopaque**. If a tissue is much less dense, e.g. lung, it will not stop the X-rays and they will pass through – the tissue is described as being **radiolucent**. The amount of absorption depends on the atomic number of the tissue. The higher the atomic number the more absorption that will occur. For example, bone is mainly composed of calcium and has a higher atomic number than lung tissue, which is composed of a high proportion of air; bone absorbs more X-rays than lung

tissue and appears white on the radiograph while lung tissue appears black (Fig. 30.5)
- **Photographic effect** – X-rays interact with the silver halides within the X-ray film to form an image. They also cause certain phosphors to emit light or fluoresce, the principle used in intensifying screens. Within radiographic film, the more X-rays that strike the silver halide crystals the greater the reaction and the whiter the appearance on the processed radiograph.

Scattered radiation

Scattered radiation or 'scatter' is the reduction in energy of the primary beam and movement of X-rays in a different direction after interaction with matter. It may have a detrimental effect on the resultant image as it darkens the film causing 'fogging' and is also a major factor in the need for radiation protection. As the X-rays have lost energy they are more likely to be absorbed than the primary beam which passes straight through with minimal absorption.

Sources of scattered radiation

Scatter is caused whenever X-rays interact with matter and this increases:

- As the patient or the region under investigation gets thicker – i.e. the thicker the body part the more chance there is for the X-rays to interact with the electrons within the patient and result in scatter
- If the collimator is not used effectively – the larger the area irradiated the more chance there is of the X-ray photons interacting and being scattered
- With the use of higher voltages – these produce X-rays with higher energy, which will have detrimental effects on the image. This scattered radiation is also more likely to travel in a forward direction and reach the film, causing fogging.

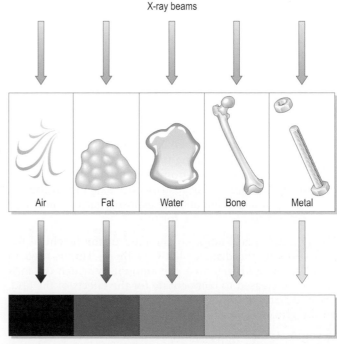

Fig. 30.5 Difference in absorption shown by different types of tissue

Control of scattered radiation

Scattered radiation should be minimized to increase radiation protection and to prevent it from affecting the film and degrading the image. This can be done in a number of ways:

- If the **thickness of a patient** is very large the area under examination can be compressed to reduce the amount of tissue that the X-rays have to pass through, reducing the chances for interaction to occur. This is especially useful in abdominal radiography of the larger patient. A compression band placed across the abdomen will reduce the thickness, improving contrast and reducing scatter
- **Collimation of the primary beam** will reduce the area exposed to radiation, which improves safety, reduces the volume of tissue exposed and reduces scatter. Collimation will improve image quality and contrast. It is achieved through the use of a collimator or light beam diaphragm, usually on the tube head mounting. This is constructed of a box containing a series of mirrors and a light source. The mirrors and light allow a beam of light to be projected on to the patient, which represents the area and position of the primary beam. The area of primary beam can be reduced using bevelled lead leaves within the collimator
- **Reducing the voltage** as much as possible, while still achieving a diagnostic image, will also reduce scatter.

As well as reducing the amount of scattered radiation produced, it is also important to reduce the amount reaching the film and thus decreasing the image quality. This can be achieved in two ways:

- **The air gap technique** – useful when imaging large animals such as horses, as scatter will result in magnification and 'unsharpness' of the image. The aim is to increase the object film distance (i.e. the distance between the patient and the film), so that the scatter generated within the patient is not able to reach the film and form an image
- **Grids** – efficient tools in the reduction of scattered radiation reaching the film. They are able to remove 85–95% of all scattered radiation, depending on the type used. A grid is constructed of alternating strips of a material able to absorb radiation, e.g. lead, and a radiolucent interspace, usually aluminium or carbon plastic fibres (Fig. 30.6) The interspacer allows the primary beam to pass through to the film but any scattered radiation hitting the lead strips will be absorbed, preventing it from reaching the film and causing fogging. The lead strips will also absorb some of the primary beam and the exposure factors must be increased to compensate for this.

The grid has a grid ratio, i.e. the ratio of the height of the lead strips to the distance between them. This is used to calculate the grid factor, i.e. the amount by which the mAs must be increased to compensate for the effects of the grid. The grid factor is usually between 2 and 6 and will be marked on the grid.

New mAs (when using a grid) = old mAs (without a grid) × grid factor.

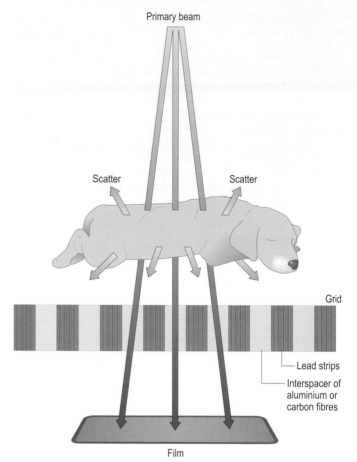

Fig. 30.6 Function of a grid

The grid must be placed between the patient and the film. There are a number of different types of grid:

- **Parallel grid** – this is the most common type in use in veterinary practice and is usually stationary, i.e. it does not move. It is the easiest to use and as long as the grid is at 90° to the primary beam and straight it will produce a good result
- **Potter–Bucky grids** – parallel grids are sometimes integrated into the X-ray table and move rapidly from side to side with the aid of a small motor. This movement eliminates the very fine lines usually visible when a stationary grid is used.

Radiation safety

Radiation can be harmful to those working with it and the use of radiation to form a diagnosis should be minimized. The risk of exposure to radiation should be balanced by the benefits of forming a diagnosis. All examinations must be clinically justified and the safety of the radiographer and anyone else around should always be the first priority.

The effects of radiation

X-rays will interact with the tissues within the human body, causing ionization in which the tissue molecules can be broken or damaged. This process may cause the cells to damage each other, or the X-ray itself may damage the cells or DNA within the body. The body is capable of repairing the damage, but sometimes it may be so severe that repair is impossible and the cells will die. Rapidly dividing and developing cells are most susceptible and most likely to be damaged, e.g. hair, nails, the cells of young people or developing fetuses. The most common effect of damage is called a **stochastic effect**. This can happen with any level of radiation but the incidence increases as the level of exposure increases and it results in damage and mutation to the cells.

Safety legislation

The use of ionizing radiation is carefully controlled in the UK and is laid down in guidelines governed by the Ionizing Radiation Regulations 1999 (IRR)(see also Ch. 3). These regulations indicate all procedures that should be adhered to when using sources of radiation, how exposure to patients should be minimized, and the measures radiographers and employers should take to ensure optimal safety at all times. The ALARP principle, i.e. ' as low as reasonably practicable', is the basis for these regulations and should be remembered at all times. If these regulations are not followed individuals may be prosecuted.

Radiation protection in practice

In practice radiation protection involves reducing the dose used to produce the radiograph and the dose to staff. Within a practice the radiation protection supervisor (RPS) will ensure that local rules described in the IRR are adhered to and that the regulations are implemented. They are helped by a radiation protection advisor (RPA), who is from outside the practice and who will set up the local rules and ensure that the practice maintains a high standard of safety.

Basic measures to reduce dose include suitable collimation at all times and the use of intensifying screens, eliminating the need for high exposure factors. The dose to staff should be reduced as much as possible and there are a number of very easy ways this can be achieved (Table 30.2).

Dosimetry

All individuals exposed to radiation should be monitored by the use of dosimeters, which measure the dose of radiation received by the body. Every radiographic procedure will result in a dose being received by the patient and potentially by the radiographer if they remain in the room. The staff dose should be monitored and recorded through the use of monitoring devices, in the form of either badges containing film or thermoluminescent dosimeters. These should always be worn on the trunk of the body, under any lead protection, and should be looked after according to the supplier's instructions. They should be returned to the supplier at regular intervals so that the dose received can be read and recorded. If an individual has received more than the maximum permissible dose, it may be recommended that that person is taken off radiography work for a few months and changes may need to be made to the practice. It is unlikely that a veterinary nurse will ever reach this dose level.

Table 30.2 Methods by which the dangers of radiation may be reduced in practice

Method of reduction	How it works
Avoid the primary beam	The primary beam is the most intense part of the X-ray beam. If you must stay in the room, you should be at least 2 m away. The primary beam should never be directed at the lead screen within the room or at the door. Even when wearing lead gloves, hands should never be placed in the primary beam
Avoid manual restraint	Patients should not be manually restrained unless there is no alternative. With the use of modern drugs for sedation or anaesthesia, pads and the use of positioning aids, a diagnostic image can be produced in most patients without the need for personnel to hold them
Lead protection	Lead aprons and thyroid shields should be used whenever an individual needs to remain in the X-ray room. Lead aprons will only protect effectively against scattered radiation and the 2 m rule should be remembered. Attempts should always be made to leave the room or use a lead screen to hide behind rather than remaining in the room during exposure
Restricting access	Always ensure that the doors to the X-ray room are closed. This will prevent people wandering into the room, disturbing the patient and potentially being exposed to radiation. By closing the doors any scattered radiation will be contained within the room

Recording the image

The image created by the X-rays passing through the patient and reaching the film must be able to be recorded for diagnostic use and stored for many years. Recording the image requires the use of film and intensifying screens.

Radiographic film

Radiographic film is sensitive to both light and X-rays. The film is used to receive X-rays that have passed through the patient and convert them into a latent image. This is then converted into a visible or radiographic image during processing. The film is also sensitive to light, which may reach the film intentionally from the intensifying screens or unintentionally from exposure to daylight.

X-ray film is made up of a number of layers, all providing a vital role in the composition and function of the film (Fig. 30.7). It may be described as being either duplitized or single-sided. In duplitized film the layers are duplicated on either side of the polyester base, which increases its efficiency, resulting in a lower radiation dose to the patient. Single-sided film has an active side and a protective, counterbalanced side to prevent curling (Table 30.3).

Care and storage of X-ray film

X-ray film should be stored for the minimum amount of time and not beyond the expiry date. Stock should be rotated

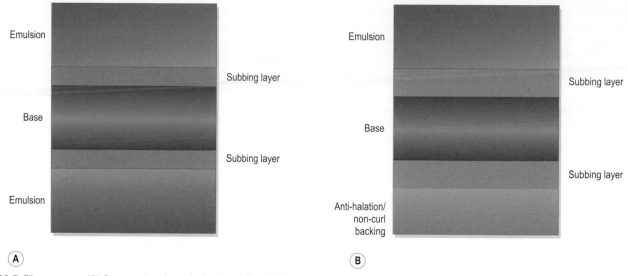

Fig. 30.7 Film structure. (**A**) Cross-section through duplitized film. (**B**) Cross-section through single-sided film

Table 30.3 Structure of radiographic film

Layer	Film type	Structure and function
Base	Single-sided Duplitized	Made of polyester Clear plastic to allow transmission of light Flexible to allow handling Does not react to chemicals
Subbing layer	Single-sided Duplitized	Provides adhesive to attach the emulsion to the base layer
Emulsion	Single-sided – one emulsion layer Duplitized – two emulsion layers on either side of the base	Composed of gelatin impregnated with silver halide crystals. Silver halides react with X-rays and light to form the latent image Liquid gelatin is used for easy application, semi-solid during processing to allow chemical penetration and solid after processing for storage
Supercoat	Single sided – one supercoat Duplitized – two supercoat layers	Thin layer of gelatin that protects the emulsion during and after processing
Anti-curl layer	Single-sided	Duplitized film has equal amounts of emulsion on both sides of the base that absorb liquid and swell equally during processing so curling is not a problem Single-sided film has an anti-curl layer to balance the curling effects of the swollen emulsion. This prevents damage to the film

so that the oldest is used first. Ideally, small orders should be placed frequently to maintain optimal film quality.

All films should be handled carefully and stored vertically to prevent pressure marks occurring. These appear as black crescents if created during handling and black lines if created during storage.

The room used for film storage should be well-ventilated, with a temperature within the range given on the film box by the manufacturers. It is not ideal to store the film in the same room as open processing chemicals or anywhere that may be exposed to radiation.

Forming the radiographic image

The radiographic image is the visible image formed from the latent image by processing. Processing involves a chain reaction that starts when the film is exposed to light and/or X-rays. The film contains silver halide crystals that are sensi-

tive to light and X-rays. In conventional film the silver halide is usually silver bromide. The manufacturers usually introduce a spot called the sensitivity speck that assists in the processing. Within the emulsion the silver and bromide ions form a lattice that becomes charged as the silver loses an electron, enabling it to bond with the bromine. During exposure the X-rays and light will cause a reaction that makes the silver migrate towards the sensitivity speck and the bromine to be released. The more silver that moves and the more bromine that is given off, the blacker the final radiograph will appear. Areas where the X-rays or light do not reach at all will have no reaction.

Film speed

Film speed is defined as the sensitivity of the film to light or radiation and is related to the density, i.e. degree of blackening of the image. Film speed is dependent on the size of the silver halide crystals in the emulsion and the thickness of the emulsion. Fast films require less exposure than slow films to produce the same density of film. As the film speed increases, so the density of the image increases. If the same density of image is required then it is the mAs that must be changed if the film speed is changed, i.e. if a faster film is used, reduce the mAs to produce a similar diagnostic image. However, fast films produce an image with poorer definition, while slow films, which require a longer exposure, produce a more highly defined image. Slower films are used for extremity radiography, e.g. feet carpus, to ensure that the necessary bone detail is shown.

Intensifying screens

Intensifying screens are designed to fluoresce, i.e. emit light, when exposed to X-rays. As the film is sensitive to both X-rays and light, use of an intensifying screen allows for a lower X-ray exposure to be used to form a diagnostic image.

Intensifying screens are contained within a cassette. In cassettes where duplitized films are used there are two separate screens, one on either side of the cassette. In single-sided cassettes there is one intensifying screen on the back of the cassette. The film is sandwiched between the intensifying screens or between the intensifying screen and the front of the cassette.

Construction of an intensifying screen

An intensifying screen (Fig. 30.8) is made up of the following layers:

1. Base (support layer):
- Back of intensifying screen
- Supports the intensifying screen
- Made of cardboard or polyester
- Moisture-resistant
- Flexible
- Does not interfere with the passage of X-rays through to the phosphor layer and film.

2. Reflecting layer:
- Made of magnesium oxide or titanium dioxide
- Redirects stray light emitted from the intensifying screen to improve image quality
- Increases effectiveness of the intensifying screen.

3. Fluorescent phosphor layer:
- Active part of the intensifying screen
- Layer of tiny phosphor crystals suspended in a binder of polyurethane

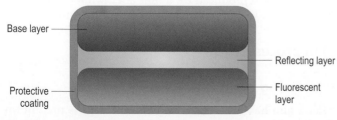

- Phosphor crystals are either rare earth or calcium tungstate
- Crystals held together and protected from moisture
- Dye to absorb stray light.

4. Protective coating:
- Outer layer of the intensifying screen
- Protects the phosphor layer against abrasions, moisture and staining
- Reduces static
- Will survive routine cleaning
- Extends around the back of the screen to prevent curling.

Luminescence

When the phosphor grain is bombarded by X-rays, fluorescence, i.e. the emission of light, and phosphorescence, i.e. the afterglow, occur. Fluorescence occurs when the X-rays pass through the phosphor layer. The interaction excites the phosphor crystals and they emit ultraviolet and visible light. The visible light is used to form the image on the radiographic film. The phosphor will emit hundreds of light photons for every X-ray photon that strikes it. Rare earth intensifying screens will convert 15–20% of all X-rays to light, while the calcium tungstate used in more old-fashioned types of screen will convert approximately 4% of all X-rays to light. This conversion ensures a reduction in the exposure needed to form a diagnostic image on the film, which in turn reduces the dose to the patient and to the staff.

Film–screen combinations

To ensure that the light emitted from an intensifying screen is utilized fully, the wavelength or colour of the light emitted from the intensifying screen must match the light sensitivity of the film. Calcium tungstate intensifying screens will emit blue light, so the film must be sensitive to blue light and these films are described as being **monochromatic**. Rare earth screens usually emit green light, although some types emit blue light, and so the film used should be sensitive to both blue and green light. This is known as **orthochromatic** film. If the film sensitivity is not matched to the light emitted by the screen the beneficial effects of the intensifying screen will be reduced.

Intensifying screen speed

The speed of an intensifying screen describes the relative exposure needed by different types of screen to produce images of a similar density (Table 30.4). The faster the screen the lower the exposure needed to form an image. The screen speed is determined by the **size of the phosphor grain**, the **thickness of the intensifying screen layer** and the **presence or absence of a reflective layer**.

Single screens

Single screens function in exactly the same way as double intensifying screens but have half the intensifying factor. They were developed for use in human mammography and

Base layer

Protective coating

Reflecting layer

Fluorescent layer

Fig. 30.8 Structure of an intensifying screen

Table 30.4 Types of intensifying screen

Intensifying screen	Speed	Uses
High-resolution	Slow (100)	Fine detail. Needs a higher exposure. Ideal for extremity work
Regular	Medium (400)	General radiography
Fast	Fast (800)	Produces a darker image for given exposure factors. Allows for a reduction in exposure time to reduce movement problems

are ideal for extremity work, where the demonstration of fine detail is essential. It should be ensured that the light emission from the intensifying screen matches the film sensitivity and also that the film emulsion is in close contact with the intensifying screen.

Film–screen contact

If a sharp image is to be achieved there must be good contact between the film and the screen. Damaged or old cassettes may have curved screens, which will result in blurring of the image where there is reduced contact. This is due to the divergence in the beam between being emitted from the intensifying screen and reaching the film. Cassettes that produce a blurred image should be checked and replaced if necessary.

Care of intensifying screens

Screens should be carefully cleaned on a regular basis. Dirt will show up as bright, white specks on the processed radiograph because the light is blocked from reaching the film after emission by the dirt and dust. Cotton wool should never be used to clean an intensifying screen and a preparatory screen cleaner should be used whenever possible. The intensifying screen should not be saturated with liquid and all cleaning movements should be gentle. The cassette should be dried thoroughly by standing it on its end before it is used again.

Radiographic cassettes

Intensifying screens are contained within a protective cassette and the film is sandwiched between the screens. The cassette ensures that light cannot reach the film and ensures good film–screen contact at all times.

Each cassette is made up of the following parts:

1. Front:
- Uniform thickness
- Conforms to BS4304/1968
- Aluminium equivalent of less than 0.2 mm
- Made from plastic or carbon
- Lightweight
- Low absorption of the primary beam, i.e. allows most of it to pass through to the film inside.

2. Back:
- Similar material to the front
- Lead strips to protect the film from back scatter
- Foam pad under the intensifying screen to hold the film in place and ensure film–screen contact.

3. Closure:
- Strong closing mechanism
- Usually a clip or plastic locking bar
- Good closure ensures light proofing and film–screen contact.

Care of cassettes

- Always treat them gently – they are expensive to replace
- Do not drop them
- They are relatively heavy so only carry a few at a time
- Avoid excessive dampness and water exposure
- Store upright to prevent bending and damage
- Use a numbering system to identify damaged or dirty cassettes.

Digital imaging

Digital imaging is becoming more common in veterinary practice, although currently cost is a limiting factor. It should be emphasized that the image is still formed by X-rays so an X-ray machine is still used and radiation safety or personnel must still be considered.

Digital imaging has a number of benefits:

- Digital sensors are used to form an image without the need for radiographic film
- Immediate image display
- High-quality images
- Images may be enhanced to overcome any incorrect exposure factors
- Images may be altered to show different windows and the windows can be varied to show, for example, just bone, just soft tissue or both
- Dose of radiation to patient and veterinary personnel is kept to a minimum
- Images can be e-mailed to other vets' computers for a second opinion without the need to post bulky films.

Diagnostic information is collected from the patient by using a charged couple device, which is placed under the patient as a cassette would be. The device detects the X-rays as they fall on to its surface and stores the pattern formed until it is placed into the reader. The data is then analysed by a computer and converted into an image, which is viewed on a monitor.

All images are stored on optical disk, zip disk or CD-ROM, which reduces storage space. If a hard copy is required, the image can be reproduced on a film laser printer to produce a radiograph, which can then be viewed in the normal way.

Film processing

Processing cycle

After a film has been exposed, a **latent image** is present on the film, but to turn this into a visible or **radiographic image** the film must be processed. Regardless of whether this is done manually or by an automatic processor, the cycle is the same (Fig. 30.9).

1. Developer

This is always the first stage:

- In the developer solution there are two active developing agents, hydroquinone and phenindone, both of which reduce exposed silver bromide crystals to metallic silver, which is deposited on the film and appears black. Unexposed silver bromide crystals will not be affected by the developer solution
- The developer also contains a preservative to slow oxidation and a lid should always be kept on the developer solution to help reduce oxidation as much as possible
- An accelerator maintains the pH of the developer. The pH is usually 9.6–10.0, i.e. it is alkaline
- Chemical fogging is reduced using a restrainer, which will improve the selectivity of the developer, ensuring that a minimal number of unexposed silver halide crystals are reduced
- As the developer is used, calcium sludge builds up, reducing the effectiveness of the developer. To reduce this a sequestering agent is added
- All the chemicals are dissolved in a solvent. In this case the solvent is water, as it is readily available and cheap. The water will also dissolve all the by-products of processing. The emulsion is softened by water and this allows the developer to penetrate the film surface more easily.

2. Wash

Between the developer and the fixer stages excess developer must be removed from the film surface. In manual processing this is done by rinsing the film in the small wash tank between the developer and the fixer tanks. In an automatic processor, developer is removed by squeegee rollers and there is usually no intermediate wash.

3. Fixer

This stops development and forms a permanent image on the film. The solution converts unexposed silver bromide

into a form that can be washed off the film. This is known as conversion:

- The fixer contains a fixing agent that will diffuse into the emulsion and react with the unexposed silver bromide crystals that remain on the film after development. The fixing agent is usually ammonium thiosulphate, which changes the unexposed areas of the film from a milky white colour to transparent
- The fixing agent is dissolved in a solvent, usually water, which allows the chemical to pass into the film emulsion
- An acidifier stops development. This neutralizes the alkaline developer and prevents further development and dichroic fog
- Sodium acetate is used as a buffer to maintain the pH to within 0.2 of the manufacturer's predetermined levels
- Decomposition of the fixer is prevented using sodium sulphite
- Damage to the film is prevented by the addition of a hardener to the fixer solution, which also helps it to dry efficiently
- The hardener produces insoluble compounds that form sludge on the bottom of the tank. This sludge formation is reduced and prevented using an antisludging agent, usually boric acid.

4. Wash

The processed film then passes through a wash tank. If the film is being manually processed, this usually consists of running water for at least 10 minutes. In an automatic processor another set of rollers takes the film through a tank of water for about 10–20 seconds. The wash prevents the continuing action of the processing chemicals and deterioration of the image quality during storage.

5. Drying

The final stage of processing is to dry the film, allowing it to be viewed and stored. During the processing cycle the film absorbs water and this makes the emulsion 'mushy'. If the emulsion were not dried this layer would be easily removed and would decrease the image quality. In an automatic processor, drying takes about 25 seconds and is usually preceded by squeegee rollers, which remove as much excess water as possible from the surface of the film. The film is then dried using hot air at 50–60°C blown on to the film. In a manual system the film has to be hung up in a clean, dry environment and steps must be taken to prevent hairs or dirt coming into contact with the film.

Automatic processors

Automatic processors carry the film through a number of tanks using a series of rollers (Fig. 30.10). The dry-to-dry time is usually 2–4 minutes, depending on the type of processor, compared with a minimum of 50 minutes with a manual processor and drying cabinet.

The film enters the processor through a film feed system. This grasps the film and takes it into the developer roller through a guide roller. The film passes through a number of

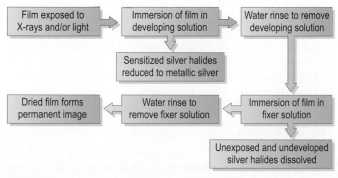

Fig. 30.9 Processing cycle from Easton 2002, page 73

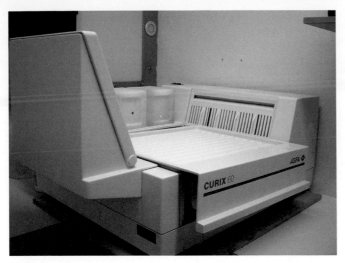

Fig. 30.10 An automatic processor

- Remove top rollers and clean
- Remove wash, developer and fixer rollers and clean thoroughly with running water
- Check movement on all sets of rollers by manually turning the roller
- Check that chemicals are being replenished by the machine's system
- Clean the drier rollers with a damp cloth
- Record all maintenance performed.

Monthly care

- Repeat daily and weekly programme
- Strip entire processor down to the basics and clean all tanks and rollers with a sponge and running water
- Close drain valves
- Check movement of rollers
- Replace all chemicals (unless using an automixer).

Replenishment

The chemicals used within a processor will become tired and less active as time progresses. To ensure that the machine is working at optimum levels, the processing chemicals should be replaced on a regular basis. At least every 6 weeks all the chemicals should be replaced with fresh solutions. As the developer and fixer work, they produce by-products, which will dilute the concentration of the processing chemicals over time. Developer solution will also oxidize in air and this further reduces its activity.

In an automatic processor the chemicals are replaced each time a film enters the machine. A small amount of solution, depending on the film size, will be removed automatically and replaced by fresh chemicals. Within the machine is either a reservoir or a series of small bottles to store a small reserve of chemical.

Maximum efficiency can be achieved by the use of an automixer which mixes stores and dispenses developer and fixer into the processor whenever required. This is ideal in situations where the throughput is large and is much cleaner and safer than the use of small bottles or a reservoir in the processor itself.

Silver recovery

During the fixing stage, metallic silver is produced and this can be recovered and recycled. There are a number of methods of recovering the silver in fixer. If used fixer is collected for disposal by a specialized firm then this process is already in place but if the fixer is disposed of down the drain then a small silver recovery unit may be installed to remove the silver before disposal. A specialist firm can then recycle the silver collected. Films also contain metallic silver that can be recycled. The process of silver recovery is not expensive and the collection and recycling charges are usually covered by the value of the silver recovered.

The darkroom

With the introduction of automatic processors that function in daylight, the need for a darkroom is decreasing. However, many practices store film, load cassettes or keep

rollers, all of which press the processing chemical into the emulsion, ensuring even and adequate coverage. To eliminate the need for a gear system the tanks are varying depths, so that the time spent in each tank is correct for the solution it contains. The developer tank is usually the deepest; the wash tank is the shallowest and the film spends the shortest time here.

The water used within the processor helps to maintain a constant temperature. If the temperature fluctuates, image quality will be low and inconsistent. Water is also used in the wash tank – usually cold, as warmer water will encourage the growth of algae, which is not ideal.

All processing chemicals should be collected in special containers and sent to a specialist company for disposal. If this is not possible, processing chemicals can be disposed of down a normal drain but care must be taken to ensure dilution and adherence to local bye-laws regarding drainage. The disposal of processing chemicals is controlled by the Deposit of Poisonous Waste Act 1972.

Care of an automatic processor

An automatic processor should be looked after carefully. Before planning a maintenance regime it is important to read the manufacturer's instructions as machines vary. A cleaning regime should be implemented to ensure it is always functioning to the highest level possible.

Daily care

- Pass an old film through an automatic processor before use to pick up any debris on the rollers
- Check levels of chemicals in tanks
- Check operating temperature
- Remove any visible chemical deposits
- Remove lid to allow circulation of air when not in use
- Wipe any rollers above the solution levels
- Insert antifungal tablet to wash tanks at the end of the day.

Weekly care

- Repeat daily programme
- Drain and scrub the wash tanks

the processor in the darkroom, so when setting one up there are several factors to be considered:

- The room should be easily accessible to all areas of the practice and should be large enough to allow safe movement when the lights are switched off
- It should not be damp or humid, as this will affect the films, and it should have a reliable source of electricity and running water
- Films and chemicals should not be stored in the same area, as the chemicals may cause fogging of the films. The darkroom should not be exposed to radiation in any way, especially if this is where film is stored
- The whole room should be painted a light colour to reflect as much light as possible into the room
- The surfaces should be washable to allow easy removal of spillages
- The room should be well-ventilated to ensure the comfort of staff and prevent deterioration of the film quality
- A method should be in place to prevent anyone entering when the room is in use and causing possible light fogging of the film, e.g. a warning light on the outside, a double-door system or a lock (but make sure the door can be opened from the outside in an emergency).

Safelights

A safelight is needed in the darkroom to prevent white light fogging the film during handling prior to processing while still allowing the radiographer to move safely around the room.

Safelights usually have a red filter but vary according to the colour sensitivity of the film. White light is a combination of red, blue and green light. A red filter allows only red light through, so if the film is sensitive to blue or green light it will be unaffected.

The safelight should be at least 2 m from the work surface and should have no more than a 15 watt bulb. There are two types:

- **Direct safelight** – sometimes known as a beehive safelight; directs light downwards on to work surfaces
- **Indirect safelight** – projects light upwards on to the ceiling; it is then reflected back down into the room.

Radiographic quality and image interpretation

Describing and viewing an image

Radiographs should always be positioned, viewed and described in a systematic and conventional manner.

There are a number of rules to remember when you are viewing a processed radiograph:

- A radiograph should be viewed on a proper viewing box – not against a window or strip light
- A lateral radiograph should always be viewed with the head to the left, the tail to the right
- Ventrodorsal and dorsoventral radiographs should be viewed as if you are shaking hands with them, i.e. the left of the animal is on your right.

- An extremity should be viewed so that the proximal end of the region is at the top of the viewing box
- Correct anatomical descriptions should be used whenever possible
- Try to describe the image so that it could be seen in the mind of someone who is not able to see the radiograph
- Use familiar objects to describe the appearance and size of areas seen on the radiograph, e.g. walnut-sized, pea-sized, appearance of a bunch of grapes.

Assessing the radiograph

When assessing the quality of a processed radiograph, consider the following points. If all these headings are examined and analysed, then low-quality, non-diagnostic radiographs will not be passed for scrutinization:

- Correct and visible identification
- Anatomical markers and legends correct and visible
- Area under examination shown
- Correct projection taken
- Suitable exposure factors used for area under examination
- Adequate contrast, density and sharpness
- Suitable collimation, accurate but not too tight
- Artefacts (lead, collar, mud, wet coat, contrast medium)
- Anatomical variants or pathology that may need an alteration of exposure factors
- Good overall image quality
- Need for further projections or repeat radiographs.

A radiograph should be assessed using the following criteria:

- **Latitude** – describes the range of exposures that will ensure that a diagnostic image is possible. If a film has wide latitude there is a greater range of exposure factors that will produce a diagnostic image. Films with wide latitude will have a longer grey scale than films with narrow latitude
- **Density** – describes the amount of blackening seen on a radiographic film. This degree of blackening is related to the specific gravity and the atomic number of the subject under examination. If the subject area has a high atomic number, e.g. the bone in the pelvis of a large dog, then the X-rays' photons will interact with the tissue and very few X-rays will reach the radiographic film, creating a white image. If the area under examination is air-filled, and thus has a low specific gravity and atomic number, there will be less interaction with the X-ray photons and more will reach the film, resulting in more blackening of the film (Table 30.5)
- **Contrast** – the difference in density, i.e. degree of blackening, between two adjacent structures. If the image has lots of grey but very little black and white, it is described as being a low-contrast image or a 'flat-film'. If there is little grey but lots of black and white, the image is said to be a high-contrast image (Fig. 30.11), often described as 'soot and whitewash'.

Table 30.5 Appearance of tissues on a radiograph related to their specific gravity and atomic number

Tissue	Specific gravity	Atomic number	Appearance on radiograph
Bone	High	High	White
Water/muscle	Medium/high	High	Grey
Fat	Low/medium	Low	Grey
Air	Low	Low	Black

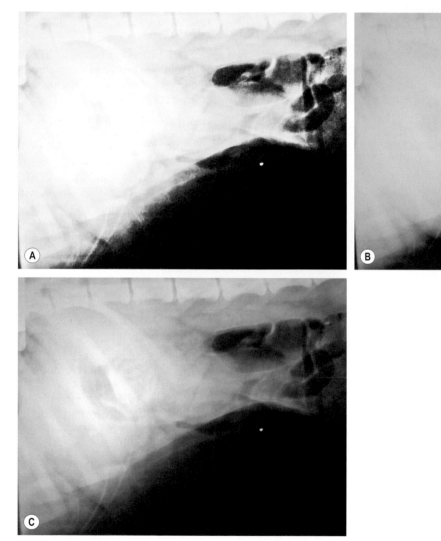

Fig. 30.11 Radiographs showing different levels of contrast. (**A**) High contrast. (**B**) Low contrast. (**C**) Acceptable

Contrast is influenced by a number of factors:

- **Tissue specific gravity and atomic number** – an increase in atomic number and specific gravity will result in more X-ray photons being absorbed. A higher voltage will ensure adequate penetration and an overall increase in contrast
- **Voltage** – low voltage will produce an image with high contrast (very black and white); as the voltage increases so the amount of contrast increases, providing a greater range of greys and less black and white

- **Object shape and thickness** – if an area is very thin it will absorb fewer X-rays and will lead to an image with minimal contrast, e.g. in abdominal radiographs of very small cats. The resultant image may demonstrate a grey abdomen with no definition of the internal organs because of the limited contrast
- **Film fogging** – fogging results in an overall greyness and a reduction in contrast and may be due to poor film storage, incorrect processing, scattered radiation or exposure to light.

Table 30.6 Most common film faults

Image problem	Description	Reason	Solution
Image is too dark	Film is overexposed Background is blackened as well as the image	Voltage and/or mAs too high Film has been fogged by light or radiation Overdevelopment caused by increased developer temperature or increased time	Reduce exposure factors Eliminate light or radiation source Check temperature of processing chemicals and the time that film remains in solution
Image is too pale	Exposed parts of background are black	The film is underexposed as it has not received enough X-rays	Increase exposure factors
	Exposed parts of the background are pale as well	The film is underdeveloped	Ensure that developer is fresh, warm enough and that the film is in solution for enough time
Film is yellow/brown	May have powdery deposits over the surface	Film is not fixed or washed properly	Check time in fixer and wash stages Replace chemicals if exhausted

Most common film faults

Film faults occur when the different radiographic techniques or protocols are not followed. They appear for many reasons and a number of remedial actions can be taken to eliminate the fault(s). Good training and effective practice procedures will reduce film faults and the need for repeated radiographs and ultimately increase radiation safety (Table 30.6).

Positioning

General principles

The following principles should be followed to ensure that the maximum benefit is gained from accurate positioning:

- All radiographs must have a clinical indication and be requested by a qualified veterinary surgeon
- Radiation safety must be understood and adhered to at all times
- Standard projections should be performed whenever possible to allow interpretation and diagnosis
- If possible, at least two views at 90° to each other should be taken of all extremities and other regions
- Careful positioning, centring and collimation should always be carried out
- If positioning will compromise the patient's condition, then alternative methods of diagnosis should be used
- Identification labels should be present to prevent the loss of films.

Restraint

To prevent production of low-quality, non-diagnostic images, all animals should be restrained. This can be in the form of chemical restraint or through the use of pads, sandbags or ties.

Chemical restraint

Spine, skull, pharynx, some contrast procedures, hip examinations and most fracture investigations should not be carried out unless the animal is anaesthetized. If it is not possible to anaesthetize the animal, then heavy sedation can be used, but accurate diagnostic images may be difficult to produce. In the case of severely dyspnoeic patients, most will tolerate sedation and this will ensure that a diagnostic radiograph with limited stress to the patient is achieved.

In veterinary medicine the patient cannot be relied upon to remain in position or to stay on the table so most radiographs will be carried out under chemical restraint. Manual positioning is not recommended (unless it is clinically essential) because it usually relies on the nurse or veterinary surgeon restraining the patient, putting them in danger of exceeding the maximum permissible dose of radiation over a period of time.

Positioning aids

These should be available for all examinations. They should be radiolucent so that they do not show up on the final radiograph. Always check any new positioning aids introduced into the practice. Care should be taken when using sandbags, which are radiopaque, to prevent them from obscuring any of the area of interest.

The list of available aids below is intended as an outline and individuals may have personal favourites:

- **Radiolucent foam or plastic troughs** for dorsoventral or ventrodorsal projections
- A selection of **radiolucent foam wedges and blocks**. These should be in a variety of shapes and sizes
- A selection of **long, floppy sandbags**
- **Hobbles or bandages**. These can be used to tie limbs out of the way or to hold the mouth open during examination of the tympanic bullae. They should not be used unless the animal is anaesthetized
- **Positioning blocks and film holders** are essential for equine examinations
- A **rope head collar** is used when imaging the equine head to prevent any metal buckles from being seen.

Markers and legends

All films should have anatomical markers that indicate the limb, the recumbency or the side of the patient. Left and right markers should be placed so that they fall just inside the primary beam and will form a permanent indication of the orientation of the patient. In equine work, the lateral aspect of the distal extremities should be marked so that lesions can be orientated. The most common form of marker is a metal clip that slides over the edge of the cassette, or plastic tablets with lead letters or markers embedded in the plastic.

All radiographs should have a permanent label incorporating the:

- Animal's and owner's names
- Date of examination.

This can be achieved using lead tape or a light marker that exposes the film with the details, after exposure but before processing.

Terminology

The term used to describe the projection describes the path of the primary beam through the patient; the side struck by the X-ray beam first is first in the description and the side through which the beam exits is second. Therefore dorsoventral means that the beam enters through the dorsal side and leaves the body through the ventral side (Table 30.7, Fig. 30.12).

BVA/KC hip dysplasia and elbow scoring schemes

For both of these schemes there are protocols available from the British Veterinary Association and the Kennel Club, which should be followed closely to produce a diagnostic image. All animals must be over 1 year of age and should be registered with the Kennel Club. The films should have no identification other than the Kennel Club number, the date and a left and right marker and this should be put on the film prior to processing, preferably during exposure, e.g. using lead tape.

Small animal positioning

Chest

Right lateral

The patient should be placed in right lateral recumbency with the forelimbs extended and held in place by sandbags. A pad should be placed under the sternum to reduce rotation. The primary beam should be centred on the caudal border of the scapula midway between the skin surfaces. Collimation should include the front of the shoulder and the diaphragm. Exposure should be made on full inspiration to give maximum inflation of the lungs.

Dorsoventral

The patient should be placed in sternal recumbency using a trough. Use sandbags to hold the forelimbs in position and the head may need to be supported with a pad. The primary beam is centred on the highest point of the scapulae, on the midline. Collimation should include the front of the shoulder and the diaphragm. Exposure should be made on full inspiration.

Abdomen

Right lateral recumbency

The patient should be placed in right lateral recumbency with the forelimbs extended and held in place by sandbags. A pad should be placed under the sternum to reduce rotation. Centring should be cranial to the last rib at the 11th/12th intercostal space, midway between the skin surfaces. Collimation should include the entire diaphragm and the hip. Exposure should be made on full expiration to allow maximum space for the organs in the abdominal cavity.

Table 30.7 Terminology used to describe radiographic positions

Full description	Abbreviation	Direction of X-ray beam or description of area
Left	L	
Right	R	
Dorsal	D	Front of lower limbs below the carpus or tarsus or upper surface of main trunk
Ventral	V	Underside of animal
Cranial	Cr	Front of lower limbs above the carpus or tarsus
Caudal	Cd	Back of lower limbs below the carpus or tarsus
Rostral	R	Towards the nose
Medial	M	Towards the centre or inside of leg
Lateral	L	Outer side of body or legs
Proximal	Pr	The end of an extremity or bone that is closest to the body
Distal	Di	The end of an extremity or bone that is furthest away from the body
Palmar	Pa or P	Undersurface of the lower forelimb below the carpus – opposite to dorsal surface
Plantar	Pl	Undersurface of lower hind limb below the tarsus – opposite to dorsal surface
Oblique	O	
Lesion orientated oblique	LOO	An oblique projection to skyline a lesion

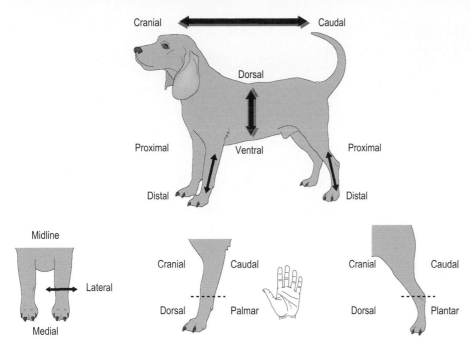

Fig. 30.12 Standard radiographic terminology

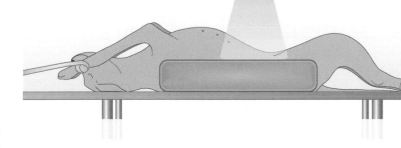

Fig. 30.13 Positioning for ventrodorsal abdomen

Ventrodorsal abdomen

The patient should be placed in dorsal recumbency in a trough if needed. The forelimbs and hind limbs should be held in position by sandbags or ties and the head may need to be supported by a pad (Fig. 30.13). The primary beam is centred to the 11th/12th intercostal space, or the umbilicus, on the midline. Collimation should include the entire liver and the top of the pelvic region. Exposure should be made on full expiration.

Head and neck

Ventrodorsal skull

The patient is placed in dorsal recumbency and the neck is extended. A foam pad is placed under the neck to ensure that the hard palate is parallel to the cassette. Centre on the midline on a point halfway along the inter-pupillary line to include the area of interest (Fig. 30.14).

Dorsoventral intraoral view

This position is used to view the nasal chambers. The patient is supported in sternal recumbency with the neck extended. A sandbag is placed over the neck to prevent rotation. A non-screen film is placed corner first as far as possible into the mouth, above the endotracheal tube. The primary beam is centred on a line midway between the external nares and a line joining the eyes (Fig. 30.15). An anatomical marker should be included.

Nasopharynx

The patient is placed in lateral recumbency. A pad supports the skull in a true lateral position and a pad is placed under the neck. The forelegs are pulled caudally against the wall of the thorax to prevent the muscle mass of the shoulder from obscuring the image. Centre on the mid-cervical area to include the pharynx and thoracic inlet. The patient should be extubated prior to exposure.

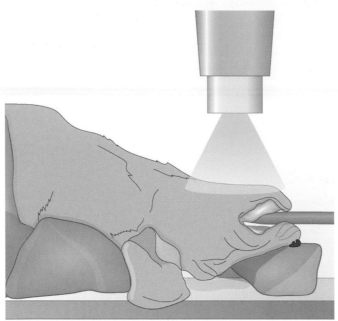

Fig. 30.14 Positioning for a ventrodorsal skull

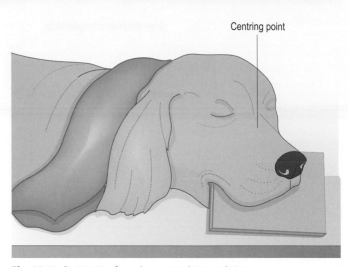

Centring point

Fig. 30.15 Positioning for a dorsoventral intraoral view

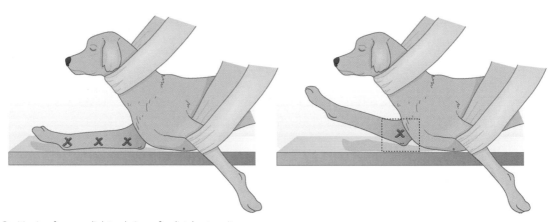

Fig. 30.16 Positioning for a mediolateral view of a distal extremity

Distal extremities

Mediolateral

The patient is placed with the side to be imaged nearest the cassette. The opposing limb is placed and supported on the flank (forelimbs pulled caudally, hind limbs pulled cranially). The limb should be parallel with the cassette; a pad may be necessary to prevent rotation (Fig. 30.16). Stifles and elbows should be flexed. Centring is at the level of the joint or mid-shaft. Collimation should include a joint above and below the long bone or a small area above and below the joint under investigation.

Dorsopalmar/plantar and caudocranial, i.e. below the level of the carpus or tarsus

The patient is placed in sternal or dorsal recumbency so that the limb under investigation is parallel with the cassette. The opposing limb may need to be lifted to rotate the limb under investigation so that it is straight (Fig. 30.17). Centring is at the level of the joint or mid-shaft. Collimation should

include the entire bone for long bones and the joint plus a small area above and below for joints.

Shoulder

Lateral

The animal is placed in lateral recumbency with the area under investigation nearest to the film. The upper limb should be extended caudally and secured in position. The limb under examination should be extended cranially and secured in place. The neck should be extended. The primary beam should be centred at the level of and caudal to the lateral tuberosity. Collimation should include the entire joint and surrounding soft tissues.

Caudocranial

The patient is placed on its back and supported with sandbags; the thorax may need to be rotated slightly. The affected limb is drawn cranially, fully extended and secured with a tie. The beam should be centred level with the acromion process of the scapula.

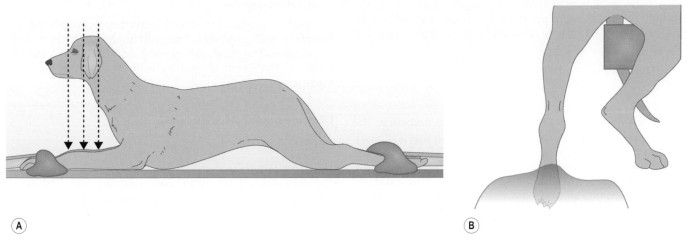

Fig. 30.17 Positioning for (**A**) craniocaudal view of the distal forelimb and (**B**) dorsoplantar view of the distal hind limb

Fig. 30.18 (**A**) Positioning for ventrodorsal pelvis. (**B**) Canine patient positioned for radiography of the pelvis

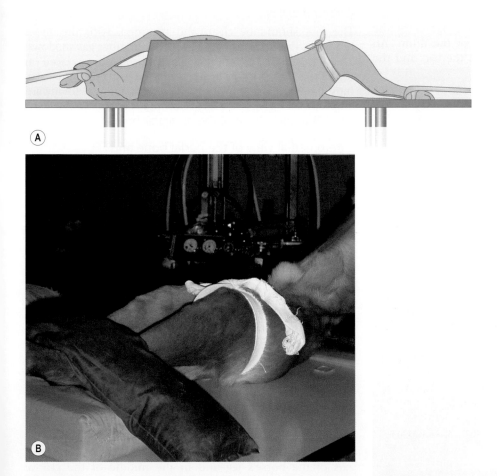

Pelvis

Ventrodorsal

The patient is placed in dorsal recumbency and supported in a trough. The forelimbs may need to be tied in an extended position (Fig. 30.18). The hind limbs are extended and internally rotated so that the femurs lie parallel to each other and the patellae are centred over the stifle joint. The legs should be supported and secured with sandbags or ties over the stifles and hocks as required. Centre on the midline, level with the greater trochanters. Collimation should include the upper third of the femur and the wings of the ilium.

This extended hip position is required for the KC/BVA hip dysplasia scheme and radiographs will be returned if the animal is not straight – look at the vertebral column and check that the obturator foramina are of equal size.

In patients that may have a damaged pelvis, e.g. as the result of a road traffic accident, the limbs should not be extended but should be allowed to flex into a 'frog leg' position.

Spine

Lateral

The patient should be placed in lateral recumbency. The spine should be supported with foam pads so that it is parallel with the tabletop. Pads should be placed under the sternum and between the limbs to prevent rotation. For the cervical spine the forelimbs should be pulled caudally. The beam should be centred over the area of interest. If the entire spine is being examined, each image should overlap with the ones on either side and each view should cover no more than 3–4 vertebrae – including too many vertebrae in one view will lead to apparent distortion of the intervertebral spaces, which may affect the diagnosis.

Lateral lumbosacral junction

The patient is placed in lateral recumbency as described in the previous position. This position has very specific positioning landmarks. Identify the greater trochanter of the femur and the cranial part of the wing of the ilium. An imaginary line should be drawn between the two and the beam centred on the midpoint of the line.

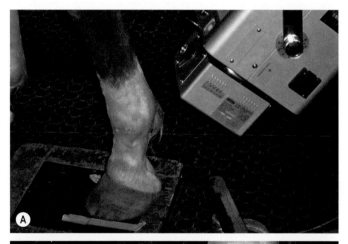

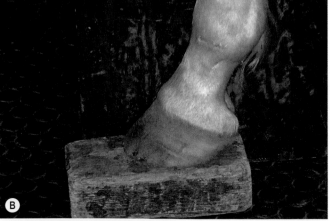

Fig. 30.19 Radiography of the equine foot. (**A**) Position to show the navicular bone. (**B**) Position for a lateral view

Ventrodorsal spine

The patient is placed in dorsal recumbency, supported in a trough or with sandbags. The patient should be as straight as possible. The hind legs should be extended to prevent rotation. The beam should be centred over the region of interest.

Large animal positioning

Foot

Dorsopalmar view of the pedal bone (DPr60°-PaDiO)

The foot should be clean and trimmed with the shoes removed. The frog should be packed with soap or play dough or other similar material to remove gas shadows. The film is placed in a film holder and the foot placed on top of this. The primary beam is centred below the coronary band on the midline of the foot with a downward angle of 60° (see Ch. 6). Collimation should include the edges of the hoof wall and the toe and heel of the foot.

Dorsopalmar view of the navicular bone (DPr60°-PaDiO)

The foot should be clean and trimmed, with the shoes removed. The frog should be packed to remove gas shadows. The film is placed in a film holder and the foot is placed on top of this. The primary beam is centred just above the coronary band on the midline of the foot, with a downward angle of 60° (Fig. 30.19A). Collimation should be large enough to include all of the navicular bone.

Lateromedial view of the pedal bone and navicular bone

The foot is prepared as for the dorsopalmar projection. The foot is placed on a block to ensure that it is high enough off the ground, and the horse should take weight on the foot (Fig. 30.19B). If laminitis is suspected, a lead strip with its top end level with the coronary band should be placed down the midline of the hoof wall. The beam is projected horizontally, parallel with the floor and centred at the level of the coronary band to include the heel and toe. Collimation should include the weight-bearing surface of the foot.

Palmaroproximal–dorsodistal oblique of the navicular bone (Pa45°P-DDiO)

The foot is cleaned and trimmed and the frog is packed to remove any gas shadows. The foot is placed on a film-holder containing the film. The foot is placed as far back as possible without the horse taking a step forward. This removes the fetlock from the area of interest. The X-ray beam is directed proximal to distal 30–40°, depending on how far back the foot is placed. The beam is centred parallel with the long axis of the horse's leg and in the middle of the groove between the bulbs of the heel. Collimation should be limited to the area of the navicular bone.

Fetlock

Dorsopalmar

The horse should stand bearing weight on all four feet. The primary beam is angled down to about 15° to the vertical to ensure that it passes through the joint space. The film is placed in a suitable container and placed behind the leg. The primary beam is centred on the fetlock joint on the midline of the leg. Collimation should include a small area above and below the joint.

Lateromedial

The horse should stand bearing weight on all four feet. The film in a suitable container is placed on the medial aspect of the leg. The primary beam is centred on the fetlock joint on the midline of the leg. Collimation should include a small area above and below the joint.

Dorsolateral–palmaromedial oblique (D45°L-PaMO) and dorsomedial–palmarolateral oblique (D45°M-PaLO)

The horse should stand bearing weight on all four feet. The primary beam is directed perpendicular to the leg:

- For the dorsolateral–palmaromedial oblique the cassette is placed midway between the medial and palmar surfaces of the leg
- For the dorsomedial–palmarolateral oblique the cassette is placed midway between the lateral and palmar surfaces of the leg.

If the horse is not cooperating then a palmarolateral–dorsomedial oblique is a safer projection to attempt as the X-ray tube and machine are not under the horse.

Cannon and splint bones

Dorsopalmar

The horse should stand bearing weight on all four feet. The film is placed in a film box or holder behind the leg. The beam is centred on the middle of the cannon bone along the midline of the leg. Collimation should include the joints above and below the cannon bone.

Lateromedial

The horse should stand bearing weight on all four feet. The cassette is placed on the medial aspect of the leg parallel with the leg. The X-ray beam is centred on the centre of the cannon bone, parallel with the film. Collimation should include the joints above and below the cannon bone.

Dorsolateral–palmaromedial oblique (D45°L-PaMO) and dorsomedial-palmarolateral oblique (D45°M-PaLO)

The horse should stand bearing weight on all four feet. The primary beam is directed perpendicular to the leg. For the dorsolateral–palmaromedial oblique the cassette is placed midway between the medial and palmar surfaces of the leg.

Hock and carpus

Dorsopalmar

The horse should stand bearing weight on all four feet. The film is placed in a film box or holder behind the leg. The beam is centred on the middle of the joint passing along the midline of the leg. Collimation should include the joint and a small area above and below.

Lateromedial

The horse should stand bearing weight on all four feet. The cassette is placed on the medial aspect of the leg parallel with the leg. If the hock is under investigation, then a slight angulation downwards (15° to the vertical) will improve image quality. The X-ray beam is centred on the middle of the joint, parallel with the film. Collimation should include a small area above and below the joint.

Dorsolateral–palmaromedial oblique (D45°L-PaMO) and dorsomedial–palmarolateral oblique (D45°M-PaLO)

The horse should stand bearing weight on all four feet. The primary beam is directed perpendicular to the leg:

- For the dorsolateral–palmaromedial oblique the cassette is placed midway between the medial and palmar surfaces of the leg
- For the dorsomedial–palmarolateral oblique the cassette is placed midway between the lateral and palmar surfaces of the leg.

The X-ray beam is centred on the middle of the joint.

Elbow

Craniocaudal

The horse should stand bearing weight on all four feet. The limb under examination is extended forwards slightly to move it away from the chest wall. A cassette is placed behind the leg, as high as possible. A slight angulation may be needed cranially to demonstrate the entire joint. The primary beam is centred on the distal margin of the humerus. Collimation should include a small amount of the radius and the humerus.

Lateral

The film should be placed in a bag on a drip stand. The leg under examination should be as close to the film as possible. The horse should stand on all feet with equal weight. The opposing foreleg is lifted and extended and held in
position. The person holding the leg should wear suitable protective clothing. The primary beam is centred on the joint on the medial aspect. Collimation should include the distal humerus and proximal radius (Fig. 30.20).

Shoulder

Lateral

The film should be placed in a bag on a drip stand. A grid should be used. The leg under examination should be as close to the film as possible. The horse should stand on all feet with equal weight. The opposing foreleg is lifted and extended and held in position. Raising the leg will place the trachea over the joint, which will improve the image quality. The person holding the leg should wear suitable protective clothing. The primary beam is centred on the joint on the medial aspect. Collimation should include the proximal humerus and the soft tissues surrounding the joint.

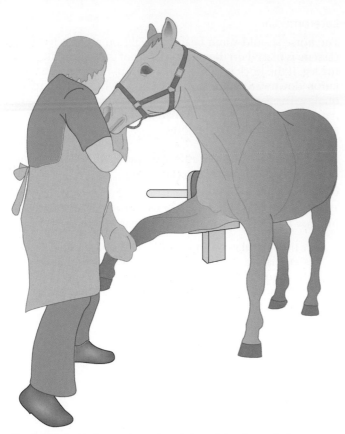

Fig. 30.20 Positioning to show a lateral view of the elbow of a horse

Stifle

Lateromedial

The horse should stand bearing weight on all four feet. The area around the stifle should be touched so that the horse is aware of contact before a cassette is inserted. A cassette is placed on the medial side of the horse's leg and rotated up as high as possible. The individual holding the cassette should wear suitable lead protection and stand as far away from the primary beam as possible. The long edge of the cassette should be visible on the cranial edge of the leg. The primary beam should be perpendicular to the leg. The beam should be centred at the base of the patella. Collimation should include the joint and surrounding soft tissue but the caudal area does not need to be included.

Caudocranial

The horse should stand bearing weight on all four feet. The area around the stifle should be touched so that the horse is aware of contact before a cassette is inserted. A cassette is placed on the cranial aspect of the horse's leg and rotated up as high as possible. The individual holding the cassette should wear suitable lead protection and stand as far away from the primary beam as possible. The long edge of the cassette should be visible on the lateral edge of the leg. The primary beam should be angled downwards about 10° to the vertical so that it passes through the joint space. The beam should be centred at the base of the patella. Collimation should include the joint and surrounding soft tissue.

Skull

Lateromedial skull and sinuses

A film should be placed in a bag on a drip stand. The horse should have a rope head collar as the buckles on a conventional collar will show on the radiograph. The horse is walked into position so that the side under investigation is closest to the film. The head is supported with a gloved hand (the nurse holding the head must wear suitable lead protection). The primary beam is centred at the base of the facial crest perpendicular to the head and film. Collimation should include all of the maxilla, the frontal sinuses and the first cheek tooth.

Contrast radiography

Types of contrast medium

Contrast media are substances that, when administered to the body, will enhance areas where radiographic contrast is low. In areas such as the gastrointestinal tract, the urogenital system and the vascular system the difference in contrast between adjacent structures is very low and so they will not always be distinguishable on a radiograph. The selected contrast medium has a higher atomic number than soft tissue and will therefore prevent more of the X-rays passing through the patient and reaching the film. The affected area appears white on the radiograph, highlighting it or increasing the contrast between it and surrounding areas.

Contrast media must:

- Be easy to administer and cause minimal discomfort or distress to the patient
- Be non-toxic
- Be a stable compound that will not alter when introduced into the patient
- Allow good, clear demonstration of the area of interest
- Be eliminated from the body as completely as possible in the shortest possible time
- Not cause further damage to the patient or be carcinogenic
- Be cost-effective.

Negative contrast media

These use gas that absorbs very little of the X-ray beam, making the area of interest appear blacker on the film. Common gases used are:

- Air – e.g. double-contrast cystogram (bladder)
- Carbon dioxide (CO_2) – e.g. barium meals
- Oxygen (O_2) – e.g. arthrograms (joints).

Negative contrast may also be seen in some injuries where gas has formed or entered an area and its presence can be used to aid diagnosis, e.g. perforations or in surgical emphysema.

Positive contrast media

These have a higher atomic number than soft tissues so X-rays are absorbed and the area under investigation appears white.

Common positive contrast media include the following:

Barium sulphate suspension

Barium sulphate (e.g. Baritop) has an atomic number of 56 and is used for barium swallows and meals. It is used to demonstrate the gastrointestinal tract because it does not react with the acid in the stomach. Other substances tend to 'clump' within the stomach, giving a strange appearance that may be mistaken for pathology. Barium sulphate is also very cheap and non-toxic. It should not be given in cases where a perforation is suspected as it can cause severe adhesions within the peritoneal cavity if it escapes from the confines of the intestine.

Iodine-based solutions

Iodine-based contrast media have an atomic number of 35 and include the water-soluble organic compounds, e.g. Omnipaque and Conray, and the non-soluble organic compounds, e.g. Lipiodol. Iodine on its own is toxic but when joined to other substances can be used within the body.

The amount of iodine within a certain type of medium is expressed in milligrams per millilitre (mg/ml); for example, Omnipaque 300 contains 300 mg of iodine per millilitre. The composition of each type of contrast medium alters the way in which it reacts within the patient to produce a diagnostic image. Contrast media can be either ionic or non-ionic. Non-ionic contrast media, e.g. Omnipaque, produce fewer reactions and are more suitable for smaller or very ill patients and in the subarachnoid or spinal areas.

Reactions to iodine-based contrast media may be:

- **Allergic (anaphylactic effects)** – this type of reaction varies from mild urticaria (skin rash) to full anaphylaxis and cardiopulmonary arrest. Whenever iodine-based contrast media are injected the patient should be anaesthetized to control the effects of a reaction
- **Chemotoxic effects** – as the dose is increased the chances of a severe reaction will increase. The type of reaction varies from patient to patient. Very sick or very young patients will be more susceptible than the average otherwise healthy patient. Effects include cerebral oedema, red blood cell damage, convulsions and renal function impairment
- **Osmotic effects** – pain may be experienced because of the osmolar shift of fluid within the tissues of the body during the introduction of contrast medium, especially when given intravenously.

Double contrast

This involves the use of both positive and negative contrast media and is used to highlight the lining epithelia of hollow structures such as the bladder, stomach and rectum. The organ is emptied as much as possible and a small amount of positive contrast medium is introduced. The patient may need to be turned to coat the lining and air is then introduced to dilate the organ (Fig. 30.21).

Use of contrast medium

All types of contrast medium are prescription only medicines (POM-V) and should only be used for the diagnosis or treatment of the prescribed patient.

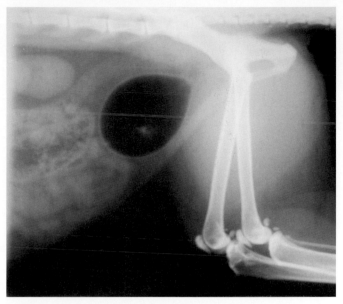

Fig. 30.21 Lateral view of the canine bladder using double-contrast technique. Note the presence of a space-filling defect in the lumen of the bladder *(Reproduced by kind permission of Richard Aspinall)*

Before using any contrast medium a number of checks and procedures should be followed:

- Check the date and type of contrast medium
- Check the quantity and concentration of contrast agent needed for the examination
- Ensure that the correct route for administration is used and is prepared
- Make sure that the contrast medium is warm so that the viscosity is reduced, making it easier to inject
- Make sure that there are no foreign particles within the contrast, especially if the container has been opened previously
- Ensure that all procedures are aseptic to prevent the introduction of infection
- Record the type of contrast and the amount given in the patient's notes for future reference.

Methods of administration

- Orally – e.g. barium swallow, barium series or follow-through (Fig. 30.22)
- Rectally – e.g. barium enema (Fig. 30.23)
- Intravenously – e.g. intravenous urography, mesenteric portal venography (Fig. 30.24)
- Mechanically – e.g. sinogram, cystogram, myelogram (Fig. 30.25)

Patients should be correctly prepared before administration and this may depend on the contrast medium being used:

- Starvation – may be recommended prior to a barium meal or swallow. If the patient is to be given a general anaesthetic for any other type of procedure, starvation will be necessary
- Enema – usually recommended prior to a barium enema or prior to intravenous urography, as a full rectum may affect the position of the ureters

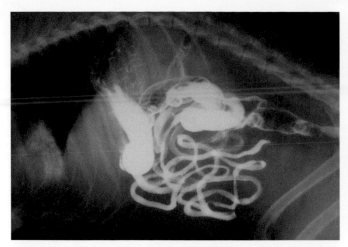

Fig. 30.22 Lateral view of the canine abdomen 2 hours after administration of a barium meal *(Reproduced by kind permission of Richard Aspinall)*

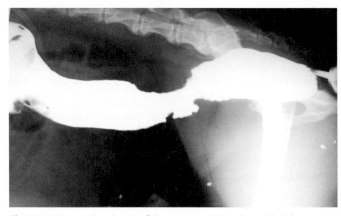

Fig. 30.23 Ventrodorsal view of the canine pelvis and caudal abdomen to demonstrate the administration of a barium enema. Note the space-occupying lesion in the descending colon *(Reproduced by kind permission of Richard Aspinall)*

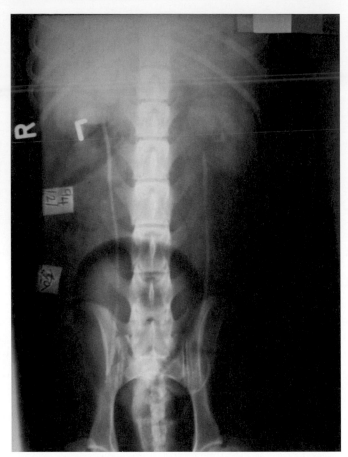

Fig. 30.24 Ventrodorsal view of the canine abdomen and pelvis to demonstrate the technique of intravenous urography. The radiograph was taken 9 minutes after administration of the contrast medium and shows the highlighted kidneys, ureters and bladder *(Reproduced by kind permission of Richard Aspinall)*

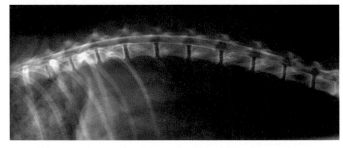

Fig. 30.25 Lateral view of the canine thoracic and lumbar spine to demonstrate the administration of contrast medium to perform a myelogram. Note the contrast medium running along the subarachnoid space of the spine *(Reproduced by kind permission of Richard Aspinall)*

- General anaesthesia – for ease of administration and positioning, anaesthesia is essential for most procedures, apart from barium studies of the gastrointestinal tract
- Plain radiographs – patients should always have preliminary radiographs taken before contrast is introduced to identify any pathology that may prevent the examination from being effective. They are also useful for comparison with the contrast radiographs.

Contrast techniques

These are listed in Table 30.8.

Alternative imaging techniques

Ultrasound

Diagnostic ultrasound uses sound waves to provide a diagnostic image of the internal organs of a patient. The sound waves have a frequency, which is measured in hertz (Hz).

The sound waves used in ultrasound are above the range of our hearing as they are supersonic and are usually between 1 and 10 megahertz (MHz)

A number of terms are used in ultrasonography:

- **Acoustic window** – the area through which the ultrasound waves will be applied. It should be as close as possible to the area under investigation
- **Acoustic impedance** – the degree of resistance to the passage of ultrasound waves

Table 30.8 Indications for and methods of using contrast media

Examination type	Indications	Area demonstrated	Contrast medium used	Quantity	Method of administration	Preliminary radiographs	Projections and time after administration
Barium swallow	Regurgitation, retching, dysphagia, suspected foreign body	Oesophagus	Barium sulphate	Dogs 5–10 ml Cats up to 5 ml	Oral	Lateral thorax	Lateral thorax immediately after administration
Barium meal and follow through	Vomiting	Stomach and small intestine	Barium sulphate	Dogs 1–3 ml/kg Cats 2–5 ml/kg	Oral. May need stomach tube	Lateral and ventrodorsal abdomen	Immediate. Four views of the abdomen then ventrodorsal and right lateral abdomen every 30 min until stomach is empty
Barium enema	Melaena, chronic diarrhoea, tenesmus	Large bowel	Barium sulphate, plus air if double-contrast examination required	10 ml/kg mixed with water 50:50	Foley catheter inserted into rectum – allow contrast to enter using the effects of gravity	Ventrodorsal and right lateral abdomen	Right and left lateral abdominal radiographs plus ventrodorsal abdomen
Intravenous urography	Incontinence, persistent haematuria, pyelonephritis, trauma	Kidneys and ureters	Ionic contrast medium (Conray 420)	1 ml/kg	Intravenously as a bolus	Right lateral and ventrodorsal abdomen	Immediate. Follow up with 5 min – ventrodorsal abdomen; 10 min – lateral abdomen; 15 min – caudal abdomen. May be followed by a vaginourethrogram
Male urethrogram	Incontinence, dysuria, persistent haematuria, trauma, bladder position	Bladder, urethra and prostate	Ionic contrast medium (Urografin 150)	2 ml/kg	Foley catheter inserted into penile urethra	Right lateral caudal abdomen to include urethra	Same position as preliminary film radiograph taken as contrast is injected
Female urethrogram	Incontinence, dysuria, persistent haematuria, trauma, position of bladder	Bladder, urethra and vagina	Ionic contrast medium (Urografin 150)	1 ml/kg to fill urethra and vagina	Foley catheter inserted into vestibule of vagina and secured to prevent leakage using Allis tissue forceps	Right lateral caudal abdomen to include urethra	Same position as preliminary film, radiograph taken as contrast is injected
Cystogram	Dysuria, persistent haematuria, trauma, position of bladder	Bladder	Ionic contrast medium (Urografin 150) Air	10 ml/kg for cystogram, then fill with air until bladder feels distended for a pneumocystogram	Bladder catheterized and urine removed; contrast and/or air introduced until resistance is felt	Right lateral caudal abdomen to include urethra	Same position as preliminary film Radiograph taken immediately after contrast and/or air is introduced
Myelogram	Spinal pain, paraplegia, quadriplegia, ataxia, trauma	Spinal column	Non-ionic contrast medium (Omnipaque 300)	0.3 ml/kg as a slow bolus	Cisternal puncture or lumbar puncture	Lateral and ventrodorsal of area of interest	Lateral radiographs of entire spine Ventrodorsal of areas of interest
Arthrography	Joint pain degeneration of articular surfaces	Joints, mainly the shoulder	Non-ionic contrast medium (Omnipaque 300)	1–1.5 ml	Injected directly into the joint space	Two projections of joint	Two projections of joint
Sinography	Demonstrate sinus tract path	Sinus tract or fistula	Ionic contrast medium (Urografin 150)	Until backflow or resistance is felt	Foley catheter inserted into opening of sinus or fistula and secured in place using Allis tissue forceps	Two projections of area of interest	Two projections of area of interest

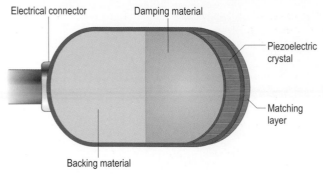

Fig. 30.26 Cross-section through a transducer

- **Acoustic interface** – the junction between two tissues of different acoustic impedance
- **Echoes** – the returning ultrasound waves picked up by the transducer and converted into the image on the screen: the brightness of the echo is determined by the acoustic impedance of the acoustic interface
- **Hyperechoic or echogenic** – bright white echoes between highly reflective interfaces, e.g. bone, gas and collagen
- **Hypoechoic or echo-poor** – sparse echoes appearing grey representing intermediate reflection or transmission of the ultrasound waves, e.g. soft tissue
- **Anechoic or echolucent** – absence of echoes so appears black, e.g. fluid.

Ultrasound interactions

The ultrasound image is formed by the reflection of the ultrasound waves within the body. As the wave travels through the patient and tissues it becomes **attenuated** and the intensity of the wave is reduced. The most common form of attenuation is absorption. The friction caused by the vibration of the molecules within the tissues of the body will cause this absorption to occur. Other causes of attenuation are scattering, reflection, refraction, diffraction, interference and divergence.

The transducer

The ultrasound transducer is the hand-held probe used during examinations and it is able to convert electrical energy to mechanical energy from the ultrasound beam and vice-versa (Fig. 30.26). The active part of the transducer is the piezoelectric crystal, which is usually made of lead zirconate titanate. It has a specific thickness for the best resolution possible, which varies depending on the wavelength produced by the crystal. The crystal will expand and contract along its shortest side as the electrical signal applied across it alternates. This electrical signal is converted into an ultrasound beam. The beam passes into the patient and is reflected back from the tissues to the transducer. The reflected echoes are detected by the transducer and converted back into an electrical signal to allow the formation of an image on a monitor. Behind the crystal is a damping material, which improves resolution. This is supported on a backing material.

Operational display modes

The ultrasound image may be displayed on the screen in one of the following ways:

1. **A-mode – amplitude mode:**
   - Echoes appear on the monitor as a series of blips
   - Used to demonstrate the depth of differences in tissues (interfaces) and their separation
   - Equipment is cheaper.
2. **B-mode – brightness mode**
   This is the most common type:
   - Shown in real time; the operator moves the transducer around and shows an image on the monitor as it happens
   - The intensity of the echo is demonstrated as a bright dot on the monitor
   - A composite image will be shown either in a rectangular format or sector view depending on the transducer type.
3. **M-mode – moving mode:**
   - Used mainly for cardiac examinations
   - Produces an image similar to that of an A-mode examination but adds in a time element
   - Being replaced by Doppler imaging and dedicated echocardiography units.

Patient preparation

Careful patient preparation is essential to produce diagnostic images. The area under examination is clipped to remove any hair and spirit is used to remove any excess oil or debris on the skin surface. A coupling gel is placed between the skin surface and the transducer to ensure good contact between the tissues and the transducer. Ultrasound waves do not travel well through air so the gel is used to ensure that the transducer is always in complete contact with the skin surface. The patient may need to be restrained and in some cases sedation may be needed; however, ultrasound is a completely painless and non-invasive technique.

Ultrasound has a number of advantages:

- Does not use radiation
- Produces real-time images
- Can be used without sedation
- Minimal patient preparation needed
- Non-invasive procedure that gives good visualization of the abdominal organs.

However, there are a number of disadvantages:

- Cannot be used in areas containing large amounts of air
- Ultrasound does not travel well through air
- Reporting of images is only possible by the operator
- Accuracy is dependent on operator experience.

Areas suitable for examination

Ultrasound is ideal for:

- Abdominal organs
- Heart
- Thyroid
- Larynx
- Tendons

- Ligaments
- Soft-tissue masses.

Nuclear medicine

This technique is sometimes known as **nuclear scintigraphy** and is used mainly in the equine field for examination of the bones and in cats for the examination of possible thyroid problems. Other areas of examination are possible and are used in specific cases.

Nuclear medicine will demonstrate the function of a tissue or organ and will show where a problem is but will not provide a specific diagnosis. It involves the use of radioactively labelled drugs or radiopharmaceuticals, which are given intravenously and are taken up by specific tissues depending on their chemical nature.

A number of terms are used in nuclear medicine:

- **Radionuclide** – an atom that disintegrates emitting gamma radiation
- **Radiopharmaceutical** – a medicinal product that is used in the examination technique
- **Half-life** – the time taken for the radioactivity to decay to half its original value. It should be long enough to allow examination but not remain unnecessarily after the examination.

Care should be taken whenever radioisotopes are used and it should be understood that all substances produced by the patient may be radioactive. Shoes should be changed before examination in case of patient urination and all urine should be collected and prevented from entering the drainage system. The patient should be isolated for at least 24 hours after examination to ensure that radiation levels are within safe limits. Contact with patients should be minimal within 24 hours of the examination.

Administration of the radioisotope

A radioisotope is attached to the radiopharmaceutical, whose type is determined by the body system under examination. If bone is to be examined then the radiopharmaceutical is methylene diphosphonate and this is attached to technetium-99m (^{99m}TcMDP). Iodine is used for thyroid imaging. The radiopharmaceutical is given intravenously and will be carried to the region under examination and then emit radiation. This is detected using a **gamma camera** or **scintillation detector** placed outside the patient in the region of interest.

Data collection

The patient is placed in front of the gamma camera, which detects any gamma radiation emitted. In a normal patient the gamma radiation emitted will demonstrate a normal distribution and will be symmetrical. Any areas that are not symmetrical or evenly distributed with the isotope are interpreted as being abnormal.

The gamma camera sends signals via a crystal that emits light and a photomultiplier tube to a computer system where acquisition, processing and storage of the data will take place. All images (Fig. 30.27) will be displayed on a TV monitor and can be manipulated and analysed. Printing can be performed on a conventional printer.

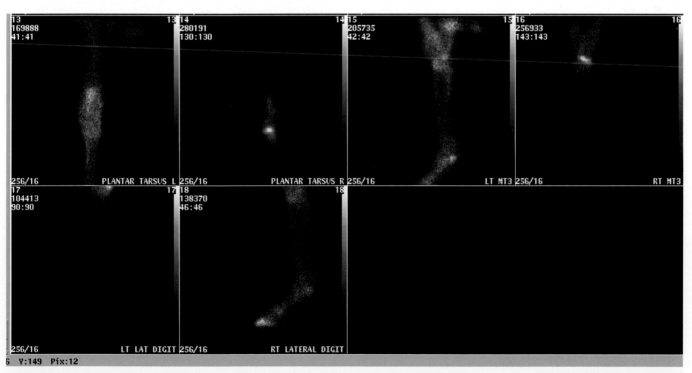

Fig. 30.27 This horse was presented with a persistent lameness that was only resolved by high leg nerve blocks. Radiography failed to identify any obvious pathology but the gamma scan (shown here) confirmed that the problem was in the region of the third tarsal bone. Subsequent radiology and surgical arthroscopic investigation confirmed a fracture of this bone *(Reproduced by kind permission of Derek Knottenbelt)*

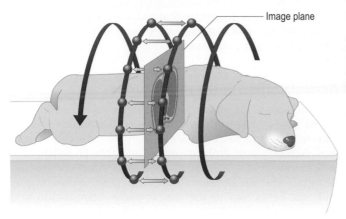

Fig. 30.28 Function of a computed tomography scanner

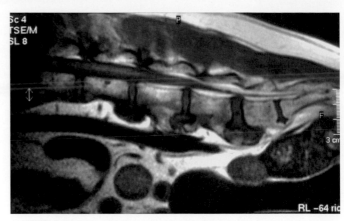

Fig. 30.29 Magnetic resonance imaging scan of the spinal cord

Computed tomography

This is also called CT or CAT (computer-aided tomography) scanning and uses an X-ray tube mounted opposite a detector. The tube emits X-rays in a fan shape that passes through the patient to reach the detector (Fig. 30.28). The X-ray tube and the detector move around the patient throughout the examination. In modern machines this is in a spiral movement. The detector then converts the X-rays into a signal that can be used by the computer system to form an image.

CT is ideal for demonstration of all organs within the body, especially the skeletal and central nervous systems, and for the demonstration of tumours. It can be used in any area to supplement the findings of a normal radiological examination.

Patient preparation and safety

As this examination takes time, the patient must be anaesthetized. A scout will be performed to provide a scan for planning and positioning. This is the most time-consuming part of the examination. Any individual remaining in the room during the scan must wear a lead apron and adhere to normal radiation safety procedures and, if possible, the patient should be on its own in the room for the very short time it takes to perform the scan. Monitoring can be performed throughout the examination so that the patient is not left unattended.

Magnetic resonance imaging

Magnetic resonance imaging or MRI is the most modern method of diagnostic imaging and does not use ionizing radiation. It was originally invented to unravel the atomic structure of chemical compounds but is now used to produce an image by mapping the location of the protons of the body tissues. This technique is ideal for demonstrating the central nervous system (Fig. 30.29) and the spinal column and for soft tissues within joints; however, it is less sensitive to calcified areas than CT scans.

Patient preparation

During an MRI scan the patient is exposed to a large magnetic field and for this reason all collars, leads and other metallic objects should be removed. An alternative method of diagnostic imaging should be used for any patients with implants or pacemakers. The scan is very noisy and takes time, so patients should be anaesthetized to reduce the distress caused by noise and having to keep still for the entire scan. Specialized equipment is required and no metallic objects should be taken into the scanner room.

An MRI scan takes place as follows:

1. The anaesthetized patient is placed on the table
2. A scout image is produced to plan the scan
3. The patient is then placed within the magnet, which has a strength of between 0.2 and 2 tesla (T). The earth's magnetic field is 0.00006 T
4. The hydrogen protons of the body align with the magnet as the patient enters the scanner. A radio frequency pulse is applied to the patient, which makes the protons 'flip' as they absorb the energy
5. After the radio pulse is turned off the protons return to their original positions and emit any excess energy
6. This energy is received by the scanner and is used to reconstruct an image, which appears on a screen in a similar format to that of a CT scan.

The magnet and detector surround a long tunnel, through which the anaesthetized patient moves very slowly. Scanning times are longer than those for CT scans.

Bibliography

Ball, J., Price, T., 1995. Chesney's Radiographic Imaging, sixth ed. Blackwell Scientific, Oxford.

Bushberg, J., Seibert, J., Leidholdt, E., Boon, J., 1994. The Essential Physics of Medical Imaging. Lippincott Williams & Wilkins, Philadelphia, PA.

Bushong, S., 1997. Radiological Science for Technologists, sixth ed. Mosby, St Louis, MO.

Easton, S., 2002. Practical Radiography for Veterinary Nurses. Butterworth-Heinemann, Oxford.

Fauber, T., 2000. Radiographic Imaging and Exposure. Mosby, St Louis, MO.

Lee, R. (Ed.), 1995. Manual of Small Animal Diagnostic Imaging. British Small Animal Veterinary Association, Cheltenham.

Mendenhall, A., Cantwell, H., 1988. Equine Radiographic Procedures. Lee & Febiger, Philadelphia, PA.

O'Meara, B., O'Neill, H., Fraser, B., 2010. Applications of nuclear scintigraphy in the investigation of equine lameness: Part 2. Thoroughbred Racehorse Companion Anim. 15 (1), 1–4.

Recommended reading

Bushong, S., 1997. Radiological Science for Technologists, sixth ed. Mosby, St Louis, MO.

This book is everything you need to know about radiographic physics. It covers all topics with clear and self-explanatory diagrams, broken down into small topic areas for easy reading.

Easton, S., 2003. Diagnostic imaging. In: Aspinall, V. (Ed.), Clinical Procedures in Veterinary Nursing. Butterworth-Heinemann, Oxford, pp. 227–264.

This text provides a step-by-step guide to radiographic procedures. Each radiographic procedure is described in stages with the theory behind the procedure provided.

Fauber, T., 2000. Radiographic Imaging and Exposure. Mosby, St Louis, MO.

Explains in detail exactly what happens when you alter exposure factors and processing conditions. There are lots of very clear diagrams and radiographs showing how exposure manipulation and equipment care and use can alter the image.

Lee, R. (Ed.), 1995. Manual of Small Animal Diagnostic Imaging. British Small Animal Veterinary Association, Gloucester.

Although this book is aimed at radiology and diagnosis it provides very clear diagrams and explanations on how positioning should be carried out. It looks at each radiographic projection in detail, with positioning and then detailed discussion on what can be seen on the resultant radiograph.

CHAPTER 31

Management and care of exotic species

Beverley Shingleton and Sarah Cottingham

Key Points

- More and more people are keeping various species of exotic pets, which have very different husbandry requirements from each other and from the more usual cats and dogs.
- The species of small mammal include the rodents and rabbits, which are omnivorous or herbivorous and are commonly kept in groups in cages, either indoors or outdoors. Ferrets are also popular; they are carnivorous and may be kept for hunting or as pets.
- Reptiles include snakes, lizards and chelonians, i.e. tortoises and terrapins. They are all cold-blooded and as such are totally dependent on their environment for their health and welfare. It is vital that the owner fully understands their husbandry requirements if they are not to suffer and die.
- Many species of bird are kept, in cages or in aviaries. They encompass several different classes of bird, each of which has differing needs in terms of diet and enclosure.
- It is essential that both the pet keeper and the veterinary nurse understand all the requirements of these animals so that they can live a long and healthy life, and if they should be admitted to the veterinary surgery they can be cared for appropriately.

Introduction

As more and more people elect to keep exotic species as 'pets', the veterinary nurse must be aware of the animal's specific needs in relation to their biology, husbandry, and general care. Nurses need to be able to rise to the challenges these animals bring and it must be highlighted that the principles applied to nursing a sick or injured dog and cat are not necessarily transferable to a small rodent, reptile or bird.

This chapter aims to provide sound practical details on how to care effectively for those usual and sometimes unusual pets that are presented for treatment in veterinary practice.

The range of animals covered includes:

- Small mammals – guinea pigs, rabbits, gerbils, mice, rats, hamsters and ferrets

- Reptiles – snakes, lizards, chelonian (shelled reptiles)
- Birds – budgies, canaries, finches, parrots, quail, etc.

Keeping exotic small mammals as pets can be just as rewarding as keeping dogs and cats and they can provide companionship and company in a similar way. However, when choosing any species of exotic animal as a pet there are advantages and disadvantages that need to be considered before purchasing the animal:

- How much time will their daily routine take?
- Will the animal need specialist veterinary care?
- Will the owner need specialist knowledge to care for the animal correctly?
- Is the animal suitable for children, adults and family?
- How much is it going to cost to look after the animal?

The veterinary nurse is frequently asked to give advice on pet selection and the advantages and disadvantages of exotic pet ownership are shown in Table 31.1.

Animal husbandry

Small mammals

Housing

Housing is obviously one of the most important factors in correct management. Housing requirements are species specific and the ethology and behaviour of the species should be understood and reflected in the choice of housing and management syle. When considering owning any small animal, the following factors should be taken into account when selecting the most appropriate environment to meet all of the animal's requirements:

- Correct levels of light/hours of daylight
- Correct temperature
- Space to exercise
- Companionship – consider the ratio of male to females
- Substrate/bedding
- Sleeping area
- Enclosure suitable for the individual species behaviour
- Safety/security requirements of species and enclosure
- Adequate and appropriate environmental stimulation
- Siting/position of enclosure.

Table 31.1 The advantages and disadvantages of keeping exotic pets

Pet	Advantages	Disadvantages
Small mammals	Relatively cheap to buy animal and initial set up are also relatively cheap. Daily management costs are low Animals require less time for daily management, e.g. hamsters, gerbils and rats do not need walking; smaller mammals do not need grooming Small mammals are good for children to learn animal management and responsible pet ownership Parent and child are able to learn to handle pet together Children should always be supervised with animals and taught correct care and consideration As most small, exotic mammals are relatively short-lived, the child has the chance to learn about grief process when the pet dies	Animal is often medically neglected due to misunderstanding/ignorance of illnesses by owners. Many owners resent veterinary costs as the animal was cheap to purchase Animals often left in cage/enclosure without adequate husbandry. As animal is in enclosure and often away from main household activity, pets often not checked, or cared for, for long periods of time Children's small hands are often unable to hold animal correctly, leading to animal being dropped and injured. Scared pets then tend to bite in anticipation of being handled Situation spirals, children become nervous of handling the pet, and the pet becomes more aggressive, culminating in the animal not being handled and then becoming neglected Often difficult to find veterinary surgery that treat exotic mammals. Many veterinary surgeons still view small mammals as non-treatable or 'specialist' Natural behaviour (many exotic mammals are prey species) and husbandry needs often neglected through incorrect advice and lack of knowledge of species requirements Pets often inappropriately chosen for children, e.g. hamsters are nocturnal and will be active and noisy at night, and not appreciate being handled during daytime sleep
Reptiles	Keeping reptiles provides an unusual and stimulating challenge. Wide variety available	Specialist knowledge of reptiles and chelonians is needed Ignorance leads to poor husbandry and inadequate housing, which results in disease and death Some species of lizard and snake grow very large and have a poor temperament, which makes them unmanageable, leading to abandonment or euthanasia Hidden costs are heating, specialist feeding and lighting requirements Some people do not understand the need to feed dead rodents or have live invertebrates as food in the house As many reptiles carry zoonotic diseases, hygiene is very important Many small reptile species purchased for young children can live in excess of 15 years – by then the novelty may have worn off!
Birds	Many species have been kept in captivity for hundreds of years and are well established as companions. Interesting, can be exhibited and readily breed in captivity Housing requirements are well documented and a range of housing is available	Some psittacines, especially the parrot family, can be challenging and suffer behavioural problems if they lack sufficient company and stimulus Many of the larger bird species are a huge monetary investment and security must be considered, as valuable birds are often stolen from aviaries Some of the housing on the market is too small and provides inadequate space for flying Aviaries can be expensive and need correct positioning and adequate space

Each species has a different behaviour pattern and therefore has different housing requirements, which should be reflected in the husbandry and environment (see Tables 31.2, 31.3). These will be discussed in more detail in the following sections.

Environmental enrichment

All caged animals should be kept in enclosures that allow them to interact with their environment and to display as many natural behaviour patterns as they would do if they were living unconfined in the wild. Environmental enrichment is not necessarily about providing a replica natural environment but about providing the animal with a variety of activities which allow natural behaviour to be expressed, e.g. foraging for hidden food rather than being given food in a bowl. Enrichment also allows the animal to 'do something' rather than have large amounts of spare time with nothing to do which the animal then fills with abnormal boredom-induced behaviours which are often repetitive and stereotypical. (Figures 31.1–31.9 provide photographic examples related to a number of commonly kept small exotic species.)

Suggestions for environmental enrichment include:

- Changing the feeding methods and routine – keeps the animal busy and rewards it for its efforts.
- Provision of appropriate toys and hiding places
- Changing the layout of a cage or enclosure increases exploratory behaviour.
- Ensuring company is available – make sure that the species is sociable and that there is an appropriate balance between the sexes.
- Provide the animal with choice and therefore a degree of control of its environment, which will reduce stress – provide the choice between hiding or being visible; hot areas and colder areas; sun or shade

Rabbits

Rabbits are active, energetic and often playful and would naturally exist in a social network, where the animals live communally in underground areas known as warrens, which are dug out of the earth. As they are a prey species, their social structure and behavioural repertoire is tailored toward

Table 31.2 Housing materials that can be used for cages/enclosures for small exotic animals

	Rats	Ferrets	Guinea pigs	Hamsters	Gerbils	Mice	Rabbits
Material suitable for construction of enclosure	Wire mesh and wood/metal-framed cage (Figs 31.5, 31.6)	Wire mesh and wood-frame cage and wooden/plastic sleeping enclosure	Plastic and wire-topped cage	Glass aquarium with multilevels. Metal mesh lid. Plastic-based cage with metal	Glass aquarium with multi levels. Metal mesh lid	Glass aquarium with multilevels. Metal mesh lid. Plastic-based cage with metal	Wooden hutch including wooden frame and wire mesh; must ensure wood is hard to resist chewing. New type of enclosure designed by Omlet is made from smooth plastic material and therefore the surfaces do not absorb moisture, unlike traditional wooden hutches that are often porus to liquid, making then hard to clean and disinfect
Construction requirements for indoor/outdoor enclosure	Not necessary	Wooden/metal frame with wire mesh sides. Chew- and escape-proof. Rest area must be waterproof and draught proof. Access to sleeping zone via a 'peep hole'. Concrete base for outdoor run – easily cleaned and known escapable	Wooden frame and wire mesh, with two wooden sides and hiding area. Include a solid roof for predator protection. Movable outside enclosure for continued grazing. Rest area must be waterproof and draught-proof. (Rabbit hutch style is suitable or new Eglu style enlosure). Access to sleeping zcne via a 'peep hole'	Not necessary	Not necessary	Not necessary	The rest area must be waterproof and draught-proof. The Eglu design has a special, twin-wall construction which insulates it against the outside temperature. So in the summer it's cool inside and in the winter the environment stays warm. Access to sleeping zone via 'pop hole'. Often tradditionally wooden frame and wire mesh, with two wooden sides and hiding area. Include a solid roof for predator protection. The wire base should be dug into the ground to prevent tunnelling and escaping; alternatively, the Eglu run is made from steel weld mesh and features Omlet's unique anti-tunnel skirt to prevent predators digging in (see Fig. 31.8). If an outdoor enclosure does have a mesh base, it also means that the rabbit cannot have tunnels built into the ground for added enrichment.
Suitable environment substrate	Newspaper lining with wood shavings/shredded paper covering the surface. Not digging or tunneling animals, therefore do not require depth of substate	Newspaper flooring, wood chip flooring for outside pen, shavings can be used for indoor pen floor covering	Wood shavings	Wood shavings. Shredded paper	Wood shavings, shredded paper or dry peat (5–10 cm depth for burrowing). Provision of a sand bath	Wood shavings, shredded paper and dry peat. Allow depth suitable for tunnelling and digging	Newspaper lining for insulation and absorption of urination, wood shavings or hay for substrate. 'Built' in 'removable' bedding trays allow easy cleaning and removal of substrate
Rest area/bedding material	Plastic or wooden boxes or tubes lined with shredded paper or shredded tissue	Wooden boxes, non-chewable plastic beds lined with towels or material for bedding. Can also use hay	Separate rest area if housed in a hutch. If housed in pen, cardboard or wooden boxes lined with shavings and hay	Shredded paper, hay or specalist hamster bedding	Shredded paper, hay or tissue	Shredded paper, hay or tissue	Hay for deep bedding providing warmth and draught reduction, shredded paper for long-haired rabbits, e.g. Angora rabbits
Provision of latrine	Not necessary	Provide litter trays, several for multi-housed animals. Wooden pellets can be used as litter material	Not necessary	Not necessary	Not necessary	Not necessary	Provide litter tray if training a house rabbit

Table 31.3 Suitable environmental enrichment and feeding facilities for small exotic animals

	Rats	Ferrets	Guinea pigs	Hamsters	Gerbils	Mice	Rabbits
Suitable environmental enrichment	Ropes for rats to climb, plastic tubing, material hammocks for playing and sleeping in. Plastic tubes to climb through, boxes to chew and hide in (see Figs 31.5, 31.6)	Plastic drainage pipes, tunnels, wooden stumps, non-chewable toys. Material hammocks for laying and sleeping in (see Fig. 31.7)	Scatter feeding hard food, fruit-tree wood for chewing and playing, large flower pots and drain pipes for hiding in (Fig. 31.12). Various grass, herbs and weeds for grazing; mental stimulation and exercise	Fruit-tree wood and cardboard boxes to chew, toilet role inners for tunnels, wheel for choice of exercise. Scatter feeding or hiding food for enrichment	Fruit-tree wood and cardboard boxes to chew, toilet role inners for tunnels, wheel for choice of exercise. Multi-layered cage for interest and to add space. Scatter feeding or hiding food for enrichment	Fruit-tree wood and cardboard boxes to chew, toilet role inners for tunnels, wheel for choice of exercise. Multi-layered cage for interest and to add space. Small ropes for climbing, millet spays hanging for enrichment. Scatter feeding or hiding food for enrichment	Large plastic tunnels dug into the ground to simulate shallow warren (see Fig. 31.3) tunnels and provide protection, mounds of soil for view points, large boxes to hide in and chew. Boxes filled with meadow hay and herbs to chew and eat. Indoor and outdoor rabbits should also have a peat box provided if they do not have access to digging facilities (see Fig. 31.8)
Feeding facilities and enrichment	Scatter feeding or food in a bowl, can also hide food in tunnels to increase activity and exploration behaviour. Water can be placed in a bottle, multiple sites if communal living	If housed communally, more than one feeding and drinking station should be provided. Water bottles rather than bowls. Hide dry food in tunnels to allow natural exploration behaviour	Plastic water bottle, change water daily as added vitamin C degrades when in contact with metal dripper. Ceramic feed bowls for hard food, but scatter feed is better for mental stimulation Also use hay balls for enrichment	Water bottle and feeding bowls, or scatter feeding for environmental stimulation	Water bottle or bowls, feeding bowls, or scatter feeding for environmental stimulation	Water bottle or bowls, feeding bowls, or scatter feeding for environmental stimulation	Water bottle or bowls, feeding bowls, or scatter feeding for environmental stimulation. Also use hay balls for enrichment (see Fig. 31.9). Placing fresh herbs and vegetables mixed in hay inside closed boxes allows rabbits to chew and rip while gaining a food source

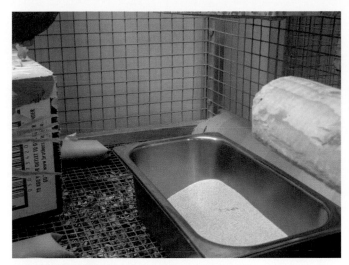

Fig. 31.1 Sand bath for small rodents *(Photo courtesy of Raystede Centre for Animal Welfare)*

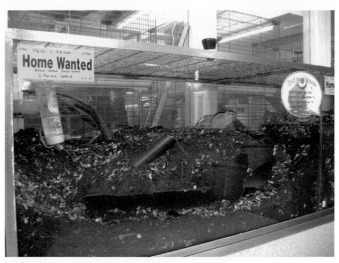

Fig. 31.2 Gerbil enclosure allowing expression of natural tunnelling behaviour *(Photo courtesy of Raystede Centre for Animal Welfare)*

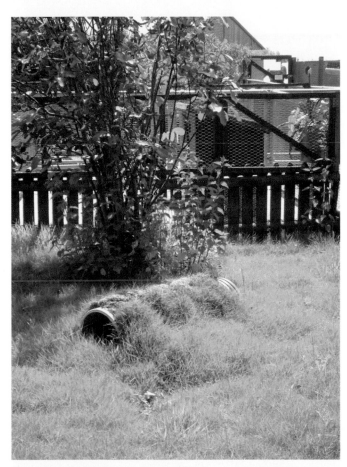

Fig. 31.3 Outdoor rabbit enclosure with built-in tunnels for hiding in *(Photo courtesy of Raystede Centre for Animal Welfare)*

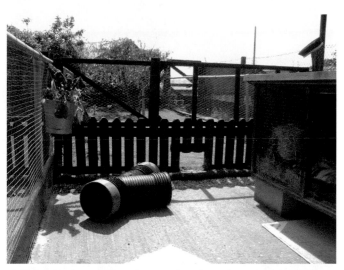

Fig. 31.4 Outdoor rabbit enclosure with traditional wooden hutch and 'pop-hole' into penned area with built-in tunnels *(Photo courtesy of Raystede Centre for Animal Welfare)*

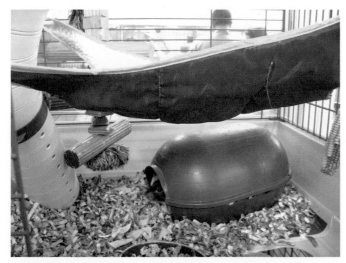

Fig. 31.5 Rat enclosure with various toys and shredded paper substrate *(Photo courtesy of Raystede Centre for Animal Welfare)*

607

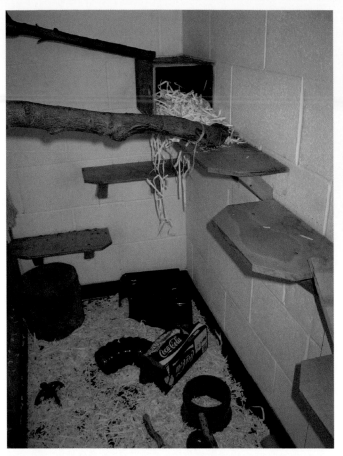

Fig. 31.6 Rat enclosure with arboreal steps allowing for 3D movement *(Photo courtesy of Plumpton College, Sussex)*

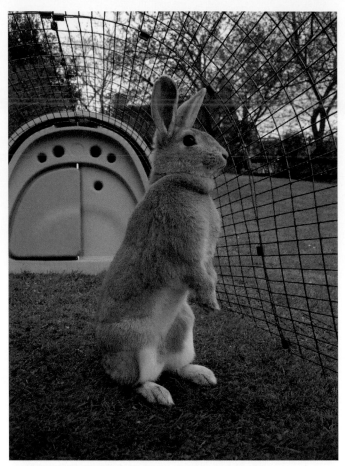

Fig. 31.8 Rabbit showing the natural tendency to stand upright, demonstrating the importance of providing sufficient height allowance in a cage – in this case the rabbit is in an Eglu™ enclosure *(Photo courtesy of Omlet™)*

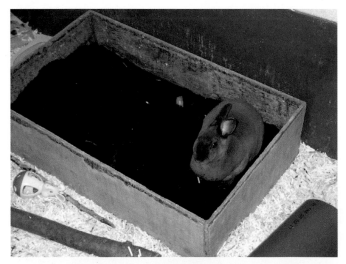

Fig. 31.7 Rabbits 'playing' in a soil box which allows for the expression of natural digging behaviour in a restricted environment *(Photo courtesy of Plumpton College Sussex)*

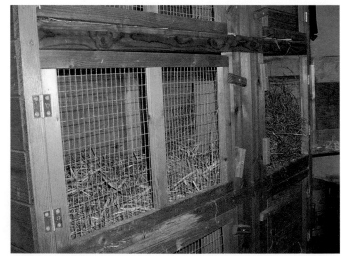

Fig. 31.9 Type of hutch suitable for a rabbit. The cage is divided into the living quarters lined with short straw and the sleeping quarters lined with softer hay *(Photo courtesy of Plumpton College, Sussex)*

survival. They spend large amounts of time grazing on grass and vegetation. The design of their housing should reflect their needs and allow rabbits to live as naturally as possible. Over the last 10 years rabbit housing has changed dramatically.

It is now common to house rabbits in two ways:

- Outdoor hutch and run
- Indoors as a house rabbit.

Both methods have their merits but whatever method is chosen it must satisfy the general requirements shown in Table 31.2.

Outdoor housing

Traditional outdoor housing usually takes the form of a wooden cage with a wire door covering half the front and a solid door covering the sleeping quarters (Fig. 31.9). The cage must be draught-proof, waterproof and vermin-proof. The doors should have good safety locks that are fox-proof. The hutch should have two areas, one for feeding and moving about and a second for sleeping:

- The feeding area should contain a water bottle, food and an ad lib hay supply
- The sleeping area should contain plenty of hay for warmth and bedding material (Table 31.2).

This type of housing is only recommended for overnight safety and the rabbit should be free to roam during the day in a fenced or penned area (Fig. 31.10). There are a variety of pens available and the common factors of all designs should include hiding places that double as shelters from the rain and heat, two opaque sides (four open sides will make the rabbit will feel vulnerable and nervous) and plenty of tunnels sunk into the ground (Fig. 31.3). Food and water must be available at all times.

Recently there has been a new rabbit/guinea pig enclosure designed known as the Eglu™. The Eglu™ for rabbits was developed in conjunction with leading animal behaviourists, Dr Anne McBride and Emma Magnus. It has two connected areas – the house and a secure outside run. The Eglu™ and run provide a living environment that the manufacturer

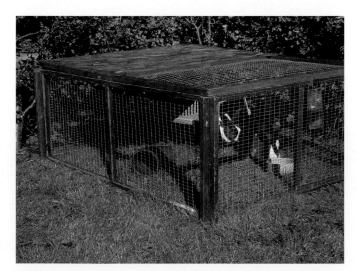

Fig. 31.10 Outdoor pen suitable for rabbits. The enclosure would benefit from more hiding areas and toys to increase mental stimulation *(Photo courtesy of Plumpton College, Sussex)*

describes as 'near to nature' (Fig. 31.8). The security of the enclosure allows the rabbit to exercise and follow its natural biological rhythms by performing and expressing natural behaviour when the need arises. The ability to control its own environment allows the animal to make choices which usually results in a more contented pet with few behavioural problems.

Rabbits should always be kept in groups or a minimum of a pair, as they are social prey animals that have evolved to live in colonies for safety and will not be able to perform normal interactive social behaviour if housed as single pets. If the owner does not wish to breed then the group should either consist of a single sex (although several bucks kept together may fight) or the rabbits should be neutered.

House rabbits

Rabbits may be kept indoors and allowed to roam freely around the house and fenced garden which provides exercise and stimulation for the rabbit. They should be provided with a low cage in which to hide and sleep and can be trained to use a litter tray. It is important to be aware that rabbits will chew electrical wiring, so care must be taken to prevent electrocution. It is also important to ensure that house plants are not in chewable proximity as many are toxic to rabbits. If an owner decides to keep a rabbit as a house pet, the species requrement for grass and exercise outside should not be forgotten. The animals should also have plenty of mental and physical stimulation. Care must be taken to ensure that house rabbits are safely managed with other family or visiting animals.

Housing rabbits within the veterinary practice

Separate accommodation should be provided for rabbits, as they are a prey species and will suffer from stress if housed with predator species such as noisy dogs, cats and ferrets. Even the smell of these animals, especially ferrets, can cause immense distress to the rabbit. Always provide a box for the rabbit to hide in while in the cage, or elect to leave them in their carriers if well ventilated. Covering the front of the cage with a clean blanket can also reduce stress, as can covering the basket when transporting them within the practice. Do not place the rabbit in a carrier on the floor as the smell of predators can be very strong and the smell from dogs being walked passed will be highly stressful.

Guinea pigs

Guinea pigs are highly social animals with a well-developed social system, so are easily housed in same-sex groups. The traditional rabbit hutch is acceptable for night-time housing, as are large, purpose-built plastic and wire cages. Guinea pigs also need access to an outdoor run for exercise and provision of fresh grass. If using this type of enclosure outdoors, a lid will be necessary to protect animals from local cats. Like rabbits, guinea pigs require hiding places, objects to chew, and items such as cardboard tubes to provide environmental enrichment (Table 31.3). Any cage designed for guinea pigs should have plenty of ventilation to reduce the build-up of ammonia levels. Guinea pigs have easily damaged toes, so a solid floor is preferable to a wire mesh. The cage should be situated out of direct sunlight, as they are susceptible to hyperthermia (Table 31.4).

Table 31.4 Optimum, minimum and maximum housing temperatures (where applicable) and siting and size of accomodation for small mammals

	Rabbits	Guinea pigs	Ferrets	Gerbils	Hamsters	Rats and mice
Optimum temperature	Prefer cooler temperatures	18–26°C	15–21°C	15–21°C	19–23°C	15–27°C
Minimum temperature	4°C	18°C	Below −7°C a heat lamp is required		Below 5°C hamsters start to enter hibernation	
Maximum temperature	28°C+ may cause heatstroke	26–30°C may cause heatstroke	32°C			30°C+ may cause heat stroke
Minimum size of accommodation	Run – minimum 1.5 m² for one rabbit, increase by half for second rabbit. Hutch – 0.3 m² for one animal, and 0.2 m² per animal if several. Rabbits should be able to stand up in enclosure and move around easily (see Fig. 31.10)	1.5 m × 1.5 m × 25 cm high for outdoor run. Hutch – 30 cm height, 0.2 m² floor area per guinea pig	1.5 m long × 0.75 m deep × 1 m high (suitable for three ferrets)	45 cm × 30 cm × 25 cm high for two-three gerbils	45 cm × 30 cm × 25 cm high for one hamster	50 cm × 30 × 50 cm high for one rat. 30 cm × 20 cm × 20 cm high for 4 mice
Siting of housing/ external enclosure	Wind-free area, with outdoor area having access to light for production of vitamin D and interesting activities for mental stimulation. Rabbits need to feel secure, so siting in a safe area where they do not feel vulnerable is essential	Wind-free area, with outdoor area having access to light and environmental stimulation. The run will need to be easily moved for continued grazing	Wind-free area, with outdoor area having access to light and environmental stimulation. Indoor area must be dry, draught-proof and heated if temperature is too cold	Place the cage in a safe area, not able to be knocked off tables or ledges. Also place where cats are unable to climb on the lid. Position cage for good ventilation but no draughts, and out of direct sunlight, but still allowing a good source of natural light	Place the cage in a safe area, not able to be knocked off tables or ledges. Also place where cats are unable to climb on the lid. Position cage for good ventilation but no draughts, and out of direct sunlight, but still allowing a good source of natural light	Rats – place the cage in a draught- and damp-free area. Good source of natural light should be available, but not direct sunlight to cause hyperthermia. Mice – place the cage in a safe area, not able to be knocked off tables or ledges. Also place where cats are unable to climb on the lid. Position cage for good ventilation but no draughts, and out of direct sunlight, but still allowing a good source of natural light

Ferrets

Ferrets are extremely active acrobatic animals and they need plenty of space and exercise. They can be housed either indoors or outdoors. The most important aspect in their housing is to ensure that the enclosure is 'ferret proof', i.e. it is free of holes and escape proof. Ferret housing should include the provision of a dark, quiet sleeping zone that can be furnished with soft bedding material such as old sheets and towels. This will allow ferrets to feel secure and perform their natural hiding behaviour. It will also protect outdoor ferrets from extreme heat and cold. More than one sleep zone is necessary for multiple-housed animals. Solid toys, tunnels and hiding places should be provided for environmental enrichment. Ferrets can be housed in wooden/wire cages (Fig. 31.11) with a solid floor but everything must be easily cleaned. Litter trays should be provided in several positions throughout the enclosure for elimination.

Mice, hamsters and gerbils

Gerbils and mice naturally live in colonies, so are much happier kept in family units, However, Syrian hamsters are naturally solitary and will fight to the death if kept with another hamster. The small Chinese and Russian hamsters can be kept in groups, providing they are introduced when young, e.g. litter mates.

Mice, hamsters and gerbils are easily housed in aquarium tanks but there must be plenty of ventilation via a metal mesh lid (Figs 31.2, 31.12). This design is preferable to cages with metal bars as they are able to accommodate a deep layer of substrate in which to burrow and dig. Gerbils in particular enjoy deep wood shavings, in which they can create a complex network of tunnels. Mice are less inclined to burrow on such a large scale. Both species enjoy having multilayered enclosures with steps or ropes connecting the areas.

Mice produce pungent-smelling urine and should be cleaned out every 2–3 days; gerbils smell less and can be cleaned less often; hamster cages need fully cleaning about once a month. All three species enjoy chewing and cardboard, small boxes and toilet roll tubes all make excellent shredding material and help to keep their teeth worn down.

Cages with different platforms and objects to supply environmental enrichment provide plenty of interest and exercise. Hamster balls are not recommended as once inside, the animal has very little control over the action of the ball. Hamsters will naturally want to move forward but the impact of hitting other objects and the vibration produced may be stressful to such a small prey species. Circular running wheels are more appropriate as the animal has a choice as to whether to use it and for how long. Sleeping zones are important and wooden or non-chewable plastic houses stuffed full of shredded paper or tissue are often used. Gerbils also enjoy sand baths and a shallow bowl filled with sand should be provided (Fig. 31.1).

Rats

Rats can be kept in large wire cages that allow vertical and horizontal movement. The enclosure needs to be situated in a dry, draught-free area with access to natural light. It is important to provide plenty of items to climb on and chew (Figs 31.6, 31.13). Plastic tunnels are useful for both running through and sleeping in. Rats enjoy comfortable bedding areas where they can curl up in. The sleeping areas can be any solid type of box with a lid (Fig. 31.5).

Nutrition and feeding

Small mammals have different nutritional requirements. Table 31.5 shows a summary of appropriate nutritional requirements and feeding methods.

Breeding

Breeding small mammals is usually easy, rapid and may result in large numbers of offspring. Most small mammals will breed during the spring and summer and slow down or stop when the day length shortens. This pattern of repeated oestrus during the spring and summer is described as being

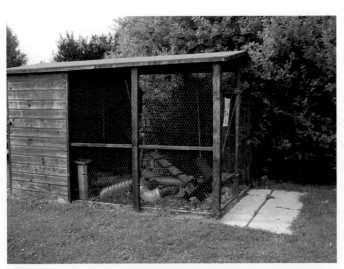

Fig. 31.11 An outdoor ferret cage that provides fresh air, entertainment and exercise (*Photo courtesy of Plumpton College, Sussex*)

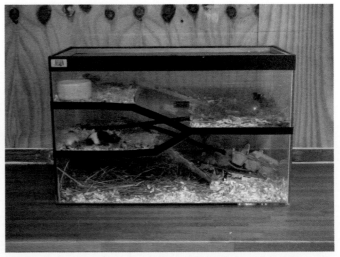

Fig. 31.12 A multilayered aquarium type of cage suitable for a colony of mice. It includes numerous boxes, ladders and tunnels for mental stimulation (*Photo courtesy of Plumpton College, Sussex*)

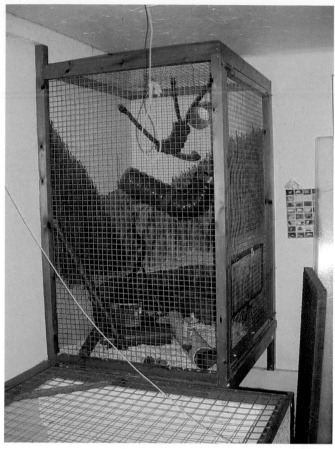

Fig. 31.13 A wooden and wire rat cage. It provides vertical and horizontal exercise and has numerous toys and tunnels for entertainment. The cage also has a bedding area containing hay *(Photo courtesy of Plumpton College, Sussex)*

seasonally polyoestrous. Non-seasonally polyoestrous animals will breed all year round regardless of the season (Table 31.6).

Small mammals may be either induced or spontaneous ovulators:

- **Induced ovulation** – the female ovulates as a result of the stimulation of coitus, e.g. ferret, rabbit
- **Spontaneous ovulation** – the female ovulates at a fixed time during the reproductive cycle, e.g. guinea pig, gerbil.

Most female mammals display a behaviour known as lordosis when they are receptive to the male, i.e. the animal flattens its back and raises the pelvis, indicating readiness to mate. Many of the small mammals display more individual behaviour around breeding and gestation periods.

Rabbits

It is normal behaviour for the doe to pull hair from her dewlap, sides and abdomen to line and soften the nest. This behaviour normally takes place a few days or hours before parturition. The young kits are altricial when born, i.e. they are blind, furless and totally dependent on the doe. The doe only feeds her young (kits) for about 3–5 minutes once a day and within this short feeding period the kits consume up to 20% of their body weight. The kits are 'held up' in the nest for 3 weeks.

Guinea pigs

Guinea pigs do not build nests to receive the young. When the pups are born, they are fully furred with their eyes open, i.e. they are precocial. Within a few hours after birth they are able to stand and, although they will start to eat solid food within 24 hours they are unable to survive alone for the first 5 days and would normally consume milk for up to 3 weeks. Guinea pig sows will also 'top and tail' the pups post feeding.

Hamsters, mice, rats and ferrets

All these species are born hairless, deaf, blind and completely reliant on the mother, i.e. they are altricial. The mother feeds her young and will wean at the appropriate time. Very little human interference is necessary once parturition is complete. If the young are rejected, which may occur if the nest is disturbed by the male or by a human, then bottle-feeding and hand-rearing is possible. The exception is young ferrets who are very difficult to hand rear when orphaned.

Common diseases and clinical conditions

Common diseases and clinical conditions of small mammals are shown in Tables 31.7–31.11.

Reptiles

The species of reptile kept as exotic pets includes various types of lizards and snakes and the shelled reptiles or chelonia, i.e. tortoises and terrapins (see also Ch. 5) (Table 31.11). They are a diverse group of animals and the large number of species available for sale and being presented for treatment in veterinary practice means that the veterinary nurse must have a good understanding of their basic housing, nutritional and breeding needs.

Housing

Reptiles are ectothermic or cold-blooded and it is important to remember that their health and well-being depend entirely on the environment in which we place them. If we get it wrong, it can lead to stress, which in turn can cause immunosuppression, ill health and death.

Reptiles are housed in **vivaria**, which are available in a variety of shapes, sizes and construction materials. Figures 31.14 and 31.15 show different types of set-up.

When selecting accommodation for a reptile or chelonian the following must be considered:

- Natural history of the species. The nurse must know the species' country of origin and from this must understand:
  - The need to house the reptile in a temperate, desert or tropical environment
  - The reptile's activity pattern, i.e. nocturnal, crepuscular or diurnal
  - The reptile's requirements for a terrestrial, arboreal, aquatic or semi-aquatic set-up.
- The size, shape and materials used in vivarium construction (Table 31.12)

Table 31.5 Nutritional requirements and feeding methods

	Rabbits	Guinea pigs	Ferrets	Hamsters	Rats	Gerbils	Mice
Classification by diet	Herbivore	Herbivore	Carnivore	Omnivore	Omnivore	Omnivore	Omnivore
Cophrophagia or caecotrophy	Caecotrophs excreted and eaten at night. They contain high levels of vitamin B and K, and twice the protein and half the fibre of hard faeces. Caecotrophs are eaten directly from the anus many times a day	Caecotrophs are eaten as with rabbit					
Special dietary needs	The digestive tract of the rabbit is designed for high fibre, and low protein, necessary for normal peristalsis, correct absorption of vitamins and prevention of dental disease. Vitamin D and calcium are necessary for development and maintenance of bones and teeth	Guinea pigs cannot synthesize vitamin C (ascorbic acid) as they do not have the necessary enzyme L-gluconolactone oxidase. Fresh green food must be given daily. Water may be supplemented with vitamin C at a dose of 10 mg/kg daily, or 1 g/l water (change daily). Pregnant sows – 30 mg/kg daily	Strict carnivores designed to eat their prey whole. Ferrets need a diet high in fat and protein, minimal fibre and carbohydrate	In the wild they will eat invertebrates and insects. Require a small proportion of animal-derived protein, e.g. cooked chicken	In the wild they will eat invertebrates and insects. Require a small proportion of animal-derived protein, e.g. cooked chicken	In the wild they will eat invertebrates and insects. Require a small proportion of animal-derived protein, e.g. cooked chicken	In the wild they will eat invertebrates and insects. Require a small proportion of animal-derived protein, e.g. cooked chicken
Foods to be avoided	Kale and spinach – may cause goitre; succulent fruit and vegetables, e.g. lettuce, may cause diarrhoea. Sugary foods	Fruits or sugary foods	Sweet sugary foods, grains	High-fat seeds, e.g. sunflower seeds, should not be fed regularly, as may exacerbate the onset of osteoporosis	High-fat seeds, e.g. sunflower seeds should not be fed regularly as rats are prone to obesity		
Diet	Ad-lib hay – high in fibre should be the main food source with a variety of vegetables. Grazing in the garden will provide much of the vegetation needed. Complementary dried feeds can be fed in addition	Grass, ad-lib hay, fresh leafy vegetables, complete food in small amounts compared to other food sources	Dead chicks, mice and rats. Raw eggs. Specially prepared dry ferret food	Can be fed a commercial complete food mix. Can also be fed table scraps	Can be fed a commercial complete food mix. Can also be fed table scraps. Rats may benefit from small pieces of cat food	Can be fed a commercial complete food mix. Can also be fed table scraps	Can be fed a commercial complete food mix. Can also be fed table scraps
Required nutritional values (Adult)	Recommended nutritional values for complete mix – fibre 16%; protein 16%	Protein 18–20%; fibre 10%	If complete dried food: fat 20%; protein 30–35%; fibre 20–25%	Minimum of: protein 16%; fat 4–5%	Minimum of: protein 16%; fat 4–5%. Pregnant females may require protein levels up to 20%	Minimum of: protein 16%; fat 4–5%. Pregnant females may require protein levels up to 20%	Minimum of: protein 16%; fat 4–5%
(Young)			Fat 20%; protein 35%				

Table 31.6 Significant information required for breeding small mammals

	Rabbits	**Guinea pigs**	**Ferrets**	**Gerbils**	**Mice**	**Rats**	**Hamsters**
Sexual maturity	Small breeds 4–5 months Medium breeds 4–6 months Large breeds 5–8 months	(M) 3 months (F) 2 months	6–12 months	(M) 9–18 weeks (F) 9–12 weeks	6 weeks	4–5 weeks	(M) 8 weeks (F) 6 weeks
Ovulation	10 h after coitus	Spontaneous	30–40 h post-coitus				
Gestation period	30–32 days	59–72 days	41–43 days	23–26 days	19–21 days	21–23 days	15–18 days
Litter size	4–5 kits (small breeds) 8–12 kits (larger breeds)	1–13 (2–4 is usual) pups/young	1–18 kits, average 8	3–8 pups	7–11 pups	6–13 pups	5–10 pups
Normal birth weight	Varies for breed of rabbit	45–115 g	6–12 g	2.5–3.5 g	1–1.5 g	4–6 g	1.5–3 g
Weaning age	By 28 days full weaning should have occurred	21 days	6–8 weeks	21–28 days	18–21 days	21 days	19–21 days

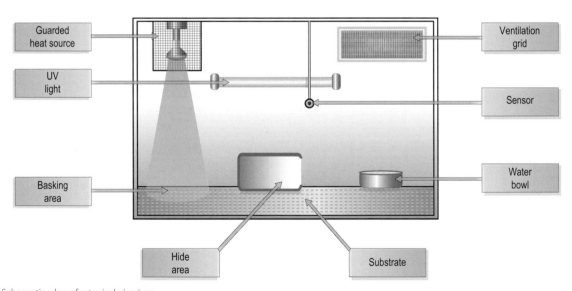

Fig. 31.14 Schematic plan of a typical vivarium

Table 31.7 Common diseases and clinical conditions of gerbils, hamsters and rats

	Disease	Causal agent	Symptoms	Age of animals affected/incubation period	Treatment	Prognosis
Hamsters	Constipation	Inappropriate diet, often due to lack of moisture in food	Swollen abdomen, pain and anorexia	Often in hamsters of 2 weeks old, just as the weaning process starts	Change diet to include green vegetables and fruit, severe cases may need an enema	Good response
Hamsters	Bacterial pneumonia	*Pasteurella pnemotropica* and *Streptococcus* spp., stressful environment can predispose animals to infection	Oculonasal discharge, anorexia, dyspnoea	Any age	Supportive treatment, warmth, antibiotics	Good response
Hamster	Impacted cheeks	Food adhering to cheeks	Swollen cheeks	Any age	Emptied and flushed with water	Good response
Mice, hamsters	Viral pneumonia	Sendai virus – parainfluenza virus type 1	Asymptomatic in adults	Any age		May cause death in younger animals
Gerbils	Swollen sebaceous glands	infection	Inflammation of large ventral abdominal sebaceous gland	Any age	Corticosteroids and antibiotics, may need surgery, or debridement in severe cases of infection	Good response
Hamsters gerbils, rats	Dental problems/ malocclusion	Insufficient wear on teeth caused by poor diet, and malocclusion often occurs as a result of bar chewing. Malocclusion is also most common inherited disease in rabbits – change in skull and jaw length	Malocclusion of teeth, problems possible with both incisors and check teeth. Teeth continue to grow and overlap causing anorexia, and drooling. In severe cases – oral lesions and teeth growing into gums	Any age	Regular clipping and food that will wear teeth down and objects to chew	Good response
Gerbils, hamsters, rats	Neoplasia	Spontaneous in gerbils over two years old	Tumours commonly found on ovaries, skin (squamous cell carcinomas), sebaceous glands, kidney and adrenal glands. In rats, common tumour sites are mammary, abdomen and shoulders	Over 2 years old. More common in males of the hamster species	No treatment	High mortality rate
Gerbils, hamsters, rats	Tyzzer's disease – intracellular bacterium, can only be confirmed via postmortem	*Clostridium piliforme* Caused by poor sanitation or deprivation of food or water	Lethargy, anorexia, loss of weight, piloerection	Weanlings are often affected. 10 days incubation period	Antibiotics are largely unsuccessful, but supportive therapy, IVFT, and rehydration solutions can be given	Usually poor
Gerbils, hamsters,	Wet tail	Multifactorial, factors include stress, possibly diet. *E. coli* and *Campylobacter* have both been isolated from samples	Severe watery diarrhoea causing staining around the anus, lethargy, anorexia, abdominal pain causing huddled appearance	Any age	Antibiotics, but are often unsuccessful, but supportive therapy, fluid therapy, and rehydration/electrolyte solutions can be given	Usually high mortality rate
Gerbils	Salmonellosis	*S. enteritidid* and *S. typhimurium* have both been isolated as possible pathogens	Moderate to severe diarrhoea, staring coat dehydration and weight loss	There is often no incubation period seen as patient often dies very quickly	Not recommended as it is a zoonotic disease and recovered patients often then become carriers	High mortality rate

Table 31.8 Common diseases and clinical conditions of guinea pigs

Disease	Causal agent	Symptoms	Age of animals affected/ incubation period	Treatment	Prognosis
Salmonellosis	*S. enteritidid* and *S. typhimurium* have both been isolated as possible pathogens	Moderate to severe diarrhoea, staring coat dehydration and weight loss. Causes septicaemia and abortions in Guinea pigs	There is often no incubation period seen as patient often dies very quickly	Not recommended as it is a zoonotic disease and recovered patients often then become carriers	High mortality rate. Sudden deaths in guinea pigs
Mites	*Trixacarus caviae* – a sarcoptid mite	Pruritus	Any age	Ivermectin (not licensed for rodents)	Good response
Barbering/alopecia	Hair loss with no obvious disease is often caused by other guinea pigs or self-inflicted due to boredom	Loss of hair from body with no pruritus	Any age, seen in female guinea pigs late in pregnancy	Separate animals if specific interactions are problematic, increase environmental enrichment.	Good response
Scurvy (hypovitaminosis C)	Lack of vitimin C in diet – management and husbandry related. Guinea pigs are unable to manufacture vitamin C and therefore need to have it provided in their diet. Vitamin C denatures easily under warm, humid conditions and direct sunlight. Old greens and vegetables may also have reduced vitamin contents	Depressed, weak and lethargic, weight loss, anorexia, anaemia, bleeding gums, gingivitis, reduced immune system and poor skin condition/ healing, pain, reluctance to walk, swollen painful joints	Various factors can affect vitamin C metabolism and usage, including life stage, pregnancy, stress, activity and environment	Supplement with 100 mg/kg vitamin C if showing symptoms	

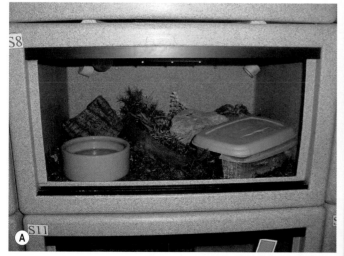

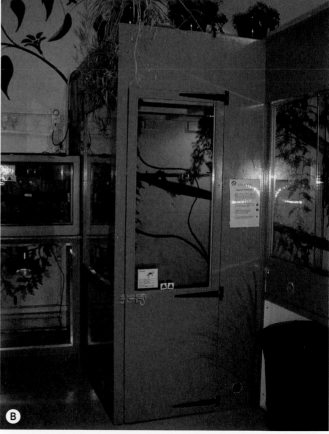

Fig. 31.15 Vivaria. (**A**) Vivarium suitable for a terrestrial snake. (**B**) Large walk-in vivarium suitable for a large arboreal lizard such as a green iguana *Iguana iguana*

Table 31.9 Common diseases and clinical conditions of rabbits

Disease	Causal agent	Symptoms	Age of animals affected/ incubation period	Treatment	Prognosis
Pododermatitis	Caused by pressure, and are often predisposed by genetically reduced amount of hair on the plantar surfaces. Also caused by wire-floored cages, poor hygiene and heavy weight of larger rabbits	Decubital ulcers on plantar surfaces of hind feet. Appearance of superficial ulcers and scabs, may become abscess if progress.	Any age, larger-sized rabbits, and those with less fur on plantar surface	Topical antibiotic application and bandages changed at a regular interval. Re-evaluate cage flooring	Good response to long-term treatment
Pasteurellosis	*Pasteurella multocida* bacterium	Respiratory disease, sneezing or snuffles, mucopurulent nasal discharge, conjunctivitis, skin abscesses, inner ear infection, pyometra, pneumonia or scepticaemia	Seen in older animals and those kept in large colonies or breeding rabbitries	Supportive therapy depending on symptoms. Antibiotics can be used for a month, but symptoms will return when drugs are stopped. Flush nares and nasolacrimal duct	Virtually impossible to rid animal of infection as very resilient. Euthanasia when symptoms causing distress or untreatable with supportive treatment
Coccidiosis	Hepatotrphic or enteric species of *Eimeria*. Vitamin E may increase coccidiosis	Diarrhoea, may cause fatal hepatic failure, icterus, hepatomegaly, and anorexia	Often seen in younger animals, especially weanlings	Treatment with sulpha drugs and reduced stress and increase in hygiene levels	Good prognosis
Gastric trichobezoars	Fur accumulation in gut possibly due to excessive grooming (possibly stress related) or diet lacking in fibre	Fur accumulation in stomach, causing blockage of the narrow pyloric lumen, leading to gut obstruction, gut dilation and anorexia.		High-fibre diets for prevention. Trichobezoars can be broken down using proteolytic enzymes, e.g. papain or bromelain (from health-food shops). Liquid paraffin is also of use	100% if not treated, otherwise good prognosis if diagnosed and treated quickly
Necrobacillosis (Schmorl's disease)	*Fusobacterium necrophorum*, associated with poor hygiene, skin abrasions and dental disease	Bacteria may cause ulceration and necrosis of skin, particularly on the face, neck and plantar areas of feet, and septicaemia	Not age-specific	Improve hygiene, debride wounds, treat with topical and oral antibiotics	Good prognosis
Myiasis (fly strike)	Due to diarrhoea (diet-related, infection, parasitic), obesity (Gosden). Poor husbandry, causing faeces-infected environment. Poor management of rabbit fur/lack of grooming. Fly eggs developing into maggots	Eggs are usually layered around the perineum area of the rabbit. They then develop into maggots and eat the skin and tissue of the animal causing lesions	Not age-specific, related to animals gut health and husbandry	Remove maggots, clean area (under sedation). Antibiotics, IVFT, wound management. Prevent with use of Rearguard (Novartis)	Prognosis dependent on severity of skin lesions and severity of infection. Rabbits are often in very poor condition when presented for treatment. If severe, euthanasia may be advised

Table 31.9 Continued

Disease	Causal agent	Symptoms	Age of animals affected/ incubation period	Treatment	Prognosis
Gastric stasis syndrome	Caused by a change in gastric motility and function, resulting in reabsorption of liquid from stomach content due to: high-carbohydrate/low-fibre diet, stress, lack of exercise, possibly ingestion of hair	Anorexia, decreased stool (faecal pellet) production, large gas-filled stomach with dough-like contents		Laxatives, paraffin oil, pineapple for bromelin (used as protein digestive enzymes). Oral rehydration – soften stomach contents, including water, fruit juices, vegetable puree, Critical Care formulae. IV/ S/C fluids. Metoclopramide to stimulate gut motility. Possibly surgical intervention if non-responsive to medical	Reduced in rabbits undergoing surgery. Patients often die due to hepatic lipidosis in surgical cases
Rabbit calicivirus disease – viral haemorrhagic disease	Caused by calicivirus, spread via faecal – oral route, via conjunctiva, nasal passages or damaged tissue , and via fomites	Acute onset, incubation 1–2 days. May show signs of depression, lethargy, anorexia, tachypnea, cyanosis, diarrhoea and constipation. Often appears asymptomatic and rabbit found dead due to such rapid onset	Older than 2 months	No suitable treatment available. Vaccination 12 monthly as prevention.	Highly infectious and high morbidity rates of 70–80% and high mortality rates of 100%
Encephalomyelitis – head tilt and ataxia	Caused by vestibular dysfunction, central (cerebellum) and peripheral (bacterial inner ear infection – otitis interna), peripheral nerve disease. Hyperaesthesia may indicate central nerve disease, and seizures and rolling may indicate brain lesions. Pasteurella multocida bacterial infection may also cause head tilt. Also caused by Encephalitozoon cuniculi (protozoal disease): signs are trauma, heat stroke	Clinical indicators include neurological signs: head tilt, nystagmus, tremors, paresis, paralysis and seizures	Any age, transmitted between rabbits, carriers may be asymptomatic	Treatment is dependent on diagnosis. Otitis media and interna should be treated with antibiotics for 4 weeks or longer, possibly flushing ear canal while under GA. If encephalitozoonosis is diagnosed, steroids to reduce inflammation, antibiotics to treat bacterial infection and sedatives to control seizures (Queensberry and Carpenter 2003). Anthelmintics for E. cuniculi	

Myxomatosis	Myxoma virus of the pox family. Transmitted via arthropod bite (usually the rabbit flea) and direct contact	Clinical signs depend on virulence of strain and genus of rabbit species infected. Wild rabbits may exhibit benign skin tumours at base of ear – if entry point. Domestic rabbits – lethargy, fever, anorexia, skin haemorrhage, and seizures	Vaccination every 6 months or annually as prevention. Treatment is possible only if strain of virus is mild, then supportive nursing care and antibacterial therapy should be implemented. To help in prevention of myxomatosis transmission, buy hay/straw from myxomatosis-free suppliers, fit fly screens to hutches, stop wild rabbits entering garden	High mortality rate
Rabbit ear mite	*Psoroptes cuniculi* (ear mites)	Clinical signs include severe otitis externa, crusting and exudate	Not age-related	Antibiotics to reduce secondary bacterial infection. Topical ear treatment, ivermectin	Good response
Abscesses	Abscesses are walled-off pockets containing bacteria	Commonly occur in the skin (secondary to injury or surgery), head, neck and secondary to dental disease (Hansen 2002). Clinical signs include swellings, pain in area of abscess, possible anorexia	Not age-specific, often due to injury or after surgery, foreign bodies – any factor which can cause localized bacterial infection	Sedation/GA to probe and clean abscess, debride necrotic tissue, pack wound cavity to prevent healing too quickly and trapping bacteria. Oral or systemic antibiotics, should be used, can also use antibiotic-impregnated beads within the wound	Abscess may burst, expelling pus externally, or bacteria may escape capsule and settle around body causing new abscesses – 'seeding' (Hansen 2002); antibiotics will not penetrate multiple abscesses that cannot be treated surgically, therefore euthanasia advised.
Uterine cancer	80% female rabbits develop uterine cancer. Adenocarcinoma – malignant tumour of the glandular tissue that metastasizes, often to the lungs	Clinical signs of advanced uterine cancer include: anaemia, decreased lethargy, swollen cystic mammary glands, weight loss, dyspnoea and increased aggression	Most common in doe's aged 5–6 years	Spay females after 5–6 months of age.	If diagnosis is made before metastasizes, possible to spay with successful recovery; otherwise, euthanasia or mobidity of affected rabbits is high
Dental problems/malocclusion	Insufficient wear on teeth caused by poor diet, and malocclusion often occurs as a result of bar chewing. Malocclusion is also most common inherited disease in rabbits – change in skull and jaw length	Malocclusion of teeth, problems possible with both incisors and cheek teeth. Teeth continue to grow and overlap causing anorexia, and drooling. Lastly, in severe cases – oral lesions and teeth growing into gums	Any age	Regular clipping and food that will wear teeth down and objects to chew	Good response

Table 31.10 Common diseases and clinical conditions of ferrets

Disease	Causal agent	Symptoms	Age of animals affected/ incubation period	Treatment	Prognosis
Canine distemper	Distemper virus	Mucopurulent ocular nasal discharge, crusty eyelids and facial lesions. Hyperkeratosis of footpads. Possibly anorexic and may be ataxic or show signs of nystagmus. Pyrexia – 40.6–41.1°C	Any age. Incubation period is 7–9 days	Can be vaccinated against using canine vaccine – Vaxitas D	100% fatal in ferrets, and if contracted, the ferret should be euthanized
Influenza	Ferrets are susceptible to several strains of the virus	Influenza causes upper respiratory disease, with symptoms including anorexia, listlessness and nasal discharge	Any age of ferret	Antibiotics may be needed if secondary infection is involved. Often recovers without the need for drugs	100% fatal in kits
Aleutian disease (AD)	Parvovirus. Immune-mediated and may also cause some immunodepression	Black tarry faeces, recurrent fevers, weight loss, behaviour changes – possibly increase in aggression or hyperaesthesia, thyroiditis, paralysis followed by death. Carriers may be asymptomatic	Any age	No specific relief, supportive therapy and antibiotics	Can be fatal
Ear mites	*Otedectes cynosis*	Black sticky discharge in one or both ears	Any age	Clean ears daily and Ivomec injections, one injection repeated in 2 weeks (not to be used in pregnant females). Can also use ear drops with active ingredient gamma BHC	Good response
Prolonged oestrus	Female ferrets are polyoestrous and induced ovulators. When in oestrus and not mated they continue to have high circulating oestrogen levels which causes bone marrow suppression	Anaemia and reduced white blood cell production.	Sexually mature entire females	Spay at 6–8 months of age if not intended for breeding. Hormone injections control oestrus. Use of vasectomized hob for coitus and completing oestrus cycle	Life-threatening

Table 31.11 Common reptilian species kept as pets in the UK

Species	Country of origin	Food	Reproductive data	Additional comments
Snakes				
Boas				
Common boa (*Boa constrictor constrictor*)	Central and South America from Mexico to northern Argentina	Depends on the size of the snake – rodents (mice, rats, gerbils); chicks (day-old); birds	Live bearers, i.e. ovoviviparous; 20–60 in a litter. Young approx. 35–60 cm in length	Heavy-bodied species average 3 m but can grow larger. Require temperature range of 28–30°C. Provide with a large ceramic water bowl, as this species likes to soak
Pythons				
Royal python (*Python regius*)	Africa	Depends on the size of the snake – mammals, rabbits, birds chicks	Oviparous; lays up to 7 eggs; incubation can last 40–80 days and young measure 40 cm	Short, stocky snake that reaches about 1.2 m in length. Although usually good-natured, can refuse to eat for periods of time – making it unsuitable for the novice. If threatened will go into a ball. Vivarium temperature range 25–30°C

Table 31.11 Continued

Species	Country of origin	Food	Reproductive data	Additional comments
Burmese python (*Python moluris bivittatus*)	Asia	As Royal python	Oviparous; reported to lay up to 100 eggs (more realistically, ~30). Incubation temperature 30°C and can last 60–80 days. Young measure 40 cm	Albino or golden Burmese have bright yellow markings on a white background. Very large snake – grows up to 6–7 m. Grows rapidly and reaches 3–4 m in 2 years. Because of potential size, feeding and space requirements, not recommended as a pet
Reticulated python (*Python reticulatus*)	South-east Asia	As above	Similar to Burmese python	Very large snake – grows up to 9 m. Not best-tempered snake and because of size and aggressive nature not recommended as a pet
Colubrids				
Corn snake (*Elaphe guttata*) – rat snake family	North America	Depends on the size of the snake: mammals, rabbits, birds chicks	Oviparous: breed snake from 2 years old. Lays 12+ eggs 1 month after mating. Incubate at 28°C for ~60–70 days	Many colour mutations. Good pet for novice keeper. Good temperament, grows to 1 m, easy to manage and eats readily in captivity
King snake (*Lampropeltis getulus*)	North America	As above	Oviparous: breed from 2 years of age. Usually produce two clutches in each breeding season. Clutch size 5–20 – subspecies vary. Incubate at 28°C for 60 days	Adults can grow to 2 m but average length 1 m. Colour usually black with yellow or white markings. Relatively easy to keep in captivity. Best kept on its own, as they have cannibalistic tendencies
Garter snakes				
Common garter snake (*Thamnophis sirtalis*)	North and Central America	Earthworms, fish, small rodents, pinkies	Ovoviviparous: clutch size 10–20; gestation period 4–5 months	Active snake and requires relatively large accommodation relative to size. Temperature range 20–30°C. Small snake: grows to 0.5–1 m. Care when feeding fish, as this must be blanched for 2 min to kill antivitamin, which causes thiamine deficiency
Lizards				
Geckos				
Leopard gecko (*Eublepharus macularis*)	Central Asia	Insects, (crickets, hoppers, locusts) neonate mammals	Oviparous. Female can lay up to five clutches per season. Eggs are laid in pairs in moistened sand, vermiculite or peat, and have soft, leathery shells. Best removed and placed in an incubator. Temperature of 27–29°C produces females, 32–33°C will produce males. If eggs stuck together do not attempt to separate. Incubate for 6–8 weeks	Good beginner's lizard – does well in captivity; friendly, easy to keep. Nocturnal temp. daytime 25–30°C. Male geckos are very territorial and will fight, so best kept on their own or with females at a ratio of 1:4.
Fat-tailed gecko (*Hemitheconyx audicinctus*)	North-east Africa			
Day gecko (*Phelsuma cepediana*)		Also offer fruit puree baby food	Oviparous: very similar to leopard geckos except that eggs have hard shells	Lively and quick, need tall, well-planted vivarium. Very colourful. Both sexes can be territorial and need a large vivarium so they can retreat to their own area

Table 31.11 Continued

Species	Country of origin	Food	Reproductive data	Additional comments
Agamas				
Water dragon (*Physignathus cocincinus*)	Indonesia	Insects, crickets, locusts, small rodents, pinkies, some fruit and vegetable matter	Oviparous: female can lay up to five clutches per breeding season of 10–15 eggs. Eggs laid in damp sand or vermiculite and should be removed and placed in an incubator at 28–30°C. Hatch in approx. 60 days. Hatchling size 15 cm. Difficult to breed in captivity	Diurnal background temperature of 25–30°C. Requires good ultraviolet and florescent lighting. Tall vivarium, as arboreal. Diurnal. Need high daytime temperature – 40°C+ in the basking area and background temperature of 25–30°C
Uromastyx or dab lizard (*Uromastyx acanthinurus*)	Arid deserts and steppe of north Africa, Middle East and northern parts of India	Fruit and vegetable matter (foliage leaf-based diet), occasional insect		
Chameleons				
Jackson's chameleon (*Chamaeleo jacksoni*)	Africa – regions around Mount Kenya	Winged insects, occasional pinky, waxworms	Oviparous or ovoviviparous depending on species. Can be difficult to breed if conditions not correct. Jackson's chameleon is ovoviviparous: up to 50 young 3 cm in length born approx. 9 months after breeding	Fascinating species. Arboreal and require tall vivarium. Can suffer from stress if housing is incorrect. As most will not drink from water bowl, foliage needs regular misting. Highly territorial, so best kept on their own or one male with females, but fighting may still occur
Panther chameleon (*Chamaeleo pardalis*)	Madagascar			
Iguanas				
Green iguana (*Iguana iguana*)	Central America to northern regions of South America	Fruit + vegetable matter (foliage – leaf-based diet). Specialist dietary requirements	Oviparous: 20–40 eggs per clutch; hatch after 10–15 weeks	Very large lizard 100–200 cm in length. Needs tall vivarium and males can be very aggressive. Not ideal pet
Monitors/tegus				
Tegu (*Tupinambis* spp.) Monitor (*Varanus* spp.)	Africa–Asia	Mammals, eggs, birds	Oviparous – limited details on captive breeding	Very large, heavy-bodied lizard; can grow to 1–3 m and has a dubious temperament. In my opinion, not suitable as a pet
Skinks				
Blue-tongued skink (*Tiligua gigas*)	Australasia	Insects, snails, mammals	Viviparous: litter size 5–10. Gestation period varies according to background temperature	Generally good-natured and can make good pets. Males can become aggressive during breeding season
Chelonia				
Mediterranean tortoises				
Spur-thigh tortoise (Greek) (*Testudo graeca*)	Four subspecies that range around Spain, Morocco, Algeria Tunisia, Turkey, Iran, Israel	Variety of leafy vegetables, salad crops, proprietary dry foods	Oviparous: gestation period 30 days to 3 years. Females can retain sperm. Female can be observed digging several holes.	With the exception of Horsfield's tortoise (*Testudo horsfieldi*), which is not truly a Mediterranean tortoise, all are protected under CITES legislation and are classified as Annex A. This means that they require DEFRA certificates in order to be bought, sold or traded
Hermann's tortoise (*Testudo hermanni*)	Two subspecies: western Hermann's range from Spain through the south of France to western Italy		Nests before finally laying 3–12 eggs. Depending on temperature and species, eggs need to be incubated for 7–20 weeks at 30–34°C. Sex can be determined by temperature – higher produces females, lower produces males	
Marginated tortoise (*Testudo marginata*)	Greece and its islands			
Horsfield's tortoise (*Testudo horsfieldi*)	Two subspecies: between them range is Iran, Afghanistan, Kazakhstan			

Table 31.11 Continued

Species	Country of origin	Food	Reproductive data	Additional comments
East and West African terrestrial chelonia				
Bell's hinge-back tortoise (*Kinixys belliana*)	Wide range in tropical and subtropical Africa and occurs in savannah habitats	Needs a diet of vegetables, fruit and meat. Foods range from those fed to Mediterranean tortoises with additions of fruits such as banana, melon peach, grapes. Will eat range of invertebrates and dog or cat food. Supplement diet with vitamins and minerals	Clutches of 1–3 eggs	These have a hinge across the rear portion of the carapace, which slopes down steeply from the middle of the fifth vertebra. Newly hatched young show no sign of a hinge. As they are a tropical species they do not hibernate – keep at temperature of 30°C+
Leopard tortoise (*Geochelone pardalis*)	East and West Africa	Mainly vegetarian – prefers green vegetables to fruit	Clutches of 5–30 eggs laid in nests dug by female. Can take 4–18 months to hatch depending on temperature	Large specimens can weigh up to 43 kg but an average is 10–15 kg. Require high temperatures – 30–35°C. Do not hibernate
North American species				
American box turtle (tortoise) (*Terrapene carolina*)	Six subspecies and range from Mexico to Florida	Eat a mixture of meats and vegetable matter. Feed tinned dog or cat food, invertebrates, fruits and leafy vegetables, plus vitamin and mineral supplementation	Mating occurs post-hibernation. Lays clutches of 2–7 eggs. Eggs need high humidity	Will hibernate for short period but must be in good health. Like to soak in dish of warm water. Size 10–12.5 cm
South American tortoises				
Red-footed tortoise (*Geochelone carbonaria*)	Tropical South America	Mixture of fruits and vegetables with added tinned dog or cat food	Lays clutches of 5–13 eggs. Eggs require high humidity. If ideal conditions maintained, hatching takes about 4 months	As they come from areas of high humidity they can easily dehydrate so need daily bathing. Vivarium temperature 28–30°C. Do not hibernate. Maturity reached at about 15 years or when animal reaches 20–30 cm in length
Yellow-footed tortoise (*Geochelone denticulata*)	Tropical South America			
Indian star tortoise (*Geochelone elegans*)	Arid lands – India, Pakistan and Sri Lanka	See information for Leopard tortoise	See information for Leopard tortoise	Very attractive tortoise with a beautifully patterned shell
Turtles and terrapins (American)				
Red-eared terrapin (*Chrysemys scripta elegans*)	Eastern USA to Mexico	Meat, fish, invertebrates, pinkies, dried cat food, some vegetable matter. Vitamin and mineral supplements	Captive-farmed in country of origin and lay up to 12 eggs	Aquatic but need access to land and basking area. Water temperature 24–30°C. Now a real problem in the UK, having been released into ponds and rivers, where they are having an effect on native species. Can carry salmonella. Grow up to 30 cm
Alligator snapping turtle (*Macrochelys temmincki*)	South-east USA	Meat, small rodents, invertebrates, fish and some vegetable matter. Requires vitamin and mineral supplement	Lay up to 50 eggs per clutch	Very large, heavy-bodied chelonian with a dubious temperament, so must be handled with care. Do not hibernate

- Any animal accommodation should:
  - Be durable
  - Be safe and secure
  - Be easy to clean
  - Have ease of access.

Durability

It is not unusual for animal accommodation to cost more than the creature to be housed and, as reptile and chelonian accommodation is specialized, prices can be high. For the accommodation to last as long as possible, to ensure human and animal safety and to maintain hygiene standards, the materials and the design of the vivarium must be robust, practical and be able to withstand the required levels of heat and humidity, and the possibility of destruction by the reptile.

Security

This is a major consideration, as all animals need to be secure and safe. Some reptiles are excellent escape artists and neighbours are never pleased to hear that there is a 14-foot reticulated python 'on the loose'. Vivarium locks should be used and all vents and joints should be sealed and securely placed. All materials should be free of rough, sharp or jagged edges to prevent injury to the reptile and the handler.

Ease of cleaning

Materials used in the construction of the vivarium should have a smooth surface, be impervious and be easy to clean. Many reptiles live in a hot, humid environment, which makes ideal conditions for pathogens to grow and multiply. To ensure good health, the ability to clean the animal's accommodation effectively is of the utmost importance.

Ease of access

It is imperative to be able to gain access to the reptile and its environment. You should not have to be a contortionist to get into the animal's accommodation and the design of the vivarium and its furnishings should allow safe handling and safe cleaning

Shape and size

Reptiles come in a variety of shapes and sizes and the chosen accommodation should reflect their physical needs. Terrestrial or ground-dwelling species require a horizontal vivarium (Fig. 31.15A); arboreal or tree-dwelling animals require a taller vivarium (Fig. 31.15B); and the burrowing species require a deep base to hold a depth of substrate.

Substrate

Table 31.12 lists the common substrates. This is the medium that sits in the bottom of the vivarium to absorb faeces and urine and, in the case of burrowing animals, allows them to display their natural behaviour. One would normally select a substrate that is both comparable with the animal's natural habitat and aesthetically pleasing.

Table 31.12 Substrates and materials suitable for vivaria

Material for vivarium construction	Substrate
Melamine chip board*	Peat†
Moulded plastics‡	Wood chip§
Glass tanks¶	Vermiculite†
Marine plywood	Bark chip§
Fibreglass‡	Corn cob§
Plastic tanks (fauna boxes)	Repti/calci sand (for desert species)‖
Small plastic tubs (hatchling snakes)	Newspaper Gravel Alfalfa pellets Wood-based cat litter§** Sphagnum moss†

*Not ideal for species requiring high humidity. †Good for retaining moisture and humidity. ‡Excellent for cleaning – can be jet-washed. §If eaten, can cause gut impaction or get stuck in mouth, so should be avoided. ¶Good for aquatic species and species requiring high humidity. Poor insulation, poor security, difficult to attach fittings. ‖Only sand produced specifically for reptiles should be used as others contain silica, which will dehydrate the animal. **Only litter free from pine oils should be used.

Cage furnishings

Furnishings are important as they:

- Provide the reptile with exercise opportunities
- Prevent boredom and behaviour problems
- Provide the reptile with security (somewhere to hide)
- Make the vivarium visually interesting.

Hides

One of the main provisions should be a series of hides. These make the reptile feel safe and secure, and reduce stress. As a guide, and to reduce stress, when a snake or lizard is in the hide it should be able to touch three sides. Most chelonians require some form of hide.

Branches

Textured branches that can support the weight of the reptile are needed for climbing and basking.

Stones

Make sure that stones or large, heavy objects in the vivarium have a flat, smooth base to prevent them from rolling on to the reptile and causing injury.

Feeding equipment

Large, heavy ceramic bowls provide drinking water and a bathing facility.

Basking and swimming areas

Aquatic and semi-aquatic species, e.g. terrapins and box tortoises, need an area in which to swim (Fig. 31.16) and an area in which to bask – this should take up approximately one-third of the tank, leaving the rest as water. There should also be a filtration system to prevent the water becoming

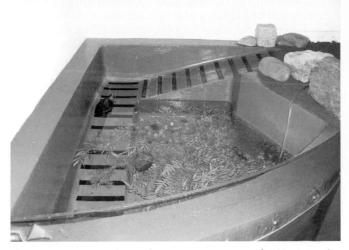

Fig. 31.16 Terrapin enclosure demonstrating provision of swimming and basking areas

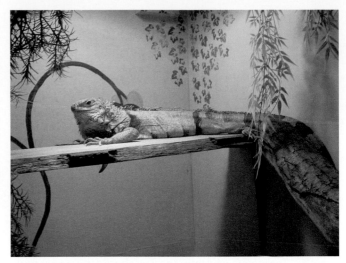

Fig. 31.17 Female green iguana (*Iguana iguana*) basking under a mercury vapour heat lamp

stagnant and polluted – if the water is not filtered it must be changed daily.

Plants

If living, these may provide humidity and a place to hide. They also look nice but are difficult to keep clean. Be warned – lizards will ingest plants and, if these are made of plastic or silk, they can cause intestinal impaction and will not show up on X-ray.

Vivarium conditions

Once a suitable vivarium has been selected there are four main factors to consider:

1. Ventilation

This is achieved by positioning holes at the back or sides of the cage. To achieve a good through-flow of air and prevent draughts, vents should be placed opposite each other but at different levels, e.g. one at the top and one at the bottom. The holes should not allow the reptile to escape and may need to be covered in wire mesh.

2. Heating

This is essential, and an understanding of reptile biology is important. As ectotherms, reptiles rely on external heat sources to warm up their internal body temperature. All reptiles have a preferred body temperature (PBT) or preferred optimum temperature zone (POTZ), which relates to the optimum temperature that the species requires for its metabolism to function correctly, i.e. movement, feeding, digestion, enzyme activity, reproduction, etc. This temperature must be achieved within the vivarium.

Vivarium temperatures must take into account the species of reptile and its POTZ. Many species require hotter or cooler temperatures depending on the time of year, so the individual species' requirements must be researched, but temperature guidelines are:

- Tropical species – 26.5–37°C
- Temperate species – 24–29.5°C.

The most common forms of heat source are:

- Ceramic and tube heaters
- Reflector bulbs with or without ultraviolet (UV)B content
- Heat mats and rocks
- Aquarium heaters (as used by fish keepers) – for aquatic and semi-aquatic chelonia. As aquatic species are very clumsy and frequently break their tank heaters, a guard should be fitted.

Most good tank heaters will be fitted with a thermostat that allows adjustments to the temperature settings. A liquid crystal thermometer can be placed on the outside of the tank to monitor the ambient temperature inside the tank.

For those species that require a basking area, such as the red-eared terrapin (*Pseudemys scripta elegans*), an incandescent light or spotlight fitted with a reflector should be positioned over an area of 'land'. This should be about 23 cm above the basking spot and reach temperatures of at least 30–35°C. The provision of such an area allows the chelonian to bask and prevents respiratory disease and shell disorders.

Make sure that all heat and light sources are guarded, as reptiles can suffer serious burns from sitting on lamps. Snakes have few nerve endings in their ventral scales and will not realize that they are roasting themselves.

The vivarium set-up must allow the reptile to thermoregulate by moving between different temperature zones, enabling it to warm up or cool down as necessary (Fig. 31.17). This is achieved by careful positioning of the heat source(s), creating a temperature gradient between hot and cool spots within the vivarium and allowing the reptile to control its body temperature at different times of the day. The temperature gradient is regulated by the use of thermostats and thermometers.

Overheating the reptile can be just as detrimental to its health as underheating. For the POTZ of individual species, refer to specialist books. Sick or injured reptiles will seek out the high ranges of their POTZ to aid their immune system. Drug absorption and utilization is influenced by the species'

POTZ, so when reptiles are receiving medication or anaesthetics the provision of heat is essential.

3. Lighting

There are three main types of lighting used for reptiles:

- Incandescent bulbs, e.g. light bulbs, coloured light bulbs
- Ultraviolet strip lights with UVB and UVA content
- Reflector bulbs (can be combined with UVA and UVB).

Lighting provides the reptile with a photoperiod, i.e. the amount of light in a normal day, and stimulates natural behaviour, e.g. basking, eating, reproduction. The amount of light depends on the species' native environment and the time of year. For example, a tropical species will require on average a 13-hour day/11-hour night summer cycle and an 11-hour day/13-hour night winter cycle, each lasting 6 months. Temperate climate species should be on a four-season cycle that provides 15 hours of daylight during the summer, 12 hours during the spring and autumn and 9 hours during the winter.

A **full-spectrum light** is one that mimics the rays produced by the sun and includes UV light. Sunlight produces UV light, which can be separated into UVA, which stimulates behavioural and physiological effects, and UVB necessary for calcium metabolism and the activation of vitamin D. UVC is not important in reptile husbandry.

A full-spectrum UV light is important for all diurnal, tropical, subtropical and desert lizards and chelonia, and also for some snakes. In an ideal situation we would allow our captive reptiles to bask in natural sunlight outdoors, but the majority of captive reptiles are kept indoors in a controlled environment and we have to supply an artificial light source. For example, Mediterranean tortoises would enjoy in excess of 14 hours of sunshine during the summer months, reducing to 12 hours in the spring and autumn, while red-eared terrapins require a full-spectrum UV light 30 cm above the basking area for effective calcium metabolism.

UVB lights do not have an infinite lifespan and, although the white light may still be seen the UVB content is generally exhausted within 6–9 months of use. For satisfactory vitamin D$_3$ synthesis the UVB light needs to be on for 10–14 hours a day and be positioned approximately 30 cm above the reptile. The height should be measured from where the rays will strike the animal, not from the base of the cage. The height should be reduced for young animals to maximize UVB utilization. Replace UVB lights every 6 months if young growing stock are kept. Mercury vapour spot or flood lamps are recommended in larger enclosures as they produce a greater intensity of UVB light.

Remember UV rays cannot pass through glass, so UV lights have to be placed inside the enclosure or provide the reptile with access to direct sunlight.

4. Humidity

This is the amount of moisture in the air. The humidity requirements will depend on the natural habitat of the species; for example, a rainforest species will require a higher humidity than a desert species. Most species do well at a relative humidity of 50–70%. The humidity can be increased by frequent spraying of the vivarium using a plant mister, or by placing damp sphagnum moss or tissue paper in a small ice cream tub or plastic sandwich container. Correct humidity is necessary to allow normal ecdysis (shedding of the skin). Decreasing ventilation should not be used as a means of increasing humidity, as this can lead to an increase in fungal disease.

When caring for a reptile within a veterinary practice it is essential to monitor the environment of the patient. Figure 31.18 shows a suggested format for a hospital chart.

Nutrition and feeding

Reptiles present a wide spectrum of nutritional challenges because there is little information about what they eat in the wild and we can only assume, rightly or wrongly, that what we offer the captive reptile goes some way to mimicking its natural diet.

Snakes

All snakes are carnivores and should be offered a whole prey item (Fig. 31.19).

Guidelines:

- Always select a food item that is as near as possible to the animal's wild diet, e.g. offer brown mice rather than white mice
- Select prey items that the snake can swallow (Fig. 31.20)
- If offering frozen foods, defrost first
- When thoroughly thawed, warm by sealing the food item in a plastic bag and then immersing the bag into warm water – reptiles do not like eating refrigerated foods!
- Offer the dead prey head first, using feeding tongs, as this will keep human smell off the food and will help to prevent the feeder from being bitten
- It may be necessary to wriggle the food item slightly in front of the snake to stimulate the strike response – this method is especially helpfully with reluctant feeders or arboreal species
- To prevent accidental cannibalism, never feed snakes together. They will try and consume the same prey item
- To prevent regurgitation, once the snake has accepted its prey item it should be left alone and not handled for 24–48 hours
- Snakes are opportunist feeders and do not require feeding every day; they may have periods of fasting
- Frequency of feeding will depend on the age of the snake and the species. As a guide, feed as much as the snake will consume in one meal then wait until the meal has been digested and faeces passed. For example, a garter snake (*Thamnophis* spp.) will require feeding every 3–7 days, depending on age and size, but a large adult Burmese python (*Python m. bivittatus*) will only require feeding once a month
- There is no need to feed live vertebrate prey in the UK, as most captive snakes will readily eat dead prey. It is probable that anyone found feeding live vertebrates could be prosecuted under the Animal Welfare Act 2006

Animal details		Owner details
Name		Name
Species and details		Address
Sex/age		
Preferred temperature zone and humidity		
Diet preference		Tel no.

Date	Temp am/pm B basking C cool end AM			PM			Humidity % Indicate if sprayed AM	PM	Food offered Amount (F) Water offered (W) F	W	Food eaten Amount	Urate faeces passed AM and PM **Comment**	Signs of shedding AM and PM **Comment**	Hygiene Spot clean Total clean	Comment signature
	B	C	B	C						4					

Fig. 31.18 Suggested husbandry sheet to monitor the environment and nutrition of the reptilian patient

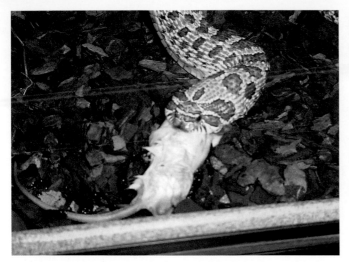

Fig. 31.19 Hognose snake eating a dead mouse

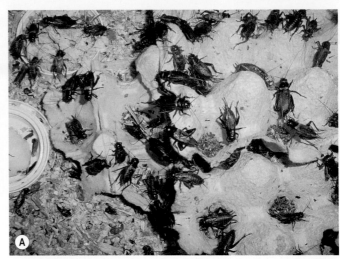

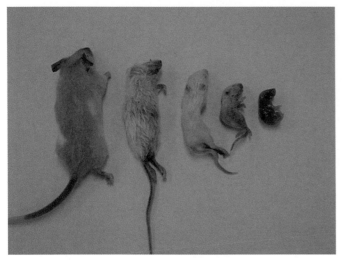

Fig. 31.20 Various sizes of dead rodent prey used to feed snakes and carnivorous lizards

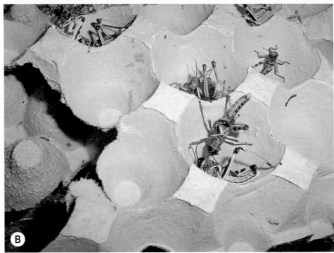

Fig. 31.21 (**A**) Black crickets suitable for insectivorous lizards; they are more nutritious and easier for the lizard to catch. (**B**) Locusts are available in various sizes; care must be taken when feeding large locusts as the barbs on their hind limbs can penetrate the mouth or digestive tract

- When feeding raw fish to snakes such as the garter snake, the fish must be blanched in hot water for approximately 10 minutes to destroy the antivitamin thiaminase. This will destroy the B vitamin thiamine and cause a deficiency presenting as convulsions and loss of the righting reflex.

Do not feed a snake …

- … before an anaesthetic
- … when it is shedding or moulting
- … when it is in brumation (hibernation) or getting ready for brumation.

Lizards

Lizards present more of a challenge when trying to meet their dietary demands and their feeding habits can be classified as:

- Carnivorous – eating whole prey items such as rodents, birds, amphibians and other small lizards (Fig. 31.20)

- Insectivorous – eating a range of invertebrates such as crickets, locusts, mealworms and waxworms (Fig. 31.21)
- Herbivorous – eating a range of plant, fruit and vegetable matter
- Omnivorous – eating a mixture of both vegetation and animal matter.

Guidelines: first investigate whether the lizard is carnivorous, herbivorous, etc. (Table 31.11).

1. **Herbivores**, e.g. green iguana (*Iguana iguana*), uromastix (*Uromastyx acanthinurus*)
   - Offer a variety of fresh, leafy vegetables, fruits, etc., to meet the lizard's needs (Table 31.11), e.g. a green iguana up to 2 years of age must be offered a diet consisting of 80% green leafy matter and 20% fruit and root vegetables; a green iguana over 2 years should be provided with a diet consisting of 95% green leafy matter and 5% fruits and roots
   - Always ensure all foods offered are fresh, free from pesticides and thoroughly washed. If food is taken

Table 31.13 Calcium to phosphorus ratio in some commonly fed vegetables and fruit

Food item	Ratio
Broccoli leaves	3:9
Cauliflower florets	0:6
Celery stalk*	1:4
Spinach raw*	2:0
Alfalfa sprouts	0:5
Broccoli stems florets chopped	0:7
Cabbage†	2:0
Chinese cabbage (Pak choi)	2:8
Red cabbage	1:2
Carrots shredded	0:6
Parsley chopped	3:3
Green peppers	0:2
Cucumber	1:1.1
Lettuce romaine	0:8
Lettuce iceberg‡	0:9
Tomatoes	0:3
Watercress	4.3:1
Apples	0.7:1.0
Bananas	0:3
Grapes	0:7
Melon (flesh)	0.6:0.9
Strawberries	0:7
Pears	1:0
Peaches	0:4

*Oxalates occur in spinach, cabbage, celery, rhubarb, peas and beet greens. They bind to calcium and trace minerals, preventing their absorption from the gut. Although these are high in calcium, they should only be offered less frequently and in smaller amounts (once a fortnight)
†Cabbage cauliflower, pak choi and kale should be fed in small amounts (once a month) as they contain goitrogens that block the production of thyroxine and utilization of iodine, causing hypothyroidism and goitre
‡Lettuce is considered not an ideal food item for many reptiles, especially tortoises and iguanas, because of its poor nutritional value, but it is no worse or better than many vegetables and better than many fruits. The mixed bag lettuces as sold ready prepared in supermarkets are probably the best choice and should be part of a varied diet.

from the fridge, allow it to reach room temperature before offering it to the lizard
- Apply necessary supplement to food (Table 31.11). A range of calcium supplements are available. It is possible to overdose and cause metabolic bone problems and calcification of soft tissues when supplementing with preparations that contain added vitamin D_3 and minerals. The frequency of supplementation depends on the frequency of feeding but, as a general rule, calcium carbonate powder can be added to each meal, whereas powders that contain vitamin D_3 and other supplements should be offered once/twice a week
- Supplementation of vitamin D_3 should not be used to overcome inadequate provision of UVB lighting – if correctly positioned UVB lighting is provided and replaced at appropriate times, vitamin D_3 synthesis should be adequate and over-supplementation of vitamin D_3 will harm the lizard
- All food should be of an appropriate size so that the animal can easily ingest it
- Take care when offering addictive foods, e.g. banana, as this encourages selective feeding, leading to dietary imbalance.

2. **Insectivores**, e.g. leopard gecko (*Eublepharus macularius*), water dragon (*Physignathus cocincinus*). These species eat a range of live invertebrate foods (Fig. 31.21):
   - When selecting foods make sure they are of appropriate size for the lizard to catch and consume
   - Before feeding newly purchased live foods, e.g. crickets and locusts, the following steps should be carried out:
     a. Place the live insects in a plastic container and offer foods such as cereals, fruit, vegetables and water. To prevent insects from drowning, offer water by soaking cotton wool and placing it in a small dish. Leave for 24–48 hours. This will allow the insects to rehydrate and be more nutritious
     b. Once live food has been nourished, it is important to dust it with a calcium or vitamin and mineral supplement by shaking it in a pot of supplement. Many invertebrate food species offered have an inverse calcium : phosphorus ratio. Ideally, calcium should be offered in the diet at a higher calcium : phosphorus ratio, otherwise calcium will be removed from the animal's own stores, causing metabolic bone disease and, in breeding animals, poorly calcified eggs and dystocia. The rules for frequency of supplementation are as for herbivore nutrition
     c. The food can then be placed in the vivarium
   - One of the problems associated with dusting live prey is that much of the supplement can fall off the prey before it is consumed and it is difficult to monitor exactly how much of the supplement the lizard ingests. A tip is to chill the live food in a refrigerator for a few minutes. This will slow the insect down and give the reptile an opportunity to catch the prey plus supplement!
   - Feed as many insects as the lizard will eat at once. Do not add too many crickets, etc., to the vivarium as the live food could actually frighten the lizard and prevent it from eating.

3. **Carnivores**, e.g. monitor (*Varanus* spp.), tegu (*Tupinambis* spp.)
   - The reptiles will eat a range of prey items ranging from rodents to other small lizards, which should be offered whole. This reduces the need to supplement unless the animal is ill

- Frozen foods must be prepared and offered as described under snake nutrition
- Caution must be taken to prevent injury when offering food to large lizards, especially the monitor family: tongs or graspers must be used (Fig. 31.22)
- Frequency of feeding will depend on the lizard's species age and size. As a guide, smaller or growing lizards should be fed daily; mature or larger species should be fed 2–3 times a week.

4. **Omnivores**, e.g. bearded dragon (*Pogona vitticeps*), skink (*Tiliqua gigas*), plated lizard (*Gerrhosaurus* spp.)

This group of lizards will eat a variety of animal and plant matter, so previous information applies.

Feeding summary

- 'Variety is the spice of life' and the reptile should be offered a varied and balanced diet. This is limited for the carnivorous species, but the common boa (*Boa constrictor*) will appreciate a dead gerbil now and again
- Always feed dead vertebrates. It is inhumane and potentially illegal to feed live ones, and live rodents could actually attack the snake or lizard, inflicting nasty wounds and causing distress to the cage occupant
- The quality of vertebrate and invertebrate prey will depend on its age, the way it has been fed and its health status
- It is not acceptable to use wild rodents as food, as they may carry disease and parasites. If collecting wild invertebrates, make sure they are non-toxic and free from pesticides
- There are a variety of commercially prepared diets on the market and these can make up part of but not the entire diet
- Non-reptilian foods are not advised because they have been manufactured for animals with different nutritional needs, metabolic processes and stress levels

- However excellent the diet provided for the reptile is, if the environmental conditions are incorrect and optimum lighting, humidity and temperature not available, the lizard or snake will not be able to reach its POTZ and its metabolic processes will be severely compromised, resulting in non-digestion of food or anorexia. Any undigested food in the gut will cause massive bacterial overgrowth, with potentially fatally consequences.

Water

Snakes and lizards require access to clean water at all times:

- For snakes, the water bowl must be large enough to allow the snake to submerge itself in the water. This also helps when the snake is shedding
- Tropical or arboreal snakes such as the Cooks tree boa (*Corallus caninus*) (Fig. 31.23) or green tree python (*Chondrophython viridis*) require daily misting with lukewarm water. The spray should be a fine mist directed toward the snake's head, allowing it to drink the water as it drips off or collects in its tight coils. Their entire body should be sprayed daily to keep them from becoming too dry, which may result in dysecdysis (difficulty in shedding)
- Non-tropical arboreal species and terrestrial species should only be misted if they are getting ready to shed
- Some lizards, e.g. arboreal species such as anoles, day geckos and some chameleons, will not drink water from a bowl, preferring to take their water in the form of droplets off a leaf. Most chameleons need to be 'rained on' daily and some species need to feel the dripping water before they will attempt to drink. There are several methods:
  - Mist the foliage in the vivarium using a hand-held spray
  - Set up an elaborate misting system
  - Adapt a drip system so that droplets fall on a leaf or branch – to prevent the substrate from becoming

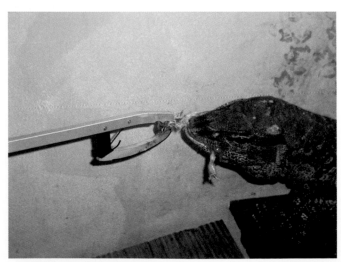

Fig. 31.22 Nile monitor lizard eating a dead rat; note the use of long graspers for the safety of the handler feeding the lizard

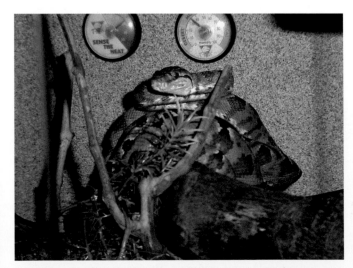

Fig. 31.23 Cooks tree boa (*Corallus caninus*). Tree pythons or boas require daily spraying as they prefer to drink water that has accumulated in their coils

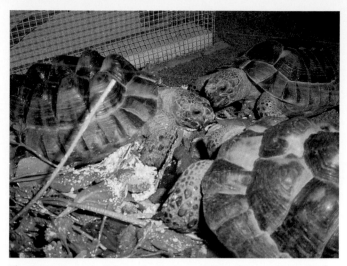

Fig. 31.24 Two subadult tortoises eating a variety of vegetables and leafy salad

saturated, place a receptacle under the drip tube to collect excess water

- No water bowl should be so deep that the species is unable to climb out; small pieces of slate can be angled in the bowl to allow small lizard a way into and out of the water
- If insects are being fed, small stones should be placed in the bottom of the bowl to prevent the insects from drowning and contaminating the water
- Water containers should be cleaned and water replenished daily, or more often if contaminated with faeces and urates.

Tortoises

Mediterranean tortoises

These common species of tortoise (Table 31.11) are opportunist feeders and their natural terrain is sparsely vegetated and infertile. Their natural diet consists of a variety of plant materials – leaves, flowers and fruits (Fig. 31.24).

In captivity the basic diet should consist of low-protein, high-fibre foods with a high mineral and vitamin content, together with a large quantity of calcium carbonate:

- Suitable wild plants – dandelions, sow thistle and clover are all favourites of the tortoise and grow widely in the UK. Grass is not digested by the tortoise, so has no nutritional valve except to add bulk and fibre to the diet
- Green vegetables – e.g. cabbage, watercress, cress, spinach, broccoli. Many cultivated vegetables are high in protein and low in fibre. Most tortoises readily take salad foods such as tomatoes, cucumber and lettuce, but their nutritional value is limited and they should be used to enhance the palatability of the food rather than making up the entire diet. Prepacked mixed salad leaves give the tortoise a range of different leaves and can help the overall nutritional value (Table 31.13)
- Proprietary foods – dried pelleted foods are available. They must be soaked in water and only offered as part of the diet

- Meat products – not recommended, as protein levels in meat are far too high and can lead to severe metabolic and organ problems
- Dairy products – not recommended: if they are offered the liver may be affected
- Vitamins and minerals – in the wild diet the levels of vitamins and mineral would be higher than in the diet provided in captivity, so supplementation is necessary:
  - Calcium should be liberally sprinkled over the diet – it is better to slightly over-supplement than under-supplement. Providing cuttlefish bone for chelonia to gnaw is a good way of getting calcium into the animal and helps to prevent the beak from overgrowing
  - Vitamin A – a deficiency may lead to swollen eyes and loss of appetite, as the animal cannot see its food
  - Vitamin D_3 – if this is deficient, calcium absorption from the intestines is affected. If in excess, it can cause excessive calcium uptake and calcification of soft tissues
- Water – a daily bath in 3–4 cm of warm water for 5–10 minutes will allow the tortoise to take in water, via either the cloaca or the mouth. A shallow bowl of water can be offered, but this is usually trampled over and spilled. Tortoises do not have a hard palate, so are unable to lap. Instead, they drop their mouths below the water line and 'siphon up' the water until they have taken in sufficient quantities.

Subadult or adult tortoises

Offer a range of salad, green leaf vegetables, fruits and wild plants (Tables 31.11 and 31.13). Wild plant material should provide at least 75% of the diet, with leafy vegetables and salad making up the remaining 25%. Fruits should be used as a treat, as too large a quantity can cause excessive dilution of dietary protein.

All foods offered should be fit for human consumption, washed and stored in a refrigerator or, in the case of wild plants, freshly picked. Foods should be offered on a flat dish or lid and should be of a size the tortoise can manage, as they prefer to bite off small pieces of food. Very large pieces of fruit or vegetables can be difficult for the tortoise to eat. If using proprietary foods, make sure they are soaked and soft before offering. All food that is offered on a daily basis should be coated in calcium carbonate powder.

Once the tortoise has had enough it will walk away to rest and digest its food. A note should be made of the amount of food offered and the amount eaten. Water should be available and a bath is the best way of providing it.

Hatchlings

Correct feeding of a hatchling tortoise is of paramount importance, as poor diet can lead to conditions such as lumpy shell, bone and shell deformities and obesity.

Various feeding regimes have been recommended but the main aim is to balance energy, protein and calcium intake and to ensure that the hatchling has access to the factors involved in calcium metabolism, i.e. heat, UVB and vitamin D:

- **Suggested regime** – feed the tortoise once a day as this allows for more thorough digestion of previously eaten meals and may help to slow rapid growth. The amount fed will depend on how much the individual consumes at each feed. Be careful not to overfeed, as this has been reported to encourage rapid growth, which can lead to the development of 'lumpy' shells. Overfed tortoises are unhealthy and can become lethargic; in fact, it is better for them to be slightly underfed than become engorged on rich unsuitable foods
- **Suggested foods** – offer a range of foods, e.g. coarse weeds such as dandelion, sow thistle, clover, mixed salad leaves, dark leaf watercress cress. Supplementation is very important and must be added at every meal – calcium and multivitamin and mineral powders can be offered on a rotational basis, e.g. every day give a calcium supplement then on every third day add a pinch of a multivitamin and mineral powder. Iceberg lettuce is a poor foodstuff and contains little or no nutritional value and indeed some tortoises can become addicted to it, causing long-term damage and difficulty in changing dietary preference
- **Water** – the hatchling must be kept hydrated and should be observed drinking while being bathed in a shallow dish of warm water at least once or twice a day for 5–10 minutes. Although low in nutritional value, iceburg lettuce is a good foodstuff for providing a dietary source of water for hatchling tortoises.

Turtles and terrapins

Note: Species of terrapin are semi-aquatic, while turtles are totally aquatic. In the USA all shelled reptiles, including tortoises, are called 'turtles'.

Terrapins and turtles range from being totally carnivorous to accepting some plant material in their diet. A range of foods should be offered:

- Proprietary terrapin and turtle pellets
- Pinkies and small mice
- Invertebrates such as locust and crickets, snails, prawns in their shells
- Cleansed earthworms (place worms in a tub for 12–24 hours to allow soil to pass through)
- Fish – whitebait, sprats
- Plant material, such as broad-leaf watercress and romaine lettuce, oxygenating water weed
- Calcium and multivitamin and mineral supplements need to be given, especially to young, growing terrapins and turtles
- Only very small quantities of the following foods should be offered if at all – raw muscle meats, crab sticks, cockles, kidney and liver. These are very low in calcium and high in phosphorus and will require supplementation
- Feed terrapins and turtles in a separate enclosure or container to reduce water pollution
- Quantity and frequency of feeding depend on the size and age of the terrapin. Young terrapins and turtles will require feeding daily, whereas adults should be fed every other day on a variety of foods from the list above.

Breeding

Most reptiles lay eggs and are described as oviparous. Some reptiles give birth to live young and can be described as either ovoviviparous or viviparous:

- **Ovoviviparous** – the egg and fetus are retained within the oviduct and nutritional support is gained through the yolk sac. Once the young are fully developed they hatch inside the female and live young are born
- **Viviparous** – the fetuses develop in the oviduct and gain nutritional support from a type of placenta.

Most newly hatched reptiles are miniature versions of their parents and are independent, receiving little if any maternal care. Table 31.11 identifies the reproductive patterns of the individual species.

Breeding regimes

To breed reptiles successfully they must be in good health and must be given the correct, balanced diet. Most reptiles have a breeding season and breeding usually follows a change to their environment. For example, a change in temperature is usually used to stimulate breeding but in some species it is the humidity (rainfall) that has to be altered.

Brumation or hibernation

Most breeding follows a period of brumation or hibernation that is brought about by slowly reducing the temperature of the vivarium. The reptile remains at this temperature for a set period depending on the species – approximately 4–12 weeks. At the end of brumation the vivarium temperature is slowly increased until the preferred temperature is reached.

Before brumation a reptile must undergo a period of fasting. If the digestive tract is full, food in the gut may rot, possibly leading to death. The fasting period is variable, e.g. snakes 2 weeks; lizards 1 week; chelonia 2–4 weeks. During brumation the reptile must be constantly monitored (once to twice weekly) and its weight monitored. If a dramatic weight loss is seen, i.e. more than 10%, the reptile must be taken out of brumation. To keep the animal hydrated, water must be available.

Gestation

Gravid or pregnant reptiles need good nutrition and optimum temperatures for both mother and offspring to thrive and survive. It is difficult to determine the length of gestation accurately but some information is included in Table 31.11. Most ovoviviparous or viviparous species will range from 1.5 to 6 months.

Before laying, an oviparous species will normally shed its skin (ecdysis). Colubrid snakes such as the corn snake (*Elaphe guttuta*) may lay 8–14 days after shedding, while pythons can range from 18 to 26 days after shedding.

Incubation

An oviparous reptile requires a 'nesting site'. This can be created in a container such as an ice cream carton with a small hole in the side, filled with moist sphagnum moss and/or vermiculite. The provision of an area to lay the eggs is very important as inadequate provision can lead to dystocia.

A healthy, fertile reptile egg is white, dry and firm. The shell varies from soft and malleable, as seen in snakes and many lizards, to firmer and less pliable, as seen in chelonian and crocodilia. Incubation periods and temperatures vary according to species (Table 31.11). Most snakes and small lizard species range from 45 to 70 days; larger lizards (iguanas and monitors) range from 90 to 130 days. Incubation temperatures range from 26 to 32°C.

Common diseases and clinical conditions

There are many conditions affecting reptiles that may be presented in a veterinary practice. The majority of them are associated with poor management and nutrition. Details are summarized in Table 31.14.

Post-hibernation anorexia

This is associated with the Mediterranean tortoises, because the climate in the UK is not suitable for these species and because the traditional methods of tortoise keeping are flawed. The majority of the wild-caught tortoises that are still alive in the UK are barely surviving and those that do survive have darker shells that absorb heat more efficiently, which maintains the body temperature closer to its preferred range.

If during hibernation the temperature rises, the tortoise will stir and burn off valuable energy reserves. The by-product of this is urea, which is stored in the kidneys in the form of uric acid or urates. If this continues, by the time the tortoise fully awakes from hibernation its energy stores are depleted. It fails to get the normal glucose boost that enables it to move, bask and find food. The increase in stored urate levels depresses the appetite, resulting in an anorexic tortoise. Normally the activity of basking, eating and drinking post-hibernation will rectify the energy imbalance and allow stored urates to be passed in the form of a creamy white paste, which is voided shortly after hibernation, usually after a bath and a long drink of water.

Post-hibernation anorexia can also be the result of a more gradual build-up of urates in the kidneys brought about by a combination of the tortoise suffering a series of poor summers and hibernation in which energy levels are slowly being reduced and urate levels increased. A healthy adult tortoise can be expected to lose about 1% of its body weight during each month of hibernation. A hatchling will lose much more and, if it loses more than 10%, must be brought out of hibernation.

Post-hibernation anorexia can be prevented by allowing only healthy tortoises to hibernate, which can be assessed using the Jackson ratio (Fig. 31.25). The use of this ratio should be limited to those tortoises of an average build and is best suited to *Testudo hermanni* (Hermann's) and *Testudo graeca* (spur thigh greek tortoise). It is not suitable for use in the *Testudo marginata* (marginated) and *Testudo horsefieldi* (Horsefields) as their body shape does not match with the original data used to formulate this ratio and will cause inaccurate results.

The ratio is measured by plotting on a graph the weight of the tortoise in grams against the length of the carapace in

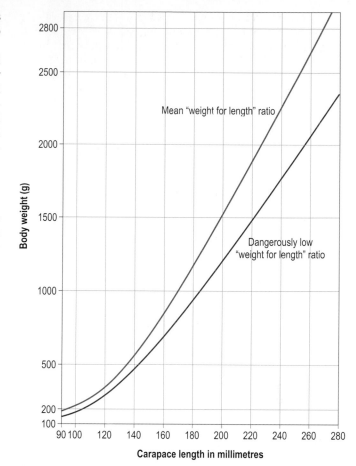

Fig. 31.25 Growth of healthy Mediterranean tortoises using the Jackson ratio

millimetres. Care should be taken to measure the carapace in a straight line rather than over the curve of the shell. Any animal falling into the 'dangerously low' area should be kept warm and awake all winter.

During hibernation the temperature should be kept between 4 and 5°C – if it rises the tortoise will begin to wake up. When the tortoise awakes after normal hibernation, it should be offered water and glucose to drink – if necessary, this may have to be given by stomach tube (see Ch. 12). It may also be necessary to give multivitamins orally or by injection.

Birds

Birds can make interesting companions and a wide variety of species are commonly kept as cage or aviary birds (Table 31.15).

Housing

Accommodation for birds kept in captivity should be designed to allow the birds to be maintained in good health and to allow them to exhibit their natural behaviour of flying. The main types of accommodation used to house birds are aviaries and cages.

The design and size depends on the numbers and species of bird but whatever type of accommodation is selected,

Table 31.14 Common diseases and clinical conditions of reptiles

Disease	Causal agent	Signs	Treatment	Additional information
Lizards and snakes				
Stomatitis (mouth rot)	Seen in both lizards and snakes. Normally caused by poor husbandry and injury to rostal (nasal) area due to fighting or running against glass front of vivarium. Bacteria, viruses and fungi invade site and set up an infection	Decrease in appetite, pinhead haemorrhages and fluid build-up on the gum. If not treated the infection will rapidly spread and pus will be seen. If untreated can lead to osteomyelitis of the jawbone	Clean mouth with povidone-iodine 2.5–5% solution applied daily to affected area. Bacteriology swab taken to determine pathogen. If severe the reptile will require an anaesthetic and area treated. Antibiotics may be given in severe cases	Look at hygiene and husbandry – environmental conditions, overcrowding
Necrotic dermatitis (scale rot)	Seen in snakes. Usually due to poor environmental conditions such as: • Vivarium temperature too low • Poor ventilation • Too much moisture in the cage • Ectoparasites	Small blisters usually appear on the ventral surface that can become infected. If left can become necrotic	Transfer reptile to a clean dry vivarium with a relative humidity of 60–70%; change substrate daily (newspaper ideal). If antibiotics needed then will have to be given by injection. Wound must be cleaned at least once or twice a day using povidone-iodine or Dermisol solution and kept as dry as possible	If reptile very sick it will require supportive therapy. Environment must be corrected before patient returns to it
Burns	Unguarded heat source hot rocks, heat pads	Signs depend on severity of burn: superficial – pain, erythema, discoloration of scales or loss of scales, wrinkling of scales, blisters and exudate. Deep – present as massive tissue damage that may slough and require surgical debridement	Treatment will depend on severity of the burn and general condition of the reptile. Bandaging may be necessary, using dressings recommended for burns patients. Fluid therapy to replace lost body fluid and electrolytes. Antibiotics if infection or septicaemia present. Surgery to debride damaged tissue	Healing by granulation can take a month to a year. Each time reptile sheds some improvement to the wound should be seen. Scarring seen, with loss of regular scale pattern. Area round scar may shed incompletely and may require soaking and manual removal Ensure all heat sources are guarded or thermostatically controlled

	Causes	Clinical signs	Treatment/intervention	Notes
Dystocia (egg binding) – snakes	Obstructive – fetal–maternal; non-obstructive – poor husbandry, poor nutrition. Lack of physical activity due to captive environment	Oviparous species: seen as a caudally located mass or able to palpate in thicker-set species (large pythons); viviparous snakes are malleable, which makes them more difficult as fetuses are malleable, which makes them difficult to locate. Prolonged straining or cloacal prolapse demonstrates unsuccessful parturition. Ultrasound can be useful in identifying the presence of fetuses in viviparous snakes	Intervention should be considered necessary 48 h after the cessation of the incomplete parturition or oviposition (egg-laying). Techniques include: • Manual manipulation – carries many risks and is not generally advised • Hormonal stimulation using oxytocin or similar agents • Aspiration of contents of egg, followed by an injection of oxytocin, snake can be left to pass the smaller egg naturally; caution must be taken not to -contaminate the coelomic cavity with egg yolk • Surgery: once snake is anaesthetized gentle manual manipulation can be attempted. If this fails a salpingotomy (making an incision into the oviduct) can be performed and eggs/fetus can be removed	Oxytocin or related drugs must not be used if a snake has an obstructive dystocia
Dystocia (egg binding) – lizards	Obstructive – fetal–maternal; non-obstructive – poor husbandry, poor nutrition. Lack of physical activity due to captive environment. Lack of suitable nesting sites common in lizards	Although anorexia is a common sign in the reproducing lizard, the lizard that is not eating and is displaying lethargy, cachexia, and loss of muscle and fat tissue from pelvic girdle, limbs and tail base suggests further investigation	Lizards do not tolerate prolonged periods of dystocia, which can cause death within several days. Prompt treatment is necessary following diagnosis, with supportive treatment given prior to any surgical procedure. Oxytocin or similar drugs can be administered to help the passage of the eggs. Surgery – salpingotomy or salpingectomy cr ovariosalpingectomy	Many lizards, including iguanas, can produce a clutch of eggs without a male present. Good pre- and postoperative care is essential for the survival of lizards or snakes undergoing surgery
Endoparasites	Mainly seen in wild-caught or farmed species, but can affect any captive snake and lizard. Numerous and varied infestations, although some are self-limiting as to complete their life cycle they need a intermediate host that captivity does not provide. The following have been seen in snakes and lizards: • Protozoans, flagellates • Coccidia • Flukes • Cestodes • Nematodes	Some infestations go unnoticed until disease or loss of a reptile occurs. Signs: eggs or oocyst are seen in faecal smears. Reptile appears listless, failure to thrive, gains weight, dull, inappetent, weight loss. Visual signs of the parasite in adult form	Anthelmintic drugs usually given orally once or twice a year. Good hygiene protocols, and do not feed wild-caught foods	Suggested drugs: metronidazole for flagellates; febendazole (Panacur) for nematodes

Table 31.14 Continued

Disease	Causal agent	Signs	Treatment	Additional information
Ectoparasites	Mainly seen in wild-caught or farmed species, but can affect any captive snake and lizard: • Ticks – *Ixodes* spp. • Mites – *Ophionyssus natricis* (mainly seen in snakes and some lizards) Both are parasitic and feed off animal's blood	*Ticks* – because of their size relatively easy to spot, but can blend in with scales; tend to favour areas near recess of ear, skin folds of the vent (lizards), cavities such as the nostrils or labial pits in some snakes. *Mites* – generally smaller than ticks and hide under scales. Colour varies from tan, reddish brown to black depending on engorgement. Common sites include between and under scales, especially around the eyes, under the chin, cloaca, axillae and inguinal regions. Other signs include the snake rubbing against furnishings in cage, spending much more time soaking in the water bowl all in an attempt to rid themselves of the mite and associated irritation. The owner may notice mites in the cage, floating in the water or crawling on to their skin. The mite causes the reptile to appear dull and listless. In severe cases can become depressed, anorexic and very sick	*Ticks* – manual removal techniques as used to remove ticks from domestic animals. *Mites* – many suggested treatments but none have proven 100% safe for reptiles and keeper. Reptile and vivarium must be isolated and vivarium totally cleaned to remove all life stages of the mite, including egg, larvae, nymphs and adults. Attention should be paid to corners, crevices, lips and all furnishings. The reptile should not be replaced until the vivarium has received a total clean. *Treatment of the reptile*: application of olive oil, the entire animal has to be covered in a thin layer of olive oil. This will suffocate the mite. Caution here because the reptile becomes very slippery and difficult to handle. Tepid baths – The animal is bathed in warm water for 30 min. This should kill most of the mites on the body but those on the head will escape. Ivermectin can be used in small doses. Fipronil can be used topically on the reptile and also to treat the vivarium (but is not licensed). Keep sprayed animal in a well-ventilated cage for 2–3 h post-spraying, as breathing fumes can be extremely damaging to the lungs. Also ensure reptile has access post-treatment to a high-humidity hide box to compensate for possible increase in cutaneous water loss. *Treatment of the vivarium*: burn any disposable or easily replaceable furnishings. Spray non-disposable items and vivarium with fipronil, paying special attention to cracks and crevices. Close vivarium and raise temperature to 40°C for 3–4 h: this will help to desiccate nymphs and stimulate hatching of eggs. Because of the alcohol vapour, frequent observation of cage is important to prevent fire. Before returning reptile to vivarium it must be ventilated (3–4 h) to ensure all traces of alcohol have dispersed. Repeat treatment on animal and vivarium three or four times at 3–4-week intervals: this will help to kill second- and third-generation mites	*Ticks* – care must be taken to remove all mouthparts, as any remaining parts can lead to formation of an abscess. *Mites* – when dealing with a lizard or snake, hygiene is essential to prevent the spread of mites to other patients. One female mite can produce 90–100 eggs in crevices in the cage. Dichlorvos (Vapona) was recommended for use in mites but has since been taken off the market. It is reportedly making a comeback – ingredients may have changed. Ivermectin and fipronil are both alcohol-based and therefore flammable. Fipronil is not licensed for treatment in reptiles. If treating the eye area with fipronil, place on a cotton wool bud and carefully apply to the scales around the eye. It has been recommended that, if spraying head (snakes), you should place ophthalmic ointment on spectacle. As the alcohol carrier in fipronil evaporates, it may chill the reptile, so the patient should be placed in a warm, well-ventilated environment. For first application, consider reducing dose. Fipronil has been used successfully on many lizards and snakes, e.g. Burmese and Royal pythons, green iguanas and monitor lizards, but adverse effects have been reported and some caution should therefore be exercised
Thiamine (vitamin B$_1$ deficiency)	Mainly seen in fish-eating snakes such as garter snakes. When these are fed thawed frozen fish, an enzyme called thiaminase, present in raw fish, destroys thiamine (vitamin B$_1$) leading to deficiency disease	Neurological signs such as incoordination, convulsions, loss of the righting reflex	Treatment is administration of vitamin B$_1$ by injection or stomach tube. Dietary correction is essential and all raw fish must be blanched/ poached before feeding (ideally taking water temperature to 80°C for 5–10 min): this will kill the antivitamin thiaminase	Fish-eating snakes should be encouraged to take other foodstuffs, e.g. pinkies, earthworms and commercially prepared diets such as 'garter grub''
Respiratory disease	• Bacterial invasion, viruses, fungi • Poor husbandry • Inadequate nutrition • Poor ventilation • Draughts • Low temperature • Endoparasites • Rhinitis (inflammation of the nasal cavity)	• Dyspnoea • Abnormal elevation of the head • Open-mouth breathing • Wheezing • Nasal discharge • Problems during sloughing • Debilitation • Severe cases – cyanotic membranes	Very sick animals will require hospitalization and much supportive therapy, such as fluids and assistance with feeding. A bacteriology swab for culture and sensitivity will aid in identification of pathogen and necessary treatment. Antimicrobial therapy is recommended. Treat endoparasites and any other suspected cause. The environment must be re-evaluated and changes made	The patient should be maintained at the higher end of its POTZ and humidity must be kept at the animal's normal range. Parenteral vitamin supplements (especially water-soluble ones) have been beneficial in some cases. In severe cases prognosis is guarded and aggressive therapy is recommended

	Cause	Signs	Treatment	Notes
Autotomy (tail loss)	Occurs as a defence mechanism in many species of lizard, geckos, green iguana, water dragons. The tail will keep wriggling to hold the predator's attention while 'lunch escapes'. In captive reptiles, usually caused by rough handling, grasping the tail or stress	Loss of tail and, if it occurs in the surgery because of poor handling, a distressed owner and embarrassed staff!	In time the tail will grow back, but it is never the same and is generally less impressive. Daily bathing in povidone-iodine solution will prevent infection until regrowth is established. If tail is sutured back on it will not regrow	
Dysecdysis (difficulty with sloughing or shedding)	Dysecdysis should be considered as a sign of a problem not the primary problem. Main causes can be attributed to poor environmental conditions: • Low temperature • Low humidity • No water bowl or bowl too small so the snake is prevented from bathing • Insufficient cage furnishings, i.e. logs or rocks for rubbing to initiate shedding • Poor nutrition	Retained flaky, dry skin over body, limbs and digits, also spectacles (snakes). If not treated, retained slough can cause infection or act as tourniquets around small limbs, tail tips and digits	The skin must be hydrated, so increase humidity in the vivarium and make sure the snake has access to a large water bowl for soaking. The snake can be placed in a bag (a pillowcase or duvet cover works well) with wet towels. The snake can rub against the towels and the moisture should help to soften the skin, allowing it to be shed. If pieces are retained, gently remove them. In snakes, if the spectacle (eye caps) are retained, leave the snake to see if they are removed during the next shed. If that fails, the spectacle should be softened using hypromellose (false tears) and gentle manipulation with a cotton wool bud. Forceps or tweezers should not be used as they may permanently damage the delicate eye tissues. Before the patient is discharged the owner must be made aware of the need to improve environmental conditions	This is a cycle that continues throughout the reptile's life. Snakes shed their skin as one single piece whereas lizards, with the exception of geckos, shed in pieces. Frequency of shedding depends on age and health status. Duration of the shedding process is between 7 and 14 days (snakes) *Signs – snakes:* • Skin lacks lustre and shine • Eyes appear cloudy • Snake will often refuse food to hide or sit for long periods of time in the water bowl (best not to handle) • Very vulnerable at this stage as vision impaired and may strike if handled • Dulling over is followed 3–4-day period where skin and eyes appear clear • When ready to shed, snake will move about cage rubbing its nose against rough objects to break skin. It will then slither out of the skin • The shed should be in one complete piece – check that spectacles and tail tip are included
Chelonia				
Metabolic bone disease	Poor environmental conditions including inadequate heating and provision of good UVB. Diet high in protein or high in phosphorus and lacking in calcium or vitamin D$_3$	• Hypocalcaemia • Soft shell • Shell deformities • Overgrown rhamphotheca (beak) and nails • Abnormal gait and movement	Correct the nutritional imbalances and environmental factors such as heat and access to good UVB	Can take on many forms according to life stage; each will be discussed separately. For more detail on specific signs and problems, see separate sections below

Table 31.14 Continued

Disease	Causal agent	Signs	Treatment	Additional information
Hypocalcaemia – common cause of death in UK-bred tortoises	Main cause is diet lacking in calcium but also associated with lack of vitamin D, high phosphorus diets and lack of good-quality UVB	*Hatchlings – acute problem* • Soft spongy shell • Edges of the mouth fail to harden, inappetence • If not treated, shell haemorrhages, lungs collapse and death • If diet too rich in protein pyramidal growth of scutes on the carapace *Juvenile tortoise – chronic problem* • Shell deformities rather than softness • Overall flattened appearance to the shell • Dip in the rear of the carapace • Scutes raised and shell feels soft and spongy • Carapace can appear too small for the chelonia • Edge of the carapace may curl dorsally • Reduced overall weight gain and growth • Deformed beak and overgrown nails • Problems with walking because of plastron deformities around the hindlimbs • X-ray shows poor mineralization of bone *Adult imported tortoise – chronic problem* • Poor shell growth, shape and hardness • Claws are curved or bent rather than straight • Beak overgrown • Shell damage prolonged poor healing or may not heal • Poor locomotion – animal tends to rub plastron against the ground; in more severe cases is unable to propel itself forward • Predispose to other disease because of depressed immune system (see text)	Depends on the signs and progression of the disease. *Hatchlings – Mild cases*, especially if being offered a high-protein diet, increase calcium uptake and slow growth (see feeding section main text) *Moderate cases* (shell is only partially soft) or *severe cases that are still bright and able to move* – aggressive dietary management necessary: increase calcium, vitamin D₃ and UVB access. Be warned: this condition can take months to rectify *Severe cases that are debilitated* – will require injections of calcium borogluconate and vitamin D₃ as well as being kept in the correct environmental conditions. As jaw will be soft, need tube feeding. If condition is very severe and some of the more terminal signs are present, euthanasia should be considered *Juvenile tortoise* – Dietary correction and environmental factors *Adult tortoise* – Dietary and environmental management Overgrown beak will need to be clipped and shaped Unfortunately, once deformities are established little can be done to alter this	*Juvenile tortoise* – If excess protein intake is a cause of the problem then the kidney and liver may be affected. Flattening of the shell can cause respiratory problems, as expansion of the lungs is hindered. Unfortunately once the deformities are established little can be done to alter this

Hypovitaminosis A	Lack of dietary vitamin A. Possible problems with vitamin A metabolism and utilization from ingested sources. Problem seen in tortoises and terrapins	The main function of vitamin A is to maintain the integrity of the skin and epithelium, especially that lining the respiratory tract and eye tissues. If deficient you may see: • Flaky skin • Poor wound healing and secondary infection • Anorexia • Lethargy • Weight loss • Swollen eyelids • Irritation around the eyes. Solid purulent matter underneath the eye lids if not treated • Respiratory problems • Renal and liver problems • Chronic condition can cause thickening of the skin	In acute cases injection of vitamin A weekly for 2–6 weeks depending on severity. Changes to dietary regime include foodstuffs rich in vitamin A, such as dark leafy greens, yellow or orange fruits and vegetables, for carnivorous species whole mice and fish, as the prey's liver will act as a good source of vitamin A. Add multivitamin supplement to the diet every other day for 2 weeks, then reduce to twice weekly for a month. In mild cases the addition of multivitamin supplement to the diet every 2–3 days may suffice, along with appropriate dietary management. If the chelonian is anorexic and very debilitated then tube feeding and fluid support will be required. Eye infections will need to, be treated with the appropriate antibiotics, as will respiratory infections	If any eye infection does not clear up with treatment, hypovitaminosis A should be considered. Care must be taken: not to overdose with vitamin A, as this can cause further problems
Runny nose syndrome – common problem in UK tortoises	Common problem in tortoises, with multifactorial aetiology, and if not treated can be fatal. Some of the more commonly identified pathogens associated with this problem are: • Gram-negative bacteria • *Pseudomonas* spp. • *Citrobacter* spp. • *Klebsiella* spp. • Fungal agents • Herpes virus. Tortoises can act as latent carriers, not showing signs but able to pass on the disease to others. For this reason, mixing tortoises from different geographical regions must be discouraged General health of the tortoise is a factor to be considered: poor diet and husbandry can lead to a susceptible immune system	A secondary bacterial infection usually intensifies the clinical signs: • Clear watery discharge from the nostrils • Occasionally sneezing • If disease progresses to the lungs, breathing becomes audible and very noisy • Open mouth and laboured breathing, lethargy, depression, anorexia	Severe cases will require supportive therapy such as fluids, supplementary heat and lots of nursing care. Assisted feeding, parenteral antibiotics, nasal drops, vitamin A injections. It may take up to 3–4 days before any significant improvement is seen	A healthy tortoise should not have a wet nose. Hypovitaminosis must also be considered here. This is a highly contagious disease and the patient should be isolated. Remember – chelonia do not possess a diaphragm and are unable to cough and swallow excess mucus produced in the lungs. This can cause these types of infection to progress and cause pneumonia. Tip – when administering nasal drops to chelonia, use a small syringe and catheter or extend head, squirt drops in the mouth and simultaneously let go of the head. As the head retracts back into the carapace it will force the fluid from the mouth down the nostrils. Terrapins seen with this disease may float on one side if one lung is more affected than the other

Table 31.14 Continued

Disease	Causal agent	Signs	Treatment	Additional information
Infectious stomatitis (mouth rot)	Common condition seen in the Mediterranean tortoise, especially if in poor condition post-hibernation. Associated with bacterial infection (Gram-negative, commonly *Pseudomonas* spp.) or viruses such as herpes virus	Early signs are often overlooked: • Reddening inside the mouth • Blistering, which commonly occurs inside lower jaw under tongue • As problem progresses, tongue becomes swollen, mouth fills with mucus and a discharge resembling cottage cheese is seen • Osteomyelitis if infection attacks jaw bone • Inappetence • Death if not treated	Mild cases – topical applications of Betadine gargle and mouthwash can be applied once a day to the affected area. More severe cases will require antibiotic treatment. Swabs can be taken to identify pathogen and treatment. Check for fungal invasion, e.g. *Candida*. Severe cases – aggressive antibiotic treatment and supportive therapy to prevent dehydration	Even if treatment is successful in severe cases where osteomyelitis is seen, the problem can reoccur
Shell rot	This problem can be seen in all chelonia. Can be due to fungal or bacterial infection, normally anaerobic Gram-negative. The fungus or bacteria gain entry as a result of shell trauma. Other contributing factors include: • Poor hygiene in both terrestrial and aquatic chelonia • High humidity • Low temperature • Lack of UV light • Inadequate diet • Overcrowding • Lack of basking sites in terrapins and turtles	Discoloration, especially around areas of shell damage. Aquatic and semi-aquatic shell appears paler. Dry flaking of shell or soft tissue. Bacterial infections – affected areas appear wet and there is an obnoxious odour, with blood and purulent discharge. Fungal infections – appear dryer and less smelly than bacterial infections. Infection can spread under scutes and lead to a deep infection with much tissue damage	Remove all affected shell until healthy tissue is seen. For at least 4–6 weeks, the area should be scrubbed for at least 5 min daily using a tooth or nailbrush, with antibacterial scrub such as chlorhexidine or povidone-iodine. Swabs may need to be taken for culture and sensitivity and antibiotic treatment administered. If abscesses form, these must be flushed out and antibiotics given. It should be noted that healing may take weeks or, in extreme cases, years. The shell can be considered free from disease when it is smooth, dry and free from odour and discharge. The animal may be permanently scarred. The very sick chelonian will need supportive therapy, including assisted feeding and fluid therapy	A common cause of trauma to the shell is oversexed males butting each other or males continually ramming the rear end of females – it is advisable to keep sexes separate. Environmental condition and diet must also be corrected before patient is discharged During hospitalization, provision of heat*, hygiene and nursing support are essential for the recovery. If untreated, septicaemia will ensue and subsequent death. Suggested antimicrobial treatments include: • *Fungal infections* – oral ketaconazole (20 mg/kg/d) • *Bacterial infections* – amikacin (Amikin paediatric) 10 mg/kg every other day for 3 days
Endoparasites	Large grey ascarids – *Angusticaecum* spp. Small, thread-like oxyurid-type nematodes	Healthy tortoise shows few physical signs apart from seeing them passed in faeces. Faecal smear will show presence of eggs. Death in hatchlings with large infestations	Oral dosage of anthelmintics: fenbendazole (Panacur) 50 mg/kg or oxfendazole (Systamex) 65 mg/kg. Two doses will need to be administered via stomach tube, with an interval of 14 days between each dose. Or use Panacur granules or paste in food	Worming should be carried out on a regular basis, especially if groups of tortoises are kept together or kept in small areas. Mediterranean tortoises should be wormed prior to hibernation. It is advisable to keep hatchlings away from pasture grazed by adults, as this is a source of infection

Condition	Aetiology	Clinical signs	Treatment	Comments
Ear abscess	Seen in tortoises, terrapins and box turtles. Bacterial infections of the middle ear gain entry via mouth and travel along eustachian tube. Poor husbandry, suboptimal temperatures and hygiene, especially poor water filtration. In aquatic species vitamin A deficiency. Depressed immune system	Large, painful swellings over ear drum (normal slightly concave). Head tilting and circling	Surgery to incise the abscess, remove pus and flush cavity. Antimicrobial therapy given by injection. In some cases 'seeding out' of the blood due to septicaemia manifests itself as abscesses and these will need to be treated using systemic antibiotics	Husbandry and diet will need to be re-evaluated. Healthy tortoises do not get abscesses
Trauma	Trauma to the shell is often caused by the chelonian being dropped or manhandled by young children, chewed by a dog (especially if young or suffering from hypocalcaemia) or coming in contact with the lawn mower or strimmer	Damage to shell. Shock makes the tortoise lethargic and lowers blood pressure. Haemorrhage – external is easy to identify; internal more problematic, so need to observe behaviour and other parameters such as mucous membrane colour. Internal organ damage is difficult to assess. Lung damage quite common Secondary infection should be considered	Stem haemorrhage. Treat shock. Fluid therapy. X-rays may be required to establish extent of damage. When patient stabilized, flush wounds using antibacterial scrub, remove debris. Antibiotics and anti-inflammatory drugs prevent infection and aid shock. Repair lung damage and consider other internal injuries. Tissue fluid will seep from wounds for a few days. Once this stops, shell repair can be performed. Use resin patches, which can be left in place for 6–12 months depending on health status of tortoise prior to injury. Very severe damage can be repaired using orthopaedic techniques	A damaged shell can take 1–2 years to heal. Chelonia that are recovering from a fractured shell should not be allowed to hibernate. Extensive trauma to the shell may never fill completely. In adult chelonia, patches can be left in place indefinitely. In young animals, to allow for growth, patches must be removed after 6 months
Penile prolapse	The penis protrudes from the cloaca for a prolonged period	Mainly seen in juvenile tortoises that have become sexually active and spend most of the day with the penis extruded	The penis can be manually replaced but usually this is only a temporary remedy. The aim is to prevent it becoming infected. Keep the penis clean and lubricated (KY Jelly and povidone-iodine). The condition will settle down in time. If penis suffers injury or becomes infected, it is important to treat the infection and keep the penis clean and lubricated as before. With the addition of systemic antibiotics the penis can be manually replaced once the inflammation has subsided. In severe infections some or all of the organ may have to be removed	It is important not to replace a dirty or infected penis. If the penis continues to prolapse then it may necessitate the need for a purse-string suture around the cloaca, which can be removed in a few days
Dystocia	Poor environmental conditions: • Lack of laying sites • Temperature too low for tortoise to lay eggs • Overcrowding: tortoise feels stressed • Poor diet, especially lack of calcium	Virtually impossible to detect without use of a radiograph but signs that may suggest problem include: • Gestation period exceeded • Depression • Anorexia • Straining • Cloacal swelling	Injection of oxytocin (5 IU/kg) should see results in approximately 1 h. During this time the tortoise must be kept at its POTZ. If this initial injection fails to stimulate the expulsion of the eggs, it is recommended that the tortoise be fed calcium supplementation for 2 days before giving a further dose at a higher rate (10 IU/kg). After receiving oxytocin, tortoise should be placed in a bath of warm water – this has proved very beneficial in helping tortoises expel their eggs. Surgical intervention must only be considered if: • Above therapy has failed and there has been a period of calcium supplementation, along with increased environmental temperature • Eggs stuck or cracked in the pelvis. If surgery is to be undertaken, a plastronotomy and celiotomy followed by a salpingotomy will have to be performed	In comparison to snakes and lizards, chelonia respond well to oxytocin injections. Problems are more commonly seen in tortoises that are due to lay in the autumn. A tortoise should not be allowed to hibernate with eggs inside her, as this will only make matters worse as the eggs become larger and more calcified, making removal more difficult

Many of the problems identified in the Mediterranean tortoise are due to the fact it is not well adapted to the UK climate: tortoises are kept in suboptimal temperatures and as a result suffer from immunosuppression.

*Sick chelonia will need to be hospitalized and kept at temperatures at the higher range of their POTZ; this will encourage metabolism of drug therapy and stimulate their own metabolism.

Table 31.15 Commonly kept species of cage and aviary birds

Species	Origin	Captive diet	General information
Order Psittaciformes			
Budgerigar (*Melopsittacus undulatus*)	Australia	Feed a good-quality proprietary seed mixture (canary seed and millet). Will eat small amount of green food, watercress, chickweed, groundsel. They need a dietary source of iodine	Can be kept on own or in groups. Males tend to be more vocal. Can be aggressive toward other smaller birds, e.g. canaries or small finches
Peach-faced lovebird (*Agapornis roseicollis*)	South-west Africa	Feed good-quality canary mix, sunflowers, safflower seeds, pine nuts, daily servings of fruit and vegetables. Hawthorn berries	Keep in pairs or small groups. Can be very aggressive to other species. Enjoy stripping bark from branches of non-poisonous trees
Cockatiel (*Nymphicus hollandicus*)	Australia	Seed mixtures – sunflower, saffron, safflower, white/red millet, canary and hemp seed, linseed, niger seed, wheat, groats. Fruits, apples green vegetables lettuce, root vegetables, raw carrot strips. Chickweed	Good aviary or cage bird. Can talk and mimic. Lives up to 10–25 years
Rosella (*Platycercus eximius*)	Australia	Similar to cockatiel diet	Keep in pairs. Aggressive toward other birds. Very vocal. Good breeders. Need to be kept in large aviary
African grey parrot (*Psittacus erithacus*)	Central Africa	Seed mixtures – sunflower, saffron, safflower, white/red millet, canary seed, wheat, oats, maize, peanuts, pine nuts, hemp. Fruits (almost any non-citrus). Green vegetables. Root vegetables, raw carrot	One of the best-talking parrots. Intelligent and sensitive and therefore prone to feather plucking if bored. Needs lots of attention and stimulation. Loves to shower in spray from plant mister
Order Passeriformes, which includes the perching birds			
Canary (*Canarius serinus*)	Canary Islands	Seed mixture – canary millet, rape maw, grass seed, hemp. Uncontaminated green stuff	Good for both cage and aviaries. Males will sing especially if on own or competition from neighbour. Nervous bird – needs careful handling
Zebra finch (*Taeniopygia (poephilia guttata)*)	Australia	Seed mixture – canary millet, rape maw, grass seed, hemp. Uncontaminated green stuff	Adaptable, hardy, sociable and easily tamed. Good for both aviaries and cages set ups
Cut throat finch (*Amadina fasciata*)	Africa	Insects, mixed seeds small amounts of uncontaminated green stuff. Soft foods, e.g. insectivorous mixtures for waxbills	Suitable for both aviary and cage. Can be kept in mixed aviary and good for those with limited experience
Hill mynah (*Gracula religiosa*)	India, south-east Asia, Indonesia	Chopped fruit. Insectivorous mixture. Mynah food. Chopped meats. Large insects such as mealworms	Great powers of mimicry. Well-balanced diet essential with adequate vitamin and mineral supplementation. Need sunlight and without access have been known to have seizures. Messy birds which will need perches and floor cleaned daily. Need heated aviary as prone to chills and respiratory problems
Order Columbiformes – pigeons and doves			
Diamond dove (*Geopelia cuneata*)	Australia	Seeds and grains according to size of bird. Chick crumb. Green foods in small amounts	Lively little birds that live well in mixed aviaries or cages. Enjoy the sun and can be seen sunbathing
Order Galliformes – domestic fowl, pheasants and quail			
Chinese painted quail (*Excalfactoria chinensis*)	India and southern China	Small seeds. Chick crumb. Finely chopped green food. Occasional mealworm	Ground-dwelling species. If in cage with flight birds, protect water and food bowls from soiling. Do not place food and water bowls at the sides of their accommodation, as they like to run along the perimeter. Cock birds will fight
Order Strigiformes – nocturnal birds of prey – the owls			
European eagle owl (*Bubo bubo*)	Europe	Meat, dead rats, quail, day-old chicks, rabbit	Large but attractive bird
Barn owl (*Tyto alba*)	Europe	Meat, dead rats, quail, day-old chicks, rabbit	Commonly kept in captivity
Order Falconiformes – diurnal birds of prey – hawks and falcons			
Harris hawk (*Circus* spp.)	South to Central America	Meat dead rats, quail, day-old chicks, rabbit	Usually kept in captivity for hunting or flying displays

once the bird is in situ it must be able to stretch out both wings fully in all directions. Accommodation should also allow the keeper to carry out general husbandry procedures, including monitoring, feeding, catching, cleaning, etc., with minimum disturbance to the birds.

Aviaries

Aviaries are divided into indoor and outdoor sections. The outdoor area or flight usually has a timber frame covered in wire mesh while the indoor area provides shelter and is normally a solid timber house with a window for light and a door for access.

When choosing an aviary consider the following:

- **Size** – depends on the ground space available, the species and the number of birds to be housed. Overstocking should be avoided, but generally 'the bigger the better' – too small an aviary will make access and cleaning difficult
- **Shape** – there are a variety of very ornate aviary designs on the market but although these look good they are usually very impractical, favouring design features over the practical needs of the bird. The best advice is keep it simple – rectangular or square shapes work well. Choose a design that allows the bird to display its natural behaviour
- **Siting** – check with the local planning office to see if planning permission is required. For security and to reduce stress, site the aviary away from roads and public access. The aviary should be south-west-facing, but whatever the position the selected site should be sheltered, not exposed to extremes of weather and away from overhanging trees. Hedges make good windbreaks
- **Materials** – these must be durable, safe and economic. Most flight areas are made of a timber, treated with an animal-safe preservative and galvanized welded mesh of a gauge suited to the size of the bird. Birds can be very destructive, especially the larger parrots, e.g. macaws, which will chew wooden frames and bite wire mesh. For these birds a 10–14 gauge mesh and a metal frame work are recommended.

At least one-third of the aviary flight area should be covered with a roof made from clear Perspex or similar plastic roof sheeting. This will protect the birds from the elements and contamination from wild birds.

A concrete base and brick surround make the ideal footing for the aviary and provides ease of cleaning and prevents rodents entering the aviary. Access should be via a double door system or by one door opening inward – both these methods prevent escape (Fig. 31.26).

The indoor area is usually a house made of timber and providing shelter. Supplementary heating and lighting can be used to help birds over the winter. Some bird keepers, especially those with extensive collections, utilize large brick-built buildings or sheds. The building is subdivided into smaller aviary units and each one provides the housed birds with access to an outdoor flight. Adjoining aviaries should have double wire partitions to prevent the birds from pecking their neighbours (Fig. 31.27).

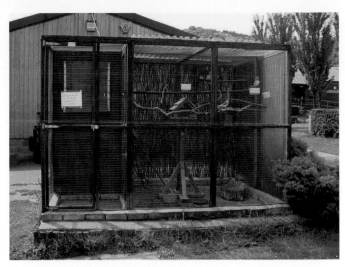

Fig. 31.26 Outside aviary. Note double entry doors and enrichment for birds

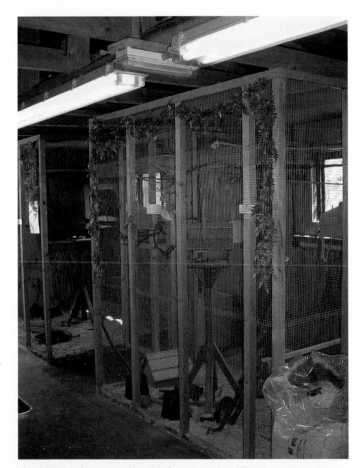

Fig. 31.27 Indoor aviary showing heating and enrichment

Furnishings

These are put into the aviary and are used to prevent boredom and subsequent behavioural problems.

- **Perches** – the outside flight area should have at least two perches, one at either end, but more can be added. Branches make the best perches as they are natural, readily available, cheap and easily replaced when soiled. Only pick branches from deciduous trees – willow and fruit trees are the best choice. Some woods are unsuitable, e.g. yew, laburnum, oak and rhododendron, as they are poisonous if eaten. Make sure that the wood has not been recently sprayed or chemically treated and that all branches are scrubbed prior to use to remove soiling from wild birds.

The perch size depends on the species of bird but a range of thicknesses and textures help to exercise the feet – the perch should be of a suitable size to allow the bird to grip without the toes overlapping. Inside the house, at least one perch should be positioned just above the level of those in the flight. This encourages the birds to roost in the most secure part of the aviary. To prevent accidents, perches should be robust and placed securely in the aviary. To prevent contamination from faecal matter perches should be placed away from food and water bowls

- **Food and water bowls** – must be correctly positioned for birds of all sizes to gain easy access
- **Toys** – there are various proprietary toys available, e.g. ropes, swings and wooden blocks. These should be used in moderation as too many can turn the aviary or cage into an obstacle course, preventing flight, and may overstimulate the birds so that they become depressed
- **Baths** – bathing is a natural activity and should be encouraged as it stimulates the bird to preen and keeps its plumage clean. Maintenance of the plumage is important for flight and for conservation of body temperature. All species love bathing and this is also

seen in wild birds. Raptors, including owls, will bathe if given the opportunity and both budgies and parrots love having a fine mist directed from a garden hose or plant sprayer on to their plumage, mimicking the rains that would fall in their native rainforests.

Birds will actively fly into the spray and enjoy preening themselves afterwards. The size and depth of the bird bath must relate to the species, e.g. for small birds fill the bath with no more than 1–2 cm of water; for larger species fill with 3–4 cm of water. Temperature of the water should be about 40°C. **Note:** Chicks should not be bathed, as the down feathers of many species give little protection.

Cages

Cages may be made from wire (Fig. 31.28) or wire and wood (Fig. 31.29). Remember that the bird must be able to stretch out both wings fully in all directions. Cages make a good base for birds that are allowed free range of the home and can be used for feeding, drinking and resting.

Consider the following:

- Wire cages are not suitable for nervous or timid birds as they are too open and the birds feel exposed and stressed
- Box-type cages must have good ventilation and be well lit
- Cages must be positioned away from draughts, windows and heaters
- Some birds enjoy being in areas of high activity where they receive lots of attention, while others seem to prefer more privacy and solitude

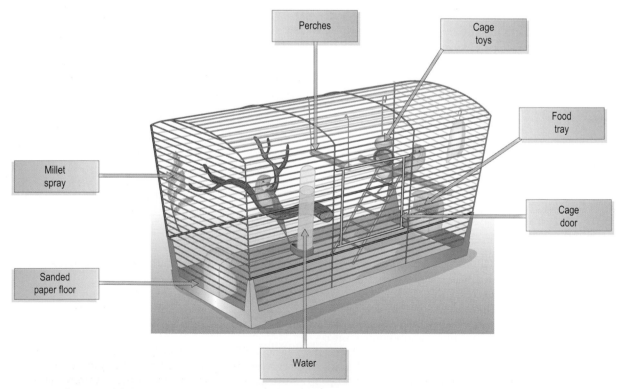

Fig. 31.28 A typical cage suitable for smaller species of bird

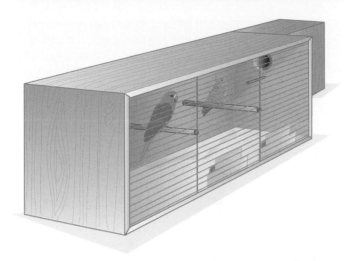

Fig. 31.29 A wooden box-type cage suitable for small species of bird

- A pet bird should never be kept in the kitchen as there are risks from cooking fumes
- Perches and furnishings should be provided. The dowelling or rigid perches often sold with cages are not suitable (see Aviaries, above)
- Food and water receptacles must be fastened securely to the sides of the cage.

Although allowing a bird to have the freedom of the house provides exercise and environmental enrichment, there are a number of dangers:

- They may eat house plants or chew electrical cables, resulting in illness or injury
- Unsupervised birds may chew and swallow carpet and other similar fabrics, resulting in crop and intestinal impactions
- Free-flying birds are more vulnerable to injury from ceiling fans, cookers, aquaria and attack by other domestic pets
- Birds may escape through open doors and windows. Bird owners often have the misguided belief that their bird would never fly away and leave them.

Cage and aviary hygiene

To prevent disease and vermin, bird accommodation must be kept scrupulously clean:

- Cages – every day clean water receptacles and food bowls; check perches for soiling and replace or clean them using a mild detergent. Rinse, dry and place back in the cage. Every week, give the accommodation a thorough clean
- Aviaries – every day clean food and water bowls, scrub soiled perches, rake soil or gravel substrate and sweep concrete to remove debris and faecal matter. Every week replace worn perches, scrub all perches, rake and hose gravel or sweep and hose concrete. Rake soil. Check wire and wooden frame for damage. At least once or twice a year change and replace substrate.

Nutrition and feeding

Good health and performance is achieved by providing a balanced palatable diet that is appropriate to the species.

This is vital in the bird, as the shape of the beak is designed to cope with a certain type of food and if the wrong food is provided the bird may be physically unable to eat it (see Ch. 12). As in reptiles, there is little scientific analysis of the nutritional needs of caged birds. Proprietary foods have been tested 'in house' with little scrutiny from outside bodies and until there is sufficient knowledge and research on the dietary needs of companion birds it is of primary importance for all bird owners to encourage their birds to eat a variety of foodstuffs.

When feeding caged birds, some consideration must be given to their different feeding, social, and migratory behaviours and the limitations of their accommodation.

Guidelines

Birds represent a large group of varied species so for nutritional purposes they can be classified as follows:

- **Hard bills** – i.e. seed eaters, e.g. parrots, parakeets, finches, doves and canaries. These eat predominantly a mixture of seeds or seeds and nuts. The size of the seed or nut must be appropriate to the size of the bird – there is no point in feeding a budgie on Brazil nuts but a large parrot would love them. Many smaller cage birds such as canaries and budgies are fed exclusively on commercial diets with little variety. This is not ideal and can have long-term effects on their longevity and health. Suggested additions to their diet include fruit, leafy vegetables and safe non-toxic plants, e.g. chickweed, groundsel and dandelion..
- **Soft bills** – i.e. fruit and or insect eaters, e.g. mynah birds, turacos, starlings. These feed on soft foods such as fruits, vegetables, proprietary soft bill mixes, insects and meat (Fig. 31.30)
- **Nectar feeders** – i.e. they eat nectar and fruit, e.g. zosterops, sugarbirds, sunbirds, hummingbirds. These eat artificial nectar mixtures, insects, small mealworms, flies, insectivorous mixture, chopped ripe fruits and soaked/chopped raisins. Design of the feeder must satisfy the species; for example, hummingbirds have long tongues that are inserted deep into certain flowers to reach the nectar.
- **Raptors (birds of prey)** – eaters of meat such as dead rodents and birds, e.g. owls, hawks and eagles (Fig. 31.31). Depending on the species, these birds will consume anything from dead day-old chicks and dead rodents to rabbit, meats and quail. To keep their beaks trim and provide minerals, bones must be offered, and many raptors will enjoy picking the meat off a rabbit skull. Raptors regurgitate to produce casts or pellets, which consist of undigested fur, feathers and bone (Fig. 31.32).

Water is an essential part of the diet; birds should not be allowed to go more than 2 hours without access to water, which is used to soak seeds in the crop and enables enzymes in the proventriculus of the stomach to work.

General feeding tips

- Nuts and seeds have a high fat and protein content and are very palatable. Overfeeding of them can lead to obesity and selective feeding. They also have low levels of carotene and iodine and provide little

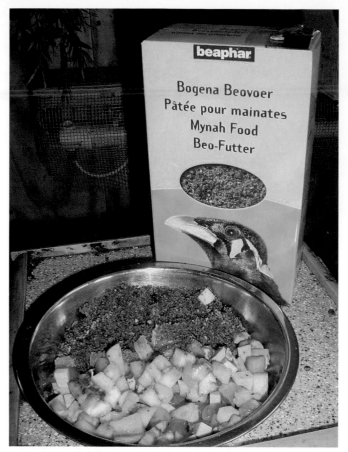

Fig. 31.30 Food prepared for a mynah bird (soft bill) that contains fruit, vegetables, soft bill mix, mealworms and a vitamin/mineral supplement

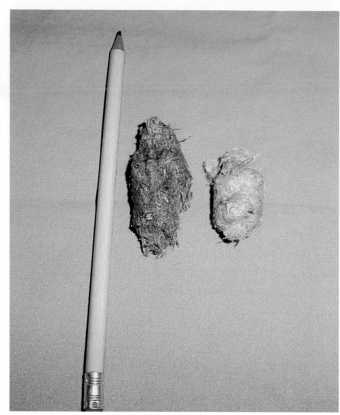

Fig. 31.32 Casts or faecal pellets from an owl

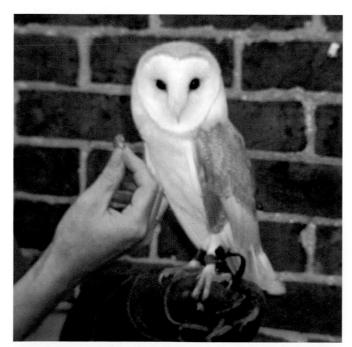

Fig. 31.31 Barn owl being fed by handler. A gauntlet is worn for the safety of the handler

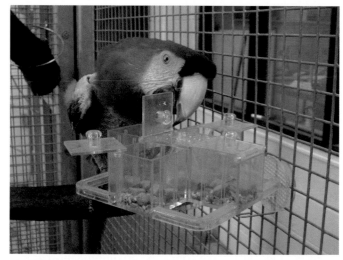

Fig. 31.33 Observe the feeding system used to stimulate a parrot suffering from boredom and demonstrating feather trauma. The parrot is being fed a proprietary complete diet.

calcium – they usually have an inverse calcium:phosphorus ratio.

• Complete diets are available that claim to prevent selective feeding and promote general health and well-being in captive birds. Although not necessarily well received by birds on initial introduction with perseverance they can be a very beneficial diet to many of the parrot family (Fig. 31.33).

- Avocados and apple seeds have been reported to be toxic to birds
- Humming birds require vitamin D and calcium supplement
- Birds can get addicted to sunflower seeds, leading to obesity and death
- As birds do not have teeth they need grit within their gizzard to to grind their food; therefore, always ensure that seed eaters have access to good-quality quartz grit
- Cuttlefish provides calcium and phosphorus in the diet and also helps to keep the beak trim
- Iodine is essential in birds, especially budgerigars, for development and maintenance of the thyroid gland
- There are a variety of bird seeds available; the type chosen depends on the condition of the bird, e.g. breeding or showing
- Examine seeds for quality and plumpness and make sure they are dust-free
- Smaller birds require ad-lib feeding while larger birds require feeding once a day
- Tonic mixes can be given to seed eaters, especially to help them stay healthy over the winter and when coming into breeding condition
- When offering fresh food, makes sure it is fit for human consumption, fresh and washed to remove traces of chemicals
- Millet sprays are a useful addition to the diet and can provide extra nutrients during moulting or to stimulate sick birds to eat
- Birds are messy eaters and will often take a bite out of a piece of fruit or vegetable and then discard it before moving on to the next food item.

Practical feeding

Seeds and nuts are generally offered in bowls that are attached to the side of the aviary or cage. The positioning of the food receptacle depends on the species being fed:

- Quail and ground-dwelling birds are fed on the floor of the aviary
- Fresh foods can be placed on a platform in the cage or aviary (Fig. 31.30)
- As birds are wasteful and will often discard food on to the floor of the aviary, hygiene is very important and all uneaten food must be removed daily
- Seed husks remaining on the top of the feed container must be removed by blowing them away to allow the birds access to the seeds underneath
- Remember not to place food bowls under perches, as they will be contaminated by faeces
- Water is best offered in a gravity-fed bottle or in water hoppers
- Water receptacles should be small to prevent birds using them as a bath.

Breeding

Over the years, interest in breeding birds has grown, which has resulted in the availability of a wide variety of captive-bred species and colour variations. Breeding is a specialized subject and within this text only a brief outline of breeding procedures and protocols is provided (Table 31.16).

Depending on the species, breeding may be a straightforward procedure with the birds readily breeding and producing healthy offspring, e.g. budgerigars, zebra finches and cockatiels, or it may be more complicated and specialized, e.g. some of the larger parrots.

Before any bird will successfully breed some fundamental requirements must be observed:

- You must have a male and female – this may sound obvious but many birds are not sexually dimorphic and sex must be determined surgically or via DNA examination (see Ch. 12)
- Accommodation and environment must be conducive to breeding
- The correct diet must be fed.

Accommodation and environment

If birds are to be bred in **an aviary** the following must be considered:

- **Siting** – the birds must be given privacy and a stress-free environment. Plants in the aviary will provide ground-dwelling birds, such as pheasants, with hiding areas
- **Freedom from vermin** – prevents disease and stops rodents destroying the eggs or killing the young
- **Sheltered flight area** – plastic sheeting on the roof and sides provides protection for nesting birds and fledglings
- **Nest boxes** should be placed in the aviary before the birds come into breeding condition (Fig. 31.26). Boxes of different sizes and securely set at different heights must be available – if the aviary contains mixed species, this will allow the birds to select the box most suitable for them.

If birds are to be bred in **a cage**, the following must be considered:

- Make sure the cage is large enough for the birds to exercise, as this will improve fitness and fertility
- Line the cage with plain paper or newspaper rather than sandpaper, as both are more absorbent and cost-effective. Many hen birds are destructive and will often chew the lining paper
- Nest boxes must be positioned according to the species being housed, but remember to leave enough space for the birds to move in and out of the nest. Budgerigar nest boxes are quite large and are best positioned on the outside of the cage.

Whether housed in indoor cages or aviaries, light and heat must also be considered:

- If the birds are housed in a cage, supplementary heating can be provided in the form of room heating, or for those housed in aviaries or in large indoor flights via tubular heaters. These heaters can be attached to the sides of the accommodation. Supplementary heating can help those birds who breed during the colder months to rear their young and sustain their own body condition, and also reduce the risk of egg binding
- As most birds tend to breed during the warmer parts of the year and are stimulated by daylight length,

Table 31.16 Breeding information for the more commonly kept species of caged bird

Species	Sexing	Clutch size	Incubation period and rearing period	Additional information
Budgerigar (*Melopsittacus undulatus*)	Cere colour – cock blue or purple; hen brown	4–6 eggs	Incubation 18 days by female. After rearing period, chicks emerge from nest at 35 days and independent by day 42	Easy to breed various colour mutations. Social birds so prefer to breed in groups. Altricial young
African grey parrot (*Psittacus erithacus*)	Difficult to sex but male may have darker wings; female is smaller	2–4 eggs	Incubation 28–29 days by female. Rearing period approx. 84 days after hatching	May not breed until their fourth year. After that will readily breed and have a long reproductive life. Males will feed young in nest. After fledging fed by both male and female. Sometimes poor parents and hand-rearing is necessary. Altricial young
Peach-faced lovebirds (*Agapornis roseicollis*)	Monomorphic – need to be surgically sexed	5 eggs	Incubation 28 days. Young fledge approx. 40–42 days after hatching	Various colour mutations. Hens carry nesting materials to line nest. Eggs white. Hatchlings fed by male for extended period. Altricial young
Cockatiels (*Nymphicus hollandicus*)	Difficult to sex until first moult at approx. 6 months Females plumage duller, especially facial markings, than male. Females have barring on under surface of the tail feathers	5+ eggs	Incubation 18–21 days. Rearing period to fledging is 30–35 days	Both parents incubate eggs. Colour variations available. Breed easily in captivity. To prevent breeding remove nest boxes especially over winter when young vulnerable to cold. Altricial young
Canary (*Canarius serinus*)	No clear distinction between male and female, although male sings during breeding season	4 eggs	Incubation period 14 days by hen. Rearing period 14 days	Altricial young
Zebra finch (*Taeniopygia (poephilia) guttata*)	Females have paler beaks and usually lack chest and flank markings of the males	6 eggs	Incubation period 12 days by hen. Rearing period – chicks start to leave nest 18 days after hatching	Fledglings will eat independently 14 days after leaving. Prolific breeders: need to limit clutches to three per year. Move nests and nesting material to prevent continuous nest building. Altricial young
Hill mynah (*Gracula religiosa*)	No visible distinction between sexes	2–4 eggs, green blue with brown spots	Incubation period 14–15 days by both parents. Fledge at 4–5 weeks, independent at 8 weeks	Supply cockatiel or starling nest boxes all year. In breeding season supply twigs leaves, straw, hay and hemp fibres as nesting materials. Altricial young
Diamond dove (*Geopelia cuneata*)	Both sexes have red eye rings but those of males are thicker during breeding season. Males have more spots on wings than females	2 eggs	Incubation period 13 days, with both parents involved in the process. After rearing period the chicks may leave nest as early as 13 days post hatching	Good parents and care for young. Altricial young
Chinese painted quail (*Excalfactoria chinensis*)	Hens have brownish overall colour and lack the cock's bluish plumage	6 eggs	Incubation period 18 days	Precocial young are virtually able to live independently after hatching providing temperature, etc., is correct. They are not fed by parents

NB. Incubation and rearing periods may vary.

controlling the provision of artificial light may stimulate the birds to breed. It also provides them with a longer period to feed, thus increasing body condition and general health. Lighting is best supplied by fluorescent lights fitted with timers.

Diet

Successful breeding and rearing of young uses a large amount of energy so the bird's diet must be of sufficient quality and quantity. Various species of parrot and soft bills can be stim-

ulated into breeding condition by increasing protein levels, and it has been shown to be of value in improving reproductive performance. A poor-quality diet will cause poor reproductive performance, egg binding and reduced numbers of offspring.

Egg laying and incubation

Signs that a hen is about to lay her eggs include:

- Spending longer periods on the nest or in the nest box, and the cock bird will often join her

- Hen's vent may appear slightly swollen
- Change in the amount and smell of hen's droppings.

The frequency of laying varies according to species. For instance, finches lay every day, budgerigars and many of the parrot family lay every other day. To prevent eggs developing at different rates, the hen will often not incubate her eggs until at least three eggs have been laid. This behaviour can alarm the novice breeder but intervention could lead to the hen abandoning her nest. During incubation the sitting bird will turn the eggs daily to prevent the embryo from sticking to the inside of the shell.

Incubation periods vary according to species (Table 31.16):

1. **Natural incubation** – eggs are incubated by either the hen alone, e.g. budgerigars, or shared between the hen and cock bird, e.g. cockatiels. In wading birds such as coots and moor hens it is the male who takes sole responsibility for incubation.
2. **Artificial incubation** – eggs are incubated in a specially designed avian incubator. There are various models available and features vary but it is advisable to purchase one that will automatically turn the eggs as this is not only time saving but reduces heat loss every time the incubator is opened. Heat is a key factor in successful hatching and a fluctuation of 0.5 °C can have quite damaging effects on the viability of the eggs. As a guide incubation temperatures range from 36.9 to 37.5 °C with a relative humidity of 40–55% depending on species.

Rearing chicks

When first hatched, chicks can be classified according to their stage of development:

- **Altricial** – blind, bald and totally dependent on the parents, e.g. budgerigars, finches
- **Precocial** – capable of living an independent life, e.g. quail, ducklings.

They may also be grouped according to when they leave the nest:

- **Nidifugous** – capable of leaving the nest soon after hatching, e.g. ducklings and goslings
- **Nidiculous** – remain in the nest until they are feathered and ready to fly, e.g. budgerigar, cockatiel, parrots.

If eggs have been incubated by the parents, then they will care for and feed the young. If they have been hatched using artificial means, then the hatchlings should be moved to a brooder and kept in a controlled environment until they are weaned and feathered. During the rearing period the accommodation and nest boxes or brooder must be kept very clean. If droppings and uneaten food remain, the nestlings' feet can become encrusted in debris, preventing them from walking and leading to disease.

Avian disease

Some bird diseases are extremely difficult to identify so if signs continue for more than 24 hours a veterinary surgeon must be consulted (Table 31.17).

General signs of ill health in a bird include:

- Lethargy
- Bird's feathers ruffled and 'puffed up'
- Sleeping with both feet on perch – especially parrots
- Poor appetite
- Regurgitating food
- Loose watery or abnormally coloured droppings
- Increased thirst
- Discharge from nostrils and eyes
- Abnormal breathing – laboured, noisy, exaggerated tail movements
- Heavy moult.

Other more specific signs include blood in the droppings, a prominent breast bone indicating severe loss of weight, gasping for breath with the beak open, uncoordinated movements and paralysis.

When dealing with an ill bird you should isolate the bird from other birds and humans as soon as possible. The isolation cage should be positioned in a quiet, well-ventilated room and have three solid sides. There should be an infrared or ceramic heat lamp to keep the cage at a temperature of at least 32 °C. If appropriate, offer food that is easily digestible and water that is lukewarm.

Welfare of captive exotic animals

Pain and distress

All the exotic species that are kept as pets are capable of feeling pain and distress and in some cases if this is not identified and is allowed to continue it may lead to the death of the animal. Even the close proximity of the human owner may be a source of distress and it is important to realize that, unlike dogs and cats, many of these exotic species do not enjoy being handled.

Definitions of pain and distress include:

- **Pain** – an unpleasant sensory and emotional experience associated with actual or potential tissue damage. This physical phenomenon may be classified as mild, moderate or substantial or depending on the duration of the pain may be described as being acute or chronic
- **Discomfort** – milder than pain and may be nothing more than an inconvenience
- **Distress** – often shortened to 'stress'. This is a psychological phenomenon and may be associated with pain. 'Stressors' include isolation (in social species), maternal separation, overcrowding, noise or lack of privacy.

It is often difficult to decide whether an animal is in pain or distress and veterinary nurses are commonly told that 'it must be very difficult to do your job because animals cannot tell you what is wrong'; however, animals cannot lie or exaggerate their situation, so the presented picture is the true one.

There are three ways of assessing the situation:

- **Subjective assessment** – using your 'gut instinct' where there are no measurable factors. If you would expect an

Table 31.17 Common diseases and clinical conditions of birds

Species	Causal agent	Symptoms	Diagnosis and treatment	Additional information
Ectoparasites				
Scaly leg and scaly face mite (cnemidocoptic mange) Budgerigars, crossbills, Passeriformes, canaries; occasionally in domestic poultry	*Cnemidocoptes* spp.	Common in budgerigar. Appears as grey white encrustations around the cere, beak, eyes, feet and legs. Seen on legs of crossbills and appears as foot lesions on canaries and other passerines	Examine a scraping of affected area. Various treatments include liquid paraffin to soften scabs, then follow up with 10% benzyl benzoate or 5% piperonyl butoxide. Ivermectin 10 mg/ml cattle injection	May infest cloaca. Mite lives and feeds on bird's beak, surrounding areas and legs. It burrows and feeds off the bird, if untreated leading to infection, rotting skin and osteomyelitis. Hygiene and isolation as mite rapidly spreads. If using ivermectin repeat dose at 10–14 days. Remember – this drug can remain in the system for prolonged periods so care not to overdose
Red mite (greyish agile mite) Seen in domestic poultry	*Dermanyssus* spp.	Bird sits restlessly on the perch, Constantly pecking and scratching at itself. If you shine a torch into the cage at night you will see the mite. Zoonotic – humans can develop a rash caused by the mite	As above	Mite lives in the dark crevices and seams of the bird's accommodation and emerges from its hiding place at night to attack and suck the blood of the sleeping bird. It is particularly difficult to treat and destroy by just disinfecting as the mite can live up to 5 months without food and reproduce at a rate of 2600 eggs per 2 months life span
Other ectoparasites: • Lice • Fleas • Feather mites • Feather follicle mites	*Mallophaga* *Siphonaptera* Various species	Irritation, feather loss Loss of condition, bird restless	Antiparasitic preparations	
• Air sac mite	*Sternostoma* spp.	Dyspnoea, loss of voice sneezing, gasping, death		Air sac mite mostly seen in passerines
Endoparasites				
Tapeworm (cestodes) Roundworms (nematodes)	Large number of different species involved	Thin, anorexic and generally lethargic birds. Diarrhoea. Screen droppings/crop smears for worm eggs	Crop tube and worm using liquid medication, or place drops in water. Use veterinary prescribed anthelmintics: *Tapeworms* – • Fenbendazole • Praziquantel *Roundworms* – • Levamisole • Fenbendazole • Ivermectin	*Tapeworms* – Worm eggs found in an intermediate host, i.e. the food they ingested infects birds. The adult worms then develop in the bird's intestine and eggs are shed in the droppings. Intermediate host ingest the worm eggs and the cycle starts again *Roundworms* – Worm eggs are passed out in the bird's droppings and are passed onto other birds by contaminating food, eggs, adhere to feathers, and feet Fenbendazole is toxic to finches. Levamisole can be toxic and deaths seen in budgerigars, pigeons and lovebirds

Enteric disease

Disease / Species	Causative agent	Clinical signs	Diagnosis / Treatment	Comments
Enteritis All species	*Escherichia coli* *Campylobacter* spp. Change in diet	Anorexia. Change in appearance to droppings yellow-green, watery. Bird listless and quiet	Histology and culture of infected tissue. Antibiotics or sulphonamides. Supportive therapy, i.e. fluid therapy	Watery green droppings suggest reduced food intake and excess bile secretion
Trichomoniasis All species	*Trichomonas gallinae*	Sometimes acute death, diarrhoea, inappetence, weight loss, lethargy dyspnoea	Microscopic examination to identify parasite. Metronidazole, good hygiene and supportive therapy	Also called 'canker' in pigeons and 'frounce' in raptors. Infections via direct contact, generally in food
Salmonellosis All species Caused by: poor hygiene, rodent infestation, wild birds, and poor quarantine	*Salmonella* spp.	Including: • Bloodstained droppings • Slimy droppings • Smelly droppings • Swelling of wings or joints • Passage of undigested food • Paralysis	Antibiotics, good hygiene, supportive therapy	Zoonosis causing enteric signs, i.e. diarrhoea and vomiting

Respiratory disease

Disease / Species	Causative agent	Clinical signs	Diagnosis / Treatment	Comments
Ornithosis Psitticosis Chlamydiosis Mainly seen in: • Psittacine birds – cockatiels, lovebirds, budgerigars, parrots • Columbiformes – doves • Anseriformes – ducks, geese and swans	*Chlamydia psittaci*	Affected bird may sit huddled up on perch, wheezing, gasping for breath, open beak and exaggerated tail movements. Respiratory signs, nasal, ocular discharge, ruffled feathers, shivering. Enteritis	Isolate affected bird. Laboratory faecal and blood tests. Keep bird warm and supportive therapy. Antibiotics, e.g. enrofloxacin; tetracyclines, chlorotetracyclines	Zoonosis causing flu-like signs, diarrhoea, shivering, pyrexia, and headaches. Never share food or allow a bird to take food from your mouth. Always wash hands after handling a bird. Disease passed on via droppings and discharges. Humans inhale causative agent. Strict hygiene protocols. Mainly seen in imported birds or smuggled birds not correctly quarantined. Most imported birds are routinely treated against *Chlamydia*. Chlorotetracyclines are bacteriocidal and require prolonged use
Avian mycoplasmosis All species	*Mycoplasma* spp.	Upper respiratory infection sneezing, sinusitis, blepharitis	Culture of causative organism. Use various antimicrobial drugs, e.g. tylosin, enrofloxacin	Seen where groups of birds kept confined and with poor ventilation
Newcastle's disease (fowl pest) – notifiable disease Affects all avians	Paramyxovirus	Variable: listlessness, green slimy droppings, neurological signs	Virus isolation. Histopathology	Highly infectious – all affected and in-contact livestock must be destroyed. Affects egg production. Major reason for avian quarantine. Vaccine available for poultry

Table 31.17 Continued

Species	Causal agent	Symptoms	Diagnosis and treatment	Additional information
Nutritional disorders				
Iodine deficiency Seen in Budgerigars	Iodine-deficient diet	Loss or change in voice, respiratory problems due to pressure from enlarged thyroid on trachea. Bird often has difficulty breathing and makes a characteristic 'click' sound. To aid respiration, bird can be observed sitting with head raised. Crop dilation as seed unable to pass into the thyroid gland into the proventriculus	Iodine supplementation. Improve diet and add iodine to drinking water	Not commonly seen because of use of packaged seeds that have been supplemented. Iodine deficiency affects thyroid hormone production, which then stimulates an increase in thyroid stimulating hormone (TSH) from the anterior pituitary. Raised levels of TSH cause hyperplasia (enlargement) of the thyroid gland (goitre)
Vitamin A deficiency Common in all species	Vitamin-A-deficient diet. Lack of fresh vegetables and fruit in diet. Overuse of sunflower seeds in the diet	Generally ill bird, lethargic, weight loss and signs of respiratory problems such as wheezing, dyspnoea and sneezing. Nasal discharge. Eyes appear swollen, with signs of conjunctivitis	Change diet, with addition of dark green vegetables and carrots. Vitamin A therapy	Psittacine birds that have been fed on an all-seed diet will not readily accept fresh fruits and vegetables, but the owner must be persuaded to persevere with this change in diet
Calcium, phosphorus and vitamin D deficiency Psittacines and those birds fed on an exclusively seed diet	High seed and nut diet, especially peanuts and sunflower seeds	Variety of skeletal problems and poor growth. Egg binding and soft shells. General signs will depend on age and duration of problem. Poor appetite, lethargy, weakness, poor feather growth, soft droppings. Bird unable to perch properly, wings held in abnormal position; in severe cases bird appears to have a hunched back. Muscle spasms and twitching. Death	Severe cases, give intravenous calcium borogluconate and intramuscular diazepam. Improve diet plus calcium supplementation	Vitamin D activated by ultraviolet light on the skin influences the uptake and usage of dietary calcium and phosphorus
Feather problems				
Feather plucking	Self-mutilation due to boredom, stress, isolation, changes in routine, over-preening during breeding season. Poor husbandry and nutrition, hormonal imbalance	Plumage on body is damaged and bald areas apart from head. Clinical history examination to rule out other feather disorders	Once established, this is very difficult to stop. Enrich cage, and bird's life. Education of the owner on how to deal with bird. Fitting of an Elizabethan collar to prevent mutilation. Drug therapy	Rule out ectoparasites by careful examination of plumage. Frequently seen in parrots. Placing another bird in the cage may seem a good idea but evidence has shown that behaviour can be passed on to new occupant
Feather cysts Certain breeds of canary; other domestic species	Genetic or due to damage to developing feather follicle or excess preening	Large, bulging swellings seen in region of the carpus (wings) but can be seen in other parts of the body – contains the remains of the undeveloped feather	Surgical removal	The wall of the follicles can become thickened and a cheesy exudates forms within it

Condition / Species	Causes	Clinical signs	Treatment	Comments
Loss of feather condition	Various pathogens and conditions that can affect the integrity of the feathers and dermis Ectoparasites Bullying Feather plucking Poor environmental conditions, especially low humidity and nutrition	Baldness Intense irritation Damage to feathers		Rule out ectoparasites. Moulting is a natural occurrence and frequency depends on species and environmental conditions. Moulting is a stressful process for the bird and nutritional demands are high, so increased nutrition and supplementation must be considered. Broken feathers will not normally regrow until the next moult. It can take 4–6 weeks for new feathers to grow
Psittacine beak and feather disease Various psittacine species, especially cockatoos	Viral: circo virus	Poor feather condition and abnormal plumage. Feathers appear small and club-like, fret lines in the vane, curled feathers. Feather loss. Feathers remain in blood-filled sheath. Beak also abnormal appearance, shiny, elongated, flaky and fault lines. Change in feather coloration	Fatal. Supportive therapy may be considered but because of its virulence and threat to bird populations, any suspected cases must be quarantined and diagnosis made rapidly	Transmission of virus via faeces, feathers and dust
Regurgitation All species	Many causes, including: • Behavioural response • Proventriculus • Dilatation disease • Ingestion of foreign body • Infections, e.g. yeast, *Trichomonas*, *Megabacterium* • Reaction to drug therapy • Ingestion of toxins, e.g. plants, insecticides • Neoplasm • Parasites • Crop stasis/necrosis • Crop impaction	Food regurgitated. Other signs depend on causative agent. Physical examination of the bird to eliminate foreign body. Check oral cavity. Palpate crop, abdomen and cloaca palpated. Faecal examination, bacteriology and blood tests to identify pathogen. Endoscopy to identify and remove foreign body	Depending on diagnosis: fluid therapy and supportive care; tube feeding	Regurgitation occurs during courtship, feeding of nestlings and weaning. Pet birds may also adopt an object or family member and regurgitate as a method of courtship or feeding

Table 31.17 Continued

Species	Causal agent	Symptoms	Diagnosis and treatment	Additional information
Other conditions				
'Going light' – megabacteriosis Budgerigars, canaries, finches, cockatiels	*Megabacterium, Toxoplasma*	Occasionally blood in faeces, chronic weight loss, lethargy, random deaths in aviary birds, dilatation of proventriculus	Supportive care, specific therapy if pathogen identified. Improve diet	Seen in large collections and where birds are frequently taken to exhibitions
Egg binding All species, particularly budgerigars and cockatiels	Multifactorial: • Size of egg • First clutch • Calcium deficiency • Obesity • Poor environmental conditions • Age of bird • Tumours	As egg laying imminent, bird appears depressed, lethargic, abdominal distension, unsteadiness on perch, squatting, straining and diarrhoea. Note: Clinical signs can vary depending on the site of the egg	Treatment varies according to position of egg, but it is important to remove the egg as soon as possible. This may be via drug therapy, manual manipulation or surgery. Keep bird warm (30–32°C)	Bird will be very distressed and it is important to keep patient warm and quiet and in a darkened room
Articular gout Poultry, waterfowl, raptors and psittacine birds, especially budgerigars, conures and lovebirds	Associated with renal disease or damage	Swollen painful joints. Bird exhibiting shifting lameness, and hanging on side of cage to take weight off painful joints. Loss of condition. Diagnosis by the muroxide test on the contents taken from one of the joint swellings	No specific treatment: only able to manage the signs, e.g. by restricting high-protein foodstuffs in diet and maintaining good state of hydration. Drug therapy to reduce uric acid production in the liver. Surgical removal of urates deposits in the joints	Water consumption can be improved by adding fruits and vegetables in the diet. Nodules of the uric acid also called tophi are creamy white in colour. They are normally seen on the intertarsals and joints of the feet. Prognosis is poor
Bumble foot Poultry, birds of prey, occasionally psittacine birds	Common microorganisms isolated: • *Staphylococcus aureus* • *Escherichia coli* • *Proteus* spp.	Septic condition of the foot leading to abscessation. Microorganism gains entry via a penetrating wound underneath the foot. Infection leads to swelling and pus-filled areas. Infection can track as far as hock. As bird is in discomfort, it can be observed resting against sides of cage	Under a general anaesthetic, lance and drain the infected area. Swab taken of area for culture and sensitivity will indicate appropriate antibiotics. Foot may be bandaged and bird kept on padded perches of varying widths	Linked with poor hygiene and perches all the same width. Also high incidence in heavy, inactive birds limited to one size of perch. Initial penetrating wound can be caused by claws growing into foot. If left untreated, area can become gangrenous

injury or disease to cause pain in humans then it probably causes pain in other species – always remember postoperative pain

- **Clinical assessment** – certain clinical signs will indicate pain, e.g. raised pulse rate or respiratory rate, raised temperature, loss of weight caused by loss of appetite or dehydration. These are quantifiable, e.g. the higher the pulse rate the greater the degree of pain
- **Behavioural assessment** – in order to assess whether an animal is behaving abnormally you must first know what is normal for that species, e.g. Is it normal for a bird to sit fluffed up on its perch with its eyes shut, for a rabbit to scream or for a mouse to sit separately from the rest of its cage mates?

Pain and distress can be reduced by:

- **Correct handling** – learn the recommended method and do it correctly the first time. Make sure that any equipment you may need is available and in good working order and, if you are likely to need assistance, make sure that help is at hand
- **Providing a high standard of animal husbandry**, i.e. appropriate housing, environment and diet
- **Making changes to the environment to reduce pain**, e.g. confine a bird with a broken wing to a small cage so that it cannot fly
- **Attending to wounds and infection** as soon as possible to minimize suffering
- **Using therapeutic agents** to reduce pain if appropriate, e.g. analgesics and anaesthetics
- **Be prepared to use euthanasia as a means of relieving suffering** if treatment is likely to cause pain or is unlikely to be successful. Euthanasia by definition is painless and very quick when performed competently and should not be overlooked as a possible course of action.

The welfare of animals should be viewed holistically, i.e. look at every aspect that affects the animal, from its environment and diet to the type of owner, which might include age and experience, employment, whether they smoke, whether they have children, where they live, etc. All these factors and many more will affect the welfare of the animal and should be taken into account when identifying problems.

There are three main areas that must be constantly reviewed by the veterinary nurse and clients should be advised upon:

- Appropriate husbandry, i.e. diet, housing, environment and their management
- Appropriate psychological and behavioural needs to avoid the development of stereotypical and other behaviour problems
- Basic health requirements of the species.

The welfare of exotic animals is also of extreme importance within the veterinary practice and as most nurses and veterinary surgeons see these animals less often, inevitably we know less about their veterinary needs and their responses to anaesthetic and analgesic drugs. Their preoperative and postoperative care is often the responsibility of the nurse, who must be aware of both normal behaviour and the significance of abnormal behaviour.

Small mammals

With the exception of the ferret, most small mammals show little evidence of pain. These are all prey species so in the wild, if they were to show pain, they would make themselves vulnerable and obvious to predators, who would then kill them. They rarely vocalize unless handled roughly, although rabbits will scream or become actively aggressive, as would a cat or dog. Table 31.18 describes both normal and abnormal behaviour patterns.

Pain should be assessed and monitored and recorded on hospital sheets at regular intervals, e.g. every 2–3 hours. This should include details of:

- Appetite – what was eaten and quantity
- Urination – quantity and appearance
- Defecation – appearance
- Demeanour – bright, lethargic, aggressive
- Body position
- Pupils – dilated or constricted.

Reptiles

Reptiles are very easily stressed and feel pain. The use of opiate-based pain relief is still an area requiring research but non-steroidal anti-inflammatory drugs can and are used with some level of effectiveness. Table 31.19 describes both normal and abnormal behaviour that may indicate pain in reptiles.

Hospitalized reptiles

Sick reptiles should be placed in hospital vivaria, ideally made from fibreglass or moulded plastic with correct controlled heating and lighting. They should be kept in a separate room away from other domestic animals and, if a lizard is very stressed and banging against the front of the vivarium, a non-reflective covering can be placed over the glass front, allowing the nurse to observe the patient without disturbing it.

Factors that can cause distress in reptiles

- Poor environmental conditions and positioning of the animal's enclosure or vivarium (see Housing, above)
- Over-handling – there is little evidence to show that reptiles enjoy constant handling and if it is incorrectly carried out some species of lizards, e.g. geckos, can carry out autotomy (tail loss). Snakes are easily bruised and can suffer spinal injuries, especially in the occipital area. **Note:** Bruising may take several weeks to show in cold-blooded species and can be a cause of death
- Inadequate nutrition (see Nutrition, above)
- Overcrowding and fighting – many lizards are territorial and males will fight to defend their territory or to claim females. Geckos, bearded dragons and water dragons are a few examples of lizards that are very territorial and must be kept either on their own or with females. Juvenile male tortoises are exceedingly 'oversexed' and bachelor groups will constantly try and mate one another, resulting in bite wounds to the

Table 31.18 Normal behaviour and abnormal behaviour as an indicator of pain and distress in small mammals

	Rabbits	Guinea pigs	Ferrets	Gerbils	Mice	Rats
Normal behaviour	Active, inquisitive, eating/foraging regularly. Copraphagia performed at night. Body posture relaxed and will often lie stretched out	Active, inquisitive, eating/foraging regularly. Copraphagia performed at night. Normal vocalization, chunter, chutt, whistles and whines. Only rodent that normally vocalizes	Active, inquisitive, sniffing ground and playing. Relaxed body posture	Active, inquisitive, eating/foraging regularly. Interacting with cage mates	Active, inquisitive, eating/foraging regularly. Interacting with cage mates	Active, inquisitive, eating/foraging regularly. Interacting with cage mates
Indication of pain/ abnormal behaviour	Hunched body posture, very still and inactive. High-pitched scream if in extreme pain or fear (usually only when attacked by predator). Anorexia. Teeth grinding, indicating pain. Will salivate if oral discomfort. Often more difficult to handle. Hiding at back of cage. Postoperatively, rabbits often interfere with wound/sutures	Hunched body posture, very still and inactive. If scared or in pain, guinea pigs will emit a very high-pitched scream. Anorexia. Teeth grinding, indicating pain. Will salivate if in oral discomfort. Hiding at back of cage	High-pitched scream, associated with fear rather than pain. May become more aggressive if in pain. Will often interfere with wound/sutures if operation site painful	May bite if handled. Fur often looks 'staring'. Quiet hunched body posture; if in communal groups, will avoid contact with other gerbils. Often ostracized by colony, may be thrown out of housing area	May bite if handled. Fur often looks 'staring'. Quiet hunched body posture; if in communal groups, will avoid contact with other mice	Quiet, reduction in exploratory behaviour. Will often interfere with wound/ sutures if operation site painful

Table 31.19 Normal and abnormal behaviour as an indicator of pain in reptiles and birds

	Snakes	Lizards	Chelonia	Birds
Normal behaviour	Hiding under furnishings or curled round branch, or basking, slowly moving round cage. Docile species accept disturbance from handler when cleaning and maintaining accommodation. Non-aggressive toward handler. Normal ecdysis. Accepting food and eating regularly. Passing normal urine and faecal matter	Lively, seen basking and moving around the accommodation. Accepting food. Docile species handled with ease. Accepts being kept in accommodation	Active, walking with shell lifted off the ground. Eating, passing urates and faecal matter. Non-aggressive, basking and thermoregulation. Quickly retreats into shell if threatened or approached. Strength in limbs	Plump and plumage in good condition and feathers held flat against the bird's body. Sits steadily on perch, greets known human companions. Able to carry out free flight. Normal relaxed respiration. Droppings appear normal white urates and brown or black faecal matter
Abnormal	Restless and moving around accommodation. Agitated by normal routine, i.e. feeding, handling and cleaning. Striking at handler. Abnormal posture head and neck raised and mouth gaping and exaggerated breathing. Contortions and twisting of body. Constantly rubbing body against furnishings. Flaccid and lethargic, problems shedding. Watery faecal matter	Quiet species may become more lively or lively species subdued. Docile species becomes aggressive and refuses food. Constantly knocking into vivarium doors, especially glass. Aggression toward fellow occupants. Not actively basking or not moving away from hot spot. Head raised and open-mouthed breathing. Flaccid and lethargic. Dark, dull colour, especially in chameleons. Iguanas males – head bobbing and knocking tail against doors and walls	Failure to retract head into shell. Limp and flaccid limbs. Slow-moving. Remains under hot spot or hidden away. Not eating. Open-mouthed breathing	Hunched or abnormal appearance on perch. Sits with eyes closed. Head under wing. Feathers ruffled and exaggerated breathing. Feather plucking, and aggression toward familiar human companions

legs and shell trauma as they constantly ram into one another. If a male and female are kept together the female will be constantly harassed by the male's amorous advances

- Poor husbandry and illness
- Wild-caught species not adjusting to a captive environment
- Prolonged transportation.

It may take weeks or months for the results of stress to become obvious and animals that have sustained long periods of stress will have a diminished immune response.

Birds

Table 31.19 shows both normal and abnormal behaviour in caged and aviary birds.

Hospitalized birds

As most birds spend most of their time above human eye-level, i.e. in aviaries or on cage perches, it makes sense to accommodate these birds in the veterinary surgery at high levels, e.g. on high shelves or in hanging cages, which will make the bird feel less threatened and reduces stress. They should be accommodated away from predator animals and excessive noise and kept in subdued light.

When handling a bird it will feel much happier if it can perch on your finger, but there is the risk of escape so steps must be taken to prevent this. Restraining a bird just around the wings causes it much distress and it will attempt to flap.

Factors that can cause distress in birds

- Siting of cages and aviaries – some birds are gregarious and enjoy being in a busy area and if deprived of human or other bird contact can become depressed and display behavioural abnormalities. To other species this would cause much distress and health problems
- Overcrowding and bullying
- Overbreeding
- Poor nutrition
- Poor environmental hygiene
- Disease and illness

Bibliography

Alderton, D., 2001. Caring for Cage and Aviary Birds. Southwater, London.

Alderton, D., 2003. Exotic Pet Handbook. Southwater, London.

Beynon, P.H., Forbes, N.A., Lawton, M.P.C. (Eds.), 1996. BSAVA Manual of Psittacine Birds. British Small Animal Veterinary Association, Cheltenham.

Coles, B.H., 1997. Avian Medicine and Surgery, second ed. Blackwell Science, Oxford.

Divers, S.J., 1997. Medical and surgical treatment of reptile dystocias. In: 21st Annual Waltham/Ohio State University Symposium (for the Treatment of Animal Diseases) Lecture Notes. College of Veterinary Medicine, Ohio State University and Waltham USA Inc, Vernon, CA, pp. 75–81.

Donoghue, S., 1997. Nutrition of companion birds and reptiles. In: 21st Annual Waltham/Ohio State University Symposium (for the Treatment of Animal Diseases) Lecture Notes. College of Veterinary Medicine, Ohio State University and Waltham USA Inc, Vernon, CA, pp. 27–33.

Fenwick, H., 1995. Taking Care of Tortoises, Their Eggs and Hatchlings. Kingston.

Frye, F.L., 1994. Reptile Clinicians Handbook. Krieger Publishing Malabar, FL.

Gosden, C., 2004. Exotics and Wildlife: a manual of veterinary nursing care. Butterworth, Oxford.

Hardcourt-Brown, N., Chitty, J.R., 2005. Manual of Psittacine Birds, second ed. BSAVA, Gloucester.

Mader, D., 1997. Approach to the anorexic reptile. In: 21st Annual Waltham/Ohio State University Symposium (for the Treatment of Animal Diseases) Lecture Notes. College of Veterinary Medicine, Ohio State University and Waltham USA Inc, Vernon, CA, pp. 71–74.

Mader, D., 1997b. Reptile urogenital system and renal disease. In: 21st Annual Waltham/Ohio State University Symposium (for the Treatment of Animal Diseases) Lecture Notes. College of Veterinary Medicine, Ohio State University and Waltham USA Inc, Vernon, CA, pp. 67–70.

Mader, D.R., et al., 2006. Reptile Medicine and Surgery, second ed. Saunders Elsevier, St Louis, Missouri.

Mara, W.P., 1997. Map Turtles and Diamondback Terrapins. TFH Publications, Havant.

Pursall, B., 1994. The Guide to Owning a Mediterranean Tortoise. TFH, Havant.

Quesenbury, K.E., Carpenter, J.W., 2004. Ferrets, Rabbits and Rodents – Clinical Medicine and Surgery, second ed. W.B. Saunders, St Louis, MO.

Recommended reading

Aspinall, V., 2008. Clinical Procedures in Veterinary Nursing. Butterworth-Heinemann. Oxford.

Excellent chapter on handling and restraint in exotic species.

Girling, S.J., Raiti, P., 2004. BSAVA Manual of Reptiles. British Small Animal Veterinary Association (BSAVA), Gloucester.

Longley, L.A., 2008. Anaesthesia of Exotic Pets. Saunders Elsevier, London.

Good for nursing and anaesthesia of exotic animals.

Meredith, A., Redrobe, S., 2002. BSAVA Manual of Exotic Pets. BSAVA, Gloucester.

Both manuals provide a wide range of information on the subject.

Quesenbury, K.E., Carpenter, J.W., 2004. Ferrets, Rabbits and Rodents – Clinical Medicine and Surgery, second ed. W B Saunders, St Louis, MO.

Excellent book covering anatomy and physiology, husbandry and clinical conditions.

Richardson, V.C.G., 1997. Diseases of Small Rodents. Blackwell Science, Oxford.

Good coverage of small 'furries'.

CHAPTER 32

Management and care of injured wildlife

Louise Minshell

Introduction

The care of sick, injured and orphaned wildlife provides the veterinary nurse with a large variety of species whose needs differ greatly from any group of animals normally presented within a veterinary practice. Wildlife casualties do not appreciate the type of care and comfort given to domestic animals and may even suffer as a result of it. Stress to the casualty is the biggest problem facing wildlife carers and this must constantly be taken into consideration.

The aim of this chapter is to provide advice on the basic care of the most common wildlife casualties based on their natural behaviour and habitat. It will also tell you how to deal with requests for help from members of the public, including how to recognize when an animal is in need of help and when it should be left alone.

Wildlife can be difficult to handle, as they are wild creatures that live in a world where humans are seen as a threat. The first thought of any carer should be how the animal's distress can be minimized and the second should be how soon can it be released back into the wild.

Wild mammals

General guidelines

Rescue and transportation

On being approached, a wild animal will do one of three things – it will freeze, run or, if cornered, defend itself. Before attempting to catch any animal, assess the situation carefully. The animal should be observed for the way it is behaving and moving and a plan should be worked out for its capture. Any additional help should be organized and then the approach, capture and confinement must be carried out swiftly and firmly but kindly. One of the most important pieces of equipment is a blanket or towel. Never use a wire basket or transparent container for wildlife. If a solid container is not available, then a cover should be provided. There is nothing more likely to cause stress and injury to an animal than for it to be put into a container it can see out of but from which it cannot escape.

The container should always be lined – newspaper and a towel or a blanket for larger casualties is ideal for providing warmth, absorbency, a place to hide and something to grip on to during transportation. The container should allow enough room for the animal to stand and turn around. If using a cardboard box it must be made secure to prevent the animal from escaping. Containers with grill-type doors must be covered to keep the animal in the dark. Badly injured individuals or those in shock may need an immediate heat source and Snuggle Pads are ideal for use during transportation. A well-wrapped hot-water bottle will suffice until the casualty is livelier.

Admission

On arrival the injured animal should go through a standard admissions procedure which should include:

- Where the animal was found – once recovered the animal should be taken back to the place it was found unless it is inappropriate, e.g. main road
- Name, address and telephone number of the finder
- Behaviour at the time of rescue – may provide an indication of the injury or condition, e.g. a fox staggering around in the road suggests a road traffic accident.

This information may reduce the need for a thorough examination, which will reduce the amount of stress.

A record card or hospital chart is then completed and remains with the casualty throughout its stay.

If the animal is in shock or particularly distressed, the carrying container should be placed in a quiet place and it should be left for 1–2 hours to calm down. There is nothing to be gained by putting an already traumatized animal through a full examination, so unless life-saving treatment is needed it should be left alone to recover. If the casualty has been transported in a sensible manner it should be able to cope with the initial examination providing it does not take too long.

It is not necessary to routinely treat for fleas and this should only be done if fleas are seen. I remember the sad case of a hedgehog that died as a result of an over-enthusiastic pyrethrin application, which was given because it was thought that all hedgehogs were infested with fleas. Fipronil can be used safely when needed, although there are reports that it may kill rabbits. Routine vitamin injections on admission are also unnecessary but long-term patients will benefit from supplements to compensate for the lack of a natural diet.

Housing

Individual housing requirements will be discussed in the sections on specific species but there are a few general guidelines:

- Each wildlife casualty should be housed according to its needs, its natural behaviour and habitat
- Mammals need a place to hide and their reaction once placed in a cage or pen is to find a suitable place out of sight
- Bedding should be put at the back of the accommodation and this is where your casualty will stay. Unlike birds, which will flap around the cage as it is opened, mammals will remain hidden away.

Heat provision should be carefully considered. Giving casualties heat that they do not need means that they will have to be weaned off it before they can be released. Remember that these are wild animals that live out in the cold, wet and windy weather. Warm bedding is all that is required. Flexible heat mats and microwavable heat pads should be well wrapped to provide a gentle heat, but they cannot be regulated and provide a constant temperature. Bedding must be kept away from the heat source in case the casualty becomes too warm and it also provides somewhere to hide. Those too sick to cool themselves must be carefully monitored to avoid overheating.

To wean an animal off heat, gradually turn the heat supply down and then off during the day, when temperatures are warmer. Once this has been achieved the process should be repeated for night-time heating.

Feeding

Wildlife species may be:

- Diurnal – active during the day
- Nocturnal – active at night
- Crepuscular – active at dawn and dusk.

Their period of natural activity must be taken into account when providing food. A nocturnal creature that is asleep all day cannot be expected to eat breakfast; dinner is far more appropriate. An uneaten meal given early in the morning may cause concern when really the animal has been fed at the incorrect time. Some animals do not eat purely because they are in captivity. One of the main problems when dealing with wildlife is knowing what to feed – the biggest myth is to give bread and milk (Table 32.1).

Orphaned mammals

Individuals in a litter of orphans must be identified in some way for their individual progress to be monitored, e.g. with blue/purple spray on different areas of their bodies so they are easily recognized. The identification mark and weight should be recorded, together with an approximate age and details of condition (Fig. 32.1).

Table 32.1 Natural diet and suitable food alternatives for captive wildlife patients

Species	Natural food	Alternative food
Hedgehog	Earthworms, insects, eggs, fruit, small mammals	Tinned cat or dog food, day-old chicks, mice
Badger	Earthworms, slugs, snails, beetles, fruit	Tinned cat or dog food, day-old chicks, mice, dog biscuits
Fox	Rabbits, rodents, earthworms, edible rubbish, carrion, birds, berries, fruit	Tinned cat or dog food, dog biscuits, day-old chicks, mice RTA victims
Bats	Flying insects	Tinned cat food mashed, chopped mealworms and maggots
Mice	Fruit, nuts, grains, seeds	As wild diet
Squirrels	Nuts, buds, foliage, berries, roots, bulbs, sometimes nestlings and small birds	Rodent mix, apple, banana, digestive biscuits, peanuts
Deer	Shrubs, brambles, grass, fruit, flowers, berries	Hay, root vegetables, apples, foliage from broad-leaf trees, brambles, rose flowers and leaves, deer pellets or lamb nuts

Species:			Date:			Patient no:			
Date	Time	ID	ml taken	Urine	Faeces	Weight	Weight gain	Comments	Initials

Fig. 32.1 Suggested format for an orphaned mammal record card

It is essential that a feeding record is completed and a check kept on weight gain. Most orphaned mammals will lose weight to begin with as they adjust to the feeding routine. The production of urine and faeces should also be monitored in order to pick up on any problem quickly. The Comments column should record any concerns or observations that other carers need to know. It is better if just one person rears the orphan as both the orphan and the carer become used to each other and the orphan will find it difficult to settle with different carers.

The orphan must be stimulated to urinate and defecate before feeding and in the wild the mother would do this by licking around the genital area. The orphan must be warm and comfortable before settling down to a feed – full bladders do not help. Use a cotton wool bud moistened with warm water or Vaseline and gently tickle around the genital area. Urine will start to drip immediately but beware, as in some species it squirts out. Faeces will also be produced but not at every session. The area should be dried thoroughly and Vaseline applied to help prevent soreness and provide protection against moisture. If the orphan becomes sore it will be necessary to bathe and dry the area thoroughly and apply cream. Once toileting is complete the orphan should be weighed – it is important that the routine of toilet, weigh and feed is kept up.

When feeding, use a formula milk such as Esbilac or goat's milk. All neonatal mammals require colostrum for the first few days and goat's colostrum may be used as a substitute if it is available. Powdered formula milk should be mixed well to ensure that all the powder has dissolved. Esbilac also comes in a ready-made liquid form that avoids the inconsistencies of mixing. The milk should be offered warm – goat's milk or a liquid formula should be poured into a jug and left to stand in a dish of very hot water to heat up; powdered formulas are best made up with boiling water and left to cool. The milk should be kept warm throughout the feed by putting the bottle into and out of the hot water as required. Vitamin and mineral supplements should be added to the first feed of the day.

Syringes are ideal for feeding orphans: a measured amount is given a drop at a time and if administered correctly the feeder has total control of the flow of the milk. During feeding the position of the orphan should be such that it can 'paddle' with its forelimbs just as it would at the mother's nipple. Hold the orphan in a towel to keep it warm, then as the feed is slowly dispensed keep an eye on the speed the milk is going down the syringe, whether the orphan is swallowing and that there is no build-up of milk in the mouth. This sounds complicated but, once mastered, the delivery of milk will synchronize with the orphan's sucking and swallowing.

When feeding is completed, clean and dry the orphan's face before it is put back to bed. Any milk that is left over should be thrown away and the syringe both washed and sterilized or thrown away. All containers used for the milk should be washed and sterilized ready for the next feed. Hands must be washed before and after each feed and in between different litters or single orphans. The volume taken by each individual should be entered on the feeding record.

Successful hand feeding depends on the age and size of the orphan and the level of patience and dedication of the carer. It is not a job to be rushed – tiny mouths need careful feeding to avoid aspiration pneumonia and distress to the orphan. If an orphan becomes unwell or develops diarrhoea the milk feeds should be replaced by a rehydrating solution, e.g. Lectade, for 24 hours, then half rehydrating solution to half milk until the orphan recovers and is back on to its usual feed.

Always have a soft toy available as a substitute 'mum', particularly for single orphans to snuggle up.

Hedgehogs (*Erinaceus europaeus*)

Hedgehogs are the wild mammal most commonly brought into a centre and seasonal changes affect the reasons and the number of admissions (Table 32.2). Hedgehogs inhabit parks and gardens, farmland, waste ground and hedgerows, where they forage for earthworms, slugs and beetles. They

Table 32.2 Hazards to hedgehogs

Hazard	Symptoms	Notes
Gardens – strimmers, mowers, forks and spades, ponds	Severe cuts, impaled on fork prongs, drowning, exhaustion	Hedgehog can swim, but not for long
Litter – plastic can or bottle rings, jars/cans, glass	Neck wounds, plastic rings around the neck, suffocation, cuts	
Poisoning	Jumpy, sensitive to slightest of sounds, stretched out and reluctant to curl. Dark faeces	Could be metaldehyde (slug bait) or other garden pesticides
Bonfires	Burns, smoke inhalation	Spines will melt in intense heat and skin and spines will slough off in time
Entangled – fruit netting/football goal nets/ tennis nets	Cuts, ligatures, exhaustion, dehydration, starvation	Hedgehogs can push forward through netting but often get stuck and cannot withdraw because of the way the spines grow
Trapped – cattle grid/drain/footings	Exhaustion, dehydration, starvation, cut and sore feet from scrabbling to escape	

will also take small mammals and eggs. Their eyesight is poor and they use their sense of smell to detect prey.

Hedgehogs are solitary creatures, seeking out the company of others only for mating. Once mating has taken place the male plays no part in the rearing of the hoglets and does not stay with the female. One litter of three to five hoglets is produced each year, usually in June, but they can be born as early as May and late litters are often seen in September.

Hedgehogs are nocturnal, so activity during the day is unusual and may suggest ill health. This is not always the case, as nursing females may come out during this time to feed and hoglets born late in the year may be seen feeding during daylight hours in an attempt to build up the necessary fat reserves for hibernation.

The hedgehog has a unique defence mechanism in that it is able to roll into a spiky ball, which protects it from danger. It can remain in this position for hours.

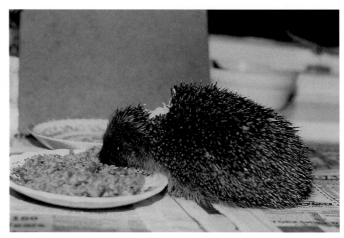

Fig. 32.2 The victim of a garden strimmer

Hibernation

Hedgehogs hibernate in winter to avoid the problem of lack of food; it is pointless to waste valuable energy endlessly searching for food in frozen ground. Instead, the hedgehog retreats to its hibernaculum (winter nest) and goes to sleep until conditions improve. People think that hedgehogs hibernate from autumn through the winter until the spring, but this is not so. Hedgehogs react to the environmental temperature and, when the temperature at ground level drops sufficiently for a prolonged period, the hedgehog goes into hibernation. In recent years this has been between January and March. The hedgehog shuts its system down almost to a standstill, the body temperature cools, breathing and heart rate slow. A hibernating hedgehog may only take a breath every 4 minutes, which enables it to conserve fat reserves. If a hedgehog is presented that is tightly curled but appears not to be breathing, it should be warmed up gently and slowly in absolute quiet. Hedgehogs may wake up during hibernation for short periods of activity, so if a hedgehog is spotted out and about in the middle of winter it is not necessarily in difficulty. Small hedgehogs may be presented in late autumn and early winter, the finder thinking

that they are too small to survive. This is due to the increasing public awareness about hibernation and the fact that a hedgehog needs to be a certain weight to survive the winter. Over-enthusiastic autumn garden tidying may result in injured hedgehogs through digging, bonfires and strimming (Fig. 32.2).

Late litters of hoglets do not always have the time to put on sufficient fat to carry them through the winter. An acceptable weight for a hoglet is 450 g (1 lb) and those that are lighter will have to be kept until they reach the acceptable weight, and then released. If temperatures are mild, hedgehogs can be released throughout the autumn and early winter period – there is little point in imprisoning a hedgehog in a cage for months on end. January is usually very cold and hedgehogs may have to be kept in during this time but as soon as the target weight is reached and the conditions in the wild are right, the hedgehog can be released.

Capture and transportation

Hedgehogs are the easiest of wildlife mammals to catch. On approach the hedgehog will either scuttle away or, more often, freeze and curl into a tight ball. Before picking up a hedgehog, some form of hand protection should be worn. Gardening gloves are ideal, or a towel folded to make several layers will protect from sharp spines. Pick the hedgehog up carefully but firmly, put it into an appropriate container and place it securely in the vehicle so that it does not move around during transportation.

Hedgehogs rarely bite as they are rolled into a ball but it should be assumed that they will. An injured animal may not curl up and if the hedgehog has just frozen it should roll up as soon as it is touched. A hedgehog may also exhibit aggression by thrusting its head upwards with its spines raised and making a huffing noise, which may be misdiagnosed as a respiratory problem.

Examination and handling

Hedgehogs are presented as casualties for a variety of reasons (Table 32.3) and should receive a full examination on arrival.

Before handling a hedgehog, put on a pair of thick gloves. Before removing the hedgehog from the container, observe it. If it is rolled into a ball this is a good sign as it is a naturally

defensive position; however, it makes examination difficult and access to the underside of the animal is impossible.

Before attempting to unroll the hedgehog, check if any of the limbs are poking out – one limb would suggest a fracture and two back limbs a spinal injury (Table 32.3). Pick up the hedgehog and look at the condition of its skin and spines; look for wounds, maggots, fly eggs and parasites (Table 32.4).

A healthy hedgehog has a rounded shape; a long hedgehog is a thin hedgehog. Infection is easily detected by smell, but its source may be hard to find unless the hedgehog is unrolled.

To unroll the hedgehog, gently jiggle it up and down with the head pointing downwards. This will make it feel insecure and it should naturally start to open up and put its feet down to locate a firm surface. Allow it to put its feet on to the examination table and hold it by its back legs so that the front feet are on the table and the back feet directly above. This will provide the opportunity to see the underside; however, touching the hedgehog, particularly on the head or face, will provoke it into curling up again. This method is not foolproof and some individuals will need to be anaesthetized.

Table 32.3 Reasons for admission of hedgehog casualties

Reason for admission	Injury/symptom	Notes
Road traffic accident	Concussion Cuts/bruises Fractures: limb/pelvis/jaw/spine	A curled hedgehog with both back legs sticking out indicates a spinal fracture
Extreme weather – prolonged hot spells	Heat exhaustion, dehydration, emaciation	Hot weather causes ground to dry out so no food or water
Extreme weather – prolonged cold spells	Hypothermia, thin and emaciated	These hedgehogs should be warmed up very slowly
Attacks	Wounds, fractures	Most commonly by dogs
Out during the day	Lethargic, half curled out in the open	Usually during not curling, staggering very hot or very cold weather or late juveniles
'Pop off' syndrome (orbicularis muscle prolapse)	The circular muscle used for curling slips up over the pelvis	Can be pulled back down under anaesthetic
'Balloon syndrome' (subcutaneous emphysema)	Build up of air under the skin, causing balloon effect	Where a wound has drawn in air under the skin during the action of curling and uncurling/or an injury to the respiratory system that leaks air
Orphan	Too young to leave the nest; no parent present	May have been taken from the nest by dog or cat

Table 32.4 Hedgehog parasites

Parasite	Symptoms	Treatment	Notes
Hedgehog flea (*Archaeopsylla erinacei*)	Easily visible between the spines	Use flea powder, (especially hoglets) or Frontline in well-ventilated situations	A very exposed habitat between spines means this flea is unique to hedgehogs
Tick (*Ixodes hexagonus*)	Easily visible, usually around ears and eyes in clusters, singly all over the body. Heavy infestations will include tiny 'pip-like' larval stages	Removal is best achieved with pointed metal tweezers	In heavy infestations on a stressed hedgehog removal by hand is unhelpful. Ivermectin is effective
Mites: Sarcoptes (*Sarcoptes scabiei*)	Spine and fur loss, crusty/flaky skin	Ivermectin, or an appropriate wash	Isolate the patient
Demodex	Crusty around follicles, small crusty lesions	Appropriate wash	Isolate the patient

Check the following:

- **Length of the claws** – hedgehogs dig and scratch around for their food, which keeps their claws trimmed. Long claws suggest a problem
- **Teeth** – check for missing and worn teeth. If present the hedgehog may be old or the poor condition of the mouth may be the reason for not feeding
- **Abscesses** – if present these are usually found around the face and neck and may discharge from the nose and eyes
- **Body temperature** – hedgehogs that are semi-curled and lying on one side are very sick and/or cold. The underside of the hedgehog should be felt to see if it is warm and the animal tested for dehydration. These individuals will respond once warmed up and given fluids
- **Faeces** – good indication of the health of the hedgehog. A normal stool is formed and brown; abnormal is anything from loose, green and mucoid to black and tar-like
- **Movement** – if a leg injury is suspected it can be difficult to assess how much the normal movement has been affected. The hedgehog will naturally curl or freeze, making movement observation very difficult. If the hedgehog is put into its accommodation it may make for a sheltered corner immediately, giving a very short opportunity for observation. After this it is more likely to freeze and not move for some time.

Once the examination is complete all observations should be recorded on the record card.

Housing

Taking into account the hedgehog's natural behaviour and habitat, a hospital cage similar in size to that used to house a cat is adequate and will provide enough room for bedding, food, water and an area in which to move around. The cage should be lined with layers of newspaper that are removed layer by layer as they become soiled. Bedding in the form of hand-shredded paper or a large towel should be placed in one of the far corners of the cage away from the door to enable the hedgehog to make a nest. Paper from a shredding machine is not suitable as it is too coarse and very thin. The hedgehog will naturally move to the back of the cage once placed inside and head for cover. As the hedgehog makes its nest it will turn around, combing the nesting material into shape. Thinly shredded paper may become tangled around the legs.

It may be necessary to cover the cage door with a towel, as the hedgehog may see this as a possible means of escape. Active hedgehogs may pace along the frontage and dig, bite and scratch at the door. This is the time to review the case: does the hedgehog need to be hospitalized further? If so, alternative housing needs to be considered, as this behaviour will lead to injury, distress and ultimately a longer stay in hospital. One that won't settle and continually 'paces' will need special provision. A few drops of lavender oil dropped into the cage will help to calm an agitated patient.

Heat – for cold hedgehogs or those unable to maintain their own body temperature, a heat or Snuggle Pad is ideal. A hedgehog that does not appear to be warm or cold would benefit from extra bedding rather than a heat pad. Use a small blanket or piece of Vetbed. Hedgehogs must be allowed to hide, so must be covered with their bedding if they are not able to burrow into it themselves.

Feeding

Hedgehogs are nocturnal and should be fed later in the day than diurnal species. Feed as close to dusk as you can unless a special feeding regime is being followed. The average hedgehog should be fed approximately one-third of a standard tin of cat or dog food per night. If the hedgehog eats all that it is offered and appears agitated, a little more should be given until an appropriate amount is reached. Similarly, if food is being left, then reduce the amount offered.

Most hedgehogs will eat any variety of cat or dog food that is offered but standard 'supermeat' is preferable and some, described as 'cuts in gravy', can lead to loose and sloppy faeces and messy cages. Varieties that are cereal-based are not favoured by any wildlife, particularly hedgehogs, and feeding this variety of food may lead to the false conclusion that there must be something wrong with the hedgehog because it is not eating.

If food is not eaten, check that the hedgehog is warm. Hedgehogs that are sick and on medication may have little or no appetite, so small tempting meals should be offered on an ad-lib basis. The food can be warmed up to increase the smell and warmed milk formula or goat's milk poured over the meaty food may also help. Strong-smelling varieties of food such as those containing tripe are popular and a chopped day-old chick mixed with the food can often do the trick. Those recovering from serious illness or hedgehogs that are very thin will need a 'little and often' regime and will benefit from warm formula or goat's milk mixed with the solid food to make it softer and easier to eat.

Fresh water should always be provided and placed in a corner of the cage to minimize the risk of spillage. Food is best offered on a saucer and the hedgehog will forage in and through the food and will push it over the sides, so the dish should be placed in the middle of the accommodation. Providing cat biscuits will break up the soft food and help to keep the teeth clean.

Pacers

These are hedgehogs that won't settle and are constantly 'on the go', pacing the cage frontage or the entire boundary. Release is the obvious answer but is not an option if they are not yet recovered. Extra feeding may help but care must be taken, as this will eventually cause the hedgehog to become overweight. Transferring to larger accommodation rarely works as it just means an increase in the area available to patrol, unless it is a run on grass, which works for a little while and then the hedgehog is back to pacing the boundary. In my experience a day-old chick will not only take the hedgehog's attention away from pacing, but will take a long time and a lot of effort to eat and even before it is finished the hedgehog may return to the nest and settle.

Orphaned hoglets

Before attempting to hand-rear orphaned hedgehogs, make sure they really are orphans. The female hedgehog will leave her young to find food and if a nest of hoglets is found it is assumed that they have been abandoned. If the hoglets seem content and sleeping, leave them alone and return to check them later. If they appear unsettled, cold or are emitting a high-pitched sound, indicating hunger, or the nest has clearly been destroyed then they will have to be picked up. A cardboard box full of warm material is adequate for transportation but if the hoglets are cold they will need a heat source, e.g. a Snuggle Pad.

On admission a general examination should also include:

- Weigh the hoglet
- Check the skin for general condition and wounds. Check for fly eggs and maggots; concentrate on folds of skin, behind the ears, in mouth, armpits and around the genital area. Clumps of fly eggs may also be found lodged between the spines and in the softer furry areas of the hedgehog. Removal of eggs is best achieved using pointed metal tweezers, or a nit or flea comb for those in the fur
- Check body temperature
- Test for dehydration
- Decide its age – this will determine the feeding regime (Table 32.5).

Once examination is complete the hoglets should be housed according to age and how warm they feel – older hoglets may just need warm bedding, very young ones will need a Snuggle Pad or heat lamp.

Feeding

This should be completed as follows (Table 32.5):

- Stimulate the hoglet to urinate and defecate
- Record results on the record sheet – the faeces of young hoglets on an all-milk diet are green and segmented. As the hoglet is weaned they change to a browner, more formed stool
- Weigh the hoglet
- Feed using goat's milk or Esbilac and a 1 ml syringe.

Hedgehogs would naturally take colostrum for up to 6 weeks in the wild, so provide it for the first month if possible.

Weaning

The weaning process can begin once the hoglets start to become active. The aim is gradually to reduce the milk feed and introduce solid food. Start with tinned puppy or kitten food. Cover the bottom of a flat dish with food, which should be mixed with goat's or formula milk until the meal is sloppy. Place the hoglets around the food dish and stand back! This is a messy business to start with as the hoglets will walk on to the plate and lick and bite at the food around them. If they show no interest in lapping at the mixture, then milk feeds should be continued for a couple for days and then the sloppy mixture can be offered again. Once the hoglets have finished feeding they may need a sponge down.

As the hoglets grow, gradually change the sloppy food to just kitten or puppy food with the milk poured over it and eventually to plain tinned cat or dog food. The hoglets should be weaned by around 6 weeks and rehabilitation can begin.

Mother hedgehogs and their babies

Occasionally a pregnant hedgehog is presented and this may only be discovered when newly born hoglets are discovered during cleaning out. This is most likely in May and June. Mothers and babies must be left alone to reduce the risk of cannibalism by the mother. Cleaning should not be done for a few days. Remove layers of soiled paper carefully and keep food and water topped up. Regular checks should be made to listen for sounds of distressed hoglets and also to make sure that they are in the nest and have not been left out in the cold. If there are any problems, the hoglets should be removed and hand-reared.

Nursing females should be given an increased amount of food and benefit from the addition of warmed goat's or formula milk.

Badgers (*Meles meles*)

Badgers live in social groups in a network of tunnels and chambers called a sett. They are nocturnal and if they are seen during the day there may be a problem. Badgers are increasingly found in urban areas and many casualties are due to road traffic accidents, but there are other reasons (Table 32.6). They are often involved in territorial fighting, where severe wounds are sustained (Fig. 32.3).

Badgers eat earthworms, insects, fruit, seeds, eggs, beetles and crane fly larvae; they will raid beehives for honey and take hedgehogs when there is competition for food.

The badger's sense of smell is very good, they have good hearing and their eyesight is adapted for night vision.

One litter of young is produced annually and the cubs are born early in the year, usually in January or February. The average litter size is two or three.

Table 32.5 Feeding regime for young hedgehogs

Age	Weight	Mount per feed	Description
Newborn	15–20 g	0.5–1 ml at 2-hourly intervals day and night	Blind, naked and deaf. Covering of white spines by 1 hour old. Not able to curl
1 week	30–50 g	2–3 ml at 2–3-hourly intervals from 6 am–12 midnight	Brown whiskers on the snout
2 weeks	50–80 g	3–4 ml at 4-hourly intervals from 7 am–11 pm	Eyes open, then ears. Now able to curl
3 weeks	80–130 g	4–7 ml at 4-hourly intervals from 7 am–11 pm	Teeth start to appear. Covering of brown hair
4 weeks	130–150 g	Start weaning	Teeth are through

Table 32.6 Reasons for the presentation of badgers as wildlife casualties

Reason	Injury/symptom	Notes
Road traffic accident (RTA)	Concussion, cuts and bruising, fractures to legs/pelvis/spine/jaw	
Prolonged hot and dry weather	Dehydration, emaciation, exhaustion	This weather affects the food and water supply
Territorial wounds	Wounds around the neck, ears and rump	Usually infected and often fly-blown
Out during the day	Out in the open, no attempt to move, lethargic, staggering	Could have fled from an RTA or be a victim of a territorial attack or extreme weather
Traps/snares	Injuries to limbs, neck or abdomen	Particularly from snares
Entangled – football goal nets, tennis nets	Cuts, ligatures, exhaustion, dehydration	
Orphan	Very young, out alone, no parent present	

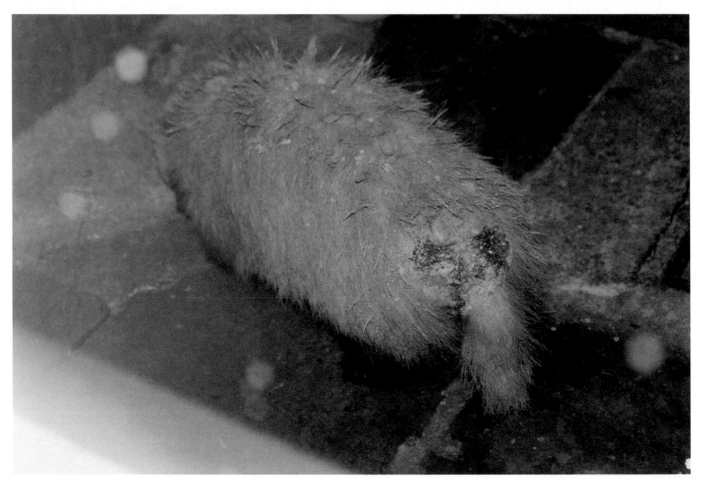

Fig. 32.3 Territorial bite wounds around the tail of a badger

Badgers do not hibernate but may stay underground during the coldest spells.

As with all other wildlife, badgers are likely to have parasites but in general these are few in number and are unlikely to be a problem unless the animal is in poor condition, sick or orphaned (Table 32.7).

Tuberculosis

A badger infected with tuberculosis (TB) will usually have no physical signs of the disease. As there is a risk of spread to other species, including humans, the utmost care should be taken with all badger casualties and orphans. Plastic gloves should be worn at all times and isolation or barrier nursing for all admitted badgers should be continued right through to release. Cubs should not be introduced to each other until they have been tested for TB. All adult casualties, once recovered, should be returned to where they were found but testing is not necessary, as the badger is taken, treated and released back into the same area, so the situation in that area has not been altered.

Table 32.7 Badger parasites

Parasite	Treatment	Notes
Badger flea (*Paracercas melis*)	Flea powder, especially in cubs. Fipronil	Treat only if infested
Badger louse (*Trichodectes melis*)	As for fleas	
Ticks	Remove with pointed metal tweezers	

Capture and transportation

Badgers are very strong animals, particularly their jaws, and they should be treated with respect. They are also sensible creatures, avoiding confrontation unless provoked. A little knowledge of natural behaviour will help to predict how a badger might react in a given situation.

Rescue in the wild can be difficult – if your casualty has a head injury, retrieval will be easy; if it has a back or rear end injury it will require more thought. Prepare the carrying basket in advance – a crush-type cage lined with a blanket is ideal. The reactions of a badger with a head injury should be tested by offering a biting stick or similar object at arm's length. If there is no reaction then push the head down with a glove on the non-leading hand and grasp the scruff with the non-gloved hand. Once the badger is restrained it should be lifted into the basket with the gloved hand supporting the bottom. Remove your hand as quickly as possible while closing the lid tightly. Secure the basket and cover it with a blanket to place the casualty in the dark. Alternatively, the badger could be wrapped in a blanket and then placed in the carrier.

Badgers that have a rear-end injury will be active at the biting end and the same procedure to test the reactions should be followed – the aim of the biting stick is that the badger will bite on it rather than the rescuer. Care must be taken, as the badger is able to shrug its shoulders and the scruff 'disappears', leaving the rescuer nothing to grasp. If the badger is able to move then the carrier (end and top opening are best) should be placed on the ground and covered apart from the entrance hole. Badgers will naturally go for a dark hidey-hole and in most cases with a little encouragement they can be lured into the basket.

It may be necessary to use a grasper but avoid them if you can. Time and care must be taken to catch the badger around one leg as well as the neck, otherwise three hands are needed: one to hold the grasper, one to grasp the scruff and one to support the bottom! Only when severely injured animals were unreachable, e.g. in brambles or dense cover at the bottom of a ditch or a pit, have I used a grasper.

Examination and handling

Examination is straightforward if the badger is concussed. A crush cage can be used to sedate it but the blanket must be removed. A muzzle may also be used. Do not to rely on the scruff as a means of restraint, as it requires a firm grip that cannot be sustained for a thorough examination. Cover the badger's head for as much of the examination as possible, as it will help to calm it.

Examine the badger, paying particular attention to the teeth. An old badger that is thin with long claws indicating that it does little digging for food, with worn and missing teeth, all mean that it is near to the end of its life and cannot be released back to the wild. Check the neck and rump for bite wounds, often sustained as a result of a territorial dispute with another badger. They are usually infected and often fly-blown (Fig. 32.3).

Housing

Suitable accommodation in a veterinary practice is similar to that used for a medium-sized dog. It should be located in the quietest area and the frontage should be covered to reduce the light – badgers are nocturnal and excessive light is distressing to them. Line the cage with a thick layer of newspaper and place bedding, e.g. hand-shredded newspaper, hay or blankets, at the back in one corner. There should be sufficient for the badger to bury itself in. Badgers will sleep all day and wake in the early evening. They can be destructive in a captive situation and 'trashed' accommodation is to be expected. By morning all the lining paper and bedding will be in a heap in one corner with the badger fast asleep underneath it.

A noisy practice is not a good place for a badger to spend any length of time and it should be transferred to more appropriate facilities as soon as possible.

Heat – the best heat source for a badger is a heat lamp unless the accommodation itself is heated. Heat pads with wires will be chewed and the microwavable Snuggle Pads will not last long against the claws or teeth of a badger.

Feeding

Use strong metal food bowls – ceramic food bowls are heavy and may be used but I have had many tossed into the air and broken by the patient and plastic will be destroyed. Put a water bowl in the corner of the cage – it will be tipped over eventually but will last longer in a corner.

As badgers are nocturnal they should be fed late in the day unless they are on a special feeding regime. They will eat most varieties of cat or dog food, but avoid those in gravy as this affects the faeces – 'supermeat' is best. Dog mixer biscuit can be added and the badger will also eat day-old chicks and mice. During eating the food will be 'dug out' of the food bowl, although this is rarely seen except in cubs, as the secretive nature of the badger does not allow for an audience.

On the first night and even for a few days the badger may refuse to eat and will simply curl up and go to sleep. Unless the badger is emaciated or dehydrated, it should not be force-fed food or fluids. There are ways to persuade a badger to eat and, as they have a sweet tooth, peanut butter or jam sandwiches or peanuts (the kind put out for birds) can be put on top of the offered meal.

Getting the patient to eat may become a vicious circle – the badger will not eat until it is released and it should not be released it until it has had a good meal. In the early days of wildlife rescue, I had a badger that had been in a road accident. He stayed a week, but did not eat. I even stuck a crust of bread with peanut butter on to the end of his nose to try and tempt him. I had made the decision to release him the next night and by morning he had eaten all the peanut butter crusts. Badgers are extremely stubborn!

For recovering sick adult badgers, Complan is a good first food – strawberry-flavoured in particular. It may be fed by 60 ml syringe while the badger is debilitated and then offered in a bowl. As the badger gains strength, small meals alongside the Complan should be provided until the badger is on a normal adult diet.

Cleaning

A hospitalized badger must be thoroughly cleaned out every day. Make up one corner of the hospital cage with a deep bed and, wearing gloves, slowly remove the bedding the badger is hiding under. The badger realizes he is being exposed, sees a pile of bedding he can hide in and scuttles across to it, allowing the corner he has just left to be cleaned. Always keep an eye on the pile of the bedding in case the badger decides to come out. There is no other casualty that I can think of that will do this or behave in this way.

An alternative way is to remove the badger to a ready made-up cage but that involves unnecessary confrontation and stress to both the patient and the nurse. If the badger is spending the night in a crush cage that becomes soiled and has to be cleaned, a clean crush cage should be prepared. Place the cages end to end (they must be end-openers). Remove the cover from over the cage that the badger is in and put it over the clean one. This will expose the badger and it will move into the dark space of the clean crush cage.

Orphaned badger cubs

A badger cub out on its own in the day indicates a problem. Most cubs start to appear above ground at about 2 months old and until this time they are in the sett. Younger cubs may have come above ground if their mother has not returned. Once a cub this young is found in difficulty, the area should be searched for others and for an injured adult. Sometimes tiny cubs are found as a result of a collapsed sett or one that has been dug out by humans (Fig. 32.4).

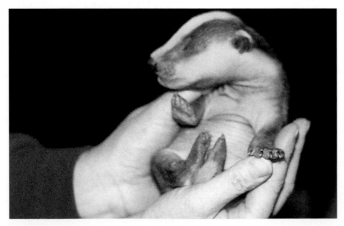

Fig. 32.4 A badger cub

Handling and transportation

Even cute and cuddly looking cubs can fight and they should be approached with care. The cub may snarl and jump and the fur will stand on end, giving the appearance of a much bigger cub (or so it thinks). Wear thick gloves and use a blanket for capturing cubs with attitude. A sickly cub must be warmed up and a Snuggle Pad is ideal for this.

Examination

Make a thorough examination, including:

- Check the skin for parasites (Table 32.7). Badger cubs often have fleas and lice and flea powder can be used on arrival. Ticks may also be found and may be removed with pointed metal tweezers
- Check the body temperature
- Check for dehydration – may need an oral rehydrating fluid
- Weigh the cub
- Assess the age.

Housing

A secure hospital cage or wire basket may be used and it should be realized that even an 8-week-old badger is very strong. The cub should be housed in a quiet area and provided with a soft toy as a substitute 'mum'. A Snuggle Pad or heat pad may be required for very young or sick cubs; older ones may just need warm bedding, but this should be monitored. As badgers take longer to wean than other mammals larger accommodation will be required for an older cub that is still being bottle-fed.

Feeding

The cub must be stimulated to urinate and defecate before being fed. The faeces of badger cubs are yellow and rather like scrambled egg, but change to browner more solid stools as the cub is weaned. The cub should then be weighed and all the information should be recorded. The amount of food and the feeding times will vary from cub to cub – exact guides do not exist and common sense is essential (Table 32.8).

Feed the cub with a kitten or puppy bottle for very young cubs and a human baby bottle for older ones. Bottle-feeding badger cubs can be difficult. Initially the cub will not suck at the bottle but will hunch its shoulders as it grips the teat with its teeth or clamps its mouth shut, and then it will maintain this position. The only way to succeed is by patience and it can take time. Shading the cub's eyes may help – remember, these cubs do not come above ground until at least 8 weeks old, so their world is a dark one. I have often reverted to a syringe and carefully dripped the milk feed in this way and tried the bottle again next feed. Once the badger has taken to the bottle, feeding is much easier until they are finally weaned around 3 months old at the earliest.

Weaning starts with soft food, e.g. tinned puppy food mixed with the milk, scrambled egg, Weetabix or a human baby cereal. Badgers are slow to wean and at first the cub may not be ready for solid food and it should be offered again in a couple of days. Once the cub is eating by itself, more foods can be added and the diet becomes a more solid one; however, the cub will still require its bottle until around the age of 3 months.

Table 32.8 Feeding young badgers

Age	Feed guide	Notes
Birth	Approx. 5 ml every 2–3 h	Blind, deaf and covered in fine white fur. A dark stripe on the head is visible. Weigh approximately 120 g
2–4 weeks	Increase the amount as appropriate. Give 3-hourly feeds from 6 am to midnight	Careful monitoring is essential as the cubs vary so much
5 weeks	Increase the amount as appropriate. Give 4-hourly feeds from 6 am–midnight	Eyes open and first teeth erupt
8–10 weeks	Offer first sloppy food, e.g. puppy food and milk, scrambled egg, Weetabix or baby cereal around 9–10 weeks. Continue milk feeds	Can be seen outside the sett in the wild
10–12 weeks	Reduce milk feeds, add chopped day-old chicks to solid food meals and leave in dish of milk	
12–14 weeks	Gradually reduce milk feeds to twice daily – morning and night	
15 weeks	Weaning complete	Have most of adult teeth

Table 32.9 Reasons for the admission of foxes as wildlife casualties

Reason for admission	Injury/symptom	Notes
Road traffic accident (RTA)	Concussion, cuts and bruising, fractures: leg/spine/jaw/pelvis	Fewer fox RTAs than other mammals
Sarcoptic mange	Bald patches around rump and tail initially, crusty skin, sores	
Trap/snare	Injuries to limbs, particularly feet	Mouth should be checked as the fox will gnaw at the snare to free itself; may even chew off a limb
Fences	General leg damage caused by hanging by one leg and constant struggling. Sometimes irreparable. Exhaustion	Happens when fox tries to clear a fence and doesn't quite manage it, often hanging and struggling for some time
Leptospirosis	Jaundice	Euthanasia
Distemper	Dribbling, sickness, diarrhoea	Euthanasia
Orphan	Alone, distressed, calling	

Tuberculosis and badger cubs

Each badger cub should be tested for TB three times during its rearing and rehabilitation. Only a cub with three negative tests can be released back into the wild. Badgers are social animals and should not be reared singly; however, cubs from different litters should not be housed together until they have been tested for TB with negative results. If cubs are housed together before all three negative results are obtained and then one tests positive, the lives of the whole group are in question. The first test should be carried out as soon after admission as possible, another during the middle part of their care and the last test as near to release date as possible.

Foxes (*Vulpes vulpes*)

There are two types of fox living alongside us these days, the country fox and the urban fox, and although they are the same species they are very different:

- The country fox eats a more natural diet consisting of small mammals, worms, beetles, fruit and rabbits

- The urban fox results from humans' development of land, trapping wildlife in small areas of 'green' and forcing them to adapt to a new way of life. Many are presented as road traffic casualties and victims of sarcoptic mange (Table 32.9). The urban fox may forage in rubbish bins, pick up food dropped from bird tables and eat discarded take-away food, as well as small mammals and birds, fruit and insects.

The fox's eye is adapted to low light levels and its sight is not very good. The fox relies on sound and touch, in the form of sensitive hairs on its face and front limbs, to locate and catch its prey. Although foxes are mainly active at night, it is not unusual to see them out during the day, particularly in quiet areas in the warm sunshine. Cubs are born annually in March and litter size is four to five cubs.

Sarcoptic mange

The most severe problem is that of sarcoptic mange, caused by the mite *Sarcoptes scabiei* (see also Ch. 27). The mite burrows into the skin and multiplies rapidly, resulting in loss of most of the fur, which takes about 4 months. The fox loses weight and many die. The lesions ooze fluid, which dries to form a crust that is full of mites. Mange is intensely irritant and the fox will scratch and gnaw at itself, often chewing a limb or its tail off. As the fox moves around and curls up with other foxes, bits of crust fall off and other foxes become infected. Caught early enough, the condition can be treated; untreated the fox will die. Sarcoptic mange is a zoonosis, so care must be taken when dealing with infected patients.

Foxes are also home to the fleas and ticks that live on other animals. Adult foxes do not usually have many internal parasites at all but in young cubs roundworms can be a problem and can be treated with fenbendazole.

Capture and transportation

The carrying basket should be prepared in advance: a crush cage with top and end openings is ideal. A fox with a head injury can be lifted as described for badgers. Make sure that you use a biting stick to test the animal's reactions and wear gloves to handle it. When the fox is injured but mobile there is no point in chasing it for miles. The person who contacted you may be able to monitor and feed the fox and so lure it into an area or shed where it is more easily caught or where a humane trap can be set.

In situations where the fox is trapped, or in dense undergrowth, or is not able to be confined in any other way, then a grasper will have to be used. It is beneficial to the casualty to loop a front leg as well as its neck through the noose and it must never be swung around on the end of a grasper by its neck.

Once secured, grasp the scruff, support the rump and put it into the basket in the usual way. Cover immediately. Foxes are very snappy and will bite and leap around to escape and they will not be lured into a carrier resembling a dark, safe, hole as a badger will.

Examination

When examining a fox it may need to be sedated, which can be achieved with the aid of a crush cage. If the fox is concussed the examination can be carried out easily but it must be remembered that it may come round quickly so a muzzle should be used. Covering the fox's head will help to keep it calm.

Housing

Foxes do not make good captive patients and they may suffer high levels of stress, throwing themselves around and constantly scratching and biting at the wire in an attempt to escape. A kennel with a secure door and a blanket covering the front is the best short-term option, but as soon as possible the fox should be transferred to somewhere with more appropriate facilities.

The fox should be given adequate bedding to enable it to hide, e.g. hay, which should be placed in one of the back corners of the cage. This will help to calm the fox – an empty pen will only fuel its anxiety and increase the manic search for a way out. A large cardboard box facing away from the door provides a good place to hide. The fox will be more active at night and the cage will have been reorganized by the morning. Plastic dog beds are not a good idea as they will be eaten.

Heat – the only practical heat source is a heat lamp, unless it is in heated accommodation. Any heat pad with a wire would be destroyed once the fox had warmed up and become more active.

Feeding

Stainless steel food bowls are best as ceramic ones may be broken and plastic ones will be chewed beyond use. Place the water bowl in a corner to help prevent it from being tipped over. Patients should have access to water at all times and, unless on a special feeding regime, food is given at the end of the day.

Foxes eat a variety of foods, e.g. tinned cat and dog food, day-old chicks, mice, rabbit and dog mixer biscuit. The fox will not eat while being watched. Warming the food and pouring goat's or formula milk over it may persuade those foxes that are reluctant to eat initially. A sick fox that is recovering should be offered food ad lib – small portions to start with, increasing the amount as appropriate and eventually reducing the amount of feeds to one meal in the evening.

Cleaning

The fox should be removed from the cage when it is being cleaned and ideally it should be moved to a ready-prepared cage to avoid over-handling, which causes stress. Unlike a badger, a fox will not tolerate its cage being cleaned around it and it will throw itself around in an attempt to escape. If a spare cage is not available then the fox should be put into a secure basket and covered while cleaning is carried out.

Orphaned fox cubs

The decision to pick up suspected orphaned fox cubs is not easy and it must be taken carefully. A search around the area may lead to facts that will help with your decision. Consider the following:

- If a group of fox cubs are seen without an adult the situation should be monitored
- A group of cubs that appear contented, asleep or playing together should be left alone and checked later
- If more than one cub is present or there is a group, but they are calling or appear to be in distress, then something may well have happened to the mother and they will need to be rescued
- If the cubs are dispersed over the area rather than together, are cold, lethargic or wet, in a flooded drain or if there are signs of a disturbance, then they should be picked up
- If a lone cub is found, out in the open, calling or appears to be distressed, it should be picked up
- If a cub is found that still has its eyes closed, then it is under 2 weeks old and at that age is not able to thermoregulate and will soon become cold and eventually die, so should be rescued.

Capture and transportation

Once the orphan or orphans have been rescued they must be approached and handled carefully. Cubs with their eyes

Table 32.10 Feeding orphaned fox cubs

Age	Feed	Guide notes
Birth (weighs approx. 100 g)	Approx. 5 ml every 2–3 h	Blind, deaf, brown fur, tail has white tip
1 week (weighs approx. 240 g)	Approx. 10 ml every 3 h	
2 weeks (weighs approx. 320 g)	15–20 ml every 3–4 h from 7 am until 11 pm	Eyes open, blue at first. Ears open, unsteady on feet
3–4 weeks	30–40 ml every 4 h Offer first solid food and start to reduce the number of milk feeds	Heat can be reduced. Weighing is more important now weaning has started
5 weeks	Dish of milk should be provided. In addition to solid food, offer day-old chicks	Eyes start to change to brown, nose and ears now more pointed
6 weeks	Weaning complete	Cubs in outside enclosure

closed will offer little resistance but an older cub will be defensive and will spit and bite. Thick gloves will help but if none are available a jumper, coat or car rug will do just as well. Holding the cub by its scruff with a hand supporting its bottom is an acceptable method of picking up a 'spitty' cub. When the mother moves them from place to place she carries them in her mouth by the scruff and in this position the cub will hang still and not struggle.

Examination

A thorough examination should be carried out, including:

- Checking through the fur and skin for wounds
- Checking for parasites – often fox cubs have ticks
- Checking body temperature – they may need supplementary heat
- Test for dehydration
- Weigh the cub
- Assess the age
- If there is more than one cub, invent a means of identifying each one.

Housing

The cub or cubs should be housed according to age and condition. A hospital cage or large wire basket will provide suitable accommodation but must be covered to provide a dark environment and should be situated in a quiet area. The very young or those that are sick will need supplementary heating. Those who are cold or wet will need gentle heat initially and then warm bedding. Older cubs will need only warm bedding. Single cubs should be provided with a soft toy as a substitute 'mum'. As the cubs grow they can be moved to larger accommodation and eventually to an outside run with a box to hide in.

Feeding

The cubs must be stimulated to urinate and defecate before being fed. Faeces of young cubs are orangey yellow and will turn brown as they are weaned on to solid food. Once toileting is complete each cub should be weighed and all the information recorded.

Feeding of very young cubs can be achieved with a 1 ml syringe or a puppy feeding bottle. Amounts fed will vary from cub to cub and there are no exact guides (Table 32.10).

Goat's milk or formula should be used with added colostrum for the first few days for very young cubs. I start feeding with a syringe and move on to a bottle when the cub settles into hand feeding and starts to suck at the syringe – if the bottle is introduced at this time the cubs take to it well. As the cub grows, and for older cubs, i.e. from about 2 weeks, a human baby bottle can be used. Fox cubs need to be 'burped', just as is done with human babies, as they are enthusiastic feeders and can take in air. The cub's back is rubbed and gently patted until the desired burp is achieved.

When the cub becomes more active, start weaning with a little mashed tinned puppy food mixed with the milk. If the cub shows no interest in the food, carry on with the hand feeding and try again a day or two later. Once the cub is taking the sloppy food well, hand feeding can be gradually reduced. Offer chopped puppy food with the milk poured over it and add day-old chicks. Eventually the milk is offered in a bowl and dishes of puppy food are placed in the cage. Weaning should be completed by 5–6 weeks, by which time the cub will be on a diet of tinned cat or dog food, day-old chicks, mice, rabbit and water. Cubs are released back into the wild after a period of rehabilitation at a wildlife centre.

Rabbits (*Oryctolagus cuniculus*) and hares (*Lepus capensis*)

Rabbits and hares are similar in many ways but there are differences that should be taken into consideration when veterinary care is needed (Table 32.11):

- **Rabbits** – live in large colonies based in a series of linked underground burrows called a warren. Their day is spent underground and they are most active outside the warren at dusk. Young are altricial, i.e. they are hairless and blind and are totally dependent on the mother until they are weaned
- **Hares** – live in scraped out hollows in the ground called forms in open countryside or woodland. They

Table 32.11 Reasons for the admission of rabbits and hares as wildlife casualties

Reason	Injury/symptom	Notes
Road traffic accident	Concussion, cuts, bruising. Fractures, usually back legs, pelvis, spine	Mostly rabbits
Victim of domestic cats	Paralysis, wounds	Mostly rabbits
Myxomatosis	Swelling on the eyes, nose, base of ears and genital area	Die within 2 weeks of catching the virus. Rabbits only. Euthanasia
Snares	Injury to neck, abdomen, sometimes limbs	Mostly rabbits
Orphan	See Orphans below	Rabbits and hares

are nocturnal but can be seen at dawn and dusk. Young are precocial, i.e. they are capable of an independent life almost from birth. Hares are becoming increasingly rare because of modern methods of farming.

Myxomatosis

Myxomatosis is a viral disease that was introduced in the 1950s to wipe out the rabbit population; it does not seem to affect hares. The rabbit flea *Spilopsyllus cuniculi* carries the virus on its blood-sucking mouthparts and passes it from one rabbit to another. A few days after becoming infected the rabbit's eyes begin to discharge a watery substance, the eyelids swell, and swellings appear on the nose, at the base of the ears and around the genital area. These swellings fill with pus and at this stage the rabbit can neither see nor hear and is often seen sitting at the roadside oblivious to its surroundings. Within approximately 2 weeks of catching the virus the rabbit dies.

Capture and transportation

Capture of most rabbit and hare casualties is easy as they are mainly road traffic casualties with severe injuries, have myxomatosis, which debilitates the rabbit, or are cat victims – a rabbit is often brought into the house by the cat. Never grasp the animal by its ears alone. Throw a towel or similar material over it and wrap it up to prevent the rescuer from being scratched. If a box is not available, the animal may be transported by being either held or put in the boot of a car. Rabbits and hares do not generally make any noise but a distressed animal may scream to deter a predator.

Examination

If the rabbit or hare is concussed the examination can be carried out easily; however, if the injury is to the rear of the animal then it is quite a different story. Hares are powerful animals and both rabbits and hares will kick out with all four limbs and must be restrained by two pairs of hands. Cover the casualty's head for as much of the examination as possible:

- In almost all rear-end injuries an X-ray is most helpful in determining the exact problem
- Where the injuries are cat-inflicted, symptoms may be due to temporary nerve damage and after a few days function may return to the limbs
- Those cat victims that sustain wounds should be treated and released as soon as possible as prolonged

captivity causes fatal stress. Antibiotics should be administered quickly to combat infection
- Testing for pain reflex is difficult in wildlife as, in the wild, to react to pain by either noise or movement may alert a predator
- Concussed patients usually recover quickly and within 24–48 hours may be released.

Housing

Rabbits and hares do not make good patients and should be housed in quiet, dark accommodation with plenty of bedding, e.g. hay, in which to hide.

Heat – should only be provided in severe cases, as rabbits in particular may suffer if kept too warm.

Feeding

Natural food should be provided where possible, e.g. dandelions, clover, grass and dock leaves. Commercial dried rabbit mix can also be offered. Food should be left in the cage at all times and the casualty left alone to eat. Always provide a source of fresh water.

Cleaning

As rabbits and hares are very nervous it is better to have a clean, prepared cage ready for transfer. Any further examination, treatment and replacing of food should be done at the same time.

Orphans

Rabbits

Rabbits are born underground and are blind, deaf and without fur, so if very young ones are seen above ground there is a problem. Mechanical diggers and dogs often dig up baby rabbits and the nests are destroyed. Rabbits are weaned at a young age and are often picked up as tiny bunnies, when really they are independent and able to care for themselves. The mother can be pregnant again 12 hours after she gives birth and so the young rabbit kittens are weaned before the next litter is born.

Hares

Baby hares or leverets are completely different and are born fully furred with their eyes and ears open. They sit motionless in their forms above ground and are often mistakenly picked up as orphans. The mother leaves them all day, returning only once in 24 hours to feed them. Unless they appear weak or injured or are wet and cold, they should be left alone.

Capture and transportation

These orphans are easily picked up and present no danger to the handler. They will need warm bedding during transportation, particularly if they are very young rabbits, but they must be completely covered so that they are in the dark, which will simulate the burrow for rabbits and provide security for leverets.

The initial examination should include:

- Check for wounds – in patients that have been picked up by dogs or cats
- Check the body temperature
- Check for dehydration
- Weigh the orphan
- Assess the age
- If there is more than one, invent a means of identifying the individuals.

As very few orphaned leverets are presented it is difficult to use past experience to age them; rabbit kittens grow very fast so there is little information on their age (Table 32.12). The advice on accommodation and feeding should be suitable for successful rearing of both rabbits and hares.

Housing

Line a cage with newspaper and a towel. Make a bed of hay with a towel over the top. The other end will be used for feeding. Cover the cage to ensure that it is dark and represents the burrow. For hares the dark will help to keep them calm and their bed can be made up of hay without the towel – they will sit in a hollow in the hay, which represents the form. As the young animals become more active, a grass run will provide more suitable accommodation, but provide a box in which to hide.

Feeding

Both rabbit and hare mothers leave their young for long periods of time in either the burrow or the form and will only return once a day, maybe twice for rabbits, allowing them to feed for a few minutes before leaving them again. As the youngsters grow, the mother will return for shorter periods of time until they are weaned. This makes a feeding regime difficult to formulate; however, one feed at each end of the day, dawn and dusk, seems to work.

Before feeding it is a good idea to try to stimulate the babies to urinate and defecate but, as the wild mums return very little to see to their youngsters, it could be that they do not need to be stimulated as often as other orphaned mammals or that they are able to defecate and urinate unaided. For this reason toileting should not be overdone: if urine is produced immediately then stimulation should be carried on until the youngster is finished but if nothing appears there is no reason to keep trying. Urine from stimulated rabbits tends to spurt out rather than dripping like that of other orphans.

Feed goat's milk using a 1 ml syringe and a lot of patience, particularly for rabbits; leverets are not quite as sensitive as baby rabbits. Orphans should be fed as much as they will take and should not be pushed to take more – rabbits in particular become very stressed. The first few feeds will be the most difficult and rabbits should be expected to lose weight over the first few days but once their feeding behaviour settles down they will gain slowly gain weight. Once their eyes open, offer a little oat and apple baby cereal mixed with the milk and a few days later solids can be introduced (Table 32.12).

During weaning, a piece of turf with the soil attached should be placed in the accommodation, allowing for nibbling and climbing over. Grated apple and carrot make good first foods, as do natural greens. Green food should always be fresh. A shallow container of goat's milk and one of water should be placed into the cage, but not in the corners as is done with other mammals as this is often where the orphans will practise their digging.

Once the orphans are feeding well on the solids, a little dried rabbit mix can be offered and release can be planned. Little rehabilitation is needed for young rabbits and hares as they are so 'stroppy' during the hand-rearing process that they never become tame, unless they have been over-handled. Anyone who successfully hand-rears rabbits is to be congratulated. In my experience they are the most difficult orphans to rear and require endless patience.

Young rabbits that are presented with their eyes open should be given the opportunity to go directly on to the first stage of weaning, making sure that goat's milk is available in a shallow container. Monitor them closely as some goat's

---

Table 32.12 Feeding wild rabbits

Age	Feed guide	Notes
Birth (approx. weight 30 g)	Goat's milk – whatever they will take – given at dawn and dusk	Blind, deaf, naked
1 week–10 days	Goat's milk – whatever they will take – given at dawn and dusk	Eyes open around 10 days, covering of velvety fur
2 weeks	Goat's milk – whatever they will take – given at dawn and dusk	Now mobile, grooming and digging
	Add grated apple and carrot, natural greens, shallow container of goat's milk	
	Oat and apple baby cereal to supplement milk feeds	
3 weeks	Should be nibbling on solid food; wean off the milk feed at dusk	
4 weeks	Should be weaned off all milk feeds. Eating solid food, offer dried rabbit mix	

Table 32.13 Reasons for the admission of bats as wildlife casualties

Reason for admission	Injury/symptom	Notes
Cat victims	Wounds/ fractures/holes and tears in the wings	Usually found on the ground, if not deposited at your feet!
Entangled, e.g. fruit netting	Cuts/fractures/torn wings	Wounds caused by the struggle to escape
Fly paper	Sticky!	Use washing up liquid to remove
Out in the day	Hanging on wall or fence in broad daylight	Usually no injuries but benefit from fluids, food and rest for 24–48 hours before release
Orphan	Small and immature, brought in by cat or found on the ground	Sometimes fall from roosts
Grounded	On the ground	As a result of trauma or attack. Benefit from fluids, food and rest for 24–48 hours before release

milk feeds by syringe may be needed initially – the older the orphan the more difficult the rearing process.

Bats

Bats are the only flying mammals in the UK. There are 14 species, and some are rarer than others. The species most commonly presented is the tiny pipistrelle bat *Pipistrellus pipistrellus*. Bats are nocturnal and hunt at night for insects using echolocation. They are also one of the few British mammals that hibernate. Bats live in a variety of places, referred to as roosts, including the roofs of houses, and the eaves and walls, in barns, stables and churches, under bridges and caves.

Many people fear bats for various reasons, many of which are old wives' tales, but they pose no threat and should be encouraged as they eat many undesirable insects. They are presented for a variety of reasons (Table 32.13), the most common of which is as victims of cats.

Capture and transportation

Capture of an injured bat is simple as it is likely to be on the ground and therefore merely requires picking up. Bats that are flying around a room, e.g. having been released by the cat, should be allowed to find their own way out. Bats that are flying do not need to be rescued and detained but rescued and released. If all the lights are turned off, all windows and outside doors to the room are opened and the room is left quiet the bat is given the opportunity to make its way out. Chasing it around the room with a net and swatting at it will increase its panic and the chance of injury.

Should the bat be discovered at night it should be picked up using gloves or a small towel and taken outside, hung as high as possible and left to fly when it is ready. If it is found during the day then it should be housed in a small box (shoe boxes are ideal for bats), lined with kitchen roll and a face flannel or similar material to enable it to hide. Push a pencil or wooden kebab skewer through one side of the box and out through the other to provide a high hanging place. The box should have small air holes and be taped shut, as bats will easily crawl out of an unsecured shoebox or the smallest of holes. A bat on the ground may be encouraged to crawl into the box.

Examination

First observe the bat in the box – is it active, is there blood on the bedding and is there anything specific that needs closer examination? Wearing latex or thicker gloves the bat should be picked up and supported with the thumb on its back and fingers under its abdomen gently but firmly. The wings should be extended to check for injuries, holes and fractures, one at a time. A bat should never be held by its wings. Check for dehydration, starvation and general bodily condition and record all results.

Housing

A shoebox as described above is sufficient for short-term housing but longer stays need more cleanable accommodation. A plastic tank with a ventilated top is ideal, with a supple twig bent into position to serve as a hanging post. The tank should be lined with kitchen roll and some sort of gauze suspended from under the lid to enable the bat to climb and hide. Cover the plastic tank to provide a dark environment. After treatment, recovery should be completed at a rescue centre with a suitable flight aviary.

Heat – bats are heterotherms, i.e. they are able to control their body temperature, regulating it to a fixed level or altering it to the ambient temperature. In times of cold weather, rather like the hedgehog, the bat will drop its temperature and enter a torpid state. This saves energy in times when food is difficult to find. When a cold or inactive bat is presented, it should be gently warmed up. A heat lamp suspended over one end of the accommodation is preferable.

Feeding

Bats eat flying insects, which they catch using echolocation. In captivity insects or moths may be offered; however, other foods will be taken that are easier to obtain. For example:

- Mealworms fed on bran and then the heads cut off, allowing the bat to suck out the soft insides.
- Maggots cut in half
- Mashed cat food mixed with insectivorous food and a little water
- Vitamin and mineral supplements should be added.

A drink should be provided before food and once the bat is warm and fully hydrated it will become more active. Supply water using a piece of clean cloth or kitchen paper. Soak it in water and squeeze it out so that it is soggy, then place it on to a jam jar lid or similar flat container. This will enable the bat to lick or suck at the cloth and avoids the risk of it drowning. Food should be offered in a shallow container, e.g. a jam jar lid.

Orphaned bats

Tiny bats sometimes fall from their roosts and where it is not possible to return them, they have to be hand reared. Many young bats that are presented are victims of cats and their original roost is unknown.

Examination

On admission a full examination should be carried out:

- Check for general condition and wounds – if the bat is thin the stomach will look indented
- Check for dehydration
- Check body temperature
- Weigh the bat
- Identify the bat if possible (information available from the Bat Conservation Trust 0171 240 0933).

Record details of the exact location in which the bat was found so that it can be released in the same place.

Housing

Orphan bats should be accommodated in the same way as adults.

Feeding

It is essential that the orphaned bat is kept warm and that the milk feed is also warm and kept at a constant temperature during feeding. This prevents fermentation of the milk inside the bat, causing problems. Use Esbilac milk formula, mixed thoroughly to dissolve it completely, and offer it on a child's paintbrush, which allows the bat to suck or lap the milk in tiny quantities. Syringes are not appropriate for these orphans as too much milk is delivered even with the smallest

drop. Care must be taken to make sure the milk is taken quickly from the brush to prevent it from becoming cold.

A newborn bat can weigh as little as 5 g depending on the species and the feeding regime should be as follows:

- Newborn bats – must be fed at 2-hourly intervals throughout the day and night
- 1 week old – feed every 2 hours between 6 am and midnight
- From 3 weeks old – feed every 3 hours between 6 am and midnight.

During weaning increase the interval between feeds. Mealworms can be used as a source of solid food by cutting off their heads and allowing the young bat to suck out the soft insides. Water and small amounts of food should be provided as with adults and replaced regularly to avoid it drying out. A rescue centre or local bat group should be contacted for access to a flight aviary and rehabilitation back to the wild.

Deer

There are seven species of deer seen in Britain; the three most often presented as casualties will be dealt with in this chapter. The majority of deer casualties are the result of road traffic accidents (Table 32.14):

- **Fallow deer** (*Dama dama*) – main times of activity are dawn and dusk but they may be seen at any time grazing on grass or browsing in deciduous forest on trees and shrubs. Their colouring varies from reddish brown with white spots to a paler brown with spots, and even black or white. The tail is black and white and the rump has distinctive black markings. One fawn is produced in June.
- **Roe deer** (*Capreolus capreolus*) – active at dawn and dusk. They feed on shrubs and the young shoots of trees. The coat is a deep red, which becomes a duller brown in the winter, the nose is black, there is a white patch on the chin and the rump is cream. Young or kids are born in May/June, often twins.
- **Muntjac deer** (*Muntiacus reevesi*) – the smallest of our deer and an introduced species from Asia. They are

Table 32.14 Reasons for admission of deer as wildlife casualties

Reason for admission	Injury/symptom	Notes
Road traffic accident (RTA)	Concussion Cuts/bruising/grazes Fractures: limbs/pelvis/spine/jaw	Most deer casualties presented are RTA victims
Trapped	No physical injuries but have become trapped in an enclosed area and in panic cannot find a way out	No need to admit but may need help in finding a way out by opening a gate, or making an opening through which the deer can pass. Often, if left alone, they will find a way out themselves
Entangled	Hanging on barbed wire/fencing, usually by a limb. Severe tear wounds and fractures	Head should be covered immediately
Dog victims	Bite/puncture wounds	Young deer
Orphans	Sitting alone in long grass	Not necessarily orphaned

active during the day and at night and are mainly browsers, feeding on shrubs and the leaves of trees. They are sometimes seen grazing. The coat is reddish brown with white around the tail. The male has fang-like teeth protruding from the upper jaw. One fawn is born at any time of the year.

Capture and transportation

Deer are not easy to capture and are equipped with lethal weapons in the form of antlers and sharp hooves. Muntjacs have tusk-like teeth as additional tools for harming humans. If a deer is able to kick, lunge, head-butt and perform other acrobatics that make capture difficult, why is an attempt being made to rescue it? If a deer is injured but can be treated by a vet at the scene, e.g. by giving antibiotics, and then released, there is nothing to be gained by adding to the animal's distress by confining it.

In those deer that are obviously injured the head should be covered as soon as it is safe to do so. Sedation should be avoided if possible, but it may be safer to sedate larger animals in order to clean the wounds and administer the antibiotics; smaller deer may be wrapped and restrained but struggling may make the injuries worse.

Injured deer that cannot be released but are not candidates for euthanasia on site should be wrapped and transported with a hood over their heads, with the nose exposed for respiration. Many rescuers tie the legs to help restraint but this is stressful to the deer and unnecessary – wrapping is preferable. The deer should be accompanied and monitored throughout the journey and care should be taken to ensure that it does not overheat in the vehicle.

Road traffic casualties found lying beside a road are usually severely injured or concussed. Any deer hit by a vehicle will, if it is able, run for cover despite having sustained fractures or internal injuries.

The approach to a deer at the roadside should include a rapid assessment of the situation. Consider the position it is in, its reactions, blood on the road, etc., all of which help to identify the injury. Those clearly awake and struggling are likely to need euthanasia on the scene. Those that appear dazed may just have received a blow to the head and be in need of a quiet place to recover.

Road traffic accidents involving deer attract bystanders and often the police are in attendance. There are vehicles, people and noise, all stressful to the casualty, and the rescuer must take charge of the situation and clear the area. Remember that the stress caused by rescuing such casualties may outweigh the possible benefits and that whatever the decision it must be made quickly.

Examination

Assessment and examination must take place at the scene of the rescue and the records must be completed after the casualty has been accommodated. Deer will not tolerate much handling and it is dangerous and exhausting for the rescuers. Recovered deer must be returned and released where they were found. In the case of road traffic casualties this should be the nearest safe place, so the exact location must be recorded on the patient's notes.

Housing

Housing deer in large practice kennels is not appropriate. Deer must be kept in isolation away from noise and the general buzz of a veterinary practice. Using outside stables or barns or even a strong shed is preferable. A smaller deer may be housed in a large kennel, but it must be dark and well away from disturbance.

Deer will rush around a pen, running into walls, and become very distressed. Absolute quiet and dark is essential for the animal to remain calm and rest. Provide a thick bed of hay and blankets for extra warmth if necessary. Be aware that on entering the pen the deer will attempt to escape and any cleaning, feeding or administering of treatments should be done at the same time, removing the need for constant disturbance.

Heat – a warm bed of hay and blankets is usually enough for an injured deer; however, severely debilitated patients may need supplementary heating. This is best provided using a heat lamp with a protective cover suspended above the animal. Close monitoring is essential and the lamp should be removed as soon as possible – I recommend that these are only used as a last resort because of health and safety implications.

Feeding

Deer patients are often distressed at being held captive and are certainly not relaxed enough to enjoy a good meal.

If they are subjected to the minimum amount of attention and the right food is offered they may feed. Deer are not usually in this situation for long and it is never worth hanging on to an animal that is ready for release just because it has not eaten – the usual reason for inappetence is captivity.

Provide water in a heavy bowl in a corner of the accommodation away from the bedding – this is unlikely to be touched in the first few days. Natural food is always better for the deer, e.g. leaves of deciduous trees, hawthorn, brambles, ivy, and the petals and leaves of roses can be offered. Also try hay, apples and root vegetables, cabbage, lettuce or spring greens and a goat mix from a farm supplier may be eaten.

Cleaning

Cleaning should be undertaken only when necessary. Take the opportunity to do anything else that needs to be done that day at the same time, e.g. injections, wound dressing, etc. Deer are usually short-stay patients and, as they are unlikely to eat or drink initially, the need for cleaning will not arise for the first day or two.

Orphaned deer

Deer may be difficult to hand-rear. They are more labour-intensive than any other orphaned mammal and are not in the least impressed by having a human mother.

In the wild, does leave their young for long periods of time, usually in long grass or areas of good cover, and often these babies are assumed to be orphaned and are picked up. The doe will usually be close by but will not return to her youngster while the human is present. It should be left alone

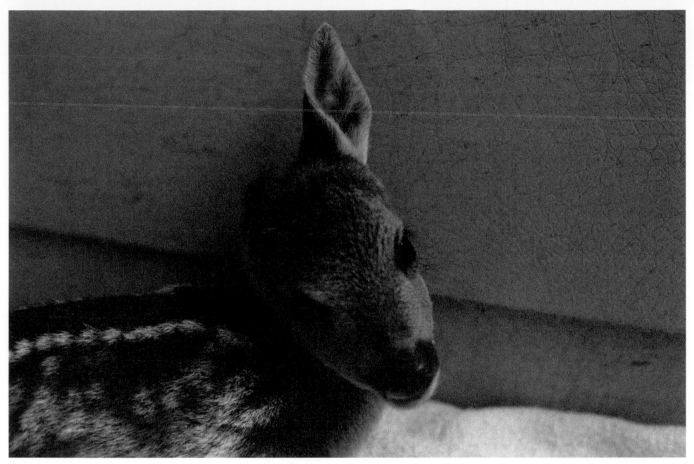

Fig. 32.5 'One Ear', a roe kid who successfully returned to the wild to breed

and checked on later. If a deer fawn or kid is presented and circumstances similar to those above are reported, it should be taken back immediately, and unless it is obviously sick or badly injured it should be left alone. Should a young animal be correctly identified as an orphan it should be transported in a large box or wire basket lined with a warm blanket and covered to keep it dark.

A few years ago we received a roe kid that had had one ear cut off by a tractor mower (Fig. 32.5). The wound was such that it had to receive veterinary treatment immediately and was taken into care. The doe was present throughout this traumatic event but the kid needed medical attention and there was no choice but to take it into our centre. Once the wounds were healed and the kid was feeding well, it was rehabilitated and released back where it came from, much to the delight of the farmer. The following year we received a call from the farmer to say that his one-eared deer had a family. Maybe this story will answer the critics of wildlife care and rehabilitation, who suggest that hand-reared animals cannot be released back into the wild – they can if it is done correctly.

Examination

Examination of a very small deer is easier than with an adult but it must not be assumed that the orphan is not distressed. It may be injured or unwell, has lost its mother, has been removed from natural surroundings and will be frightened and will also put up a fight. Make sure that the initial examination is carried out as quickly as possible and that the youngster is then accommodated and left to rest. No attempt should be made at this stage to feed it, unless it needs life-saving fluids.

A general examination should include:

- Check for wounds, and fly eggs or maggots
- Check for dehydration
- Assess the age – this can be difficult unless evidence of the umbilicus is present
- Check for normal/abnormal palate
- Check the general bodily condition.

An appropriate-sized kennel or large basket should be lined with warm blankets and the orphan should be left to rest. If supplementary heat is needed a Snuggle Pad can be used under the blankets to provide gentle warmth.

Feeding

Feed Esbilac or a lamb milk replacer using a lamb or human baby feeding bottle depending on the size of the fawn. The formula should be thoroughly mixed using boiled water cooled to the correct temperature for feeding. Newly admitted orphans are often reluctant to feed and it may take some time. In some cases it may be necessary to stomach tube the fawn until it is ready to suck on the bottle. Four feeds per day are adequate for deer fawns and once they have taken to the bottle, feed them until they have had enough.

Deer need to be stimulated to defecate and urinate and this is best achieved while feeding is under way. Using one hand to hold the bottle, the other hand is used to gently stimulate the genital area with a warm, damp cloth.

Weaning takes place gradually and from about 1 week of age the fawn will nibble on fresh food, and a tray of soil should be provided along with young shoots and leaves as described in feeding adults. Rose petals and leaves are a popular first food and goat mix and lamb pellets, brambles and hawthorn can also be given, If the fawn is reluctant to take the solid food, try offering sliced apples and carrots, cabbage, lettuce and spring greens, but once the deer is feeding well these should be reduced until natural food and the dried preparations are all that is offered. Weaning should be complete by 10–12 weeks of age and the young deer will need time in an enclosure at a wildlife rehabilitation centre in preparation for release back into the wild.

Grey squirrels (*Sciurus carolinensis*)

The grey squirrel is seen both in urban areas in parks and gardens and in the country, where it often seems to be dicing with death on our roads and this is the reason most are presented as casualties (Table 32.15).

Squirrels are active by day and use their sense of smell and eyesight to survey their surroundings and search for food. They eat nuts, bark, leaves, shoots, acorns, buds and flowers and nest in dreys high up in the trees. Young are born early in the spring – the average litter size is three and late litters may be seen in September. They are independent by about 2 months old and are reared exclusively by the female. Squirrels are extremely agile and are able to scale vertical walls, poles and trees, hanging on with sharp claws.

Capture and transportation

Squirrels who have sustained head injuries are the easiest to capture, while those with severe injuries to the hindquarters are usually still very active at the biting end and should be handled with extreme caution. Squirrels are very agile and have the kind of gnawing teeth that cause nasty wounds.

Approach the casualty with a pair of thick gloves and a towel. Drop the towel over the squirrel, scoop it up and place both towel and animal into a secure carrier for transportation. For those that are still mobile (usually those with a back or hind leg injury) you may need a net. It must be remembered that a squirrel's teeth are such that they may penetrate the glove, but the towel provides additional protection.

Examination

For squirrels that show no obvious sign of injury, examination of the squirrel is a four-handed job. One person should restrain the squirrel and keep the head under control while the second person completes the examination safely. For those with obvious injuries, sedation may be required for a detailed examination. Always try to keep the head covered to reduce stress.

Housing

The squirrel's ability to gnaw has already been established, and this must be considered when providing suitable accommodation. Cardboard and thin plastic are not advisable; a small wire kennel with a metal door is ideal. Line the kennel with newspaper and warm bedding; cover it so that the squirrel is in the dark and place it in a quiet room.

Heat – a microwavable Snuggle Pad is excellent to provide heat for seriously sick or injured squirrels as it avoids the use of anything with chewable wires! As soon as the squirrel becomes more active, the heat supply should be removed and replaced with warm bedding. Synthetic fleece such as Vetbed is ideal.

Feeding

Squirrels are rodents, so for adults offer a basic diet of commercial rodent or rat mix. Plain digestive biscuits, apple and peanuts can be added. Water in a small ceramic bowl should be placed in a corner of the cage to avoid spillage.

Cleaning

When cleaning, remove the food and water bowls first, but only if it is safe to do so. Then tip the cage up on to its end so the squirrel is at the bottom and the door now at the top. Wearing thick gloves and armed with a towel, transfer the squirrel to a clean, ready-prepared cage. This saves over-handling of a difficult species and ensures that the ordeal is over quickly for the squirrel.

Table 32.15 Reasons for grey squirrels being admitted as wildlife casualties

Reason for admittance	Injury/symptom	Notes
Road traffic casualty	Concussion Cuts/bruising/grazes Fractures: pelvis/spinal/limbs/jaw	Sometimes impaled on the front grilles of vehicles
Attacks	Bite wounds	Usually young squirrels. Often by dogs or cats
Orphans	Very young squirrel, no parent present, eyes shut	Often found by a cat or dog, or lying on the ground
Stuck!	Up a telegraph pole, on the roof of a house	No rescue needed; usually been frightened up there by a cat or dog. Will come down when safe to do so but may not be until nightfall

Orphaned squirrels

Always make sure that the squirrel is an orphan before rescuing it. Because the squirrel's drey is high up in trees, it is difficult to return orphans to the nest, even if you knew which hole was the right one. The fact that a young squirrel has been found indicates that all is not well. Other examples include young squirrels found in lofts after the parent has been evicted, either by the homeowner or by pest control. There are legal issues attached to some wildlife casualties and none more so than squirrels (see relevant legislation below).

Hungry orphans will emit a high-pitched and insistent whistle, which may be the reason they are discovered in the first place. A cardboard box filled with warm bedding may be used for transportation and a prewarmed Snuggle Pad should be provided for very young orphans.

Examination

The orphan should be examined thoroughly, including:

- Check for wounds, bite marks and grazes
- Check the body temperature
- Check for dehydration
- Assess the age of the squirrel
- Weigh the squirrel.

Squirrels are born naked, blind and deaf, so if very young or newly born ones are presented heat should be provided. To identify the orphan as a young squirrel, look for the long tail and if in doubt check the claws, which look as if they have been painted with black nail varnish. Ageing is an inexact science but the eyes open at around 3 weeks and at this stage the fur forms a short but thick covering and the tail is furry but not bushy.

Feeding

Before being fed the squirrel should be stimulated to urinate and defecate and then weighed. The faeces of milk-fed squirrels are tiny yellowy/orange pellets, which change to brown when weaned. Feed using a 1 ml syringe and goat's milk or Esbilac.

Once the eyes open, a little solid food can be introduced. Human baby cereal is ideal, a particular favourite is oat and apple flavour, made up with whichever milk you are using to feed and mixed to a sloppy consistency. Start the feed with the usual milk, giving slightly less than usual, and then offer the cereal. I have never known a squirrel refuse it – in fact it is important to offer the milk first otherwise the squirrel will take just the cereal – the oat and apple is just too nice! At this stage a broken digestive biscuit should be left in the cage and water provided. Reducing the milk feeds can begin when the biscuit is being eaten. Weighing is important to monitor the squirrel's progress. Reduce heat in the cage to night time only for a few days and then turn it off completely.

Once the squirrel is nibbling well at the biscuit, more solids can be added, e.g. chunks of peeled apple, peanuts, sultanas and rat mix. It is important to provide vitamins and minerals for those animals not receiving a natural diet, as squirrels in captivity can develop metabolic bone disease. Once weaned, the squirrel should move into an aviary or enclosure such as a wildlife rescue centre can offer.

Birds

Birds are admitted as casualties for a variety of reasons, including:

- **Road traffic accidents** – affects owls in particular but small birds are less commonly affected
- **Cat and dog attacks** – affects mainly small birds and may cause septicaemia, puncture of the air sacs or feather damage
- **Litter** – may wind itself around legs and beaks and if the bird is not released it will die
- **Oiled birds** – from garage waste or polluted water. Oil is removed by washing with detergent but it takes time for the bird's natural oils to return
- **Damage caused by fishing line and hooks and the lead weights attached to them** – hooks may become fixed in the mouth or oesophagus while lead poisoning may present as loss of weight, lethargy, weakness, the head resting over the back or crooked, green faeces and a change in natural behaviour
- **Fledglings that have fallen from the nest**
- **Small birds that have flown into windows** and are concussed.

Birds have their own species of parasites (Table 32.16). They are not routinely treated for nematode worms unless a problem is suspected. Good hygiene in the accommodation should prevent their spread and break life cycles. Gapeworm (*Syngamus trachea*) is a roundworm that may be seen in

Table 32.16 Ectoparasites found on the bird

Parasite	Appearance	Treatment	Notes
Ticks	Resemble tiny pips before feeding, and grapes after. Can be white, grey, bluish grey	Remove with tweezers by grasping base of tick near host's skin and tug sharply. Do not grab body of tick	Blood-sucking parasites, becoming more common and in greater numbers on birds
Lice	Long, thin parasites easily seen on feathers, particularly around the neck	Mite spray for birds	Parasite that chews feathers and skin debris. Plumage looks as if it has been cut
Flat flies	Like a large housefly, but flat for moving under feathers, with feet that grip on to and run along the bird's plumage	Can be removed by hand, but difficult to kill – should be crushed. Use mite spray if the host is infested, but most flat flies leave the body when disturbed	Blood-sucking parasite

starlings; it causes coughing or sneezing sounds that can resemble breathing difficulties. Canker, however, is more common and appears as a creamy substance growing in the mouth, throat and crop. Untreated, the bird will die as the throat closes and it is unable to feed.

Capture and transportation

Any wild bird that is easily caught has something wrong with it. Sometimes these casualties have an injury but are still very active, e.g. a duck with an injured leg can still fly and a pigeon with an injured wing can run!

On approach the bird will either freeze, run or, if cornered, defend itself. Before attempting to catch any bird in the wild, the situation should be carefully assessed. Observe the way that the bird is moving and behaving and work out a plan for its capture. The approach, capture and confinement should be carried out swiftly and firmly.

Capture of most birds is best achieved with a towel, light blanket, coat, car rug, etc. Do not chase the casualty around, as the shock could be fatal. It is much better to lure the bird into a corner, shed or area where there is no escape. Throw the towel over the bird and then gently but firmly scoop it up and place it into a cardboard box or carrier for transportation. Do not remove the towel at this stage as it almost always results in the casualty escaping. If a box or carrying container is not available then the bird should remain loosely but safely contained in its wrap.

Larger more aggressive birds, e.g. birds of prey, can be captured in the same way, but extra care must be taken because talons and beaks are likely to be used as weapons. Most birds, once confined with their heads covered, will not struggle but the rescuer should always be prepared for the unexpected.

Water birds will almost certainly make for the water as their means of escape so rescuers must place themselves between the water and the bird before moving in for the capture. When catching swans and geese it is important to restrain the wings, as the blow from an adult swan's wings is sufficient to fracture human bones! Grab the neck first and then wrap the bird in a large towel or blanket with the head and neck exposed to secure the wings and prevent them from flapping.

Never use a wire basket or transparent container for wild bird casualties. If a solid container is not available then cover the basket. The bird will become distressed and may injure itself if it can see out but cannot escape. The container should be lined with newspaper and a towel or a blanket for larger casualties. The bedding provides warmth and absorbency, a place to hide and something to grip on to during transportation.

Whatever type of container is used it should allow enough room for the bird to stand and stretch out its wings. If using a cardboard box it must be made secure to prevent the casualty from escaping during transportation. Containers with grill-type doors must be covered to keep the casualty in the dark and prevent birds from pushing their beaks through the holes in their attempt to free themselves.

Examination

If the bird is in shock or distressed after transportation, it should be left for a while in a dark quiet environment to calm down, unless it needs life-saving attention.

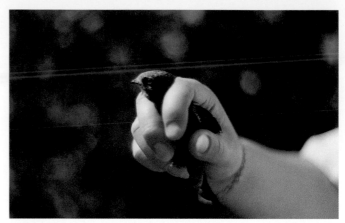

Fig. 32.6 The correct way to restrain a small bird, in this case a young swift

Observe the bird before examination. A great deal can be learned by watching the way the bird is moving, e.g. whether it is lame, has any deformities, or wings hanging or sticking up at an odd angle, how it is breathing, the state of its plumage and general behaviour. These are important observations that can be followed up during the examination, and mean less time handling a distressed, struggling patient.

Restraint for examination can be difficult and depends on the size of the bird:

- When restraining small birds, be aware that applying too much pressure to the body can cause asphyxia. The correct method is to create a 'net' with the fingers of your hand to control the wings and allow the head to poke out between the second and third fingers (Fig. 32.6). The underside of the bird and its legs can be examined by turning it over and the wings can be gently extended on each side
- Larger birds, such as members of the crow family and seagulls, have strong beaks. For examination, they may need to have their beaks taped or an elastic band placed around them to prevent pecking, taking care not to cover the nares or nostrils. One person should hold the bird around the wings while another carries out the examination.
- Birds of prey should be held with a gloved hand on either side of the bird and are more likely to strike out with their talons, which can be kept under control by holding the legs between the first two fingers of one hand. If the head is covered the bird is more likely to remain calm. Another person should then make the examination.
- Ducks and game birds are very strong and should also be held by two hands restraining the wings. Swans are best examined on the floor with one person restraining the wings while the other carries out the examination.

A general examination should include checking the following:

- Feet and legs – fractures, wounds, fly eggs and maggots, frost bite, fungal lesions
- Wings – hanging down or sticking up
- Beak – fractures, splits, top and bottom do not meet

- Mouth – general colour, fly eggs, canker, smelly breath – a garlicky smell in owls indicates poisoning
- Nares – discharge, blockage
- Eyes – discharge, swelling, dilated pupils, unequal pupils, prolapse
- Crop – torn, impacted
- Keel – sharp keel bone indicates thin bird
- Cloaca – dirty, blocked, fly eggs and maggots, prolapse
- Plumage – should be sleek with no ruffled feathers. Chewed or cut appearance indicates feather mites, white feathers on a black bird suggest a deficiency
- Respiration – gasping or panting, gurgling, laboured
- Parasites – (Table 32.16)
- Skin – wounds, flaky, fly eggs or maggots, crusty and feather loss may indicate ringworm
- Dehydration.

Patient records should include:

- Species
- Date
- Details of condition
- Name, address and telephone number of finder
- Details of the exact spot where the casualty was found – this is essential because when the bird recovers it should be returned to the area from where it came
- Any other useful information, e.g. it was lying on its back struggling to stand up. This is important because it may lead to a diagnosis, reducing the need for examination.

There is no need to give routine flea or worm treatment unless such parasites are obvious. Routine vitamin injections are also unnecessary but long term patients will benefit from supplements to compensate for the lack of a natural diet. These birds are wild and must be returned to their natural habitats with as little interference as possible.

Housing

Each bird should be housed according to its needs, its natural behaviour and its habitat:

- Birds must have sufficient room to stretch their wings and be able to preen
- Perching birds need the correct size of perch, e.g. a perch for a sparrow could be a twig while a buzzard needs a small branch. Incorrect perch size result in difficulties in perching and infections such as bumble foot, which occurs when the claws pierce the underside of the foot. Perch positioning is also important to make best use of the space and to encourage exercise as the bird hops or flies between them
- Place natural foliage in a cage to provide places to hide. There is a noted change in behaviour when greenery is present in the cage
- Do not place the cage close to domestic animals, especially cats, or in noisy areas. Some bird species are more susceptible to stress than others and may throw themselves around when first introduced to a hospital cage. This may be helped by placing a towel over the front.
- Many birds will make for the door as soon as it is opened, in an attempt to escape
- Sometimes after handling and replacing in the cage a bird may remain flat on the bottom or on its back,

'playing dead'. This may take you by surprise when you open the cage to check! Owls, particularly chicks, often sleep lying down.

Heat – the need for heat should be carefully considered. If heat is provided the bird must be weaned off it before release. These are wild birds that naturally live out in cold, wet and windy weather. Heat boxes, brooders, incubators and heat lamps can be regulated and are the best option, but the bird is unable to get away from the heat source so careful monitoring is needed.

Feeding

The period of major activity, including feeding, in the day varies with the species of bird. Some are diurnal, others nocturnal and a few are crepuscular, i.e. active mainly at dawn and dusk. There will be some patients that are on a special feeding regime and will not be keeping to their natural hours of activity. Some wild birds may refuse to eat because they are captive.

One of the many problems is knowing what to feed and this is made easier by correct identification of the species. This will then allow you to find out their natural food and if necessary find an acceptable substitute (Table 32.17).

The shape of a bird's beak will give an idea as to the diet of the bird even if you are unable to identify the species (Fig. 32.7). A robin's beak is small and thin for eating insects; finches and sparrows have shorter, stubbier beaks for cracking seeds; a blackbird's beak is longer for probing soil for earthworms. Every veterinary practice would benefit from a basic bird identification book – those that contain photographs rather than drawings or paintings will make identification much easier.

It is a myth that bread and milk is good for wildlife and in no way does it resemble a natural diet. Casualties that are confined for more than a few days should receive vitamin and mineral supplements to compensate for deficiencies in the captive diet.

Cleaning

Accommodation should be cleaned thoroughly once a day. Layers of newspaper should line the cage so that soiled layers can be easily and quickly removed, preventing the build-up

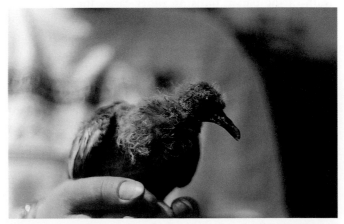

Fig. 32.7 A common error is to identify young wood pigeons as hawks or vultures

Table 32.17 Suggested diets for wild birds

Species	Natural food	Alternative food
Finch, sparrow	A variety of seeds, nuts, grains and berries	Seed–finch mix
Blackbird, thrush, robin, starling	Earthworms, grubs, insects, fruit, berries, snails, slugs	Mealworms, earthworms in soil, cat food mashed with insectivorous food, fruit
Swallows, swifts, house martins	Insects caught on the wing and insect grubs	Maggots cut in half, insectivorous mix. Need hand feeding
Woodpeckers	Insects	Smear food on to bark. Suet, peanut butter, cat food mashed with insectivorous food, grated cheese
Pigeons, doves, game birds	Grain and seeds. Insects for the game birds	Corn, chick crumb. Mealworms for the game birds
Ducks and geese	Insects, worms and grubs, aquatic plants, grain and graze on grass	Chick crumb, corn, mealworms, grass
Swans	Aquatic plants and insects, graze on grass	Chick crumb and corn in water with grass mixed in
Crows, jackdaws, rooks, magpies, jays	Insects, grubs, worms, eggs, small birds, mammals, seed, grain, berries, nuts, fruit, carrion	Tinned cat or dog meat, day-old chicks, RTA victims scraped from road, fruit, mealworms
Kestrel	Small rodents	Mice and day-old chicks
Sparrow hawk	Small birds, doves and pigeons	Mice and day-old chicks
Buzzard	Small mammals, rabbits, worms and beetles	Rabbit with fur, mice, rats, day-old chicks
Barn and tawny owls	Small mammals, moths, beetles	Mice, rats, day-old chicks
Little owl	Mostly insects, voles, mice	Mice and day-old chicks
Gulls	At sea, freshly caught fish. Town gulls eat anything, worms and grubs	Tinned cat or dog food, day-old chicks, sprats floating in water
Heron	Fish, frogs	Trout or sprats in water
Coots, moorhens	Insects and larvae, worms, water weeds, grains	Mashed cat food mixed with water and insectivorous food to form a paste. Finely chopped sprats in water, cress in water, maggots

of faeces. Handling can be reduced by having clean accommodation ready for the bird to be moved into. Any other tasks such as feeding or treatment should be carried out at the same time to avoid unnecessary distress caused by repeated disturbance. Use a towel to move birds from cage to cage. Food and water containers should not be placed near to or under perches as they will become soiled with faeces.

Orphaned birds

Orphans or fledgling birds most commonly result from the death of the parent birds. In other cases, they are not so much orphaned as 'rescued' and taken away from their parents for their own good:

- The nest may have been exposed by hedge trimming or tree felling. If it is possible to find a suitable new site for the nest it is worth a try as the parents may continue to care for their young
- Nests may be built in unused farm machinery or cars, which are then put into use and the nestlings are discovered
- Ducklings may become separated from their mother – often a single duckling is lost
- Birds may have been caught in a storm and are wet and cold. Even though the parent is still present, the bird needs more help than the parent can offer. Sometimes after a night in care it is possible to put them back in the nest

- The most common case is the fledgling caught by a cat. Even those uninjured and apparently well cannot be returned unless their nest site is known. There is also a risk of septicaemia from the cat's teeth. Some of these fledglings are older and can become very distressed. In many cases the best course of action is to retrieve the bird from the cat and, if it is active and protesting, lock the cat in and release the bird.

All cases should be judged on an individual basis as every case is slightly different.

There are two types of fledgling:

- **Altricial** – fledglings remain in the nest and are fed by one or both parents. They are blind, deaf and have few or no feathers or down when they hatch. Examples are blackbirds, thrushes, sparrows, finches, robins, starlings, crows, jackdaws, jays, swallows, swifts, house martins, tits, pigeons, doves, woodpeckers, owls and birds of prey
- **Precocial** – birds that hatch as active chicks, most of which feed themselves. Examples are ducklings, swans, geese and pheasants. Some, e.g. moorhens and herons, are fed by the parents.

Identification of the species of a baby bird is difficult because there are so many species and the juvenile plumage (if they have any) is different from that of the adult. A good bird book with photographs of both adult and juvenile plumage is essential. Most veterinary practices will be willing to provide initial care and feeding and then usually pass the fledgling on to a wildlife centre.

Housing

Fledglings must be kept warm until they have feathers and should be provided with a brooder or heat lamp. Create a 'nest' in the form of a ceramic feeding bowl or similar vessel, lined with kitchen paper. This provides a familiar, temporary home that allows the fledglings to behave normally and is easy to clean.

Once the fledgling becomes more active, low perches can be arranged around the nest pot and a little foliage provided. As the feathers develop the heat can be gradually reduced until it is only provided at night and then turned off completely. As the bird grows, move it to a nursery cage lined with paper, which gives more room to move around. The bird will spend more time out of the nest pot and food can be introduced into the cage so that the bird can start to feed itself. Higher perches and more foliage create a natural environment. Once the bird's tail feathers have grown and it is feeding itself, it is time to move it to an aviary for flight practice and muscle building prior to release.

Feeding

There are a variety of diets and ways of administering the food to the fledgling, which depend on the species (Table 32.18).

Suggested recipes for feeding orphaned birds:

- **Baby bird mix:**
  2 parts puppy or kitten food to 1 part insectivorous mix
  Pinch of vitamin and mineral supplement
  Pinch of probiotic
  Water to mix.
  All the ingredients should be mixed well to ensure that there are no lumps, as little birds may choke. The water should be added until the mixture is sloppy – not dripping wet and not too dry. It will dry out over time, so more water may need to be added. Baby bird mix can be made up in large batches and stored in the refrigerator. It must be taken out prior to feeding and food should be offered at room temperature.

- **Scrambled egg mix:** (a prepared dry food is available to buy from good pet stores called 'egg biscuit'; this just requires the addition of water)
  Soft scrambled egg
  Crumbled digestive biscuit
  Pinch of vitamin and mineral supplement
  Pinch of probiotic
  Goat's milk to mix.
  The scrambled egg should be soft and mashed finely. Add the dry ingredients and mix together. Add the goat's milk to make a sloppy consistency.

  This is administered using an adapted 1-ml syringe. The scrambled egg mix is sucked up into the syringe and must be pushed out again without air bubbles or lumps. The narrow end of the syringe should be trimmed off and filed until smooth. This makes a simple but essential tool for delivering a measured amount of food when crop feeding fledgling pigeons and doves. A 60-ml syringe saves time when the technique has been perfected as long as it is the wide-ended design as a large amount can be deposited in the crop in one go.

Baby birds must be given vitamin and mineral supplements because they are not being fed a natural diet. Fledglings will not feed if they are cold – if the bird does not open its mouth or gape to begin with, make sure it is warm.

There are a few ways in which to encourage a fledgling to gape:

- By touching the beak
- Tapping the nest pot
- Passing your hand over the nest, which mimics the parent returning to the nest
- Whistling may have heads popping up with the beaks open. The whistle imitates bird song and, although it sounds strange, it really does work.

Once the bird is gaping, small amounts of food can be placed at the back of the mouth using tweezers. Once feeder and fledgling have got used to each other, the bird will

Table 32.18 Feeding orphaned birds

Species	Rearing food	How to feed
Finch/sparrow	Chopped white maggots and baby bird mix	Tweezers
Blackbird/thrush/robin/starling	Baby bird mix	Tweezers
Swallows/swifts/house martins/tits	Chopped white maggots, baby bird mix, moistened raw minced beef	Tweezers
Pigeons and doves	Scrambled egg mix/Egg biscuit	Adapted 1-ml/60-ml syringe
Ducklings	Rearing chick crumbs	Self-feeding
Cygnets	Rearing chick crumb, chopped grass	Offer in water, self-feeding
Crow/jackdaw/rook/jay/magpie	Baby bird mix, cat food chunks in jelly, chopped day-old chicks	Tweezers
Kestrel/sparrowhawk/owl	Chopped day-old chicks and mice	Tweezers
Buzzard	Chopped day-old chicks, mice, rats, pieces of rabbit with fur	Tweezers
Gulls	Sprats/whitebait/chopped day-old chicks/tinned cat food chunks in jelly	Tweezers
Moorhen	Finely chopped sprats covered in water, baby bird mix, soaked insectivorous food and chick crumb, cress floating on water, live white maggots	

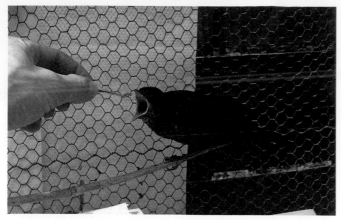

Fig. 32.8 Blackbird fledgling being fed using tweezers

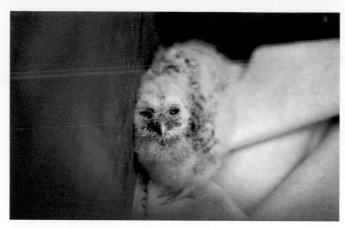

Fig. 32.9 Owl chick displaying its fluff

readily take food off the tweezers and swallow each time it is offered (Fig. 32.8).

Sometimes new arrivals and some more difficult cases have to be fed by forcibly opening the beak. This must be done by carefully squeezing the hinged part of the mouth on either side – the tip of the beak should never be forced open. Once food has been placed in the mouth, the beak often flies open ready to receive more – sometimes it takes a bit longer. Fledglings should be fed at least every 30 minutes from dawn until dusk. In the wild they wake up at first light and go to roost at dusk and these times should be adhered to unless the bird is very sick.

Once the birds become more active and are spending more time out of the nest pot, solid food can be introduced. A small flat container of whatever they are used to should be placed in the cage with a shallow container of water. Hand feeding can be reduced as the fledglings start to feed them-selves and an adult diet gradually introduced, decreasing the baby food.

Food and water containers should be an appropriate size so the birds can drink but not drown and can reach the food easily. Place the food and water containers in an area that is easily accessible but not on one of the main 'runways', as it will be walked through or flapped in, resulting in the cage and the bird's plumage become soiled.

When first taken into captivity older fledglings are more reluctant to tolerate being hand-fed and they will become distressed and throw themselves around the cage. Restrain-ing the bird gently and offering it food on tweezers may work, as older fledglings will often peck at whatever comes near to them. As it tastes the food it may open its beak and allow itself to be fed. If not, then one half of the cage should be covered to provide a place to hide, the food and water should be placed in this half and the fledgling should be left in peace. It may respond to hand feeding later or may have started to feed itself.

Specific species of bird

Owls and birds of prey

Housing

Chicks of these species hatch covered in down and need supplementary heating in the form of a heat lamp or brooder (Fig. 32.9).

The cage should be lined with layers of newspaper and a towel for warmth and should contain a low perch of the correct size for their feet. A mixing or pudding bowl of the appropriate size, lined with warm material, will suit a very young bird that would have naturally come from a nest. (**Note:** not all birds of prey have nests.) It is rare for birds of this age to be brought in. Foliage should be used to create hiding places. As the youngster grows, reduce the heat and raise the perches. Birds that are neither newly nor recently hatched will not need supplementary heating unless debilitated.

Feeding

Most birds of prey are fed on mice and day-old chicks and larger species such as buzzards are fed on rabbit as well. It is important that these birds are given fur, feathers and bones, as they need the whole animal. Vitamin and mineral supplements are added. Food should be offered in small pieces using tweezers. In cases where a little persuasion is needed, the beak should be touched with the food, or it should be offered from above. If neither method works, then the mouth will have to be opened manually, which can be achieved by carefully prising open the beak at each side.

Once it is open, the food is placed at the back of the mouth and the bird should then swallow. This may have to be repeated a few times until the bird starts to grab the food from the tweezers.

Small meals are offered every 2–3 hours. Birds of prey will regurgitate a pellet that contains the indigestible fur, feathers and bone (see also Ch. 31). As the bird grows it should be offered larger pieces of food, which it will stand on and tear with its talons. Eventually it should be given whole food. These birds must be taken to a rescue centre for rehabilitation.

Swallows, swifts and house martins

These species of bird are aerial feeders and spend their whole lives in flight. They will not feed themselves from a dish of food and, although swallows and house martins may take advantage of a perch to sit on by the time the hand-rearing process is almost finished, swifts will not. A swift should be provided with something to hang on to and may use the bars of the cage, a piece of bark or even a bit of material to grip on to and climb.

Precocial fledglings, e.g. swans, ducks, geese, game birds, coots and moorhens, gulls

Housing

When these birds first hatch they should be given a heat source to replace their mother. The best kind is a heat lamp or brooder, as these chicks are active and need space to run around and a warm place to huddle together. If a single orphan is presented it will need a 'mum', which could be a soft toy or a stringy mop head – these chicks hatch in broods and it is unnatural for them to be alone; a substitute 'mum' might make the difference between surviving or not.

At one end of the cage, suspend a heat lamp over warm bedding such as a towel. At the other end place the food and water containers. At this end there should be several layers of newspaper that can be removed one by one to keep the cage clean.

This type of fledgling is more susceptible to stress and the accommodation should be partially covered to provide an area in which to hide. Once weaned off the heat lamp, the youngsters can be transferred to a run on grass. Provide a box to hide in. They must be brought inside at night and may need gentle heat for the first few nights or if the temperature drops too low.

Feeding

Some of these fledglings, e.g. gulls, may need to be fed by hand initially. However, most will feed themselves once they have settled in and are left in peace. Food and water should be available from dawn until dusk.

Euthanasia

Any wildlife casualty that is too severely injured or sick to recover and be able to sustain itself in the wild is a candidate for euthanasia. Very often the decision is made to keep the animal alive because it is easier for the human being, although it may be severely disabled or unable to behave normally, e.g. a bird that will never fly. The length of time the casualty is likely to be in captivity and receiving treatment must also be considered, because it will cause immense stress and may result in a certain amount of humanization, i.e. becoming used to humans, which may be dangerous in the wild. There may even be a degree of kudos involved with possessing the animal, but the saying 'Where there is life there is hope' is not always the case.

Where there is unlikely to be a positive outcome, where there is suffering and recovery is uncertain or the amount of time in care is going to be lengthy, euthanasia is the humane option. However, each case must be judged on its merits and there will be some situations where a suitable permanent home that provides a good quality of life is appropriate.

Relevant legislation

The **Wildlife and Countryside Act 1981 (WCA)** is the principal source of information for anyone working in wildlife rescue and rehabilitation. The complete document is available from the Stationery Office, or from their website www.tso.co.uk. The Act is extensive but the main points in respect to the animals discussed in this chapter are as follows:

- A species that has protection under the Act can only be taken from the wild in order to give it the necessary care it needs to be able to return it to the wild or for humane destruction where appropriate. These creatures should be cared for in a way that ensures their return to the wild, should not be tamed and should be housed appropriately
- Mammals that do not have protection under the WCA have provision to protect them against cruelty under the **Wild Mammals (Protection) Act 1996**, e.g. it is an offence to 'cruelly kick, beat, impale, burn, drown or crush any wild mammal'
- Grey squirrels are non-indigenous species and it is an offence under the WCA to release a grey squirrel back into the wild or to allow it to escape, although it is permitted to take it from the wild and euthanase it if it is sick or injured
- All species of bat and their roosts are protected
- **The Protection of Badgers Act 1992** protects badgers and their setts
- **The Deer Act 1991** details how and when deer maybe taken
- Protection of birds – 'a person cannot kill, injure or take any wild bird, take, damage or destroy the nest of any wild bird that contains chicks or eggs or is being built, or take or destroy any egg of any wild bird'. There are exceptions where birds have no protection or may be taken outside the close season, or may be taken by authorized persons:
  - Game birds have no protection under this Act apart from during the close season, but there are rules governing the way they may be killed or taken. The hunting season for:

    Pheasant – 1 October to 1 February;
    Canada goose and mallard duck – 1 September to 20 February;
    Moorhen – 1 September to 31 January
  - Part of the Wildlife and Countryside Act 1981 used to include Schedule 2 Part II, which listed 13 'pest' species, e.g. magpie, jay, feral pigeon, that were allowed to be killed or taken by authorized persons at any time. In 1993 this part of the act was removed and was replaced by general licences allowing the taking of certain 'pest' species by authorized persons. These licences were designed to protect other wild birds and agricultural interests from damage or pollution and to protect the air, safety and public health. Full details of these licences and what they refer to can be obtained from the DEFRA website, www.defra.gov.uk/wildlife-country. Licenses are issued by DEFRA annually in England and similar ones can be obtained for Scotland and Wales.

Bibliography

Best, R., Cooper, J.E., Mullineaux, E. (Eds.), 2003. BSAVA Manual of Wildlife Casualties. British Small Animal Veterinary Association, Gloucester.

Cooper, J.E., Ely, J.T., 1979. First Aid Care of Wild Birds. David & Charles, Newton Abbot.

Recommended reading

Best, R., Cooper, J.E., Mullineaux, E. (Eds.), 2003. BSAVA Manual of Wildlife Casualties. British Small Animal Veterinary Association, Gloucester.

Provides essential information for dealing with all the injured wildlife that may be presented in the practice. It is written mainly for veterinary surgeons and therefore focuses on diagnosis and treatment, but also covers care during recovery.

Normal values

(from various sources)

Dog, cat and horse

Table A.1 Normal clinical parameters

Parameter	Dog	Cat	Horse
Body temperature (°C)	38.3–8.7	38.0–38.5	38.0–38.2
Pulse rate (beats/min)	60–180	110–180	32–44
Respiratory rate (breaths/min)	10–30	20–30	8–12

Table A.2 Normal haematological values

Parameter	Dog	Cat	Horse
Total red blood cell count ($\times 10^{12}$/l)	5.5–8.5	5.0–10.0	7.0
Total white blood cell count ($\times 10^9$/l)	6–17	5.5–19.5	8–11
Differential white cell count (%)			
Neutrophils	65–70	45–75	50–60
Eosinophils	2–5	4–12	2–5
Basophils	<1	<1	<1
Monocytes	5	0–4	5–6
Lymphocytes	20–25	20–25	30–40
Thrombocyte count ($\times 10^9$/l)	200–500	200–600	113–299
Packed cell volume (%)	37–55	24–45	42
Haemoglobin (g/dl)	12–18	8–15	12.5
Blood pH	7.35–7.45	7.35–7.45	7.35–7.43
Clotting time (min)	2.5	2.5	11.5

Table A.3 Normal urine values

Parameter	Dog	Cat	Horse
pH	5.2–6.8	6.0–7.0	7.5–8.5
Specific gravity	1.015–1.045	1.020–1.040	1.008–1.040
Daily volume (ml/kg bodyweight)	20–100	10–12	20–50

Table A.4 Normal values for blood biochemistry

Parameter	Dog	Cat	Horse
Total serum protein (g/l)	50–78	60–82	55–71
Serum albumin (g/l)	22–35	25–39	28–36
Cholesterol (mmol/l)	2.7–9.5	1.5–6.0	2.1–3.6
Total bilirubin (μmol/l)	0–6.8	0–6.8	11–48
Calcium (mmol/l)	2.20–2.90	2.20–2.90	2.7–3.2
Blood urea nitrogen (mmol/l)	3.0–9.0	5.0–10.0	4.0–8.0
Creatinine (μmol/l)	Up to 120	Up to 180	86–204
Fasting plasma glucose (mmol/l)	3.5–5.5	3.5–6.5	3.6–6.4

Small mammals

Table A.5 Normal clinical parameters for small mammals

Parameter	Rabbit	Guinea pig	Ferret	Gerbil	Mouse	Rat	Hamster
Weight (g)							
Male	Varies according to breed	900–1200	1000–2000	46–131	20–40	267–500	87–130
Female	Varies according to breed	700–900	600–1000	50–55	22–63	225–325	95–130
Life span	7 years (average)	5–6 years	5–11 years	24–39 months	12–36 months	26–40 months	18–36 months
Body temperature (°C)	37–39.4	37.2–39.5	37.8–40	38.2	37.1	37.7	37.6
Pulse rate (beats/min)	198–330	240–310	200–300	85–160	427–697	313–493	310–471
Respiratory rate (breaths/min)	35–60	40–80	33–36	85–160	91–216	71–146	38–110

Table A.6 Serum biochemical reference values for gerbils, hamsters, mice, rats and guinea pigs

Value	Gerbil	Hamster	Mouse	Rat	Guinea pig
Total protein (g/dl)	4.6–14.7	5.5–7.2	59–103	5.9–7.8	4.2–6.8
Albumin (g/dl)	1.8–5.8	2.0–4.2	2.5–4.8	3.3–4.6	2.1–3.9
Globulin (g/dl)	0.8–10.0	2.5–4.9	0.6	2.2 3.5	1.7–2.6
Glucose (mg/dl)	47–137	60–160	73–183	74–163	60–125
Cholesterol (mg/dl)	90–141	65–148	59–103	44–138	16–43
Urea nitrogen (mg/dl)	17–30	14–27	18–31	12–22	9.0–31.5
Creatinine (mg/dl)	NA	0.4-1.0	0.48–1.1	0.38–0.8	0.6–2.2
Creatine kinase (IU/l)	NA	366–776	155	111–334	NA
Aspartate aminotransferase (IU/l)	NA	43–134	101–214	54–192	26–68
Alanine aminotransferase (IU/l)	NA	22–63	44–87	52–144	25–59
Alkaline phosphatase (IU/l)	NA	6–14.2	43–71	40–191	55–108
Lactate dehydrogenase (IU/l)	NA	134–360	366	225–275	NA
Total bilirubin (mg/dl)	0.8–1.6	0.24–0.72	0.3–0.8	0.23–0.48	0.0–0.9
Sodium (mEq/l)	143–147	124–147	143–164	142–150	120–152
Potassium (mEq/l)	3.6–5.9	3.9–6.8	6.3–8.0	4.3–6.3	3.8–7.9
Chloride (mEq/l)	93-118	92–103	105–118	100–109	90–115
Phosphorus (mg/dl)	3.7–11.2	4.0–8.2	5.2–9.4	5.3–8.4	3.0–7.6
Calcium (mg/dl)	3.7–6.1	8.4–12.3	4.6–9.6	7.6–12.6	8.2–12.0
Magnesium (mg/dl)	NA	1.9–2.9	1.4–3.1	2.6–3.2	NA

Source: from Quesenbury, K.E., Carpenter, J.W., 2004. Ferrets, Rabbits and Rodents. Clinical Medicine and Surgery, second ed. W B Saunders, St Louis, MO.

Table A.7 Haematological reference values for gerbils, hamsters, mice, rats and guinea pigs

Parameter	Gerbil	Hamster	Mouse	Rat	Guinea pig
Red blood cells ($\times 10^6$/µl)	7.0–10.0	5–9.2	7.9–10.1	5.4–8.5	3.2–8.0
Haemoglobin (g/dl)	12.1–16.9	14.6–20	11.0–14.5	11.5–16.0	10.0–17.2
Haematocrit (%)	41–52	46–52	37–46	37–49	32–50
Platelets ($\times 10^3$/µl)	400–600	300–570	600–1200	450–885	260–740
White blood cells ($\times 10^3$/µl)	4.3–21.6	5.0–10.0	5.0–13.7	4.0–10.2	5.5–17.5
Neutrophils (%)	5–34	10–42	10–40	6–17	22–48
Lymphocytes (%)	60–95	50–95	55–95	9–34	39–72
Eosinophils (%)	0–4	0–4.5	0–4	0–6	0–7
Monocytes (%)	0–3	0–3	0.1–3.5	0–5	0–1
Basophils (%)	0–1	0–1	0–0.3	0–1.5	0–2.7
Total blood volume (ml/kg)	60–85	65–80	70–80	50–65	NA

Source: from Quesenbury, K.E., Carpenter, J.W., 2004. Ferrets, Rabbits and Rodents. Clinical Medicine and Surgery, second ed. W B Saunders, St Louis, MO.

Table A.8 Reference ranges for serum biochemistry values in the rabbit

Parameter	Value
Serum protein	5.4–8.3 g/dl
Albumin	2.4–4.6 g/dl
Globulin	1.5–2.8 g/dl
Glucose	75–155 g/dl
Blood urea nitrogen	13–29 mg/dl
Creatinine	0.5–2.5 mg/dl
Total bilirubin	0.0–0.7 mg/dl
Cholesterol	10–80 mg/dl
Total lipids	243–390 mg/dl
Calcium	5.6–12.5 mg/dl
Phosphorus	4.0–6.9 mg/dl
Sodium	131–155 mEq/l
Potassium	3.6–6.9 mEq/l
Chloride	92–112 mEq/l
Bicarbonate	16–38 mEq/l
Amylase	166.5–314.5 U/l
Alkaline phosphatase	4–16 U/l
Alanine aminotransferase	48–80 U/l
Aspartate aminotransferase	14–113 U/l
Lactic dehydrogenase	34–129 U/l

Source: from Quesenbury, K.E., Carpenter, J.W., 2004. Ferrets, Rabbits and Rodents. Clinical Medicine and Surgery, second ed. W B Saunders, St Louis, MO.

Table A.9 Reference ranges for haematological values in the rabbit

Parameter	Value
Erythrocytes	$5.1–7.9 \times 10^6/\mu l$
Haematocrit	33–50%
Haemoglobin	10.0–17.4 g/dl
Mean corpuscular volume	$57.8–66.5\ \mu m^3$
Mean corpuscular haemoglobin	17.1–23.5 pg
Mean corpuscular haemoglobin concentration	29–37%
Platelets	$250–650 \times 10^3/\mu l$
Leucocytes	$5.2–12.5 \times 10^3/\mu l$
Neutrophils	20–75%
Lymphocytes	30–85%
Monocytes	1–4%
Eosinophils	1–4%
Basophils	1–7%

Source: from Quesenbury, K.E., Carpenter, J.W., 2004. Ferrets, Rabbits and Rodents. Clinical Medicine and Surgery, second ed. W B Saunders, St Louis, MO.

Table A.10 Serum biochemical values in the ferret

Parameter	Albino	Fitch
Total protein (g/dl)	5.1–7.4	5.3–7.2
Albumin (g/dl)	2.6–3.8	3.3–4.1
Glucose (mg/dl)	94–207	62.5–134
Fasting glucose (mg/dl)	–	90–125
Blood urea nitrogen (mg/dl)	10–45	12–43
Creatinine (mg/dl)	0.4–0.9	0.2–0.6
Sodium (mmol/l)	137–162	146–160
Potassium (mmol/l)	4.5–7.7	4.3–5.3
Chloride (mmol/l)	106–125	102–121
Calcium (mg/dl)	8.0–11.8	8.6–10.5
Phosphorus (mg/dl)	4.0–9.1	5.6–8.7
Alanine aminotransferase (U/l)	–	82–289
	–	78–149
Aspartate aminotransferase (U/l)	28–120	57–248
Alkaline phosphatase (U/l)	9–84	30–120
	–	31–66
Bilirubin (mg/dl)	< 1.0	0–0.1
Cholesterol (mg/dl)	64–296	119–209
Carbon dioxide (mmol/l)	16.5–28	16–28

Source: from Quesenbury, K.E., Carpenter, J.W., 2004. Ferrets, Rabbits and Rodents. Clinical Medicine and Surgery, second ed. W B Saunders, St Louis, MO.

Essential calculations

Pip Millard

This is a summary of all the calculations that may be used in veterinary practice, including:

- Anaesthetic flow rates
- Fluid therapy flow rates
- Percentages of solutions
- Drug dosages
- Calorific requirements
- Radiographic exposures.

Each section provides an explanation of how to approach the calculation, a worked example, and then some questions to do on your own with the answers included at the end.

Useful measurements

- 1 kilogram (kg) = 2.2 lb
- 1 kg = 1000 grams (g)
- 1 g = 1000 milligrams (mg)
- 1 mg = 1000 micrograms (μg, mcg)
- 1 litre (l) = 1000 millilitres (ml)
- 1 teaspoon = 5 ml
- 1 metre (m) = 100 centimetres (cm) = 1000 millimetres (mm)
- 1 cm = 10 mm

Anaesthetic flow rates

The formula required to calculate an anaesthetic flow rate is:

Bodyweight (kg) × Minute volume (ml/min) × Circuit factor

We must first calculate the minute volume of the patient and in order to do this we need to know the patient's tidal volume and respiratory rate.

1. **Tidal volume** – this is the amount of air which is inhaled or exhaled in each respiration. It is estimated at 10–15 ml/kg:
   - Cats/small dogs = 15 ml/kg
   - Medium/large dogs = 10 ml/kg.
2. **Minute volume** – this is the amount of air passing in and out of the lungs in 1 minute.

The formula to calculate minute volume is:

Tidal volume × Respiratory rate.

If accurate figures are unavailable, a minute volume of 200 ml/kg can be used. This is an average minute volume, based on 10 ml/kg tidal volume and 20 breaths per minute respiratory rate.

3. **Circuit factor** – this is the factor by which the minute volume must be increased to prevent rebreathing. This is used to calculate the correct settings for the anaesthetic machine in relation to the particular patient.

Ayre's T-piece	2.5–3 × minute volume
Bain	2.5–3 × minute volume
Magill	1–1.5 × minute volume
Lack	1–1.5 × minute volume
Circle – closed	No circuit factor: calculate using a flow rate of 10 ml/kg
To-and-fro – partial rebreathing	No circuit factor: calculate using a flow rate of 25 ml/kg

Example

What is the required anaesthetic flow rate for a 30 kg dog with a respiratory rate of 20 breaths/minute on a Magill circuit?

Bodyweight × minute volume × circuit factor
30 kg × (10 ml tidal volume × 20 breaths/min) × 1–1.5
30 kg × 200 ml × 1–1.5

Answer: 6000 ml (6 l) or 9000 ml (9 l) per min

Example

Calculate the anaesthetic flow rate required to maintain anaesthesia in a 15 kg dog on a Bain circuit with a respiratory rate of 20 breaths/minute:

Bodyweight × minute volume × circuit factor
15 kg × (10 ml tidal volume × 20 breaths/min) × 2.5–3
15 kg × 200 ml × 2.5–3

Answer: 7500 ml (7.5 l) or 9000 ml (9 l)

Respiratory/cutaneous losses:	20 ml/kg – these are described as **inevitable losses**
Faecal losses (normal faeces):	10–20 ml/kg
Urinary losses (normal range):	20 ml/kg
Further losses include:	
Vomit: approximately	4 ml/kg/vomit

With an accurate history the fluid deficit can be calculated.

Fluid therapy flow rates

Giving sets

These usually have the number of drops per millilitre stated on the packaging, so check before calculating the drip rate. A standard giving set will deliver approximately 15–20 drops/ml. For smaller patients, a paediatric giving set can be used, which gives 60 drops/ml – this faster rate is useful to administer small volumes more accurately. Automated infusion pumps are also available, which can deliver a set amount of fluid over a given period of time.

Example

An 8 kg dog has been anorexic for 3 days and has vomited three times daily for the last 2 days. It has not produced urine for 24 hours. Calculate the total fluid deficit for this animal

Inevitable water losses:	20 ml × 8 kg × 3 days = 480 ml
Urinary water losses:	20 ml × 8 kg × 2 days = 320 ml
Vomiting:	4 ml × 8 kg × 3 vomits × 2 days = 192 ml

Answer: Total water deficit: 480 + 320 + 192 = 992 ml

Estimating fluid loss

There are three main ways to estimate fluid loss:

- Using percentage dehydration of the animal
- Calculating the water deficit from the patient's history
- Using the packed cell volume (PCV).

1. Percentage dehydration method

A clinical examination should enable the veterinary surgeon to estimate the percentage by which the patient is dehydrated.

Example

A 20 kg dog is found to be 9% dehydrated. Calculate the total fluid deficit for this animal:

20 kg × % dehydration × 10
20 kg × 9% × 10

Answer: 1800 ml fluid deficit

---

3. Using the packed cell volume (PCV)

For every 1% increase in PCV, there is a 10 ml/kg water deficit. In most cases, the patient's normal PCV is unlikely to be known so the following average figures are used:

Dog: 45%
Cat: 37%.

Example

A 15 kg dog has a PCV of 54%. Calculate the total fluid deficit:

Bodyweight (kg) × 10 ml for every 1% increase in PCV
15 kg × (54% − 45%) × 10 ml = 15 kg × 9% × 10 ml

Answer: 1350 ml fluid deficit

Intravenous fluid therapy

Once fluid deficit has been calculated it must be added to the daily maintenance fluid requirement – 50–60 ml/kg. This will give the total amount of fluid to be replaced. Ideally, half of the total amount should be replaced in the first 8 hours.

2. Calculating the water deficit from the history

The volume of fluid required to maintain a healthy animal is calculated at 50–60 ml/kg/24 hours, which compensates for normal fluid losses during the day – these are made up as follows:

Example

A 20 kg dog has a fluid deficit of 1800 ml. A standard giving set delivering 20 drops/ml is used. Calculate the fluid flow rates over 24 hours:

Maintenance:

50 ml/24 h × 20 kg =	1000 ml/24 hours
1000 ml ÷ 24 h =	41.67 ml/hours

Replacing deficit:

Half in first 8 hours:	1800 ml ÷ 2= 900 ml
	900 ÷ 8 h = 112.5 ml/hours
Total ml/hour:	Maintenance + Deficit
	41.67 ml + 112.5 ml/hour = 154.17 ml/hour
Total ml/min:	154.17 ml ÷ 60 min = 2.57 ml/min
Drops/min:	2.57 ml × drip factor
	2.57 ml × 20 = 51.4 drops/min
Seconds/drop:	60 seconds ÷ 51.4 drops/min

Answer: 1 drop every 1.17 seconds for first 8 hours

Replacing deficit:

Last 16 hours:	1800 ml ÷ 2 = 900 ml
	900 ÷ 16 h = 56.25 ml/hour
Total ml/hour:	Maintenance + Deficit
	41.67 ml + 56.25 ml = 97.92 ml/hour
Total ml/min:	97.92 ml ÷ 60 min = 1.63 ml/min
Drops/min:	1.63 ml × 20 = 32.6 drops/min
Seconds/drop:	60 seconds ÷ 32.6 drops/min

Answer: 1 drop every 1.84 (2) seconds for remaining 16 hours

Example

A 21 kg dog requires 1000 ml of fluid over a 6-hour period at a rate of 5 ml/kg/hour. A standard giving set is used delivering 20 drops/ml. Calculate the flow rate:

Flow rate:	5 ml × 21 kg = 105 ml/hour
ml/min:	105 ml ÷ 60 min = 1.75 ml/min
Drops/min:	1.75 ml × 20 drops = 35 drops/min
Seconds/drop:	60 s ÷ 35 drops/min

Answer: 1 drop every 1.71 (2) seconds

Questions

6. A 16 kg dog requires fluids at a rate of 10 ml/kg/hour. A standard giving set is used delivering 15 drops/ml. Calculate the flow rate
7. A 3 kg cat requires a total of 60 ml of fluids at a rate of 5 ml/kg/hour. A paediatric giving set is used. Calculate the flow rate
8. A 20 kg dog with a PCV of 50% requires fluid therapy to replace fluid deficit. A standard giving set delivering 20 drops/ml is used. Calculate the fluid therapy flow rates over 24 hours
9. A 15 kg dog requires 750 ml fluid over 24 hours. Using a giving set that delivers 15 drops/ml, calculate the flow rate
10. Calculate the fluid rate for a 5 kg cat requiring 125 ml Hartmann's over 10 hours. A paediatric giving set is used.

Percentage solutions

The percentage of a solution is expressed as the weight (w) of a drug per volume (v) of a solution:

1 g (w) in 100 ml (v) = 1% solution
2 g (w) in 100 ml (v) = 2% solution

and so on.

It is, however, more useful to express the percentage in terms of mg/ml when calculating doses:

2.5% solution	= 2.5 g/100 ml
÷ 100	= 0.025 g/ml
convert g to mg – 1000 mg in 1 g	
so to convert 0.025 g to mg	
multiply by 1000	= 25 mg/ml.

Formulae for calculating volume, percentage solution and weight of a drug

$$\text{Volume (ml)} = \frac{\text{weight (g)} \times 100}{\% \text{ solution}}$$

$$\text{Weight (g)} = \frac{\% \text{ solution} \times \text{volume (ml)}}{100}$$

$$\% \text{ solution} = \frac{\text{weight (g)} \times 100}{\text{volume (ml)}}$$

Example 1

Calculate the percentage solution that could be made up with 125 mg glucose and 50 ml water, using all the glucose and water:

Convert mg to g: 125 mg ÷1000 = 0.125 g

Apply formula:

$$\% \text{ solution} = \frac{\text{weight (g)} \times 100}{\text{volume (ml)}}$$
$$= \frac{0.125\,g \times 100}{50\,ml}$$

Answer: 0.25%

Example 2

A 44 lb dog requires injections every 8 hours at a drug rate of 25 mg/kg/24 hour. The injection is produced as a 5% solution. Calculate the volume of solution to be given at each injection.

(1 kg = 2.2 lb)	
Convert 44 lb to kg:	44 ÷ 2.2 = 20 kg
(1 g = 1000 mg)	
Convert mg to g:	25 ÷ 1000 = 0.025 g
Total drug required per 24 hour:	20 kg × 0.025 g = 0.5 g/24 hours

Apply formula:

$$\text{Volume} = \frac{\text{weight (g)} \times 100}{5\%} = 10\,ml$$

Given every 8 hours, i.e. three times per day: 10 ml ÷ 3

Answer: 3.33 ml per injection

Example 3

Calculate the amount of thiopentone (thiopental) required to produce 20 ml of a 2.5 % solution:

Apply formula:

$$\text{Weight (g)} = \frac{\% \text{ solution} \times \text{volume (ml)}}{100}$$
$$= \frac{2.5\% \times 20 \text{ ml}}{100}$$

Answer: 0.5 g

Questions

11. An antibiotic is supplied as a 15% suspension. If the dose for a dog is 10 mg/kg, calculate the volume required for a 30 kg labrador

12. A 20 kg dog is to be given an intravenous injection of a 5% solution. The dose rate of the drug is 15 mg/kg. Calculate the volume of the solution to be given

13. Calculate the percentage solution achieved when mixing 500 mg of a drug in 100 ml sterile water

14. Calculate the amount of dextrose required to produce 1 litre of a 2.5% solution

15. An 11 lb rabbit requires antibiotic injections twice daily. Calculate the volume required for each injection of a 5% solution at a dose rate of 15 mg/kg.

Drug dosages

In order to calculate a drug dose, the following information is required:

- Bodyweight of the animal in kilograms
- Daily dose rate – this may need to be divided throughout the day
- Strength of each tablet.

Example

A 10 kg dog requires antibiotic tablets for 14 days. The recommended dose is 5 mg/kg every 6 hour. The tablets contain 200 mg antibiotic each. Calculate the number to be dispensed.

Total dose required:	10 kg × 5 mg = 50 mg every 6 hours
Number of tablets required:	50 mg ÷200 mg = 0.25 tablet = ¼ tablet every 6 hours
Number of tablets daily:	24 hours ÷ 6 hours = 4
	4 times × ¼ tablet = 1 tablet daily
Total number of tablets dispensed: 1 daily × 14 days.	

Answer: 14 tablets dispensed

Questions

16. A cat weighing 4 kg requires antibiotics by mouth as a tablet for 5 days. The recommended dose is 24 mg/kg/24 hours and should ideally be divided into two or three equal doses throughout the day. The tablets are available in the following strengths: 50 mg, 100 mg and 250 mg. Calculate the strength and number dispensed.

17. Antibiotic tablets are to be dispensed to a 4 kg cat at a dose rate of 25 mg/kg/day. The tablets are presented as 50 mg and should be given in divided doses. Calculate the number to be given per day.

18. A 7 kg dog requires tablets at a rate of 1.5 mg/kg twice daily for 7 days. The tablets are available as 10 mg, 15 mg, 50 mg and 150 mg. Calculate the correct tablet size to dispense, the number to dispense and the instructions for dosing.

19. A 8.8 lb rabbit requires oral antibiotics twice daily for 10 days. The dose rate is 5 mg/kg. The tablets are available in 5 mg, 10 mg and 20 mg blister packs. Calculate the total number of tablets to be dispensed and of which strength.

20. A 33lb dog requires antibiotics for 21 days. The recommended dose is 5 mg/kg every 12 hours. Each capsule is 25 mg. Calculate the number dispensed.

Calorific requirements

Calculating the calorific requirement of a patient involves working out the basal energy requirement (BER), and then multiplying this by the disease factor:

BER × Disease factor = Kilocalories required in 24 hours

Basal energy requirement

For dogs over 5 kg	BER = (30 × bodyweight (kg)) + 70
For small dogs and cats	BER = 60 × bodyweight (kg)

Disease factors

The disease factor is the proportion of extra kilocalories (kcal) required in certain stressful or disease situations:

Cage rest	1.2
Surgery/trauma	1.3
Multiple surgery/trauma	1.5
Sepsis/neoplasia	1.7
Burns	2.0
Growth	2.0

Example

Calculate the calorific requirement of a 25 kg dog following routine surgery:

Calculate BER:	(30 × Bodyweight kg) + 70
	(30 × 25 kg) + 70 = 820 kcal
Disease factor (Surgery):	1.3
Total kcal:	1.3 × 820 kcal

Answer: 1066 kcal required

Radiographic exposures

There are a number of different calculations that are encountered in radiography:

- Amperage (in milliamps, mA) and exposure time (mAs)
- Voltage (in kilovolts, kV)
- Film focal distance (FFD)
- Grid factor.

mAs

$$mAs = Amperage\,(mA) \times Time\,(s)$$

Provided the mAs and mA are given, the exposure time in seconds can be calculated:

$$mAs \div mA = time\,(s)$$

Example

The radiographic exposure required for a dog's chest is 70 kV and 50 mAs. Calculate the exposure time if the machine has an output of 200 mA:

$Time\,(s) = mAs \div mA$
$\qquad = 50\,mAs \div 200\,mA.$

Answer: 0.25 seconds

kV

The rule when calculating voltage is:

If the voltage is raised by 10 kV, then the mAs should be halved
If the voltage is lowered by 10 kV, then the mAs should be doubled.

Thus

60 kV @ 16 mAs
70 kV @ 8 mAs
50 kV @ 32 mAs

are all the same!

Example

An exposure for a dog's abdomen has been found to be satisfactory at 75 kV and 40 mAs. Calculate the new mAs if the voltage were increased to 85 kV:

The kV has been increased by 10 so the mAs should be halved:

$40\,mAs \div 2$

Answer: 20 mAs

Film focal distance (FFD)

The inverse square law applies when altering the FFD: 'The intensity of the beam varies inversely as the square of the distance from the source', i.e.:

$$New\,mAs = \frac{old\,mAs \times new\,FFD^2}{old\,FFD^2}$$

Example

An exposure is found to be satisfactory for a dog's abdomen at 60 kV, 20 mAs and a FFD of 40 cm. Calculate the new mAs if the FFD were increased to 80 cm:

$New\,mAs = \dfrac{old\,mAs \times new\,FFD^2}{old\,FFD^2}$
$\qquad = \dfrac{20 \times 80^2}{40^2}$
$\qquad = \dfrac{20 \times 6400}{1600}$

Answer: 80 mAs

Grid factor

The grid factor is the amount by which the exposure (mAs) must be increased to compensate for the use of the grid. It is usually written on the grid:

$$New\,mAs = Old\,mAs \times Grid\,factor$$

Example

A radiograph requires an exposure of 20 mAs when taken at a FFD of 90 cm without a grid. Calculate the new mAs if a grid with a grid factor of 4 is used:

$Old\,mAs \times Grid\,factor$
$20\,mAs \times 4$

Answer: 80 mAs

Questions

26. If the mAs is 50 and the amperage is 200 mA, calculate the correct exposure time.

27. A dog is radiographed using a FFD of 50 cm with an mAs of 5. A decision is made to increase the FFD to 100 cm to minimize geometric distortion. Calculate the new mAs.

28. A radiograph requires an exposure of 30 mAs without the use of a grid. Calculate the new mAs when a grid is introduced with a grid factor of 3.

29. A radiograph has been taken at 60 kV and 35 mAs. Calculate the new mAs if the voltage were changed to 50 kV.

30. Calculate the mAs for a radiograph with a time of 0.4 second and a mA of 180.

Answers to questions

Now let's see how much you have understood!

1. Calculate the gas flow rate for a dog weighing 20 kg when using a Lack system, at a respiratory rate of 20 breaths per minute:

   Bodyweight × Minute volume × Circuit factor
   20 kg × (10 ml × 20 breaths per minute) × 1–1.5
   20 kg × 200 ml × 1–1.5 = **4000 ml (4 l)** or **6000 ml (6 l)**

2. A 30 kg dog is anaesthetized and maintained on a Magill circuit. Calculate the flow rate required if the dog is breathing 20 times per minute:

   Bodyweight × Minute volume × Circuit factor
   30 kg × (10 ml × 20 breaths per minute) × 1–1.5
   30 kg × 200 ml × 1–1.5 = **6000 ml (6 l)** or **9000 ml (9 l)**

3. Calculate the flow rate for a 5 kg dog on an Ayre's T-piece anaesthetic circuit breathing at a rate of 15 breaths per minute:

   Bodyweight × Minute volume × Circuit factor
   5 kg × (15 ml × 15 breaths per minute) × 2.5–3
   5 kg × 225 ml × 2.5–3 = **2812.5 ml (2.8 l)**
        or **3375 ml (3.4 l)**

4. Calculate the flow rate required for a 35 kg dog maintained on a circle circuit, breathing 15 times per minute:

   35 kg × 10 ml = **350 ml**

5. Calculate the flow rate for a 3 kg cat on an Ayre's T-piece anaesthetic circuit with a respiratory rate of 25 breaths/minute.

   Bodyweight × Minute volume × Circuit factor
   3 kg × (15 ml × 25 breaths/min) × 2.5–3
   3 kg × 375 ml × 2.5–3 = **2812.5 ml (2.8 l)**
        or **3375 ml (3.4 l)**

6. A 16 kg dog requires fluids at a rate of 10 ml/kg/h. A standard giving set is used delivering 15 drops/ml. Calculate the flow rate:

   16 kg × 10 ml = 160 ml/h
   160 ml ÷ 60 min = 2.67 ml/min
   2.67 ml × 15 drops = 40.05 drops/min
   60 s ÷ 40.05 = **1 drop every 1.5 seconds**

7. A 3 kg cat requires a total of 60 ml of fluids at a rate of 5 ml/kg/h. A paediatric giving set is used. Calculate the flow rate:

   3 kg × 5 ml = 15 ml/h
   15 ml ÷ 60 min = 0.25 ml/min
   0.25 ml × 60 drops = 15 drops/min
   60 s ÷ 15 drops = **1 drop every 4 seconds**

8. A 20 kg dog with a PCV of 50% requires fluid therapy to replace fluid deficit. A standard giving set delivering 20 drops/ml is used. Calculate the fluid therapy flow rates over 24 hours:

   Bodyweight (kg) × 10 ml for every 1% increase in PCV
   20 kg × (50–45%) × 10 ml
   20 kg × 5% × 10 ml = 1000 ml fluid deficit/24 hours

Maintenance: ÷24 hours	50 ml/ 24 h × 20 kg = 1000 ml 1000 ml ÷24 hours= 41.67 ml/h
Replacing deficit: Half in first 8 hours: Total ml/h:	1000 ml ÷ 2 ÷ 8= 62.5 ml/h *Maintenance + Deficit* 41.67 ml/h + 62.5 ml/h = 104.17 ml/h
Total ml/min:	104.17 ml ÷ 60 min = 1.74 ml/min
Drops/min:	1.74 ml × Drip factor 1.75 ml × 20 = 34.8 drops/min
Seconds/drop:	60 s ÷ 34.8 drops = **1 drop every 1.72 seconds for first 8 hours**
Replacing deficit: Last 16 hours:	1000 ml ÷ 2 ÷ 16 h = 31.25 ml/h
Total ml/h:	*Maintenance + Deficit* 41.67 ml + 31.25 ml = 72.92 ml/h
Total ml/min: Drops/min: Seconds/drop:	72.92 ml ÷ 60 = 1.22 ml/min 1.22 ml × 20 = 24.4 drops/min 60 s ÷ 24.4 drops = **1 drop every 2.46 seconds for remaining 16 hours**

9. A 15 kg dog requires 750 ml fluid over 24 hours. Using a giving set that delivers 15 drops/ml, calculate the flow rate:

$$750 \text{ ml} \div 24 \text{ h} = 31.25 \text{ ml/h}$$
$$31.25 \text{ ml} \div 60 \text{ min} = 0.52 \text{ ml/min}$$
$$0.52 \text{ ml} \times 15 \text{ drops} = 7.8 \text{ drops/min}$$
$$60 \text{ s} \div 7.8 \text{ drops} = \textbf{1 drop every 7.7 seconds}$$

10. Calculate the fluid rate for a 5 kg cat requiring 125 ml Hartmann's over 10 hours. A paediatric giving set is used.

$$125 \text{ ml} \div 10 \text{ h} = 12.5 \text{ ml/h}$$
$$12.5 \text{ ml} \div 60 \text{ min} = 0.21 \text{ ml/min}$$
$$0.21 \text{ ml} \times 60 \text{ drops} = 12.6 \text{ drops/min}$$
$$60 \text{ s} \div 12.6 \text{ drops} = \textbf{1 drop every 5 seconds}$$

11. An antibiotic is supplied as a 15% suspension. If the dose for a dog is 10 mg/kg, calculate the volume required for a 30 kg labrador:

$$\text{Dose} = (30 \text{ kg} \times 10 \text{ mg}) \div 1000 \text{ (to convert to grams)} = 0.3 \text{ g}$$
$$\text{Volume (ml)} = \frac{\text{Weight of drug (g)} \times 100}{\% \text{ solution}}$$
$$= \frac{0.3 \times 100}{15}$$
$$= \textbf{2 ml}$$

12. A 20 kg dog is to be given an intravenous injection of a 5% solution. The dose rate of the drug is 15 mg/kg. Calculate the volume of the solution to be given:

$$\text{Dose} = 20 \text{ kg} \times 15 \text{ mg} = \frac{300 \text{ mg}}{1000} = 0.3 \text{ g}$$
$$\text{Volume (ml)} = \frac{\text{Weight of drug (g)} \times 100}{\% \text{ solution}}$$
$$= \frac{0.3 \times 100}{5\%}$$
$$= \textbf{6 ml}$$

13. Calculate the percentage solution achieved when mixing 500 mg of a drug in 100 ml sterile water:

$$\frac{500 \text{ mg}}{1000} = 0.5 \text{ g}$$
$$\% = \frac{\text{Weight (g)} \times 100}{\text{volume (ml)}}$$
$$= \frac{0.5 \times 100}{100}$$
$$= \textbf{0.5\%}$$

14. Calculate the amount of dextrose required to produce 1 litre of a 2.5% solution:

$$\text{Weight (g)} = \frac{\text{Volume (ml)} \times \% \text{ solution}}{100}$$
$$= \frac{1000 \text{ ml} \times 2.5\%}{100}$$
$$= \textbf{25 g}$$

15. An 11 lb rabbit requires antibiotic injections twice daily. Calculate the volume required for each injection of a 5% solution at a dose rate of 15 mg/kg.

Convert lb to kg: 11 lb ÷ 2.2 = 5 kg
                      5 kg × 15 mg = 75 mg
Convert mg to g: 75 mg ÷ 1000 = 0.075 g

$$\text{Volume (ml)} = \frac{\text{Weight of drug (g)} \times 100}{\% \text{ solution}}$$
$$= \frac{0.075 \text{ g} \times 100}{5\%}$$
$$= 1.5 \text{ ml}$$

Divide into two doses: = 1.5 ml ÷ 2
                       = **0.75 ml**

16. A cat weighing 4 kg requires antibiotics by mouth as a tablet for 5 days. The recommended dose is 24 mg/kg/24 hours and should, ideally, be divided into two or three equal doses throughout the day. The tablets are available in the following strengths: 50 mg, 100 mg and 250 mg. Calculate the strength and number dispensed:

Dose/24 hour   = 4 kg × 24 mg = 96 mg
Twice-daily dose   = 96 mg ÷ 2 = 48 mg = 1 × 50 mg tablet
Two tablets daily × 5 days   = **10 × 50 mg tablets dispensed**

17. Antibiotic tablets are to be dispensed to a 4 kg cat at a dose rate of 25 mg/kg/day. The tablets are presented as 50 mg and should be given in divided doses. Calculate the number to be given per day:

Daily dose   = 4 kg × 25 mg = 100 mg
Number of tablets = 100 mg/50 mg = 2
1 tablet to be given twice daily

18. A 7 kg dog requires tablets at a rate of 1.5 mg/kg twice daily for 7 days. The tablets are available as 10 mg, 15 mg, 50 mg and 150 mg. Calculate the correct tablet size to dispense, the number to dispense and the instructions for dosing:

Twice-daily dose   = 7 kg × 1.5 mg = 10.5 mg = 1 × 10 mg tablet
Two tablets × 7 days   = 14 tablets
14 × 10 mg tablets dispensed to be given twice daily

19. An 8.8lb rabbit requires oral antibiotics twice daily for 10 days. The dose rate is 5 mg/kg. The tablets are available in 5 mg, 10 mg and 20 mg blister packs. Calculate the total number of tablets to be dispensed and of which strength.

Convert lb to kg:	8.8 lb ÷ 2.2 = 4 kg
Dose/24 hours:	4 kg × 5 mg = 20 mg
Twice-daily dose:	20 mg ÷ 2 = 10 mg = 1 × 10 mg tablet twice daily
Total number dispensed:	(2 × 10 kg daily) × 10 days 2 × 10 = **20 of the 10 mg tablets**

20. A 33 lb dog requires antibiotic capsules for 21 days. The recommended dose is 5 mg/kg every 12 hours. Each capsule is 25 mg. Calculate the number dispensed.

Dog's weight (kg)	= 33 ÷ 2.2 = 15 kg
12-hourly dose	= 15 × 5 mg = 75 mg
Number of tablets	= 75 mg ÷ 25 mg = 3 tablets
3 tablets every 12 hours	= 6 tablets /day

6 tablets × 21 days = 126 tablets dispensed

21. Calculate the calorific requirement of a 55 kg Great Dane that is hospitalized after parturition with a disease factor of 1.2:

$$\text{Daily requirement (kcal)} = (30 \times \text{Bodyweight (kg)}) + 70) \times \text{Disease factor}$$
$$= ((30 \times 55) + 70) \times 1.2$$
$$= \textbf{2064 kcal}$$

22. Calculate the calorific requirement of a 1 kg kitten who is recovering from severe burns:

$$\text{Daily requirement (kcal)} = \text{Bodyweight (kg)} \times 60 \times \text{disease factor}$$
$$= 1 \times 60 \times 2$$
$$= \textbf{120 kcal}$$

23. Calculate the calorific requirement of a 10 kg dog fitted with a nasogastric tube. Then calculate the amount of food required if the energy density of the food is 0.8 kcal/ml:

$$\text{Daily requirement (kcal)} = (\text{Bodyweight (kg)} \times 30) + 70$$
$$= (10 \text{ kg} \times 30) + 70$$
$$= 370 \text{ kcal}$$
$$\text{Amount of food required at 0.8 kcal/ml} = 370 \div 0.8$$
$$= \textbf{462.5 ml}$$

24. Calculate the calorific requirement of a 32 kg dog. Using your answer, calculate the amount of food required if the food has an energy density of 420 kcal per 100 g tin:

$$\text{Daily requirement (kcal)} = (\text{Bodyweight (kg)} \times 30) + 70$$
$$= (32 \text{ kg} \times 30) + 70$$
$$= 1030 \text{ kcal}$$
$$\text{Amount of food required at 420 kcal/100 g} = 1030 \div 420$$
$$= 245 \text{ g}$$
$$\text{Number of tins at 100 g per tin} = 245 \div 100 \text{ g}$$
$$= \textbf{2.45 tins required}$$

25. Calculate the daily calorie requirement of a 5 kg Yorkshire terrier.

$$\text{Daily requirement (kcal)} = \text{Bodyweight (kg)} \times 60$$
$$= 5 \text{ kg} \times 60$$
$$= \textbf{300 kcal}$$

26. If the mAs is 50 and the amperage is 200 mA, calculate the correct exposure time:

$$\text{Time (s)} = \frac{\text{mAs}}{\text{mA}}$$
$$= \frac{50 \text{ mAs}}{200} = \textbf{0.25 second}$$

27. A dog is radiographed using an FFD of 50 cm with an mAs of 5. A decision is made to increase the FFD to 100 cm to minimize geometric distortion. Calculate the new mAs:

$$\text{New mAs} = \frac{\text{Old mAs} \times \text{New FFD}^2}{\text{Old FFD}^2}$$
$$= \frac{5 \times 100^2}{50^2}$$
$$= \frac{5 \times 10000}{2500}$$
$$= 5 \times 4$$
$$= \textbf{20 mAs}$$

28. A radiograph requires an exposure of 30 mAs without the use of a grid. Calculate the new mAs when a grid is introduced with a grid factor of 3:

$$\text{New mAs} = \text{mAs without grid} \times \text{Grid factor}$$
$$= 30 \text{ mAs} \times 3$$
$$= \textbf{90 mAs}$$

29. A radiograph has been taken at 60 kV and 35 mAs. Calculate the new mAs if the voltage were changed to 50 kV:

If the voltage is lowered by 10 kV, then the mAs should be doubled:

$$35 \text{ mAs} \times 2 = \textbf{70 mAs}$$

30. Calculate the mAs for a radiograph with a time of 0.4 second and an mA of 180.

$$\text{mAs} = \text{mA} \times \text{s}$$
$$= 180 \text{ mA} \times 0.4 \text{ s}$$
$$= \textbf{72 mAs}$$

Index

Page numbers followed by "f" indicate figures, "t" indicate tables, and "b" indicate boxes.

A